Handbook of Neurosurgery

Sixth edition

Mark S. Greenberg, M.D.
Assistant Professor
Department of Neurosurgery
University of South Florida
Tampa, Florida

With contributions by:
Nicolas Arredondo, M.D.
Edward A. M. Duckworth, M.D.
Tann A. Nichols, M.D.
Justin Whitlow
Ashraf Samy Youssef, M.D., Ph.D.

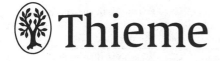

Thieme

2006
Greenberg Graphics, Inc.
Lakeland, Florida

Thieme Medical Publishers
New York, New York

The exclusive distributor in the Americas and Canada is
Thieme New York
333 Seventh Avenue
New York, NY 10001
United States of America
(800) 782-3488

The exclusive distributor outside the Americas is
Thieme International
Rudigerstrasse 14
Stuttgart, Germany
+49 (0) 711-8931-126

Library of Congress Cataloging-in-Publication Data is available from the publisher

HANDBOOK OF NEUROSURGERY
Mark S. Greenberg

ISBN 1-58890-457-1   (Thieme New York)
ISBN 3-13-110886-X   (Georg Thieme Verlag Stuttgart)

Copyright © 2006
Mark S. Greenberg. All rights reserved.

First edition, 1990   Third edition, 1994   Fifth edition, 2001
Second edition, 1991   Fourth edition, 1997

Greenberg Graphics, Inc.
Lakeland, FL
e-mail: editor@grgraphics.com
www.grgraphics.com

Important note: Medical knowledge is ever-changing. As new research and clinical experience broaden our knowledge, changes in treatment and drug therapy may be required. The authors and editors of the material contained herein have consulted sources believed to be reliable in their efforts to provide information that is complete and in accord with the standards accepted at the time of publication. However, in view of the possibility of human error by the authors, editors, or publisher of the work herein, or changes in medical knowledge, neither the authors, editors, publisher, nor any other party who has been involved in the preparation of this work, warrants that the information contained herein is in every respect accurate or complete, and they are not responsible for any errors or omissions or for the results obtained from use of such information. Readers are encouraged to confirm the information contained herein with other sources. For example, readers are advised to check the product information sheet included in the package of each drug they plan to administer to be certain that the information contained in this publication is accurate and that changes have not been made in the recommended dose or in the contraindications for administration. This recommendation is of particular importance in connection with new or infrequently used drugs.

Some of the product names, patents, and registered designs referred to in this book are in fact registered trademarks or proprietary names even though specific reference to this fact is not always made in the text. Therefore, the appearance of a name without designation as proprietary is not to be construed as a representation by the publisher that it is in the public domain.

Cover illustration by the author depicting the anterolateral brainstem and its vasculature, modified with permission from: Lewis SB, Chang DJ, Peace DA, Lafrentz PJ, Day AL. Distal posterior inferior cerebellar artery aneurysms: clinical features and management. J Neurosurg 2002; 97(4): 756-66. For a labeled illustration of the anatomy, *see page 80* herein.

Printed in Ontario, Canada.   Printer: Webcom, Limited.

Printing: 5   4   3   2   1

DEDICATION

The sixth edition of the Handbook of Neurosurgery book is dedicated to the memory of my mother, Mary, to the continued gift of my father, Louis, to the present of my darling wife, Debbie, and to the future of my children, Shaina, Alexa, Leah and Michael.

CONVENTIONS

Cross references are utilized extensively for ease of use. The terms *see below* and *see above* are normally used when the referenced item is on the same page, or at most on the following (or preceding) page. When further excursions are needed, the page number will usually be included.

Σ Paragraphs with this symbol summarize or synthesizes key points from the associated text.

EVIDENCE BASED MEDICINE

The following configuration is used to call attention to practice parameter guidelines developed by authoritative committees. The definitions employed are in accordance with generally accepted current usage. The relevant document will be cited. A standard of care is not implied, and does not preclude selective deviation from guidelines to individualize care for specific and unique circumstances of a particular case. For an up-to-date listing of some guidelines, visit www.guidelines.gov. For a listing of practice parameters contained in this book, see the *Index* under *practice parameter*.

PRACTICE PARAMETER: DEFINITIONS

Standards Practice *Standards* indicate a high degree of clinical certainty and are generally based on **Class I evidence** (one or more well-designed, randomized controlled studies) or strong Class II evidence especially when circumstances preclude randomized clinical trials

Guidelines Practice *Guidelines* reflect a moderate degree of clinical certainty and are recommended when the reviewers felt there was insufficient information to create a *Standard*, and are usually based on **Class II evidence** (one or more well-designed comparative clinical studies or less well-designed randomized studies) or a preponderance of Class III evidence

Options Practice *Options* of unclear clinical certainty and are recommended when the reviewers felt there was insufficient information to create a *Standard* or *Guideline*, and are generally based on **Class III evidence** (case series, historical controls, case reports and expert opinion)

Recommendations Some references use this term generically and then specify the strength of the data. For these, the nature of the data will be given.

ACKNOWLEDGMENTS

I would like to acknowledge all the sources used for the material in this book. This includes the many people involved in my medical and neurosurgical training. Special appreciation is expressed to John M. Tew, Jr., M.D., under whose guidance I received my neurosurgical training. It also includes those who generously granted permission to use figures and tables previously published.

ABBREVIATIONS

Abbreviations used only locally are defined in that section using boldface type. Where appropriate, page numbers for the main section relevant to that topic is given.

a.	artery	ACh	acetycholine (neurotransmitter)
AA	anaplastic astrocytoma - 412	AChA	anterior choroidal artery
Abx.	antibiotics	ACoA	anterior communicating artery
AC	arachnoid cyst - 94	ACTH	adrenocorticotropic hormone
ACA	anterior cerebral artery	ADH	antidiuretic hormone - 12
ACAS	asymptomatic carotid artery stenosis - 872 or Asymptomatic Carotid Atherosclerosis Study - 873	ADI	atlantodental interval - 140
		AED	anti-epileptic drug - 268
		Ag	antigen
ACDF	anterior cervical discectomy & fusion - 319	AHCPR	Agency for Health Care Policy and Research (of the U. S. Public Health Service)
ACE	angiotensin-converting enzyme		

AICA	anterior inferior cerebellar artery	DACA	distal anterior cerebral artery
AIDS	acquired immunodeficiency syndrome - 230	DAI	diffuse axonal injury - 632
		D/C	discontinue
AKA	also known as	DDx	differential diagnosis - 902
ALIF	anterior lumbar interbody fusion	DI	diabetes insipidus - 16
A-line	arterial line	DIND	delayed ischemic neurologic deficit - 791
ALL	anterior longitudinal ligament	DISH	diffuse idiopathic skeletal hyperostosis -
ALS	amyotrophic lateral sclerosis - 52		346
AN	acoustic neuroma - 429	DKA	diabetic keto-acidosis
ANA	antinuclear antibodies	DOC	drug of choice
AOD	atlanto-occipital dislocation - 717	DM	diabetes mellitus
AP	antero-posterior	DMZ	dexamethasone
APAG	antipseudomonal aminoglycoside	DNT	(or DNET) dysembryoplastic neuroepithe-
APAP	acetaminophen - 28		lial tumors - 409
APTT	activated partial thromboplastin time (or PTT)	DPL	diagnostic peritoneal lavage
		DREZ	dorsal root entry zone lesion - 395
ARDS	adult respiratory distress syndrome	DSA	digital subtraction angiogram
ASA	American Society of Anesthesiologists *or* aspirin (acetylsalicylic acid)	DSD	degenerative spine - 323
		DST	dural sinus thrombosis - 888
ASAP	as soon as possible	DTs	delerium tremens - 151
ASHD	atherosclerotic heart disease	DVT	deep-vein thrombosis - 25
AVM	arteriovenous malformation - 835	DWI	diffusion-weighted imaging (MRI) - 136
BA	basilar artery	EAC	external auditory canal
BBB	blood-brain barrier - 84	EAM	external auditory meatus
BCP	birth control pills	EBRT	external beam radiation therapy
BG	basal ganglia	ECM	erythema chronicum migrans - 234
BMD	bone mineral density - 749	EDH	epidural hematoma - 669
BMP	bone morphogenetic protein - 627	EHL	extensor hallicus longus
BOB	benign osteoblastoma - 511	ELISA	enzyme-linked immunosorbent assay
BP	blood pressure	EM	electron microscope (microscopy)
BR	bed rest (activity restriction)	ENG	electronystagmography - 432
BSF	basal skull fracture - 665	ENT	ear, nose and throat (otolaryngology)
BSG	brainstem glioma - 420	EOM	extra-ocular muscles
Ca	cancer	EOO	external oculomotor ophthalmoplegia
CA	cavernous angioma - 841	ESR	erythrocyte sedimentation rate
CAA	cerebral amyloid angiopathy - 853	EtOH	ethyl alcohol (ethanol)
CABG	coronary artery bypass graft	ET tube	endotracheal tube
CAD	coronary artery disease	EVD	external ventricular drain (ventriculostomy)
CBF	cerebral blood flow - 763	FIM	Functional Impairment Measure™ - 901
CBV	cerebral blood volume	FLAIR	fluid-attenuated inversion recovery (on
CBZ	carbamazepine - 273		MRI) - 135
CCB	calcium-channel blocker	FM	face mask
CCF	carotid-cavernous (sinus) fistula - 845	FMD	fibromuscular dysplasia - 63
CCHD	congenital cyanotic heart disease	F/U	follow-up
CEA	carotid endarterectomy - 874 *or* carcinoembryonic antigen - 501	FUO	fever of unknown origin
		GABA	gamma-aminobutyric acid
cf	(Latin: confer) compare	GBM	glioblastoma multiforme - 412
cGy	centi-Gray (1cGy = 1 rad)	GBS	Guillain-Barré syndrome - 53
CHF	congestive heart failure	GCA	giant cell arteritis - 58
CIDP	chronic inflammatory demyelinating polyra-diculoneuropathy - 54	GCS	Glasgow coma scale - 154
		GD	Grave's disease
CJD	Creutzfeldt-Jakob disease - 227	GDC	Guglielmi detachable coils - 803
CM	cavernous malformation - 841	GFAP	glial fibrillary acidic protein - 500
CMRO$_2$	cerebral metabolic rate of oxygen con-sumption - 763	GGT	gamma glutamyl transpeptidase
		GMH	germinal matrix hemorrhage - 861
CMT	Charcot-Marie-Tooth - 554	GNR	gram negative rods
CMV	cytomegalovirus	GSW	gunshot wound
CNS	central nervous system	GTC	generalized tonic-clonic (seizure)
cCO	continuous cardiac output	H/A	headache - 44
CO	cardiac output	H&H	Hunt and Hess (SAH grade) - 785
CPA	cerebellopontine angle	HBsAg	hepatitis B surface antigen
CPM	central pontine myelinolysis - 12	HCD	herniated cervical disc - 318
CPN	common peroneal nerve - 575	HCP	hydrocephalus - 180
CPP	cerebral perfusion pressure - 647	HDT	hyperdynamic therapy - 797
Cr. N.	cranial nerve(s)	HGB	hemangioblastoma - 459
CSM	cervical spondylotic myelopathy - 331	Hgb-A1C	hemoglobin A1C
CRP	C-reactive protein	hGH	human growth hormone
CRPS	complex regional pain syndrome - 396	HHT	hereditary hemorrhagic telangiectasia -
CSO	craniosynostosis - 99		841
CSW	cerebral salt wasting - 14	HIV	human immunodeficiency virus
CTE	chronic traumatic encephalopathy - 683	HLD	herniated lumber disc - 302
CTS	carpal tunnel syndrome - 565	HLA	human leukocyte antigen
CVA	cerebrovascular accident, stroke - 763	H.O.	house officer
CVP	central venous pressure	HNP	herniated nucleus pulposus (herniated
CVVT	cerebrovascular venous thrombosis - 888		disc) - 302
CVR	cerebrovascular resistance - 763	HNPP	hereditary neuropathy with liability to pres-
CVS	cerebral vasospasm - 791		sure palsies - 554
CXR	chest x-ray	HOB	head of bed

HPA	hypothalamic-pituitary-adrenal axis	NCD	neurocutaneous disorders - 502
HSE	herpes simplex encephalitis - 225	NCV	nerve conduction velocity
HTN	hypertension	NEC	necrotizing enterocolitis
IAC	internal auditory canal	NFT	neurofibromatosis - 502
IASDH	infantile acute subdural hematoma - 674	NG tube	nasogastric tube
ICA	internal carotid artery	NMBA	neuromuscular blocking agent - 38
ICH	intracerebral hemorrhage - 849	NPH	normal pressure hydrocephalus - 199
IC-HTN	intracranial hypertension (increased ICP)	NPS	neuropathic pain syndrome - 387
ICP	intracranial pressure - 647	NS	normal saline
ICU	intensive care unit	NSAID	non-steroidal anti-inflammatory drug - 28
IDDM	insulin-dependent diabetes mellitus	NSCLC	non-small cell cancer of the lung - 486
IDET	intradiscal endothermal therapy - 307	NTP	nitroprusside - 3
IEP	immune electrophoresis	N/V	nausea and vomiting
IGF-I	insulin-like growth factor-I (AKA somatome-din-C) - 441	OALL	ossification of the anterior longitudinal ligament - 346
IIH	idiopathic intracranial hypertension (pseudotumor cerebri) - 493	OCB	oligoclonal bands (in CSF) - 51
		OCF	occipital condylae fracture - 721
IIHWOP	idiopathic intracranial hypertension without papilledema - 495	OFC	occipital-frontal (head) circumference
		OMO	open-mouth odontoid (C-spine x-ray view)
INO	internuclear ophthalmoplegia - 585	OMP	oculomotor (third nerve) palsy
INR	international normalized ratio - 23	ONSF	optic nerve sheath fenestration - 498
IPA	idiopathic paralysis agitans (Parkinson's disease) - 47	OP	opening pressure (on LP)
		OPG	ocular pneumoplethysmography - 871
ISAT	International Subarachnoid Hemorrhage Aneurysm Trial - 803	OPLL	ossification of the posterior longitudinal ligament - 345
IVC	intraventricular catheter	ORIF	open reduction/internal fixation
IVP	intravenous push (medication route), or intravenous pyelogram (x-ray study)	OTC	over the counter (i.e. without prescription)
		PACU	post-anesthesia care unit (AKA recovery room, PAR)
JPS	joint position sense	PAN	poly- (or peri-) arteritis nodosa - 61
LBP	low back pain	PBPP	perinatal brachial plexus palsy - 562
LE	lower extremity	PCA	pilocytic astrocytoma - 417 or posterior cerebral artery
LFTs	liver function tests		
LGG	low-grade glioma - 408	PCB	pneumatic compression boot
LMD	low molecular weight dextran	PCC	prothrombin complex concentrate - 24
LMN	lower motor neuron	PCN	penicillin
LMW	low-molecular-weight (e.g. heparins)	PCNSL	primary CNS lymphoma - 461
LOC	loss of consciousness	P-comm	posterior communicating artery
LP	lumbar puncture - 615	PCV	procarbazine, CCNU & vincristine (chemotherapy)
LSO	lumbo-sacral orthosis		
MAOI	monoamine oxidase inhibitor	PCWP	pulmonary capillary wedge pressure
MAP	mean arterial pressure	PDA	patent ductus arteriosus
MAST®	military anti-shock trousers	PDN	painful diabetic neuropathy - 376
MBI	modified Barthel index - 900	PDR	Physicians Desk Reference®
MBS	medulloblastoma - 473	peds	pediatrics (infants & children)
MCA	middle cerebral artery	PET	positron emission tomography (scan)
mcg	microgram	p-fossa	posterior fossa
μg	microgram	PFT	pulmonary function test
MCP	mean carotid pressure	PHN	postherpetic neuralgia - 387
mg	milligram	PHT	phenytoin (Dilantin®) - 271
MI	myocardial infarction	PICA	posterior inferior cerebellar artery
MIC	minimum inhibitory concentration (for antibiotics)	PLEDs	periodic lateralizing epileptiform discharges
		PLIF	posterior lumbar interbody fusion
MID	multi-infarct dementia	PML	progressive multifocal leukoencephalopathy - 231
MDMA	methylenedioxymethamphetamine - 48		
MLF	medial longitudinal fasciculus	PMR	polymyalgia rheumatica - 61
MM	myelomeningocele - 115; or multiple myeloma - 514	PMV	pontomesencephalic vein
		PNET	primitive neuroectodermal tumor - 472
MMPI	Minnesota Multiphasic Personality Inventory	PR	per rectum
		PRN	as needed
mos	months	PRSP	penicillinase resistant synthetic PCN
MPTP	1-methyl-4-phenyl-1,2,3,6-tetrahydropyridine - 47	PSNP	progressive supra-nuclear palsy - 48
		PSR	percutaneous stereotactic rhizotomy (for trigeminal neuralgia) - 380
MRS	MRI spectroscopy - 137		
MRSA	methicillin resistant staphylococcus aureus	pt	patient
MS	multiple sclerosis - 49	PT	physical therapy; or prothrombin time
MSO₄	morphine sulfate	PTR	percutaneous trigeminal rhizotomy
MVA	motor vehicle accident	PTT	partial thromboplastin time (or APTT)
MVD	microvascular decompression - 385	PUD	peptic ulcer disease
MW	molecular weight	PVP	percutaneous vertebroplasty - 750
Na or Na⁺	sodium	PWI	perfusion-weighted imaging (MRI) - 136
N₂O	nitrous oxide - 1	q	(Latin: quaque) every
NAA	N-acetyl aspartate - 137	RA	rheumatoid arthritis
NASCET	North American Symptomatic Carotid Endarterectomy Trial - 874	REZ	root entry zone
		RFR	radiofrequency rhizotomy
NB	(Latin: nota bene) note well	rFVIIa	recombinant (activated) factor VII
NC	nasal cannula		

RH	recurrent artery of Heubner	TM	tympanic membrane
RIND	reversible ischemic neurologic deficit - 869	TMB	transient monocular blindness (amaurosis fugax) - 869
R/O	rule out	t-PA	tissue plasminogen activator
RTOG	Radiation Therapy Oncology Group	TR	time to repetition (on MRI) - 134
rt-PA	recombinant tissue plasminogen activator (AKA tissue plasminogen activator)	TRH	thyrotropin releasing hormone; AKA TSH-RH
RTX	(or XRT) radiation therapy	TS	tuberous sclerosis - 504 *or* transverse sinus
S/S	signs and symptoms		
SAH	subarachnoid hemorrhage - 781	TSH	thyroid-stimulating hormone; AKA thyrotropin
SBE	subacute bacterial endocarditis		
SBP	systolic blood pressure	TSV	thalamostriate vein
SCA	superior cerebellar artery	TTP	thrombotic thrombocytopenic purpura
SCLC	small cell lung cancer - 486	TVO	transient visual obscurations - 495
SCD	sequential compression device	Tx.	treatment
SCI	spinal cord injury - 698	UBOs	unidentified bright objects (on MRI)
SCM	sternocleidomastoid (muscle)	UE	upper extremity
SD	standard deviation	UMN	upper motor neuron
SDE	subdural empyema - 223	UTI	urinary tract infection
SDH	subdural hematoma - 672	URI	upper respiratory tract infection
SE	status epilepticus (for seizures) - 264)	U/S	ultrasound
SEA	spinal epidural abscess - 240	VA	vertebral artery *or* ventriculoatrial
SEP	(or SSEP) somatosensory evoked potential	VB	vertebral body
SG	specific gravity	VHL	von Hippel-Lindau (disease) - 459
SIADH	syndrome of inappropriate antidiuretic hormone (ADH) secretion - 13	VMA	vanillylmandelic acid
		VP	ventriculoperitoneal
SIDS	sudden infant death syndrome	VZV	(herpes) varicella zoster virus
SLAD	surgical laser aiming device	WBRT	whole brain radiation therapy
SLE	systemic lupus erythematosus	WHO	World Health Organization
SOMI	sternal-occipital-mandibular immobilizer - 741	wks	weeks
		WNL	within normal limits
S/P	status-post	XRT	x-ray treatment (or RTX, radiation therapy)
SPEP	serum protein electrophoresis		
SQ	subcutaneous injection		
SRS	stereotactic radiosurgery - 537		———— SYMBOLS————
SSEP	(or SEP) somatosensory evoked potential	*Rx*	prescribing information
SSPE	subacute sclerosing panencephalitis - 145	→	causes or leads to
SSRI	selective serotonin reuptake inhibitors	Δ	change
SSS	superior sagittal sinus	↑	increased
STA	superficial temporal artery	↓	decreased
STICH	Surgical Trial in Intracerebral Haemorrhage - 859	≈	approximately
		⸙	key features
STIR	short tau inversion recover (MRI image)	⋏	innervates (nerve distribution)
SVR	systemic venous resistance	⇒	supplies (used in describing vascular territories)
SVT	supraventricular tachycardia		
Sz.	seizure - 256	➡	a branch of the preceding nerve
T1WI	T1 weighted image (on MRI) - 134	★	crucial point
T2WI	T2 weighted image (on MRI) - 135	❏	post-op check item
TBI	traumatic brain injury	✶	caution; possible danger…
TCA	tricyclic antidepressants	Σ	summary
TCD	transcranial doppler		
TDL	tumefactive demyelinating lesions - 51	∴	therefore
TE	time to echo (on MRI) - 134	www.net	an internet URL address
TEN	toxic epidermal necrolysis		
TENS	transcutaneous electrical nerve stimulation		medical pearls
TGN	trigeminal neuralgia - 378		
T-H lines	Taylor-Haughton lines - 70		
TIA	transient ischemic attack - 869		
TL	transverse (atlantoaxial) ligament - 719		
TLIF	transforaminal lumbar interbody fusion		
TLSO	thoracolumbar-sacral orthosis		

Contents

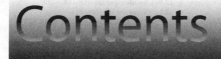

CONTENTS

CONTENTS

1. General

1.1. Neuroanesthesia

INHALATIONAL AGENTS

Most reduce cerebral metabolism (except nitrous oxide, *see below*) by suppressing neuronal activity. These agents disturb cerebral autoregulation and cause cerebral vasodilatation which increases cerebral blood volume **(CBV)** and can increase ICP. With administration > 2 hrs they increase CSF volume which can also potentially contribute to increased ICP. Most agents increase the CO_2 reactivity of cerebral blood vessels. All of these agents affect intra-operative EP monitoring (*see above*).

halothane (Fluothane®) DRUG INFO

Increases CBF and CBV, and decreases CSF absorption, all of which can increase ICP. Autoregulation is disrupted. Affects EEG and EP (*see above*), and produces isoelectric EEG at concentration of ≈ 4.5%. Produces cerebrotoxic effects at lower levels (≈ 2%).

enflurane (Ethrane®) DRUG INFO

A poor agent for neuroanesthesia. ✖ Lowers seizure threshold at therapeutic levels (further exacerbated by hypocapnia). CSF production increases and absorption decreases both of which contribute to increased intracranial volume and thus increased ICP.

nitrous oxide (N₂O) DRUG INFO

A potent vasodilator that markedly increases CBF and minimally *increases* cerebral metabolism.

Nitrous oxide concerns with pneumocephalus and air embolism: " The solubility of nitrous oxide **(N₂O)** is ≈ 34 times that of nitrogen[1],. When N_2O comes out of solution in an airtight space it can increase the pressure which may convert pneumocephalus to "tension pneumocephalus". It may also aggravate air embolism. Thus caution must be used especially in the sitting position where significant post-op pneumocephalus and air embolism are common. The risk of tension pneumocephalus may be reduced by filling the cavity with fluid in conjunction with turning off N_2O about 10 minutes prior to completion of dural closure. See *Pneumocephalus* on page 667.

Halogenated agents that may provide cerebral protection
All of these agents suppress EEG activity.

isoflurane (Forane®) DRUG INFO

Can produce isoelectric EEG without metabolic toxicity. Improves neurologic outcome in cases of incomplete global ischemia (although in experimental studies on rats, the amount of tissue injury was greater than with thiopental[2]).

desflurane (Suprane®) DRUG INFO

A cerebral vasodilator, increases CBF and ICP. Decreases $CMRO_2$ which tends to cause a compensatory vasoconstriction.

Mildly increases CBP and ICP, and reduces CMRO$_2$. Mild negative inotrope, cardiac output not as well maintained as with isoflurane or desflurane.

INTRAVENOUS AGENTS

BARBITURATES IN ANESTHESIA

Produce significant reduction in CMRO$_2$ and scavenge free radicals among other effects (*see page 807*). Produce dose-dependent EEG suppression which can be taken all the way to isoelectric. Minimally affect EP. Most are anticonvulsant, but methohexital (Brevital®) can *lower* the seizure threshold (*see page 36*). Myocardial suppression and peripheral vasodilatation from barbiturates may cause hypotension and compromise CPP, especially in hypovolemic patients.

NARCOTICS IN ANESTHESIA

Increase CSF absorption and minimally reduce cerebral metabolism. They slow the EEG but will <u>not</u> produce an isoelectric tracing. ✖ All narcotics cause dose-dependent respiratory depression which can result in hypercarbia and concomitant increased ICP in non-ventilated patients.

Morphine: does not significantly cross the BBB.
✖ Disadvantages in neuro patients:
1. causes histamine release which
   A. may produce hypotension
   B. may cause cerebrovascular vasodilation → increased ICP[3] (p 1593)
   C. the above together may compromise CPP
2. in renal or hepatic insufficiency, the metabolite morphine-6-glucuronide can accumulate which may cause confusion

Meperidine (Demerol®): has negative inotropic effects, and its neuroexcitatory metabolite nor-meperidine can cause hyperactivity or seizures (*see footnote, page 32*). Also causes histamine release.

Synthetic narcotics
These do <u>not</u> cause histamine release, unlike morphine and meperidine.

★ **Fentanyl**: crosses the BBB. Reduces CMRO$_2$, CBV and ICP.

Sufentanil: more potent then fentanyl. Does not increase CBF, but ✖ raises ICP and is thus often not appropriate for neurosurgical cases.

Alfentanil: the most rapid onset and the shortest duration of the narcotics. ✖ NB: also raises ICP.

BENZODIAZEPINES IN ANESTHESIA

These drugs are GABA agonists and decrease cerebral metabolism. They also provide anticonvulsant action and produce amnesia. See *page 35* for agents and reversal.

MISCELLANEOUS DRUGS IN ANESTHESIA

Etomidate: used primarily for induction. Also described for cerebral protection during aneurysm surgery (*see page 808*). A cerebrovasoconstrictor, it reduces CBF and ICP. Does not suppress brainstem activity. Suppresses cortisol production with prolonged administration, and may induce seizures.

Propofol: a sedative hypnotic. Reduces cerebral metabolism, CBF and ICP. Has been described for cerebral protection (*see page 808*) and for sedation (*see page 37*). Useful for cortical mapping where rapid recovery from anesthesia is needed (recovery is not as rapid as with methohexital). Not analgesic.

Lidocaine: suppresses laryngeal reflexes which may help blunt ICP rises that normally follow endotracheal intubation or suctioning. Anticonvulsant at low doses, may provoke seizures at high concentrations.

REVERSAL OF COMPETITIVE MUSCLE BLOCKADE
It can take up to ≈ 20 minutes for full reversal of pancuronium (Pavulon®) (depending on the amount of time since the last dose). Reversal is usually not attempted until patient has at least 1 twitch to a train of 4 stimulus, otherwise reversal may be incomplete if patient is profoundly blocked and blockade may reoccur as the reversal wears off.
♦ neostigmine (Prostigmin®): 2.5 mg (minimum) to 5 mg (maximum) IV (start low, no efficacy from > 5 mg and can produce severe weakness especially if the maximum dose is exceeded in the absence of neuromuscular blockade)
PLUS (to prevent bradycardia...), EITHER
      • 0.5 mg atropine for each mg of neostigmine
OR
      • 0.2 mg glycopyrrolate (Robinul®) for each mg of neostigmine

EVOKED POTENTIAL MONITORING

Anesthesia requirements for intra-operative monitoring of evoked potentials **(EPs)**:
1. if inhalational anesthetic agents have to be used
   A. avoid halothane, isoflurane (both reduce the amplitude and increase the latency of EPs and slow the EEG) and Ethrane®
   B. agents should be used at concentrations < 0.25%
   C. recommend: e.g. Forane® at < 1 MAC (ideally < 0.5 MAC)
2. nitrous/narcotic technique preferred
3. muscle relaxants are permissible
4. avoid benzodiazepines
5. minimize pentothal at induction, or use etomidate (expect ≈ 30 minutes of suppression of EPs after induction due to medication)
6. continuous infusion of fentanyl is preferred over intermittent injections

1.2.   Critical care

1.2.1.   Hypertension

PARENTERAL AGENTS

Table 1-1 shows some parenteral agents for acute control of hypertension grouped based on their effect on ICP[5, 6].

Table 1-1   Effect of antihypertensives on ICP

Agents that may raise ICP (mostly vasodilators)	Agents that do **not** raise ICP
nitroglycerin (NTG)	trimethaphan (Arfonad®)
nitroprusside (NTP) (Nipride®)	methyldopa (Aldomet®)
	labetalol (Normodyne®...)
	nicardipine (Cardene®)

★   nicardipine (Cardene®)   DRUG INFO

Calcium channel blocker **(CCB)** that may be given IV. Unlike NTP, does not require arterial line, <u>does not raise ICP</u>, and no cyanide toxicity. Does not reduce heart rate, but may be used in conjunction with e.g. labetalol or esmolol if that is desired. SIDE EFFECTS: H/A 15%, nausea 5%, hypotension 5%, reflex tachycardia 3.5%.

Rx start at 5 mg/hr IV (off label: 10 mg/hr may be used in situations where urgent reduction is needed). Increase by 2.5 mg/hr every 5-15 minutes up to a maximum of 15 mg/hr.

Raises ICP in patients with intracranial mass lesions[7] due to direct vasodilatation, arterial > venous (small coronaries > large). May preferentially dilate peripheral vessels before cerebral vessels, thus producing a "cerebral steal" phenomenon. Acts in seconds, duration 3-5 min.

SIDE EFFECTS: thiocyanate and cyanide toxicity (may cause neurologic deterioration[8] or hypotension) (follow thiocyanate levels if used > 24 hrs, at a rate ≥ 10 µg/kg/min, or in renal failure; D/C if thiocyanate levels > 10 mg%), tachycardia, tachyphylaxis, hypotension which can extend an MI, "coronary steal". Avoid in pregnancy.

Rx IV drip 0.25-8 µg/kg/min (ave. = 3). To reduce risk of cyanide toxicity, start at very low rate of 0.3 µg/kg/min, and do not give maximum rate of 10 µg/kg/min for more than 10 minutes. To prepare: put 50 mg in 500 ml D5W (can only be mixed in D5W; solution can be double concentrated to reduce fluid or glucose load) = 100 µg/ml; cover bottle with foil (light sensitive).

Raises ICP (less than with nitroprusside due to preferential venous action[7]). Vasodilator, venous > arterial (large coronaries > small). Result: decreases LV filling pressure (pre-load). Does not cause "coronary steal" (cf nitroprusside).

Rx 10-20 µg/min IV drip (increase by 5-10 µg/min q 5-10 min). For angina pectoris: 0.4 mg SL q 5 min x 3 doses, check BP before each dose.

Blocks α_1 selective, ß non-selective (potency < propranolol). ICP reduces or no change[9]. Pulse rate: decreases or no change. Cardiac output does not change. Does not exacerbate coronary ischemia. May be used in controlled CHF, but not in overt CHF. Contraindicated in asthma. Renal failure: same dose. SIDE EFFECTS: fatigue, dizziness, orthostatic hypotension.

Intravenous (IV)

Onset 5 mins, peak 10 mins, duration 3-6 hrs.

Rx IV: patient supine; check BP q 5 min; give each dose slow IVP (over 2 min) q 10 minutes until desired BP achieved; dose sequence: 20, 40, 80, 80, then 80 mg (300 mg total). Once controlled, use ≈ same total dose IVP q 8 hrs.

Rx IV drip (alternative): add 40 ml (200 mg) to 160 ml of IVF (result: 1 mg/ml); run at 2 ml/min (2 mg/min) until desired BP (usual effective dose = 50-200 mg) or until 300 mg given; then titrate rate (bradycardia limits dose, increase slowly since effect takes 10-20 minutes).

Oral (PO)

Undergoes first pass liver degradation, therefore requires higher doses PO. PO onset: 2 hrs, peak: 4 hrs.

Rx PO: to convert IV → PO, start with 200 mg PO BID. To start with PO, give 100 mg BID, and increase 100 mg/dose q 2 day; max. = 2400 mg/day.

An angiotensin-converting enzyme (ACE) inhibitor. The active metabolite of the orally administered drug enalapril (*see below*). Acts within ≈ 15 mins of administration. SIDE EFFECTS: hyperkalemia occurs in ≈ 1%. Do not use during pregnancy.

Rx IV: start with 1.25 mg slow IV over 5 mins, may increase up to 5 mg q 6 hrs PRN.

Cardioselective short-acting beta blocker[10]. Being investigated for hypertensive emergencies. Metabolized by RBC esterase. Elimination half-life: 9 mins. Therapeutic response (> 20% decrease in heart rate, HR < 100, or conversion to sinus rhythm) in 72%. SIDE EFFECTS: dose related hypotension (in 20-50%), generally resolves within 30 mins of

D/C. Bronchospasm less likely than other beta blockers. Avoid in CHF.

Rx 500 µg/kg loading dose over 1 min, follow with 4 min infusion starting with 50 µg/kg/min. Repeat loading dose and increment infusion rate by 50 µg/kg/min q 5 mins. Rarely > 100 µg/kg/min required. Doses > 200 µg/kg/min add little.

fenoldopam (Corlopam®) — DRUG INFO

Vasodilator. Onset of action < 5 minutes, duration 30 mins.

Rx IV infusion (no bolus doses): start with 0.1-0.3 mcg/kg/min, titrate by 0.1 mcg/kg/min q 15 min up to a maximum of 1.6 mcg/kg/min.

propranolol (Inderal®) — DRUG INFO

Main use IV is to counteract tachycardia with vasodilators (usually doesn't lower BP acutely when used alone).

Rx IV: load with 1-10 mg slow IVP, follow with 3 mg/hr. PO: 80-640 mg q d in divided doses.

ORAL AGENTS

For less urgent control of HTN (exception: sublingual nifedipine (*see below*)).

clonidine (Catapres®) — DRUG INFO

Acts on cardiovascular control receptors in medulla oblongata, inhibits sympathetic outflow. Less confusion than Aldomet, but still sedating. Tachycardia rare. Onset: < 30 min.

SIDE EFFECTS: fluid retention (which may reduce effectiveness, counter with diuretic) dry mouth, sedation (minimize by slow dose increments), constipation, decreased CO & HR (by increased vagal tone), rebound HTN if withdrawn rapidly (caution in unreliable patients; treatment for rebound HTN: clonidine and labetalol, *see page 4*). Rebound is less likely and less severe with clonidine patches (Catapres TTS®), applied once per week.

Rx Rapid control: 0.2 mg PO, then 0.1 mg PO q 1 hr, stop at 0.8 mg total or if orthostatic. Maintenance dose: 0.1 mg PO BID or TID, increase slowly to max. 2.4 mg/day (usual 0.2-0.8 mg/day).

propranolol (Inderal®) — DRUG INFO

Beta blocker. Use in HTN: blunts reflex tachycardia from vasodilators.

SIDE EFFECTS: CHF, symptomatic bradycardia, bronchospasm (avoid in asthmatics), rapid withdrawl → reflex tachycardia → exacerbates myocardial ischemia in CAD.

Rx 40 mg PO BID (usually with diuretic), titrate up to 640 mg/day in 2-3 divided doses. Or, Inderal-LA, 80 mg PO q d. **SUPPLIED:** 10, 20 40, 60 & 80 mg scored tabs. Inderal-LA (long acting) 60, 80, 120 & 160 mg capsules.

nifedipine (Procardia®, Adalat®) — DRUG INFO

Short-acting calcium channel blocker **(CCB)**. Decreases systemic vascular resistance. Increases cardiac index, CBF (by 10-20%), GFR, and Na excretion. Response somewhat variable. Onset: 1-15 mins. Duration: 3-5 hrs.

SIDE EFFECTS: flushing H/A, palpitation, edema; reflex tachycardia, caution with beta blocker as negative inotropy may be additive. May cause severe hypotension in volume depleted patients (thus use with caution with mannitol or furosemide). May increase serum phenytoin (Dilantin®) levels. Use of short-acting CCBs may be associated with cardiac risk, thus long-acting agents should be used unless specific benefit outweighs the risk.

Rx 10-20 mg PO, faster onset with sublingual or buccal administration (puncture capsule), or if chewed (patient expels capsule after chewing). Note: the beneficial effects of the drug results from swallowing the capsule contents, the medication is <u>not</u> absorbed through the mucosa. If no response after 20-30 min, give additional 10 mg.

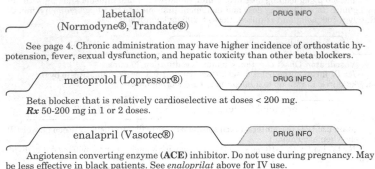

labetalol
(Normodyne®, Trandate®)
DRUG INFO

See page 4. Chronic administration may have higher incidence of orthostatic hypotension, fever, sexual dysfunction, and hepatic toxicity than other beta blockers.

metoprolol (Lopressor®)
DRUG INFO

Beta blocker that is relatively cardioselective at doses < 200 mg.
Rx 50-200 mg in 1 or 2 doses.

enalapril (Vasotec®)
DRUG INFO

Angiotensin converting enzyme **(ACE)** inhibitor. Do not use during pregnancy. May be less effective in black patients. See *enaloprilat* above for IV use.
Rx initial dose 2.5-5 mg in one dose; maintenance 5-40 mg in 1 or 2 doses.

1.2.2.   Hypotension (shock)

Classification:
1. hypovolemic: first sign usually tachycardia. > 20-40% of blood volume loss must occur before perfusion of vital organs is impaired. Includes:
   A. hemorrhage (external or internal)
   B. bowel obstruction (with third spacing)
2. septic: most often due to gram negative sepsis
3. cardiogenic: includes MI, cardiomyopathy, dysrhythmias (including A-fib)
4. neurogenic: e.g. paralysis due to spinal cord injury. Blood pools in venous capacitance vessels
5. miscellaneous
   A. anaphylaxis
   B. insulin reaction

CARDIOVASCULAR AGENTS FOR SHOCK

Plasma expanders. Includes:
1. crystalloids: normal saline has less tendency to promote cerebral edema than others (see *IV fluids*, page 657 under control of elevated ICP)
2. colloids: e.g. hetastarch (Hespan®). ✖ CAUTION: repeated administration over a period of days may prolong PT/PTT and clotting times and may increase the risk of rebleeding in aneurysmal SAH[11] (*see page 787*)
3. blood products: expensive. Risk of transmissible diseases or transfusion reaction

PRESSORS

phenylephrine
(Neo-Synephrine®)
DRUG INFO

Pure alpha sympathomimetic. Useful in hypotension associated with tachycardia (atrial tachyarrhythmias). Elevates BP by increasing SVR via vasoconstriction, causes reflex increase in parasympathetic tone (with resultant slowing of pulse). Lack of ß action means non-inotropic, no cardiac acceleration, and no relaxation of bronchial smooth muscle. Cardiac output and renal blood flow may decrease. Avoid in spinal cord injuries (*see page 703*).
Rx pressor range: 100-180 µg/min; maintenance: 40-60 µg/min. To prepare: put 40 mg (4 amps) in 500 ml D5W to yield 80 µg/ml; a rate of 8 ml/hr = 10 µg/min.

dopamine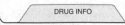

See *Table 1-2* for a summary of the effects of dopamine (**DA**) at various dosages. DA is primarily a vasoconstrictor (ß₁ effects usually overridden by α-activity). 25% of dopamine given is rapidly converted to norepinephrine (**NE**). At doses > 10 μg/kg/min one is essentially giving NE. May cause significant hyperglycemia at high doses.

Rx Start with 2-5 μg/kg/min and titrate.

Table 1-2 Dopamine dosage

Dose (μg/kg/min)	Effect	Result
0.5-2.0 (sometimes up to 5)	dopaminergic	renal, mesenteric, coronary, & cerebral vasodilatation, (+) inotrope
2-10	ß₁	positive inotrope
> 10	α, ß & dopaminergic	releases nor-epi (vasoconstrictor)

dobutamine (Dobutrex®) DRUG INFO

Vasodilates by ß₁ (primary) and by increased CO from (+) inotropy (ß₂); result: little or no fall in BP, less tachycardia than DA. No alpha release nor vasoconstriction. May be used synergistically with nitroprusside. Tachyphylaxis after ≈ 72 hrs. Pulse increases > 10% may exacerbate myocardial ischemia, more common at doses > 20 μg/kg/min. Optimal use requires hemodynamic monitoring. Possible platelet function inhibition.

Rx usual range 2.5-10 μg/kg/min; rarely doses up to 40 used (to prepare: put 50 mg in 250 ml D5W to yield 200 μg/ml).

amrinone (Inocor®) DRUG INFO

Nonadrenergic cardiotonic. Phosphodiesterase inhibitor, effects similar to dobutamine (including exacerbation of myocardial ischemia). 2% incidence of thrombocytopenia.

Rx 0.75 mg/kg initially over 2-3 min, then drip 5-10 μg/kg/min.

norepinephrine DRUG INFO

Primarily vasoconstrictor (? counterproductive in cerebral vasospasm, ? decreases CBF). ß-agonist at low doses. Increases pulmonary vascular resistance.

epinephrine DRUG INFO

Rx 0.5-1.0 mg of 1:10,000 solution IVP; may repeat q 5 minutes (may bolus per ET tube). Drip: start at 1.0 μg/min, titrate up to 8 μg/min (to prepare: put 1 mg in 100 ml NS or D5W).

isoproterenol (Isuprel®) DRUG INFO

Positive chronotropic and inotropic, → increased cardiac O₂ consumption, arrhythmias, vasodilatation (by ß₁ action) skeletal muscle > cerebral vessels.

levophed DRUG INFO

Direct ß stimulation (positive inotropic and chronotropic).

Rx start drip at 8-12 μg/min; maintenance 2-4 μg/min (0.5-1.0 ml/min) (to prepare: put 2 mg in 500 ml NS or D5W to yield 4 μg/cc).

1.2.3. Neurogenic pulmonary edema

A rare condition associated with a variety of intracranial pathologies, including:

subarachnoid hemorrhage, generalized seizures, and head injury.

Pathophysiology

Two possibly synergistic mechanisms. Sudden increased ICP or hypothalamic injury may produce a salvo of sympathetic discharge causing redistribution of blood to the pulmonary circulation, resulting in elevation of pulmonary capillary wedge pressures (**PCWP**) and increased permeability. Secondly, the associated surge of catecholamines directly disrupts the capillary endothelium which increases alveolar permeability.

Treatment

Supportive, using measures such as positive pressure ventilation with <u>low</u> levels of PEEP (*see page 659*) and treatment to normalize ICP. A PA-catheter is usually helpful.

There may be some efficacy in using a dobutamine infusion[12] supplemented with furosemide as needed. The theoretical advantage of dobutamine over previously attempted alpha- and beta-blockers is that dobutamine does <u>not</u> reduce cerebral perfusion. Nitroprusside may help dilate the pulmonary vasculature.

1.3. Endocrinology

1.3.1. Steroids

1.3.1.1. Replacement therapy

Under normal, basal conditions, the adrenal cortex secretes 15-25 mg/day of **hydrocortisone** (AKA cortisol), and 1.5-4 mg/day of **corticosterone**. Cortisol has a half-life of ≈ 90 minutes.

In primary adrenocortical insufficiency (Addison's disease), both glucocorticoids and mineralocorticoids must be replaced. In secondary adrenal insufficiency caused by deficient corticotropin (**ACTH**) release by the pituitary, mineralocorticoid secretion is usually normal and only glucocorticoids need to be replaced.

Table 1-3 shows equivalent daily corticosteroid doses for replacement therapy.

Table 1-3   Equivalent corticosteroid doses*

Steroid: generic (proprietary)	Equiv dose (mg)	Route	Dosing	Mineralo-corticoid potency	Oral dosing forms
cortisone (Cortone®)	25	PO, IM	2/3 in AM, 1/3 in PM	2+	tabs: 5, 10 & 25 mg
hydrocortisone AKA cortisol (Cortef®)	20	PO	2/3 in AM, 1/3 in PM	2+	tabs: 5, 10 & 20 mg
(Solu-Cortef®)		IV, IM†			
prednisone (Deltasone®)	5	PO only	BID-TID	1+	tabs: 1, 2.5, 5, 10, 20, 50 mg‡
methylprednisolone (Solumedrol®)	4	PO, IV, IM		0	tabs§: 2, 4, 8, 16, 24, 32 mg
dexamethasone (Decadron®)	0.75	PO, IV	BID-QID	0	scored tabs: 0.25, 0.5, 0.75, 1.5, 4, 6 mg

*   doses given are <u>daily</u> doses. Steroids listed are used primarily as glucocorticoids: equivalent <u>glucocorticoid</u> PO or IV dose is given; IM may differ

†   IM route recommended only for emergencies where IV access cannot be rapidly obtained

‡   Sterapred Uni-Pak® contains 21 tabs of 5 mgs prednisone and tapers dosage from 30 to 5 mgs over 6 days; "DS" contains 10 mg tabs and tapers from 60 mg to 10 mg over 6 days; "DS 12-Day" contains 48 10 mg tabs and tapers from 60 mg to 20 mg over 12 days

§   Medrol Dosepak® contains 21 tabs of 4 mgs methylprednisolone and tapers dosage from 24 to 4 mgs over 6 days

Physiologic replacement (in the absence of stress) can be accomplished with either:
1.   hydrocortisone: 20 mg PO q AM and 10 mg PO q PM
2.   or prednisone: 5 mg PO q AM and 2.5 mg PO q PM

Cortisol and cortisone are useful for chronic primary adrenocortical insufficiency or for Addisonian crisis. Because of mineralocorticoid activity, use for chronic therapy of other conditions (e.g. hypopituitarism) may result in salt and fluid retention, hypertension and hypokalemia.

HYPOTHALAMIC-PITUITARY-ADRENAL AXIS SUPPRESSION

Chronic steroid administration suppresses the hypothalamic-pituitary-adrenal (HPA) axis, and eventually causes adrenal atrophy. If steroids are abruptly stopped or if acute illness develops, symptoms of adrenocortical insufficiency (AI) may ensue (see Table 1-4), which if severe may progress to Addisonian crisis (see page 11). Recovery of adrenal cortex lags behind the pituitary, so basal ACTH levels increase before cortisol levels do.

HPA suppression depends on the specific glucocorticoid used, the route, frequency, time, and duration of treatment. Suppression is unlikely with < 40 mg prednisone (or equivalent) given in the morning for less than ≈ 7 days, or with every-other-day therapy of < 40 mg for ≈ 5 weeks[13]. Some adrenal atrophy may occur after 3-4 days of high dose steroids, and some axis suppression will almost certainly occur after 2 weeks of 40-60 mg hydrocortisone (or equivalent) daily. After a month or more of steroids, the HPA axis may be depressed for as long as one year.

Table 1-4 Symptoms of adrenal insufficiency

• fatigue	• orthostatic dizziness
• weakness	• hypoglycemia
• arthralgia	• dyspnea
• anorexia	• Addisonian crisis (if
• nausea	severe; with risk of
• hypotension	death, see page 11)

Measuring morning plasma hydrocortisone can evaluate the degree of recovery of basal adrenocortical function, but does not assess adequacy stress response.

STEROID WITHDRAWAL[13]

In addition to the above dangers of hypocortisolism in the presence of HPA suppression, too rapid a taper may cause a flare-up of the underlying condition for which steroids were prescribed.

When the risk of HPA suppression is low (as is the case with short courses of steroids for less than ≈ 5-7 days[14] generally prescribed for most neurosurgical indications) abrupt discontinuation usually carries a low risk of AI. For up to≈ 2 weeks of use, steroids are usually safely withdrawn by tapering over 1-2 weeks. For longer treatment, or when withdrawal problems develop, use the following conservative taper:
1. make small decrements (equivalent to 2.5-5 mg prednisone) every 3-7 d. Patient may experience mild withdrawal symptoms of[15]:
    A. fatigue
    B. anorexia
    C. nausea
    D. orthostatic dizziness
2. "backtrack" (i.e. increase the dose and resume a more gradual taper) if any of the following occur:
    A. exacerbation of the underlying condition for which steroids were used
    B. evidence of steroid withdrawal symptoms (see Table 1-4)
    C. intercurrent infection or need for surgery (see Stress doses below)
3. once "physiologic" doses of glucocorticoid have been reached (about 20 mg hydrocortisone/day or equivalent (see Table 1-3)):
    A. the patient is switched to 20 mg hydrocortisone PO q AM (do not use long acting preparations)
    B. after ≈ 2-4 weeks, a morning cortisol level is checked (prior to the AM hydrocortisone dose), and the hydrocortisone is tapered by 2.5 mg weekly until 10 mg/d is reached (lower limits of physiologic)
    C. then, every 2-4 weeks, the AM cortisol level is drawn (prior to AM dose) until the 8 AM cortisol is > 10 µg/100 ml, indicating return of baseline adrenal function
    D. when this return of baseline adrenal function occurs:
        1. daily steroids are stopped, but stress doses must still be given when needed (see below)
        2. monthly cosyntropin stimulation tests (see page 444) are performed until normal. The need for stress doses of steroids ceases when a positive test is obtained. The risk for adrenal insufficiency persists ≈ 2 years after cessation of chronic steroids (especially the first year)

STRESS DOSES

During physiologic "stress" the normal adrenal gland produces ≈ 250-300 mg hydrocortisone/day. With chronic glucocorticoid therapy (either at present, or in last 1-2 yrs), suppression of the normal "stress-response" necessitates supplemental doses.

In patients with a suppressed HPA axis:
- for mild illness (e.g. UTI, common cold), single dental extraction: double the daily dose (if off steroids, give 40 mg hydrocortisone BID)
- for moderate stress (e.g. flu), minor surgery under local anesthesia (endoscopy, multiple dental extractions…): give 50 mg hydrocortisone BID
- for major illness (pneumonia, systemic infections, high fever), severe trauma, or emergency surgery under general anesthesia: give 100 mg hydrocortisone IV q 6-8 hrs for 3-4 days until the stress is resolved
- for elective surgery, see Table 1-5 for guidelines

Table 1-5 Steroid stress doses for elective surgery

On day of surgery, 50 mg cortisone acetate IM, followed by 200 mg hydrocortisone IV infused over 24 hrs

Post-op day	Hydrocortisone (mg)		
	8 AM	4 PM	10 PM
1	50	50	50
2	50	25	25
3	40	20	20
4	30	20	10
5	25	20	5
6	25	15	–
7	20	10	–

POSSIBLE DELETERIOUS SIDE EFFECTS OF STEROIDS

Although these side effects are more common with prolonged administration[16], some can occur even with short treatment courses. Possible side effects include[15, 17]:
- cardiovascular and renal
  - ♦ hypertension
  - ♦ sodium and water retention
  - ♦ hypokalemic alkalosis
- CNS
  - ♦ progressive multifocal leukoencephalopathy (**PML**) (see page 231)
  - ♦ mental agitation or "steroid psychosis"
  - ♦ spinal cord compression from spinal epidural lipomatosis: rare (see page 903)
  - ♦ pseudotumor cerebri (see Idiopathic intracranial hypertension, page 493)
- endocrine
  - ♦ caution: because of growth suppressant effect in children, daily glucocorticoid dosing over prolonged periods should be reserved for the most urgent indications
  - ♦ secondary amenorrhea
  - ♦ suppression of hypothalamic-pituitary-adrenal axis: reduces endogenous steroid production → risk of adrenal insufficiency with steroid withdrawal (see above)
  - ♦ Cushingoid features with prolonged usage (iatrogenic Cushing's syndrome): obesity, hypertension, hirsutism…
- GI: risk increased only with steroid therapy > 3 weeks duration and regimens of prednisone > 400-1000 mg/d or dexamethasone > 40 mg/d[18]
  - ♦ gastritis and steroid ulcers: incidence lowered with the use of antacids and/or H_2 antagonists (e.g. cimetidine, ranitidine…)
  - ♦ pancreatitis
  - ♦ intestinal or sigmoid diverticular perforation[19]: incidence ≈ 0.7%. Since steroids may mask signs of peritonitis, this should be considered in patients on steroids with abdominal discomfort, especially in the elderly and those with a history of diverticular disease. Abdominal x-ray usually shows free intraperitoneal air
- inhibition of fibroblasts
  - ♦ impaired wound healing or wound breakdown
  - ♦ subcutaneous tissue atrophy
- metabolic
  - ♦ glucose intolerance (diabetes) and disturbance of nitrogen metabolism
  - ♦ hyperosmolar nonketotic coma
  - ♦ hyperlipidemia
- ophthalmologic
  - ♦ posterior subcapsular cataracts
  - ♦ glaucoma
- musculoskeletal
  - ♦ avascular necrosis (**AVN**) of the hip or other bones: usually with prolonged administration → cushingoid habitus and increased marrow fat within the bone[20]

- osteoporosis: may predispose to vertebral compression fractures which occur in 30-50% of patients on prolonged glucocorticoids(*see page 748*). Steroid induced bone loss may be reversed with cyclical administration of etidronate[21] in 4 cycles of 400 mg/d **x** 14 days followed by 76 days of oral calcium supplements of 500 mg/d (not proven to reduced rate of VB fractures, *see page 748*)
  - muscle weakness (steroid myopathy): often worse in proximal muscles
- infectious
  - immunosuppression: with possible superinfection, especially fungal, parasitic
  - possible reactivation of TB, chickenpox
- hematologic
  - hypercoagulopathy from inhibition of tissue plasminogen activator
  - steroids cause demargination of white blood cells, which may artifactually elevate the WBC count even in the absence of infection
- miscellaneous
  - hiccups: may respond to chlorpromazine (Thorazine®) 25-50 mg PO TID-QID **x** 2-3 days (if symptoms persist, give 25-50 mg IM)
  - steroids readily cross the placenta, and fetal adrenal hypoplasia may occur with the administration of large doses during pregnancy

1.3.1.2. Addisonian crisis

An adrenal insufficiency emergency.

Symptoms: mental status changes (confusion, lethargy, or agitation), muscle weakness.

Signs: postural hypotension or shock, hyponatremia, hyperkalemia, hypoglycemia, hyperthermia (as high as 105° F).

TREATMENT OF ADDISONIAN CRISIS

If possible, draw serum for cortisol determination (do **not** wait for these results to institute therapy). Give fluids sufficient for dehydration and shock.

For "glucocorticoid emergency"
- hydrocortisone sodium succinate (Solu-Cortef®): 100 mg IV STAT and then 50 mg IV q 6 hrs
- AND cortisone acetate 75-100 mg IM STAT, and then 50-75 mg IM q 6 hrs

For "mineralocorticoid emergency"
Usually not necessary in secondary adrenal insufficiency (e.g. panhypopituitarism)
- desoxycorticosterone acetate (Doca®): 5 mg IM BID
- OR fludrocortisone (Florinef®): 0.05- 0.2 mg PO q d

NOT recommended for emergency treatment
- ✖ methylprednisolone

1.4.   Fluids and Electrolytes

SERUM OSMOLALITY

Clinical significance of various serum osmolarity values is shown in *Table 1-6*.

Approximate value may be calculated using using *Eq 1-1*.

Table 1-6 Clinical correlates of serum osmolality

Value (mOsm/L)	Comment
282-295	normal
< 240 or > 321	panic values
> 320	risk of renal failure
> 384	produces stupor
> 400	risk of generalized seizures
> 420	usually fatal

$$\text{Osmolality (mOsm/L)} = 2 \times \{[Na^+] + [K^+]\} + \frac{[BUN]}{2.8} + \frac{[glucose]}{18}$$ **Eq 1-1**

NB: terms in square brackets [] represent serum concentrations (in mEq/L for electrolytes)

1.4.1. Electrolyte abnormalities

1.4.1.1. Sodium

Antidiuretic hormone

The major source of the nanopeptide arginine vasopressin, AKA antidiuretic hormone (**ADH**) is the magnocellular portion of the supraoptic nucleus of the hypothalamus. It is conveyed along axons in the supraoptic-hypophyseal tract to the posterior pituitary gland (neurohypophysis) where it is released into the systemic circulation. All actions of ADH result from binding of the hormone to specific membrane bound receptors on the surface of target cells[22]. One of the major effects of ADH is to increase the permeability of the distal renal tubules resulting in increased reabsorption of water, diluting the circulating blood and producing a concentrated urine. The most powerful physiologic stimulus for ADH release is an increase in serum osmolality, a less potent stimulus is a reduction of intravascular volume. ADH is also released in glucocorticoid deficiency, and is inhibited by exogenous glucocorticoids and adrenergic drugs. ADH is also a potent vasoconstrictor.

HYPONATREMIA

Hyponatremia may occur in conditions of volume overload such as congestive heart failure. However, hyponatremia in neurosurgical patients is chiefly seen in:
* syndrome of inappropriate antidiuretic hormone secretion (**SIADH**, *see below*): dilutional hyponatremia with normal or elevated intravascular volume. Usually treated with fluid restriction
* cerebral salt wasting (**CSW**): inappropriate natriuresis with volume depletion. Treated with sodium and volume replacement (opposite to SIADH), symptoms from derangements due to CSW may be *exacerbated* by fluid restriction[23] (*see page 14*)
* postoperative hyponatremia: a rare condition usually described in young, otherwise healthy women undergoing elective surgery[24]

Due to slow compensatory mechanisms in the brain, a gradual decline in serum sodium is better tolerated than a rapid drop. Symptoms of mild or gradual hyponatremia include anorexia, headache, irritability, and muscle weakness. Severe hyponatremia (< 120 mmol/L) or a rapid drop (> 0.5 mmol/hr) can cause neuromuscular excitability, cerebral edema, muscle twitching and cramps, nausea/vomiting, confusion, seizures, respiratory arrest and possibly permanent neurologic injury, coma or death.

Central pontine myelinolysis

Whereas excessively slow correction of hyponatremia is associated with increased morbidity and mortality[25], inordinately rapid treatment has been associated with central pontine myelinolysis (**CPM**), AKA osmotic demyelination syndrome, a rare disorder of pontine white matter[26] as well as other areas of cerebral white matter, first described in alcoholics[27], producing insidious flaccid quadriplegia, mental status changes, and cranial nerve abnormalities with a pseudobulbar palsy appearance. In one review[28], no patient developed CPM when treated slowly as outlined below. And yet, the rate of correction correlates poorly with CPM; it may be that the magnitude is the critical variable[29]. Features common to patients who develop CPM are[28]:
* delay in the diagnosis of hyponatremia with resultant respiratory arrest or seizure with probable hypoxemic event
* rapid correction to normo- or hyper-natremia (> 135 mEq/L) within 48 hours of initiation of therapy
* increase of serum sodium by > 25 mEq/L within 48 hours of initiation of therapy
* over-correcting serum sodium in patients with hepatic encephalopathy
* NB: many patients developing CPM were victims of chronic debilitating disease,

malnourishment, or alcoholism and never had hyponatremia. Many had an episode of hypoxia/anoxia[30]
- presence of hyponatremia > 24 hrs prior to treatment[29]

TREATMENT OF HYPONATREMIA

Patients with hyponatremia of unknown duration probably have chronic hyponatremia if minimally symptomatic, and should be treated slowly, preferably with fluid restriction. Those with acute symptomatic hyponatremia (convulsions, stupor or coma) should be treated promptly since the presence of CNS symptoms has been shown to be associated with brain edema (radiographically and at necropsy) and may herald impending herniation and cardiorespiratory arrest.

Symptomatic patients with hyponatremia of unknown duration are the ones at risk of neurologic sequelae, and one should start off with a 10% correction, followed by a more gradual treatment as outlined below[29]. The following method for correcting hyponatremia ([Na^+] < 125 mEq/L) is associated with low risk of developing CPM (although it may not be possible to define a rate of correction that is consistently free of risk):

1. ✖ CAUTION: avoid normo- or hyper-natremia during correction, check frequent serum [Na^+] levels and modulate therapy as follows:
   - stop if serum [Na^+] ≥ 126 mEq/L over a period of ≈ 17 ± 1 hours
   - stop if the <u>change</u> in serum [Na^+] is ≥ 10 mEq/L in 24 hours[31]
   - do not exceed a rate of correction of ≈ 1.3 ± 0.2 mEq/L/hr
2. slowly administer 3% (513 mEq/L) or 5% (856 mEq/L) NaCl to adhere to the above criteria (start with 25-50 cc/hr of the 3% solution and follow [Na^+] closely)
3. simultaneously administer furosemide (Lasix®)[32] to prevent volume overload with subsequent increase in atrial natriuretic factor and resultant urinary dumping of the extra Na^+ being administered
4. measure K^+ lost in urine and replace accordingly

SYNDROME OF INAPPROPRIATE ANTIDIURETIC HORMONE SECRETION
❢ Key features
- release of ADH in the absence of physiologic (osmotic) stimuli
- results in hyponatremia with high urine osmolality
- usually accompanied by hypervolemia (occasionally with euvolemia)
- may be seen with certain malignancies and many intracranial abnormalities
- critical to distinguish from cerebral salt wasting which produces <u>hypo</u>volemia

SIADH, AKA Schwartz-Bartter syndrome, was first described with bronchogenic cancer. It is the release of antidiuretic hormone **(ADH)** in the absence of physiologic (osmotic) stimuli. This produces elevated urine osmolality, and expansion of the extracellular fluid volume leading to a dilutional hyponatremia, which can produce fluid overload (hypervolemia) but SIADH may also occur with euvolemia. For reasons that are unclear, edema does not occur.

Etiologies of SIADH
The hyponatremia of SIADH must be differentiated from that due to cerebral salt wasting **(CSW)** (*see below*). SIADH may be seen in the following settings (see reference[33] for more extensive list):

1. malignant tumors: especially bronchogenic
2. numerous intracranial processes including:
   A. meningitis: especially in pediatric patients, also with TB meningitis
   B. trauma: seen in 4.6% of head trauma patients
   C. increased ICP
   D. tumors
   E. post craniotomy
   F. SAH (NB: rule-out CSW, which requires different treatment, *see below*)
3. numerous pulmonary disorders
   A. malignancy
   B. pulmonary TB
   C. aspergillosis
4. may sometimes occur secondary to anemia
5. with stress, severe pain, nausea or hypotension (all can stimulate ADH release)
6. occasionally seen with acute intermittent porphyria **(AIP)**
7. drugs:
   A. chlorpropramide (Diabinese®): may cause a "relative" SIADH by increasing

the renal sensitivity to endogenous ADH
  B. oxytocin: has some "cross activity" with ADH, and may also be contaminat-
      ed with ADH
  C. thiazide diuretics: hydrochlorothiazide... (see page 18)
  D. carbamazepine (Tegretol®)

DIAGNOSIS OF SIADH
  In general, 3 diagnostic criteria are: hyponatremia, inappropriately concentrated
urine, and no evidence of renal or adrenal dysfunction. In more detail:
  1. low serum sodium (hyponatremia): usually < 134 mEq/L
  2. low serum osmolality: < 280 mOsm/L
  3. high urinary sodium[A] (salt wasting): at least > 18 mEq/L, often 50-150
  4. high ratio of urine:serum osmolality: often 1.5-2.5:1, but may be 1:1
  5. normal renal function (check BUN & creatinine): BUN commonly < 10
  6. normal adrenal function (no hypotension, no hyperkalemia)
  7. no hypothyroidism
  8. no signs of dehydration or overhydration (in many patients with acute brain dis-
      ease, there is significant hypovolemia often due to CSW (see below) and as this is
      a stimulus for ADH secretion, the ADH release may be "appropriate"[34])

  If further testing is required, the **water-load test** is considered to be the definitive
test[35]. The patient is asked to consume a water load of 20 ml/kg up to 1500 ml. In the absence of adrenal or renal insufficiency, the failure to excrete 65% of the water load in 4
hrs or 80% in 5 hrs indicates SIADH. ✖ CAUTION: this test is dangerous if the starting
serum [Na⁺] is ≤ 124 mEq/L or if the patient has symptoms of hyponatremia.

  Alternatively, one may measure serum or urinary levels of ADH which is normally
undetectable in hyponatremia of other causes. In SIADH, it is often detectable and, in
the context of the low serum sodium, excessive.

Symptoms of SIADH
  Symptoms of SIADH are those of hyponatremia (confusion, lethargy, N/V, coma, seizure) and possibly fluid overload. If mild, or if descent of [Na⁺] is gradual, it may be tolerated. [Na⁺] < 120-125 mEq/L is almost always symptomatic. These patients often have
a paradoxical (inappropriate) thirst.

TREATMENT
Be sure that hyponatremia is not due to CSW (see below) before restricting fluids.

Treatment of acute SIADH
  • if caused by anemia: usually responds to transfusion
  • if mild and asymptomatic: fluid restriction < 1 L/day (peds: 1 L/m²/day) (caution
     in SAH: see Hyponatremia following SAH, page 788
  • if severe or symptomatic: use hypertonic saline and, if necessary, furosemide (see
     page 13). CAUTION: CPM may be associated with excessively rapid correction
     (see page 12)

Treatment of chronic SIADH
  • long-term fluid restriction: 1200-1800 ml/d
  • **demeclocycline**: 150-300 mg PO q 6 hrs, a tetracycline antibiotic found to par-
     tially antagonize the effects of ADH on the renal tubules[36-38]
  • **furosemide** (Lasix®): ≈ 40 mg PO q d (once daily) along with high dietary sodium
     intake and monitoring for hypochloremic alkalosis[39]
  • **phenytoin** (Dilantin®): may inhibit ADH release
  • **lithium**: not very effective and many side effects

CEREBRAL SALT WASTING
  Cerebral salt wasting (CSW): renal loss of sodium as a result of intracranial disease, producing hyponatremia and a decrease in extracellular fluid volume[35]. CAUTION:
patients with aneurysmal SAH may have CSW with hyponatremia which mimics
SIADH, however there is usually also hypovolemia in CSW. In this setting, fluid restriction may exacerbate vasospasm induced ischemia[35, 40-42].

A. there has not been an adequate explanation of the high urinary sodium in SIADH

The mechanism whereby the kidneys fail to conserve sodium in CSW is not known, and may be either a result of an as yet unidentified natriuretic factor or direct neural control mechanisms (see *Hyponatremia following SAH*, page 788).

Laboratory tests (serum and urinary electrolytes and osmolalities) may be identical with SIADH and CSW[43]. Furthermore, hypovolemia in CSW may stimulate ADH release. To differentiate: CVP, PCWP, and plasma volume (a nuclear medicine study) are low in hypovolemia (i.e. CSW). *Table 1-7* compares some features of CSW and SIADH, the two most important differences being extracellular volume and salt balance. An elevated serum $[K^+]$ with hyponatremia is incompatible with the diagnosis of SIADH.

Treatment of CSW

Goals: volume replacement and positive salt balance. Hydrate patient with 0.9% NS or sometimes hypertonic 3% NaCl. Salt may also be replaced orally. Blood products may be needed if anemia is present. Rapid correction of hyponatremia has been associated with CPM and care should be taken to avoid overcorrection (*see page 13*).

Fludrocortisone acetate acts directly on the renal tubule to increase sodium absorption. Benefits of giving 0.2 mg IV or PO q d in CSW have been reported[44], but significant complications of pulmonary edema, hypokalemia and HTN may occur.

Table 1-7   CSW vs. SIADH[35]*

Parameter	CSW	SIADH
★ Plasma volume	↓ (< 35 ml/kg)	↑
★ Salt balance	negative	variable
Signs & symptoms of dehydration	present	absent
Weight	↓	↑ or no Δ
PCWP	↓ (< 8 mm Hg)	↑ or WNL
CVP	↓ (< 6 mm Hg)	↑ or WNL
Orthostatic hypotension	+	±
Hematocrit	↑	↓ or no Δ
Serum osmolality	↑ or WNL	↓
Ratio of serum [BUN]:[creatinine]	↑	WNL
Serum [protein]	↑	WNL
Urinary $[Na^+]$	↑↑	↑
Serum $[K^+]$	↑ or no Δ	↓ or no Δ
Serum [uric acid]	WNL	↓

*   abbreviations: ↓ = decreased, ↑ = increased, ↑↑ = significantly increased, WNL = within normal limits, no Δ = no change, [] = concentration, + = present, ± = may or may not be present

An alternative treatment using urea may be applicable to the hyponatremia of either SIADH *or* CSW, and therefore may be used before the cause has been ascertained: urea (Ureaphil®) 0.5 grams/kg (dissolve 40 gm in 100-150 ml NS) IV over 30-60 mins q 8 hrs[45]. Use NS + 20 mEq KCl/L at 2 ml/kg/hr as the main IV until the hyponatremia is corrected (unlike mannitol, urea does not increase ADH secretion).

HYPERNATREMIA

Definition: serum sodium > 150 mEq/L. In neurosurgical patients, most often seen in the setting of diabetes insipidus (**DI**) (*see below*).

Since normal total body water (**TBW**) is ≈ 60% of the patient's normal body weight, the patient's current TBW may be estimated by *Eq 1-2*.

$$TBW_{current} = \frac{[Na^+]_{normal} \times TBW_{normal}}{[Na^+]_{current}}$$

$$= \frac{140 \text{ mEq/L} \times 0.6 \times \text{usual body wt (kg)}}{[Na^+]_{current}}$$

Eq 1-2

The free water deficit to be replaced is given by *Eq 1-3*. Correction must be made slowly to avoid exacerbating cerebral edema. <u>One half</u> the water deficit is replaced over 24 hours, and the remainder is given over 1-2 additional days. Judicious replacement of deficient ADH in cases of true DI must also be made (*see below*).

$$\text{free water deficit} = 0.6 \times \text{usual body wt (kg)} - TBW_{current}$$

$$= \frac{[Na^+]_{current} - 140 \text{ mEq/L}}{140 \text{ mEq/L}} \times 0.6 \times \text{usual body wt (kg)}$$

Eq 1-3

DIABETES INSIPIDUS

❦ Key features
- due to low levels of ADH (or, rarely, renal insensitivity to ADH)
- high output of dilute urine (< 200 mOsmol/L or SG < 1.003) with normal or high serum osmolality
- often accompanied by craving for water, especially ice-water
- danger of severe dehydration if not managed carefully

Diabetes insipidus **(DI)** is due to insufficient ADH, and results in the excessive renal loss of water and electrolytes. DI may be produced by two different etiologies:
- central or neurogenic DI: subnormal levels of ADH caused by hypothalamic-pituitary axis dysfunction. This is the type most often seen by neurosurgeons
- **"nephrogenic DI"**: due to relative resistance of the kidney to normal or supranormal levels of ADH. Seen with some drugs (*see below*)

Etiologies of DI[22]:
1. (neurogenic) diabetes insipidus
   A. familial (autosomal dominant)
   B. idiopathic
   C. posttraumatic (including surgery)
   D. tumor: craniopharyngioma, metastasis, lymphoma...
   E. granuloma: neurosarcoidosis, histiocytosis
   F. infectious: meningitis, encephalitis
   G. autoimmune
   H. vascular: aneurysm, Sheehan's syndrome (rarely causes DI)
2. nephrogenic diabetes insipidus
   A. familial (X-linked recessive)
   B. hypokalemia
   C. hypercalcemia
   D. Sjögren's syndrome
   E. drugs: lithium, demeclocycline, colchicine...
   F. chronic renal disease: pyelonephritis, amyloidosis, sickle cell disease, polycystic kidney disease, sarcoidosis

CENTRAL DI
85% of ADH secretory capacity must be lost before clinical DI ensues. Characteristic high urine output (polyuria) with low urine osmolality, and (in the conscious patient) craving for water (polydipsia), especially ice-water.

Differential diagnosis of DI:
1. (neurogenic) diabetes insipidus
2. nephrogenic diabetes insipidus
3. psychogenic
   A. idiopathic: from resetting of the osmostat
   B. psychogenic polydipsia
4. osmotic diuresis: e.g. following mannitol, or with renal glucose spilling
5. diuretic use: furosemide, hydrochlorothiazide...

Central DI may be seen in the following situations:
1. following transsphenoidal surgery or removal of craniopharyngioma: (usually transient, therefore avoid long-acting agents until it can be determined if long-term replacement is required). Injury to the posterior pituitary or stalk usually causes one of three patterns of DI[46]:
   A. transient DI: supra-normal urine output **(UO)** and polydipsia which normalizes ≈ 12-36 hrs post-op
   B. "prolonged" DI: UO stays supra-normal for prolonged period (may be months) or even permanently: only about one third of these patients will not return to near-normal at one year post-op
   C. **"triphasic response"**: least common
      - phase 1: injury to pituitary reduces ADH levels for 4-5 days → DI (polyuria/polydipsia)
      - phase 2: cell death liberates ADH for the next 4-5 days → transient normalization or even SIADH-like water retention (<u>NB</u>: there is a danger of inadvertently continuing vasopressin therapy beyond the initial DI phase into this phase causing significant hemodilution)
      - phase 3: reduced or absent ADH secretion → either transient DI (as in "A" above) or a "prolonged" DI (as in "B" above)

2. following brain death (hypothalamic production of ADH ceases)
3. with certain tumors (e.g. craniopharyngioma, often postoperatively): rare, since damage to pituitary or lower stalk does not prevent production and release of ADH by hypothalamic nuclei
4. with other mass lesions pressing on hypothalamus: e.g. a-comm aneurysm
5. following head injury: primarily with basal (clival) skull fractures (*see page 666*)
6. with encephalitis or meningitis
7. drug induced:
   A. ethanol and phenytoin can inhibit ADH release
   B. exogenous steroids may seem to "bring out" DI because they may correct adrenal insufficiency (see *Diagnosis* below) and they inhibit ADH release
8. Wegener's granulomatosis: a vasculitis (*see page 61*)
9. inflammatory: lymphocytic hypophysitis[47] (*see page 928*) or lymphocytic infundibuloneurohypophysitis[48] (distinct conditions)

DIAGNOSIS

The following are usually adequate to make the diagnosis of DI, especially in the appropriate clinical setting:
1. dilute urine:
   A. urine **osmolality < 200** mOsm/L (usually 50-150)[A] or specific gravity (**SG**) < **1.003** (may be 1.001 to 1.005)
   B. or the inability to concentrate urine to > 300 mOsm/L in the presence of clinical dehydration
   C. NB: large doses of mannitol as may be used in head trauma can mask this by producing a more concentrated urine
2. urine output (**UO**) > 250 cc/hr (peds: > 3 cc/kg/hr)
3. normal or above-normal serum sodium
4. normal adrenal function: DI cannot occur in primary adrenal insufficiency because a minimum of mineralocorticoid activity is needed for the kidney to make free water, thus steroids may "bring out" underlying DI by correcting adrenal insufficiency

In uncertain cases, plot simultaneous urine and serum osmolality on the graph in *Figure 1-1*
1. low serum osmolality: the patient has polydipsia
2. if the point falls in the "normal" range, a super-vised water deprivation test is needed to determine if the patient can concentrate their urine with dehydration (caution: *see below*)
3. high serum osmolality: diagnosis of DI is established, and further testing is not needed (except to differentiate central from nephrogenic DI, if desired)
   • to differentiate central from nephrogenic DI, give aqueous Pitressin® 5 U SQ: in central DI the urine osmolality should double within 1-2 hours
4. plotting more than one data point may help as some patients tend to "vacillate" around the border zones

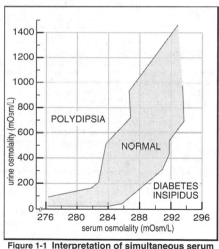

Figure 1-1 Interpretation of simultaneous serum vs. urine osmolality
(Provided by Arnold M. Moses, M.D., used with permission)

A. normally, urine osmolality averages between 500-800 mOsm/L (extreme range: 50-1400)

Water deprivation test

If still unclear, the diagnosis of DI is confirmed by a water deprivation test (✖ CAUTION: perform only under close supervision as rapid and potentially fatal dehydration may ensue in DI). This test is rarely necessary if serum osmolality > 298 mOsm/L[A]. Stop IVs and make the patient NPO; check urine osmolality q hr.

1. continue the test until one of the following occurs:
    A. normal response occurs: urine output decreases, and urine osmolality rises to 600-850 mOsm/L
    B. 6-8 hours lapse
    C. urine osmolality plateaus (i.e. changes < 30 mOsm in 3 consecutive hours)
    D. patient loses 3% of body weight
2. if patient fails to demonstrate the normal response, then:
    A. give exogenous ADH (5 U aqueous Pitressin® SQ), which normally increases urine osmolality to > 300 mOsm/L
    B. check urine osmolality 30 and 60 minutes later
    C. compare highest urine osmolality after Pitressin® to the osmolality just before Pitressin® according to *Table 1-8*

Table 1-8 Highest urinary osmolality after Pitressin in water deprivation test

Δ in urinary Osm	Interpretation
< 5% increase	normal
6-67% increase	partial ADH deficiency
> 67% increase	severe ADH deficiency

TREATMENT OF DI

See*Table 1-9* and *Table 1-10* for dosing forms and duration of action of various vasopressin preparations.

Table 1-9 Available preparations of vasopressin

Generic name	Trade name	Route	Concentration	Availability	Manufacturer
desmopressin	DDAVP®	SQ, IM, IV	4 µg/ml	1 & 10 ml	Aventis
desmopressin	DDAVP® Nasal Spray	nasal spray	100 µg/ml, each spray delivers 10 µg	50 doses per bottle	Aventis
desmopressin	DDAVP® Tablets	PO		0.1 & 0.2 mg	Aventis
arginine vasopressin	aqueous Pitressin®	SQ, IM	20 U/ml (50 µg/ml)	0.5 and 1 ml	Parke-Davis
posterior pituitary powder in oil	Pitressin tannate in oil	IM (poor absorption)	5 U/ml	1 ml	Parke-Davis

In conscious ambulatory patient

If DI is mild, and natural thirst mechanism is intact, instruct patient to drink only when thirsty and they usually "keep up" with losses and will not become overhydrated. If severe, patient may not be able to continue adequate intake of fluid (and constant trips to bathroom), in this case administer either:

1. desmopressin (DDAVP®)
    A. PO: 0.1 mg PO BID, adjust up or down PRN urine output (typical dosage range: 0.1-0.;8 mg/d in divided doses)
    B. nasal spray: 2.5 µg (0.025 ml) by nasal insufflation BID, titrate up to 20 µg BID as needed (the nasal *spray* may be used for doses that are multiples of 10 µg)
OR
2. ADH enhancing medications (works primarily in chronic partial ADH deficiency. Will not work in total absence of ADH)
    A. clofibrate (Atromid S®) 500 mg PO QID
    B. chlorpropramide: increases renal sensitivity to ADH
    C. hydrochlorothiazide: thiazide diuretics may act by depleting Na+ which increases reabsorption in proximal tubules and shifting fluid away from distal tubules which is where ADH works. *Rx*: e.g. Dyazide® 1 PO q d (may increase up to 2 per day PRN)

In conscious ambulatory patient with impaired thirst mechanisms

If thirst mechanisms are not intact in conscious ambulatory patient, they run the risk of dehydration or fluid overload. For these patients:

1. have patient follow UO and daily weights, balance fluid intake and output using

---

A. in compensated DI serum osmolality is more likely to be lower and to overlap with normals[49]

antidiuretic medication as needed to keep UO reasonable

2. check serial labs (approximately q weekly) including serum sodium, BUN

In non-ambulatory, comatose/stuporous, or brain-dead patient
(also see *Management after brain death for organ donation*, page 169)

1. follow I's & O's q 1 hr, with urine specific gravity **(SG)** q 4 hrs and whenever urine output **(UO)** > 250 ml/hr
2. labs: serum electrolytes with osmolality q 6 hrs
3. IV fluid management:
   BASE IV: D5 1/2 NS + 20 mEq KCl/L at appropriate rate (75-100 ml/hr)
   PLUS: replace UO above base IV rate ml for ml with 1/2 NS

   NB: for post-op patients, if the patient received significant intraoperative fluids, then they may have an appropriate post-op diuresis, in this case use 1/2 NS to replace only ≈ 2/3 of UO that exceeds the basal IV rate

Table 1-10 Mean time of hypertonic urine*
(relative to plasma)†

Generic name	Route	Dose	Mean duration of action‡
desmopressin	SQ, IM, IV	0.5 µg	8 hrs
	SQ, IM, IV	1.0 µg§	12 hrs
	SQ, IM, IV	2.0 µg	16 hrs
	SQ, IM, IV	4.0 µg	20 hrs
	intranasal	10 µg (0.1 ml)	12 hrs
	intranasal	15 µg (0.15 ml)	16 hrs
	intranasal	20 µg (0.2 ml)	20 hrs
arginine vasopressin	SQ, IM	5 U (12.5 µg)	4 hrs (range: 4-8)
posterior pituitary powder in oil	IM	5 U	48-72 hrs

* provided by Arnold M. Moses, M.D., used with permission

† onset of antidiuretic action of these preparations is 30-45 minutes following administration (except pituitary powder in oil which takes 2-4 hrs to start working)

‡ times may vary from patient to patient, but are usually consistent in any individual

§ Note: 1 µg BID of desmopressin is as effective as 4 µg q d, but would obviously be less expensive

4. if unable to keep up with fluid loss with IV (or NG) replacement (usually with UO > 300 ml/hr), then EITHER
   - 5 U arginine vasopressin (aqueous Pitressin®) IVP/IM/SQ q 4-6 hrs (avoid tannate oil suspension due to erratic absorption and variable duration)
   OR
   - vasopressin IV drip: start at 0.2 U/min & titrate (max: 0.9 U/min)
   OR
   - desmopressin injection SQ/IV titrated to UO, usual adult dose: 0.5-1 ml (2-4 µg) daily in 2 divided doses

1.5. Hematology

1.5.1. Blood component therapy

PLATELETS

Normal platelet count **(PC)** is 150K-400K[A]. Bleeding (spontaneous or with invasive procedures) is rarely a problem with PC > 50K. Spontaneous hemorrhage is very likely with PC < 5K. 1 unit contains 5.5×10^{10} (minimum) to 10×10^{10} platelets. The volume of 6 units is 250-300 ml. Platelets may be stored up to 5 days.

Recommended transfusion criteria[50]:

1. thrombocytopenia due to ↓ production (with or without increased destruction) (the most common causes are aplastic anemia and leukemia)
   A. PC < 10K even if no bleeding (prophylactic transfusion to prevent bleeding)
   B. PC < 20K and bleeding
   C. PC < 30K and patient at risk for bleeding: complaints of H/A, has confluent

---

A. abbreviation used here: $150K = 150,000/mm^3 = 150 \times 10^9/L$

(c.f. scattered) petechiae, continuous bleeding from a wound, increasing retinal hemorrhage
  D. PC < 50K *AND*
     1. major surgery planned within 12 hours
     2. PC rapidly falling
     3. patient < 48 hours post-op
     4. patient requires lumbar puncture
     5. acute blood loss of > 1 blood volume in < 24 hours
  2. platelet transfusions have limited usefulness when thrombocytopenia is due to platelet destruction (e.g. by antibodies as in ITTP) or consumption (if production is adequate or increased, platelet transfusion usually will not be useful)
  3. documented platelet dysfunction in a patient scheduled for surgery or in a patient with advanced hepatic and/or renal insufficiency (consider pharmacologic enhancement of platelet function, e.g. desmopressin[51])

Other indications for platelet transfusion:
  1. patients who have been on Plavix® or aspirin who nee urgent surgery that cannot be postponed for ≈ 5 days to allow new platelets to be synthesized

Dosage
  Approximately 25% of platelets are lost just with transfusion.
  Peds: 1 U/m^2 raises PC by ≈ 10K, usually give 4 U/m^2.
  Adult: 1 U raises platelet count by ≈ 5-10K. Typical dose for thrombocytopenic bleeding adult: 6-10 U (usual order: "8-pack"). Alternatively, 1 U of pheresed platelets may be given (obtained from a single donor by apheresis, equivalent to 8-10 U of pooled donor platelets).
  Check PC 1-2 hrs after transfusion. The increase in PC will be less in DIC, sepsis, splenomegaly, with platelet antibodies, or if the patient is on chemotherapy. In the absence of increased consumption, platelets will be needed q 3-5 days.

PLASMA PROTEINS

FFP (FRESH FROZEN PLASMA)
  1 bag = 200-250 ml (usually referred to as a "unit", not to be confused with 1 unit of *factor activity* which is defined as 1 ml). FFP is plasma separated from RBCs and platelets, and contains all coagulation factors and natural inhibitors. FFP has an out-date period of 12 months. The risk of AIDS and hepatitis for each unit of FFP is equal to that of a whole unit of blood.

Recommended transfusion criteria (modified[50]):
  1. history or clinical course suggestive of coagulopathy due to congenital or acquired coagulation factor deficiency with active bleeding or pre-op, with PT > 18 sec or APTT > 1.5 **x** upper limit of normal (usually > 55 sec), fibrinogen functioning normally and level > 1 g/L, and coagulation factor assay < 25% activity
  2. proven coagulation factor deficiency with active bleeding or scheduled for surgery or other invasive procedure
     A. congenital deficiency of factor II, V, VII, X, XI or XII
     B. deficiency of factor VIII or IX if safe replacement factors unavailable
     C. von Willebrand's disease unresponsive to DDAVP
     D. multiple coagulation factor deficiency as in hepatic dysfunction, vitamin K depletion or DIC
  3. reversal of warfarin (Coumadin®) effect (PT > 18 sec, or INR > 1.6) in patient actively bleeding or requiring emergency surgery or procedure with insufficient time for vitamin K to correct (which usually requires > 6-12 hrs) (*see page 24*)
  4. deficiency of antithrombin III, heparin cofactor II, or protein C or S
  5. massive blood transfusion: replacement of > 1 blood volume (≈ 5 L in 70 kg adult) within several hours with evidence of coagulation deficiency as in (1) and with continued bleeding
  6. treatment of thrombotic thrombocytopenic purpura, hemolytic uremic syndrome
  7. ✖ because of associated hazards and suitable alternatives, the use of FFP as a volume expander is relatively contraindicated

Dosage: Usual starting dose is 2 bags of FFP (400-600 ml). If PT is 18-22 secs or APTT is 55-70 secs, 1 bag may suffice. Doses as high as 10-15 ml/kg may be needed for some patients. Monitor PT/PTT (or specific factor assay) and clinical bleeding. Since factor VII has a shorter half-life (≈ 6 hrs) than the other factors, PT may become prolonged before

APTT.
Remember: if patient is also receiving platelets, that for every 5-6 units of platelets the patient is also receiving coagulation factors equivalent to ≈ 1 bag of FFP.

ALBUMIN AND PLASMA PROTEIN FRACTION (PPF, AKA PLASMANATE®)

Usually from outdated blood, treated to inactivate hepatitis B virus. Ratio of albumin:globulin percentage in "albumin" is 96%:4%, in PPF it is 83%:17%. Available in 5% (oncotically and osmotically equivalent to plasma) and 25% (contraindicated in dehydrated patients). 25% albumin may be diluted to 5% by mixing 1 volume of 25% albumin to 4 volumes of D5W or 0.9% NS (✖ caution: mixing with sterile water will result in a hypotonic solution that can cause hemolysis and possible renal failure).

Expensive for use simply as a volume expander (≈ $60-80 per unit). Indicated only when total protein < 5.2 gm% (otherwise, use crystalloid which is equally effective). Rapid infusion (> 10 cc/min) has been reported to cause hypotension (due to Na-acetate and Hegeman factor fragments) Use in ARDS is controversial. In neurosurgical patients, may be considered as an adjunct for volume expansion (along with crystalloids) for hyperdynamic therapy (see page 797) when the hematocrit is < 40% following SAH where there is concern about increasing the risk of rebleeding e.g. with the use of hetastartch (see page 787).

CRYOPRECIPITATE

Recommended transfusion criteria:
1. hemophilia A
2. von Willebrand disease
3. documented fibrinogen/factor VIII deficiency
4. documented disseminated intravascular coagulation (DIC): along with other modes of therapy

1.5.2. Coagulation

1.5.2.1. Anticoagulation

ANTICOAGULANT CONSIDERATIONS IN NEUROSURGERY

Contraindications to heparin therapy

Many traditional contraindications are being reconsidered and challenged. Massive PE producing hemodynamic compromise should be treated with anticoagulation in most cases despite intracranial risks. Contraindications to heparin include:
- recent severe head injury
- recent craniotomy: see below
- patients with coagulopathies
- hemorrhagic infarction
- bleeding ulcer or other inaccessible bleeding site
- uncontrollable hypertension
- severe hepatic or renal disease
- immediately before invasive procedure (see below for angiography or myelography)
- brain tumor: see below

In patients with unruptured (incidental) cerebral aneurysms

Anticoagulation may not increase the risk of hemorrhage (i.e. rupture), however, should rupture occur, anticoagulation would most likely increase volume of hemorrhage and thus increase morbidity and mortality.

In patients with brain tumor

Some authors are reluctant to administer heparin to any patient with a brain tumor[52], although a number of studies found no higher risk in these patients when treated with heparin or oral anticoagulation [53-55] (PT should be followed very closely, one study recommended maintaining PT ≈ 1.25 x control[55]).

Post-operatively following craniotomy

Requires individualization based on the reason for craniotomy (i.e. tumor, AVM, aneurysm, etc.). However, most neurosurgeons would probably not fully anticoagulate patients < 3-5 days following craniotomy[56], and some recommend at least 2 weeks (one study found no increased incidence of bleeding when anticoagulation was resumed 3 days post craniotomy[57]).

Safe levels of PT/INR to perform neurosurgical procedures

Patients on warfarin who must be anticoagulated as long as possible (e.g. mechanical heart valves) need to be admitted to the hospital and converted to heparin. Most can stop warfarin at home, and then be admitted 2-3 days later and started on heparin as PT begins to normalize. Patients with less critical needs for anticoagulation (e.g. chronic a-fib) can usually be taken off of the warfarin at least 4-5 days before the procedure, and a PT/INR is then checked on admission to the hospital. Patients need to be aware that during the time that they are not anticoagulated, that they are at risk of possible complications from the condition for which they are receiving the agents (annual risk for mechanical valve is ≈ 6%, for a-fib it is ≈ 1.5%).

In patients needing angiography or myelography: In all patients, stop heparin 4 hrs prior to the study.

For non-emergent neurosurgical procedures: For procedures where post-op mass effect from bleeding would pose serious risk (which includes most neurosurgical operations), it is recommended that the **PT should be** ≈ ≤ **13.5 sec** (i.e. ≤ upper limits of normal) or the **INR should be** ≈ ≤ **1.4** (e.g. for reference, this INR is considered safe for performing a percutaneous needle liver biopsy). To reverse anticoagulants, *see page 24.*

For emergent neurosurgical procedures: For emergency situations, give FFP (start with 2 units) and vitamin K (10-20 mg IV at ≤ 1 mg/min) as soon as possible (*see page 24* for reversal of anticoagulation). The timing of surgery is then based on the urgency of the situation and the nature of the procedure (e.g. the decision might be to evacuate a spinal epidural hematoma in an acutely paralyzed patient before anticoagulation is fully reversed).

Antiplatelet drugs and neurosurgical procedures

Plavix® (clopidogrel) (*see page 872*) and aspirin cause permanent inhibition of platelet function that persists ≈ 5 days after discontinuation of the drug and can increase the risk of bleeding. For elective cases, 5-7 days off these drugs is recommended. For emergency surgery, platelets may be given (*see page 20*), however, with Plavix the drug persists in the system for up to a couple of days after the last dose, and can actually inhibit platelets given *after* the drug is discontinued (the half-life of aspirin is lower and should not be an issue after 1 day). In cases with continued oozing in the first day or so after discontinuing Plavix, use the following regimen:

1. recombinant activated coagulation factor VII **(rFVIIa)**: even though the defect is in the platelets, rFVIIa works, via a mechanism not mediated by protein clotting factors. Very expensive (≈ $10,000 per dose), but this must be balanced against the cost of repeat craniotomy, increased ICU stay and additional morbidity
   A. initial dose[58]: 90-120 mcg/kg
   B. same dose 2 hrs later
   C. 3rd dose 6 hrs after initial dose
2. platelets every 8 hours for 24 hours, either
   A. 6 U of regular platelets
   B. 1 unit of pheresed platelets (if pt. is on fluid or volume restriction)

ANTICOAGULANTS

heparin
DRUG INFO

Rx: Administered as IV drip or sub-Q bolus. To anticoagulate average weight patient, give 5000 U bolus IV, follow with 1000 U/hr IV drip. Titrate to therapeutic anticoagulation of APTT = 2-2.5 **x** control (for DVT, some recommend 1.5-2 **x** control[61]).

SIDE EFFECTS: (see *Anticoagulant considerations in neurosurgery* above): hemorrhage, thrombosis[62] (heparin activates anti-thrombin III and can cause platelet aggregation) which can result in MIs, CVAs, DVTs, PEs, etc. Thrombocytopenia: transient mild thrombocytopenia is fairly common in the first few days after initiating heparin therapy, however severe thrombocytopenia occurs in 1-2% of patients receiving heparin > 4 days (usually has a delayed onset of 6-12 days, and is due to consumption in heparin-induced thrombosis or to antibodies formed against a heparin-platelet protein complex). Consider use of lepirudin (*see below*) in thrombocytopenic patients. Chronic therapy may cause osteoporosis.

Low molecular weight heparins[63, 64]

Low molecular weight heparins **(LMWH)** (average molecular weight = 3000-8000 daltons) are derived from unfractionated heparin (average MW = 12,000-15,000 daltons). LMWHs differ from unfractionated heparin because they have a higher ratio of anti-factor Xa to anti-factor IIa (antithrombin) activity which theoretically should produce antithrombic effects with fewer hemorrhagic complications. Realization of this benefit has been very minor in clinical trials. LMWH have greater bioavailability after sub-Q injection leading to more predictable plasma levels which eliminates the need to monitor biologic activity (such as APTT). LMWH have a longer half-life and therefore require fewer doses per day.

Drugs include:
- dalteparin (Fragmin®): **Rx** 2500 anti-Xa U SQ q d
- enoxaparin (Lovenox®): **Rx** dosage established following hip replacement is 30 mg SQ BID **x** 7-14 days. Alternative: 100 U/kg SQ BID
- ardeparin (Normiflo®): **Rx** 50 anti-Xa U/kg SQ q 12 hrs
- danaparoid (Orgaran®): a heparinoid. Even higher anti-Xa:anti-IIa ratio than LMWHs. Does not require laboratory monitoring. **Rx** 750 anti-Xa U SQ BID
- tinzaparin (Logiparin®, Innohep®): not available in U.S. **Rx** 175 anti-Xa U per kg SQ once daily

Spinal epidural hematomas: There have been a number of case reports of spinal epidural hematomas occurring in patients on LMWH (primarily enoxaparin) who also underwent spinal/epidural anesthesia or lumbar puncture, primarily in elderly women undergoing orthopedic surgery. Some have had significant neurologic sequelae, including permanent paralysis[65]. The risk is further increased by the use of NSAIDs, platelet inhibitors, or other anticoagulants, and with traumatic or repeated epidural or spinal puncture.

Fondaparinux (Arixtra®)[66]

Increases factor Xa inhibition without affecting factor IIa (thrombin). Unfractionated & LMW heparins bind platelet factor 4 and can cause immune-mediated heparin-induced thrombocytopenia **(HIT)**. Fondaparinux does not bind platelet factor 4, and has not caused HIT. May be more effective than enoxaparin (Lovenox®) for preventing post-op DVTs. **SIDE EFFECTS:** Bleeding is the most common side effect (may be increased by concurrent NSAID use).

Rx: 2.5 mg SQ injection q d. **SUPPLIED:** 2.5 mg single-dose syringes.

Lepirudin (Refludan®)[67]

A direct thrombin inhibitor which blocks the thrombogenic activity of thrombin, and, unlike heparin, also acts on clot-bound thrombin. It is FDA approved for anticoagulation in patients with heparin-induced thrombocytopenia.

Rx: loading dose of 0.4 mg/kg (up to 44 mg) IV, followed by continuous infusion of 0.15 mg/kg/hr for 2-10 days. The dose is titrated to a target aPTT ratio of 1.5-2.5. **SUPPLIED:** 1 ml vials containing 50 mg.

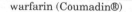

warfarin (Coumadin®)   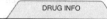 DRUG INFO

To anticoagulate average weight patient, give 10 mg PO q d **x** 2-4 days, then ≈ 5 mg q d. Follow coagulation studies, titrate to PT **=** 1.2-1.5 **x** control (or INR ≈ 2-3) for most conditions (e.g. DVT, single TIA). Higher PT ratios of 1.5-2 **x** control (INR ≈ 3-4) may be needed for recurrent systemic embolism, mechanical heart valves... (the recommended ranges for the **International Normalized Ratio (INR)** are shown in *Table 1-11*).

NB: Warfarin should not be started until a therapeutic PTT has been achieved on heparin to reduce the risk of "Coumadin necrosis." During the first ≈ 3 days of warfarin therapy, patients are actually <u>hypercoagulable</u> (secondary to reduction of vitamin-K dependent anticoagulation factors protein C and protein S), therefore, continue heparin during the first few days.

SUPPLIED: scored tabs of 1, 2, 2.5, 5, 7.5 and 10 mg. IV form: 5mg/vial.

Table 1-11 Recommended INRs[59]

Indication	INR
• mechanical prosthetic heart valve • prevention of recurrent MI	2.5-3.5
antiphospholipid antibody syndrome[60] (*see page 775*)	≥ 3
all other indications (DVT prophylaxis and treatment, PE, atrial fibrillation, recurrent systemic embolism, tissue heart valves)	2-3

1.5.2.2. Coagulopathies

CORRECTION OF COAGULOPATHIES OR REVERSAL OF ANTICOAGULANTS
For recommended normal values for coagulation studies in neurosurgery, *see page 22*.

Platelets
See page 19 for indications and administration guidelines.

Fresh frozen plasma
To reverse warfarin anticoagulation, use the following as a starting point and recheck PT/PTT afterwards:
- when patient is "therapeutically anticoagulated" start with 2-3 units FFP (approximately 15 ml/kg is usually needed)
- for severely prolonged PT/PTT, start with 6 units FFP

Prothrombin complex concentrate
Warfarin induced anticoagulation may be reversed up to 4 or 5 times more quickly with prothrombin complex concentrate (**PCC**) (contains coag factors II, IX, and X) than with FFP[68]. Patient may become hyperthrombotic with this.

vitamin K (Aquamephyton®) DRUG INFO

To reverse elevated PT from <u>warfarin</u>, give aqueous colloidal solution of vitamin K_1 (phytonadione, Aquamephyton®). Doses > 10 mg may produce warfarin resistance for up to 1 week. FFP may be administered concurrently for more rapid correction (*see above*). For recommended levels of PT, *see page 22*.
Rx **adult**: start with 10-15 mg IM; the effect takes 6-12 hrs (in absence of liver disease). Repeat dose if needed. The average total dose needed to reverse therapeutic anticoagulation is 25-35 mg.
IV administration has been associated with severe reactions (possibly anaphylactic), including hypotension and even fatalities (even with proper precautions to dilute and administer slowly), therefore IV route is reserved only for situations where other routes are not feasible and the serious risk is justified. *Rx* **IV** (when IM route not feasible): 10-20 mg IV at a rate of injection not to exceed 1 mg/min (e.g. put 10 mg in 50 ml of D5W and give over 30 minutes).

protamine sulfate DRUG INFO

1 mg reverses approximately 100 U <u>heparin</u> (give slowly, not to exceed 50 mg in any 10 min period). Therapy should be guided by coagulation studies. Protamine can also reverse ≈ 60% of Lovenox.

desmopressin (DDAVP®) DRUG INFO

Causes an increase in factor III coagulant activity and von Willebrand factor which helps coagulation and platelet activity in hemophilia A and in von Willebrand's disease Type I (where the factors are normal in makeup but low in concentration, ✖ but may cause thrombocytopenia in von Willebrand's disease Type IIB where factors may be abnormal or missing).
Rx 0.3 µg/kg (use 50 ml of diluent for doses ≤ 3 µg, use 10 ml for doses > 3 µg) given over 15-30 minutes 30 minutes prior to a surgical procedure.

ELEVATED PRE-OP PTT
In a patient with no history of coagulopathy, a significantly elevated pre-op PTT is commonly due to either a factor deficiency or to lupus anticoagulant. Workup:
1. mixing study
2. lupus coagulant

If the mixing study corrects the elevated PTT, then there is probably a factor deficiency. Consult a hematologist.

Lupus anticoagulant: If the test for lupus anticoagulant is positive, then the major risk to the patient with surgery is <u>not</u> bleeding, rather it is thromboembolism. Management recommendations:

1. as soon as feasible post-op, start patient on heparin (*see page 22*) or LMW heparin (*see page 23*), e.g. Lovenox
2. at the same time start warfarin, and maintain therapeutic anticoagulation for 3-4 weeks (the risk of DVT/PE is actually highest in the first few weeks post-op)
3. mobilize as soon as possible post-op
4. consider vena-cava interruption filter in patients for whom anticoagulation is contraindicated

THROMBOEMBOLISM IN NEUROSURGERY

Deep-vein thrombosis (DVT) is of concern primarily because of the potential for material (clot, platelet clumps...) to dislodge and form emboli (including pulmonary emboli, **(PE)**) which may cause pulmonary infarction, sudden death (from cardiac arrest), or cerebral infarction (from a so called paradoxical embolus, which may occur in the presence of a patent foramen ovale, see *Cardiogenic brain embolism*, page 773). The reported mortality from DVT in the LEs ranges from 9-50%[69]. DVT limited to the calf has a low threat (< 1%) of embolization, however, these clots later extend into the proximal deep veins in 30-50% of cases[69], from where embolization may occur (in 40-50%), or they may produce postphlebitic syndrome.

Neurosurgical patients are particularly prone to developing DVTs (estimated risk: 19-50%) due at least in part to the relative frequency of the following:
1. long operating times of some procedures
2. prolonged bed rest
3. paralyzed limbs (e.g. in spinal cord injuries or stroke patients)
4. alterations in coagulation status
   A. in patients with brain tumors (*see below*) or head injury[70]
      1. related to the condition itself
      2. due to release of brain thromboplastins during brain surgery
   B. increased blood viscosity with concomitant "sludging"
      1. from dehydration therapy sometimes used to reduce cerebral edema
      2. from volume loss following SAH (cerebral salt wasting)
   C. use of high-dose glucocorticoids

Specific "neurological" risk factors for DVT and PE include[69]:
1. spinal cord injury (*see page 705*)
2. brain tumor: autopsy prevalence of DVT = 28%, of PE = 8.4%. Incidence using ^{125}I-fibrinogen[71]: meningioma 72%, malignant glioma 60%, metastasis 20%. Risk may be reduced by pre-op use of aspirin[72]
3. subarachnoid hemorrhage
4. head trauma
5. stroke: incidence of PE = 1-19.8%, with mortality of 25-100%
6. patients undergoing neurosurgical operation

PROPHYLAXIS AGAINST DVT
Options include:
1. general measures
   A. passive range of motion
   B. ambulate appropriate patients as early as possible
2. mechanical techniques (minimal risk of complications):
   A. pneumatic compression boots[73] **(PCBs)** or sequential compression devices **(SCDs)**: reduces the incidence of DVTs and probably PEs. Do not use if DVTs already present. Continue use until patient able to walk 3-4 hrs per day
   B. TED Stockings®[A]: **(TEDS)** applies graduated pressure, higher distally. As effective as PCB. No evidence that the benefit is additive[69]. Care should be taken to avoid a tourniquet effect at the proximal end
   C. electrical stimulation of calf muscles
   D. rotating beds
3. anticoagulation[B]
   A. full anticoagulation is associated with perioperative complications[74]

A. TEDS® is a registered trademark. "TED" stands for thromboembolic disease
B. for contraindications and considerations of anticoagulation in neurosurgery, *see page 21*

B. "low-dose" anticoagulation[75] ("mini-dose" heparin): 5000 IU SQ q 8 or 12 hrs, starting 2 hrs pre-op or on admission to hospital. Potential for hazardous hemorrhage within brain or spinal canal has limited its use

C. low molecular weight heparins and heparinoids (see page 23): not a homogeneous group. Efficacy in neurosurgical prophylaxis has not been determined

D. aspirin: role in DVT prophylaxis is limited because ASA inhibits platelet aggregation, and platelets play only a minor role in DVT

4. combination of PCBs and "mini-dose" heparin starting on the morning of post-op day 1 (with no evidence of significant complications)[76]

Recommendations

Recommended prophylaxis varies with the risk of developing DVT, as illustrated in Table 1-12 [69]. Also see page 705 for details of prophylaxis in cervical spinal cord injuries.

Table 1-12   Risk & prophylaxis of DVT in neurosurgical patients*

Risk group	Estimated risk of calf DVT	Typical neurosurgical patients	Treatment recommendation
low risk	< 10%	age < 40 yrs, minimal general risk factors, surgery with < 30 minutes general anesthesia	no prophylaxis, or PCB/TEDS
moderate risk	10-40%	age ≥ 40 yrs, malignancy, prolonged bed rest, extensive surgery, varicose veins, obesity, surgery > 30 minutes duration (except simple lumbar discectomy), SAH, head injury	PCB/TEDs; or for patients without ICH or SAH, mini-dose heparin
high risk	40-80%	history of DVT or PE, paralysis† (para- or quadriplegia or hemiparesis), brain tumor (especially meningioma or malignant glioma)	PCB/TEDS + (in patients without ICH or SAH) mini-dose heparin

*   abbreviations: DVT = deep venous thrombosis, PCB = pneumatic compression device, TEDS = TED (thromboembolic disease) Stockings®, ICH = intracerebral hemorrhage, SAH = subarachnoid hemorrhage

†   see page 705 for specifics regarding DVT prophylaxis in cervical SCI

DIAGNOSIS OF DVT

The clinical diagnosis of DVT is very unreliable. A patient with the "classic signs" of a hot, swollen, and tender calf, or a positive Homans' sign (calf pain on dorsiflexion of the ankle) will have a DVT only 20-50% of the time[69]. 50-60% of patients with DVT will not have these findings.

Laboratory tests

- contrast venography: the "gold standard", however it is invasive and carries risk of iodine reaction, occasionally produces phlebitis, not readily repeated
- Doppler ultrasound with B-mode imaging: 95% sensitive and 99% specific for proximal DVT. Less effective for calf DVT[77]. May be used in immobilized or casted LE (unlike IPG). Widely accepted as the non-invasive test of choice for DVT[78]
- impedance plethysmography (**IPG**): looks for reduced electrical impedance produced by blood flow from the calf following relaxation of a pneumatic tourniquet. Good in detecting proximal DVT, not sensitive for calf DVT. A positive study indicates DVT that should be treated, a negative study can occur with non-occlusive DVT or with good collaterals, and should be repeated over a 2 week period
- ^{125}I-fibrinogen: radiolabeled fibrinogen is incorporated into the developing thrombus. Better for calf DVT than proximal DVT. Expensive, and many false positives. Risk of HIV transmission has resulted in withdrawal of use
- **D-dimer** (a specific fibrin degradation product): high levels are associated with DVT and PE[79]

TREATMENT OF DVT

1. bed rest, with elevation of involved leg(s)
2. unless anticoagulation is contraindicated (see page 21), start heparin (as outlined in Anticoagulation on page 21, aim for APTT = 1.5-2 **x** control) or fixed dose of LMW heparinoids (e.g. tinzaparin (Logiparin®[80], or in the U.S. enoxaparin (Lovenox®) see page 23): simultaneously initiate warfarin therapy. Heparin can be stopped after ≈ 5 days[81]
3. in patients where anticoagulation is contraindicated, consider inferior vena cava interruption or placement of a filter (e.g. Greenfield filter)
4. in non-paralyzed patients, cautiously begin to ambulate after ≈ 7-10 days

5. wear anti-embolic stocking on affected LE indefinitely (limb is always at risk of recurrent DVT)

1.5.3. Extramedullary hematopoiesis

In chronic anemias (especially thalassemia major, AKA Cooley's anemia), low hematocrit results in chronic over-stimulation of bone marrow to produce RBCs. This results in systemic bony abnormalities, cardiomyopathy (due to hemochromatosis caused by increased breakdown of defective RBCs).

Pertinent to the CNS, there are three sites where extramedullary hematopoiesis (**EMH**) can cause findings:
- skull: produces "hair-on-end" appearance on skull x-ray
- vertebral bodies: may result in epidural cord compression[82] (*see below*)
- choroid plexus

EPIDURAL CORD COMPRESSION FROM EMH

The exuberant tissue is very radiosensitive, however, the patient may be somewhat dependent on the hematopoietic capacity of the tissue.

Treatment

Surgical excision followed by radiation therapy has been the recommended treatment. Repeated blood transfusions may help reduce EMH and may be useful post-op instead of RTX except for refractory cases[82].

Surgery on these patients is difficult because of:
1. low platelet count
2. poor condition of bone
3. cardiomyopathy: increased anesthetic risk
4. anemia, coupled with the fact that most of these patients are "iron-toxic" from multiple previous transfusions
5. total removal of the mass is not always possible

1.6. Pharmacology

1.6.1. Analgesics

For a discussion of types of pain and pain procedures, *see page 376.*

GENERAL PRINCIPLES

The key to good pain control is the early use of adequate levels of effective analgesics. For cancer pain, scheduled dosing is superior to PRN dosing, and "rescue" medication should be available[83] Nonopioid analgesics should be continued as more potent medications and invasive techniques are utilized.

ANALGESICS FOR SOME SPECIFIC TYPES OF PAIN

Visceral or deafferentation pain

May sometimes be effectively treated with tricyclic antidepressants (*see page 33*). Tryptophan may be effective (*see page 33*).

Carbamazepine (Tegretol®) may be useful for paroxysmal, lancinating pain.

Pain from metastatic bone disease

Steroids, aspirin, or NSAIDs are especially helpful, probably by reducing prostaglandin mediated sensitization of A-delta and C fibers, and therefore may be preferred to APAP.

1.6.1.1. Nonopioid analgesics

ACETAMINOPHEN

Table 1-13   Acetaminophen dosing

Medication	Dosage
acetaminophen (APAP) (Tylenol®)	adult dose: 650 or 1000 mg PO/PR q 4-6 hrs, not to exceed 4000 mg/day* pediatric dose: infants: 10-15 mg/kg PO/PR q 4-6 hrs children: 1 grain/yr age (= 65 mg/yr up to 650 mg) PO/PR q 4-6 hrs not to exceed 15 mg/kg q 4 hrs

*   hepatic toxicity from APAP: usually with doses $\geq$ 10 gm/day, rare at doses < 4000 mg. However, may occur at lower doses (even at high therapeutic doses) in alcoholics, fasting patients, and those taking cytochrome P-450 enzyme-inducing drugs

NONSTEROIDAL ANTI-INFLAMMATORY DRUGS (NSAIDS)

The anti-inflammatory properties of NSAIDs is primarily due to inhibition of the enzyme cyclooxygenase (COX) which participates in the synthesis of prostaglandins and thromboxanes[84].

Characteristics of nonselective nonsteroidal anti-inflammatory drugs:
- all are given orally except ketorolac tromethamine (Toradol®) (see below)
- no dependence develops
- additive effect improves the pain relief with opioid analgesics
- NSAIDs (and APAP) demonstrate a **ceiling effect**: a maximum dose above which no further analgesia is obtained. For aspirin and APAP, this is usually between 650-1300 mg, and is often higher for other NSAIDs which may also have a longer duration of action
- risk of GI upset is common, more serious risks of hepatotoxicity[85], or GI ulceration, hemorrhage, or perforation are less common
- taking medication with meals or antacids has not been proven effective in reducing GI side effects. **Misoprostol** (Cytotec®), a prostaglandin, may be effective in mitigating NSAID-induced gastric erosion or peptic ulcer. Contraindicated in pregnancy. *Rx* 200 µg PO QID with food as long as patient is on NSAIDs. If not tolerated, use 100 µg. ✖ CAUTION: an abortifacient. Should not be given to pregnant women or women of childbearing potential
- most reversibly inhibit platelet function and prolong bleeding time (nonacetlyated salicylates have less antiplatelet action, e.g. salsalate, trisalicylate, nabumetome). Aspirin, unlike all other NSAIDS, <u>irreversibly</u> binds to cyclooxygenase and thus inhibits platelet function for the 8-10 day life of the platelet
- all cause sodium and water retention and carry the risk of NSAID-induced nephrotoxicity[86] (renal insufficiency, interstitial nephritis, nephrotic syndrome, hyperkalemia)

Table 1-14   Nonsteroidal anti-inflammatory drugs (NSAIDs)

Generic name	Proprietary (®)	Typical adult oral dose*	Tabs/caps availability (mg)†	Daily maximum (mg)
aspirin‡	(many)	500-1000 mg PO q 4-6 hrs (ceiling dose $\approx$ 1 gm)	325, 500	4000
bromfenac[87]	Duract	25 mg PO q 6-8 hrs on empty stomach up to 10 d	25	150
diclofenac	Voltaren, Cataflam	start at 25 mg QID; additional dose q hs PRN; increase up to 50 mg TID or QID, or 75 mg BID	25, 50, 75	200
diflunisol	Dolobid	1000 mg initial; then 500 mg BID	250, 500	1500
etodolac	Lodine	for acute pain: 200-400 mg q 6-8 hrs	200, 300 caps, 400 tabs	1200
fenoprofen	Nalfon	200 mg q 4-6 hrs; for rheumatoid arthritis 300-600 mg TID-QID	200, 300, 600	3200

Table 1-14 Nonsteroidal anti-inflammatory drugs (NSAIDs) (continued)

Generic name	Propri-etary (®)	Typical adult oral dose*	Tabs/caps availability (mg)†	Daily maximum (mg)
flurbiprofen	Ansaid	50 mg TID-QID or 100 mg TID	50, 100	300
ketoprofen	Orudis	start at 75 mg TID or 50 mg QID, ↑to 150-300 mg daily DIV TID-QID	25, 50, 75	300
	Oruvail	extended release capsule 150 mg q d	ER† 150	
ketorolac	Toradol	*see below*	*see below*	
ibuprofen§	Motrin	400-800 mg QID (ceiling dose: 800 mg)	300, 400, 600, 800	3200
indomethacin	Indocin	25 mg TID, ↑ by 25 mg total per day PRN	25, 50, SR 75	150-200
meclofenamate	Meclomen	50 mg q 4-6 hrs; ↑ to 100 mg QID if needed	50, 100	400
mefenamic	Ponstel	500 mg initial; then 250 mg q 6 hrs	250	
nabumetomeΔ	Relafen	1000-2000 mg/d given in 1 or 2 doses	500, 750	2000
naproxen	Naprosyn	500 mg, then 250 mg q 6-8 hrs	250, 375, 500	<1250
naproxen sodium	Anaprox	550 mg, followed by 275 mg q 6-8 hrs	275, DS = 550	1375
oxaprozin	Daypro	1200 mg q d (1st day may take 1800)	600	1800
phenylbutazone	Butazolidin	high incidence of agranulocytosis. Not first DOC, and not a simple analgesic		
piroxicam	Feldene	10-20 mg q d (steady state takes 7-12 d)	10, 20	
sulindac	Clinoril	200 mg BID; ↓ to 150 BID when pain controlled	150, 200	400
salsalate	Disalcid	3000 mg divided BID-TID (e.g. 500 mg 2-tabs TID)	500, 750	
tolmetin	Tolectin	400 mg TID (bioavailability is reduced by food)	200, DS = 400, 600	1800
trisalicylate	Trilisate	2000-3000 mg/d usually divided BID (but may be divided TID)	500, 750, 1000, liquid 500mg/5ml	

* when dosage ranges are given, use the smallest effective dose

† abbreviations: DS = double strength; SR = slow release; ER = extended release; DOC = drug of choice

‡ aspirin: has unique effectiveness in pain from bone metastases

§ ibuprofen: is available as a suspension (PediaProfen®) 100 mg/ml; dose for children 6 mos to 12 yrs age is 5-10 mg/kg with a maximum of 40 mg/kg/day (not FDA approved for children because of possible Reye's syndrome)

Δ unlike most NSAIDs, nabumetome does not interfere with platelet function

ketorolac tromethamine (Toradol®)

DRUG INFO

The only parenteral NSAID approved for use in pain control in the U.S. Analgesic effect is more potent than anti-inflammatory effect. Half-life ≈ 6 hrs. May be useful to control pain in the following situations:

1. where the avoidance of sedation or respiratory depression is critical
2. when constipation cannot be tolerated
3. for patients who are nauseated by narcotics
4. where narcotic dependency is a serious concern
5. when epidural morphine has been used and further analgesia is needed without risk of respiratory depression (agonist type narcotics are contraindicated)
6. cautions:
   A. not indicated for use > 72 hrs (complications have been reported primarily with prolonged use of the oral form)
   B. use with caution in postoperative patients since (as with most NSAIDs) bleeding time is prolonged by platelet function inhibition (risk of GI or op-site hemorrhage is small, but is increased in patients > 75 yrs old, when used > 5 days, and when used in higher doses[88])
   C. even though IM dosing circumvents the GI system, gastric mucosal irritation and erosions may occur as with all NSAIDs (avoid use with PUD)
   D. as with all NSAIDs, use with caution in patients at risk for renal side effects

***Rx* Parenteral:** For single dose administration: 30 mg IV or 60 mg IM in healthy adult. For multiple dosing: 30 mg IV or IM q 6 hrs PRN. Maximum dosage: 120 mg/day.

For patient weight < 50 kg, age > 65 yrs, or reduced renal function (creatinine clearance < 50 ml/min), all of the above dosages are halved (max daily dose: 60 mg).
Parenteral use should not exceed 5 days (3 days may be a better guideline).

Rx **PO:** Indicated only as a continuation of IV or IM therapy, not for routine use as an NSAID. Switching from IM to PO: start with 10 mg PO q 4-6 hrs (combined PO and IM dose should be ≤ 120 mg on the day of transition). SUPPLIED: 10 mg tablets.

1.6.1.2.   Opioid analgesics

Narcotics are most commonly used for moderate to severe acute pain or cancer pain (some experts characterize cancer pain as recurrent acute pain and not chronic pain).

Characteristics of narcotics:
- <u>no</u> **ceiling effect** (*see page 28*): i.e. increasing dosage increases the effectiveness (although with weak opioids for moderate pain, side effects may limit dosages to relatively low levels[83])
- with chronic use, tolerance develops (physical and psychological)
- overdose possible, with the potential for respiratory depression with all, and seizures with some (*see page 151*)

MILD TO MODERATE PAIN
Some useful medications are shown in *Table 1-15*.

Table 1-15   Weak opioids for mild to moderate pain

Medication	Dosage
codeine	usual adult dose: 30-60 mg IM/PO q 3 hrs PRN; (30 mg PO is equivalent to 300 mg aspirin) pediatric dose: 0.5-1 mg/kg/dose q 4-6 hrs PO or IV PRN
propoxyphene (Darvon®...)	usually used as propoxyphene napsylate with acetaminophen (Darvocet-N)* Darvocet-N 100 *Rx*: 1-2 PO q 4-6 hrs PRN
pentazocine	pentazocine is a mixed agonist-antagonist
(Talwin®,	→ 12.5 mg pentazocine, 325 mg ASA. *Rx*: 2 PO TID-QID PRN
Talwin® Nx,	→ 50 mg pentazocine, 0.5 mg naloxone. *Rx*: 1-2 PO q 3-4 hrs PRN up to 12 tabs/day
Talacen®)	→ 25 mg pentazocine, 650 mg APAP. *Rx*: 1 PO q 4-6 hrs PRN up to 6 tabs/day
tramadol (Ultram®)	(*see below*)

*   CAUTION: propoxyphene can cause dangerous elevations of carbamazepine levels

Codeine and its congeners, propoxyphene and pentazocine, are usually no more effective that ASA or APAP and are usually combined with these drugs.

tramadol (Ultram®)   DRUG INFO

An oral opioid agonist that binds to μ-opioid receptors, and is also a centrally acting analgesic that inhibits reuptake of norepinephrine and serotonin. For acute pain, 100 mg is comparable to codeine 60 mg with ASA or APAP[89, 90]. There has been no report of respiratory depression when oral dosing recommendations are followed. Seizures and opioid-like dependence have been reported[90].

Rx 50 to 100 mg PO q 4-6 hrs PRN pain up to a maximum of 400 mg/day (or 300 mg/d for older patients). For moderately severe acute pain, an initial dose of 100 mg followed by 50 mg doses may suffice. SUPPLIED: 50 mg tabs.

Table 1-16 Opioids for moderate to severe pain

Medication	Dosage
hydrocodone	(Vicodin®, Lorcet®, Lortab®...): 5 mg hydrocodone + 500 mg acetaminophen; (Vicodin ES®, Lortab 7.5/500®): 7.5 mg hydrocodone + 500 mg APAP; *Rx* 1 PO q 6 hrs PRN (may increase up to 2 tabs PO q 3-4 hrs not to exceed 8 pills/24 hrs).
	(Lorcet® Plus, Lorcet® 10/650): 7.5 or 10 mg hydrocodone (respectively) + 650 mg APAP; *Rx* 1 tab PO q 6 hrs PRN (not to exceed 6 tabs in 24 hrs).
	(Lortab® 10/500: 10 mg. hydrocodone + 500 mg APAP); *Rx*: 1-2 PO q 4 hrs PRN up to 6 tabs/day.
	(Norco®): 10 mg hydrocodone + 325 mg APAP scored tabs; *Rx*: 1 PO q 4 hrs PRN up to 6 tabs/day.
oxycodone	SUPPLIED: usually available in combination as: aspirin 325 mg with oxycodone 5 mg (Percodan®) or acetaminophen (APAP) (Tylox® = APAP 500 mg + oxycodone 5 mg) (Percocet® = oxycodone/APAP in 2.5/325, 5/325, 7.5/500, 10/650) dose: 1 PO q 3-4 hrs PRN (may increase up to 2 PO q 3 hrs*) SUPPLIED: also available alone as **OxyIR®** 5 mg, OxyFast® oral solution of 20 mg/ml, or in controlled-<u>release</u> tablets as **OxyContin®** 10, 20, 40, 80† & 160† mg (which last 12 hours, achieving steady state in 24-36 hours). *Rx* Adult: OxyContin® tablets are taken whole and are not to be divided, chewed or crushed. It is intended for management of moderate to severe pain when continuous around-the-clock analgesic is needed for an extended period of time and is not intended for use as a PRN analgesic. For opiate naive patients, start with 10 mg PO q 12 hrs. For patients on narcotic medications, a conversion table is provided below for some medications. Titrate dose every 1-2 days, increasing dose by 25-50% q 12 hrs.

Conversion table for starting OxyContin®		
Preparation currently being used	Dose	Suggested starting dose of OxyContin®
oxycodone combination pills (Tylox, Percodan...) or Lortab, Vicodin or Tylenol #3	1-5 pills/day	10-20 mg PO q 12 hrs
	6-9 pills/day	20-30 mg PO q 12 hrs
	10-12 pills/day	30-40 mg PO q 12 hrs
IV PCA morphine	determine total MSO4 dose used per 24 hrs	multiply total MSO4 dose in 24 hrs X 1.3 for total OxyContin dose in 24 hrs

Medication	Dosage
hydromorphone	Dilaudid®: (*see Table 1-17*)
morphine	used in low doses (*see Table 1-17*)
levorphanol	Levo-Dromoran®: 2 mg IM ≈ 10 mg morphine; long half-life (*see Table 1-17*)

* not to exceed 4000 mg of acetaminophen/24 hrs (see footnote to *Table 1-13* on *page 28*)
† for use only in opioid-tolerant patients

SEVERE PAIN

Table 1-17 Equianalgesic doses for SEVERE pain, AGONIST opioids
(parenteral route is referenced to 10 mg IM morphine)

Drug name: generic (proprietary®)	Route	Dose (mg)	Peak (hrs)	Duration (hrs)	Comments
morphine	IM	10	0.5-1	4-6	respiratory depression
	PO	20-60*	1.5-2	4-7	long acting PO forms: MS Contin®, Avinza® (*see below*)
codeine	IM	130		3-5	these high doses cause unacceptable side effects
	PO	200			
meperidine† (Demerol®)	IM	75	0.5-1	4-5	avoid prolonged use†, irritating to tissues
	PO	300-400	1-2	4-6	
methadone‡ (Dolophine®)	IM	10	0.5-1	4-6	long half-life‡
	PO	20	1.5-2	4-7	

Drug name: generic (proprietary®)	Route	Dose (mg)	Peak (hrs)	Duration (hrs)	Comments
levorphanol‡ (Levo-Dromoran®)	IM	1.5-2.5		4-6	long half-life‡
	PO	2-4			
oxycodone (e.g. Tylox®§) (OxyContin®)	IM	15			
	PO	30	1	2-3	combination (Tylox®) or liquid
	PO	30-40		12	see Table 1-16
oxymorphone (Numorphan®)	IM	1		3-5	available as suppository
	PR	10			
hydromorphone (Dilaudid®)	IM	1.5	0.5-1	3	
	PO	7.5	1.5-2	3	supplied: 1, 2, 3, & 4 mg tabs
transdermal fentanyl patch (Duragesic®)Δ	transdermal			12-24	72	patches delivering 25, 50, 75 or 100 µg/hr (use lowest effective)

*   IM:PO potency ratio for morphine is 1:6 for single doses, but changes to 1:2-3 with chronic dosing

†   high doses or long-term use is not recommended because meperidine is metabolized to nor-meperidine, a stimulant with a 15-20 hour half-life, that may accumulate and cause agitation or other CNS hyperactivity (including delerium and seizures), may also manifest when given agonist/antagonist drugs. Meperidine may also cause severe encephalopathy and death when given with MAOIs

‡   due to long half-life, repeated dosing can lead to accumulation and CNS depression (must reduce dose after ≈ 3 days, even though the analgesic half-life does not change), especially in the elderly or debilitated patient. Use should be limited to physicians with experience using these drugs

§   may not be practical for use in severe pain since 1 Tylox® contains only 5 mg oxycodone (the acetaminophen limits the dosage), may use OxyContin® for higher doses of oxycodone

Δ   ✖ should not be used as routine post-op analgesic (risk of respiratory depression). Apply 1 patch to upper torso, replace q 72 hrs PRN.

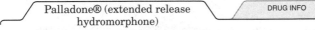

Avinza® (extended release morphine)

Once daily oral morphine formulation using a spherical oral drug absorption system (**SODAS**) (numerous ammonio-methacrylate copolymer beads, ≈ 1 mm dia.).

Rx: Dosage is titrated based on patient's opioid tolerance and degree of pain. Taken as 1 capsule p.o. q d. Not to be taken "PRN". Not for post-op pain. ✖ CAUTION: To prevent potentially fatal doses of morphine, capsules are to be swallowed whole, and are not to be chewed, crushed or dissolved. However, the contents of the capsule (the beads) may be sprinkled on apple-sauce for those unable to swallow the capsules, but the beads are not to be chewed or crushed. SIDE EFFECTS: Due to the potentially nephrotoxic effect of fumaric acid used in SODAS, the maximum dose of Avinza is 1600 mg/d. Doses ≥ 60 mg are for opioid tolerant patients only.

SUPPLIED: 30, 60, 90 & 120 mg capsules.

Palladone® (extended release hydromorphone)

Once daily extended release hydromorphone HCl (immediate release forms include Dilaudid®), a semisynthetic congener of morphine and active metabolite of hydrocodone. Risk for abuse or accidental overdosage by violating capsule or concurrent use of alcohol. Recommended only for opioid tolerant patients who have failed other therapies[91].

Rx A schedule II drug. For opioid tolerant patients only, start with 12-32 mg PO q 24 hours. Titrate upward by 25-50% increments every 2-3 days PRN. ✖ Capsules are not to be opened, broken, chewed, dissolved or crushed or taken with alcohol. Do not use if severe hepatic insufficiency.

SUPPLIED: 12, 16, 24 & 32 mg capsules.

Table 1-18 Equianalgesic doses for SEVERE pain, AGONIST/ANTAGONIST opioids (referenced to 10 mg IM morphine)

Drug name: generic (proprietary®)	Route	Dose (mg)	Peak (hrs)	Duration (hrs)	Comments
buprenorphine (Buprenex®)	IM	0.4			partial agonist
	SL	0.3			
MIXED AGONIST/ANTAGONIST*					
butorphanol (Stadol®)	IM	2	0.5-1	4-6	
nalbuphine (Nubain®)	IM	10	1	3-6	no sigma receptor occupation†
	IV	140 µg/kg	0.5	2-5	
pentazocine (Talwin®‡)	IM†	20-40	0.5-1	4-6	
	PO†	180 (start @ 50)	1.5-2	4-7	
dezocine (Dalgan®)	IM	10		3-6	

*   all can precipitate withdrawal symptoms in patients physically dependent on agonists

†   most agonist/antagonist drugs occupy sigma receptors (Stadol > Nubain), which may cause hallucinations

‡   Talwin injectable (for IM use) contains only pentazocine. Talwin® Compound tablets contain ASA, therefore for high PO doses, use Talwin Nx which contains no ASA (see *Table 1-15*, page 30)

1.6.1.3.   Alpha-2 adrenoreceptor agonists

Alpha-2 agonists have some sedative and analgesic properties and dramatically reduce the risk of respiratory depression and the amount of narcotic analgesics required.

Procedex™ (dexmedetomidine)   *DRUG INFO*

Rx: usual loading dose is 1 mcg/kg over 10 minutes, followed by continuous IV infusion of 0.2-0.7 mcg/kg/hr titrated to desired effect, not to exceed 24 hours.

SIDE EFFECTS: clinically significant bradycardia and sinus arrest have occurred in young, healthy volunteers with increased vagal tone (anticholinergics such as atropine 0.2 mg IV or glycopyrrolate 0.2 mg IV may help). Use with caution in patients with advanced heart block.

SUPPLIED:2 ml vials of 100 mcg/ml for IV use.

1.6.1.4.   Adjuvant pain medications

The following may have efficacy in enhancing the effectiveness of opioid analgesics (and thereby may reduce the required dose).

Tricyclic antidepressants: *see page 376.*

Tryptophan: an amino acid and a precursor of serotonin, may work by increasing serotonin levels. Requires high doses and has hypnotic effects, therefore 1.5-2 gm given usually q hs. Must give daily MVI as chronic tryptophan therapy depletes vitamin B_6.

Antihistamines: histamines play a role in nociception. Antihistamines, which are also anxiolytic, antiemetic, and mildly hypnotic, are effective as analgesics or as adjuvants. Hydroxyzine (Atarax®, Vistaril®): *Rx* start with 50 mg PO q AM and 100 mg PO q hs. May increase up to ≈ 200 mg daily.

Anticonvulsants: carbamazepine, clonazepam, phenytoin or gabapentin may be effective in neuropathic pain from diabetic neuropathy, trigeminal neuralgia, post-herpetic neuralgia, glossopharyngeal neuralgia, and neuralgias due to nerve injury or infiltration with cancer[90].

Phenothiazines: some cause mild reduction in nociception. Most are tranquilizing and antiemetic. Best known for this use is fluphenazine (Prolixin®), usually given with a tricyclic antidepressant for neuropathic pain, see *Diabetic neuropathy*, *Treatment* on page 556. Phenothiazines may reduce the seizure threshold.

Corticosteroids: in addition to the reduction of toxic effects of radiation or chemotherapy, they may potentiate narcotic analgesics. There are also a number of nonspecific beneficial effects: increased appetite, sense of well being, antiemetic. Side effects may limit usefulness (see *Possible deleterious side effects of steroids*, page 10).

Caffeine: although it possesses no intrinsic analgesic properties, doses of 65-200 mg enhance the analgesic effect of APAP, ASA or ibuprofen in H/A, oral surgery pain and post-partum pain.

1.6.2.   Antispasmodics/muscle relaxants

Oral centrally-acting muscle relaxants have a sedating effect on the central nervous system, and there is little evidence of any other beneficial effect. Efficacy of use in patients with acute low back problems is dubious[92] (*see page 297*). Only doses are listed below. Be familiar with approved indications and precautions.

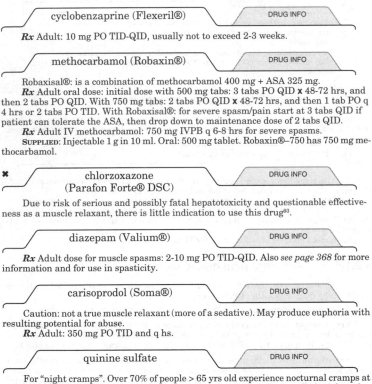

cyclobenzaprine (Flexeril®)   DRUG INFO

Rx Adult: 10 mg PO TID-QID, usually not to exceed 2-3 weeks.

methocarbamol (Robaxin®)   DRUG INFO

Robaxisal®: is a combination of methocarbamol 400 mg + ASA 325 mg.
Rx Adult oral dose: initial dose with 500 mg tabs: 3 tabs PO QID **x** 48-72 hrs, and then 2 tabs PO QID. With 750 mg tabs: 2 tabs PO QID **x** 48-72 hrs, and then 1 tab PO q 4 hrs or 2 tabs PO TID. With Robaxisal®: for severe spasm/pain start at 3 tabs QID if patient can tolerate the ASA, then drop down to maintenance dose of 2 tabs QID.
Rx Adult IV methocarbamol: 750 mg IVPB q 6-8 hrs for severe spasms.
SUPPLIED: Injectable 1 g in 10 ml. Oral: 500 mg tablet. Robaxin®–750 has 750 mg methocarbamol.

✖ chlorzoxazone
(Parafon Forte® DSC)   DRUG INFO

Due to risk of serious and possibly fatal hepatotoxicity and questionable effectiveness as a muscle relaxant, there is little indication to use this drug[93].

diazepam (Valium®)   DRUG INFO

Rx Adult dose for muscle spasms: 2-10 mg PO TID-QID. Also *see page 368* for more information and for use in spasticity.

carisoprodol (Soma®)   DRUG INFO

Caution: not a true muscle relaxant (more of a sedative). May produce euphoria with resulting potential for abuse.
Rx Adult: 350 mg PO TID and q hs.

quinine sulfate   DRUG INFO

For "night cramps". Over 70% of people > 65 yrs old experience nocturnal cramps at some time (usually in the legs, sometimes in the hands). No well-controlled trials to document effectiveness. Meta-analysis suggested that the frequency of cramps can be reduced by ≈ 25% over 2 weeks of treatment, and by more over 4 weeks, but there was no change in severity or duration[94]. Avoid in pregnancy (abortifacient). Caution: even low dose can cause TTP in sensitive patients, repeated doses can cause cinchoism (watch for tinnitus, H/A, N/V, hearing loss) [95]. Rule-out uremic neuropathy before treating (*see page 560*).
Rx Adult: 200 or 300 mg PO q hs PRN (better efficacy seen with regular dosing).

1.6.3. Benzodiazepines

Also see *Sedatives & paralytics*, page 36. All are effective for treating anxiety and insomnia, and vary only in pharmacokinetics or site of metabolism. Those with shorter duration of action are less likely to sedate, but are more prone to cause rebound depression or withdrawl syndrome (may include tachycardia, HTN, tremulousness, diaphoresis, dysphoria, confusion, muscle twitching, and seizures) upon discontinuation. Those with long duration of action are more likely to result in cumulative sedation, and impairment of psychomotor and intellectual function[96]. Lower doses are used for elderly patients. May be reversed with flumazenil (*see below*).

SIDE EFFECTS: ventilatory depression and hypotension exacerbated by opioids, worse in patients with COPD. All contraindicated in first trimester of pregnancy (cause congenital malformations)[97].

Table 1-19 Comparisons of oral benzodiazepines
(Taken from **The Medical Letter**, Vol. 30, pp. 28, 1988, with permission)

Generic name	Proprietary	Rapidity of onset	Duration	Typical daily dose
alprazolam	Xanax®	intermediate	intermediate	0.25-0.5 mg TID
chlordiazepoxide	Librium®	intermediate	long	5-10 mg TID-QID
clorazepate	Tranxene®	rapid	long	15-60 mg/d divided
diazepam	Valium®	rapid	long	2-10 mg BID-QID
lorazepam	Ativan®	intermediate	intermediate	1 mg BID-TID
halazepam	Paxipam®	intermediate	long	20-40 mg TID-QID
prazepam	Centrax®	slow	long	20-60 mg/d divided
oxazepam	Serax®	intermediate to slow	intermediate to short	10-15 mg TID-QID
flurazepam	Dalmane®	rapid to intermediate	long	30 mg
temazepam	Restoril®	intermediate to slow	intermediate	15-30 mg

---

oxazepam (Serax®) — DRUG INFO

Thought not to be metabolized in liver.
Rx Adult: 10-15 mg PO TID-QID (increase to 30 mg TID-QID for EtOH withdrawl or severe anxiety).

alprazolam (Xanax®) — DRUG INFO

May have antidepressant effects similar to tricyclics, with more rapid onset.
Rx Adult: start at 0.25-0.5 mg PO TID, titrate to max of 4 mg/day divided; comes in 0.25, 0.5 & 1 mg tabs.

midazolam (Versed®) — DRUG INFO

3 to 4 times as potent as diazepam (Valium®). Dissolves in aqueous solution, thus less burning and phlebitis than diazepam. At physiologic pH, is lipid soluble and readily crosses BBB. Greater amnestic effect than diazepam. Excellent anticonvulsant properties. Given IM, onset occurs at 15 min, peak at 30 min, duration 1-2 hrs[98].

Rx:
1. for **conscious sedation** (slow IVP): 1-2 mg over 2 min (do not exceed 2.5 mg with initial dose), wait 2-3 mins, and repeat up to total of 0.1-0.15 mg/kg. Reduce by at least 25% if opioids are also being used or in patients > 60 yrs. To maintain sedation, repeat doses of 25% of initial. Caution: midazolam has been associated with respiratory arrest (even in young patients). Monitor patient continuously, use extra caution in elderly
2. for IM **pre-op**: 0.07-0.08 mg/kg (5 mg/70 kg) about 1 hr pre-op.
3. for induction for general anesthesia:
   A. initial dose (slow IVP) of:
      1. for unpremedicated average adult age ≤ 55 yrs: 0.25 mg/kg
      2. > 55 yrs, ASA class I or II: 0.2 mg/kg

3. ASA III or IV: 0.15 mg/kg
  B. to maintain: repeat 25% of initial dose.

Midazolam <u>drip</u>:
  Dilute 50 mg midazolam in 100 cc IV fluid (only <u>glass</u> bottle recommended, as plastic adsorbs midazolam); start at 1-2 mg/hr and titrate to desired level of sedation.

BENZODIAZEPINE REVERSAL

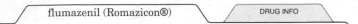
flumazenil (Romazicon®) DRUG INFO

Competitively inhibits benzodiazepines **(BDZ)** at receptor sites. Since duration of action is shorter than most BDZs, resedation may occur, especially with large doses of BDZs given over a long procedure. BDZ antagonism begins < 2 mins after IV dose, peaks in 6-10 mins, and lasts ≈ 60 mins. Sedation is only partially reversed in some patients. Reversal of BDZ induced respiratory depression is partial or nil[99].

Contraindicated in patients chronically treated with BDZs (for seizures or for other indications) where antagonism may provoke a withdrawal syndrome and/or seizures. May provoke a panic attack. Not approved for use in pregnancy.

Rx To reverse BDZs used for conscious sedation or general anesthesia: 0.2 mg (2 ml) IV over 15 seconds; repeat at 1 minute intervals if level of reversal is inadequate up to a maximum of 1 mg (total of 5 doses). If resedation occurs, may repeat dosing at 20 minute intervals, keeping within a maximum of 3 mg per hour. For suspected overdosage, give 0.2 mg over 30 secs, wait 30 secs, then give 0.3 mg over 30 secs at 1 minute intervals up to 3 mg or until patient arouses.

1.6.4. Sedatives & paralytics

The modified Ramsay sedation scale[100] is shown in *Table 1-20*. This is useful e.g. for quantitating the desired level of sedation when prescribing sedatives for an agitated patient.

1.6.4.1. Conscious sedation

- midazolam (Versed®): *see page 35*
- pentobarbital (Nembutal®): a barbiturate. ***Rx*** for 70 kg adult: 100 mg slow IVP
- chloral hydrate: sedation dose is 25 mg/kg (*see below*)

Table 1-20 Modified Ramsay sedation scale

Awake levels	1	anxious and agitated or restless or both
	2	cooperative, oriented and tranquil
	3	responds to commands only
Response to light glabellar tap or loud auditory stimulus		
Asleep levels	4	brisk response
	5	sluggish response
	6	no response

1.6.4.2. Sedatives for procedures

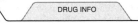
thiopental (Pentothal®) DRUG INFO

A short acting barbiturate. 1st dose causes unconsciousness in 20-30 secs (circulation time), depth increases up to 40 secs, duration = 5 mins (terminated by redistribution), consciousness returns over 20-30 mins.
  SIDE EFFECTS: dose related respiratory depression, irritation if extravassated, intra-arterial injection → necrosis, agitation if injected slowly, an <u>antianalgesic</u>, myocardial depressant, hypotension in hypovolemic patients.
  Rx Adult: initial concentration should not exceed 2.5%, give 50 mg test dose moderately rapid IVP, then if tolerated give 100-200 mg IVP over 20-30 secs (500 mg may be required in large patient).

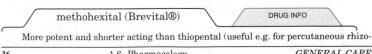
methohexital (Brevital®) DRUG INFO

More potent and shorter acting than thiopental (useful e.g. for percutaneous rhizotomy where patient needs to be sedated and awakened repeatedly). Lasts 5-7 min. Similar cautions with the added problem that methohexital may <u>induce</u> seizures.

Rx Adult: 1 gm% solution (add 50 ml diluent to 500 mg to yield 10 mg/ml), 2 ml test dose, then 5-12 ml IVP at rate of 1 ml/5 secs, then 2 to 4 ml q 4-7 min PRN.

---

fentanyl (Sublimaze®)   DRUG INFO

Narcotic, potency ≈ 100 **x** morphine. In small doses, lasts 20-30 min. Unlike morphine and meperidine, does not cause histamine release. Lowers ICP. SIDE EFFECTS: dose dependent respiratory depression, large doses given rapidly may cause chest wall rigidity.

Rx Adult: 25-100 μg (0.5-2 ml) IVP, repeat q 1-2 hrs PRN. SUPPLIED: 50 μg/ml, requires refrigeration.

---

propofol (Diprivan®)   DRUG INFO

A sedative hypnotic. Also useful in high doses during aneurysm surgery as a neuroprotectant (*see page 808*). Protection seems to be less than with barbiturates.

Rx for sedation: start at 5-10 μg/kg/min. Increase by 5-10 μg/kg/min q 5-10 minutes PRN desired sedation (up to a max of 50 μg/kg/min).

SUPPLIED: 500 mg suspended in a 50 ml bottle of fat emulsion. The bottle and tubing must be changed every 12 hours since it contains no bacteriostatic agent.

---

haloperidol (Haldol®)   DRUG INFO

SIDE EFFECTS: rare neuroleptic malignant syndrome. ✖ Contraindicated in Parkinson's disease. Anticholinergic effects may exacerbate urinary retention.

Rx For "rapid sequence tranquilization" (to sedate acutely agitated patient): 5-10 mg haloperidol IM q 15 minutes until patient controlled.

PEDIATRIC SEDATION

The following agents may be used to sedate patients for procedures (e.g. CT or MRI). Above 1 year, any of these may be used. For children < 1 year age, use chloral hydrate at 50 mg/kg (*see below*).
- pentobarbital (Nembutal®): 2 mg/kg IV q 4 hrs PRN
OR
- fentanyl (Sublimaze®): 1 μg/kg IVP
OR
- diazepam (Valium®): 0.1-0.5 mg/kg (not to exceed 10 mg) <u>or</u> midazolam (Versed®) 0.1 mg/kg IVP

---

chloral hydrate   DRUG INFO

- takes 30-60 minutes after oral dose to work
- SUPPLIED: suspension 100 mg/ml (= 500 mg/5 ml which is 500 mg/teaspoon) or 500 mg capsules

Table 1-21 Chloral hydrate dosage for pediatrics

Description	Dosage
sedative dose	25 mg/kg
hypnotic dose	50 mg/kg PO, if ineffective in 30-60 minutes may give additional 25 mg/kg; sometimes up to 100 mg/kg is needed
repeat dosing	may repeat whole dose after 6 hrs

"DPT" (DEMEROL, PHENERGAN & THORAZINE)
AKA "lytic cocktail". Combine in 1 syringe and give as deep IM injection:
- meperidine (Demerol®): 2 mg/kg (max dose 50 mg)
+ promethazine (Phenergan®): 1 mg/kg (✖ contraindicated in patients < 2 yrs age)
+ chlorpromazine (Thorazine®): 1 mg/kg

1.6.4.3.   Paralytics (neuromuscular blocking agents)

CAUTION: requires ventilation (intubation or Ambu-bag/mask). Reminder: para-lyzed patients may still be conscious and therefore able to feel pain, the simultaneous use of sedation is thus required for conscious patients.

Early routine use in head-injured patients lowers ICP (e.g. from suctioning[101]) and mortality, but does not improve overall outcome[102].

Neuromuscular blocking agents (NMBAs) are classified clinically by time to onset and duration of paralysis as shown in *Table 6-22*. Additional information for some agents follows the table along with some considerations for neurosurgical patients.

Table 6-22   Onset and duration of muscle relaxants

Clini-cal class	Agent	Trade name (®)	On-set (min)	Dura-tion (min)	Spontane-ous recov-ery (min)	Comment
Ultra-short	succinylcho-line	Anectine	1	5-10	20	shortest onset and duration; plasma cho-linesterase dependent; many side effects
	rapacuronium	Raplon	1.5	15	33	closest to succinylcholine in onset
Short	mivacurium	Mivacron	2-2.5	15-20	25-30	plasma cholinesterase dependent
	rocuronium	Zemuron	1-1.5	20-35	40-60	close to succinylcholine in onset in large dos-es; some vagolytic action in children
Inter-mediate	atracurium	Tracrium	3-5	20-35	40-60	no renal or hepatic metabolism; histamine re-lease in larger doses
	vecuronium	Norcuron	3-5	20-35	40-60	minimal cardiovascular side effects (brady-cardia reported); no histamine release
	cisatracurium	Nimbex	1.5-2	40-60	60-80	no histamine release at recommended doses
Long	d-tub-ocurarine		4-6	45-60	60-180	histamine release; ↑ ICP; ganglion block
	metocurine	Metubine	4-6	45-60	60-180	fewer side effects than d-tubocurarine*
	pancuronium	Pavulon	4-6	45-60	60-180	cardiovascular side effects; vagolytic
	doxacurium	Nuromax	4-6	45-60	60-180	minimal cardiovascular side effects*
	pipecuronium	Arduan	3-5	45-60	60-180	minimal cardiovascular side effects

*   not commonly used in ICU due to lack of clinical experience

ULTRA-SHORT ACTING PARALYTICS

succinylcholine (Anectine®)   DRUG INFO

The only depolarizing ganglionic blocker (the rest are competitive blockers). Rapidly inactivated by plasma pseudocholinesterases. A single dose produces fasciculations then paralysis. Onset: 1 min. Duration of action: 5-10 min.

Indications

Due to significant side effects (*see below*), use is now limited primarily to the follow-ing indications. Adults: generally recommended only for emergency intubations where the airway is not controlled. In children: only when intubation is needed with a full stom-ach, or if laryngospasm occurs during attempted intubation using other agents.

Side effects

✖ CAUTIONS: usually increases serum K^+ by 0.5 mEq/L (on rare occasion causes severe hyperkalemia ($[K^+]$ up to 12 mEq/L) in patients with neuronal or muscular pathol-ogy, causing cardiac complications which cannot be blocked), therefore contraindicated in acute phase of injury following major burns, multiple trauma or extensive denervation of skeletal muscle or upper motor neuron injury. Do not use for routine intubations in adolescents and children (may cause cardiac arrest even in apparently healthy young-sters, many of whom have undiagnosed myopathies). Linked to malignant hyperthermia.

May cause dysrhythmias, especially sinus bradycardia (treat with atropine). May get autonomic stimulation from ACh-like action → HTN, and brady- or tachycardia (es-pecially in peds with repeated doses). The fasciculations may increase ICP, intragastric pressure, and intraocular pressure (contraindicated in penetrating eye injury, especially to anterior chamber; OK in glaucoma).

Precurarization with a "priming dose" of a nondepolarizing blocker (usually ≈ 10% of the intubating dose, e.g. pancuronium 0.5-1 mg IV 3-5 minutes prior to succinylcholine) in patients with elevated ICP or increased intraocular pressure (to ameliorate further pressure increases during fasciculation phase) and in patients who have eaten recently (controversial[103]). Phase II block (similar to nondepolarizing blocker) may develop with excessive doses or in patients with abnormal pseudocholinesterase.

Dosing

***Rx* Adult**: 0.6-1.1 mg/kg (2-3 ml/70 kg) IVP (err on high side to allow time for procedure & to avoid multi-dosing complications), may repeat this dose **x** 1.

***Rx* Peds** (CAUTION: <u>Not</u> recommended for routine use, *see above*) <u>Children</u>: 1.1 mg/kg. <u>Infants</u> (< 1 mos): 2 mg/kg.

SUPPLIED: 20 mg/ml concentration.

---

rapacuronium (Raplon®)   DRUG INFO

The shortest acting nondepolarizing (competitive) NMBA. Duration of action and histamine release are both dose dependent.

***Rx* Adult**: for intubation, 1.5 mg/kg.

SHORT ACTING PARALYTICS

mivacurium (Mivacron®)   DRUG INFO

Metabolism is by plasma pseudocholinesterase, independent of kidneys or liver. Patients with pseudocholinesterase deficiency may experience prolonged paralysis lasting for hours.

***Rx* Adult**: for intubation, to avoid hypotension, give 0.15 mg/kg over 5-15 secs, or 0.20 mg/kg over 30 secs, or 0.15 mg/kg followed 30 seconds later by 0.1 mg/kg.

rocuronium (Zemuron®)   DRUG INFO

In large doses, has speed of onset that approaches succinylcholine. However, in these doses, paralysis usually lasts ≈ 1-2 hrs. Expensive.

***Rx* Adult**: initial dose 0.6-1 mg/kg. May be used as infusion of 10-12 µg/kg/min.

INTERMEDIATE ACTING PARALYTICS

★   vecuronium (Norcuron®)   DRUG INFO

Nondepolarizing (competitive) NMBA. Adequate paralysis for intubation within 2.5-3 minutes of administration. About one third more potent than pancuronium, shorter duration of action (lasts ≈ 30 minutes after initial dose). Unlike pancuronium, very little vagal (i.e. cardiovascular) effects. No CNS active metabolites. Does not affect ICP or CPP. Hepatically metabolized. Due to active metabolites, paralysis has been reported to take 6 hrs to 7 days to recede following discontinuation of the drug after ≥ 2 days use in patients with renal failure[104]. Must be mixed to use.

Dosing

SUPPLIED: 10 mg freeze-dried cakes requiring reconstitution. Use within 24 hrs.

***Rx* Adult and children** > 10 years age: 0.1 mg/kg (for most adults use 8-10 mg as initial dose). May repeat q 1 hr PRN. Infusion: 1-2 µg/kg/min.

***Rx* Pediatric**: <u>children</u> (1-10 yrs) require slightly higher dose and more frequent dosing than adult. <u>Infants</u> (7 weeks - 1 yr): slightly more sensitive on a mg/kg basis than adults, takes ≈ 1.5 **x** longer to recover. Use in neonates and continuous infusion in children is insufficiently studied.

★ **cisatracurium (Nimbex®)** DRUG INFO

Nondepolarizing (competitive) blocker. This isomer of atracurium does not release histamine unlike its parent compound (*see below*). Provides about 1 hour of paralysis. Also undergoes Hofmann degradation, with laudanosine as one of its metabolites.

Rx Adult and children > 12 years age: 0.15 or 0.2 mg/kg as part of propofol/nitrous oxide/oxygen induction-intubation technique produces muscle paralysis adequate for intubation within 2 or 1.5 minutes, respectively. Infusion: 1-3 µg/kg/min.

Rx Pediatric: <u>children</u> (2-12 yrs): 0.1 mg/kg given over 5-10 seconds during halothane or opioid anesthesia.

atracurium (Tracrium®) DRUG INFO

Nondepolarizing (competitive) blocker. After IV bolus: onset 2-2.5 mins, peak 3-5 mins, duration 15-20 mins (initial dose may last up to 30 minutes). Undergoes nonenzymatic Hofmann degradation and ester hydrolysis at normal physiologic pH and temperature, inactivating the drug in ≈ 30 minutes. Therefore useful in patients with liver or renal failure. Reversible with neostigmine. Causes histamine release which can produce hypotension (consider cisatracurium instead, *see above*). A metabolite, laudanosine, is neuroexcitatory, and accumulation could theoretically cause seizures (no documented cases)[103].

Dosing
SUPPLIED: 5 & 10 ml ampules of 10 mg/ml concentration.

Rx <u>Adult & children</u> > 2 yrs age: 0.4-0.5 mg/kg IVP. Reduce subsequent doses to 0.02 mg/kg.

Rx <u>Neonates</u> (1 month - 2 yrs): 0.3-0.4 mg/kg.

LONG ACTING PARALYTICS

pancuronium (Pavulon®) DRUG INFO

"Prototype" nondepolarizing (competitive) paralytic. Peak: 3-5 mins, duration up to 60 mins. Reversible with anticholinesterases such as neostigmine. Renal elimination.

SIDE EFFECTS: usefulness is limited because the drug is <u>vagolytic</u> and an indirect sympathomimetic which increases cardiac output, pulse rate and ICP. Consider vecuronium as an alternative (*see above*).

Dosing
Rx <u>Adult & children</u>: 0.04-0.10 mg/kg IVP (start with 3 mg). Reduce subsequent doses to 0.02 mg/kg.

Rx <u>Neonates</u>: especially sensitive, test dose 0.02 mg/kg.

1.6.5.   Acid inhibitors

Stress ulcers in neurosurgery[18]
The risk of stress ulcers (**SU**) is high in critically ill patients with CNS pathology. 17% of SUs produce clinically significant hemorrhage. CNS risk factors include intracranial pathology: brain injury (especially Glasgow Coma scale score < 9), brain tumors, intracerebral hemorrhage, SIADH, CNS infection, ischemic CVA, as well as spinal cord injury. The odds are increased with the coexistence of extra-CNS risk factors including: long-term use of steroids (usually > 3 weeks), burns > 25% of body surface area, hypotension, respiratory failure, coagulopathies, renal or hepatic failure and sepsis.

CNS pathology, especially that involving the diencephalon or brain stem, can lead to reduction of vagal output which leads to hypersecretion of gastric acid and pepsin. There is a peak in acid and pepsin production 3-5 days after CNS injury.

Prophylaxis for stress ulcers
There is strong evidence that reduction of gastric acid (whether by antacids or agents that inhibit acid secretion) reduces the incidence of GI bleeding from stress ulcers

in critically ill patients. Elevating gastric pH > 4.5 also inactivates pepsin.

Other therapies that don't involve alterations of pH that may be effective include sucralfate and enteral nutrition (controversial)[18]. Titrated antacids or sucralfate appear to be superior to H_2 antagonists in reducing the incidence of SUs.

Routine prophylaxis when steroids are used is not warranted unless one of the following risk factors are present: prior PUD, concurrent use of NSAIDs, hepatic or renal failure, malnourishment, or prolonged steroid therapy > 3 weeks.

1.7.   References

1.   Raggio J F, Fleischer A S, Sung Y F, *et al.*: Expanding pneumocephalus due to nitrous oxide anesthesia. Case report. **Neurosurgery** 4: 261-3, 1979.

2.   Drummond J C, Cole D J, Patel P M, *et al.*: Focal cerebral ischemia during anesthesia with etomidate, isofluorane, or thiopental: A comparison of the extent of cerebral injury. **Neurosurgery** 37: 742-9, 1995.

3.   Shapiro H M: *Neurosurgical anesthesia and intracranial hypertension*. In **Anesthesia**, Miller R D, (ed.). Churchill Livingstone, New York, 2nd ed., 1986, Vol. 2: pp 1563-620.

4.   Nelson T E, Flewellen E H: The malignant hyperthermia syndrome. **N Engl J Med** 309: 416-8, 1983.

5.   Drugs for hypertensive emergencies. **Med Letter** 29: 18-20, 1987.

6.   Ferguson R K, Vlasses P H: Hypertensive emergencies and urgencies. **JAMA** 255: 1607-13, 1986.

7.   Cottrell J E, Patel K, Turndorf H, *et al.*: ICP changes induced by sodium nitroprusside in patients with intracranial mass lesions. **J Neurosurg** 48: 329-31, 1978.

8.   Ram Z, Spiegelman R, Findler G, *et al.*: Delayed postoperative neurological deterioration from prolonged sodium nitroprusside administration. **J Neurosurg** 71: 605-7, 1989.

9.   Orlowski J P, Shiesley D, Vidt D G, *et al.*: Labetalol to control blood pressure after cerebrovascular surgery. **Crit Care Med** 16: 765-8, 1988.

10.   Esmolol - A short-acting IV beta blocker. **Med Letter** 29: 57-8, 1987.

11.   Trumble E R, Muizelaar J P, Myseros J S: Coagulopathy with the use of hetastarch in the treatment of vasospasm. **J Neurosurg** 82: 44-7, 1995.

12.   Knudsen F, Jensen H P, Petersen P L: Neurogenic pulmonary edema: Treatment with dobutamine. **Neurosurgery** 29: 269-70, 1991.

13.   Byyny R L: Withdrawal from glucocorticoid therapy. **N Engl J Med** 295: 30-2, 1976.

14.   Szabo G C, Winkler S R: Withdrawal of glucocorticoid therapy in neurosurgical patients. **Surg Neurol** 44: 498, 1995.

15.   Kountz D S: An algorithm for corticosteroid withdrawal. **Am Fam Physician** 39: 250-4, 1989.

16.   Marshall L F, King J, Langfitt T W: The complication of high-dose corticosteroid therapy in neurosurgical patients: A prospective study. **Ann Neurol** 1: 201-3, 1977.

17.   Braughler J M, Hall E D: Current application of "high-dose" steroid therapy for CNS injury: A pharmacological perspective. **J Neurosurg** 62: 806-10, 1985.

18.   Lu W Y, Rhoney D H, Boling W B, *et al.*: A review of stress ulcer prophylaxis in the neurosurgical intensive care unit. **Neurosurgery** 41: 416-26, 1997.

19.   Weiner H L, Rezai A R, Cooper P R: Sigmoid diverticular perforation in neurosurgical patients receiving high-dose corticosteroids. **Neurosurgery** 33: 40-3, 1993.

20.   Zizic T M, Marcoux C, Hungerfold D S, *et al.*: Corticosteroid therapy associated with ischemic necrosis of bone in systemic lupus erythematosus. **Am J Med** 79: 597-603, 1985.

21.   Struys A, Snelder A A, Mulder H: Cyclical etidronate reverses bone loss of the spine and proximal femur in patients with established corticosteroid-induced osteoporosis. **Am J Med** 99: 235-42, 1995.

22.   Thibonnier M: *Antidiuretic hormone: Regulation, disorders, and clinical evaluation*. In **Neuroendocrinology**, Barrow D L and Selman W, (eds.). Concepts in neurosurgery. Williams and Wilkins, Baltimore, 1992, Vol. 5: pp 19-30.

23.   Diringer M, Ladenson P W, Borel C, *et al.*: Sodium and water regulation in a patient with cerebral salt wasting. **Arch Neurol** 46: 928-30, 1989.

24.   Arieff A I: Hyponatremia, convulsions, respiratory arrest and permanent brain damage after elective surgery in healthy women. **N Engl J Med** 314: 1529-35, 1986.

25.   Ayus J C, Krothapalli R K, Arieff A I: Changing concepts on treatment of severe symptomatic hyponatremia. Rapid correction and possible relation to central pontine myelinolysis. **Am J Med** 78: 879-902, 1985.

26.   Fraser C L, Arieff A I: Symptomatic hyponatremia: Management and relation to central pontine myelinolysis. **Sem Neurol** 4: 445-52, 1984.

27.   Adams R D, Victor M, Mancall E L: Central pontine myelinolysis: A hitherto undescribed disease occurring in alcoholic and malnourished patients. **Arch Neurol Psychiatr** 81: 154-72, 1959.

28.   Ayus J C, Krothapalli R K, Arieff A I: Treatment of symptomatic hyponatremia and its relation to brain damage. **N Engl J Med** 317: 1190-5, 1987.

29.   Berl T: Treating hyponatremia: What is all the controversy about? **Ann Intern Med** 113: 417-9, 1990.

30.   Arieff A I: Hyponatremia associated with permanent brain damage. **Adv Intern Med** 32: 325-44, 1987.

31.   Laureno R, Karp B I: Myelinolysis after correction of hyponatremia. **Ann Intern Med** 126: 57-62, 1997.

32.   Hantman D, Rossier B, Zohlman R, *et al.*: Rapid correction of hyponatremia in SIADH: An alternative treatment to hypertonic saline. **Ann Intern Med** 78: 870-5, 1973.

33.   Lester M C, Nelson P B: Neurological aspects of vasopressin release and the syndrome of inappropriate secretion of antidiuretic hormone. **Neurosurgery** 8: 725-40, 1981.

34.   Kröll M, Juhler M, Lindholm J: Hyponatremia in acute brain disease. **J Int Med** 232: 291-7, 1992.

35.   Harrigan M R: Cerebral salt wasting syndrome: A review. **Neurosurgery** 38: 152-60, 1996.

36.   De Troyer A, Demanet J C: Correction of antidiuresis by demeclocycline. **N Engl J Med** 293: 915-8, 1975.

37.   Perks W H, Mohr P, Liversedge L A: Demeclocycline in inappropriate ADH syndrome. **Lancet** 2: 1414, 1976 (letter).

38.   Forrest J N, Cox M, Hong C, *et al.*: Superiority of demeclocycline over lithium in the treatment of chronic syndrome of inappropriate secretion of an-

tidiuretic hormone. **N Engl J Med** 298: 173-7, 1978.

39. Decaux G, Waterlot Y, Genette F, *et al.*: Treatment of the syndrome of inappropriate secretion of antidiuretic hormone with furosemide. **N Engl J Med** 304: 329-30, 1981.

40. Maroon J C, Nelson P B: Hypovolemia in patients with subarachnoid hemorrhage: Therapeutic implications. **Neurosurgery** 4: 223-6, 1979.

41. Wijdicks E F M, Vermeulen M, Hijdra A, *et al.*: Hyponatremia and cerebral infarction in patients with ruptured intracranial aneurysms: Is fluid restriction harmful? **Ann Neurol** 17: 137-40, 1985.

42. Wijdicks E F M, Vermeulen M, ten Haaf J A, *et al.*: Volume depletion and natriuresis in patients with a ruptured intracranial aneurysm. **Ann Neurol** 18: 211-6, 1985.

43. Nelson P B, Seif S M, Maroon J C, *et al.*: Hyponatremia in intracranial disease. Perhaps not the syndrome of inappropriate secretion of antidiuretic hormone (SIADH). **J Neurosurg** 55: 938-41, 1981.

44. Hasan D, Lindsay K W, Wijdicks E F M, *et al.*: Effect of fludrocortisone acetate in patients with subarachnoid hemorrhage. **Stroke** 20: 1156-61, 1989.

45. Reeder R F, Harbaugh R E: Administration of intravenous urea and normal saline for the treatment of hyponatremia in neurosurgical patients. **J Neurosurg** 70: 201-6, 1989.

46. Verbalis J G, Robinson A G, Moses A M: Postoperative and post-traumatic diabetes insipidus. **Front Horm Res** 13: 247-65, 1985.

47. Abe T, Matsumoto K, Sanno N, *et al.*: Lymphocytic hypophysitis: Case report. **Neurosurgery** 36: 1016-9, 1995.

48. Imura H, Nakao K, Shimatsu A, *et al.*: Lymphocytic infundibuloneurohypophysitis as a cause of central diabetes insipidus. **N Engl J Med** 329: 683-9, 1993.

49. Miller M, Dalakos T, Moses A M, *et al.*: Recognition of partial defects in antidiuretic hormone secretion. **Ann Intern Med** 73: 721-9, 1970.

50. Fresh-Frozen Plasma Cryoprecipitate and Platelets Administration Practice Guidelines Development Task Force of the College of American Pathologists: Practice parameter for the use of fresh-frozen plasma, cryoprecipitate, and platelets. **JAMA** 271: 777-81, 1994.

51. Mannucci P M: Desmopressin: A nontransfusion form of treatment for congenital and acquired bleeding disorders. **Blood** 72: 1449-55, 1988.

52. So W, Hugenholtz H, Richard M T: Complications of anticoagulant therapy in patients with known central nervous system lesions. **Can J Surg** 26: 181-3, 1983.

53. Ruff R, Posner J: Incidence and treatment of peripheral thrombosis in patients with glioma. **Ann Neurol** 13: 334-6, 1983.

54. Olin J W, Young J R, Graor R A, *et al.*: Treatment of deep vein thrombosis and pulmonary emboli in patients with primary and metastatic brain tumors: Anticoagulants or inferior vena cava filter? **Arch Intern Med** 147: 2177-9, 1987.

55. Altschuler E, Moosa H, Selker R G, *et al.*: The risk and efficacy of anticoagulant therapy in the treatment of thromboembolic complications in patients with primary malignant brain tumors. **Neurosurgery** 27: 74-7, 1990.

56. Stern W E: *Preoperative evaluation: Complications, their prevention and treatment*. In **Neurological surgery**, Youmans J, (ed.). W. B. Saunders, Philadelphia, 2nd ed., 1982, Vol. 2: pp 1051-116.

57. Kawamata T, Takeshita M, Kubo O, *et al.*: Management of intracranial hemorrhage associated with anticoagulant therapy. **Surg Neurol** 44: 438-43, 1995.

58. Novoseven for non-hemophilia hemostasis. **Med Letter** 46: 33-4, 2004.

59. Hirsh J, Dalen J E, Deykin D, *et al.*: Oral anticoagulants: Mechanism of action, clinical effectiveness, and optimal therapeutic range. **Chest** 102 (Suppl):

312-26, 1992.

60. Khamashta M A, Cuadrado M J, Mujic F, *et al.*: The management of thrombosis in the antiphospholipid-antibody syndrome. **N Engl J Med** 332: 993-7, 1995.

61. Hyers T M, Hull R D, Weg J G: Antithrombotic therapy for venous thromboembolic disease. **Chest** 95: 37S-51S, 1989.

62. Atkinson J L D, Sundt T M, Kazmier F J, *et al.*: Heparin-induced thrombocytopenia and thrombosis in ischemic stroke. **Mayo Clin Proc** 63: 353-61, 1988.

63. Dalteparin - another low-molecular-weight heparin. **Med Letter** 37: 115-6, 1995.

64. Ardeparin and danaparoid for prevention of deep vein thrombosis. **Med Letter** 39 (1011): 94-5, 1997.

65. **FDA public health advisory**, Food and Drug Administration, Public Health Service. Rockville, MD. December 15, 1997.

66. Fondaparinux (arixtra), a new anticoagulant. **Med Letter** 44: 43-4, 2002.

67. Lepirudin for heparin-induced thrombocytopenia. **Med Letter** 40: 94-5, 1998.

68. Fredriksson K, Norrving B, Stromblad L G: Emergency reversal of anticoagulation after intracerebral hemorrhage. **Stroke** 23: 972-7, 1992.

69. Hamilton M G, Hull R D, Pineo G F: Venous thromboembolism in neurosurgery and neurology patients: A review. **Neurosurgery** 34: 280-96, 1994.

70. Olson J D, Kaufman H H, Moake J, *et al.*: The incidence and significance of hemostatic abnormalities in patients with head injuries. **Neurosurgery** 24: 825-32, 1989.

71. Sawaya R, Zuccarello M, El-Kalliny M: Brain tumors and thromboembolism: Clinical, hemostatic, and biochemical correlations. **J Neurosurg** 70: 314A, 1989 (abstract).

72. Quevedo J F, Buckner J C, Schmidt J L, *et al.*: Thromboembolism in patients with high-grade glioma. **Mayo Clin Proc** 69: 329-32, 1994.

73. Black P M, Baker M F, Snook C P: Experience with external pneumatic calf compression in neurology and neurosurgery. **Neurosurgery** 18: 440-4, 1986.

74. Snyder M, Renaudin J: Intracranial hemorrhage associated with anticoagulation therapy. **Surg Neurol** 7: 31-4, 1977.

75. Cerrato D, Ariano C, Fiacchino F: Deep vein thrombosis and low-dose heparin prophylaxis in neurosurgical patients. **J Neurosurg** 49: 378-81, 1978.

76. Frim D M, Barker F G, Poletti C E, *et al.*: Postoperative low-dose heparin decreases thromboembolic complications in neurosurgical patients. **Neurosurgery** 30: 830-3, 1992.

77. Rose S C, Zwiebel W J, Murdock L E, *et al.*: Insensitivity of color Doppler flow imaging for detection of acute calf deep venous thrombosis in asymptomatic postoperative patients. **J Vasc Interv Radiol** 4: 111-7, 1993.

78. Wells P S, Anderson D R, Bormanis J, *et al.*: Value of assessment of pretest probability of deep-vein thrombosis in clinical management. **Lancet** 350: 1795-8, 1997.

79. Ginsberg J S, Wells P S, Kearon C, *et al.*: Sensitivity and specificity of a rapid whole-blood assay for D-dimer in the diagnosis of pulmonary embolism. **Ann Intern Med** 129: 1006-11, 1998.

80. Hull R D, Raskob G E, Pineo G F, *et al.*: Subcutaneous low-molecular-weight heparin compared with continuous intravenous heparin in the treatment of proximal-vein thrombosis. **N Engl J Med** 326: 975-82, 1992.

81. Hull R D, Raskob G E, Rosenbloom D, *et al.*: Heparin for five days as compared with ten days in the initial treatment of proximal venous thrombosis. **N Engl J Med** 322: 1260-4, 1990.

82. Mann K S, Yue C P, Chan K H, *et al.*: Paraplegia due to extramedullary hematopoiesis in thalassemia: Case report. **J Neurosurg** 66: 938-40, 1987.

83. Marshall K A: Managing cancer pain: Basic principles and invasive treatment. **Mayo Clin Proc** 71: 472-7, 1996.

84. Celecoxib for arthritis. **Med Letter** 41: 11-2, 1999.

85. Helfgott S M, Sandberg-Cook J, Zakim D, *et al*.: Diclofenac-associated hepatotoxicity. **JAMA** 264: 2660-2, 1990.

86. Henrich W L: Analgesic nephropathy. **Am J Med Sci** 295: 561-8, 1988.

87. Bromfenac for analgesia. **Med Letter** 39: 93-4, 1997.

88. Strom B L, Berlin J A, Kinman J L, *et al*.: Parenteral ketorolac and risk of gastrointestinal and operative site bleeding. **JAMA** 275: 376-82, 1996.

89. Tramadol - A new oral analgesic. **Med Letter** 37: 59-60, 1995.

90. Drugs for pain. **Med Letter** 40: 79-84, 1998.

91. Palladone for chronic pain. **Med Letter** 47: 21-3, 2005.

92. Bigos S, Bowyer O, Braen G, *et al*.: **Acute low back problems in adults. Clinical pratice guideline no.14. AHCPR publication no. 95-0642**. Agency for Health Care Policy and Research, Public Health Service, U.S. Department of Health and Human Services, Rockville, MD, 1994.

93. Chlorzoxazone hepatotoxicity. **Med Letter** 38: 46, 1996.

94. Man-Son-Hing M, Wells G: Meta-analysis of efficacy of quinine for treatment of nocturnal leg cramps in elderly people. **BMJ** 310: 13-7, 1995.

95. Quinine for 'night cramps'. **Med Letter** 28: 110, 1986.

96. Choice of benzodiazepines. **Med Letter** 30: 26-8, 1988.

97. Drugs for psychiatric disorders. **Med Letter** 28: 99-100, 1986.

98. Midazolam. **Med Letter** 28: 73-4, 1986.

99. Flumazenil. **Med Letter** 34: 66-8, 1992.

100. Ramsay M A E, Savege T M, Simpson B R J, *et al*.: Controlled sedation with alphaxalone-alphadolone. **Br Med J** 2: 656-9, 1974.

101. Werba A, Weinstabi C, Petricek W, *et al*.: Vecuronium prevents increases in intracranial pressure during routine tracheobronchial suctioning in neurosurgical patients. **Anaesthetist** 40: 328-31, 1991.

102. Hsiang J K, Chesnut R M, Crisp C D, *et al*.: Early, routine paralysis for intracranial pressure control in severe head injury: Is it necessary? **Crit Care Med** 22: 1471-6, 1994.

103. Ohlinger M J, Rhoney D H: Neuromuscular blocking agents in the neurosurgical intensive care unit. **Surg Neurol** 49: 217-21, 1998.

104. Segredo V, Caldwell J E, Matthay M A, *et al*.: Persistent paralysis in critically ill patients after long-term administration of vecuronium. **N Engl J Med** 327: 524-8, 1992.

2. Neurology

2.1. Dementia

Definition: loss of intellectual abilities previously attained (memory, judgement, abstract thought, and other higher cortical functions) severe enough to interfere with social and/or occupational functioning[1]. Memory deficit is the cardinal feature, however, the DSM-IV definition requires impairment in at least one other domain (language, perception, visuospatial function, calculation, judgement, abstraction, problem-solving skills). Affects 3-11% of community-dwelling adults > 65 yrs of age, with a greater presence among institutionalized residents[2].

Risk factors: advanced age, family history of dementia, and apolipoprotein E-4 allele.

Delerium: AKA acute confusional state. Distinct from dementia, however, patients with dementia are at increased risk of developing delerium[3, 4]. A primary disorder of attention that subsequently affects all other aspects of cognition[5]. Often represents life-threatening illness, e.g. hypoxia, sepsis, uremic encephalopathy (also *see page 64*), electrolyte abnormality, drug intoxication, MI. 50% of patients die within 2 yrs of this diagnosis.

Unlike dementia, delerium has acute onset, motor signs (tremor, myoclonus, asterixis), slurred speech, altered consciousness (hyperalert/agitated or lethargic, or fluctuations), hallucinations may be florid. EEG → pronounced diffuse slowing.

Brain biopsy for dementia

Clinical criteria are usually sufficient for the diagnosis of most dementias. Biopsy should be reserved for cases of a chronic progressive cerebral disorder with an unusual clinical course where all other possible diagnostic methods have been exhausted and have failed to provide adequate diagnostic certainty[6]. Biopsy may disclose CJD, low grade astrocytoma, and AD among others. The high incidence of CJD among patients selected for biopsy under these criteria necessitates appropriate precautions (see *Creutzfeldt-Jakob disease*, page 227). In a report of 50 brain biopsies performed to assess progressive neurodegenerative disease of unclear etiology[7], the diagnostic yield was only 20% (6% were only suggestive of a diagnosis, 66% were abnormal but nonspecific, 8% were normal). The yield was highest in those with focal MRI abnormalities. Among the 10 patients with diagnostic biopsies, the biopsy result led to a meaningful therapeutic intervention in only 4.

Recommendations: Based on the above, the following recommendations are made for patients with an otherwise unexplained neurodegenerative disease:
1. those with a focal abnormality on MRI: stereotactic biopsy
2. those without focal abnormality (possibly including SPECT or PET scan): brain biopsy should only be performed within an investigative protocol

2.2. Headache

Headache **(H/A)** may be broadly categorized as follows:
1. chronic recurring headaches
   A. vascular type (migraine): *see below*
   B. muscle contraction (tension) headaches
2. headache due to pathology
   A. systemic pathology
   B. intracranial pathology: a wide variety of etiologies including:
      1. subarachnoid hemorrhage: <u>sudden</u> onset, severe, usually with vomiting, apoplexy, focal deficits possible (*see page 782* for differential diag-

nosis of paroxysmal H/A)
2. increased intracranial pressure from any cause (tumor, communicating hydrocephalus, inflammation, pseudotumor cerebri...)
3. irritation or inflammation of meninges: meningitis
4. tumor: with or without elevated ICP (*see page 405*)
C. local pathology of the eye, nasopharynx, or extracranial tissues (including giant cell arteritis, *see page 58*)
D. following head trauma (postconcussive syndrome): *see page 682*
E. following craniotomy ("syndrome of the trephined"): *see page 612*

A severe new H/A, or a change in the pattern of a longstanding or recurrent H/A (including developing associated N/V, or an abnormal neurologic exam) warrants further investigation with CT or MRI[8].

2.2.1. Migraine

Migraine attacks usually occur in individuals predisposed to the condition, and may be activated by factors such as bright light, stress, diet changes, trauma, administration of radiologic contrast media (especially angiography) and vasodilators.

CLASSIFICATION
See also index under *Headache*, e.g. for: crash migraine (thunderclap headache) *page 782*, post-myelogram headache *page 46*...

COMMON MIGRAINE
Episodic H/A with N/V and photophobia, without aura or neurologic deficit.

CLASSIC MIGRAINE
Common migraine + aura. May have H/A with occasional focal neurologic deficit(s) that resolve completely in ≤ 24 hrs.
Over half of the transient neurologic disturbances are visual, and usually consist of positive phenomena (spark photopsia, stars, complex geometric patterns, fortification spectra) which may leave negative phenomena (scotoma, hemianopia, monocular or binocular visual loss...) in their wake. The second most common symptoms are somatosensory involving the hand and lower face. Less frequently, deficits may consist of aphasia, hemiparesis, or unilateral clumsiness. A slow march-like progression of deficit is characteristic. The risk of stroke is probably increased in patients with migraine[9].

COMPLICATED MIGRAINE
Occasional attacks of classic migraine with minimal or no associated H/A, and complete resolution of neurologic deficit in ≤ 30 days.

MIGRAINE EQUIVALENT
Neurologic symptoms (N/V, visual aura, etc.) without H/A (acephalgic migraine). Seen mostly in children. Usually develops into typical migraine with age. Aura may be shortened by opening and swallowing contents of a 10 mg nifedipine capsule[10].

HEMIPLEGIC MIGRAINE
H/A typically precedes hemiplegia which may persist even after H/A resolves.

CLUSTER HEADACHE
AKA histaminic migraine. Actually a neurovascular event, distinct from true migraine. Recurrent unilateral attacks of severe pain. Usually oculofrontal or oculotemporal with occasional radiation into the jaw, usually recurring on the same side of the head. Ipsilateral autonomic symptoms (conjunctival injection, nasal congestion, rhinorrhea, lacrimation, facial flushing) are common. Partial Horner's syndrome (ptosis and miosis) sometimes occurs. Male:female ratio is ≈ 5:1. 25% of patients have a personal or family history of migraine.
Headaches characteristically have no prodrome, last 30-90 minutes, and recur one or more times daily usually for 4-12 weeks, often at a similar time of day, following which there is typically a remission for an average of 12 months[11].

Essentially restricted to adolescence. Recurrent episodes lasting minutes to hours of transient neurologic deficits in distribution of vertebrobasilar system. Deficits include: vertigo (most common), gait ataxia, visual disturbance (scotomata, bilateral blindness), dysarthria, followed by severe H/A and occasionally nausea and vomiting[12]. Family history of migraine is present in 86%.

2.2.2.   Post LP (myelogram) H/A

AKA "postspinal headache" or "spinal headache". May also follow procedures other than LP/myelogram, such as dural opening (*see page 308*). Can also occur with spontaneous intracranial hypotension (*see page 178*).

Clinical features
Important distinctive characteristic: H/A occurs when patient is erect, and is completely or partially (but significantly) relieved when recumbent. May be associated with nausea, vomiting, dizziness, or visual disturbances.

Time course: Most post-LP headaches **(PLPHA)** have a delayed onset 24-48 hrs after the LP, and although they may occur weeks post-LP, most also develop within 3 days. The duration of PLPHA varies, with a mean of 4 days[13], and reports of duration of months[14] and even > 1 year[15].

Pathophysiology
Thought to be due to continued CSF leakage through the hole in the dura[16], which reduces the CSF "cushion" of the brain. In the upright position, the pull of gravity on the brain produces traction on the blood vessels and any structures tethering the brain to the pain-sensitive dura. CSF may sometimes be demonstrable in the epidural space.

Epidemiology following LP
Reported incidence range is 2-40% (typically ≈ 20%), higher after diagnostic LP than for epidural anesthesia[13].
For variables in LP that impact upon the risk of PLPHA, *see page 617*

TREATMENT FOR H/A FOLLOWING LP
Initial "conservative" measures include:
1. flat in bed for at least 24 hrs
2. hydration (PO or IV)
3. analgesics for H/A
4. tight abdominal binder
5. desoxycortisone acetate 5 mg IM q 8 hrs[13]
6. caffeine sodium benzoate 500 mg in 2 cc IV q 8 hrs up to 3 d max (70% of patients had relief with 1 or 2 injections)[17]
7. high-dose steroids: report of success in a case of intracranial hypotension associated with spontaneous slit ventricles tapering down from a starting dose of dexamethasone 20 mg/day[18]
8. blood patch if refractory (*see below*)

EPIDURAL BLOOD PATCH
For refractory post-lumbar puncture or post-myelogram H/A. Works in one application in over 90% of cases, may be repeated if ineffective[14]. Theoretical risks: infection, cauda equina compression, failure to relieve H/A.

Technique
Accessing epidural space (one of several techniques): proceed as routine LP. When ligaments are traversed, and needle tip is nearing spinal canal, stylet is removed. Then, either place drop of sterile saline in hub (hanging drop technique) and advance while watching for it to be drawn into needle as epidural space is entered, or gently try injecting air with small syringe (preferably glass) while advancing, when the epidural space is entered, resistance to injection disappears, but CSF cannot be aspirated.

A venipuncture site is prepared aseptically. 10 ml of the patient's blood is withdrawn. After verifying CSF cannot be aspirated through the spinal needle, the blood is injected into the epidural space. After 30 minutes supine, patient may ambulate ad lib.

2.3.   Parkinsonism

Parkinsonism may be primary (idiopathic paralysis agitans **(IPA)**, classical Parkinson's disease) or secondary to other conditions. All result from a relative loss of the dopamine mediated inhibition of the effects of acetylcholine in the basal ganglia.

IDIOPATHIC PARALYSIS AGITANS

Classical Parkinson's disease, AKA shaking palsy.

Clinical

Affects ≈ 1% of Americans > age 50 yrs[19]. Male:female ratio is 3:2. Not clearly environmentally or genetically induced, but may be influenced by these factors.

The classic triad is shown in *Table 2-1*. Other signs may include: postural instability, micrographia, mask-like facies. Gait consists of small, shuffling steps (marche á petits pas) or festinating gait.

Table 2-1   Classic triad of Parkinson's disease

• tremor (resting, 4-7/second)
• rigidity (cogwheel)
• bradykinesia

Clinically distinguishing IPA from secondary parkinsonism (*see below*): May be difficult early. IPA generally exhibits gradual onset of bradykinesia with tremor that is often asymmetrical, and initially responds well to levodopa. Other disorders are suggested with rapid progression of symptoms, when the initial response to levodopa is equivocal, or when there is early midline symptoms (ataxia or impairment of gait and balance, sphincter disturbance…) or the presence of other features such as early dementia, sensory findings, profound orthostatic hypotension, or abnormalities of extraocular movements[20, 21].

Pathophysiology

Degeneration primarily of pigmented (neuromelanin-laden) dopaminergic neurons of the pars compacta of the substantia nigra, resulting in reduced levels of dopamine in the neostriatum (caudate nucleus, putamen, globus pallidus). This decreases the activity of inhibitory neurons with predominantly D2 class of dopamine receptors which project directly to the internal segment of the globus pallidus **(GPi)**, and also increases (by loss of inhibition) activity of neurons with predominantly D1 receptors which project indirectly to the globus pallidus externa **(GPe)** and subthalamic nucleus[22]. The net result is increased activity in GPi which has inhibitory projections to the thalamus which then suppresses activity in the supplemental motor cortex among other locations.

Histologically: **Lewy bodies** (eosinophilic intraneuronal hyaline inclusion) are the hallmark of IPA.

SECONDARY PARKINSONISM

The differential diagnosis includes the following etiologies of secondary parkinsonism or Parkinson-like conditions (some referred to as "Parkinson plus"):

1. **olivopontocerebellar degeneration (OPC)**
2. striato-nigral degeneration **(SND)**: more aggressive than parkinsonism
3. postencephalitic parkinsonism: followed an epidemic of encephalitis lethargica (von Economo disease) in the 1920's, victims are no longer living. Distinguishing features: oculogyric crisis, tremor involves not only extremities but also trunk and head, asymmetrical, no Lewy bodies
4. progressive supranuclear palsy **(PSNP)**: impaired vertical gaze (*see below*)
5. multiple system atrophy (Shy-Drager syndrome): *see below*
6. drug induced: includes:
   A. prescription drugs (elderly females seem more susceptible)
      1. antipsychotics (AKA neuroleptics): haloperidol (Haldol®) which works by blocking postsynaptic dopamine receptors
      2. phenothiazine antiemetics: prochlorperazine (Compazine®)
      3. metoclopramide (Reglan®)
      4. reserpine
   B. MPTP (1-methyl-4-phenyl-1,2,3,6-tetrahydropyridine): a commercially available chemical intermediate which is also a by-product of the synthesis of MPPP (a meperidine analog) that was synthesized and self-injected by a

graduate student[23], and later produced by illicit drug manufacturers to be sold as "synthetic heroin" and unwittingly injected by some IV drug abusers in northern California in 1983[24]. MPTP was subsequently discovered to be a potent neurotoxin for dopaminergic neurons. As a rule, the response to levodopa is dramatic, but short-lived

   C. there is an as yet unproven assertion that methylenedioxymethamphetamine **(MDMA)** AKA Ecstasy (on the street), may hasten the onset of Parkinsonism

7. toxic: poisoning with carbon monoxide, manganese...
8. ischemic (lacunes in basal ganglia): produces so-called **arteriosclerotic parkinsonism** AKA vascular parkinsonism: "lower-half" parkinsonism (gait disturbance predominates[25]). Also causes pseudobulbar deficits, emotional lability. Tremor is rare
9. posttraumatic: parkinsonian symptoms may occur in chronic traumatic encephalopathy (dementia pugilistica, *see page 683*). There are usually other features not normally present in IPA (e.g. cerebellar findings)
10. normal pressure hydrocephalus **(NPH)**: urinary incontinence... (*see page 199*)
11. neoplasm in the region of the substantia nigra
12. Riley-Day (familial dysautonomia)
13. parkinson-dementia complex of Guam: classic IPA + amyotrophic lateral sclerosis **(ALS)**. Pathologically has features of parkinsonism and Alzheimer's disease but no Lewy bodies nor senile plaques
14. Huntington's disease **(HD)**: whereas adults typically show chorea, when HD manifests in a young person it may resemble IPA
15. (spontaneous) intracranial hypotension may present with findings mimicking IPA (*see page 178*)

MULTIPLE SYSTEM ATROPHY **(MSA)**

AKA Shy-Drager syndrome. Parkinsonism (indistinguishable from IPA), *PLUS* idiopathic orthostatic hypotension, *PLUS* other signs of autonomic nervous system **(ANS)** dysfunction (ANS findings may precede parkinsonism and may include urinary sphincter disturbance and hypersensitivity to noradrenaline or tyramine infusions). Degeneration of preganglionic lateral horn neurons of thoracic spinal cord. NB: classic IPA may eventually produce orthostatic hypotension from inactivity or as a result of progressive autonomic failure. Unlike IPA, most do not respond to dopa therapy.

PROGRESSIVE SUPRANUCLEAR PALSY **(PSNP)**

AKA Steele-Richardson-Olszewski syndrome[26].

Triad:
1. progressive supranuclear ophthalmoplegia (chiefly vertical gaze): paresis of voluntary vertical eye movement, but still moves to vertical doll's eyes maneuver
2. pseudobulbar palsy (mask-like facies with marked dysarthria and dysphagia, hyperactive jaw jerk, emotional incontinence usually mild)
3. axial dystonia (especially of neck and upper trunk)

Associated findings: subcortical dementia (inconstant), motor findings of pyramidal, extrapyramidal and cerebellar systems. Average age of onset: 60 yrs. Males comprise 60%. Response to anti-parkinson drugs is usually very short lived. Average survival after diagnosis: 5.7 yrs.

Differentiating from Parkinson's disease (IPA):
Patients with PSNP have a pseudo-parkinsonism. They have mask facies, but do not walk bent forward (they walk erect), and they do not have a tremor. They tend to fall backwards.

Course
1. early:
   A. many falls: due to dysequilibrium + downgaze palsy (can't see floor)
   B. eye findings may be normal initially, subsequently may develop difficulty looking down (especially to command, less to following), calorics have normal tonic component but absent nystagmus (cortical component)
   C. slurred speech
   D. personality changes
   E. difficulty eating: due to pseudobulbar palsy + inability to look down at food on plate

2. late:
   A. eyes fixed centrally (no response to oculocephalics or oculovestibulars): ocular immotility is due to frontal lobe lesions
   B. neck stiffens in extension (retrocollis)

SURGICAL TREATMENT FOR PARKINSON'S DISEASE

Before the introduction of L-dopa in the late 1960's, stereotactic thalamotomy was widely used for Parkinson's disease. The location ultimately targeted for lesioning was the ventrolateral nucleus. The procedure worked better for relieving the tremor than for the bradykinesia, however it was the latter symptom that was most disabling. This procedure cannot be done bilaterally without significant risk to speech function. The procedure fell out of favor when more effective drugs became available[27].

See *Surgical treatment of Parkinson's disease* on page 365 for further information.

2.4. Multiple sclerosis

A demyelinating disease (affecting only white matter) of the cerebrum, optic nerves, and spinal cord (especially corticospinal tracts and the posterior columns). Produces multiple plaques of various age in diffuse locations in the CNS, especially in the periventricular white matter. Lesions initially evoke an inflammatory response with monocytes and lymphocytic perivascular cuffing, but with age settle down to glial scars.

EPIDEMIOLOGY
Usual age of onset: 10-50 years, with the greatest peak between ages 20-40 years. Male to female ratio: 1.5:1.

Prevalence varies with latitude, and is < 1 per 100,000 near the equator, and is ≈ 30-80 per 100,000 in the northern U.S. and Canada.

CLINICAL
Causes exacerbations and remissions in various locations in the CNS (dissemination in space and time). Common symptoms: visual disturbances (diplopia, blurring, field cuts or scotoma), spastic paraparesis, and bladder disturbances. Nomenclature for the time course of MS is shown in *Table 2-2*[28]. Relapsing-remitting MS is the most common pattern at onset, and has the best response to therapy, but > 50% of cases eventually become secondary progressive MS. Only 10% have primary progressive MS, and these patients tend to be older at onset (40-60 years) and frequently develop progressive myelopathy[29]. Progressive relapsing MS is very uncommon.

Table 2-2 Clinical categories of MS

Category	Definition
relapsing-remitting	episodes of acute worsening with recovery and a stable course between relapses
secondary progressive	gradual neurologic deterioration ± superimposed acute relapses in a patient who previously had relapsing-remitting MS
primary progressive	gradual, nearly continuous neurologic deterioration from the onset of symptoms
progressive relapsing	gradual neurologic deterioration from the onset of symptoms, but with subsequent superimposed relapses

Deficits present > 6 months usually persist.

Differential diagnosis
The plethora of possible signs and symptoms in MS causes the differential diagnosis to extend to almost all conditions causing focal or diffuse dysfunction of the CNS. Conditions that may closely mimic MS clinically and on diagnostic testing include:
1. acute disseminated encephalomyelitis (**ADEM**): may also have CSF-OCB, generally monophasic
2. CNS lymphoma: *see page 462*
3. other closely related demyelinating diseases: e.g. Devic syndrome (*see page 904*)

Signs and symptoms

Visual disturbances: Disturbances of visual acuity may be caused by optic or retrobulbar neuritis which is the presenting symptom of MS in 15% of cases, and which occurs at some time in 50% of MS patients. The percentage of patients with an attack of optic neuritis and no prior attack that will go on to develop MS ranges from 17-87% depending on the series[30]. Symptoms: acute visual loss in one or both eyes with mild pain (often on eye movement).

Diplopia may be due to internuclear ophthalmoplegia **(INO)** from a plaque in the MLF. INO is an important sign because it rarely occurs in other conditions besides MS.

Motor findings: Extremity weakness (mono, para, or quadriparesis) and gait ataxia are among the most common symptoms of MS. Spasticity of the LEs is often due to pyramidal tract involvement. Scanning speech results from cerebellar lesions.

Sensory findings: Posterior column involvement often causes loss of proprioception. Paresthesias of extremities, trunk, or face occur. Lhermitte's sign (electric shock-like pain radiating down the spine on neck flexion) is common, but is not pathognomonic. Trigeminal neuralgia occurs in ≈ 2%, and is more often bilateral and occurs at a younger age than the population in general[31].

Mental disturbances:
Euphoria (la belle indifference) and depression occur in ≈ 50% of patients.

Reflex changes: Hyperreflexia and Babinski signs are common. Abdominal cutaneous reflexes disappear in 70-80%.

GU symptoms: Urinary frequency, urgency, and incontinence are common. Impotence in males and reduced libido in either sex is often seen.

DIAGNOSTIC CRITERIA

No single clinical feature or diagnostic test is adequate for the accurate diagnosis of MS. Therefore, clinical information is integrated with additional data. Diagnosing MS after a single, acute remitting clinically isolated syndrome **(CIS)** is very risky. 50-70% of patients with a CIS suggestive of MS will have multifocal MRI abnormalities characteristic of MS. The presence of these MRI abnormalities increases the risk of developing MS in 1-3 years (with greater prognostic significance than CSF-OCB). The more MRI lesions, the higher the risk[32]. Criteria for the diagnosis of MS[33] follows.

The terms "clinically definite MS" and "clinically probable MS" are no longer recommended. Preferred terms: MS, possible MS (at risk for MS but diagnosis is equivocal), or not MS[33].

Table 2-3 Diagnostic criteria for MS

Clinical presentation	Additional data needed to diagnose MS
≥ 2 attacks; objective clinical evidence of ≥ 2 lesions	none*
≥ 2 attacks; objective clinical evidence of 1 lesion	demonstrate dissemination in *space* by: • MRI† or • ≥ 2 MS-compatible lesions on MRI PLUS positive CSF‡ or • await additional clinical attack implicating another site
1 attack; objective clinical evidence of ≥ 2 lesions	demonstrate dissemination in *time* by • MRI§ or • second clinical attack
1 attack; objective clinical evidence of 1 lesion (monsymptomatic presentation; clinically isolated syndrome)	demonstrate dissemination in *space* by: • MRI† or • ≥ 2 MS-compatible lesions on MRI PLUS positive CSF‡ or and demonstrate dissemination in *time* by: • MRI§ or • second clinical attack
insidious neurological progression suggestive of MS	positive CSF‡ and demonstrate dissemination in *space* by A. ≥ 9 T2WI lesions on MRI or B. ≥ 2 lesions in spinal cord or C. 4-8 brain + 1 spinal cord lesion or D. abnormal VEPΔ + (4-8 brain lesions or< 4 brain lesions + 1 spinal cord lesion on MRI) and demonstrate dissemination in *time* by A. MRI§ or B. continued progression for 1 year

*	additional tests not required. If MRI or CSF tests are done and are negative, apply extreme caution in diagnosing MS
†	must meet criteria in *Table 2-4*
‡	positive CSF showing oligoclonal bands, see *Table 2-6*
§	dissemination in *time* on MRI must meet the criteria in *Table 2-5*
Δ	abnormal visual evoked potential as seen in MS (delay with well-preserved wave-form)

Diagnostic criteria are shown in *Table 2-3*[33].

Definitions[33]

1. attack (exacerbation, relapse): neurologic disturbance lasting > 24 hrs[34] typical of MS when clinicopathological studies determine that the cause is demyelinating or inflammatory lesions
2. typical of MS: signs & symptoms **(S/S)** known to occur frequently in MS. Thus excludes gray matter lesions, peripheral nervous system lesions, non-specific complaints such as H/A, depression, convulsive seizures, etc.
3. separate lesions: S/S cannot be explained on basis of single lesion (optic neuritis of both eyes simultaneously or within 15 days represents single lesion)

MRI

MRI is the preferred imaging study in evaluating MS[35] and can demonstrate dissemination of lesions in time and space. Recommended[33] brain MRI criteria for diagnosing MS are shown in *Table 2-4*[36, 37]. Lesions are normally > 3 mm diameter[33]. MRI shows multiple white matter abnormalities in 80% of patients with MS (compared to 29% for CT)[38, 39]. Lesions are high signal on T2WI, and acute lesions tend to enhance with gadolinium more than old lesions do. Periventricular lesions may blend in with the signal from CSF in the ventricles on T2WI, these lesions are shown to better advantage on proton density images as higher intensity than CSF. Spinal cord lesions normally show little or no swelling, should be ≥ 3 mm but < 2 vertebral segments, occupy on a portion of the cross-section of the cord, and must be hyperintense on T2WI[40]. Specificity of MRI is ≈ 94%[41], however, encephalitis as well as UBOs seen in aging may mimic MS lesions.

Focal **tumefactive demyelinating lesions (TDL)** may occur in isolation or, more commonly, in patients with established MS. TDL may represent an intermediate position between MS and ADEM[42]. TDLs may enhance, and show perilesional edema and thus be mistaken for neoplasms. Biopsy results may be confusing. MRS may not be able to differentiate from neoplasm[43].

CSF

CSF analysis can support the diagnosis in some cases, but cannot document dissemination of lesions in time or space. The CSF in MS is clear and colorless. The OP is normal. Total CSF protein is < 55 mg/dl in ≈ 75% of patients, and < 108 mg/dl in 99.7% (values near 100 should prompt a search for an alternative diagnosis). The WBC count is ≤ 5 cells/µl in 70% of patients, and only 1% have a count > 20 cells/µl (high values may be seen in the acute myelitis).

In ≈ 90% of patients with MS, CSF-IgG is increased relative to other CSF proteins, and a characteristic pattern occurs. Agarose gel electrophoresis shows a few IgG bands in the gamma region (**oligoclonal bands (OCB)**) that are not present in the serum. CSF-OCB are not specific for MS, and can occur in CNS infections and less commonly with CVAs or tumors. The pre-

Table 2-4 Brain MRI criteria for MS

3 of the following 4 criteria*
1. 1 gadolinium-enhancing lesion or, if no gadolinium enhancing lesions, then 9 T2WI lesions
2. ≥ 1 infratentorial lesion
3. ≥ 1 juxtacortical lesion (i.e. involving subcortical u fibers)
4. ≥ 3 periventricular lesions

* 1 spinal cord lesion canbe substituted for 1 brain lesion

Table 2-5 MRI criteria for dissemination of lesions in time

1. if first MRI occurs ≥ 3 months after the onset of the clinical event, then a gadolinium enhancing lesion in a different location than that implicated by the event meets the criteria. If there is no enhancing lselon, a follow-up MRI is required*. A new enhancing or T2WI lesion meets the criteria
2. if first MRI is < 3 months from onset, a second MRI ≥ 3 months from onset showing a new gadolinium enhancing lesion meets the criteria. If no enhancing lesion, a 3rd MRI ≥ 3 months from the first showing a new enhancing or T2WI lesion meets the criteria

* timing not critical, but 3 months is recommended[44]

Table 2-6 CSF criteria for MS

1. qualitative assessment of IgG is the most informative analysis
2. analysis should be performed on unconcentrated CSF and must be compared to simultaneously run serum sample in the same assay
3. quantitative analysis should be made in terms of one of the 5 recognized staining patterns for OCB
4. all other tests performed on the CSF (including WBC, protein & glucose, lactate) should be taken into consideration
5. if clinical suspicion is high but CSF results are equivocal, negative or show only a single band, consider repeating the LP
6. quantitative IgG is a complementary test, but is not a substitute for qualitative IgG testing

dictive value of the absence of IgG in a patient with suspected MS has not been satisfactorily elucidated.

Recommended criteria have been published[45], most of which pertain to specifics of laboratory analysis, pertinent clinical excerpts are shown in *Table 2-6*.

2.5.   Amyotrophic lateral sclerosis

❦ Key features
- a mixed upper and lower motor neuron disease (UMN → mild spasticity in LEs; LMN → atrophy and fasciculations in UEs)
- no cognitive, sensory, nor autonomic dysfunction
- caused by degeneration of neurons in the cervical spine and medulla (bulb)

In the U.S. amyotrophic lateral sclerosis (**ALS**) is AKA Lou Gehrig's disease.

EPIDEMIOLOGY[30]
Prevalence: 4-6/100,000. Incidence: 0.8-1.2/100,000.

Familial in 8-10% of cases. Familial cases usually follow autosomal dominant inheritance, but occasionally demonstrate a recessive pattern.

Onset usually after 40 years of age.

PATHOLOGY
Degeneration of anterior horn alpha-motoneurons (in the spinal cord <u>and</u> in brain stem motor nuclei) and corticospinal tracts (hence AKA motor neuron disease). This produces a mixed upper and lower motor neuron disease, with a great deal of variability depending on which predominates at any given time.

The etiology of ALS is still not known with certainty.

CLINICAL
Involvement is of voluntary muscles, sparing the voluntary eye muscles and urinary sphincter.

Classically, presents initially with weakness and atrophy of the hands (lower motor neuron) with spasticity and hyperreflexia of the lower extremities (upper motor neuron). However, LEs may be hyporeflexic if the lower motor neuron deficits predominate.

Dysarthria and dysphagia are caused by a combination of upper and lower motor neuron pathology. Tongue atrophy and fasciculations may occur.

Although cognitive deficits are generally considered to be absent in ALS, in actuality 1-2% of cases are associated with dementia, and cognitive changes may occasionally predate the usual features of ALS[46].

DIFFERENTIAL DIAGNOSIS
It is important for the neurosurgeon to be able to distinguish ALS from cervical spondylotic myelopathy. See *page 333* for a discussion of differentiating features.

DIAGNOSTIC STUDIES
EMG: Not absolutely necessary to make diagnosis in most cases. Fibrillations and positive sharp waves are found in advanced cases (may be absent early, especially if upper motor neuron pathology predominates). LMN findings in the LE in the absence of lumbar spine disease, or fibrillation potentials in the tongue are suggestive of ALS.

LP (CSF): May have slightly elevated protein.

TREATMENT
Ongoing trials with riluzole (Rilutek®), which inhibits the presynaptic release of glutamate, indicate that doses of 50-200 mg/d increases tracheostomy-free survival at 9 & 12 months, but the improvement is more modest or may be non-existent by ≈ 18 months[47-49]. At the time of this writing, the drug is available only for premarketing trials, and cannot be procured commercially.

Much of care is directed towards minimizing disability:
1. aspiration may be treated with

A. tracheostomy
B. gastrostomy tube to allow continued feeding
C. vocal cord injection with Teflon
2. spasticity that occurs when upper motor neuron deficits predominate may be treated (usually with short-lived response) with:
A. baclofen: also may relieve the commonly occurring cramps (*see page 368*)
B. diazepam

PROGNOSIS
Most patients die within 5 years of onset (median survival: 3-4 yrs). Those with prominent oropharyngeal symptoms may have a shorter life-span usually due to complications of aspiration.

2.6. Guillain-Barré syndrome

❢ Key features
- acute onset of peripheral neuropathy with progressive muscle weakness (more severe proximally) with areflexia, reaches maximum over 3 days to 3 weeks
- cranial neuropathy: also common, may include facial diplegia, ophthalmoplegia
- little or no sensory involvement (paresthesias are not uncommon)
- onset often 3 days-5 weeks following viral URI, immunization, or surgery
- pathology: focal segmental demyelination with endoneurial monocytic infiltrate
- elevated CSF protein without pleocytosis (albuminocytologic dissociation)

AKA acute idiopathic polyradiculoneuritis. The most common acquired demyelinating neuropathy. Incidence is ≈ 1/100,000. The lifetime risk for any one individual getting Guillain-Barré syndrome (GBS) is ≈ 1/1,000.

Mild cases of GBS may present only with ataxia, whereas fulminant cases may ascend to paralyze respiratory muscles and cranial nerves.

Frequent (but not essential) preceding events: viral infection, surgery, immunization, mycoplasma infection. May follow infection with *Campylobacter jejuni* (≈ 4 days of intense diarrhea). Higher frequency in the following conditions than in general population: Hodgkin's disease, lymphoma, lupus.

The actual cause is not known. May be due to antibodies to peripheral myelin.

DIAGNOSTIC CRITERIA[50]
1. features required for diagnosis:
   A. progressive motor weakness of more than 1 limb (from minimal weakness ± ataxia to paralysis, may include bulbar or facial or EOM palsy). Unlike most neuropathies, proximal muscles are affected more than distal
   B. areflexia (usually universal, but distal areflexia with definite hyporeflexia of biceps and knee jerks suffices if other features consistent)
2. features strongly supportive of diagnosis:
   A. clinical features (in order of importance)
      1. progression: motor weakness peaks at 2 wks in 50%, by 3 wks in 80%, and by 4 wks in > 90%
      2. relative symmetry
      3. mild sensory symptoms/signs (e.g. mild paresthesias in hands or feet)
      4. cranial nerve involvement: facial weakness in 50%, usually bilateral. GBS presents initially in EOMs or other Cr. N. in < 5% of cases. Oropharyngeal muscles may be affected
      5. recovery usually by 2-4 wks after progression stops, may be delayed by months (most patients recover functionally)
      6. autonomic dysfunction (may fluctuate): tachycardia and other arrhythmias, postural hypotension, HTN, vasomotor symptoms
      7. afebrile at onset of neuritic symptoms
      8. variants (not ranked):
         a. fever at onset of neuritic symptoms
         b. severe sensory loss with pain
         c. progression > 4 wks
         d. cessation of progression without recovery
         e. sphincter dysfunction (usually spared): e.g. bladder paralysis

      f.   CNS involvement (controversial): e.g. ataxia, dysarthria, Babin-
         ski signs
  B. CSF findings: **albuminocytologic dissociation** (elevated CSF protein
     without pleocytosis)
     1.   protein: elevated after 1 wk of symptoms, > 55 mg/dl
     2.   cells: 10 or fewer mononuclear leukocytes/ml
     3.   variants
         a.   no CSF protein rise 1-10 wks after onset (rare)
         b.   11-50 monocytes/ml
         c.   electrodiagnostics: 80% have NCV slowing or block at some time
            (may take several weeks in some). NCV usually < 60% of nor-
            mal, but not in all nerves
3. features casting doubt on diagnosis:
  A. marked, persistent, asymmetry of weakness
  B. persistent bowel or bladder dysfunction
  C. > 50 monocytes/ml CSF
  D. PMNs in CSF
  E. sharp sensory level
4. features that rule out diagnosis (findings that suggest the presence of one of the
    conditions in the differential diagnosis, e.g. see *Myelopathy*, page 902):
  A. current hexacarbon use: volatile solvents (n-hexane, methyl n-butyl ke-
     tone), glue sniffing
  B. **acute intermittent porphyria (AIP)**: a disorder of porphyrin metabo-
     lism. CSF protein is not elevated in AIP. Recurrent painful abdominal cri-
     ses are common. Check urine delta-aminolevulinic acid or porphobilinogen
  C. recent diphtheritic infection: diphtheritic polyneuropathy has a longer la-
     tency and a slower crescendo of symptoms
  D. lead neuropathy: UE weakness with wrist drop. May be asymmetrical
  E. purely sensory syndrome
  F. poliomyelitis: usually asymmetric, has meningeal irritation
  G. hypophosphatemia (may occur in chronic IV hyperalimentation)
  H. botulism: difficult to distinguish clinically from GBS. Normal NCV and a fa-
     cilitating response to repetitive nerve stimulation on electrodiagnostics
  I. toxic neuropathy (e.g. from nitrofurantoin, dapsone, thallium or arsenic)
  J. tick paralysis: may cause an ascending motor neuropathy without sensory
     impairment. Careful examination of the scalp for tick(s)
  K. long time course: may indicate **chronic immune demyelinating polyra-
     diculoneuropathy (CIDP)** AKA chronic relapsing GBS, chronic relapsing
     polyneuritis[51]. Similar to GBS, however symptoms must be present > 2 mos.
     CIDP produces progressive, symmetrical, proximal & distal weakness, de-
     pression of muscle stretch reflexes, and variable sensory loss. Cranial
     nerves are usually spared (facial muscles may be involved). Balance diffi-
     culties are common. Need for respiratory support is rare. Peak incidence:
     age 40-60 yrs. Electrodiagnostics and nerve biopsy findings are indicative of
     demyelination. CSF findings are similar to GBS (*see above*). Most respond
     to immunosuppressive therapy (especially prednisolone & plasmapheresis)
     but relapses are common. Refractory cases may be treated with IV gamma-
     globulin, cyclosporin-A[52], total body lymphoid irradiation or interferon-α[53]

The Miller-Fisher variant of GBS includes ataxia, areflexia and ophthalmoplegia.

TREATMENT

    Immunoglobulins may be helpful. In severe cases, early plasmapheresis hastens the
recovery and reduces the residual deficit. Its role in mild cases is uncertain. Steroids are
not helpful[54]. Mechanical ventilation and measures to prevent aspiration are used as appropriate. In cases of facial diplegia, the eyes must be protected from exposure keratitis.

OUTCOME

    Recovery may not be complete for several months. 35% of untreated patients have
residual weakness and atrophy. Recurrence of GBS after achieving maximal recovery occurs in ≈ 2%.

2.7.   Myelitis

AKA acute transverse myelitis **(ATM)**. The terminology is confusing: myelitis overlaps with "myelopathy". Both are pathologic conditions of the spinal cord. Myelitis indicates inflammation, and includes infectious, post-infectious, autoimmune, and idiopathic. Myelopathy is generally reserved for compressive, toxic, or metabolic etiologies[55].

ETIOLOGY

Many so-called "causes" remain unproven. Immunologic response against the CNS (most likely via cell mediated component) is the probable common mechanism. Animal model: experimental allergic encephalomyelitis (requires myelin basic protein of CNS, not peripheral).

Generally accepted etiologies include:
1. infectious and post-infectious
   A. primary infectious myelitis
      1. viral: poliomyelitis, myelitis with viral encephalomyelitis, herpes zoster, rabies
      2. bacterial: including tuberculoma of spinal cord
      3. spirochetal: AKA syphilitic myelitis. Causes syphilitic endarteritis
      4. fungal (aspergillosis, blastomycosis, cryptococcosis)
      5. parasitic (Echinococcus, cysticercosis, paragonimiasis, schistosomiasis)
   B. post-infectious: including post-exanthematous, influenza
2. post-traumatic
3. physical agents
   A. decompression sickness (dysbarism)
   B. electrical injury*
   C. post-irradiation
4. paraneoplastic syndrome (remote effect of cancer): most common primary is lung, but prostate, ovary and rectum have also been described[56]
5. metabolic
   A. diabetes mellitus*
   B. pernicious anemia*
   C. chronic liver disease*
6. toxins
   A. cresyl phosphates*
   B. intra-arterial contrast agents*
   C. spinal anesthetics
   D. myelographic contrast agents
   E. following chemonucleolysis[57]
7. arachnoiditis
8. autoimmune
   A. multiple sclerosis **(MS)**, especially Devic syndrome (*see page 904*)
   B. following vaccination (smallpox, rabies)
9. collagen vascular disease
   A. systemic lupus erythematosus
   B. mixed connective tissue disease

*   items with an asterisk may be more properly associated with myelopathy rather than myelitis

Table 2-7   Presenting symptoms in myelitis

Symptom	Series A*	Series B†
pain (back or radicular)	35%	35%
muscle weakness	32%	13%
sensory deficit or paresthesias	26%	46%
sphincter disturbance	12%	6%

*   series A: 34 patients with ATM[58]

†   series B: 52 patients with acute or subacute transverse myelitis[59]

CLINICAL

PRESENTATION

34 patients with ATM[58]: age of onset ranged 15-55 yrs, with 66% occurring in 3rd and 4th decade. 12 patients (35%) had a

viral-like prodrome. Presenting symptoms are shown in *Table 2-7*, with other presenting symptoms of unspecified frequency including[60]: fever and rash.

Presenting level
The levels at presentation in 62 patients with ATM are shown in *Table 2-8*[60]. The thoracic level is the most common sensory level. ATM is rarely the presenting symptom of MS (≈ 3-6% of patients with ATM develop MS).

Table 2-8 Level of sensory deficit

Level	%
cervical	8%
high thoracic	36%
low thoracic	32%
lumbar	8%
unknown	16%

PROGRESSION
Progression is usually rapid, with 66% reaching maximal deficit by 24 hrs, however the interval between first symptom and maximal deficit varies from 2 hrs-14 days[60]. Findings at the time of maximal deficit are shown in *Table 2-9*.

EVALUATION
Myelogram, CT & MRI: no characteristic finding. One paper reports 2 patients with fusiform cord enlargement[61]. High resolution MRI with thin cuts may be able to demonstrate area of involvement within the cord. Patient should have imaging to R/O compressive lesion.
CSF: normal during acute phase in 38% of LPs. Remainder (62%) had elevated protein (usually > 40 mg%) or pleocytosis (lymphocytes, PMNs, or both) or both.

Table 2-9 Symptoms at time of maximal deficit
(62 patients with ATM[60])

Symptom	%
sensory deficit or paresthesias	100%
muscle weakness	97%
sphincter disturbance (hesitancy, retention, overflow incontinence)	94%
pain in back, abdomen, or limbs	34%
fever	27%
nuchal rigidity	13%

EVALUATION SCHEME
In a patient developing acute myelopathy/paraplegia, especially when ATM is considered likely, the first test of choice is an emergency MRI. If not readily available, a myelogram (with CT to follow) directed at the region of the sensory level is performed (CSF may be sent in this circumstance once block is ruled out).

TREATMENT
Suggested efficacy of high-dose steroid treatment in 1 patient with ATM[62] (methylprednisolone 250 mg IV q 6 hrs **x** 24 hrs, 125 mg IV q 6 hrs **x** 24 hrs, 125 mg IV q 12 hrs **x** 48 hrs, then 30 mg PO q 6 hrs, tapered gradually). Regimen should probably be individualized based on response).

PROGNOSIS
In a series of 34 ATM patients with ≥ 5 yrs follow-up **(F/U)**[58]: 9 patients (26%) had good recovery (ambulate well, mild urinary symptoms, minimal sensory and UMN signs); 9 (26%) had fair recovery (functional gait with some degree of spasticity, urinary urgency, obvious sensory signs, paraparesis); 11 (32%) poor (paraplegic, absent sphincter control); 5 (15%) died within 4 mos of illness. 18 patients (62% of survivors) became ambulatory (in these cases, all could walk with support by 3-6 mos).
In a series of 59 patients[60] (F/U period unspecified): 22 (37%) had good recovery; 14 (24%) poor; 3 died in acute stage (respiratory insufficiency in 2, sepsis in 1). Recovery occurred between 4 weeks and 3 mos after onset (no improvement occurred after 3 mos).

2.8.   Neurosarcoidosis

Sarcoidosis is a granulomatous disease that is usually systemic, and may include the CNS (so-called **neurosarcoidosis**). Only 3% of cases have CNS findings without systemic manifestations[63]. The cause of the disease is unknown. An infectious agent is possible. Organs commonly involved include lungs, skin, lymph nodes, bones, eyes, muscles, and parotid glands[30].

PATHOLOGY

CNS sarcoidosis primarily involves the leptomeninges, however parenchymal invasion often occurs. Adhesive arachnoiditis with nodule formation may also occur (nodules have a predilection for the posterior fossa). Diffuse meningitis or meningoencephalitis may occur, and may be most pronounced at the base of the brain (basal meningitis) and in the subependymal region of the third ventricle (including the hypothalamus).

Constant microscopic features of neurosarcoidosis include noncaseating granulomas with lymphocytic infiltrates. Langhans giant cells may or may not be present.

EPIDEMIOLOGY

Incidence of sarcoidosis is ≈ 3-50 cases/100,000 population; neurosarcoidosis occurs in ≈ 5% of cases (reported range: 1-27%). In one series, the median age of onset of neurologic symptoms was 44 years.

CLINICAL FINDINGS

Clinical findings include multiple cranial nerve palsies, peripheral neuropathy, and myopathy[64]. Occasionally the lesions may produce mass effect[65], and hydrocephalus may result from adhesive basal arachnoiditis. Patients may have low grade fever. Intracranial hypertension is common and may be dangerous.

Hypothalamic involvement may produce disorders of ADH (diabetes insipidus, disordered thirst).

LABORATORY

CBC: mild leukocytosis and eosinophilia may occur.

Serum angiotensin-converting enzyme (ACE): abnormally elevated in 83% of patients with active pulmonary sarcoidosis, but in only 11% with inactive disease[66]. False positive rate: 2-3%; may also be elevated in primary biliary cirrhosis.

CSF: similar to any subacute meningitis: elevated pressure, mild pleocytosis (10-200 cells/mm³) mostly lymphocytes, elevated protein (up to 2,000 mg/dl), mild hypoglycorrhachia (15-40 mg/dl), CSF ACE is elevated in ≈ 55% of cases with neurosarcoidosis (normal in patients with sarcoidosis not involving the CNS)[67]. No organisms are recovered on culture or gram stain.

DIAGNOSIS

Differentiating granulomatous angiitis (GA) from neurosarcoidosis that involves only the CNS can be done on histologic criteria: the inflammatory reaction in sarcoidosis is not limited to the region immediately surrounding blood vessels as it is in GA, where extensive disruption of the vessel wall may occur.

Making the diagnosis is relatively easy when systemic involvement occurs: characteristic findings on CXR, biopsy of skin or liver nodules, muscle biopsy, serum ACE assay.

Isolated neurosarcoidosis may be more difficult to diagnose, and may require biopsy (*see below*).

Table 2-10 Differential diagnosis of neurosarcoidosis

1. Hodgkin's disease
2. chronic granulomatous meningitis:
A. Hansen's disease (leprosy)
B. syphilis
C. cryptococcosis
D. tuberculosis
3. multiple sclerosis
4. CNS lymphoma
5. pseudotumor cerebri
6. granulomatous angiitis

BIOPSY

In uncertain cases, biopsy may be indicated. Whenever possible, MRI should be used to localize a supratentorial region of involvement, and biopsy should include all layers of meninges and cerebral cortex. Cultures and stains for fungus and acid-fast bacteria (TB) should be performed in addition to microscopic examination.

TREATMENT

Antibiotics have not been proven to be of benefit. Steroids are beneficial for systemic as well as neurologic involvement. Therapy with cyclosporine may allow a reduction in steroid dosage in refractory cases[68]. Other less well studied treatments: methotrexate, cytoxan. CSF shunting is indicated if hydrocephalus develops.

PROGNOSIS

Usually a benign disease. Peripheral and cranial nerve palsies recover slowly.

2.9. Vasculitis and vasculopathy

The vasculitides are a group of disorders characterized by inflammation and necrosis of blood vessels. Vasculitis may be primary or secondary. Those that may affect the CNS are listed in *Table 2-11*, all of these cause tissue ischemia (even after the inflammation is quiescent) that may range in effect from neuropraxia to infarction.

Table 2-11   Vasculitides that may affect the CNS[73]

Vasculitis	Frequency of neuro involvement	—TYPE OF CNS INVOLVEMENT*—				
		Acute encephalopathy	Seizure	Cranial nerve	Spinal cord	ICH or SAH
periarteritis nodosa† (PAN)‡	20-40%	++	++	+	+	+
hypersensitivity vasculitis†	10%	+	+	0	0	+
giant cell (temporal) arteritis†	10%	+	0	++	0	0
Takayasu's arteritis	10-36%	+	++	++	+	+
Wegener's granulomatosis†	23-50%	+	++	++	+	+
lymphomatoid granulomatosis†	20-30%	++	+	++	+	0
isolated angiitis of the CNS†	100%	++	+	++	++	+
Behçet's disease†	10-29%	++	+	++	+	+

*   KEY: 0 = uncommon or unreported; + = not uncommon; ++ = common; ICH = intracerebral hemorrhage; SAH = subarachnoid hemorrhage
†   see section that follows for these topics
‡   PAN: a group of disorders, frequencies may vary by subgroup

---

2.9.1.   Giant cell arteritis (GCA)

⁊ Key features
  • formerly often referred to as temporal arteritis
  • a chronic vasculitis of large and medium caliber vessels, primarily involving cranial branches of the arteries arising from the aortic arch
  • age > 50 years; affects women twice as often as men
  • important possible late complications: blindness, stroke, thoracic aortic aneurysms and aortic dissections
  • temporal artery biopsy is recommended for all patients suspected of GCA
  • corticosteroids are the drug of choice for treatment

AKA **temporal arteritis (TA)**, AKA cranial arteritis. A chronic granulomatous arteritis of unknown etiology involving primarily the cranial branches of the aortic arch (especially the external carotid artery **(ECA)**)[74], which if untreated, may lead to blindness. Takayasu's arteritis is similar to GCA, but tends to affect large arteries in young women.

EPIDEMIOLOGY

Seen almost exclusively in Caucasians > 50 yrs age (mean age of onset is 70). Incidence: 17.8 per 100,000 people ≥ 50 years old[75] (range: 0.49-23). Prevalence: ≈ 223 (autopsy incidence may be much higher)[76]. More common in northern latitudes and among individuals of Scandinavian descent[74]. Female:male ratio is ≈ 2:1 (reported range: 1.05-7.4:1). 50% of GCA patients also have polymyalgia rheumatica (**PMR**) (*see page 61*).

PATHOLOGY

Discontinuous (so-called "skip lesions") inflammatory reaction of lymphocytes, plasma cells, macrophages, ± giant cells (if absent, intimal proliferation may be prominent); predominantly in media of involved arteries. Arteries preferentially involved include the ophthalmic and posterior ciliary branches and the entire distribution of the external carotid system (of which the STA is a terminal branch). Other arteries in the body may be involved (reported involvement of abdominal aorta, femoral, brachial and mesenteric arteries are rarely symptomatic). Unlike PAN, GCA generally spares the renal arteries.

CLINICAL

Various combinations of symptoms of giant cell arteritis are listed in *Table 2-12*. Onset is usually insidious, although occasionally it may be abrupt[78].

Details of some findings:
1. H/A: the most common presenting symptom. May be nonspecific or located in one or both temporal areas, forehead, or occiput. May be superficial or burning with paroxysmal lancinating pain

Table 2-12 Signs and symptoms of GCA[74, 77]

Frequent (> 50% of cases)	Occasional (10-50% of cases)	Rare (< 10% of cases)
H/A: 66% temporal artery tenderness	visual symptoms weight loss fever (low grade) proximal myalgias jaw claudication facial pain scalp tenderness	blindness extremity claudication tongue claudication ear pain synovitis stroke angina

2. symptoms relating to ECA blood supply (strongly suggestive of GCA, but not pathognomonic[79]): jaw claudication, tongue, or pharyngeal muscles
3. ophthalmologic symptoms: due to arteritis and occlusion of branches of ophthalmic artery or posterior ciliary arteries
   A. symptoms include: amaurosis fugax (precedes permanent visual loss in 44%), blindness, visual field cuts, diplopia, ptosis, ocular pain, corneal edema, chemosis
   B. blindness: incidence is ≈ 7%, and once it occurs, recovery of sight is unlikely
4. systemic symptoms
   A. nonspecific constitutional symptoms: fever (may present as FUO in 15% of cases), anorexia, weight loss, fatigue, malaise
   B. 30% have neurologic manifestations. 14% are neuropathies including mononeuropathies and peripheral polyneuropathies of the arms or legs[80]
   C. musculoskeletal symptoms
      1. PMR is the most common (occurs in 40% of patients): *see page 61*
      2. peripheral arthritis, swelling & pitting edema of hands & feet in 25%
      3. arm claudication from stenosis of subclavian and axillary arteries
   D. thoracic aortic aneurysms: 17 times as likely in GCA. Annual CXRs are adequate for screening
5. temporal arteries on physical examination may exhibit tenderness, swelling, erythema, reduced pulsations, or nodularity. Normal in 33%
6. the presence of systemic symptoms correlates with a <u>lower</u> incidence of blindness or stroke

Differential diagnosis:
1. periarteritis nodosa (PAN): *see page 61*
2. hypersensitivity vasculitis
3. atherosclerotic occlusive disease
4. malignancy: symptoms of low grade fever, malaise and weight loss
5. infection
6. trigeminal neuralgia: *see page 378*
7. ophthalmoplegic migraine
8. dental problems

EVALUATION

Laboratory studies

1. ESR > 40 mm/hr (usually > 50) by Westergren method (if > 80 mm/hr with above clinical syndromes, highly suggestive of GCA). ESR is normal in up to 22.5%[81]
2. C-reactive protein: another acute phase reactant that is more sensitive than ESR. Has the advantage that it can be performed on frozen sera
3. CBC: may show mild normochromic anemia[82]
4. rheumatoid factor, ANA, and serum complement usually normal
5. LFTs abnormal in 30% (usually elevated alkaline phosphatase)
6. tests for rheumatoid factor and ANA are usually negative
7. temporal artery angiography not helpful (angiography elsewhere indicated if suspicion of large artery involvement exists)
8. CT: usually not helpful, one report described calcified areas corresponding to the temporal arteries[83]
9. temporal artery biopsy: *see below*

TEMPORAL ARTERY BIOPSY

Sensitivity and specificity are shown in *Table 2-13*.

Indications and timing

Current recommendations: temporal artery biopsy in all patients suspected of having GCA[74].

Preferably, biopsy should be done before treatment is initiated[74]. However, pathologic changes be seen after more than 2 weeks of therapy[85], therefore do not withhold steroids to await biopsy.

Table 2-13 Temporal artery biopsy

sensitivity	≈ 90% (reported range[77, 84] is 9-97%)
specificity	near 100%
predictive value	≈ 94%

Technique of temporal artery biopsy

Biopsy of the contralateral side if the first side is negative in cases where clinical suspicion is high increases the yield by 5-10%.

TREATMENT

No known cure. Steroids can produce symptomatic relief and usually prevent blindness (progression of ocular problems 24-48 hrs after institution of adequate steroids is rare). Totally blind patients or those with longstanding partial visual loss are unlikely to respond to any treatment.
1. for most cases:
   A. start with <u>prednisone</u>, 40-60 mg/d PO divided BID-QID (qod dosing is usually not effective in initial management)
   B. if no response after 72 hrs, and diagnosis certain, ↑ to 10-25 mg QID
   C. once response occurs (usually within 3-7 days), give entire dose as q AM dose for 3-6 weeks until symptoms resolved and ESR normalizes (occurs in 87% of patients within ≈ 4 weeks) or stabilizes at < 40-50 mm/hr
   D. once quiescent, a gradual taper is performed to prevent exacerbations: reduce by 10 mg/d q 2-4 weeks to 40 mg/d, then by 5 mg/d q 2-4 wks to 20 mg/d, then 2.5 mg/d q 2-4 wks to 5-7.5 mg/d which is maintained for several months, followed by 1 mg/d decrements q 1-3 mos (usual length of treatment is 6-24 mos; do <u>not</u> D/C steroids when ESR normalizes)
   E. if symptoms recur during treatment, prednisone dose is temporarily increased until symptoms resolve (isolated rise in ESR is not sufficient reason to increase steroids[74])
   F. patients should be followed closely for ≈ 2 years
2. in severely ill patients: methylprednisolone, 15-20 mg IV QID
3. anticoagulant therapy: controversial
4. acute blindness (onset within 24-36 hrs) in a patient with giant cell arteritis:
   A. consider up to 500 mg methylprednisolone IV over 30-60 mins (no controlled studies show reversal of blindness)
   B. some have used intermittent inhalation of 5% carbon dioxide and oxygen

OUTCOME

Complications of steroid therapy occur in ≈ 50% of patients (most are not life threatening, and include vertebral compression fractures in ≈ 36%, peptic ulcer disease in

~ 12%, proximal myopathy, cataracts, exacerbation of diabetes; also see *Possible deleterious side effects of steroids*, page 10).

30-50% of patients will have spontaneous exacerbations of GCA (especially during the first 2 years) regardless of the corticosteroid regimen[74].

Survival parallels that of the general population. Onset of blindness after initiation of steroid therapy is rare.

2.9.2. Polymyalgia rheumatica

Polymyalgia rheumatica **(PMR)** and giant cell arteritis **(GCA)** *(see page 58)* may be different points on a continuum of the same disease.

Epidemiology[74]

Both GCA & PMR occur in people ≥ 50 years old. The incidence increases with age and peaks between 70-80 years and is higher at higher latitudes[74].

Polymyalgia rheumatica (PMR)[74]
• an inflammatory condition of unknown etiology
• clinical characteristics
   A. aching and morning stiffness in the cervical region and shoulder & pelvic girdles lasting > 1 month. The pain usually increases with movement
      1. shoulder pain: present in 70-95% of patients. Radiates toward elbow
      2. hip & neck pain: 50-70%. Hip pain radiates towards knees
   B. age ≥ 50 years
   C. ESR ≥ 40 mm/hr (7-20% have normal ESR[86])
   D. usually responds rapidly to low dose corticosteroids (≤ 20 mg prednisone/day) *see below*
   E. systemic symptoms (present in ~ 33%): fever, malaise or fatigue, anorexia and weight loss
• prevalence: more common than GCA
   A. 500/100,000)[87]
   B. 1 case per 133 people ≥ age 50[88]
• favorable prognosis

Treatment

PMR responds to either to low doses of steroids[87] (10-20 mg prednisone/day) or sometimes to NSAIDs (response to steroids is much more rapid). The initial dose of steroids is maintained for 2-4 weeks, and then by ≤ 10% of the daily dose every 1-2 weeks[74] while observing for signs of GCA.

2.9.3. Other vasculitides

PERIARTERITIS NODOSA

AKA polyarteritis nodosa. Actually a group of necrotizing vasculitides, including:
• classic periarteritis nodosa **(PAN)**: a multisystem disease with inflammatory necrosis, thrombosis (occlusion), and hemorrhage of arteries and arterioles in every organ except lung & spleen. Nodules may be palpated along medium sized muscular arteries. Commonly produces mononeuritis multiplex, weight loss, fever, and tachycardia. Peripheral nerve manifestations are attributed to arteritic occlusion of vasa nervorum. CNS manifestations are uncommon and include H/A, seizures, SAH, retinal hemorrhages, and CVA in ~ 13%
• allergic angiitis and granulomatosis (Churg-Strauss syndrome)
• systemic necrotizing vasculitis

These patients do better when treated with cyclophosphamide rather than steroids.

WEGENER'S GRANULOMATOSIS

A systemic necrotizing granulomatous vasculitis involving the respiratory tract (lung → cough/hemoptysis, and/or nasal airways → serosanguinous nasal drainage ± septal perforation → characteristic "saddle nose deformity") and frequently the kidneys (no reported cases of kidney involvement without respiratory)[89].

Nasal obstruction and crusting are the usual initial findings. Arthralgia (not true arthritis) is present in > 50%.

Neurologic involvement usually consists of cranial nerve dysfunction (usually II, III, IV, & VI; less often V, VII, & VIII; and least commonly IX, X, XI, & XII) and peripheral neuropathies, with diabetes insipidus (occasionally preceding other symptoms by up to 9 months). Focal lesions of the brain and spinal cord occur less frequently.

Differential diagnosis includes:

* **"lethal midline granuloma"** (may be similar or identical to polymorphic reticulosis) may evolve into lymphoma. May cause fulminant local destruction of the nasal tissue. Differentiation is crucial as this condition is treated by radiation; one should avoid immune suppression (e.g. cyclophosphamide). Probably does not involve true granulomas. Renal and tracheal involvement do not occur
* fungal disease: *Sporothrix schenckii* & Coccidioides may cause identical syndrome
* other vasculitides: especially Churg-Strauss syndrome (asthma and peripheral eosinophilia usually seen), and PAN (granulomas usually lacking)

LYMPHOMATOID GRANULOMATOSIS
Rare; affects mainly the lungs, skin (erythematous macules or indurated placques in 40%) and nervous system (CNS in 20%, peripheral neuropathies in 15%). Sinuses, lymph nodes, and spleen are usually spared.

BEHÇET'S SYNDROME
Relapsing ocular lesions and recurrent oral and genital ulcers, with occasional skin lesions, thrombophlebitis, and arthritis [73]. H/A occur in > 50%. Neurologic involvement includes pseudotumor, cerebellar ataxia, paraplegia, seizures, and dural sinus thrombosis. Only 5% have neurologic symptoms as the presenting complaint.

86% have CSF pleocytosis and protein elevation. Cerebral angiography is usually normal. CT may show focal areas of enhancing low density.

Steroids usually ameliorate ocular and cerebral symptoms, but usually have no effect on skin and genital lesions. Uncontrolled trials of cytotoxic agents → some benefit. Thalidomide may be effective (uncontrolled studies), but carries risk of serious adverse effects (teratogenicity, peripheral neuropathy…)[90].

Although painful, the disease is usually benign. Neurologic involvement portends a worse prognosis.

ISOLATED CNS VASCULITIS
AKA **isolated angiitis of the CNS**. Rare (≈ 20 cases reported[91] as of 1983); limited to vessels of CNS. Small vessel vasculitis is ≈ always present → segmental inflammation and necrosis of small leptomeningeal and parenchymal blood vessels with surrounding tissue ischemia or hemorrhage[73].

PRESENTATION
Combinations of H/A, confusion, dementia, and lethargy. Occasionally seizures. Focal and multifocal brain disturbance occurs in > 80%. Visual symptoms are frequent (secondary either to involvement of choroidal and retinal arteries, or to involvement of visual cortex → visual hallucinations).

EVALUATION
ESR & WBC count are usually normal. CSF may be normal or have pleocytosis and/or elevated protein. CT may show enhancing areas of low density.

Angiography (required for diagnosis): characteristically shows multiple areas of symmetrical narrowing ("string of pearls" configuration). If normal, it does not exclude diagnosis.

Histological diagnosis (recommended): all biopsy material should be cultured. Brain parenchyma biopsy infrequently shows vasculitis. Leptomeningeal biopsy invariably shows involvement.

HYPERSENSITIVITY VASCULITIS
Neurologic involvement is not a prominent feature of this group of vasculitides, which include:
* drug induced allergic vasculitis
* cutaneous vasculitis
* serum sickness: may → encephalopathy, seizures, coma, peripheral neuropathy and brachial plexopathy
* Henoch-Schönlein purpura

DRUG INDUCED VASCULITIS
A number of drugs are associated with the development of cerebral vasculitis. These include methamphetamines ("speed"), cocaine (frank vasculitis occurs[92] but is rare), heroin and ephedrine.

2.9.4. Fibromuscular dysplasia

A vasculopathy (angiopathy) affecting primarily branches of the aorta, with renal artery involvement in 85% of cases (the most common site) and commonly associated with hypertension. The disease has an incidence of ≈ 1%, and results in multifocal arterial constrictions and intervening regions of aneurysmal dilatation.

The second most commonly involved site is the cervical internal carotid (primarily near C1-2), with fibromuscular dysplasia (**FMD**) appearing on 1% of carotid angiograms, making FMD the second most common cause of extracranial carotid stenosis[93]. Bilateral cervical ICA involvement occurs in ≈ 80% of cases. 50% of patients with carotid FMD have renal FMD. Patients with FMD have an increased risk of intracranial aneurysms and neoplasms, and are probably at higher risk of carotid dissection.

ETIOLOGY
The actual etiology remains unknown, although congenital defects of the media (muscular layer) and internal elastic layer of the arteries has been identified which may predispose the arteries to injury from otherwise well-tolerated trauma. A high familial rate of strokes, HTN, and migraine have supported the suggestion that FMD is an autosomal dominant trait with reduced penetrance in males[94].

ANEURYSMS AND FIBROMUSCULAR DYSPLASIA
The reported incidence of aneurysms with FMD[95] ranges from 20-50%.

PRESENTATION
Most patients have recurrent, multiple symptoms shown in *Table 2-14*.

Up to 50% of patients present with episodes of transient cerebral ischemia or infarction. However, FMD may also be an incidental finding and some cases have been followed for 5 years without recurrence of ischemic symptoms suggesting that FMD may be a relatively benign condition.

Headaches are commonly unilateral and may be mistaken for typical migraine. Syncope may be caused by involvement of the carotid sinus.

Horner's syndrome occurs in ≈ 8% of cases. T-wave changes on EKG may be seen in up to one third of cases, and may be due to involvement of the coronary arteries.

Table 2-14 Previous symptoms in 37 cases of aortocranial FMD[94]

Symptom	%
H/A	78%
mental distress	48%
tinnitus	38%
vertigo	34%
cardiac arrhythmia	31%
TIA	31%
syncope	31%
carotidynia	21%
epilepsy	15%
hearing impairment	12%
abdominal angina	8%
angina/MI	8%

DIAGNOSIS
The "gold-standard" for the diagnosis of FMD is the angiogram. The three angiographic types of FMD[96] are shown in *Table 2-15*.

TREATMENT
Medical therapy including antiplatelet medication (e.g. aspirin) has been recommended.

Direct surgical treatment is problem ridden due to the difficult location (high carotid artery, near the base of the skull), and the friable nature of the vessels making anastamosis or arteriotomy closure difficult.

Transluminal angioplasty has achieved some degree of success. Carotid cavernous fistulas and arterial rupture have been reported as complications.

Table 2-15   Angiographic classification of FMD

Type	Findings
1	most common (80-100% of reported cases). Multiple, irregularly spaced, concentric narrowings with normal or dilated intervening segments giving rise to the so-called **"string of pearls"** appearance. Corresponds with arterial medial fibroplasia
2	focal tubular stenosis, seen in ≈ 7% of cases. Less characteristic for FMD than Type 1, and may also be seen in Takayasu's arteritis and other conditions
3	"atypical FMD". Rare. May take on various appearances, most commonly consisting of diverticular outpouchings of one wall of the artery

2.9.5.   Miscellaneous vasculopathies

CADASIL
† Key features
  • clinical: migraines, dementia, TIAs, psychiatric disturbances
  • MRI: white matter abnormalities
  • autosomal dominant inheritance
  • anticoagulants controversial, generally discouraged

An acronym for Cerebral Autosomal Dominant Arteriopathy with Subcortical Infarcts and Leukoencephalopathy[97]. A familial disease with onset in early adulthood (mean age at onset: 45 ± 11 yrs), mapped to chromosome 19. Clinical and neuroradiologic features are similar to those seen with multiple subcortical infarcts from HTN, except there is no evidence of HTN. The vasculopathy is distinct from that seen in lipohyalinosis, arteriosclerosis and amyloid angiopathy, and causes thickening of the media of leptomeningeal and perforating arteries measuring 100-400 μm in diameter.

Clinical involvement: recurrent subcortical infarcts (84%), progressive or stepwise dementia (31%), migraine with aura (22%), and depression (20%). All symptomatic and 18% of asymptomatic patients had prominent subcortical white-matter and basal ganglia hyperintensities on T2WI MRI.

Treatment: Coumadin® is used by some.

2.10.   Vascular dysautoregulatory encephalopathy

This section encompasses a group of encephalopathies that may be related to disordered vascular autoregulation[69]. Etiologies and findings include:
1. those due to <u>subacute</u> blood pressure elevations: imaging studies show symmetric confluent lesions with mild mass effect and patchy enhancement primarily in the subcortical white matter of the <u>occipital lobes</u>[69] (possibly because of limited sympathetic innervation in the <u>posterior circulation</u>) which may produce cortical blindness
    A. hypertensive encephalopathy (as may occur with malignant hypertension)
    B. peripartum: associated with cerebral edema[70]. Often temporary, but (permanent) infarctions also occur
       1. may present (e.g. with blindness) <u>during</u> pregnancy complicated by preeclampsia or eclampsia[71]
       2. may develop 4-9 days post-partum and may be associated with vasospasm[72]
    C. cyclosporine toxicity
2. uremic encephalopathies: imaging studies show multiple areas of symmetric edema in the basal ganglia, with severe cases developing focal infarcts with or without hemorrhage[69]. These disorders are associated with elevated BUN and include:
    A. uremia

B. glomerulonephritis
C. hemolytic-uremic syndrome (HUS)
D. thrombotic thrombocytic purpura (TTP)

These patients may present with headache, seizures, mental status changes and focal neurologic deficit. Intracerebral hemorrhage **(ICH)** may occur.

Treatment

Disordered autoregulation mandates tight control of blood pressure to avoid hypertension to reduce the risk of ICH.

2.11. References

1. Consensus Conference: Differential diagnosis of dementing diseases. **JAMA** 258: 3411-6, 1987.
2. Fleming K C, Adams A C, Petersen R C: Dementia: Diagnosis and evaluation. **Mayo Clin Proc** 70: 1093-107, 1995.
3. Lipowski Z J: Delerium (acute confusional States). **JAMA** 258: 1789-92, 1987.
4. Pompei P, Foreman M, Rudberg M A, et al.: Delerium in hospitalized older persons: Outcomes and predictors. **J Am Geriatr Soc** 42: 809-15, 1994.
5. Petersen R C: Acute confusional state: Don't mistake it for dementia. **Postgrad Med** 92: 141-8, 1992.
6. Hulette C M, Earl N L, Crain B J: Evaluation of cerebral biopsies for the diagnosis of dementia. **Arch Neurol** 49: 28-31, 1992.
7. Javedan S P, Tamargo R J: Diagnostic yield of brain biopsy in neurodegenerative disorders. **Neurosurgery** 41: 823-30, 1997.
8. Forsyth P A, Posner J B: Headaches in patients with brain tumors: A study of 111 patients. **Neurology** 43: 1678-83, 1993.
9. Welch K M A, Levine S R: Migraine-related stroke in the context of the international headache society classification of head pain. **Arch Neurol** 47: 458-62, 1990.
10. Lance J W: Treatment of migraine. **Lancet** 339: 1207-9, 1992.
11. Kittrelle J P, Grouse D S, Seybold M E: Cluster headache: Local anesthetic abortive agents. **Arch Neurol** 42: 496-8, 1985.
12. Lapkin M L, Golden G S: Basilar artery migraine: A review of 30 cases. **Am J Dis Child** 132: 278-81, 1978.
13. DiGiovanni A J, Dunbar B S: Epidural injections of autologous blood for postlumbar-puncture headache. **Anesth and Analg** 49: 268-71, 1970.
14. Seebacher J, Ribeiro V, Le Guillou J L, et al.: Epidural blood patch in the treatment of post dural puncture headache: A double blind study. **Headache** 29: 630-2, 1989.
15. Lance J W, Branch G B: Persistent headache after lumbar puncture. **Lancet** 343: 414, 1994 (letter).
16. Gass H, Goldstein A S, Ruskin R, et al.: Chronic postmyelogram headache. **Arch Neurol** 25: 168-170, 1971.
17. Sechzer P H, Abel L: Post-spinal anesthesia headache treated with caffeine: Evaluation with demand method. Part 1. **Cur Ther Res** 24: 307-12, 1978.
18. Murros K, Fogelholm R: Spontaneous intracranial hypotension with slit ventricles. **J Neurol Neurosurg Psychiatry** 46: 1149-51, 1983.
19. Mitchell S L, Kiely D K, Kiel D P, et al.: The epidemiology, clinical characteristics, and natural history of older nursing home residents with a diagnosis of Parkinson's disease. **J Am Geriatr Soc** 44: 394-9, 1996.
20. Koller W C, Silver D E, Lieberman A: An algorithm for the management of Parkinson's disease. **Neurology** 44 (Suppl 10): S5-52, 1994.
21. Young R: Update on Parkinson's disease. **Am Fam Physician** 59: 2155-67, 1999.
22. Kondziolka D, Bonaroti E A, Lunsford L D: Pallidotomy for Parkinson's disease. **Contemp Neurosurg** 18 (6): 1-6, 1996.
23. Davis G C, Williams A C, Markey S P, et al.: Chronic parkinsonism secondary to intravenous injection of meperidine analogues. **Psychiatry Res** 1, 249-54, 1979.
24. Langston J W, Ballard P, Tetrud J W, et al.: Chronic parkinsonism in humans due to a product of meperidine-analog synthesis. **Science** 219: 979-80, 1983.
25. Lang A E, Lozano A M: Parkinson's disease. First of two parts. **N Engl J Med** 339: 1044-53, 1998.
26. Kristensen M O: Progressive supranuclear palsy - 10 years later. **Acta Neurol Scand** 71: 177-89, 1985.
27. Gildenberg P L: Whatever happened to stereotactic surgery? **Neurosurgery** 20: 983-7, 1987.
28. Lublin F D, Reingold S C: Defining the clinical course of multiple sclerosis: Results of an international survey. **Neurology** 46: 907-11, 1996.
29. Rudick R A, Cohen J A, Weinstock-Guttman B, et al.: Management of multiple sclerosis. **N Engl J Med** 22: 1604-11, 1997.
30. Rowland L P, (ed.) **Merritt's textbook of neurology**. 8th ed., Lea and Febiger, Philadelphia, 1989.
31. Jensen T S, Rasmussen P, Reske-Nielsen E: Association of trigeminal neuralgia with multiple sclerosis. **Arch Neurol** 65: 182-9, 1982.
32. Filippi M, Horsfield M A, Morrissey S P, et al.: Quantitative brain MRI lesion load predicts the course of clinically isolated syndromes suggestive of multiple sclerosis. **Neurology** 44: 635-41, 1994.
33. McDonald W I, Compston A, Edan G, et al.: Recommended diagnostic criteria for multiple sclerosis: Guidelines from the international panel on the diagnosis of multiple sclerosis. **Ann Neurol** 50: 121-7, 2001.
34. Poser C M, Paty D W, Scheinberg L, et al.: New diagnostic criteria for multiple sclerosis: Guidelines for research protocols. **Ann Neurol** 13: 227-31, 1983.
35. Swanson J W: Multiple sclerosis: Update in diagnosis and review of prognostic factors. **Mayo Clin Proc** 64: 577-86, 1989.
36. Barkhof F, Filippi M, Miller D H, et al.: Comparison of MR imaging criteria at first presentation to predict conversion to clinically definite multiple sclerosis. **Brain** 120: 2059-69, 1997.
37. Tintore M, Rovira A, Martinez M, et al.: Isolated demyelinating syndromes: Comparison of different MR imaging criteria to predict conversion to clinically definite multiple sclerosis. **AJNR** 21: 702-6, 2000.
38. Stewart J M, Houser O W, Baker H L, et al.: Magnetic resonance imaging and clinical relationships in multiple sclerosis. **Mayo Clin Proc** 62: 174-84, 1987.
39. Mushlin A I, Detsky A S, Phelps C E, et al.: The ac-

40. Kidd C, Thorpe J W, Thompson A J, *et al.*: Spinal cord imaging MRI using multi-array coils and fast spin echo . II. Findings in multiple sclerosis. **Neurology** 43: 2632-7, 1993.

41. Kent D L, Larson E B: Magnetic resonance imaging of the brain and spine. **Ann Intern Med** 108: 402-24, 1988.

42. Kepes J J: Large focal tumor-like demyelinating lesions of the brain: Intermediate entity between multiple sclerosis and acute disseminated encephalomyelitis? A study of 31 patients. **Ann Neurol** 33 (1): 18-27, 1993.

43. Law M, Meltzer D E, Cha S: Spectroscopic magnetic resonance imaging of a tumefactive demyelinating lesion. **Neuroradiology** 44 (12): 986-9, 2002.

44. Brex F A, Miszkiel K A, O'Riordan J I, *et al.*: Asessing the risk of early ms in patients with clinically isolated syndromes: The role of follow-up MRI. **J Neurol Neurosurg Psychiatry** 70: 390-3, 2001.

45. Freedman M S, Thompson E J, Deisenhammer D, *et al.*: Recommended standard of cerebrospinal fluid analysis in the diagnosis of multiple sclerosis: A consensus statement. **Arch Neurol** 62: 865-70, 2005.

46. Peavy G M, Herzog A G, Rubin N P, *et al.*: Neuropsychological aspects of dementia of motor neuron disease: A report of two cases. **Neurology** 42: 1004-8, 1992.

47. Bensimon G, Lacomblez L, Meininger V, *et al.*: A controlled trial of riluzole in amyotrophic lateral sclerosis. **N Engl J Med** 24: 585-91, 1994.

48. Riluzole for amyotrophic lateral sclerosis. **Med Letter** 37: 113-4, 1995.

49. Lacomblez L, Bensimon G, Guillet P, *et al.*: Riluzole: A double-blind randomized placebo-controlled dose-range study in amyotrophic lateral sclerosis (ALS). **Electroenceph Clin Neurophysiol** 97: S68, 1995 (abstract).

50. Asbury A K, Arnaso B G W, Karp H R, *et al.*: Criteria for diagnosis of Guillain-Barre syndrome. **Ann Neurol** 3: 565-6, 1978.

51. Mendell J R: Chronic inflammatory demyelinating polyradiculoneuropathy. **Annu Rev Med** 44: 211-9, 1993.

52. Mahattanakul W, Crawford T O, Griffin J W, *et al.*: Treatment of chronic inflammatory demyelinating polyneuropathy with cyclosporin-A. **J Neurol Neurosurg Psychiatry** 60: 185-7, 1996.

53. Gorson K C, Ropper A H, Clark B D, *et al.*: Treatment of chronic inflammatory demyelinating polyneuropathy with interferon-α 2a. **Neurology** 50: 84-7, 1998.

54. Guillain-Barré Syndrome Steroid Trial Group: Double-blind trial of intravenous methylprednisolone in Guillain-Barré syndrome. **Lancet** 341: 586-90, 1993.

55. Kincaid J C, Dyken M L: *Myelitis and myelopathy.* In **Clinical neurology**, Baker A B and Joynt R J, (eds.). Harper and Row, Hagerstown, 1984: pp 1-32.

56. Altrocchi P H: Acute transverse myelopathy. **Arch Neurol** 9: 111-9, 1963.

57. Eguro H: Transverse myelitis following chemonucleolysis: Report of a case. **J Bone Joint Surg** 65A: 1328-9, 1983.

58. Lipton H L, Teasdall R D: Acute transverse myelopathy in adults: A follow-up study. **Arch Neurol** 28: 252-7, 1973.

59. Ropper A H, Poskanzer D C: The prognosis of acute and subacute transverse myelopathy based on early signs and symptoms. **Ann Neurol** 4: 51-9, 1978.

60. Berman M, Feldman S, Alter M, *et al.*: Acute transverse myelitis: Incidence and etiologic considerations. **Neurology** 31: 966-71, 1981.

61. Merine D, Wang H, Kumar A J, *et al.*: CT myelography and MRI of acute transverse myelitis. **J Comput Assist Tomogr** 11: 606-8, 1987.

62. Dowling P C, Bosch V V, Cook S D: Possible beneficial effect of high-dose IV steroid therapy in acute demyelinating disease and transverse myelitis. **Neurology** 30: 33-6, 1980.

63. Stern B J, Krumholz A, Johns C, *et al.*: Sarcoidosis and its neurological manifestations. **Arch Neurol** 42: 909-17, 1985.

64. Oksanen V: Neurosarcoidosis: Clinical presentation and course in 50 patients. **Acta Neurol Scand** 73: 283-90, 1986.

65. de Tribolet N, Zander E: Intracranial sarcoidosis presenting angiographically as a subdural hematoma. **Surg Neurol** 9: 169-71, 1978.

66. Rohrbach M S, DeRemee R A: Pulmonary sarcoidosis and serum angiotensin-converting enzyme. **Mayo Clin Proc** 57: 64-6, 1982.

67. Oksanen V: New cerebrospinal fluid, neurophysiological and neuroradiological examinations in the diagnosis and follow-up of neurosarcoidosis. **Sarcoidosis** 4: 105-10, 1987.

68. Stern B J, Schonfeld S A, Sewell C, *et al.*: The treatment of neurosarcoidosis with cyclosporine. **Arch Neurol** 49: 1065-72, 1992.

69. Port J D, Beauchamp N J: Reversible intracerebral pathologic entities mediated by vascular autoregulatory dysfunction. **Radiographics** 18: 353-67, 1998.

70. Schaefer P W, Buonanno F S, Gonzalez R G, *et al.*: Diffusion-weighted imaging discriminates between cytotoxic and vasogenic edema in a patient with eclampsia. **Stroke** 28: 1082-5, 1997.

71. Beeson J H, Duda E E: Computed axial tomography scan demonstration of cerebral edema in eclampsia preceded by blindness. **Obstet Gynecol** 60: 529-32, 1982.

72. Raps E C, Galetta S L, Broderick M, *et al.*: Delayed peripartum vasculopathy: Cerebral eclampsia revisited. **Ann Neurol** 33: 222-5, 1993.

73. Moore P M, Cupps T R: Neurologic complications of vasculitis. **Ann Neurol** 14: 155-67, 1983.

74. Salvarani C, Cantini F, Boiardi L, *et al.*: Polymyalgia rheumatica and giant-cell arteritis. **N Engl J Med** 347: 261-71, 2002.

75. Salvarani C, Gabriel S E, O'Fallon W M, *et al.*: The incidence of giant cell arteritis in Olmstead county, Minnesota: Apparent fluctuations ina cyclic pattern. **Ann Intern Med** 123: 192-4, 1995.

76. Machado E B, Michet C J, Ballard D J, *et al.*: Trends in incidence and clinical presentation of temporal arteritis in Olmstead county, Minnesota, 1950-1985. **Arthritis Rheum** 31: 745-9, 1988.

77. Allen N B, Studenski S A: Polymyalgia rheumatica and temporal arteritis. **Med Clin N Amer** 70: 369-84, 1986.

78. Hunder G G: Giant cell (temporal) arteritis. **Rheum Dis Clin N Amer** 16: 399-409, 1990.

79. Hall S, Hunder G G: Is temporal artery biopsy prudent? **Mayo Clin Proc** 59: 793-6, 1984.

80. Caselli R J, Danube J R, Hunder G G, *et al.*: Peripheral neuropathic syndromes in giant cell (temporal) arteritis. **Neurology** 38: 685-9, 1988.

81. Salvarani C, Hunder G G: Giant cell arteritis with low erythrocyte sedimentation rate: Frequency of occurrence in a population-based study. **Arthritis Rheum** 45: 140-5, 2001.

82. Baumel B, Eisner L S: Diagnosis and treatment of headache in the elderly. **Med Clin N Amer** 75: 661-75, 1991.

83. Karacostas D, Taskos N, Nikolaides T: CT findings in temporal arteritis: A report of two cases. **Neurorad** 28: 373, 1986.

84. McDonnell P J, Moore G W, Miller N R, *et al.*: Temporal arteritis: A clinicopathologic study. **Ophthalmology** 93: 518-30, 1986.

85. Achkar A A, Lie J T, Hunder G G, *et al.*: How does previous corticosteroid treatment affect the biopsy

findings in giant cell (temporal) arteritis? **Ann Intern Med** 120: 987-92, 1994.

86. Cantini F, Salvarani C, Olivieri I, *et al.*: Erythrocyte sedimentation rate and C-reactive protein in the evaluation of disease activity and severity in polymyalgia rheumatica: A prospective follow-up study. **Semin Arthritis Rheum** 30: 17-24, 2000.

87. Chuang T Y, Hunder G G, Ilstrup D M, *et al.*: Polymyalgia rheumatica: A 10-year epidemiologic and clinical study. **Ann Intern Med** 97: 672-80, 1982.

88. Salvarani C, Gabriel S E, O'Fallon W M, *et al.*: Epidemiology of polymyalgia rheumatica in Olmstead county, Minnesota, 1970-1991. **Arthritis Rheum** 38: 369-73, 1995.

89. McDonald T J, DeRemee R A: Wegener's granulomatosis. **Laryngoscope** 93: 220-31, 1983.

90. New uses of thalidomide. **Med Letter** 38: 15-6, 1996.

91. Cupps T R, Moore P M, Fauci A S: Isolated angitis of the central nervous system: Prospective diagnostic and therapeutic experience. **Am J Med** 74: 97-105, 1983.

92. Kaye B R, Fainstat M: Cerebral vasculitis associated with cocaine abuse. **JAMA** 258: 2104-6, 1987.

93. Hasso A N, Bird C R, Zinke D E, *et al.*: Fibromuscular dysplasia of the internal carotid artery: Percutaneous transluminal angioplasty. **AJR** 136: 955-60, 1981.

94. Mettinger K L, Ericson K: Fibromuscular dysplasia and the brain: Observations on angiographic, clinical, and genetic characteristics. **Stroke** 13: 46-52, 1982.

95. Mettinger K L: Fibromuscular dysplasia and the brain II: Current concept of the disease. **Stroke** 13: 53-8, 1982.

96. Osborn A G, Anderson R E: Angiographic spectrum of cervical and intracranial fibromuscular dysplasia. **Stroke** 8: 617-26, 1977.

97. Chabriat H, Vahedi K, Iba-Zizen M T, *et al.*: Clinical spectrum of cadasil: A study of seven families. **Lancet** 346: 934-9, 1995.

3. Anatomy

3.1. Surface anatomy

3.1.1. Cortical surface anatomy

Figure 3-1 shows some important cortical surface landmarks. This may be helpful in correlating with MRI to determine the location of lesions[1]. The MFG is usually more sinuous than the IFG or SFG, and it often connects to the pre-central gyrus via a thin isthmus. The central sulcus joins the Sylvian fissure in only 2% of cases (i.e. in 98% of cases there is a "subcentral" gyrus). The interparietal sulcus (**ips**) separates the superior and inferior parietal lobules. The IPL is composed primarily of the AG and SMG. The Sylvian fissure terminates in the SMG (Brodmann's area 40). The superior temporal sulcus terminates in the AG.

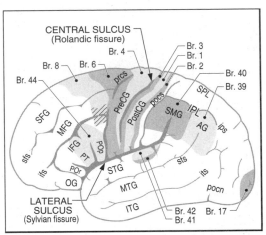

Figure 3-1 Cerebral cortical surface anatomy*

* Br. = Brodmann's area (shaded). See *Table 3-1* and *Table 3-2* for abbreviations.

Brodmann's areas

Figure 3-1 also identifies the clinically significant areas of Brodmann's (**Br.**) map of the cytoarchitectonic fields of the human brain. Functional significance of these areas is as follows:

- Br. areas 3,1,2: primary somatosensory cortex
- Br. areas 41 & 42: primary auditory areas (transverse gyri of Heschl)
- Br. area 4: precentral gyrus, primary motor cortex (AKA "**motor strip**"). Large concentration of giant pyramidal cells of Betz
- Br. area 6: premotor area or supplemental motor area. Immediately anterior to motor strip, it plays a role in contralateral motor programming
- Br. area 44: (dominant hemisphere) **Broca's area** (motor speech)[A]

Table 3-1 Cerebral sulci

prcs	pre-central sulcus
pocs	post-central sulcus
sfs, ifs	superior, inferior frontal sulcus
sts, its	superior, inferior temporal sulcus
ips	interparietal sulcus
pocn	pre-occipital notch

- Br. area 17: primary visual cortex
- **Wernicke's area** (language)[A]: in the dominant hemisphere, most of Br. area 40 and a portion of Br. area 39 (may also include ≈ posterior third of STG)
- Br. area 8: the striped portion in *Figure 3-1* (frontal eye field) initiates voluntary eye movements to the opposite direction

Table 3-2　Cerebral gyri

SFG, MFG	superior & middle frontal gyrus
IFG	inferior frontal gyrus
POp	pars opercularis of the IFG
PT	pars triangularis of the IFG
POr	pars orbitalis of the IFG
STG, MTG, ITG	superior, middle and inferior temporal gyrus
SPL, IPL	superior and inferior parietal lobule
PreCG, PostCG	pre and post-central gyrus
SMG	supramarginal gyrus
AG	angular gyrus
OG	orbital gyrus

3.1.2.　Surface anatomy of the cranium

CRANIOMETRIC POINTS

Craniometric points are shown in *Figure 3-2*.

Pterion: region where the following bones are approximated: frontal, parietal, temporal and sphenoid (greater wing). Estimated as 2 finger-breadths above the zygomatic arch, and a thumb's breadth behind the frontal process of the zygomatic bone.

Asterion: junction of lambdoid, occipitomastoid and parietomastoid sutures. Overlies the junction of transverse and sigmoid sinuses.

Vertex: the topmost point of the skull.

Lambda: junction of the lambdoid and sagittal sutures.

Stephanion: junction of the coronal suture and the superior temporal line.

Glabella: the most forward projecting point of the forehead at the level of the supraorbital ridge in the midline.

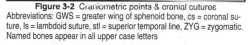

Figure 3-2 Craniometric points & cranial sutures
Abbreviations: GWS = greater wing of sphenoid bone, cs = coronal suture, ls = lambdoid suture, stl = superior temporal line, ZYG = zygomatic. Named bones appear in all upper case letters

Opisthion: the posterior margin of the foramen magnum in the midline.

Bregma: the junction of the coronal and sagittal sutures.

A. language function cannot be reliably localized on anatomic grounds due to individual variability in its exact location; in order to perform maximal brain resections with minimal risk of aphasia, techniques such as intra-operative brain mapping[2] or looking for phase reversal on intraoperative cortical SSEP[3] should be employed

Taylor-Haughton lines

Taylor-Haughton (T-H) lines can be constructed on an angiogram, CT scout film, or skull x-ray, and can then be reconstructed on the patient in the O.R. based on visible external landmarks[4]. T-H lines are shown as dashed lines in *Figure 3-3*.

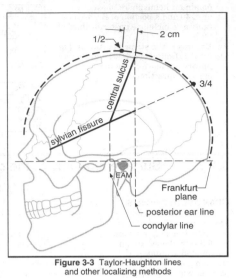

Figure 3-3 Taylor-Haughton lines and other localizing methods

1. **Frankfurt plane**, AKA baseline: line from inferior margin of orbit through the upper margin of the external auditory meatus (**EAM**) (as distinguished from **Reid's base line**: from inferior orbital margin through the *center* of the EAM)[5 (p 313)]
2. the distance from the nasion to the inion is measured across the top of the calvaria and is divided into quarters (can be done simply with a piece of tape which is then folded in half twice)
3. posterior ear line: perpendicular to the baseline through the mastoid process
4. condylar line: perpendicular to the baseline through the mandibular condyle
5. T-H lines can then be used to approximate the sylvian fissure (*see below*) and the motor cortex (also *see below*)

Sylvian fissure AKA lateral fissure

Approximated by a line connecting the lateral canthus to the point 3/4 of the way posterior along the arc running over convexity from nasion to inion (T-H lines).

Angular gyrus

Located just above the pinna, important on the dominant hemisphere as part of Wernicke's area. Note: there is significant individual variability in the location[2].

Angular artery

Located 6 cm above the EAM.

Motor cortex

Numerous methods utilize external landmarks to locate the motor strip (pre-central gyrus) or the central sulcus (Rolandic fissure) which separates motor strip anteriorly from primary sensory cortex posteriorly. These are just approximations since individual variability causes the motor strip to lie anywhere from 4 to 5.4 cm behind the coronal suture[6]. The central sulcus cannot even be reliably identified visually at surgery[7].

*   method 1: the superior aspect of the motor cortex is almost straight up from the EAM near the midline
*   method 2[8]: the central sulcus is approximated by connecting:
    A. the point 2 cm posterior to the midposition of the arc extending from nasion to inion (illustrated in *Figure 3-3*), to
    B. the point 5 cm straight up from the EAM
*   method 3: using T-H lines, the cerebral sulcus is approximated by connecting:
    A. the point where the "posterior ear line" intersects the circumference of the skull (*see Figure 3-3*) (usually about 1 cm behind the vertex, and 3-4 cm behind the coronal suture), to
    B. the point where the "condylar line" intersects the line representing the sylvian fissure

- method 4: a line drawn 45° to Reid's base line starting at the pterion points in the <u>direction</u> of the motor strip[9 (p 584-5)]

RELATIONSHIP OF VENTRICLES TO SKULL

Figure 3-4 shows the relationship of non-hydrocephalic ventricles to the skull in the lateral view. Some dimensions of interest are shown in *Table 3-3*[10].

In the non-hydrocephalic adult, the lateral ventricles lie 4-5 cm below the outer skull surface. The center of the body of the lateral ventricle sits in the midpupillary line, and the frontal horn is intersected by a line passing perpendicular to the calvaria along this line[11]. The anterior horns extend 1-2 cm anterior to the coronal suture.

Average length of third ventricle ≈ 2.8 cm.

The midpoint of Twining's line (• in *Figure 3-4*) should lie within the 4th ventricle.

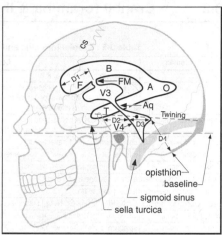

Figure 3-4 Relationship of ventricles to skull landmarks*

* Abbreviations: (F = frontal horn, B = body, A = atrium, O = occipital horn, T = temporal horn) of lateral ventricle. FM = foramen of Monro. Aq = sylvian aqueduct. V3 = third ventricle. V4 = fourth ventricle. cs = coronal suture. Dimensions D1-4 → *see Table 3-3*

Table 3-3   Dimensions from *Figure 3-4*

Dimension (see Figure 3-4)	Description	Lower limit (mm)	Average (mm)	Upper limit (mm)
D1	length of frontal horn anterior to FM		25	
D2	distance from clivus to floor of 4th ventricle at level of fastigium*	33.3	36.1	40.0
D3	length of 4th ventricle at level of fastigium*	10.0	14.6	19.0
D4	distance from fastigium* to opisthion	30.0	32.6	40.0

* the fastigium is the apex of the 4th ventricle within the cerebellum

3.1.3.   Surface landmarks of cervical levels

Estimates of cervical levels for anterior cervical spine surgery may be made using the landmarks shown in *Table 3-4*. Intra-operative C-spine x-rays are essential to verify these estimates.

Table 3-4   Cervical levels[12]

Level	Landmark
C1-2	angle of mandible
C3-4	1 cm above thyroid cartilage (≈ hyoid bone)
C4-5	level of thyroid cartilage
C5-6	crico-thyroid membrane
C6	carotid tubercle
C6-7	cricoid cartilage

3.2. Cranial foramina & their contents

Table 3-5 Cranial foramina and their contents*

Foramen	Contents
nasal slits	anterior ethmoidal nn., a. & v
superior orbital fissure	Cr. Nn. III, IV, VI, all 3 branches of V1 (ophthalmic division divides into nasociliary, frontal, and lacrimal nerves); superior ophthalmic vv.; recurrent meningeal br. from lacrimal a.; orbital branch of middle meningeal a.; sympathetic filaments from ICA plexus
inferior orbital fissure	Cr. N. V-2 (maxillary div.), zygomatic n.; filaments from pterygopalatine branch of maxillary n.; infraorbital a. & v.; v. between inferior ophthalmic v. & pterygoid venous plexus
foramen lacerum	usually nothing (ICA traverses upper portion, 30% have vidian a.)
carotid canal	internal carotid a., ascending sympathetic nerves
incisive foramen	descending septal a.; nasopalatine nn.
greater palatine foramen	greater palatine n., a., & v.
lesser palatine foramen	lesser palatine nn.
internal acoustic meatus	Cr. N. VI I (facial); Cr. N. VI I I (stato-acoustic)
hypoglossal canal	Cr. N. XI I (hypoglossal); a meningeal branch of the ascending pharyngeal a.
foramen magnum	spinal cord (medulla oblongata); Cr. N. XI (spinal accessory nn.) <u>entering</u> the skull; vertebral aa.; anterior & posterior spinal arteries
foramen cecum	occasional small vein
cribriform plate	olfactory nn.
optic canal	Cr. N. I I (optic); ophthalmic a.
foramen rotundum	Cr. N. V2 (maxillary div.), a. of foramen rotundum
foramen ovale	Cr. N. V3 (mandibular div.) + portio minor (motor for CrN V)
foramen spinosum	middle meningeal a. & v.
jugular foramen	internal jugular v. (beginning); Cr. Nn. IX, X, XI
stylomastoid foramen	Cr. N. VI I (facial); stylomastoid a.
condyloid foramen	v. from transverse sinus
mastoid foramen	v. to mastoid sinus; branch of occipital a. to dura mater

*   Abbreviations: a. = artery, aa. = arteries, v. = vein, vv. = veins, n. = nerve, nn. = nerves, br. = branch, Cr. N. = cranial nerve, fmn. = foramen, div. = division

Porus acusticus

(*see Figure 3-5*)

The filaments of the acoustic portion of VIII penetrate the tiny openings of the lamina cribrosa of the cochlear area[13].

Transverse crest separates superior vestibular area and facial canal (above) from the inferior vestibular area and cochlear area (below)[13].

Vertical crest: separates superior vestibular area from meatus to facial canal.

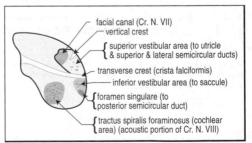

facial canal (Cr. N. VII)
vertical crest
{ superior vestibular area (to utricle & superior & lateral semicircular ducts)
transverse crest (crista falciformis)
inferior vestibular area (to saccule)
{ foramen singulare (to posterior semicircular duct)
{ tractus spiralis foraminosus (cochlear area) (acoustic portion of Cr. N. VIII)

Figure 3-5 Right internal auditory canal (porus acusticus)

3.3.   Spinal cord anatomy

3.3.1.   Spinal cord tracts

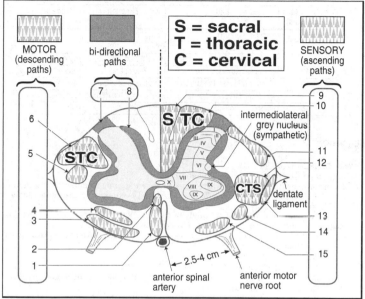

Figure 3-6 Schematic cross-section of cervical spinal cord

Figure 3-6 depicts a cross-section of a typical spinal cord segment, combining some elements from different levels (e.g. the intermediolateral grey nucleus is only present from T1 to ≈ L1 or L2 where there are sympathetic (thoracolumbar outflow) nuclei). It is schematically divided into ascending and descending halves, however, in actuality, ascending and descending paths coexist on both sides.

Figure 3-6 also depicts some of the laminae according to the scheme of Rexed. Lamina II is equivalent to the substantia gelatinosa. Laminae III and IV are the nucleus proprius. Lamina VI is located in the base of the posterior horn.

Table 3-6   Descending (motor) tracts (↓) in *Figure 3-6*

Number (see Figure 3-6)	Path	Function	Side of body
1	anterior corticospinal tract	skilled movement	opposite
2	medial longitudinal fasciculus	?	same
3	vestibulospinal tract	facilitates extensor muscle tone	same
4	medullary (ventrolateral) reticulospinal tract	automatic respirations?	same
5	rubrospinal tract	flexor muscle tone	same
6	lateral corticospinal (pyramidal) tract	skilled movement	same

Table 3-7 Bi-directional tracts in *Figure 3-6*

Number (see Figure 3-6)	Path	Function
7	dorsolateral fasciculus	
8	fasciculus proprius	short spinospinal connections

Table 3-8 Ascending (sensory) tracts (↑) in *Figure 3-6*

Number (see Figure 3-6)	Path	Function	Side of body
9	fasciculus gracilis	joint position, fine touch, vibration	same
10	fasciculus cuneatus		
11	posterior spinocerebellar tract	stretch receptors	same
12	lateral spinothalamic tract	pain & temperature	opposite
13	anterior spinocerebellar tract	whole limb position	opposite
14	spinotectal tract	unknown, ? nociceptive	opposite
15	anterior spinothalamic tract	light touch	opposite

SENSATION

PAIN & TEMPERATURE: BODY

Receptors: free nerve endings (probable).

1st order neuron: small, finely myelinated afferents; soma in dorsal root ganglion (no synapse). Enter cord at dorsolateral tract (zone of Lissauer). Synapse: substantia gelatinosa (Rexed II).

2nd order neuron axon cross obliquely in the anterior white commisure ascending ≈ 1-3 segments while crossing to enter the lateral spinothalamic tract.

Synapse: VPL thalamus. 3rd order neurons pass through IC to postcentral gyrus (Brodmann's areas 3, 1, 2).

FINE TOUCH, DEEP PRESSURE & PROPRIOCEPTION: BODY

Fine touch AKA discriminative touch. Receptors: Meissner's & pacinian corpuscles, Merkel's disks, free nerve endings.

1st order neuron: heavily myelinated afferents; soma in dorsal root ganglion (no synapse). Short branches synapse in nucleus proprius (Rexed III & IV) of posterior gray; long fibers enter the ipsilateral posterior columns without synapsing (below T6: fasciculus gracilis; above T6: fasciculus cuneatus).

Synapse: nucleus gracilis/cuneatus (respectively), just above pyramidal decussation. 2nd order neuron axons form internal arcuate fibers, decussate in lower medulla as **medial lemniscus**.

Synapse: VPL thalamus. 3rd order neurons pass through IC primarily to postcentral gyrus.

LIGHT (CRUDE) TOUCH: BODY

Receptors: as fine touch (*see above*), also peritrichial arborizations.

1st order neuron: large, heavily myelinated afferents (Type II); soma in dorsal root ganglion (no synapse). Some ascend uncrossed in post. columns (with fine touch); most synapse in Rexed VI & VII.

2nd order neuron axons cross in anterior white commisure (a few don't cross); enter anterior spinothalamic tract.

Synapse: VPL thalamus. 3rd order neurons pass through IC primarily to postcentral gyrus.

3.3.2.   Dermatomes and sensory nerves

Figure 3-7 shows anterior and posterior view, each schematically separated into sensory dermatomes (segmental) and peripheral sensory nerve distribution.

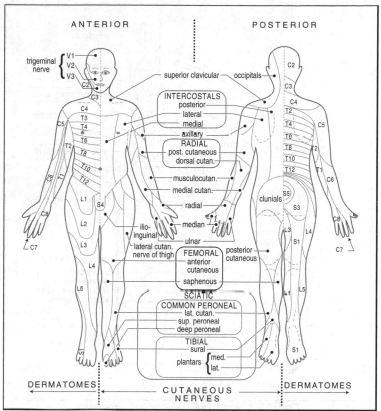

Figure 3-7 Dermatomal and sensory nerve distribution
(Redrawn from "Introduction to Basic Neurology", by Harry D. Patton, John W. Sundsten, Wayne E. Crill and Phillip D. Swanson, © 1976, pp 173, W. B. Saunders Co., Philadelphia, PA, with permission)

3.3.3. Spinal cord vasculature

Although a radicular artery from the aorta accompanies the nerve root at many levels, most of these contribute little flow to the spinal cord itself. The major blood supply to the anterior spinal cord is from 6-8 radicular arteries at the following levels ("radiculomedullary arteries", the levels listed are fairly consistent, but the side varies[14 (p 1180-1)]):

- C3 - arises from vertebral artery
- C6 - usually arises from deep cervical artery ⎫ ≈ 10% of population lack an anterior
- C8 - usually from costocervical trunk ⎭ radicular artery in lower cervical spine[15]

- T4 or T5
- Adamkiewicz (*see below*)

The paired posterior spinal arteries are less well defined than the anterior spinal artery, and are fed by 10-23 radicular branches.

The midthoracic region has a tenuous vascular supply ("watershed zone"), possessing only the above noted artery at T4 or T5. It is thus more susceptible to vascular insults.

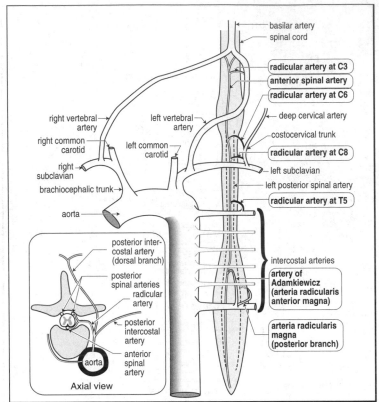

Figure 3-8 Schematic diagram of spinal cord arterial supply
(Modified from **Diagnostic Neuroradiology**, 2nd ed., Volume II, pp. 1181, Taveras J M, Woods E H, editors,
© 1976, the Williams and Wilkins Co., Baltimore, with permission)

Artery of Adamkiewicz AKA arteria radicularis anterior magna
- the main arterial supply for the spinal cord from ≈ T8 to the conus
- located on the left in 80%
- occurs between T9 & L2 in 85% (between T9 & T12 in 75%); in remaining 15% between T5 & T8 (in these latter cases, there may be a supplemental radicular artery further down)
- usually fairly large, gives off cephalic and caudal branch (latter is usually larger) giving a characteristic hair-pin appearance on angiography

3.4.   Cerebrovascular anatomy

3.4.1.   Cerebral vascular territories

Figure 3-9 depicts approximate vascular distributions of the major cerebral arteries.

There is considerable variability of the major arteries[16] as well as the central distribution (the lenticulostriates, recurrent artery of Heubner **(RH)** (AKA medial striate artery), etc. have varying distributions and may have origins off of different segments of the middle or anterior cerebral artery).

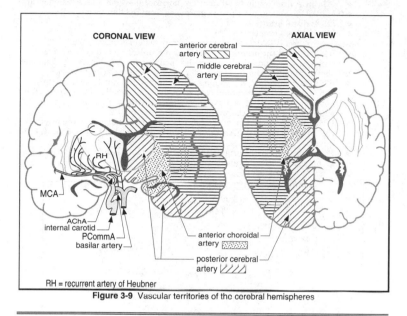

CORONAL VIEW

anterior cerebral artery

middle cerebral artery

RH

MCA

AChA
internal carotid
PCommA
basilar artery

AXIAL VIEW

anterior choroidal artery

posterior cerebral artery

RH = recurrent artery of Heubner

Figure 3-9 Vascular territories of the cerebral hemispheres

3.4.2. Cerebral arterial anatomy

The symbol "⇒" is used to denote a region supplied by the indicated artery. See *Angiography (cerebral)* on page 130 for angiographic diagrams of the following anatomy.

CIRCLE OF WILLIS

A balanced configuration of the Circle of Willis is present in only 18% of the population. Hypoplasia of 1 or both p-comms occurs in 22-32%, absent or hypoplastic A1 segments occurs in 25%.

Anatomical segments of intracranial cerebral arteries

- carotid artery: the traditional numbering system[17] was from rostral to caudal (counter to the direction of flow, and to the numbering scheme of the other arteries). A number of systems have been described to addresses this inconsistency and also to identify anatomically important segments of the ICA that were not originally delineated (e.g. *see Table 3-9*[18]). Also *see below* for more detail
- anterior cerebral[19]:
  - ◆ A1: ACA from origin to ACoA
  - ◆ A2: ACA from ACoA to branch-point of callosomarginal
  - ◆ A3: from branch-point of callosomarginal to superior surface of corpus callosum

Table 3-9   Segments of the ICA

Proposed system	System of Fischer
C1 (cervical)	not
C2 (petrous)	described
C3 (lacerum)	C5
C4 (cavernous)	C4 + part of C5
C5 (clinoid)	C3
C6 (ophthalmic)	C2
C7 (communicating)	C1

3 cm posterior to the genu
- ◆ A4: pericallosal
- ◆ A5: terminal branch
- • middle cerebral[19]:
  - ◆ M1: MCA from origin to bifurcation (horizontal segment on AP angiogram)
  - ◆ M2: MCA from bifurcation to emergence from Sylvian fissure
  - ◆ M3-4: distal branches
  - ◆ M5: terminal branch
- • posterior cerebral (PCA) (several nomenclature schemes exist[20, 21]):
  - ◆ P1: PCA from the origin to posterior communicating artery (AKA mesencephalic, precommunicating, circular, peduncular, basilar…). The long and short circumflex and thalamoperforating arteries arise from P1
  - ◆ P2: PCA from origin of p-comm to the origin of inferior temporal arteries (AKA ambient, postcommunicating, perimesencephalic), P2 traverses the ambient cistern, Hippocampal, anterior temporal, peduncular perforating and medial posterior choroidal arteries arise from P2
  - ◆ P3: PCA from the origin of the inferior temporal branches to the origin of the terminal branches (AKA quadrigeminal segment). P3 traverses the quadrigeminal cistern
  - ◆ P4: segment after the origin of the parieto-occipital and calcarine arteries, includes the cortical branches of the PCA

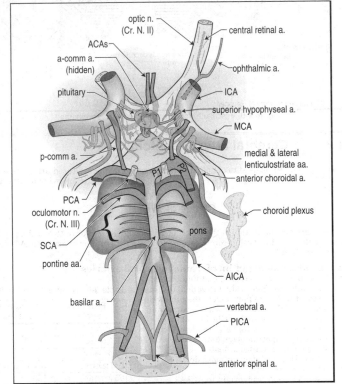

Figure 3-10 Circle of Willis viewed from in front of and below the brain

Key point: the anterior cerebral arteries pass over the superior surface of the optic chiasm.

ANTERIOR CIRCULATION

INTERNAL CAROTID (ICA)
Acutely occluding one carotid artery will cause a stroke in 15-20% of people.

Segments of the ICA and its branches
"**Carotid siphon**": begins at the posterior bend of the cavernous ICA, and ends at the ICA bifurcation (thus incorporating the cavernous, ophthalmic and communicating segments)[18].

- **C1 (cervical)**: begins at carotid bifurcation. Travels in carotid sheath with IJV and vagus nerve, encircled with postganglionic sympathetic nerves **(PGSN)**. Lies posterior & medial to the external carotid. Ends where it enters carotid canal of petrous bone. No branches
- **C2 (petrous)**: still surrounded by PCSNs. Ends at the posterior edge of the foramen lacerum (**f-Lac**) (inferomedial to the edge of the Gasserian ganglion in Meckel's cave). Three segments:
  - A. vertical segment: ICA ascends then bends as the...
  - B. **posterior loop**: anterior to cochlea, bends antero-medially becoming the...
  - C. horizontal segment: deep and medial to greater and lesser superficial petrosal nerves, anterior to tympanic membrane (TM)
- **C3 (lacerum)**: the ICA passes over (but not through) the f-Lac forming the lateral loop. Ascends in the canalicular portion of the f-Lac to juxtasellar position, piercing the dura as it passes the petrolingual ligament to become the cavernous segment. Branches (usually not visible angiographically):
  - A. caroticotympanic (inconsistent) ⇒ tympanic cavity
  - B. pterygoid (vidian) branch: passes through foramen lacerum, present in 30%, may continue as artery of pterygoid canal
- **C4 (cavernous)**: covered by vascular membrane lining sinus, still surrounded by PGSNs. Passes anteriorly then supero-medially, bends posteriorly (**medial loop** of ICA), travels horizontally, and bends anteriorly (part of **anterior loop** of ICA) to anterior clinoid process. Ends at the proximal dural ring (incomplete encircles ICA). Many branches, main ones include:
  - A. meningohypophyseal trunk (largest & most proximal)
    1. a. of tentorium (AKA **artery of Bernasconi & Cassinari**)
    2. dorsal meningeal a.
    3. inferior hypophyseal a. (⇒ posterior lobe of pituitary): occlusion causes pituitary infarcts in post-partum Sheehan's necrosis, however, DI is rare because the stalk is spared
  - B. anterior meningeal a.
  - C. a. to inferior portion of cavernous sinus (present in 80%)
  - D. capsular aa. of McConnell (in 30%): supply the capsule of the pituitary[22]
- **C5 (clinoid)**: ends at the distal dural ring (completely encircles ICA) where the ICA becomes intradural
- **C6 (ophthalmic)**: begins at distal dural ring, ends just proximal to p-comm
  - A. ophthalmic a.: the origin from the ICA is distal to the cavernous sinus in 89% (intracavernous in 8%, absent in 3%[20]). Passes through the optic canal into the orbit. Has a characteristic bayonet-like "kink" on lateral angiogram.
  - B. superior hypophyseal a. branches ⇒ anterior lobe of pituitary & stalk (1st branch of supraclinoid ICA)
  - C. posterior communicating a. (p-comm)
    1. few anterior **thalamoperforators** (⇒ optic tract, chiasm & posterior hypothalamus): see *Posterior circulation* below
  - D. **anterior choroidal artery**[24]: takeoff 2-4 mm distal to p-comm ⇒ (variable) portion of optic tract, medial globus pallidus, genu of internal capsule (**IC**) (in 50%), inferior half of posterior limb of IC, uncus, retrolenticular fibers (optic radiation), lateral geniculate body (see *page 778* for occlusion syndromes)
    1. plexal segment: enters supracornual recess of temporal horn, ⇒ only this portion of choroid plexus
    2. cisternal segment: passes through crural cistern
- **C7 (communicating)**: begins just proximal to p-comm origin, travels between Cr. N. II & III, terminates just below anterior perforated substance where it bifurcates into the ACA & MCA

ANTERIOR CEREBRAL (ACA)

Passes between Cr. N. II and anterior perforated substance. See *Figure 5-2*, page 132 for angiogram and branches.

MIDDLE CEREBRAL (MCA)

See*Figure 5-3*, page 132 for angiogram and branches.

POSTERIOR CIRCULATION

See *Figure 5-5*, page 133 for angiogram and branches.

VERTEBRAL ARTERY (VA)

The VA is the first and usually the largest branch of the subclavian artery. Variant: the left VA arises off the aortic arch in ≈ 4%. Diameter ≈ 3 mm. Mean blood flow ≈ 150 ml/min. The left VA is dominant in 60%. The right VA will be hypoplastic in 10%, and the left will be hypoplastic in 5%. The VA is atretic and does not communicate with the BA on the left in 3%, and on the right in 2%.

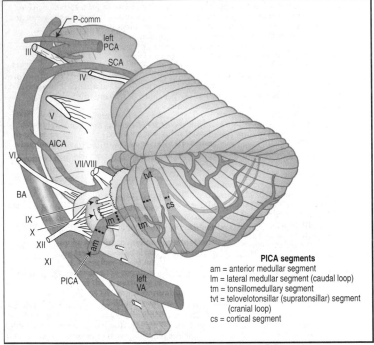

Figure 3-11 Lateral diagram showing intradural VA and PICA segments

Modified with permission from: Lewis SB, Chang DJ, Peace DA, Lafrentz PJ, Day AL. Distal posterior inferior cerebellar artery aneurysms: clinical features and management. J Neurosurg 2002; 97(4): 756-66.

Four segments:
- first segment: courses superiorly and posteriorly and enters the foramen transversarium, usually of the 6th vertebral body
- second segment: ascends vertically within the transverse foramina of the cervical vertebrae accompanied by a network of sympathetic fibers (from the stellate gan-

glion) and a venous plexus. It turns laterally within the transverse process of the axis
- third segment: exits the foramen of the axis and curves posteriorly and medially in a groove on the upper surface of the atlas and enters the foramen magnum
- fourth segment: pierces the dura and immediately enters subarachnoid space. Joins contralateral VA at the **vertebral confluens** located at the lower pontine border to form the basilar artery **(BA)**

Branches:
1. anterior meningeal: arises at body of C_2 (axis), may feed chordomas or foramen magnum meningiomas, may also act as collateral in vascular occlusion
2. posterior meningeal
3. medullary (bulbar) aa.
4. posterior spinal
5. PICA (largest branch): (*see Figure 3-11*) arises ≈10 mm distal to point where VA becomes intradural, ≈ 15 mm proximal to the vertebrobasilar junction (in 5-8% the PICA has an extradural origin)
    A. 5 segments[25] (some systems some describe only 4). During surgery, the first three must be preserved, but the last 2 may usually be sacrificed with minimal deficit[26]:
        1. anterior medullary: from PICA origin to inferior olivary prominence. 1 or 2 short medullary short circumflex branches ⇒ ventral medulla
        2. lateral medullary: to origin of nerves IX, X & XI. Up to 5 branches that supply brainstem
        3. tonsillomedullary: to tonsillar midportion (contains caudal loop on angio)
        4. telovelotonsillar (supratonsillar): ascends in tonsillomedullary fissure (contains cranial loop on angio)
        5. cortical segments
    B. 3 branches
        1. **choroidal** a. (BRANCH 1) arises from cranial loop (choroidal point), ⇒ choroid plexus of 4th ventricle
        2. terminal branches:
            a. **tonsillohemispheric** (BRANCH 2)
            b. **inferior vermian** (BRANCH 3) inferior inflection = copular point on angio
6. anterior spinal

BASILAR ARTERY (BA)

Formed by the junction of the 2 vertebral arteries. Branches:
1. AICA: from lower part of BA, runs posterolaterally anterior to VI, VII & VIII. Often gives off a loop that runs into the IAC and gives off the labyrinthine artery and then emerges to supply the anterolateral inferior cerebellum and then anastamoses with PICA
2. internal auditory (labyrinthine)
3. pontine branches
4. superior cerebellar a. **(SCA)**
    A. sup. vermian
5. **posterior cerebral**: joined by p-comms ≈ 1 cm from origin (the p-comm is the major origin of the PCA in 15% and is termed "fetal" circulation, bilateral in 2%). 3 segments (named for surrounding cistern) and their branches:
    A. peduncular segment (P1)
        1. mesencephalic perforating aa. (⇒ tectum, cerebral peduncles, and these nucleii: Edinger-Westphal, oculomotor and trochlear)
        2. interpeduncular **thalamoperforators** (1st of 2 groups of posterior thalamoperforating aa.)
        3. medial post. choroidal (most from P1 or P2)
    B. ambient segment (P2)
        1. lateral post. choroidal (most from P2)
        2. thalamogeniculate **thalamoperforators** (2nd of 2 groups of posterior thalamoperforating aa.) ⇒ geniculate bodies + pulvinar
        3. anterior temporal (anastamoses with anterior temporal br. of MCA)
        4. posterior temporal
        5. parieto-occipital

        6. calcarine
C. quadrigeminal segment (P3)
        1. quadrigeminal & geniculate branches ⇒ quadrigeminal plate
        2. post. pericallosal (splenial) (anastamoses with pericallosal of ACA)

EXTERNAL CAROTID

1. superior thyroid: 1st anterior branch
2. ascending pharyngeal
3. lingual
4. facial: branches anastamose with ophthalmic (key in collateral flow)
5. occipital
6. posterior auricular
7. superficial temporal
    A. frontal branch
    B. parietal branch
8. maxillary - initially within parotid gland
    A. middle meningeal
    B. accessory meningeal
    C. inferior alveolar
    D. infra-orbital
    E. others: distal branches of which may anastomose with branches of ophthalmic artery in the orbit

---

3.4.3.   Cerebral venous anatomy

SUPRATENTORIAL VENOUS SYSTEM
See *Figure 5-4*, page 133 for angiogram and branches.
    The left and right internal jugular veins **(IJVs)** are the major source of outflow of blood from the intracranial compartment. The <u>right</u> IJV is usually dominant. Other sources of outflow include orbital veins and the vertebral venous plexus. Diploic and scalp veins may act as collateral pathways, e.g. with superior sagittal sinus obstruction[27]. The following outline traces the venous drainage back from the IJVs.
A. inferior petrosal sinus
B. sigmoid sinus
    1. superior petrosal sinus
    2. transverse sinus (R > L in 65%)
        A. v. of Labbe (inferior anastomotic v.)
        B. confluens of sinuses (torcular herophili)
            1. occipital sinus
            2. superior sagittal sinus
                a. v. of Trolard (superior anastomotic v.): the prominent superficial vein on the <u>non-dominant</u> side (Labbé is more prominent on the dominant side)
            3. straight sinus
                a. inferior sagittal sinus
                b. great cerebral v. (of Galen)
                    i.   pre-central cerebellar v.
                    ii.   basal vein of Rosenthal
                    iii. internal cerebral v.: joined at the foramen of Monro (venous angle) by:
                        1. anterior septal v.
                        2. thalamostriate v.

CAVERNOUS SINUS
    Although classical teaching depicts the cavernous sinus as a large venous space with multiple trabeculations, injection studies[28] and surgical experience[29] supports the concept of the cavernous sinus as a plexus of veins.
    1. contributing veins:

A. superior & inferior ophthalmic veins
B. superficial middle cerebral veins
C. sphenoparietal sinus
D. superior & inferior petrosal sinus

2. contents[30]
- Oculomotor n. (III)
- Trochlear n. (IV)
- Ophthalmic division of trigeminal (V1)
- Maxillary division of trigeminal (V2): the only nerve of the cavernous sinus that doesn't exit the skull through the superior orbital fissure (it exits through foramen rotundum)
- Carotid
- Abducens n. (VI): the only nerve NOT attached to lateral dural wall

3. **triangular space** (of Parkinson): superior border formed by Cr. N. III & IV, and the lower margin formed by V$_1$ & VI (a landmark for surgical entrance to the cavernous sinus)[31, 32 (p 3007)]

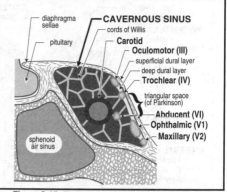

Figure 3-12 Right cavernous sinus (coronal section)
(Modified from the **Journal of Neurosurgery**, F. Umansky and H. Nathan, Vol. 56, pp. 228-34, 1982, with permission)

3.5. Internal capsule

Vascular supply of the internal capsule (IC)

1. anterior choroidal: ⇒ all of retrolenticular part (includes optic radiation) and ventral part of posterior limb of IC
2. lateral striate branches (AKA capsular branches) of middle cerebral artery: ⇒ most of anterior AND posterior limbs of IC
3. genu usually receives some direct branches of the internal carotid artery

Most IC lesions are caused by vascular accidents (thrombosis or hemorrhage).

Table 3-10 Four Thalamic "subradiations" (AKA thalamic peduncles)
(labeled A-D in *Figure 3-13*)

Radiation	Connection		Comments
anterior (A)	medial & anterior thalamic nucleus	↔ frontal lobe	
superior (B)	rolandic areas	↔ ventral thalamic nuclei	general sensory fibers from body & head to terminate in postcentral gyrus (areas 3,1,2)
posterior (C)	occipital & posterior parietal	↔ caudal thalamus	
inferior (D)	transverse temporal gyrus of Heschl	↔ MGB	(small) includes auditory radiation

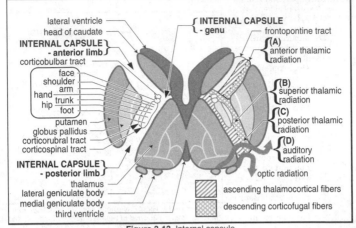

Figure 3-13 Internal capsule

3.6. Miscellaneous

OBERSTEINER-REDLICH ZONE (ORZ)

AKA root entry zone. Transition from CNS myelin to peripheral myelin of cranial nerves = area where root entry zone pressure from intracranial structures can cause cranial nerve symptoms (trigeminal neuralgias, hemifacial spasm, disabling positional vertigo, etc.)[33]. Also, zone where neoplasms tend to occur, especially acoustic neuroma. On Cr. N. VIII, the ORZ is 8-12 mm distal to exit point from brainstem, and is close to porus acusticus (especially common on vestibular division)[9 (p 695)].

DENTATE LIGAMENT

The spinal accessory nerve is dorsal to the dentate ligament. The dentate ligament separates dorsal from ventral nerve roots in the spinal nerves.

3.7. Neurophysiology

3.7.1. Blood-brain barrier

The passage of water-soluble substances from the blood to the CNS is limited by tight junctions (zonulae occludentes) which are found between cerebral capillary endothelial cells, limiting penetration of the cerebral parenchyma (blood-brain barrier, **(BBB)**), as well as between choroid plexus epithelial cells (blood-CSF barrier)[34]. A number of specialized mediated transport systems allow transmission of, among other things, glucose and certain amino acids (especially precursors to neurotransmitters).

The efficacy of the BBB is compromised in certain pathological states (e.g. tumor, infection, trauma, stroke, hepatic encephalopathy...), and can also be manipulated pharmacologically (e.g. hypertonic mannitol increases the permeability, whereas steroids reduce the penetration of small hydrophilic molecules).

The BBB is absent in the following areas: choroid plexus, hypophysis, tuber cinereum, area postrema, pineal and preoptic recess.

CEREBRAL EDEMA

Three basic types (diffusion-weighted MRI may be able to differentiate, *see page 136*):

1. **cytotoxic**: BBB is closed, therefore no protein extravassation, therefore no enhancement on CT or MRI. Cells swell then shrink. Seen e.g. in head injury
2. **vasogenic**: BBB disrupted. Protein (serum) leaks out of vascular system, and therefore may enhance on imaging. Extracellular space (**ECS**) expands. Cells are stable. Responds to corticosteroids (e.g. dexamethasone). Seen e.g. surrounding metastatic brain tumor
3. **ischemic**: a combination of the above. BBB closed initially, but then may open. ECS shrinks then expands. Fluid extravassates late. May cause delayed deterioration following intracerebral hemorrhage (*see page 855*)

3.7.2. Regional brain syndromes

This section serves to briefly describe typical syndrome associated with lesions in various areas of the brain. Unless otherwise noted, lesions considered are destructive.

1. frontal lobe
   A. unilateral injury:
      1. may produce few clinical findings except with very large lesions
      2. bilateral or large unilateral lesions: apathy, abulia
      3. the frontal eye field (for contralateral gaze) is located in the posterior frontal lobe (Br. area 8, shown as the striped area in *Figure 3-1*, page 68). Destructive lesions impair gaze to the contralateral side (patient looks <u>towards</u> the side of the lesion), whereas irritative lesions (i.e. seizures) cause the center to activate, producing contralateral gaze (patient looks <u>away</u> from the side of the lesion). Also *see page 584*
   B. bilateral injury: may produce apathy, abulia
   C. olfactory groove region: may produce Foster-Kennedy syndrome (*see below*)
   D. prefrontal lobes control "executive function": planning, prioritizing, organizing thoughts, suppressing impulses, understanding the consequences of decisions
2. parietal lobe: major features (*see page 87* for details)
   A. either side: cortical sensory syndrome, sensory extinction, contralateral homonymous hemianopia, contralateral neglect
   B. *dominant* parietal lobe lesion (left in most): language disorders (aphasias), Gerstmann's syndrome (*see page 87*), bilateral astereognosis
   C. *non-dominant* parietal lobe lesions: topographic memory loss, anosognosia and dressing apraxia
3. occipital lobe: homonymous hemianopia
4. cerebellum
   A. lesions of the cerebellar *hemisphere* cause ataxia in the <u>ipsilateral</u> limbs
   B. lesions of the cerebellar vermis cause truncal ataxia
5. brainstem: usually produces a mixture of cranial nerve deficits and long tract findings (*see below* for some specific brainstem syndromes)
6. pineal region
   A. Parinaud's syndrome: *see page 86*

FOSTER-KENNEDY SYNDROME

Usually from olfactory groove or medial third sphenoid wing tumor (usually meningioma). Now rare due to earlier detection by CT scan. Classic triad:

1. ipsilateral anosmia
2. <u>ipsilateral</u> central scotoma (with optic <u>atrophy</u> due pressure on optic nerve)
3. <u>contralateral</u> papilledema (from elevated ICP)

Occasionally ipsilateral proptosis will also occur due to orbital invasion of tumor.

3.7.2.1. Brain stem and related syndromes

WEBER'S SYNDROME

Cr. N. III palsy with contralateral hemiparesis (also see *Lacunar strokes*, page 776). Third nerve palsies from parenchymal lesions may be relatively pupil sparing.

BENEDIKT'S SYNDROME

Similar to Weber's, plus red nucleus lesion. Cr. N. III palsy with contralateral hemiparesis except arm which has hyperkinesia, ataxia, and a coarse intention tremor. Lesion: midbrain tegmentum involving red nucleus, brachium conjunctivum, and fascicles of III.

MILLARD-GUBLER SYNDROME

Facial (VII) & abducens (VI) palsy + contralateral hemiplegia (corticospinal tract) from lesion in base of pons (usually ischemic infarct, occasionally tumor).

PARINAUD'S SYNDROME

Convergence, accommodation and supranuclear upward gaze palsy (i.e. upgaze palsy with normal response to vertical doll's eyes) with lid retraction (upgaze palsy + lid retraction = "**setting sun sign**"). May have fixed pupils, dissociated light-near response, convergence spasm and nystagmus retractorius. Skew deviation may be a unilateral variant. When combined with downgaze palsy, Parinaud's syndrome (**PS**) is known as the **syndrome of the Sylvian aqueduct**.

Etiologies
1. masses pressing directly on quadrigeminal plate (e.g. pineal region tumors)
2. elevated ICP: secondary to compression of mesencephalic tectum by dilated suprapineal recess, e.g. in hydrocephalus

Differential diagnosis
Conditions affecting ocular motility that could mimic the upgaze palsy of PS:
1. Guillain-Barré syndrome
2. myasthenia gravis
3. botulism
4. hypothyroidism
5. there may be a gradual benign loss of upgaze with senescence

3.7.3. Jugular foramen syndromes

Contents of jugular foramen (**JF**): Cr. N. IX, X, XI, petrosal sinus, sigmoid sinus, some meningeal branches from the ascending pharyngeal and occipital arteries[35].

Nearby: Cr. N. XII passes through the hypoglossal canal in the occipital condyle. The carotid artery with the sympathetic plexus enters the carotid canal.

See *Table 3-11* for a summary and *Figure 3-14* for a schematic diagram of deficits in various JF syndromes.

Vernet's syndrome: AKA syndrome of the jugular foramen. Damage of nerves in JF itself, more likely due to intracranial lesion.

Collet-Sicard syndrome: More likely with lesion outside skull. If caused by an intracranial lesion, it would have to be of such a large size that it would usually produce brain stem compression → long tract findings.

Villaret's syndrome: Posterior retropharyngeal syndrome.

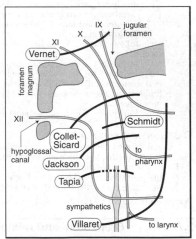

Figure 3-14 Schematic diagram of jugular foramen syndromes
(solid line through a nerve indicates a deficit)
(dashed line indicates ± involvement)

Table 3-11 Cranial nerve dysfunction in jugular foramen syndromes

Nerve	Result of lesion	――――――― SYNDROME* ―――――――					
		Vernet	Collet Sicard	Villaret	Tapia	Jackson	Schmidt
IX	loss of taste and sensation in posterior third of tongue	✖	✖	✖			
X	paralysis of vocal cords & palate, anesthesia of pharynx & larynx	✖	✖	✖	✖	✖	✖
XI	weak trapezius & SCM	✖	✖	✖	±	✖	✖
XII	tongue paralysis & atrophy		✖	✖	✖	✖	
sympathetics	Horner's syndrome			✖	±		

* KEY:✖ indicates dysfunction of that nerve; ± indicates involvement may or may not occur

3.7.4.   Parietal lobe syndromes[36 (p 308-12)]

PARIETAL LOBE ANATOMY
The parietal lobe is located behind the central sulcus, above the Sylvian fissure, merging posteriorly into the occipital lobe (the border on the medial surface of brain is defined by a line connecting the parieto-occipital sulcus to the pre-occipital notch).

PARIETAL LOBE NEUROPHYSIOLOGY
- either side: anterior parietal cortex organizes tactile precepts (probably contralateral) and integrates with visual and auditory sensation to build awareness of body and its spatial relations
- dominant side (on left in 97% of adults): understanding language, includes "cross-modal matching" (auditory-visual, visual-tactile, etc.). Dysphasia present with dominant lobe lesions often impedes assessment
- non-dominant side (right in most): integrates visual and proprioceptive sensation to allow manipulation of body and objects, and for certain constructional activities

CLINICAL SYNDROMES OF PARIETAL LOBE DISEASE

1. unilateral parietal lobe disease (dominant or non-dominant):
   A. cortical sensory syndrome (*see below*) and sensory extinction (neglecting 1 of 2 simultaneously presented stimuli). Large lesion → hemianesthesia
   B. congenital injury → mild hemiparesis & contralateral muscle atrophy
   C. homonymous hemianopia or visual inattentiveness
   D. occasionally: anosognosia
   E. neglect of contralateral half of body and visual space (more common with right side lesions)
   F. abolition of optokinetic nystagmus to one side
2. additional effects of *dominant* parietal lobe lesion (left in most):
   A. language disorders (aphasias)
   B. speech-related or verbally mediated functions, e.g. cross-modal matching (e.g. patient understands spoken words and can read, but cannot understand sentences with elements of relationships)
   C. **Gerstmann's syndrome**, classically:
       1. agraphia without alexia (patients can read but cannot write)
       2. left-right confusion
       3. digit agnosia: inability to identify finger by name
       4. acalculia
   D. tactile agnosia (bilateral astereognosis)
   E. bilateral ideomotor apraxia (inability to carry out verbal commands for activities that can otherwise be performed spontaneously with ease)
3. additional effects of *non-dominant* parietal lobe lesions (usually right):
   A. topographic memory loss
   B. anosognosia and dressing apraxia

Lesion of postcentral gyrus, especially area that maps to hand.
* sensory deficits:
    A. loss of position sense and of passive movement sense
    B. inability to localize tactile, thermal, and noxious stimuli
    C. astereognosis (inability to judge object size, shape, and identity by feel)
    D. agraphesthesia (cannot interpret numbers written on hand)
    E. loss of two point discrimination
* preserved sensations: pain, touch, pressure, vibration, temperature
* other features
    A. easy fatigability of sensory perceptions
    B. difficulty distinguishing simultaneous stimulations
    C. prolongation of superficial pain with hyperpathia
    D. touch hallucinations

ASOMATAGNOSIAS

ANTON-BABINSKI SYNDROME

Unilateral asomatagnosia. May seem more common with non-dominant (right) parietal lesions because it may be obscured by the aphasia that occurs with dominant (left) sided lesions.
1. anosognosia (indifference or unawareness of deficits, patient may deny that paralyzed extremity is theirs)
2. apathy (indifference to failure)
3. allocheiria (one-sided stimuli perceived contralaterally)
4. dressing apraxia: neglect of one side of body in dressing and grooming
5. extinction: contralaterally to double-sided simultaneous stimulation
6. inattention to an entire visual field (with or without homonymous hemianopia), with deviation of head, eyes, and torsion of body to unaffected side

APHASIAS

As related to parietal lobe lesions:
1. **Wernicke's aphasia**: lesion of auditory association areas or their separation from angular gyrus and primary auditory cortex. A fluent aphasia (normal sentence length & intonation, devoid of meaning). May include paraphasias. Lesion in region of Wernicke's area (Brodmann areas 40 & 39, see *Figure 3-1*, page 68)
2. **Broca's (motor) aphasia**: in reality, "apraxia" of motor sequencing for speech (speech and phonation muscles aren't paralyzed, and function for other activities), producing faltering, dysarthric speech. Lesion in region of Broca's area (Brodmann area 44, see *Figure 3-1*, page 68)
3. **global aphasia**: usually due to lesion that destroys large portion of language center; all aspects of speech and language affected
    A. unable to speak except for some clichés, habitual phrases, or expletives
    B. anomia (inability to name objects or parts of objects)
    C. verbal and motor perseveration
    D. unable to understand all except for a few words
    E. inability to read or write
4. conduction aphasia: due to disruption of connections between frontal and temporal speech areas, usually involving supramarginal gyrus. Similar to Wernicke's (fluent spontaneous speech and paraphasias), but patients understand spoken or written words, and are aware of their deficit. Repetition is severely affected
5. pure word blindness: AKA **alexia without agraphia** (rare) due to lesion in parieto-occipital lobe that interrupts connections between left angular gyrus and both occipital lobes. Patients can write, but are unable to read what they've written, and frequently seem unconcerned about this. Often accompanied by loss of ability to name colors. Reading and naming numbers usually preserved

3.7.5.   Babinski sign

Although regarded as the most famous sign in neurology, there is still disagreement over what constitutes a normal response and when abnormal responses should occur[37]. The following represents one interpretation.

The **plantar reflex (PR)** (AKA Babinski sign) is a primitive reflex, present in infancy, consisting of extension of the great toe in response to a noxious stimulus applied to the foot. The small toes may fan, but this is not consistent nor clinically important. The PR disappears usually at ≈ 10 months age (range: 6 mos to 12 yrs), presumably under inhibitory control as myelination of the CNS occurs, and the normal response then converts to plantarflexion of the great toe. An upper motor neuron **(UMN)** lesion anywhere along the pyramidal (corticospinal) tract from the motor strip down to ≈ L4 will result in a loss of inhibition, and the PR will be "unmasked" producing *extension* of the great toe. With such an UMN lesion, there may also be exaggeration of flexor synergy resulting in dorsiflexion of the ankle, and flexion of the knee and hip (AKA **triple flexor response**).

Neuroanatomy

The afferent limb of the reflex originates in cutaneous receptors restricted to the first sacral dermatome (S1) and travels proximally via the tibial nerve. The spinal cord segments involved in the reflex-arc lie within L4-S2. The efferent limb to the toe extensors travels via the peroneal nerve.

Etiologies

Lesions producing a PR need not be structural, but may be functional and reversible. etiologies are listed in *Table 3-12*.

Eliciting the PR, and variations

The optimal stimulus consists of stimulation of the lateral plantar surface and transverse arch in a single movement lasting 5-6 seconds[38]. Other means for applying noxious stimuli may also elicit the plantar reflex (even outside the S1 dermatome, although these do not produce toe flexion in normals). Described maneuvers include: **Chaddock** (scratch the lateral foot; positive in 3% where plantar stimulation was negative), **Schaeffer** (pinch the Achilles tendon), **Oppenheim** (slide knuckles down shin), **Gordon** (momentarily squeeze lower gastrocnemius), **Bing** (light pinpricks on dorsolateral foot), **Gonda** or **Stronsky** (pull the 4th or 5th toe down and out and allow it to snap back).

Hoffmann's sign

May signify a similar UMN interruption to the upper extremities. Elicited by snapping the distal phalanx of the middle finger: a pathologic response consists of thumb flexion (may be weakly present in normals). Can sometimes be seen as normal in young individual with diffusely brisk reflexes & positive jaw jerk, usually symmetric. When present pathologically, represents disinhibition of a C8 reflex, ∴ indicates lesion above C8.

Table 3-12 Differential diagnosis of the PR
• spinal cord injuries*
• cervical spinal myelopathy
• lesions in motor strip or internal capsule (CVA, tumor, contusion...)
• subdural or epidural hematoma
• hydranencephaly
• toxic-metabolic coma
• seizures
• trauma
• TIAs
• hemiplegic migraine
• motor neuron disease (ALS)

* in spinal cord injuries, the PR may initially be absent during the period of spinal "shock" (*see page 698*)

3.7.6.   Bladder neurophysiology

CENTRAL PATHWAYS

The primary coordinating center for bladder function resides within the nucleus locus coeruleus of the pons. This center synchronizes bladder contraction with relaxation of the urethral sphincter during voiding[39].

Voluntary cortical control primarily involves inhibition of the pontine reflex, and originates in the anteromedial portion of the frontal lobes and in the genu of the corpus callosum. In an uninhibited bladder (e.g. infancy) the pontine voiding center functions without cortical inhibition and the

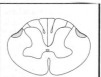

Figure 3-15 Location of spinal cord bladder efferents

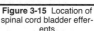

detrusor muscle contracts when the bladder reaches a critical capacity. Voluntary suppression from the cortex via the pyramidal tract may contract the external sphincter and may also inhibit detrusor contraction. Cortical lesions in this location → urgency incontinence with inability to suppress the micturition reflex[32 (p 1031)].

Efferents to the bladder travel in the dorsal portion of the lateral columns of the spi-

---

nal cord (shaded areas in *Figure 3-15*).

MOTOR

There are two sphincters that prevent the flow of urine from the bladder: internal (autonomic, involuntary control), and external (striated muscle, voluntary control).

Parasympathetics (PSN): the detrusor muscle of the bladder contracts and the internal sphincter relaxes under PSN stimulation. PSN preganglionic cell bodies reside in the intermediolateral grey of spinal cord segments S2-4. Fibers exit as ventral nerve roots and travel via pelvic splanchnic nerves (**nervi erigentes**) to terminate on ganglia within the wall of the detrusor muscle in the body and dome of the bladder.

Somatic nerves: somatic voluntary control descends in the pyramidal tract to synapse on motor nerves in S2-4, and then travels via the **pudendal nerve** to the external sphincter. This sphincter may be voluntarily contracted, but relaxes reflexly with opening of the internal sphincter at the initiation of micturition. Primarily maintains continence during ↑ vesical pressure (e.g. valsalva).

Sympathetics: sympathetic cell bodies lie within the intermediolateral gray column of lumbar spinal cord from segments T12 - L2. Preganglionic axons pass through the sympathetic chain (without synapsing) to the inferior mesenteric ganglion. Postganglionic fibers pass through the inferior hypogastric plexus to the bladder wall and internal sphincter. Sympathetics heavily innervate the bladder neck and trigone.
Sympathetics have little effect on bladder motor activity, but alpha adrenergic stimulation results in bladder neck closure which is necessary for bladder filling.

Pelvic nerve stimulation → increased sympathetic tone → detrusor relaxation & increased bladder neck tone (allowing larger volume to be accommodated).

SENSORY

Less well understood than motor innervation. Bladder wall stretch receptors sense bladder filling and send afferent signals via pelvic, pudendal and hypogastric nerves to spinal cord segments T10-L2 & S2-4. Fibers ascend primarily in the spinothalamic tract.

URINARY BLADDER DYSFUNCTION

The term **neurogenic bladder** describes bladder dysfunction due to lesions within the central or peripheral nervous systems. Some use the term synonymously with detrusor areflexia.

Dorsal (sensory) roots lesions interrupt the afferent limb, producing an atonic bladder that fills until dribbling and overflow incontinence occur. No sensation of bladder fullness is appreciated. Voluntary voiding is still possible, but is usually incomplete.

Detrusor hyperreflexia: Can result from interruption of efferents anywhere from cortex to sacral cord. When a critical volume is attained, reflex bladder emptying occurs. Clinically associated with frequent, uncontrollable, precipitous voiding. Cerebral lesions include: CVA, head injury, brain tumors, hydrocephalus, Parkinson's disease, various dementias, and MS. Cord lesions include anything that causes myelopathy (see *Myelopathy*, page 902).

Detrusor areflexia: Clinically correlates with difficulty initiating micturition, interrupted flow, and significant residual urine. Incontinence may result from over-distention of the bladder (**overflow incontinence**), or may be associated with absence of sphincter tone. Etiologies include: chronic infection, long-term bladder catheterization, certain drugs (especially phenothiazines), injury or tumor of the cauda equina or conus medullaris, myelomeningocele, and diabetes mellitus (autonomic neuropathy).

In general, regarding discrete neurologic lesions affecting the bladder[40]:
   1. **supraspinal** (lesions above the brain stem): loss of centrally mediated inhibition of the pontine voiding reflex. Usually produces involuntary bladder contractions with smooth and striated sphincter synergy, often with preserved sensation and voluntary striated sphincter function. Symptoms: urinary frequency or urgency, urgency incontinence, and nocturia[39]. If sensory pathways are interrupted, unconscious incontinence occurs (incontinence of the unawares type). Since muscles are coordinated, normal bladder pressures are maintained and there is low risk of high-pressure related renal dysfunction. Voluntary bladder emptying is usually maintained, and timed voiding together with anticholinergic medications are used in management. Areflexia may sometimes occur
   2. complete (or near complete) **spinal cord lesions**:

A. **suprasacral** (lesion <u>above</u> the S2 spinal <u>cord</u> level, which is ≈ T12/L1 vertebral body level in an adult): the sacral voiding center is located in the conus medullaris. Etiologies: spinal cord injuries (after spinal shock has subsided[A]), tumors, transverse myelitis. Usually develop <u>detrusor hyperreflexia</u> → involuntary bladder contractions without sensation (**automatic bladder**), smooth sphincter synergy, but striated dyssynergy (involuntary contraction of the external sphincter during voiding which produces a functional outlet obstruction with poor emptying and high vesical pressures). Bladder fills and empties spontaneously (or in response to lower extremity cutaneous stimulation). Bladder compliance is often reduced. Managed by intermittent catheterizations + anticholinergics

B. **infrasacral lesions** (lesion below the S2 spinal cord level): includes injury to conus medullaris, cauda equina or peripheral nerves (formerly referred to as lower motor neuron lesions). Etiologies: large HLD, trauma with compromise of spinal canal. Usually develop detrusor areflexia, and do not have involuntary bladder contractions. Reduced urinary flow rate or retention results, and voluntary voiding may be lost. Overflow incontinence develops. There may be reduced compliance during filling, and paralysis of the smooth sphincter. Usually associated with loss of bulbocavernosus and anal wink reflex (preserved in suprasacral lesions) and perineal sensory loss

3. **interruption of the peripheral reflex arc**: may produce disturbances similar to low spinal cord injury with detrusor areflexia, low compliance and inability to relax the striated sphincter

4. herniated lumbar disc: (*see page 302*) most consist initially of difficulty voiding, straining, or urinary retention. Later, irritative symptoms may develop

5. spinal stenosis (lumbar or cervical): urologic symptoms vary, and depend on the spinal level(s) involved and the type of involvement

6. cauda equina syndrome: usually produces urinary retention, although sometimes incontinence may occur (some cases are overflow incontinence) (*see page 305*)

7. peripheral neuropathies: such as with diabetes, usually produce impaired detrusor activity

8. neurospinal dysraphism: most myelodysplastic patients have an areflexic bladder with an open bladder neck. The bladder usually fills until the resting residual fixed external sphincter pressure is exceeded and the leakage occurs

9. **multiple sclerosis**: 50-90% of patients develop voiding symptoms at some time. The demyelination primarily involves the posterior and lateral columns of the cervical spinal cord. Detrusor hyperreflexia is the most common urodynamic abnormality (in 50-99% of cases), with bladder areflexia being less common (5-20%)

URINARY RETENTION

Etiologies of urinary retention:
1. bladder outlet obstruction (a brief differential diagnosis list is presented here)
   A. urethral stricture: retention tends to be progressive over time
   B. prostatic enlargement in males:
      1. benign prostatic hypertrophy (**BPH**) & prostate cancer: retention tends to be progressive over time
      2. acute prostatitis: onset of retention may be sudden
      3. rare: extruded prostatic stone
   C. women may develop a cystocele which can produce a urethral kink
   D. rare: urethral cancer
2. detrusor areflexia (*see page 90*) or hypotonia
   A. spinal cord injury
   B. cauda equina syndrome (*see page 305*)
   C. chronic infection
   D. long-term bladder catheterization
   E. certain drugs (narcotics, phenothiazines)
   F. injury of the cauda equina or conus medullaris, or of the spinal cord at or below the sacrum
      1. trauma
      2. tumor
      3. myelomeningocele

A. during spinal shock (*see page 698*), the bladder is acontractile and areflexic (detrusor areflexia); sphincter tone usually persists and urinary retention is the rule (urinary incontinence generally does not occur except with overdistention)

G. diabetes mellitus (autonomic neuropathy)

H. herpes zoster at the level of the sacral dorsal root ganglia[40 (p 967)]

I. incomplete opening of the bladder neck: occurs almost exclusively in young males with longstanding obstructive and irritative symptoms[40 (p 968)]

J. following severe bladder over distention from any of the above

3. postoperative retention: well-recognized but poorly understood. More common after lower urinary tract, perineal, gynecologic and anorectal operations. Anesthesia and analgesia may contribute to a number of factors[40 (p 969)]

4. psychogenic

EVALUATION OF BLADDER FUNCTION

URODYNAMICS

Usually combined with x-ray (cystometrogram (**CMG**)) or fluoro (videourodynamics). Measures intravesicular pressures during retrograde bladder filling through a urethral catheter, usually combined with sphincter electromyography. Presence or absence (detrusor areflexia, *see below*) of detrusor reflex is detected. If present, procedure is repeated, asking patient to suppress the urge to void. Inability to suppress is called an uninhibited detrusor reflex (AKA detrusor hyperreflexia, *see above*).

SPHINCTER ELECTROMYOGRAPHY (**EMG**)

Either via needle electrodes, or with externally mounted surface electrodes. Voluntary sphincter contraction tests intactness of supraspinal innervation. When combined with CMG, detects electrical activity in sphincters during associated phases of detrusor contraction.

VOIDING CYSTOURETHROGRAM AND INTRAVENOUS PYELOGRAPHY (**IVP**)

Voiding cystourethrogram (**VCUG**) detects urethral pathology (diverticula, strictures...), abnormalities of bladder (diverticula, detrusor trabeculations associated with longstanding contractions against high resistance...), and vesical-ureteral reflux.

TREATMENT

Goals are to preserve renal function (which usually involves prevention of UTIs, renal calculi, and ureteral reflux due to high intravesicular pressures) and optimization of urinary continence. Patients with inadequate emptying or increased bladder pressure are often managed by intermittent catheterizations and anticholinergics. Anticholinergics and behavioral therapy are used for patients with maintained voluntary bladder emptying with urinary frequency or urgency incontinence.

3.8. References

1. Naidich T P: MR imaging of brain surface anatomy. **Neuroradiology** 33 (Suppl): S95-9, 1991.

2. Ojemann G, Ojemann J, Lettich E, *et al.*: Cortical language localization in left, dominant hemisphere. An electrical stimulation mapping investigation in 117 patients. **J Neurosurg** 71: 316-26, 1989.

3. Suzuki A, Yasui N: Intraoperative localization of the central sulcus by cortical somatosensory evoked potentials in brain tumor: Case report. **J Neurosurg** 76: 867-70, 1992.

4. Willis W D, Grossman R G: *The brain and its environment*. In **Medical neurobiology**. C V Mosby, St. Louis, 3rd ed., 1981: pp 192-3.

5. Warwick R, Williams P L, (eds.): **Gray's anatomy**. 35th ed., W.B. Saunders, Philadelphia, 1973.

6. Kido D, LeMay M, Levinson A, *et al.*: Computed tomographic localization of the precentral gyrus. **Radiology** 135: 373-7, 1980.

7. Martin N, Grafton S, Viñuela F, *et al.*: Imaging techniques for cortical functional localization. **Clin**

8. Anderson J E: **Grant's atlas of anatomy**. Vol. 7, Williams and Wilkins, Baltimore, 1978.

9. Wilkins R H, Rengachary S S, (eds.): **Neurosurgery**. McGraw-Hill, New York, 1985.

10. Lusted L B, Keats T E: **Atlas of roentgenographic measurement**. 3rd ed. Year Book Medical Publishers, Chicago, 1972.

11. Ghajar J B G: A guide for ventricular catheter placement: Technical note. **J Neurosurg** 63: 985-6, 1985.

12. Watkins R G: *Anterior cervical approaches to the spine*. In **Surgical approaches to the spine**. Springer-Verlag, New York, 1983: pp 1-6.

13. Rhoton A L, Jr.: The cerebellopontine angle and posterior fossa cranial nerves by the retrosigmoid approach. **Neurosurgery** 47 (3 Suppl): S93-129, 2000.

14. Taveras J M, Wood E H: **Diagnostic neuroradiology**. 2nd ed. Williams and Wilkins, Baltimore, 1976.

15. Turnbull I M, Breig A, Hassler O: Blood supply of

Neurosurg 38: 132-65, 1990.

the cervical spinal cord in man. A microangiograph-
ic cadaver study. **J Neurosurg** 24: 951-65, 1966.

16. van der Zwan A, Hillen B, Tulleken C A F, *et al.*:
Variability of the territories of the major cerebral arteries. **J Neurosurg** 77: 927-40, 1992.

17. Fischer E: Die lageabweichungen der vorderen hir-
narterie im gefässbild. **Zentralbl Neurochir** 3: 300-
13, 1938.

18. Bouthillier A, van Loveren H R, Keller J T: Segments of the internal carotid artery: A new classification. **Neurosurgery** 38: 425-33, 1996.

19. Krayenbühl H, Yasargil M G: *Rontgenanatomie und
topographie der hirngefasse.* In **Zerebrale angiog-
raphie fur klinik und praxis**, Huber P, (ed.). Georg
Thieme Verlag, Stuttgart, 1979: pp 38-246.

20. Ecker A, Riemenschneider P A: In **Angiographic
localization of intracranial masses**, Charles C. Thomas, Springfield, Illinois, 1955: pp 433.

21. Krayenbühl H A, Yasargil M G: In **Cerebral angiography**. Butterworths, London, 2nd ed., 1968: pp
80-1.

22. Gibo H, Lenkey C, Rhoton A L: Microsurgical anatomy of the supraclinoid portion of the internal carotid artery. **J Neurosurg** 55: 560-74, 1981.

23. Renn W H, Rhoton A L: Microsurgical anatomy of
the sellar region. **J Neurosurg** 43: 288-98, 1975.

24. Rhoton A L., Jr.: The supratentorial arteries. **Neurosurgery** 51 (4 Suppl): S53-120, 2002.

25. Lister J R, Rhoton A L, Matsushima T, *et al.*: Microsurgical anatomy of the posterior inferior cerebellar
artery. **Neurosurgery** 10: 170-99, 1982.

26. Getch C C, O'Shaughnessy B A, Bendok B R, *et al.*:
Surgical management of intracranial aneurysms involving the posterior inferior cerebellar artery. **Contemp Neurosurg** 26 (9): 1-7, 2004.

27. Schmidek H H, Auer L M, Kapp J P: The cerebral
venous system. **Neurosurgery** 17: 663-78, 1985.

28. Taptas J N: The so-called cavernous sinus: A review
of the controversy and its implications for neurosurgeons. **Neurosurgery** 11: 712-7, 1982.

29. Sekhar L N: *Operative management of tumors involving the cavernous sinus.* In **Tumors of the cranial base: Diagnosis and treatment**, Sekhar L N
and Schramm V L, (eds.). Futura Publishing, Mount
Krisco, 1987: pp 393-419.

30. Umansky F, Nathan H: The lateral wall of the cavernous sinus: With special reference to the nerves related to it. **J Neurosurg** 56: 228-34, 1982.

31. van Loveren H R, Keller J T, El-Kalliny M, *et al.*:
The Dolenc technique for cavernous sinus exploration (cadaveric prosection). **J Neurosurg** 74: 837-
44, 1991.

32. Youmans J R, (ed.) **Neurological surgery**. 2nd ed.,
W. B. Saunders, Philadelphia, 1982.

33. Jannetta P J, Moller M B, Moller A R: Disabling positional vertigo. **N Engl J Med** 310: 1700-5, 1984.

34. Neuwelt E A, Barnett P A, McCormick C I, *et al.*:
Osmotic blood brain barrier modification: Monoclonal antibody, albumin, and methotrexate delivery
to cerebrospinal fluid and brain. **Neurosurgery** 17:
419-23, 1985.

35. Svien H J, Baker H L, Rivers M H: Jugular foramen
syndrome and allied syndromes. **Neurology** 13:
797-809, 1963.

36. Adams R D, Victor M: **Principles of neurology**.
2nd ed. McGraw-Hill, New York, 1981.

37. Marcus J C: Flexor plantar responses in children
with upper motor neuron lesions. **Arch Neurol** 49:
1198-9, 1992.

38. Dohrmann G J, Nowack W J: The upgoing great toe:
Optimal method of elicitation. **Lancet** 1: 339-41,
1973.

39. MacDiarmid S A: The ABCs of neurogenic bladder
for the neurosurgeon. **Contemp Neurosurg** 21 (4):
1-8, 1999.

40. Wein A J: *Neuromuscular dysfunction of the lower
urinary tract and its treatment.* In **Campbell's urology**, Walsh P C, Retik A B, Vaughan E D, *et al.*,
(eds.). W.B. Saunders, Philadelphia, 7th ed., 1998,
Vol. 1, Chapter 29: pp 953-1006.

4. Developmental

4.1. Arachnoid cysts

4.1.1. Arachnoid cysts, intracranial

AKA **leptomeningeal cysts**, distinct from *posttraumatic* leptomeningeal cysts (AKA growing skull fractures, *see page 668*), and unrelated to infection. Arachnoid cysts **(AC)** are congenital lesions that arise during development from splitting of arachnoid membrane (thus they are technically *intra-arachnoid* cysts).

"Temporal lobe agenesis syndrome" is a label that had been used to describe the findings with middle cranial fossa ACs. This term is now obsolete since brain volumes on each side are actually the same[1], bone expansion and shift of brain matter account for the parenchyma that appears to be replaced by the AC.

Incidence is 5 per 1000 in autopsy series.

Two types of histological findings[2]:
1. "simple arachnoid cysts": arachnoid lining with cells that appear to be capable of active CSF secretion. Middle fossa cysts seem to be exclusively of this type
2. cysts with more complex lining which may also contain neuroglia, ependyma, and other tissue types

PRESENTATION

Most ACs that become symptomatic do so in early childhood[3]. The presentation varies with location of the cyst, and oftentimes appear mild considering the large size of some.

Typical presentations are shown in *Table 4-1*[3] and include:

Table 4-1   Typical presentations of arachnoid cysts

Middle fossa cysts	Suprasellar cysts with hydrocephalus	Diffuse supra- or infratentorial cysts with hydrocephalus
seizures headache hemiparesis	intracranial hypertension craniomegaly developmental delay visual loss precocious puberty bobble-head doll syndrome	intracranial hypertension craniomegaly developmental delay

1. symptoms of intracranial hypertension (elevated ICP): H/A, N/V, lethargy
2. seizures
3. sudden deterioration:
    A. due to hemorrhage (into cyst or subdural compartment): middle fossa cysts are notorious for hemorrhage due to tearing of bridging veins. Some sports organizations do not allow participation in contact sports for these patients
    B. due to rupture of the cyst
4. as a focal protrusion of the skull
5. with focal signs/symptoms of a space occupying lesion
6. incidental finding discovered during evaluation for unrelated condition
7. suprasellar cysts may additionally present with[4]:
    A. hydrocephalus (probably due to compression of the third ventricle)
    B. endocrine symptoms: occurs in up to 60%. Includes precocious puberty
    C. head bobbing (the so-called "bobble-head doll syndrome"[5]): considered suggestive of suprasellar cysts, but occurs in as few as 10%

D. visual impairment

DISTRIBUTION

Almost all occur in relation to an arachnoid cistern (exception: intrasellar, the only one that is extradural, *see Table 4-2*). Retrocerebellar arachnoid cysts may mimic Dandy-Walker malformation (*see page 110*).

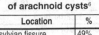

Table 4-2 Distribution of arachnoid cysts[6]

Location	%
sylvian fissure	49%
CPA	11%
supracollicular	10%
vermian	9%
sellar & suprasellar	9%
interhemispheric	5%
cerebral convexity	4%
clival	3%

EVALUATION

Routine evaluation with CT or MRI is usually satisfactory. Further evaluation with CSF contrast or flow studies (cisternograms, ventriculograms) are only occasionally necessary for the diagnosis of midline suprasellar and posterior fossa lesions[3] (for Differential diagnosis, *see Intracranial cysts*, page 928). See *Figure 4-1* for classification for middle fossa cysts.

CT SCAN

Smooth bordered non-calcified extraparenchymal cystic mass with density similar to CSF and no enhancement with IV contrast. Expansion of nearby bone by remodelling is usually seen, confirming their chronic nature. Often associated with ventriculomegaly (in 64% of supratentorial and 80% of infratentorial cysts).

Convexity or middle fossa cysts exert mass effect on adjacent brain and may compress ipsilateral lateral ventricle and cause midline shift. Suprasellar, quadrigeminal plate, and midline posterior-fossa cysts may compress the third and fourth ventricle and cause hydrocephalus by obstructing the foramina of Monro or the Sylvian aqueduct.

MRI

Better than CT in differentiating the CSF contained in arachnoid cysts from the fluid of neoplastic cysts. May also show cyst walls.

CISTERNOGRAMS AND/OR VENTRICULOGRAMS

Using either iodinated contrast or radionuclide tracers. Variable rate of opacification has resulted in difficulty correlating results with operative findings. Some cysts are actually diverticula, and may fill with radiotracer or contrast.

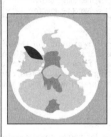

Type I: small, biconvex, located in anterior temporal tip. No mass effect. Communicates with subarachnoid space on water-soluble contrast CT cisternogram **(WS-CTC)**

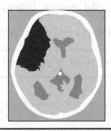

Type II: involves proximal and intermediate segments of Sylvian fissure. Completely open insula gives rectangular shape. Partial communication on WS-CTC

Type III: involves entire Sylvian fissure. Marked midline shift. Bony expansion of middle fossa (elevation of lesser wing of sphenoid, outward expansion of squamous temporal bone). Minimal communication on WS-CTC. Surgical treatment usually does not result in total reexpansion of brain (may approach type II lesion)

Figure 4-1 CT Classification of Sylvian fissure cysts[7]

Many (but not all) authors recommend not treating arachnoid cysts that do not cause mass effect or symptoms, regardless of their size and location. Surgical treatment options are summarized in *Table 4-3*.

Table 4-3   Surgical treatment options for arachnoid cysts

Procedure	Advantages	Disadvantages
drainage by needle aspiration or burr hole evacuation	• simple • quick	• high rate of recurrence of cyst and neurologic deficit
craniotomy, excising cyst wall and fenestrating it into basal cisterns	• permits direct inspection of cyst (may help with diagnosis) • loculated cysts (rare) treated more effectively • avoids permanent shunt (in some cases) • allows visualization of bridging vessels (small advantage)	• subsequent scarring may block fenestration allowing reaccumulation of cyst • flow through subarachnoid space may be deficient; many patients develop shunt dependency post-op • significant morbidity and mortality (may be due to abrupt decompression)
endoscopic cyst fenestration through a burr hole[8]	• as above	• as above
shunting of cyst into peritoneum or into vascular system	• definitive treatment • low morbidity/mortality • low rate of recurrence	• patient becomes "shunt dependent" • risk of infection of foreign body (shunt)

CYST SHUNTING
Probably the best overall treatment. For shunting into peritoneum, use a low pressure valve. If there is concurrent ventriculomegaly, one may simultaneously place a ventricular shunt (e.g. through a "Y" connector). Ultrasound, ventriculoscope, or image guidance may assist in locating suprasellar cysts. Shunting of middle fossa ACs may also be accomplished through the lateral ventricle, thus shunting both compartments[9].

SUPRASELLAR CYSTS
Treatments proposed include:
1. transcallosal cystectomy[10]
2. percutaneous ventriculo-cystostomy: procedure of choice of Pierre-Kahn et al.[4]. Performed via a paramedian coronal burr hole through the lateral ventricle and foramen of Monro (may be facilitated by using a ventriculoscope[8])
3. subfrontal approach (for fenestration or removal): dangerous and ineffective[4]
4. ✘ ventricular drainage: ineffective (actually promotes cyst enlargement)

OUTCOME
Even following successful treatment a portion of the cyst may remain due to the remodeling of the bone and chronic shift of brain contents. Hydrocephalus may develop following treatment. Endocrinopathies tend to persist even after successful treatment of suprasellar cysts.

4.1.2.   Arachnoid cysts, intraspinal

Almost always dorsal. With a ventral cyst, consider a neurenteric cyst (*see below*).

4.2.   Intracranial lipomas

Intracranial and intraspinal lipomas are felt to be of maldevelopmental origin[11 (p 706)] and may arise from failure of involution of the primitive meninges[12].

Epidemiology of intracranial lipomas
Incidence: 8 in 10,000 autopsies. Usually found in or near the midsagittal plane, particularly over the corpus callosum (lipomas in this region are frequently associated

with agenesis of the corpus callosum, *see page 114*). The tuber cinereum and quadrigeminal plate are less frequently affected[13]. Rarely, the CP angle or cerebellar vermis may be involved. May occur in isolation, but also has been described in association with a number of congenital anomalies, including: trisomy 21, Pai's syndrome, frontal encephalocele, facial anomalies.... Other midline abnormalities may also be found: agenesis of the corpus callosum, myelomeningocele, and spina bifida[12].

Evaluation
May be diagnosed by CT, MRI (study of choice), and by ultrasound in infants.

CT: Low density, may have peripheral calcification (difficult to appreciate on MRI)[12]. Differential diagnosis on CT: primarily between dermoid cyst, teratoma[14] and germinoma[12].

MRI: characteristic finding is a midline lesion with signal characteristics of fat (high intensity on T1WI, low intensity on T2WI).

Presentation
Often discovered incidentally. Large lipomas may be associated with seizures, hypothalamic dysfunction, or hydrocephalus (possibly from compression of the aqueduct). Associated findings that may or may not be directly related: mental retardation, behavioral disorders and headache.

Treatment
Direct surgical approach is seldom necessary for intracranial lipomas[14]. Shunting may be required for cases where hydrocephalus results from obstruction of CSF circulation[14].

4.3.   Hypothalamic hamartomas

Hypothalamic hamartomas are rare non-neoplastic congenital malformations consisting of masses of ectopic neuronal tissue that arise from the inferior hypothalamus or tuber cinereum.

Clinical manifestations include:
1. specific types of seizures:
   A. gelastic (laughing) seizures: the most characteristic type. Resistant to medical management, and can lead to cognitive and behavioral deficits later
   B. later development of complex partial seizures, drop attacks, tonic seizures, tonic-clonic seizures, and secondarily generalized seizures
2. behavioral disturbances: aggressive behavior, rage attacks...
3. precocious puberty
4. mental retardation
5. visual impairment

Two subtypes of hypothalamic hamartomas[15]:
1. pedunculated or parahypothalamic: narrower base attached to the floor of the hypothalamus (not arising within hypothalamus). Tend to produce precocious puberty more than they produce gelastic seizures
2. sessile or intrathalamic: broad attachment to hypothalamus. More often associated with gelastic seizures

Treatment
Treatment alternatives:
1. medical treatment for precocious puberty
2. stereotactic radiosurgery
3. surgical resection

Indications for surgery:
1. precocious puberty that fails to respond to medical therapy
2. gelastic seizures: no effective medical therapy[16]
3. neurologic deficit from mass effect of the tumor

Surgical options:
1. pterional approach
2. transcallosal anterior interforniceal[17]
3. neuroendoscopic approach: difficult because ventricles are rarely dilated

---

4.4.   Neurenteric cysts

No uniformly accepted nomenclature. Working definition: a CNS cyst lined by endothelium primarily resembling that of the GI tract, or less often, the respiratory tract. Not true neoplasms. The most common alternate term is **enterogenous cyst**, with less common terms including: teratomatous cyst, intestinoma, archenteric cyst[18], enterogene cyst, and endodermal cyst. Usually affect the upper thoracic and cervical spine, and other associated developmental vertebral anomalies are common[19]. May also occur intracranially, including 6 reported cases in the cerebellopontine angle **(CPA)**[18]. Spinal neurenteric cysts **(NEC)** may have a fistulous or fibrous connection to the GI tract and some call these **endodermal sinus cysts**. These are thought to occur as a result of incomplete developmental separation of the notochord from the primitive gut. This is distinct from isolated intracranial enterogenous cysts.

Clinical
Most commonly present during the first decade of life[19]. Pain or myelopathy from the intraspinal mass are the most common presentations in older children and adults. Neonates and young children may present with cardiorespiratory compromise from an intrathoracic mass or cervical spinal cord compression[19]. Meningitis may occur from the fistulous tract, especially in newborns and infants.

Histology
Most are simple cysts lined by cuboidal-columnar epithelium and mucin secreting goblet cells. Less common types of epithelium described include: stratified squamous and pseudostratified columnar, and ciliated epithelial cells. Mesodermal components may be present, including smooth muscle and adipose tissue, and some have called these teratomatous cysts[20, 21] which is not to be confused with teratomas which are true germinal cell neoplasms.

Treatment
Complete removal of spinal NECs usually reverses the symptoms. An adherent capsule may prevent complete resection of intracranial lesions, which predisposes to delayed recurrence and mandates long-term follow-up.

4.5.   Craniofacial development

4.5.1.   Normal development

FONTANELLES
Anterior fontanelle: the largest fontanelle. Diamond shaped, 4 cm (AP) x 2.5 cm (transverse) at birth. Normally closes by age 2.5 yrs.

Posterior fontanelle: triangular. Normally closes by age 2-3 mos.

Sphenoid and mastoid fontanelles: small, irregular. Normally, former closes by age 2-3 mos, latter by age 1 yr.

CRANIAL VAULT
Growth: largely determined by growth of brain; 90% of adult head size is achieved by age 1 yr; 95% by age 6 yrs. Growth essentially ceases at age 7 yrs. By end of 2nd yr, bones have interlocked at sutures and further growth occurs by accretion and absorption.
Skull is unilaminar at birth. Diplöe appear by 4th yr and reach a maximum by age 35 yrs (when diploic veins form).
Mastoid process: formation commences by age 2 yrs, air cell formation occurs during 6th yr.

4.5.2.   Craniosynostosis

Originally called craniostenosis. Incidence: ≈ 0.6/1000 live births.

Primarily a prenatal deformity, postnatal craniosynostosis (**CSO**) occurs uncommonly (postnatal causes consist primarily of positional alterations which may not represent true synostosis). CSO is rarely associated with hydrocephalus (**HCP**)[22]. The assertion that CSO may follow CSF shunting for HCP is unproven (*see page 199*). Other causes for failure of normal skull growth include lack of brain growth due to any of the causes of arrested development of the cerebral hemispheres (lissencephaly, micropolygyria, some cases of hydranencephaly...).

Treatment is usually surgical. In most instances, the indication for surgery is for cosmesis and to prevent the severe psychological effects of having a disfiguring deformity. However, with multiple CSO, brain growth may be impeded by the unyielding skull. Also, ICP may be pathologically elevated, and although this is more common in multiple CSO[23], elevated ICP occurs in ≈ 11% of cases with a single stenotic suture. Coronal synostosis can cause amblyopia. Most cases of single suture involvement can be treated with linear excision of the suture. Involvement of multiple sutures or the skull base usually requires the combined efforts of a neurosurgeon and craniofacial surgeon, and may need to be staged in some cases. Risks of surgery include: blood loss, seizures, stroke.

DIAGNOSIS

Many cases of "synostosis" are really due to positional flattening (e.g. "lazy lambdoid", *see below*). If this is suspected, instruct parents to keep head off of flattened area and recheck patient in 6-8 weeks: if it was positional, it should be improved, if it was CSO then it usually declares itself. The diagnosis of CSO may be aided by:

1. palpation of a bony prominence over the suspected synostotic suture (exception: lambdoidal synostosis, *see below*)
2. gentle firm pressure with the thumbs fails to cause relative movement of the bones on either side of the suture
3. plain skull x-rays:
   A. lack of normal lucency in center of suture. Some cases with normal x-ray appearance of the suture (even on CT) may be due to focal bony spicule formation[24]
   B. beaten copper calvaria (*see page 101*), sutural diastasis and erosion of the sella may be seen in cases of increased ICP[25]
4. CT scan:
   A. helps demonstrate cranial contour
   B. may show thickening and/or ridging at the site of synostosis
   C. will demonstrate hydrocephalus if present
   D. may show expansion of the frontal subarachnoid space[26]
   E. three-dimensional CT may help better visualize abnormalities
5. in questionable cases, a technetium bone scan can be performed[27]:
   • there is little isotope uptake by any of the cranial sutures in the first weeks of life
   • in prematurely closing sutures, increased activity compared to the other (normal) sutures will be demonstrated
   • in completely closed sutures, no uptake will be demonstrated
6. MRI: usually reserved for cases with associated intracranial abnormalities. Often not as helpful as CT
7. measurements, such as occipito-frontal-circumference may <u>not</u> be abnormal even in the face of a deformed skull shape

Increased ICP

Evidence of increased ICP in the newborn with craniosynostosis include:
1. radiographic signs (on plain skull x-ray or CT, *see above*)
2. failure of calvarial growth (unlike the non-synostotic skull where increased ICP causes macrocrania in the newborn, here it is the synostosis that *causes* the increased ICP and lack of skull growth)
3. papilledema
4. developmental delay

TYPES OF CRANIOSYNOSTOSIS

SAGITTAL SYNOSTOSIS

The most common CSO affecting a single suture; 80% male. Results in **dolichocephaly** or **scaphocephaly** (boat shaped skull) with frontal bossing, prominent occiput, palpable keel-like sagittal ridge. OFC remains close to normal, but the biparietal diameter is markedly reduced.

Surgical treatment

Skin incision may be longitudinal or transverse. A linear "strip" craniectomy is performed, excising the sagittal suture from the coronal to the lambdoid suture, preferably within the first 3-6 months of life. The width of the strip should be at least 3 cm, no proof exists that interposing artificial substances (e.g. silastic sheeting over the exposed edges of the parietal bone) retards the recurrence of synostosis. Great care is taken to avoid dural laceration with potential injury to the underlying superior sagittal sinus. The child is followed and reoperated if fusion recurs before 6 months age. After ≈ 1 yr age, more extensive cranial remodelling is usually required.

CORONAL SYNOSTOSIS

Accounts for 18% of CSO, more common in females. In **Crouzon's syndrome** this is accompanied by abnormalities of sphenoid, orbital and facial bones (hypoplasia of midface), and in Apert's syndrome is accompanied by syndactyly[28]. Unilateral coronal CSO → **plagiocephaly** with forehead on affected side flattened or concave above eye (normal side falsely appears to bulge abnormally), supra-orbital margin higher than normal side (on skull x-ray → **harlequin eye sign**). The orbit rotates out on the abnormal side, and can produce amblyopia. Without treatment, flattened cheeks develop and the nose deviates to the normal side (root of nose tends to rotate towards deformity).

Bilateral coronal CSO (usually in craniofacial dysmorphism with multiple suture CSO, e.g. Apert's) → **brachycephaly** with broad, flattened forehead (**acrocephaly**). When combined with premature closure of frontosphenoidal and frontoethmoidal sutures, results in foreshortened anterior fossa with maxillary hypoplasia, shallow orbits, progressive proptosis.

Surgical treatment

Simple strip craniectomy of the involved suture has been used, often with excellent cosmetic result. However, some argument that this may not be adequate has been presented. Therefore, a more current recommendation is to do frontal craniotomy (uni- or bilateral) with lateral canthal advancement by taking off orbital bar.

METOPIC SYNOSTOSIS

At birth, the frontal bone consists of two halves separated by the frontal or metopic suture. Abnormal closure results in a pointed forehead with a midline ridge (**trigonocephaly**). Many of these have a 19p chromosome abnormality and are retarded.

LAMBDOID SYNOSTOSIS

Epidemiology

Long considered a clinical rarity with a reported incidence of 1-9% of CSO[29], recent reports suggest a higher incidence of 10-20%[30] which may be due to an actual increased incidence, or simply to increased awareness or changing diagnostic criteria. More common in males (male:female = 4:1), and the right side is involved in 70% of cases. Usually presents between 3-18 months of age, but may be seen as early as 1-2 months of age.

Controversy exists regarding the criteria for this condition, and some authors differentiate between those cases which appear to have a primary abnormality of the lambdoid suture from those which may be due to positional flattening, the so-called "lazy lambdoid". Others do not make this distinction, and sometimes refer to the condition as occipital plagiocephaly to avoid the need to implicate abnormalities of the lambdoid suture.

Positional flattening (or molding) may be produced by:
1. decreased mobility: patients who constantly lie supine with the head to the same side, e.g. cerebral palsy, mental retardation, prematurity, chronic illness
2. abnormal postures: <u>congenital torticollis</u>[31], congenital disorders of the cervical spine
3. intentional positioning: trend since 1992 to place newborns in a supine sleeping position to reduce the risk of sudden infant death syndrome (**SIDS**)[32], sometimes

with a foam wedge to tilt the child to one side to reduce the risk of aspiration
4. intrauterine etiologies[33]: intrauterine crowding (e.g. from multiparous births or large fetal size), uterine anomalies

Clinical findings

Flattening of the occiput. May be unilateral or bilateral. If unilateral, it is sometimes termed **lambdoid plagiocephaly** which when severe also produces bulging of the ipsilateral forehead resulting in a "rhomboid" skull with the ipsilateral ear located anterior and inferior to the contralateral ear. The contralateral orbit and forehead may also be flattened. This may be confused with hemifacial microsomia or with plagiocephaly seen in unilateral coronal craniosynostosis. Bilateral lambdoid synostosis produces brachycephaly with both ears displaced anteriorly and inferiorly[29]. Unlike the palpable ridge of sagittal or coronal synostosis, an <u>indentation</u> may be palpated along the synostotic lambdoid suture (although a perisutural ridge may be found in some).

Diagnostic evaluation

The physical exam is the most important aspect of diagnosis. Skull x-ray may help differentiate (*see below*). If the skull x-ray is equivocal, prevent the infant from laying on the affected side for several weeks. A bone scan should be obtained if no improvement occurs (*see below*). In definite cases of synostosis, and for some cases of refractory positional flattening (which usually corrects with time, but may take up to 2 years) surgical treatment may be indicated.

Skull x-ray: Shows a sclerotic margin along one edge of the lambdoid suture in 70% of cases. Local "beaten copper cranium" (**BCC**) occasionally may be seen due to indentations in the bone from underlying gyri which may be due to locally increased ICP. BCC produces a characteristic mottled appearance of the bone with lucencies of varying depth having round and poorly marginated edges. BCC correlates with generalized ↑ ICP only when it is seen with sellar erosion and sutural diastasis[25].

CT scan: Bone windows may show eroded or thinned inner table in the occipital region in 10-20% of cases[30], > 95% are on the side of the involvement. The suture may appear closed. Brain windows show parenchymal brain abnormalities in < 2% (heterotopias, hydrocephalus, agenesis of the corpus callosum; but ≈ 70% will have significant expansion of the frontal subarachnoid space (may be seen in synostosis of other sutures, *see above*).

Bone scan: Isotope uptake in the lambdoid suture increases during the first year, with a peak at 3 months of age[34] (following the usual inactivity of the first weeks of life). The findings with synostosis are those typical for CSO (*see page 99*).

Treatment

Early surgical treatment is indicated in cases with severe craniofacial disfigurement or those with evidence of increased ICP. Otherwise, children may be managed nonsurgically for 3-6 months. The majority of cases will remain static or will improve with time and simple nonsurgical intervention. Approximately 15% will continue to develop a significant cosmetic deformity.

Nonsurgical management[36]:
Although improvement can usually be attained, some degree of permanent disfigurement is frequent.
Repositioning will be effective in ≈ 85% of cases. Patients are placed on the unaffected side or on the abdomen. Infants with occipital flattening from torticollis should have aggressive physical therapy and resolution should be observed within 3-6 months.
More severe involvement may be treated with a trial of molding helmets[36] (however, no controlled study has proven the efficacy).

Surgical treatment:
Required in only ≈ 20% of cases. The ideal age for surgery is between 6 and 18 months. The patient is positioned prone on a well-padded cerebellar headrest (the face should be lifted and gently massaged every ≈ 30 minutes by the anesthesiologist to prevent pressure injuries).
Surgical options range from simple unilateral craniectomy of the suture to elaborate reconstruction by a craniofacial team.
Linear craniectomy extends from the sagittal suture to the asterion is often adequate for patients ≤ 12 weeks of age without severe disfigurement. Great care is taken to avoid dural laceration near the asterion which is in the region of the transverse sinus. The excised suture demonstrates an <u>internal</u> ridge. Better results are obtained with earlier surgery, more radical surgery may be necessary after the age of 6 months.
Average blood loss for uncomplicated cases is 100-200 ml and therefore transfusion

is often required.

MULTIPLE SYNOSTOSES

Fusion of many or all cranial sutures → **oxycephaly** (tower skull with undeveloped sinuses and shallow orbits). These patients have elevated ICP.

CRANIOFACIAL DYSMORPHIC SYNDROMES

Over 50 syndromes have been described, *Table 4-4*, shows a few selected ones.

A number of craniosynostosis syndromes are due to mutations in the FGFR (fibroblast growth factor receptor) genes. FGFR gene-related craniosynostosis syndromes include some classic syndromes (Apert, Crouzon, Pfeiffer…) as well as several newer entities (Beare-Stevenson, Muenke, Jackson-Weiss syndromes). All exhibit autosomal dominant inheritance.

Table 4-4 Selected craniofacial dysmorphic syndromes (modified[37 (p 123-4)])

Syndrome	– – – Genetics – – –		Craniofacial findings	Associated findings
	Sporadic	Inherited		
Crouzon (craniofacial dysostosis)	yes (25%)	FGFR AD*	CSO of coronal & basal skull sutures, maxillary hypoplasia, shallow orbits, proptosis	HCP rare
Apert (acrocephalosyndactyly)	yes (95%)	FGFR AD	same as Crouzon	syndactyly of digits 2,3,4; shortened UE, HCP common
Kleeblattschadel	yes	AD	CSO with trilobular skull	isolated, or with Apert's or thanatophoric dwarfism

* abbreviations: AD = autosomal dominant; FGFR = fibroblast growth factor receptor gene-related; CSO = craniosynostosis; HCP = hydrocephalus; UE = upper extremities

4.5.3. Encephalocele

Cranium bifidum is a defect in the fusion of the cranial bone, it occurs in the midline, and is most common in the occipital region. If meninges and CSF herniate through the defect, it is called a meningocele. If meninges and cerebral tissue protrude, it is called an encephalocele.

Encephalocele AKA **cephalocele** is an extension of intracranial structures outside of the normal confines of the skull. One case was seen for every five cases of spinal myelomeningoceles[38]. A nasal polypoid mass in a newborn should be considered an encephalocele until proven otherwise. See also *Differential diagnosis,* page 938.

CLASSIFICATION

System based on Suwanwela and Suwanwela[39]:
1. occipital: often involves vascular structures
2. cranial vault: comprises ≈ 80% of encephaloceles in Western hemisphere
   A. interfrontal
   B. anterior fontanelle
   C. interparietal: often involves vascular structures
   D. temporal
   E. posterior fontanelle
3. fronto-ethmoidal: AKA sincipital; 15% of encephaloceles; external opening into face in one of the following 3 regions:
   A. nasofrontal: external defect in the nasion
   B. naso-ethmoidal: defect between nasal bone and nasal cartilage
   C. naso-orbital: defect in the antero-inferior portion of medial orbital wall
4. basal: 1.5% of encephaloceles; (*see below*)
   A. transethmoidal: protrudes into nasal cavity through defect in cribriform plate
   B. spheno-ethmoidal: protrudes into posterior nasal cavity
   C. transsphenoidal: protrudes into sphenoid sinus or nasopharynx through patent craniopharyngeal canal (foramen cecum)
   D. fronto-sphenoidal or spheno-orbital: protrudes into orbit through superior

orbital fissure

5. posterior fossa: usually contains cerebellar tissue and ventricular component

BASAL ENCEPHALOCELE

The only group that does not produce a visible soft tissue mass. May present as CSF leak or recurrent meningitis. May be associated with other craniofacial deformities, including: cleft lip, bifid nose, optic-nerve dysplasia, coloboma and microphthalmia, hypothalamic-pituitary dysfunction.

Iniencephaly is characterized by defects around the foramen magnum, rachischisis and retrocollis. Most are stillborn, some survive up to age 17.

ETIOLOGY

Two main theories:

1. arrested closure of normal confining tissue allows herniation through persistent defect
2. early outgrowth of neural tissue prevents normal closure of cranial coverings

TREATMENT

Occipital encephalocele

Surgical excision of the sac and its contents with water-tight dural closure. It must be kept in mind that vascular structures are often included in the sac. Hydrocephalus is often present and may need to be treated separately.

Basal encephalocele

Caution: a transnasal approach to a basal encephalocele (even for biopsy alone) may be fraught with intracranial hemorrhage, meningitis, or persistent CSF leak. Usually a combined intracranial approach (with amputation of the extracranial mass) and transnasal approach is used.

OUTCOME

Occipital encephalocele

The prognosis is better in occipital meningocele than in encephalocele. The prognosis is worse if a significant amount cerebral tissue is present in the sac, if the ventricles extend into the sac, or if there is hydrocephalus. Less than ≈ 5% of infants with encephalocele develop normally.

4.6. Chiari malformation

The term "Chiari malformation" (after pathologist, Hans Chiari) is preferred for type 1 malformations, with the term "Arnold-Chiari malformation" reserved for type 2 malformation.

The Chiari malformations consists of four types of hindbrain abnormalities, probably unrelated to each other. The majority of Chiari malformations are types 1 or 2 (*see Table 4-5*), a very limited number of cases comprise the remaining types.

Table 4-5 Comparisons of Chiari type 1 and 2 anomalies (adapted[40])

Finding	Chiari type 1	Chiari type 2
caudal dislocation of medulla	unusual	yes
caudal dislocation into cervical canal	tonsils	inferior vermis, medulla, 4th ventricle
spina bifida (myelomeningocele)	may be present	rarely absent
hydrocephalus	may be absent	rarely absent
medullary "kink"	absent	present in 55%
course of upper cervical nerves	usually normal	usually cephalad
usual age of presentation	young adult	infancy
usual presentation	cervical pain, suboccipital H/A	progressive hydrocephalus, respiratory distress

TYPE 1 CHIARI MALFORMATION

❢ Key features:
- a heterogeneous entity with the common feature of impaired CSF circulation through the foramen magnum
- cerebellar tonsillar herniation: variable, > 5 mm below the foramen magnum is common, but is not essential nor diagnostic of the condition
- treatment, when indicated, is surgical, but aspects of what that surgery should entail are controversial (enlargement of foramen magnum is usually involved)
- associated with syringomyelia in 30-70% which almost always improves with treatment of the Chiari malformation

AKA primary cerebellar ectopia[41], AKA adult Chiari malformation (since it tends to be diagnosed in the 2nd or 3rd decade of life). A heterogeneous group of conditions, with the underlying commonality of disruption of normal CSF flow through the foramen magnum (**FM**). Some cases are congenital, but others are acquired.

Classically described as a rare abnormality restricted to caudal displacement of cerebellum with tonsillar herniation below the foramen magnum (see *MRI* below for criteria) and "peg-like elongation of tonsils". Unlike Chiari type 2, the medulla is not caudally displaced (some authors disagree on this point[42]), the brainstem is not involved, lower cranial nerves are not elongated, and upper cervical nerves do not course cephalad. Syringomyelia[A] of the spinal cord is present in 30-70%[43]. Hydrocephalus occurs in 7-9% of patients with Chiari type 1 malformation and syringomyelia[43].

Cerebellar tonsil descent below FM with impaction, while common, is no longer a sine qua non of diagnosis.

Etiology: may be associated with
1. a small posterior fossa
   A. underdevelopment of the occipital bone
   B. low lying tentorium (the roof of the p-fossa)
   C. thickened or elevated occipital bone (the floor of the p-fossa)
   D. space occupying lesion in p-fossa: arachnoid, cyst, tumor (e.g. FM meningioma or cerebellar astrocytoma), hypervascular dura
2. has been described with just about anything that takes up intracranial space
   A. chronic subdural hematomas
   B. hydrocephalus
3. following lumboperitoneal shunt (*see page 189*) or multiple (traumatic) LPs[44]: acquired Chiari 1 malformation (usually asymptomatic)
4. arachnoid web or scar or fibrosis around brainstem and tonsils near FM
5. abnormalities of the upper cervical spine
   A. hypermobility of the craniovertebral junction
   B. Klippel-Feil syndrome
   C. occipitalization of the atlas
   D. anterior indentation at foramen magnum: e.g. basilar invagination or retroversion of the odontoid process
6. Ehlers-Danlos syndrome
7. craniosynostosis: especially cases involving all sutures
8. retained rhomboid roof: rare

EPIDEMIOLOGY

Average age at presentation is 41 years (range: 12-73 yrs). Slight female preponderance (female:male = 1.3:1). Average duration of symptoms clearly related to Chiari malformation is 3.1 yrs (range: 1 month-20 yrs); if nonspecific complaints, e.g. H/A, are included, this becomes 7.3 years[45]. This latency is probably lower in the MRI era.

CLINICAL

Patients with Chiari type 1 malformation may present due to any or all of the following:
1. compression of brain stem at the level of the foramen magnum
2. hydrocephalus

A. True hydromyelia probably doesn't occur. CSF flow has not been documented in man, and it is generally not possible to find communication between the syrinx and the central canal in Chiari 1 patients

3. syringomyelia
4. isolation of the intracranial pressure compartment from the spinal compartment causing transient elevations of intracranial pressure
5. 15-30% of patients with adult Chiari malformation are asymptomatic[46]

SYMPTOMS

The most common symptom is pain (69%), especially headache which is usually felt in the suboccipital region (*see Table 4-6*). H/A are often brought on by neck extension or valsalva maneuver. Weakness is also prominent, especially unilateral grasp. Lhermitte's sign may also occur. Lower extremity involvement usually consists of bilateral spasticity.

SIGNS

See *Table 4-7*. Three main patterns of clustering of signs[42]:
1. foramen magnum compression syndrome (22%): ataxia, corticospinal and sensory deficits, cerebellar signs, lower cranial nerve palsies. 37% have severe H/A
2. central cord syndrome (65%): dissociated sensory loss (loss of pain & temperature sensation with preserved touch & JPS), occasional segmental weakness, and long tract signs (syringomyelic syndrome[47]), 11% have lower cranial nerve palsies
3. cerebellar syndrome (11%): truncal and limb ataxia, nystagmus, dysarthria

Downbeat nystagmus is considered a characteristic of this condition. 10% will have a normal neurologic exam with occipital H/A as their only complaint. Some patients may present primarily with spasticity.

NATURAL HISTORY

The natural history is not known with certainty (only 2 reports on "natural history"). A patient may remain stable for years, with intermittent periods of deterioration. Rarely, spontaneous improvement may occur (debated).

EVALUATION

Plain x-rays

Of 70 skull x-rays, only 36% were abnormal (26% showed basilar impression, 7% platybasia, and 1 patient each with Paget's and concave clivus); in 60 C-spine x-rays, 35% were abnormal (including assimilation of atlas, widened canal, cervical fusions, agenesis of posterior arch of atlas).

MRI

Diagnostic test of choice. Easily shows many of the classic abnormalities described earlier, including tonsillar herniation, as well as hydrosyringomyelia which occurs in 20-30% of cases. Also demonstrates ventral

Table 4-6 Presenting symptoms in Chiari 1 malformation (71 cases[42])

Symptom	%
pain	69%
H/A	34%
neck (suboccipital, cervical)	13%
girdle	11%
arm	8%
leg	3%
weakness (1 or more limbs)	56%
numbness (1 or more limbs)	52%
loss of temperature sensation	40%
painless burns	15%
unsteadiness	40%
diplopia	13%
dysphasia	8%
tinnitus	7%
vomiting	5%
dysarthria	4%
miscellaneous	
dizziness	3%
deafness	3%
fainting	3%
facial numbness	3%
hiccough	1%
facial hyperhidrosis	1%

Table 4-7 Presenting signs in Chiari I malformation (127 patients[45])

Sign	%
hyperactive lower extremity reflexes	52%
nystagmus*	47%
gait disturbance	43%
hand atrophy	35%
upper extremity weakness	33%
"cape" sensory loss	31%
cerebellar signs	27%
hyperactive upper extremity reflexes	26%
lower cranial nerve dysfunction	26%
Babinski sign	24%
lower extremity weakness	17%
dysesthesia	17%
fasciculation	11%
Horner's sign	6%

* classically: downbeat nystagmus on vertical movement, and rotatory nystagmus on horizontal movement; also includes oscillopsia[48]

brain stem compression when present.

Tonsillar herniation: Criteria for the descent of the tonsillar tips below the foramen magnum **(FM)** to diagnose Chiari type 1 malformation have gone through a number of reconsiderations.

Σ | Tonsillar herniation identified radiographically is of limited prognostic value to diagnose Chiari malformation, and requires clinical correlation.

Initially, > **5 mm** was defined as clearly pathologic[49] (with 3-5 mm being borderline). Barkovich[50] found tonsillar positions as shown in *Table 4-8*, and *Table 4-9* shows the effect of utilizing 2 vs. 3 mm as the lowest normal position.

Table 4-8 Location of cerebellar tonsils below foramen magnum[50]

Group	Mean*	Range
normal	1 mm above	8 mm above to 5 mm below
Chiari I	13 mm below	3-29 mm below

* based on measurements in 200 normals and 25 Chiari I patients taken in relation to the lower part of the foramen magnum

Table 4-9 Criteria for Chiari I[50]

Criteria for lowest extent of tonsils accepted as normal	Sensitivity for Chiari I	Specificity for Chiari I
2 mm below FM	100%	98.5%
3 mm below FM	96%	99.5%

The tonsils normally ascend with age[51] as shown in *Table 4-10*.

Patients with syringohydromyelia without hindbrain herniation that responded to p-fossa decompression have been described[52] (so-called "**Chiari zero malformation**"). Conversely, 14% of patients with tonsillar herniation > 5 mm are asymptomatic[53] (average extent of ectopia in this group was 11.4 ± 4.86 mm).

Potentially more significant than the absolute tonsillar descent is the amount of compression of the brainstem at the FM, best appreciated on axial T2WI MRI though the FM. Complete obliteration of CSF signal and compression of the brainstem at the FM by impacted tonsils is a common significant finding.

Cine MRI: May demonstrate blockage of CSF flow at FM.

Myelography

Only 6% false negative. Must run dye all the way up to the foramen magnum.

CT

CT has difficulty evaluating the foramen magnum region due to bony artifact. When combined with intrathecal water-soluble contrast (myelogram), reliability improves. Findings: tonsillar descent and/or ventricular dilatation.

Table 4-10 Tonsillar descent below FM related to age[51]

Age (years)	2 S.D.* (mm)
0-9	6
10-29	5
30-79	4
80-89	3

* S.D. = standard deviation. Descent > 2 S.D. beyond normal is suggested as a criteria for tonsillar ectopia

TREATMENT

Indications for surgery

Since patients respond best when operated on within 2 years of the onset of symptoms (see *Operative results* below), early surgery is recommended for symptomatic patients. Asymptomatic patients may be followed and operated upon if and when they become symptomatic. Patients who have been symptomatic and stable for years may be considered for observation, with surgery indicated for signs of deterioration.

Surgical techniques

The most frequently performed operation is posterior fossa decompression (suboccipital craniectomy), with or without other procedures (usually combined with dural patch grafting and cervical laminectomy of C1, sometimes to C2 or C3).

Some authors advocate performing a transoral clivus-odontoid resection in cases with ventral brain-stem compression, as they feel these patients may potentially deteriorate with posterior fossa decompression alone[54]. Since this deterioration was reversible with odontoidectomy, it may be reasonable to perform this procedure on patients who show signs of deterioration or progression of basilar impression on serial MRIs after posterior fossa decompression.

OPERATIVE FINDINGS

See *Table 4-11*. Tonsillar herniation is present in all cases (by definition); the most common position being at C1 (62%). Fibrous adhesions between dura, arachnoid and tonsils with occlusion of foramina of Luschka and Magendie in 41%. The tonsils separated easily in 40%.

SURGICAL COMPLICATIONS

After suboccipital craniectomy plus C1-3 laminectomy in 71 patients, with dural patch grafting in 69, one death due to sleep apnea occurred 36 hrs post-op. Respiratory depression was the most common post-op complication (in 10 patients), usually within 5 days, mostly at night. Close respiratory monitoring is therefore recommended[42]. Other risks of the procedure include: CSF leak, herniation of cerebellar hemispheres, vascular injuries (to PICA...).

Table 4-11 Operative findings in Chiari I
(71 patients[42])

Finding	%
tonsillar descent	
below foramen magnum	4%
C1	62%
C2	25%
C3	3%
unspecified level	6%
total	100%
adhesions	41%
syringomyelia	32%
dural band (at foramen magnum or C1 arch)	30%
vascular abnormalities*	20%
skeletal abnormalities	
inverted foramen magnum	10%
keel of bone	3%
C1 arch atresia	3%
occipitalization of C1 arch	1%
cervicomedullary "hump"	12%

*   vascular abnormalities: PICA dilated or abnormal course in 8 patients (PICA often descends to lower margin of tonsils[47]), large dural venous lakes in 3

OPERATIVE RESULTS

See *Table 4-12*. Patients with pre-op complaints of pain generally respond well to surgery. Weakness is less responsive to surgery, especially when muscle atrophy is present[54]. Sensation may improve when the posterior columns are unaffected and the deficit is due to spinothalamic involvement alone.

Rhoton feels that the main benefit of operation is to arrest progression.

The most favorable results occurred in patients with cerebellar syndrome (87% showing improvement, no late deterioration). Factors that correlate with a worse outcome are the presence of atrophy, ataxia, scoliosis, and symptoms lasting longer than 2 years[54].

Table 4-12 Long-term follow-up after surgery for Chiari I malformation
(69 patients, 4 years mean follow-up[42])

early improvement of pre-op symptoms	82%
percent of above that relapsed*	21%
early improvement of pre-op signs	70%
no change from pre-op status	16%
worse than pre-op	0

*   these patients deteriorated to pre-op status (none deteriorated further) within 2-3 years of surgery; relapse occurred in 30% with foramen magnum compression syndrome, and in 21% with central cord syndrome

TYPE 2 (ARNOLD)-CHIARI MALFORMATION

Usually associated with myelomeningocele (**MM**), or rarely spina bifida occulta.

PATHOPHYSIOLOGY

Probably does not result from tethering of the cord by the accompanying MM. Primary dysgenesis of the brainstem with multiple other developmental anomalies is more likely[55].

Major findings

Caudally dislocated cervicomedullary junction, pons, 4th ventricle and medulla. Cerebellar tonsils located at or below the foramen magnum. Replacement of normal cervicomedullary junction flexure with a "kink-like deformity".

Other possible associated findings:
1. beaking of tectum
2. absence of the septum pellucidum with enlarged interthalamic adhesion: absence of the septum pellucidum is thought to be due to necrosis with resorption secondary to hydrocephalus, and not a congenital absence[56 (p 178)]
3. poorly myelinated cerebellar folia
4. hydrocephalus: present in most
5. heterotopias
6. hypoplasia of falx
7. microgyria
8. degeneration of lower cranial nerve nuclei
9. bony abnormalities:
    A. of cervicomedullary junction
    B. assimilation of atlas
    C. platybasia
    D. basilar impression
    E. Klippel-Feil deformity: *see page 119*
10. hydromyelia
11. craniolacunia of the skull (*see below*)

PRESENTATION

Findings are due to brain stem and lower cranial nerve dysfunction. Onset is rare in adulthood. The presentation of neonates differs substantially from older children, and neonates were more likely to develop rapid neurological deterioration with profound brain stem dysfunction over a period of several days than were older children in whom symptoms were more insidious and rarely as severe[57].

Findings include[57, 58]:
1. swallowing difficulties (neurogenic dysphagia) (69%)[59]. Manifests as poor feeding, cyanosis during feeding, nasal regurgitation, prolonged feeding time, or pooling of oral secretions. Gag reflex often decreased. More severe in neonates
2. apneic spells (58%): due to impaired ventilatory drive. More common in neonates
3. stridor (56%): more common in neonates, usually worse on inspiration (abductor and occasionally adductor vocal cord paralysis seen on laryngoscopy) due to 10th nerve paresis; usually transient, but may progress to respiratory arrest
4. aspiration (40%)
5. arm weakness (27%) that may progress to quadriparesis[60]
6. opisthotonos (18%)
7. nystagmus: especially downbeat nystagmus
8. weak or absent cry
9. facial weakness

DIAGNOSTIC EVALUATION

Skull films

May demonstrate cephalofacial disproportion from congenital HCP. **Craniolacunia** (AKA **lückenschädel**) in 85% (round defects in the skull with sharp borders, separated by irregularly branching bands of bone). Low lying internal occipital protuberance (foreshortened posterior fossa). Enlarged foramen magnum in 70%; elongation of upper cervical lamina[40].

CT and/or MRI findings

(* items with an asterisk are best appreciated on MRI)
- primary findings
    A. "Z" bend deformity of medulla*
    B. cerebellar peg
    C. tectal fusion ("tectal beaking")
    D. enlarged massa intermedia (interthalamic adhesion)*
    E. elongation/cervicallization of medulla
    F. low attachment of tentorium
- associated findings
    A. hydrocephalus
    B. syringomyelia in the area of the cervicomedullary junction (reported incidence in pre MRI era[54] ranges from 48-88%)
    C. trapped fourth ventricle
    D. agenesis/dysgenesis of corpus callosum*

E.   cerebellomedullary compression

Laryngoscopy

Performed in patients with stridor to rule out croup or other upper respiratory tract infection.

TREATMENT

*   insert CSF shunt for hydrocephalus (or check function of existing shunt)
*   if neurogenic dysphagia, stridor, or apneic spells occur, expeditious posterior fossa decompression is recommended (*see below*) (required in 18.7% of MM patients[58]); before recommending decompression, always make sure the patient has a functioning shunt!

Surgical decompression

NB. it has been argued that part of the explanation for the poor operative results in infants is that many of the neurological findings may be due in part to intrinsic (uncorrectable) abnormalities which surgical decompression cannot improve[61, 62]. A dissenting view is that the histologic lesions are due to chronic brain stem compression and concomitant ischemia, and that expeditious brain stem decompression should be carried out when any of the following critical warning signs develop: neurogenic dysphagia, stridor, apneic spells[57].

Surgical technique:

Decompression of cerebellar tonsils, usually with dural graft to decompress dura. Patients is placed prone, with the neck flexed. A suboccipital craniectomy is combined with a cervical laminectomy which must be carried down to the bottom of the tonsillar tip[60]. A thick constricting dural band is usually found between the C1 arch and foramen magnum. The dura is opened in a "Y" shaped incision. Caution when opening the dura above the level of the foramen magnum in infants as they have a well developed occipital sinus and may have large dural lakes[58]. DO NOT attempt to dissect tonsils from underlying medulla. In cases with a significant syringomyelia cavity, a syringo-subarachnoid shunt is placed[57].

Tracheostomy (usually temporary) is recommended if stridor and abductor laryngeal palsy were present pre-op. Close post-op respiratory monitoring is needed for obstruction and reduced ventilatory drive (mechanical ventilation is indicated for hypoxia or hypercarbia).

OUTCOME

68% had complete or near complete resolution of symptoms, 12% had mild to moderate residual deficits, and 20% had no improvement (in general, neonates fared worse than older children)[57].

Respiratory arrest is the most common cause of mortality (8 of 17 patients who died), with the rest due to meningitis/ventriculitis (6 patients), aspiration (2 patients), and biliary atresia (1 patient)[58].

In follow-up ranging 7 mos-6 yrs, 37.8% mortality in operated patients.

Pre-op status and the rapidity of neurologic deterioration were the most important prognosticators. Mortality rate is 71% in infants having cardiopulmonary arrest, vocal cord paralysis or arm weakness within 2 weeks of presentation; compared to 23% mortality in patients with a more gradual deterioration. Bilateral vocal cord paralysis was a particularly poor prognosticator for response to surgery[57].

OTHER CHIARI MALFORMATIONS

CHIARI TYPE 3

Rare. The most severe form. Displacement of posterior fossa structures, with cerebellum herniated through foramen magnum into cervical canal, often with a high cervical or suboccipital encephalomeningocele. Usually incompatible with life.

CHIARI TYPE 4

Cerebellar hypoplasia without cerebellar herniation.

4.7.   Dandy-Walker malformation

Atresia of foramina of Magendie and Luschka[63]. This results in agenesis of the cerebellar vermis with a large posterior fossa cyst communicating with an enlarged 4th ventricle (some retrocerebellar arachnoid cysts mimic Dandy-Walker, but these do not have vermian agenesis and the cyst does not open into the 4th ventricle).

Hydrocephalus occurs in 90% of cases, and Dandy-Walker malformation is present in 2-4% of all cases of hydrocephalus.

Associated abnormalities
CNS abnormalities include agenesis of the corpus callosum in 17%[64], and occipital encephalocele in 7%. Other findings include heterotopias, spina bifida, syringomyelia, microcephaly, dermoid cysts, porencephaly, and Klippel-Feil deformity. Most have an enlarged posterior fossa with elevation of the torcular herophili.

Systemic abnormalities include[64]: facial abnormalities (e.g. angiomas, cleft palates, macroglossia, facial dysmorphia), ocular abnormalities (e.g. coloboma, retinal dysgenesis, microphthalmia), and cardiovascular anomalies (e.g. septal defects, patent ductus arteriosus, aortic coarctation, dextrocardia). Note: be aware of the likelihood of a cardiac abnormality when considering surgery on these patients.

Treatment
In the absence of hydrocephalus, these may be followed. When treatment is necessary, shunt the posterior fossa cyst. In the rare patient with aqueductal stenosis, shunt the lateral ventricles also. Shunting the ventricles alone is contraindicated because of the risk of upward herniation.

Prognosis
75-100% chance of survival. Only 50% have normal IQ. Ataxia, spasticity, and poor fine motor control are common. Seizures occur in 15%.

4.8.   Aqueductal stenosis

Aqueductal stenosis (AqS) produces what is sometimes called **triventricular hydrocephalus**, characterized by a normal sized 4th ventricle and enlarged third and lateral ventricles on MRI or CT. Most cases occur in children, however some present for the first time in adulthood.

ETIOLOGIES
1. a congenital malformation: may be associated with Chiari malformation or neurofibromatosis
2. acquired
    A. due to inflammation (following hemorrhage or infection, e.g. syphilis, T.B.)
    B. neoplasm: especially brainstem astrocytomas (including tectal gliomas, *see page 422*), lipomas
    C. quadrigeminal plate arachnoid cysts

IN INFANCY
AqS is a frequent cause of congenital hydrocephalus (HCP) (up to 70% of cases[37]), but occasionally may be the result of HCP. Patients with congenital AqS usually have HCP at birth or develop it within ≈ 2-3 mos. Congenital AqS may be due to an X-linked recessive gene[38]. Four types of congenital AqS described by Russell (summarized[65]):
1. forking: multiple channels (often narrowed) with normal epithelial lining that do not meet, separated by normal nervous tissue. Usually associated with other congenital abnormalities (spina bifida, myelomeningocele)
2. periaqueductal gliosis: luminal narrowing due to subependymal astrocytic proliferation
3. true stenosis: aqueduct histologically normal
4. septum

AqS may be an overlooked cause of "normal pressure hydrocephalus" in the adult[66]. It is unknown why some cases of AqS would remain occult, and manifest only in adulthood. In one series of 55 cases[67], 35% had duration of symptoms < 1 year, 47% for 1-5 years; the longest was 40 yrs. Although most follow this longstanding benign course, there are reports of elevated ICP and sudden death.

Symptoms

See *Table 4-13*. Headache was the most common symptom, and had characteristics of H/A associated with elevated ICP. Visual changes were next, and usually consisted of blurring or loss of acuity. Endocrine changes included menstrual irregularities, hypothyroidism, and hirsutism.

Signs

Papilledema was the most common finding (53%). Visual fields were normal in 78%, the remainder having reduced peripheral vision, increased blind spots, quadrantic or hemianopic field cuts, or scotomata. Intellectual impairment was present in at least 36%. Other signs included: ataxia (29%), "pyramidal tract signs" in 44% (mild hemi- or paraparesis (22%), spasticity (22%), or Babinski's (20%)), anosmia (9%).

Table 4-13 Symptoms of aqueductal stenosis presenting in adulthood
(55 patients > 16 years age[67])

Symptom	No.	%
H/A	32	58%
visual disturbances	22	40%
mental deterioration	17	31%
gait disturbance	16	29%
frequent falling	13	24%
endocrine disturbance	10	18%
nausea/vomiting	9	16%
seizures	8	15%
incontinence	7	13%
vertigo	6	11%
LE weakness	4	7%
hemiparesis or hemianesthesia	4	7%
diplopia	3	5%
dysarthria	1	
deafness	1	

EVALUATION

MRI is the test of choice. MRI will show the absence of the normal flow void in the Sylvian aqueduct. Contrast should be given to rule-out tumor.

TREATMENT (OF NON-TUMORAL AqS)

Although treatments of the primary lesion have been attempted (e.g. lysis of aqueductal septum), this has fallen into disfavor with the improved efficacy of CSF shunting. CSF is usually shunted to the peritoneum or the vascular system, however shunting to subarachnoid space is also feasible (once obstruction at the level of the arachnoid granulations has been ruled out). A Torkildson shunt may work in adult cases[65], however pediatric patients with obstructive hydrocephalus may not have an adequately developed subarachnoid space for this to function properly.

Follow-up of at least two years to rule-out tumor is recommended.

4.9. Neural tube defects

CLASSIFICATION

Various classification systems exist, this one is adapted from Lemire[68].
1. neurulation defects: non-closure of the neural tube results in open lesions
    A. craniorachischisis: total dysraphism. Many die as spontaneous abortion
    B. **anencephaly**: AKA exencephaly. Due to failure of fusion of the anterior neuropore. Neither cranial vault nor scalp covers the partially destroyed brain. Uniformly fatal. Risk of recurrence in future pregnancies: 3%
    C. meningomyelocele: most common in lumbar region
        1. myelomeningocele (**MM**): *see page 115*
        2. myelocele
2. postneurulation defects: produces skin-covered (AKA closed) lesions (some may also be considered "migration abnormalities", *see below*)
    A. cranial

1. microcephaly: *see below*
2. **hydranencephaly**: loss of significant portion of cerebral hemispheres which are replaced by CSF. Must be differentiated from maximal hydrocephalus (*see page 180*)
3. holoprosencephaly: *see below*
4. **lissencephaly**: *see below*
5. porencephaly: *see below* to distinguish from schizencephaly
6. agenesis of corpus callosum: *see below*
7. cerebellar hypoplasia/Dandy-Walker syndrome: *see page 110*
8. macroencephaly AKA megalencephaly: *see below*

B. spinal
1. diastematomyelia, diplomyelia: see *Split cord malformation*, page 122
2. hydromyelia/syringomyelia: *see page 349*

Migration abnormalities

A slightly different classification scheme defines the following as abnormalities of neuronal migration (some are considered postneurulation defects, *see above*):
1. **lissencephaly**: The most severe neuronal migration abnormality. Maldevelopment of cerebral convolutions (probably an arrest of cortical development at an early fetal age). Infants are severely retarded and usually don't survive > 2 yrs
   A. **agyria**: completely smooth surface
   B. **pachygyria**: few broad & flat gyri with shallow sulci
   C. **polymicrogyria**: small gyri with shallow sulci. May be difficult to diagnose by CT/MRI, and may be confused with pachygyria
2. **heterotopia**: abnormal foci of gray matter which may be located anywhere from the subcortical white matter to the subependymal lining of the ventricles
3. **schizencephaly**:
   A. cleft that communicates with the ventricle (as may be demonstrated on CT cisternogram)
   B. lined with cortical grey matter. This is the key to differentiate from **porencephaly**, a cystic lesion lined with connective or glial tissue that may communicate with the ventricular system, often caused by vascular infarcts or following intracerebral hemorrhage or penetrating trauma (including repeated ventricular punctures)
   C. pia and arachnoid fuse
   D. two forms: open lipped (large cleft to ventricle) and close lipped (walls fused)

HOLOPROSENCEPHALY

AKA **arhinencephaly**. Failure of the telencephalic vesicle to cleave into two cerebral hemispheres. The degree of cleavage failure ranges from the severe alobar (single ventricle, no interhemispheric fissure) to semilobar and lobar (less severe malformations). The olfactory bulbs are usually small and the cingulate gyrus remains fused. Median faciocerebral dysplasia is common, and the degree of severity parallels the extent of the cleavage failure (*see Table 4-14*). Trisomy is often the cause of this malformation, although normal karyotypes are common. Survival beyond infancy is uncommon, most survivors are severely retarded, a minority are able to function in society. Shunt dependent hydrocephalus develops in some of these children. The risk of holoprosencephaly is increased in subsequent pregnancies of the same couple.

Table 4-14   The five facies of severe holoprosencephaly[69]

Type of face	Facial features	Cranium and brain findings
cyclopia	single eye or partially divided eye in single orbit; arhinia with proboscis	microcephaly; alobar holoprosencephaly
ethmocephaly	extreme orbital hypotelorism; separate orbits; arhinia with proboscis	microcephaly; alobar holoprosencephaly
cebocephaly	orbital hypotelorism; proboscis-like nose; no median cleft lip	microcephaly; usually has alobar holoprosencephaly
with median cleft lip	orbital hypotelorism; flat nose	microcephaly; sometimes has trigonocephaly; usually has alobar holoprosencephaly
with median philtrum-premaxilla anlage	orbital hypotelorism; bilateral lateral cleft lip with median process representing philtrum-premaxillary anlage; flat nose	microcephaly; sometimes has trigonocephaly; semilobar or lobar holoprosencephaly

MICROCEPHALY

Definition: head circumference more than 2 standard deviations below the mean for sex and gestational age. Terms that are sometimes used synonymously: microcrania, microcephalus. Not a single entity, many of the conditions in *Table 4-14* may be associated with microcephaly. It may also result from maternal cocaine abuse[70]. It is important to differentiate microcephaly from a small skull resulting from craniosynostosis in which surgical treatment may provide opportunity for improved cerebral development.

MACROENCEPHALY[37 (PP 109)]

AKA macrencephaly, AKA megalencephaly (not to be confused with *macrocephaly*, which is enlargement of the skull (*see page 919*)). Not a single pathologic entity. An enlarged brain which may be due to: hypertrophy of gray matter alone, gray and white matter, presence of additional structures (glial overgrowth, diffuse gliomas, heterotopias, metabolic storage diseases...). May be seen in neurocutaneous syndromes (especially neurofibromatosis).

Brains may weigh up to 1600-2850 grams. IQ may be normal, but developmental delay, retardation, spasticity and hypotonia may occur. Head circumference is 4-7 cm above mean. The usual signs of hydrocephalus (frontal bossing, bulging fontanelle, "setting sun" sign, scalp vein engorgement) are absent. Imaging studies (CT or MRI) show normal sized ventricles and can be used to rule out extra-axial fluid collections.

RISK FACTORS

1. early administration of prenatal vitamins (especially 0.4 mg of folic acid daily[71-73]) may <u>reduce</u> the incidence of neural tube defects (**NTDs**) (confirm that vitamin B_{12} levels are normal, *see page 904*)
2. maternal heat exposure in the form of hot-tubs, saunas or fever (but not electric blankets) in the first trimester was associated with an increased risk of NTDs[74]
3. use of valproic acid (Depakene®) during pregnancy is associated with a 1-2% risk of NTD[75]
4. obesity (before and during pregnancy) increases the risk of NTD[76, 77]
5. maternal cocaine abuse may increase the risk of microcephaly, disorders of neuronal migration, neuronal differentiation and myelination[70]

PRENATAL DETECTION OF NEURAL TUBE DEFECTS

Serum alpha-fetoprotein (AFP)

(See *Alpha-fetoprotein* on page 501 for background). A high maternal serum AFP (≥ 2 multiples of the median for the appropriate week of gestation) between 15-20 weeks gestation carries a relative risk of 224 for neural tube defects, and an abnormal value (high or low) was associated with 34% of all major congenital defects[78]. The sensitivity of maternal serum AFP for spina bifida was 91% (10 of 11 cases), it was 100% for 9 cases of anencephaly. However, other series show a lower sensitivity. Closed lumbosacral spine defects, accounting for ≈ 20% of spina bifida patients[79], will probably be missed by serum AFP screening, and may also be missed on ultrasound. Since maternal serum AFP rises during normal pregnancy, an overestimate of gestational age may cause an elevated AFP to be interpreted as normal, and an underestimate may cause a normal level to be interpreted as elevated[80].

Ultrasound

Prenatal ultrasound will detect 90-95% of cases of spina bifida, and thus in cases of elevated AFP, it can help differentiate NTDs from non-neurologic causes of elevated AFP (e.g. omphalocele), and can help to more accurately estimate gestational age.

Amniocentesis

For pregnancies subsequent to a MM, if prenatal ultrasound does not show spinal dysraphism, then amniocentesis is recommended (even if abortion is not considered, it may allow for optimal post-partum care if MM is diagnosed). <u>Amniotic</u> fluid AFP levels are elevated with open neural tube defects, with a peak between weeks 13-15 of pregnancy. Amniocentesis also carries a ≈ 6% risk of fetal loss in this population.

4.9.1.   Agenesis of the corpus callosum

A failure of commissuration occurring ≈ 2 weeks after conception. The corpus callosum **(CC)** forms from rostrum (genu) to splenium[81], thus in most cases there may be an anterior portion (genu) with no splenium (the converse occurs less frequently). Results in expansion of the third ventricle and separation of the lateral ventricles (which develop dilated occipital horns and atria, and concave medial borders).

Incidence
1 in 2,000-3,000 neuroradiological examinations.

Associated neuropathologic findings[13]
* porencephaly
* microgyria
* interhemispheric lipomas and lipomas of the corpus callosum (*see page 96*)
* arhinencephaly
* optic atrophy
* colobomas
* hypoplasia of the limbic system
* bundles of Probst: aborted beginnings of corpus callosum, bulge into lateral ventricles
* loss of horizontal orientation of cingulate gyrus
* schizencephaly (*see page 112*)
* anterior and hippocampal commissures may be totally or partially absent[82]
* hydrocephalus
* cysts in the region of the corpus callosum
* spina bifida with or without myelomeningocele
* absence of the septum pellucidum: *see page 122*

Possible presentation
* hydrocephalus
* microcephaly
* seizures (rare)
* precocious puberty
* disconnection syndrome: more likely with acquired CC defect than in congenital

May be an incidental finding, and by itself may have no clinical significance. However, may be occur as part of a more complex clinical syndrome or chromosomal abnormality (e.g. Aicardi syndrome: agenesis of CC, seizures, retardation, patches of retinal pigmentation).

4.9.2.   Spinal dysraphism (spina bifida)

DEFINITIONS[38]

spina bifida occulta	Congenital absence of a spinous process and variable amounts of lamina. No visible exposure of meninges or neural tissue (*see below*).

The following two entities are grouped together under the term **spina bifida aperta** (*aperta* from the Latin for "open") or **spina bifida cystica**.

meningocele	Congenital defect in vertebral arches with cystic distension of meninges, but no abnormality of neural tissue. One third have some neurologic deficit.
myelomeningocele	Congenital defect in vertebral arches with cystic dilatation of meninges and structural or functional abnormality of spinal cord or cauda equina (*see below*).

SPINA BIFIDA OCCULTA

Occurs in ≈ 20-30% of North Americans. Often an incidental finding, usually of no clinical importance when it occurs alone. However, it may occasionally be associated with diastematomyelia, tethered cord, lipoma, or dermoid tumor.

When symptomatic from one of the associated conditions, the presentation is that of tethered cord (gait disturbance, leg weakness and atrophy, urinary disturbance, foot deformities..., see *Tethered cord syndrome*, page 120). The defect may be palpable, and there may be overlying cutaneous manifestations (see *cutaneous stigmata of dysraphism* in *Table 4-17*, page 121).

MYELOMENINGOCELE

EPIDEMIOLOGY/GENETICS
Incidence of spina bifida with meningocele or myelomeningocele (**MM**) is 1-2/1000 live births (0.1-0.2%). Risk increases to 2-3% if there is one previous birth with MM, and 6-8% after two affected children. The risk is also increased in families where close relatives (e.g. siblings) have given birth to MM children, especially when on the mother's side of the family. Incidence may increase in times of war, famine or economic disasters, but it may be gradually declining overall[83]. Transmission follows non-Mendelian genetics, and is probably multifactorial.

Hydrocephalus in myelomeningocele
Hydrocephalus (**HCP**) develops in 65-85% of patients with MM, and 5-10% of MM patients have clinically overt HCP at birth[84]. Over 80% of MM patients who will develop HCP do so before age 6 mos. Most MM patients will have an associated Chiari type 2 malformation (see *Type 2 (Arnold)-Chiari malformation*, page 107). Closure of the MM defect may convert a latent HCP to active HCP by eliminating a route of egress of CSF.

PRENATAL DIAGNOSIS
See *Prenatal detection of neural tube defects* on page 113.

MANAGEMENT

ADMISSION
1. assessment and management of lesion:
    A. measure size of defect
    B. assess whether lesion is ruptured or unruptured
        1. ruptured: start antibiotics (e.g. nafcillin and gentamicin; D/C 6 hrs after MM closure, or continue if shunt anticipated in next 5 or 6 days)
        2. unruptured: no antibiotics necessary
    C. cover lesion with telfa, then sponges soaked in lactated ringers or normal saline (form a sterile gauze ring around the lesion if it is cystic and protruding) to prevent desiccation
    D. Trendelenburg position, patient on stomach (keeps pressure off lesion)
    E. perform surgical closure within 36 hrs unless there is a contraindication to surgery (simultaneous shunt if overt hydrocephalus (**HCP**) at birth): see *Timing of MM closure* below
2. neurological assessment and management:
    A. items related to spinal lesion
        1. watch for spontaneous movement of the LEs (good spontaneous movement correlates with better later functional outcome[85])
        2. assess lowest level of neurologic function (see *Table 4-15*) by checking response of LEs to painful stimulus: although some infants will have a clear demarcation between normal and abnormal levels, at least 50% show some mixture of normal, reflex, and autonomous activity (arising from uninhibited anterior horn motor neurons)[85]
            a. differentiating reflex movement from voluntary may be difficult. In general, voluntary movement is not stereotyped with repetitive stimulus and reflex movement usually only persists as long as the noxious stimulus is applied
    B. items related to the commonly associated Chiari type 2 malformation:
        1. measure OFC: risk of developing hydrocephalus (see *above*). Use OFC graphs (see *page 184*), and also look for abnormal rate of growth (e.g. > 1 cm/day)
        2. head U/S within ≈ 24 hrs

3.   check for inspiratory stridor, apneic episodes
3. ancillary assessment and management:
   A. evaluation by neonatologist to assess for other abnormalities, especially those that may preclude surgery (e.g. pulmonary immaturity). There is an average incidence of 2-2.5 additional anomalies in MM patients
   B. bladder: start patient on regular urinary catheterizations, obtain urological consultation (non-emergent)
   C. AP & lat spine films: assess scoliosis (baseline)
   D. orthopedic consultation for severe kyphotic or scoliotic spine deformities and for hip or knee deformities

Table 4-15   Findings in various levels of MM lesion[86]

Paraly-sis below	Findings
T12	complete paralysis of all muscles in LEs
L1	weak to moderate hip flexion, palpable contraction in sartorius
L2	strong hip flexion and moderate hip adduction
L3	normal hip adduction & almost normal knee extension
L4	normal hip adduction, knee extension & dorsiflexion/inversion of foot; some hip abduction in flexion
L5	normal adduction, flexion & lateral rotation of hip; moderate abduction; normal knee extension, moderate flexion; normal foot dorsiflexion; hip extension absent; • produces dorsiflexed foot and flexed thigh
S1	normal hip flexion & abduction/adduction, moderate extension and lateral rotation; strong knee flexion & inversion/eversion of foot; moderate plantarflexion of foot; extension of all toes, but flexion only of terminal phalanx of great toe; normal medial & lateral hip rotation; complete paralysis of foot intrinsic (except abductor and flexor hallicus brevis); • produces clawing of toes and flattening of sole of foot
S2	difficult to detect abnormality clinically; • with growth this produces clawing of the toes due to weakness of intrinsic muscles of sole of foot (innervated by S3)

SURGICAL CONSIDERATIONS

TIMING OF MM CLOSURE
Early closure of MM defect is not associated with improvement of neurologic function, but evidence supports lower infection rate with early closure. MM should be closed within 24 hrs whether or not membrane is intact (after ≈ 36 hrs the back lesion is colonized and there is increased risk of postoperative infection).

Simultaneous MM repair and VP shunting
In patients without hydrocephalus, most surgeons wait at least ≈ 3 days after MM repair before shunting. In MM patients with clinically overt HCP at birth (ventriculomegaly with enlarged OFC and/or symptoms), MM repair and shunting may be performed in the same sitting without increased incidence of infection, and with shorter hospitalization[87, 88]. It may also reduce the risk of MM repair breakdown previously seen during the interval before shunting. Patient is positioned prone, head turned to right (to expose the right occiput), right knee and thigh flexed to expose right flank (consider using left flank to prevent confusion with appendectomy scar later in life).

POST-OP MANAGEMENT OF MM REPAIR
1. keep patient off all incisions
2. bladder catheterization regimen
3. daily OFC measurements
4. if not shunted
   A. regular head U/S (twice weekly to weekly)
   B. keep patient flat to ↓ CSF pressure on incision

LATE PROBLEMS
Include:
1. hydrocephalus: may mimic ≈ anything listed below. ALWAYS RULE OUT

SHUNT MALFUNCTION when a MM patient deteriorates
2. syringomyelia (and/or syringobulbia): *see page 349*
3. tethered cord (see *Tethered cord syndrome*, page 120): ≈ all patients with MM closures have a tethered cord radiographically, but only a minority are symptomatic. Unfortunately there is no good test to check for symptomatic retethering (SSEPs may deteriorate)[89]
   A. scoliosis: early untethering of cord may improve scoliosis (see *Scoliosis in tethered cord*, page 120)
   B. symptomatic tethering is often manifested as neurological deterioration of delayed onset[90]
4. medullary compression at foramen magnum (symptomatic Chiari II malformation, *see page 107*)

OUTCOME

Without any treatment, only 14-30% of MM infants survive infancy; these usually represent the least severely involved; 70% will have normal IQ's. 50% are ambulatory. With modern treatment, ≈ 85% of MM infants survive. The most common cause of early mortality are complications from the Chiari malformation (respiratory arrest, aspiration...), where late mortality is usually due to shunt malfunction. 80% will have normal IQ. Mental retardation is most closely linked to shunt infection. 40-85% are ambulatory with bracing, however, most choose to use wheelchairs for ease. 3-10% have normal urinary continence, but most may be able to remain dry with intermittent catheterization.

LIPOMYELOSCHISIS

Dorsal spinal dysraphism with lipoma. Six forms are described[91], the following 3 are clinically important as possible causes of progressive neurologic dysfunction via tethering (see *Tethered cord syndrome*, page 120) and/or compression:
1. (intra)dural lipoma
2. lipomyelomeningocele (*see below*)
3. fibrolipoma of the filum terminale

LIPOMYELOMENINGOCELE

A subcutaneous lipoma that passes through a midline defect in the lumbodorsal fascia, vertebral neural arch, and dura, and merges with an abnormally low tethered cord[91]. These may be terminal, dorsal, or transitional (between the two).

The intradural fatty tumor may also be known as **lipoma of the cauda equina**. In addition to being abnormally low, the conus medullaris is split in the midline dorsally usually at the same level as the bifid spine, and this dorsal myeloschisis may extend superiorly under intact spinal arches[92]. There is a thick fibrovascular band that joins the lamina of the most cephalic vertebrae with the bifid lamina. This band constricts the meningocele sac and neural tissue, causing a kink in the superior surface of the meningocele.

The dura is dehiscent at the level of the dorsal myeloschisis, and reflects onto the placode. The lipoma passes through this dehiscence to become attached to the dorsal surface of the placode, and may continue cephalad under intact arches with the possibility of extension into the central canal superiorly to levels without dorsal myeloschisis. The lipoma is distinct from the normal epidural fat which is looser and more areolar. The subarachnoid space typically bulges to the side contralateral to the lipoma. These lipomas account for 20% of covered lumbosacral masses.

PRESENTATION

In a pediatric series, 56% presented with a back mass, 32% with bladder problems, and 10% because of foot deformities, paralysis or leg pain[93].

PHYSICAL EXAMINATION

Almost all patients have cutaneous stigmata of the associated spina bifida: fatty subcutaneous pads (located over the midline and usually extends asymmetrically to one side) with or without dimples, port-wine stains, abnormal hair, dermal sinus opening, or skin appendages[94]. Clubbing of the feet (talipes equinovarus) may occur.

The neurologic exam may be normal in up to 50% of patients (most presenting with skin lesion only). The most common neurologic abnormality was sensory loss in the sacral dermatomes.

EVALUATION

Plain LS spine x-rays will show spina bifida in most cases (present in almost all by definition, but some may have segmentation anomalies instead such as butterfly vertebrae). Abnormalities of fusion and sacral defects may also be seen.

The abnormally low conus can be demonstrated on myelogram/CT or on MRI. MRI also demonstrates the lipomatous mass (high signal on T1WI, low signal on T2WI).

All patients should have pre-op urological evaluation to document any deficit.

TREATMENT

Since symptoms are due to (1) tethering of the spinal cord, especially during growth spurts, and (2) compression due to progressive deposition of fat, especially during periods of rapid weight gain; the goals of surgery are to release the tethering and reduce the bulk of fatty tumor. Simple cosmetic treatment of the subcutaneous fat pad does not prevent neurologic deficit, and may make later definitive repair more difficult or impossible.

Surgical treatment is indicated when the patient reaches 2 months of age, or at the time of diagnosis if the patient presents later in life. Adjuncts to surgical treatment include evoked potential monitoring and laser. Overall, with surgery, 19% will improve, 75% will be unchanged, and 6% will worsen. Foot deformities often progress regardless.

DERMAL SINUS

A tract beginning at the skin surface, lined with epithelium. Usually located at either end of neural tube: cephalic or caudal; most common location is lumbosacral. Probably results from failure of the cutaneous ectoderm to separate from the neuro-ectoderm at the time of closure of the neural groove[38].

SPINAL DERMAL SINUS

May appear as a dimple or as a sinus, with or without hairs, usually very close to midline, with an opening of only 1-2 mm. Surrounding skin may be normal, pigmented ("port wine" discoloration), or distorted by an underlying mass.

The sinus may terminate superficially, may connect with the coccyx, or may traverse between normal vertebrae or through bifid spines to the dural tube. It may widen at any point along its path to form a cyst; called an **epidermoid cyst** if lined with stratified squamous epithelium and containing only keratin from desquamated epithelium, or called a **dermoid cyst** if also lined with dermis (containing skin appendages, such as hair follicles and sebaceous glands) and also containing sebum and hair.

Although innocuous in appearance, they are a potential pathway for intradural infection which may result in meningitis (sometimes recurrent) and/or intrathecal abscess. Less serious, a local infection may occur. The lining dermis contains normal skin appendages which may result in hair, sebum, desquamated epithelium and cholesterol, within the tract. As a result, the contents of the sinus tract are irritating and can cause a sterile (chemical) meningitis with possible delayed arachnoiditis if it enters the dural space.

Incidence of a presumed sacral sinus (a dimple whose bottom could not be seen on skin retraction): 1.2% of neonates[95].

Dermal sinuses are similar but distinct from **pilonidal cysts** which may also be congenital (although some authors say they are acquired), contain hair, are located superficial to the postsacral fascia, and may become infected.

If the tract expands intrathecally to form a cyst, the mass may present as a tethered cord or as an intradural tumor. Bladder dysfunction is usually the first manifestation.

The tract from a spinal dermal sinus always courses cephalad as it dives inward. An occipital sinus may penetrate the skull and can communicate with dermoid cysts as deep as the cerebellum or fourth ventricle.

EVALUATION

These tracts are NOT to be probed or injected with contrast as this can precipitate infection or sterile meningitis.

Exam is directed towards detecting abnormalities in sphincter function (anal and urinary), lumbosacral reflexes, and lower extremity sensation and function.

Radiologic evaluation

When seen at birth, ultrasound is the best means to evaluate for spina bifida and a possible mass inside the canal.

If seen initially following birth, an MRI should be obtained. Sagittal images may demonstrate the tract and its point of attachment. MRI also optimally demonstrates masses (lipomas, epidermoids...) within the canal.

Plain x-rays and CT are unable to demonstrate the fine tract which may exist between the skin and the dura.

Plain x-rays must be done when embarking on surgery as part of operative planning, as preparation for the possibility of a complete laminectomy.

TREATMENT

Sinuses above the lumbosacral region should be surgically removed. More caudally located sinuses are slightly controversial. Although ≈ 25% of presumed sacral sinuses seen at birth will regress to a deep dimple on follow-up (time not specified), it is recommended that all dermal sinuses should be surgically explored and fully excised prior to the development of neurologic deficit or signs of infection. The results following intradural infection are never as good as when undertaken prior to infection. Surgery within the week of diagnosis is appropriate. Sinuses that terminate on the tip of the coccyx rarely penetrate the dura, and may not need to be treated unless local infection occurs.

Surgical technique

CRANIAL DERMAL SINUS

Stalk begins with a dimple in the occipital or nasal region. Cutaneous stigmata of hemangioma, subcutaneous dermoid cyst, or abnormal hair formation may occur. Occipital sinuses extend caudally, and if they enter the skull, they do so caudal to the torcular herophili. Presentation may include recurrent bacterial (usually *S. aureus*) or aseptic meningitis. Evaluation should include MRI to look for intracranial extension and associated anomalies, including an intracranial dermoid cyst.

Treatment

When operating on a cranial dermal sinus, use a sagittally based incision to permit deep exploration. The tract must be followed completely. Be prepared to enter the posterior fossa.

4.10.   Klippel-Feil syndrome

Congenital fusion of two or more cervical vertebrae. Ranges from fusion of only the bodies (congenital **block vertebrae**) to fusion of the entire vertebrae (including posterior elements). Results from failure of normal segmentation of cervical somites between 3-8 weeks gestation. Involved vertebral bodies are often flattened and associated disc spaces are absent or hypoplastic. Hemivertebrae may also occur. Neural foramina are smaller than normal and oval. Cervical stenosis is rare. Complete absence of the posterior elements with an enlarged foramen magnum and fixed hyperextension posture is called **iniencephaly** and is rare. Incidence of Klippel-Feil is unknown due to its rarity and the fact that it is frequently asymptomatic.

Classic clinical triad (all 3 are present in < 50%): low posterior hairline, shortened neck (**brevicollis**), and limitation of neck motion (may not be evident if < 3 vertebrae are fused, if fusion is limited only to the lower cervical levels[96], or if hypermobility of non-fused segments compensates). Limitation of movement is more common in rotation than flexion-extension or lateral bending.

May occur in conjunction with other congenital cervical spine anomalies such as basilar impression and atlanto-occipital fusion. Other clinical associations include scoliosis in 60%, facial asymmetry, torticollis, webbing of the neck (called **pterygium colli** when severe), **Sprengel's deformity** in 25-35% (raised scapula due to failure of the scapula to properly descend from its region of formation high in the neck to its normal position about the same time as the Klippel-Feil lesion occurs), **synkinesis** (mirror mo-

---

tions, primarily of hands but occasionally arms also) and less commonly facial nerve palsy, ptosis, cleft or high arched palate. Systemic congenital abnormalities may also occur including: genitourinary (the most frequent being unilateral absence of a kidney), cardiopulmonary, CNS, and in ≈ 30% deafness[97] (due to defective development of the osseous inner ear).

No symptoms have ever been directly attributed to the fused vertebrae, however symptoms may occur from nonfused segments (less common in short-segment fusions) which may be hypermobile possibly leading to instability or degenerative arthritic changes.

TREATMENT

Usually directed at detecting and managing the associated systemic anomalies. Patients should have cardiac evaluation (EKG), CXR, and a renal ultrasound. Serial examinations with lateral flexion-extension lateral C-spine x-rays to monitor for instability. Occasionally, judicious fusion of an unstable nonfused segment may be needed at the risk of further loss of mobility. Also *see page 742*, for recommendations regarding athletic competition.

4.11. Tethered cord syndrome

Abnormally low conus medullaris associated with a short, thickened filum terminale, or with an intradural lipoma (other lesions, e.g. as lipoma extending through dura, or diastematomyelia are considered as separate entities). Most common in myelomeningocele (**MM**). Diagnosis must be made clinically in MM, as almost all of these patients will have tethering radiographically.

Table 4-16 Presenting signs and symptoms[98]

Finding	%
cutaneous findings	54%
hypertrichosis	22%
sub-Q lipoma (no intraspinal extension)	15%
miscellaneous (hemangiomatous discoloration, dermal sinus, multiple manifestations)	17%
gait difficulty with LE weakness	93%
visible muscle atrophy, short limb, or ankle deformity	63%
sensory deficit	70%
bladder dysfunction	40%
bladder dysfunction as only deficit	4%
pain in back, leg, or foot arches	37%
scoliosis or kyphosis*	29%
posterior spina bifida (lumbar or sacral)	98%

*   high incidence of scoliosis and kyphosis due to inclusion of series by Hoffman

PRESENTATION

Presenting signs and symptoms in patients with tethered cord are shown in *Table 4-16*.

MYELOMENINGOCELE PATIENTS

If a MM patient has increasing scoliosis, increasing spasticity, worsening gait (in those previously ambulatory), or deteriorating urodynamics[99]:

- always make sure that there is a working shunt with normal ICP
- if painful, should be considered tethered cord until proven otherwise
- if painless, should be considered syringomyelia until proven otherwise
- may be due to brainstem compression (symptomatic Chiari II malformation, *see page 107*) requiring posterior fossa decompression

Scoliosis in tethered cord

Progressive scoliosis may be seen in conjunction with tethered cord; early untethering of the cord may result in improvement of scoliosis, however, untethering must be done when the scoliosis is mild. When cases of ≤ 10° scoliosis were untethered, 68% had neurologic improvement and the remaining 32% were stabilized, whereas when scoliosis is severe (≥ 50°) ≈ 16% deteriorated.

TETHERED CORD IN ADULTS

Although most cases of tethered cord present in childhood, cases of adult tethered cord have been reported (≈ 50 published cases as of 1982). For comparison of adult and childhood forms, *see Table 4-17*.

Table 4-17 Comparison of childhood and adult tethered cord syndrome[100]

(from J Neurosurg, D. Pang and J.E. Wilberger, Vol. 57, pp. 40, 1982, with permission)

Finding	Childhood tethered cord	Adult tethered cord
pain	uncommon; usually in back and legs, not peri-anal nor perineal	present in 86%, often peri-anal & perineal; diffuse & bilateral; occasionally shock-like
foot deformities	common early; usually progressive cavovarus deformity (club foot)	not seen
progressive spinal deformity	common; usually progressive scoliosis	uncommon (< 5%)
motor deficits	common; usually gait abnormalities & regression of gait training	usually presents as leg weakness
urological symptoms	common; usually continuous urinary dribbling, delayed toilet training, recurrent UTIs, enuresis	common; usually urinary frequency, urgency, sensation of incomplete emptying, stress incontinence, overflow incontinence
trophic ulcerations	relatively common in LEs	rare
cutaneous stigmata of dysraphism	present in 80-100% (tuft of hair, dimple, capillary angioma (**naevus flammeus**)	present in < 50%
aggravating factors	growth spurts	trauma, maneuvers associated with stretching conus, lumbar spondylosis, disc herniation, spinal stenosis

EVALUATION

Radiographically: low conus medullaris (below L2) and thickened filum terminale (normal diameter < 1 mm; diameters > 2 mm are pathological). NB: apparent filum diameter on CT-myelogram may vary with concentration of contrast material.

It is difficult to differentiate a tethered cord from a congenitally low lying cord (filum diameter is generally normal in latter).

Pre-op evaluation

Pre-operative cystometrogram is strongly recommended, especially if the patient seems continent (postoperative changes in bladder function are not uncommon, possibly due to stretching of the lower fibers of the cauda equina).

TREATMENT

If the only abnormality is a thickened, shortened filum, then a limited lumbosacral laminectomy may suffice, with division of the filum once identified.

If a lipoma is found, it may be removed with the filum if it separates easily from neural tissues.

Distinguishing features of the filum terminale

The filum is differentiated from nerve roots by presence of characteristic squiggly vessel on surface of filum. Also, under the microscope, the filum has a distinctively whiter appearance than the nerve roots, and ligamentous-like strands can be seen running through it. NB: intra-op electrical stimulation and recording of anal sphincter EMG are more definitive.

OUTCOME

In MM, it is usually impossible to permanently untether a cord, however, in a growing MM child, it may be that after 2-4 untetherings that the child will be finished growing and tethering may cease to be a problem. Cases that are untethered early in childhood may recur later, especially during the adolescent growth-spurt. Incidence of post-op CSF leak: 15%.

Adult form: surgical release is usually good for pain relief. However, it is poor for return of bladder function.

4.12.   Split cord malformation

There is no uniformly accepted nomenclature for malformations characterized by duplicate or split spinal cords. Pang et al.[101] have proposed the following.

The term split cord malformation **(SCM)** should be used for all double spinal cords, all of which appear to have a common embryologic etiology.

Type I SCM

Defined as two hemicords, each with its own central canal and surrounding pia, each within a separate dural tube separated by a dural-sheathed rigid osseocartilaginous (bony) median septum. This has often (but not consistently) been referred to as **diastematomyelia**. There are abnormalities of the spine at the level of the split (absent disc, dorsal hypertrophic bone where the median "spike" attaches)[102]. Two-thirds have overlying skin abnormalities including: nevi, hypertrichosis (tuft of hair), lipomas, dimples or hemangiomas. These patients often have and an orthopedic foot deformity (neurogenic high arches).

Treatment: symptoms are most commonly due to tethering of the cord; and are usually improved by untethering. In addition to untethering, the bony septum must be removed and the dura reconstituted as a single tube (these spines are often very distorted and rotated, therefore start at normal anatomy and work towards defect). ✖ DO NOT cut the tethered filum until after the median septum is removed to avoid having the cord retract up against septum.

Type II SCM

Consists of two hemicords within a single dural tube, separated by a nonrigid fibrous median septum. This has sometimes been referred to as **diplomyelia**. Each hemicord has nerve roots arising from it. There is usually no spine abnormality at the level of the split, but there is usually spina bifida occulta in the lumbosacral region.

Treatment: consists of untethering the cord at the level of the spina bifida occulta, and occasionally at the level of the split[102].

4.13.   Miscellaneous developmental anomalies

Some anomalies that may be seen by the neurosurgeon include the following.

Septo-optic dysplasia[56 (p 175-8), 103]

AKA de Morsier syndrome. Incomplete early morphogenesis of anterior midline structures produces hypoplasia of the optic nerves and possibly optic chiasm (affected patients are blind) and pituitary infundibulum. The septum pellucidum is absent in about half the cases. About half the cases also have schizencephaly (*see page 112*).

Presentation may be due to secondary hypopituitarism manifesting as dwarfism, isolated growth hormone deficiency, or panhypopituitarism. Occasionally hypersecretion of growth hormone, corticotropin or prolactin may occur, and sexual precocity may occur. Most patients are of normal intelligence although retardation may occur. Septo-optic dysplasia may be a less severe form of holoprosencephaly, and occasionally may occur as part of this anomaly (with its attendant poorer prognosis for function or survival, *see page 112*). The ventricles may be normal or dilated. May be seen by the neurosurgeon because of concerns of possible hydrocephalus.

Absence of the septum pellucidum[56 (p 178)]

Absence of the septum pellucidum may occur in:
1. holoprosencephaly: *see page 112*
2. schizencephaly: *see page 112*
3. agenesis of the corpus callosum: *see page 114*
4. Chiari type 2 malformation: *see page 107*
5. basal encephalocele
6. porencephaly/hydranencephaly
7. may occur in severe hydrocephalus: thought to be due to necrosis with resorption
8. septo-optic dysplasia: *see above*

4.14. References

1. Van Der Meche F, Braakman R: Arachnoid cysts in the middle cranial fossa: Cause and treatment of progressive and non-progressive symptoms. **J Neurol Neurosurg Psychiatry** 46: 1102-7, 1983.
2. Mayr U, Aichner F, Bauer G, et al.: Supratentorial extracerebral cysts of the middle cranial fossa: A report of 23 consecutive cases of the so-called temporal lobe agenesis syndrome. **Neurochirugia** 25: 51-6, 1982.
3. Harsh G R, Edwards M S B, Wilson C B: Intracranial arachnoid cysts in children. **J Neurosurg** 64: 835-42, 1986.
4. Pierre-Kahn A, Capelle L, Brauner R, et al.: Presentation and management of suprasellar arachnoid cysts: Review of 20 cases. **J Neurosurg** 73: 355-9, 1990.
5. Altschuler E M, Jungreis C A, Sekhar L N, et al.: Operative treatment of intracranial epidermoid cysts and cholesterol granulomas: Report of 21 cases. **Neurosurgery** 26: 606-14, 1990.
6. Rengachary S S, Watanabe I: Ultrastructure and pathogenesis of intracranial arachnoid cysts. **J Neuropathol Exp Neurol** 40: 61-83, 1981.
7. Galassi E, Tognetti F, Gaist G, et al.: CT scan and metrizamide CT cisternography in arachnoid cysts of the middle cranial fossa. **Surg Neurol** 17: 363-9, 1982.
8. Hopf N J, Perneczky A: Endoscopic neurosurgery and endoscope-assisted microneurosurgery for the treatment of intracranial cysts. **Neurosurgery** 43: 1330-7, 1998.
9. Page L K: Comment on Albright L: Treatment of bobble-head doll syndrome by transcallosal cystectomy. **Neurosurgery** 8: 595, 1981.
10. Albright L: Treatment of bobble-head doll syndrome by transcallosal cystectomy. **Neurosurgery** 8: 593-5, 1981.
11. Russell D S, Rubenstein L J: **Pathology of tumours of the nervous system**. 5th ed. Williams and Wilkins, Baltimore, 1989.
12. Rubio G, Garcci Guijo C, Mallada J J: MR and CT diagnosis of intracranial lipoma. **AJR** 157: 887-8, 1991 (letter).
13. Atlas S W, Zimmerman R A, Bilaniuk L T, et al.: Corpus callosum and limbic system: Neuroanatomic MR evaluation of developmental anomalies. **Radiology** 160: 355-62, 1986.
14. Kazner E, Stochdorph O, Wende S, et al.: Intracranial lipoma. Diagnostic and therapeutic considerations. **J Neurosurg** 52: 234-45, 1980.
15. Arita K, Ikawa F, Kurisu K, et al.: The relationship between magnetic resonance imaging findings and clinical manifestations of hypothalamic hamartoma. **J Neurosurg** 91 (2): 212-20, 1999.
16. Striano S, Meo R, Bilo L, et al.: Gelastic epilepsy: Symptomatic and cryptogenic cases. **Epilepsia** 40 (3): 294-302, 1999.
17. Ng Y, Rekate H L, Kerrigan J F, et al.: Transcallosal resection of a hypothalamic hamartoma: Case report. **BNI Quarterly** 20: 13-7, 2004.
18. Enyon-Lewis N J, Kitchen N, Scaravilli F, et al.: Neurenteric cyst of the cerebellopontine angle. **Neurosurgery** 42: 655-8, 1998.
19. LeDoux M S, Faye-Petersen O M, Aronin P A: Lumbosacral neurenteric cyst in an infant. **J Neurosurg** 78: 821-5, 1993.
20. Morita Y: Neurenteric cyst or teratomatous cyst. **J Neurosurg** 80: 179, 1994 (letter).
21. Hes R: Neurenteric cyst or teratomatous cyst. **J Neurosurg** 80: 179-80, 1994 (letter).
22. Golabi M, Edwards M S B, Ousterhout D K: Cran-

23. iosynostosis and hydrocephalus. **Neurosurgery** 21: 63-7, 1987.
23. Renier D, Sainte-Rose C, Marchac D, et al.: Intracranial pressure in craniostenosis. **J Neurosurg** 57: 370-7, 1982.
24. Burke M J, Winston K R, Williams S: Normal sutural fusion and the etiology of single suture craniosynostosis: The microspicule hypothesis. **Pediatr Neurosurg** 22: 241-6, 1995.
25. Tuite G F, Evanson J, Chong W K, et al.: The beaten copper cranium: A correlation between intracranial pressure, cranial radiographs, and computed tomographic scans in children with craniosynostosis. **Neurosurgery** 39: 691-9, 1996.
26. Chadduck W M, Chadduck J B, Boop F A: The subarachnoid spaces in craniosynostosis. **Neurosurgery** 30: 867-71, 1992.
27. Gates G F, Dore E K: Detection of craniosynostosis by bone scanning. **Radiology** 115: 665-71, 1975.
28. Renier D, Arnaud E, Cinalli G, et al.: Prognosis for mental function in Apert's sydrome. **J Neurosurg** 85: 66-72, 1996.
29. Muakkassa K F, Hoffman H J, Hinton D R, et al.: Lambdoid synostosis: Part 2: Review of cases managed at the hospital for sick children, 1972-1982. **J Neurosurg** 61: 340-7, 1984.
30. Keating R F, Goodrich J T: Lambdoid plagiocephaly. **Contemp Neurosurg** 18 (8): 1-7, 1996.
31. Morrison D L, MacEwen G D: Congenital muscular torticollis: Observations regarding clinical findings, associated conditions, and results of treatment. **J Pediatr Orthop** 2: 500-5, 1982.
32. American Academy of Pediatrics Task Force on Infant Positioning and SIDS: Positioning and SIDS. **Pediatrics** 89: 1120-6, 1992.
33. Higginbottom M C, Jones K L, James H E: Intrauterine constraint and craniosynostosis. **Neurosurgery** 6: 39, 1980.
34. Hinton D R, Becker L E, Muakkassa K F, et al.: Lambdoid synostosis: Part 1: The lambdoid suture: Normal development and pathology of 'synostosis'. **J Neurosurg** 61: 333-9, 1984.
35. McComb J G: Treatment of functional lambdoid synostosis. **Neurosurg Clin North Am** 2. 665, 1991.
36. Clarren S K: Plagiocephaly and torticollis: Etiology, natural history, and helmet treatment. **J Pediatr** 98: 92, 1981.
37. Section of Pediatric Neurosurgery of the American Association of Neurological Surgeons, (ed.) **Pediatric neurosurgery**. 1st ed., Grune and Stratton, New York, 1982.
38. Matson D D: **Neurosurgery of infancy and childhood**. 2nd ed. Charles C Thomas, Springfield, 1969.
39. Suwanwela C, Suwanwela N: A morphological classification of sincipital encephalomeningoceles. **J Neurosurg** 36: 201-11, 1972.
40. Carmel P W: Management of the Chiari malformations in childhood. **Clinical Neurosurg** 30: 385-406, 1983.
41. Spillane J D, Pallis C, Jones A M: Developmental abnormalities in the region of the foramen magnum. **Brain** 80: 11-52, 1957.
42. Paul K S, Lye R H, Strang F A, et al.: Arnold-Chiari malformation: Review of 71 cases. **J Neurosurg** 58: 183-7, 1983.
43. Guinto G, Zamorano C, Dominguez F, et al.: Chiari I malformation: Part I. **Contemp Neurosurg** 26 (25): 1-7, 2004.
44. Sathi S, Stieg P E: "Acquired" Chiari I malformation after multiple lumbar punctures: Case report. **Neu-**

45. Levy W J, Mason L, Hahn J F: Chiari malformation presenting in adults: A surgical experience in 127 cases. **Neurosurgery** 12: 377-90, 1983.

46. Bejjani G K, Cockerham K P: Adult Chiari malformation. **Contemp Neurosurg** 23 (26): 1-7, 2001.

47. Rhoton A L: Microsurgery of Arnold-Chiari malformation in adults with and without hydromyelia. **J Neurosurg** 45: 473-83, 1976.

48. Gingold S I, Winfield J A: Oscillopsia and primary cerebellar ectopie: Case report and review of the literature. **Neurosurgery** 29: 932-6, 1991.

49. Aboulezz A O, Sartor K, Geyer C A, *et al.*: Position of cerebellar tonsils in the normal population and in patients with Chiari malformation: A quantitative approach with MR imaging. **J Comput Assist Tomogr** 9: 1033-6, 1985.

50. Barkovich A J, Wippold F J, Sherman J L, *et al.*: Significance of cerebellar tonsillar position on MR. **AJNR** 7: 795-9, 1986.

51. Mikulis D J, Diaz O, Egglin T K, *et al.*: Variance of the position of the cerebellar tonsils with age: Preliminary report. **Radiology** 183 (3): 725-8, 1992.

52. Iskandar B J, Hedlund G L, Grabb P A, *et al.*: The resolution of syringohydromyelia without hindbrain herniation after posterior fossa decompression. **J Neurosurg** 89 (2): 212-6, 1998.

53. Meadows J, Kraut M, Guarnieri M, *et al.*: Asymptomatic Chiari type I malformations identified on magnetic resonance imaging. **J Neurosurg** 92 (6): 920-6, 2000.

54. Dyste G N, Menezes A H, VanGilder J C: Symptomatic Chiari malformations: An analysis of presentation, management, and long-term outcome. **J Neurosurg** 71: 159-68, 1989.

55. Peach B: The Arnold-Chiari malformation. Morphogenesis. **Arch Neurol** 12: 527-35, 1965.

56. Taveras J M, Pile-Spellman J: **Neuroradiology**. 3rd ed. Williams and Wilkins, Baltimore, 1996.

57. Pollack I F, Pang D, Albright A L, *et al.*: Outcome following hindbrain decompression of symptomatic Chiari malformations in children previously treated with myelomeningocele closure and shunts. **J Neurosurg** 77: 881-8, 1992.

58. Park T S, Hoffman H J, Hendrick E B, *et al.*: Experience with surgical decompression of the Arnold-Chiari malformation in young infants with myelomeningocele. **Neurosurgery** 13: 147-52, 1983.

59. Pollack I F, Pang D, Kocoshis S, *et al.*: Neurogenic dysphagia resulting from Chiari malformations. **Neurosurgery** 30: 709-19, 1992.

60. Hoffman H J, Hendrick E B, Humphreys R P: Manifestations and management of Arnold-Chiari malformation in patients with myelomeningocele. **Childs Brain** 1: 255-9, 1975.

61. Gilbert J N, Jones K L, Rorke L B, *et al.*: Central nervous system anomalies associated with myelomeningocele, hydrocephalus, and the Arnold-Chiari malformation: Reappraisal of theories regarding the pathogenesis of posterior neural tube closure defects. **Neurosurgery** 18: 559-64, 1986.

62. Bell W O, Charney E B, Bruce D A, *et al.*: Symptomatic Arnold-Chiari malformation: Review of experience with 22 cases. **J Neurosurg** 66: 812-6, 1987.

63. Raimondi A J, Samuelson G, Yarzagaray L, *et al.*: Atresia of the foramina of Luschka and Magendie: The Dandy-Walker cyst. **J Neurosurg** 31: 202-16, 1969.

64. Hirsch J F, Pierre-Kahn A, Renier D, *et al.*: The Dandy-Walker malformation: A review of 40 cases. **J Neurosurg** 61: 515-22, 1984.

65. Nag T K, Falconer M A: Non-tumoral stenosis of the aqueduct in adults. **Brit Med J** 2: 1168-70, 1966.

66. Vanneste J, Hyman R: Non-tumoral aqueduct stenosis and normal pressure hydrocephalus in the elderly. **J Neurol Neurosurg Psychiatry** 49: 529-35, 1986.

67. Harrison M J G, Robert C M, Uttley D: Benign aqueduct stenosis in adults. **J Neurol Neurosurg Psychiatry** 37: 1322-8, 1974.

68. Lemire R J: Neural tube defects. **JAMA** 259: 558-62, 1988.

69. DeMyer W, Zeman W, Palmer C G: The face predicts the brain: Diagnostic significance of median facial anomalies for holoprosencephaly (arhinencephaly). **Pediatrics** 34: 256-63, 1964.

70. Volpe J J: Effect of cocaine use on the fetus. **N Engl J Med** 327: 399-407, 1992.

71. Werler M M, Shapiro S, Mitchell A A: Periconceptual folic acid exposure and risk of occurent neural tube defects. **JAMA** 269: 1257-61, 1993.

72. Centers for Disease Control: Recommendations for use of folic acid to reduce number of spina bifida cases and other neural tube defects. **MMWR** 41: RR-14, 1992.

73. Daly L E, Kirke P N, Molloy A, *et al.*: Folate levels and neural tube defects. **JAMA** 274: 1698-1702, 1995.

74. Milunsky A, Ulcickas M, Rothman J, *et al.*: Maternal heat exposure and neural tube defects. **JAMA** 268: 882-5, 1992.

75. Oakeshott P, Hunt G M: Valproate and spina bifida. **Br Med J** 298: 1300-1, 1989.

76. Werler M M, Louik C, Shapiro S, *et al.*: Prepregnant weight in relation to risk of neural tube defects. **JAMA** 275: 1089-92, 1996.

77. Shaw G M, Velie E M, Schaffer D: Risk of neural tube defect-affected pregnancies among obese women. **JAMA** 275: 1093-6, 1996.

78. Milunsky A: Predictive values, relative risks, and overall benefits of high and low maternal serum alpha-fetoprotein screening in singleton pregnancies. **Surg Obstet Gynecol** 161: 291-7, 1989.

79. Burton B K: Alpha-fetoprotein screening. **Adv Pediatr** 33: 181-96, 1986.

80. Bennett M J, Blau K, Johnson R D, *et al.*: Some problems of alpha-fetoprotein screening. **Lancet** 2: 1296-7, 1978.

81. Davidson H D, Abraham R, Steiner R E: Agenesis of the corpus callosum: Magnetic resonance imaging. **Radiology** 155: 371-3, 1985.

82. Loeser J D, Alvord E C: Agenesis of the corpus callosum. **Brain** 91: 553-70, 1968.

83. Lorber J, Ward A M: Spina bifida - A vanishing nightmare? **Arch Dis Child** 60: 1086-91, 1985.

84. Stein S C, Schut L: Hydrocephalus in myelomeningocele. **Childs Brain** 5: 413-9, 1979.

85. Sharrard W J W: *Assessment of the myelomeningocele child*. In **Myelomeningocele**, McLaurin R L, (ed.). Grune and Stratton, New York, 1977: pp 389-410.

86. Sharrard W J W: The segmental innervation of the lower limb muscles in man. **Ann R Coll Surgeons (Engl)** 34: 106-22, 1964.

87. Epstein N E, Rosenthal R D, Zito J, *et al.*: Shunt placement and myelomeningocele repair: Simultaneous versus sequential shunting. **Childs Nerv Syst** 1: 145-7, 1985.

88. Hubballah M Y, Hoffman H J: Early repair of myelomeningocele and simultaneous insertion of VP shunt: Technique and results. **Neurosurgery** 20: 21-3, 1987.

89. Larson S J, Sances A, Christenson P C: Evoked somatosensory potentials in man. **Arch Neurol** 15: 88-93, 1966.

90. Heinz E R, Rosenbaum A E, Scarff T B, *et al.*: Tethered spinal cord following meningomyelocele repair. **Radiology** 131: 153-60, 1979.

91. Emery J L, Lendon R G: Lipomas of the cauda equina and other fatty tumors related to neurospinal dysraphism. **Dev Med Child Neurol** 11 (Suppl): 62-70, 1969.

---

92. Naidich T P, McLone D G, Mutluer S: A new understanding of dorsal dysraphism with lipoma (lipomyeloschisis): Radiologic evaluation and surgical
correction. **AJNR** 4: 103-16, 1983.
93. Bruce D A, Schut L: Spinal lipomas in infancy and
childhood. **Childs Brain** 5: 192-203, 1979.
94. Sato K, Shimoji T, Sumie H, *et al*.: Surgically confirmed myelographic classification of congenital intraspinal lipoma in the lumbosacral region. **Childs
Nerv Syst** 1: 2-11, 1985.
95. Powell K R, Cherry J D, Horigan T J, *et al*.: A prospective search for congenital dermal abnormalities
of craniospinal axis. **J Pediatr** 87: 744-50, 1975.
96. Gray S W, Romaine C B, Skandalakis J E: Congenital fusion of the cervical vertebrae. **Surg Gynecol
Obstet** 118: 37385, 1964.
97. Hensinger R N, Lang J R, MacEwen G D: Klippel-
Feil syndrome: A constellation of associated anomalies. **J Bone Joint Surg** 56A: 124653, 1974.

98. Youmans J R, (ed.) **Neurological surgery**. 2nd ed.,
W. B. Saunders, Philadelphia, 1982.
99. Park T S, Cail W S, Maggio W M, *et al*.: Progressive
spasticity and scoliosis in children with myelomeningocele: Radiological investigation and surgical
treatment. **J Neurosurg** 62: 367-75, 1985.
100. Pang D, Wilberger J E: Tethered cord syndrome in
adults. **J Neurosurg** 57: 32-47, 1982.
101. Pang D, Dias M S, Ahab-Barmada M: Split cord
malformation: Part I: A unified theory of embryo-
genesis for double spinal cord malformations. **Neurosurgery** 31: 451-80, 1992.
102. Hoffman H J: Comment on Pang D, et al.: Split cord
malformation: Part I: A unified theory of embryo-
genesis for double spinal cord malformations. **Neurosurgery** 31: 480, 1992.
103. Jones K L: **Smith's recognizable patterns of human malformation**. 4th ed. W.D. Saunders, Phila
delphia, 1988.

5. Neuroradiology

5.1. Contrast agents in neuroradiology

Also see *Intraoperative dyes*, page 599 for visible dyes useful in the operating room.

IODINATED CONTRAST AGENTS

Water-soluble contrast agents have superseded older non-water-soluble ones such as Pantopaque® (ethyl iodophenylundecylate or iophendylate meglumine).

✖ Caution: iodinated contrast (IV or intra-arterial) may delay excretion of **metformin** (Glucophage®, Avandamet®), an oral hypoglycemic agent used in diabetes type II, and can be associated with lactic acidosis and renal failure. The manufacturer recommends withholding metformin 48 hrs prior to and following contrast administration (or longer if there is evidence of declining renal function following use of contrast). Metformin should also be held ≈ 48 hours before any surgery, and should not be restarted post-op until the patient has fully recovered and is eating and drinking normally.

INTRATHECAL CONTRAST AGENTS

The primary approved agent employed for intrathecal use today is iohexol (Omnipaque®) (*see below*).

Inadvertent intrathecal injection of ionic contrast agents

✖ Caution: serious reactions can occur with inadvertent intrathecal injection (e.g. for myelography, cisternography, ventriculography…) of iodinated contrast media that are not specifically indicated for intrathecal use (including ionic contrast agents as well as some non-ionic agents (e.g. Optiray®, Reno-60…)). This can cause uncontrollable seizures, intracerebral hemorrhage, cerebral edema, coma, paralysis, arachnoiditis, myoclonus (tonic-clonic muscle spasms), rhabdomyolysis with subsequent renal failure, hyperthermia, and respiratory compromise, with a significant fatality rate[1].

Management suggestions include:
1. immediately remove CSF + contrast if the error is recognized when the opportunity is available (e.g. withdraw fluid through myelography needle)
2. elevate head of bed ≈ 45° (to keep contrast out of head)
3. if there is a question about what may have occurred (i.e. it is not certain if an inappropriate contrast agent was used) send blood and CSF with contrast for high-performance liquid chromatography for identification of agent[2]
4. antihistamines: e.g. diphenhydramine (Benadryl®) 50 mg deep IM
5. respiration: supplemental oxygen, and if needed, intubation
6. control HTN
7. IV hydration
8. IV steroids
9. sedation if patient is agitated
10. treat fever with acetaminophen and if needed with a cooling blanket
11. pharmacologic paralysis if necessary to manage muscle activity (e.g. etomidate)
12. anticonvulsant medication: more than one agent may be required (e.g. phenytoin + phenobarbital + a benzodiazepine)
13. consider unenhanced brain CT scan: may help assess if contrast has diffused intracranially, but this requires placing patient flat and may not be advisable
14. insertion of lumbar subarachnoid drain
15. monitor: electrolytes, anticonvulsant levels, creatine kinase **(CK)**
16. repeat EEGs to assess seizure activity while sedated/paralyzed

Iohexol (Omnipaque®)

A non-ionic triiodinated compound. It has replaced metrizamide. Concentrations expressed as follows: e.g. Omnipaque 300 contains the equivalent of 300 mg of organic iodine per ml of media (300 mgI/ml).

Usually reserved for IV contrast CT scan of brain primarily for patients with previous dye reaction, e.g. to Reno-60. Uses and concentrations are shown in *Table 5-1*.

Intrathecal use: NB: only Omnipaque 180, 210, 240 and 300 are labeled for intrathecal use. 140 and 350 are not FDA approved for intrathecal use, however, some neuroradiologists will use Omnipaque 140 or diluted 180 e.g. for CT ventriculography.

Consider discontinuing neuroleptic drugs (including: phenothiazines, e.g. chlorpromazine, prochlorperazine, and promethazine) at least 48 hours prior to procedure. Elevate HOB ≥ 30° for the first few hours after the procedure. Hydrate orally or IV.

Use with caution in patients with seizure history, severe cardiovascular disease, chronic alcoholism or multiple sclerosis.

Iohexol undergoes slow diffusion from the intrathecal space to the systemic circulation and is eliminated by renal excretion with no significant metabolism or deiodination.

Maximum dosage: a total dose of 3060 mg iodine should not be exceeded in an adult during a single myelogram (some say up to 4500 mg is OK) (e.g. 15 cc of Omnipaque 300 = 15 ml **x** 300 mgI/ml= 4500 mg of iodine).

Table 5-1 Iohexol concentrations for adults

Procedure	Concentration (mgI/ml)	Volume (ml)
lumbar myelography via LP	180 / 240	10-17 / 7-12.5
thoracic myelography via LP or cervical injection	240 / 300	6-12.5 / 6-10
cervical myelography via LP	240 / 300	6-12.5 / 6-10
cervical myelography via C1-2 puncture	180 / 240 / 300	7-10 / 6-12.5 / 4-10
complete myelography via LP	240 / 300	6-12.5 / 6-10
cerebral arteriography*	300	≈ 6-12 ml/vessel
IV contrast enhanced CT scan of the brain	240 / 350	120-250 ml IV drip / 70-150 ml bolus†
CT cisternography via LP or C1-2 puncture	300 / 350	12 / 12
CT ventriculography via ventricular catheter	180‡	2-3
plain film ventriculography via ventricular catheter	180	2-3
plain film "shunt-o-gram" injected via shunt into ventricles	180	2-3
plain film "shunt-o-gram" injected via shunt distal to valve so as not to enter into ventricles (to check distal shunt function)	300 / 350	10-12 / 10-12

* most centers use Optiray®, *see text*

† follow with 250 ml bolus of 0.45% NS to rehydrate patient

‡ 180 will be very dense on CT, and some use 1-3 ml of 140 or diluted 180%(dilute approximately 2 parts contrast to 1 part preservative-free normal saline)

NON-INTRATHECAL CONTRAST AGENTS

For inadvertent intrathecal injection of contrast agents not intended for intrathecal use, *see above*.

Diatrizoate meglumine (e.g. Reno-60®, Reno-dip®)

✖ Not for intrathecal use (*see above*).

A tri-iodinated benzine derivative similar to Conray. Both have been available for a long time. Due to the fact that it ionizes, it is ionic and hyperosmolar. Widely used IV, in neuroradiology for IV contrast enhanced CAT scan when there is no history of prior reaction to IV contrast agents (use iohexol in patients with previous reaction, *see above*).

• IV contrast enhanced CT scan of the brain in adult patient with no history of previous dye reaction:
  A. 300 ml IV drip of Reno-dip® (30% solution, i.e. 300 mg/ml) over ≈ 15 mins
  B. 50-150 ml of Reno-60 (60% solution). Typically: 150 ml is used

• body CT: bolus of 150 ml of Reno-60® (3 vials of 50 ml each), followed e.g. by 250 ml of 0.45% NS to help prevent dehydration. Usually given more slowly to diabetics and the elderly where there is increased risk of renal failure

Ioversol (Optiray®)

✖ Not for intrathecal use (*see above*).

Uses and concentrations include:

- arteriography: Optiray 300 (ioversol 64%) or Optiray 320 (ioversol 68%). Total procedural dose should not usually exceed 200 ml
- IV contrast enhanced CT scan of brain:
  - A. adult: 50-150 ml of Optiray 300, 320, or 100-250 ml of Optiray 240. Typically: 100 ml of Optiray 320
  - B. pediatrics: 1-3 ml/kg of Optiray 320

5.1.1.   Iodinated contrast allergy prep

Indicated for patients with previous history of reaction to IV iodinated contrast material. Minor previous reactions such as hives and itching should merit preparation with this regimen whenever possible. Patients with anaphylactic shock or severe edema causing compromise of the airway should probably not receive IV iodine even with this prep, unless absolutely necessary. Caution: the patient may still have serious reaction (modified[3]).

- utilize non-ionic contrast medium (e.g. iohexol) whenever possible
- steroid (*see page 8* for further details of steroid dosing)
  - ♦ prednisone 50 mg PO: 20-24 hrs, 8-12 hrs & 2 hrs before study
  - ♦ equivalent dose of Solumedrol® (methylprednisolone) for IV use would be ≈ 25 mg
- diphenhydramine (Benadryl®) 50 mg, *EITHER* IM 1 hr before, *OR* IV 5 min before study
- optional: H_2 antagonist, e.g. cimetidine 300 mg PO or IV 1 hr before study
- have emergency equipment available during study

5.1.2.   Reactions to intravascular contrast media

BETA BLOCKERS
Beta blockers can increase the risk of contrast media reactions, and may mask some manifestations of an anaphylactoid reaction.

They also make use of epinephrine inadvisable since the alpha effects of epinephrine will predominate (bronchospasm, vasoconstriction, increased vagal tone). If treatment is required for hypotension, may try **glucagon** 2-3 mg IV bolus, followed by 5 mg IV drip over 1 hour (glucagon has positive inotropic and chronotropic effect that is not mediated through adrenergic pathways).

IDIOSYNCRATIC REACTIONS AND TREATMENT
For treatment of inadvertent intrathecal injection of ionic contrast agents, *see page 126*.

HYPOTENSION WITH TACHYCARDIA (ANAPHYLACTOID REACTION)
1. mild: Trendelenburg position. IV fluids
2. if no response but remains mild:
   epinephrine (use with caution in patients with coronary artery disease, limited cardiac reserve, hypertension, or unclipped cerebral aneurysm)
   A. 0.3-0.5 ml of 1:1000 SQ (0.3-0.5 mg) q 15-20 mins (peds: 0.01 mg/kg)
   B. OR, ASEP recommendations (especially for elderly or patients in shock): 10 ml of 1:100,000 IV over 5 to 10 min (put 0.1 ml of 1:1000 in 10 ml of NS, or dilute 1 amp of 1:10,000 to 10 ml with NS)
3. moderate to severe or worsening (anaphylaxis): add:
   A. IV colloidal fluids, e.g. hetastarch (Hespan®) 6% (colloids are required since there is extravascular shift of fluids due to seepage, these agents also carry a small risk of allergic reaction)
   B. epinephrine (*see above*). May repeat x 1
   C. O_2 2-6 L/min per NC. Intubate if necessary
   D. EKG to R/O ischemic changes
4. if shock develops: add dopamine, start at 5 µg/kg/min (*see page 7*)

HYPOTENSION WITH BRADYCARDIA (VASOVAGAL REACTION)
1. mild:
   A. Trendelenburg position

B. IV fluids
2. if no response, add:
   A. atropine 0.75 mg IV, may repeat up to 2-3 mg over 15 mins PRN. Use with caution in patients with underlying heart disease
   B. EKG and/or cardiac monitor: especially if atropine or dopamine are used
3. if no response: add dopamine, start at 5 µg/kg/min (*see page 7*)

URTICARIA
1. mild: self limited. No treatment necessary
2. moderate:
   A. **diphenhydramine** (Benadryl®) 50 mg PO or deep IM (avoid IV, can cause anaphylaxis itself)
   B. **cimetidine** (Tagamet®) 300 mg PO or IV diluted to 20 ml and given over 20 mins. H_2 receptors contribute to wheal and flare of reaction
3. severe: treat as above for moderate reaction, and add:
   A. epinephrine (*see above*)
   B. maintain IV line

FACIAL OR LARYNGEAL ANGIOEDEMA
1. epinephrine: *see above*. May repeat up to 1 mg
2. if respiratory distress: O_2 2-6 L/min. Intubate if necessary
3. diphenhydramine: *see above*
4. cimetidine: *see above*
5. if angioedema is accessible, add ice pack
6. maintain IV line

BRONCHOSPASM
1. mild to moderate:
   A. epinephrine: *see above*. May repeat up to 1 ml
   B. if respiratory distress: O_2 2-6 L/min. Intubate if necessary
   C. maintain IV line
   D. inhalational therapy with a ß-adrenergic agonist, e.g. albuterol (Proventil®) if respiratory therapy is available, otherwise, metered dose inhaler e.g. pirbuterol (Maxair®) or metaproterenol (Metaprel®), 2 puffs
2. severe: treat as above for moderate reaction, and add:
   A. aminophylline 250-500 mg in 10-20 cc NS slow IV over 15-30 mins. Monitor for hypotension and arrhythmias
   B. intubate
3. prolonged: add the following (will not have immediate effect):
   A. hydrocortisone 250 mg IV
   B. diphenhydramine: *see above*
   C. cimetidine: *see above*

PULMONARY EDEMA
1. O_2 2-6 L/min per NC. Intubate if necessary
2. raise head and body
3. furosemide (Lasix®) 40 mg IV
4. EKG
5. if hypoxia develops (may manifest as agitation or combativeness), add:
   A. morphine 8-15 mg IV. May cause respiratory depression, be prepared to intubate
   B. epinephrine: *see above*. ✖ CAUTION: use only if MI can be R/O as cause of the pulmonary edema. Patients with acute intracranial pathology may be at risk of neurogenic pulmonary edema (*see page 7*)

SEIZURES
If seizure is not self limited, start with lorazepam (Ativan®) 2-4 mg IV for an adult. Take precautions for status epilepticus (*see page 265*) and proceed to other drugs as indicated (*see page 266*).

5.2.   CAT scan

Attenuation of the x-ray beam on a CT scan is defined in Hounsfield units. These units are not absolute, and vary between CT scanner models, with a sample being shown in *Table 5-2*.

If there are no calibration marks on scan, one can estimate average adult globe (eyeball) is 25 mm diameter (through its equator).

Table 5-2 Hounsfield units for a sample CT scanner

DEFINITIONS	Hounsfield units	Comment
no attenuation (air)	−1000	definition
water	0	definition
dense bone	+1000	definition
CRANIAL CT		
brain (grey matter)	30 to 40	
brain (white matter)	20 to 35	
cerebral edema	10 to 14	
CSF	+5	
bone	+600	
blood clot*	75 to 80	e.g. fresh SAH
fat	−35 to −40	
calcium	100 to 300	
enhanced vessels	90-100	
SPINE CT		
disc material	55-70	disc density is
thecal sac	20-30	≈ 2 x thecal sac

*   Hct < 23% will cause an acute SDH to be isodense with brain

5.3.   Angiography (cerebral)

Risks
Risk varies with the nature of the pathology being investigated and with the experience of the angiography team. Overall risk of a complication resulting in a permanent neurologic deficit[4, 5]: 0.1%. In ACAS, there was a 1.2% complication rate (*see page 873*).

General information[6]
In general: non-vascular deep lesions cause changes in venous structures, superficial lesions affect arterial structures. The classic feature of a malignant neoplasm (e.g. glioblastoma multiforme) on angiography is an early draining vein.

Bovine circulation: anatomic variant where the common carotids arise from a common trunk off the aorta.

Hypoid: having only one anterior cerebral artery (as in a horse).

Allcock test: evaluates flow through the posterior communicating arteries by vertebral angiography during common carotid compression.

Fetal circulation: 15-35% of patients supply their posterior cerebral artery on one or both sides from the carotid (via p-comm) instead of via the vertebrobasilar system.

To help find the middle meningeal artery on lateral ECA angio, follow the anterior sweep of the sphenoid air sinus.

Carotid-basilar anastamoses
A **persistent primitive trigeminal artery (PPTA)** is seen in ≈ 0.6% of cerebral angiograms, and is the most common of the persistent carotid-basilar anastamoses. Arises from the ICA proximal to the origin of the meningohypophyseal trunk and connects to the upper basilar artery. The VAs are usually small. Occasionally the p-comms may be hypoplastic and the PPTA may provide significant blood supply to the distributions of the distal basilar artery, the posterior cerebral artery and the superior cerebellar arteries, particularly if the basilar artery is also hypoplastic (Saltzman type I anatomy). A PPTA

may be associated with vascular anomalies, such as aneurysms or AVMs. Rarely, aneurysms may directly involve these vessels. May also be associated with trigeminal neuralgia (*see page 379*).

Anterior Circulation

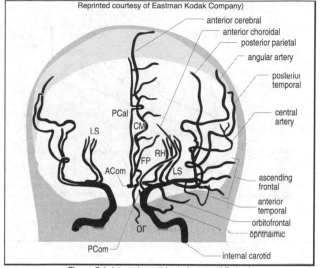

Reprinted courtesy of Eastman Kodak Company)

anterior cerebral
anterior choroidal
posterior parietal
angular artery
posterior temporal
central artery
ascending frontal
anterior temporal
orbitofrontal
ophthalmic
internal carotid

PCal
LS
CM
RH
FP
ACom
LS
OF
PCom

Figure 5-1 Internal carotid arteriogram (AP view)

Anterior Cerebral Artery (ACA)
See *Figure 5-2*. Branches:
1. recurrent artery (of **Heubner**): 80% arise from A1 (one of the larger medial lenticulostriates, remainder of lenticulostriates may arise from this artery) ⇒ head of caudate, putamen, and anterior internal capsule
2. medial orbitofrontal artery
3. frontopolar artery
4. callosomarginal
   A. internal frontal branches
      1. anterior
      2. middle
      3. posterior
   B. paracentral artery
5. pericallosal artery (continuation of ACA)
   A. superior internal parietal (precuneate) artery
   B. inferior internal parietal artery

Abbreviations from *Figure 5-1*

ACom	anterior communicating artery
CM	callosomarginal artery
FP	frontopolar artery
LS	lenticulostriate arteries
OF	orbitofrontal artery
PCal	pericallosal artery
PCom	posterior communicating artery
RH	recurrent artery of Heubner

Middle Cerebral Artery (MCA)
See *Figure 5-3*. Branches vary widely, 10 relatively common ones:
1. medial (3-6 per side) and lateral lenticulostriate arteries
2. anterior temporal
3. posterior temporal
4. lateral orbitofrontal

5. ascending frontal (candelabra)
6. precentral (prerolandic)
7. central (rolandic)
8. anterior parietal (postrolandic)
9. posterior parietal
10. angular

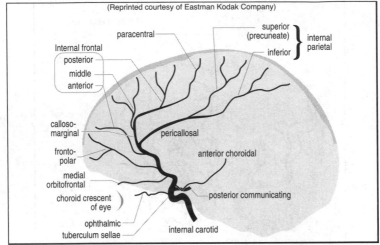

Figure 5-2 Anterior cerebral arteriogram (lateral view)

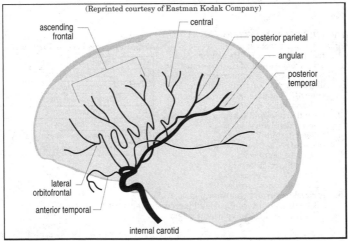

Figure 5-3 Middle cerebral arteriogram (lateral view)

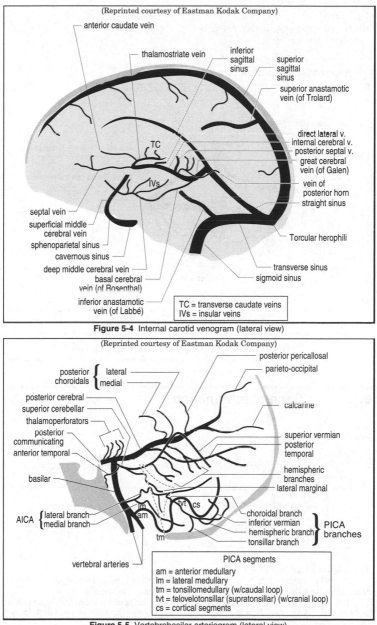

anterior caudate vein

thalamostriate vein

inferior sagittal sinus

superior sagittal sinus

superior anastamotic vein (of Trolard)

direct lateral v.
internal cerebral v.
posterior septal v.
great cerebral vein (of Galen)

vein of posterior horn
straight sinus

TC

IVs

septal vein

superficial middle cerebral vein

sphenoparietal sinus

cavernous sinus

deep middle cerebral vein

basal cerebral vein (of Rosenthal)

inferior anastamotic vein (of Labbé)

Torcular herophili

transverse sinus
sigmoid sinus

TC = transverse caudate veins
IVs = insular veins

Figure 5-4 Internal carotid venogram (lateral view)

posterior pericallosal
parieto-occipital

posterior choroidals { lateral / medial }

posterior cerebral
superior cerebellar
thalamoperforators
posterior communicating
anterior temporal

basilar

calcarine

superior vermian
posterior temporal

hemispheric branches
lateral marginal

AICA { lateral branch / medial branch }

lm
am
tvt cs
tm

choroidal branch
inferior vermian
hemispheric branch } PICA branches
tonsillar branch

vertebral arteries

PICA segments
am = anterior medullary
lm = lateral medullary
tm = tonsillomedullary (w/caudal loop)
tvt = telovelotonsillar (supratonsillar) (w/cranial loop)
cs = cortical segments

Figure 5-5 Vertebrobasilar arteriogram (lateral view)

POSTERIOR CEREBRAL ARTERY (PCA)
See *Figure 5-5*.

POSTERIOR FOSSA VENOUS ANATOMY

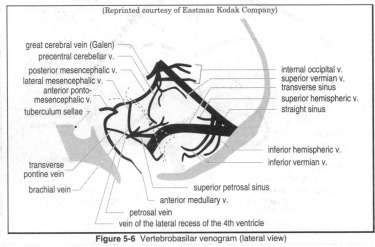

(Reprinted courtesy of Eastman Kodak Company)

great cerebral vein (Galen)
precentral cerebellar v.
posterior mesencephalic v.
lateral mesencephalic v.
anterior ponto-
mesencephalic v.
tuberculum sellae

internal occipital v.
superior vermian v.
transverse sinus
superior hemispheric v.
straight sinus

inferior hemispheric v.
inferior vermian v.

transverse
pontine vein

brachial vein

superior petrosal sinus
anterior medullary v.
petrosal vein
vein of the lateral recess of the 4th ventricle

Figure 5-6 Vertebrobasilar venogram (lateral view)

5.4. Magnetic resonance imaging (MRI)

5.4.1. General information

DEFINITIONS[7]

Abbreviations

TR	time to repetition
TE	time to echo
T_i	time to inversion
T_1	spin-lattice relaxation time ("time to magnetize") (regrowth)
T_2	spin-spin relaxation time ("time to demagnetize") (decay)

Table 5-3 Range of acquisition data

	short TE (te < 50)	long TE (te > 80)
short TR (TR < 1000)	T1WI	
long TR (TR > 2000)	proton density or spin density	T2WI

T_1 weighted image (T1WI)

Short $T_1 \rightarrow$ high signal (bright). "Anatomic image", somewhat resembles CT. Shorter acquisition time than T2WI. Proton rich tissue (e.g. H_2O) has long T_1.

The only objects that appear white on T1WI are fat, melanin, and subacute blood (> 48 hrs old). White matter is higher signal than grey matter (myelin has a high fat content). Most pathology is low signal on T1WI.

fat (including bone marrow), blood > 48 hrs old, melanin	white matter	grey matter	calcium	CSF, bone
(note: grey-bar illustrates direction of intensity change and does <u>not</u> show actual grey on MRI)

T_2 weighted image (T2WI)

Long T_2 → high signal (bright). "Pathological image". Most pathology shows up as high signal, including surrounding edema.

brain edema/water	CSF	grey matter	white matter	bone, fat
(note: grey-bar illustrates direction of intensity change and does <u>not</u> show actual grey on MRI)

KEY POINT: both fat and 7-14 day-old blood (see *Table 29-4*, page 856) are high signal on T1WI. On T2WI blood remains high signal but fat "drops out" and becomes black.

Spin density image

AKA balanced image, AKA proton density image. Partway between T1WI and T2WI. CSF = grey, approximately isodense with brain (useful in white matter demyelinating disease).

FLAIR

Acronym for FLuid-Attenuated Inversion Recovery. CSF appears dark. Most lesions including MS plaques, other white matter lesions, tumors, edema, and acute infarcts appear bright. Periventricular lesions such as MS plaques become more conspicuous.

Echo train (AKA fast spin echo (FSE))

tr is held constant, te is progressively increased utilizing multiple echoes (8-16) rather than 1. Image approaches T2WI but with substantially reduced acquisition time (fat is brighter on FSE, which may be rectified by fat suppression techniques).

"GRASS" image

Acronym for "Gradient Recalled Acquisition in a Steady State". A "fast" T2WI utilizing a partial flip angle. GRASS is a GE trademark, other manufacturers use different names, e.g. FISP. CSF appears white, bone is black, and flowing vessels are white. Typical acquisition data: TR = 22, TE = 11, angle 8°. Used e.g. in cervical MRI to produce a "myelographic" image, improves MRI's ability to delineate bony spurs.

"STIR" image

Acronym for "short tau inversion recovery". Summates T_1 & T_2 signals. Causes fat to drop out (sometimes also called **fat suppression** image), allows gadolinium enhancement to show up better in areas of fat. Useful primarily in spine and orbit.

CONTRAINDICATIONS TO MRI

An authoritative reference[8] details safety issues. Web sites for MRI safety include: www.MRIsafety.com and www.IMRSER.org. Some issues that come up frequently in neurosurgical patients follows.

Pregnancy and MRI: During the first trimester, MRI can cause reabsorption of products of conception (miscarriage). There are no studies to determine the long term effects of MRI on a fetus after the first trimester (the low risk of MRI in this situation is probably preferable to the known dangers of ionizing radiation of x-rays (including CT)[9]). Gadolinium contrast is contraindicated during all of pregnancy, and is not approved for use in age < 2 years. Breast-feeding must be interrupted for 2 days after administration of gadolinium to the mother.

Contraindications to MRI:
1. cardiac pacemaker, implanted neurostimulators, cochlear implants: may cause temporary or permanent malfunction
2. ferromagnetic aneurysm clips (*see below*): some centers exclude *all* patients with any type of aneurysm clip
3. metallic implants or foreign bodies with large component of iron or cobalt (may move in field, may heat up)
4. metallic fragments within the eye
5. placement of a vascular stent, coil or filter within the past 6 weeks
6. shrapnel: BB's (some bullets are OK)
7. relative contraindications:
   A. claustrophobic patients: may be able to sedate adequately to perform study
   B. critically ill patients: ability to monitor and access to patient are impaired. Specially designed non-magnetic ventilator may be required. Cannot use most brands of electronic IV pumps/regulators
   C. obese patients: may not physically fit into many closed bore MRI scanners. Open bore scanners may circumvent this but many utilize lower field strength magnets and produce inferior quality images in large patients
   D. metal implants in the region of interest (or previous surgery with high speed drills which may leave metal filings): may produce susceptibility artifact which can distort the image in that area

ANEURYSM CLIPS AND MRI

MRI considerations in patients with a cerebral aneurysm clip:
1. the danger of the MRI magnetic field causing the aneurysm clip to be pulled or torqued off of the aneurysm or to tear the neck
2. the artifact produced by the metal of the clip in the magnetic field
3. heat generated in the region of the clip: not clinically significant

The more ferromagnetic the clip, the larger the force exerted on it by the magnetic field and the greater the image distortion near the clip.

Stainless steel (**SS**) is classified as **martensitic** (ferromagnetic) or **austenitic** (non-ferromagnetic). Co-balt-based superalloys are non-ferromagnetic and include Elgiloy (Sugita clips), Phynox (Yasargil), and Vari-Angle (McFadden).

Table 5-4 shows the magnetic remnance of various clips which is related to their ferromagnetic properties. If in doubt at the time of aneurysm surgery, apply the following simple test: non-ferromagnetic clips cannot be lifted or dragged with a small magnet.

Table 5-4   Magnetic remnance of aneurysm clips[10]

Clip	Type of steel	Magnetic remnance (no units)	MRI compatible?
Drake DR 12	martensitic SS	100	no
Heifetz	17-7PH	44	no
Mayfield	martensitic SS	74	no
Scoville	EN-58J	64	no
Olivecrona		0	yes
Sugita	Elgiloy	0	yes
Sugita with loop	gold plated	1	yes
McFadden	Vari-Angle	0	yes
Yasargil	316	0	yes
Yasargil	Phynox	0	yes
Yasargil (old)		1	yes
silver clip		0	yes

HEMORRHAGE ON MRI

One of the most complex lesions to interpret on MRI. *See page 856.*

5.4.2.   Diffusion-weighted imaging (DWI) and perfusion-imaging (PWI)

Gaining usage in ischemic brain disease (some MRI machines do not yet have the necessary gradients for diffusion weighting or the speed needed for both DWI and PWI).

Diffusion-weighted imaging: DWI is sensitive to random Brownian motion of water molecules, and an apparent diffusion coefficient (**ADC**) is determined for each area based on a number of variables (time, slice orientation...)[11].

Freely diffusing water (e.g. in CSF) appears dark on DWI. Areas of acute brain ischemia show up as increased signal intensity on DWI within minutes[11, 12]. DWI may also be able to distinguish cytotoxic from vasogenic **edema**[13, 14] (*see page 85*). However, factors other than focal ischemia (e.g. global ischemia, hypoglycemia, status epilepticus...) can produce ADC decline and the DWI images must therefore be interpreted in relation to the clinical setting[11]. Some, but not all[15], TIAs are associated with abnormalities on DWI. Diffusion defects do not indicate irreversible injury, but indicates tissue that is near cell death.

Perfusion imaging: Provides information related to the perfusion status of the microcirculation. There are several methods currently in use, with the bolus-contrast approach being the most widely employed[11]. Ultrafast gradient imaging is used to follow the gradual reduction to normal following administration of contrast (usually gadolinium). A signal wash-out curve is derived and is compared to contrast in an artery.

Use

In theory, DWI and PWI may be combined to locate areas of perfusion deficit on PWI that exceeds the zone of diffusion deficit on DWI, thus identifying salvageable brain tissue at risk of infarction ("**penumbra**", *see page 806*) e.g. to screen for potential candidates for thrombolytic therapy[16].

5.4.3.   Magnetic resonance spectroscopy (MRS)

This section specifically covers proton (H+) MRS which can be performed on almost any MRI scanner (especially units ≥ 1.5 T) with the appropriate software. Spectroscopy of other nuclei (e.g. phosphorous) can be evaluated only with specialized equipment.

SINGLE VOXEL MRS

A small area is selected on the "scout" MRI and the spectroscopic peaks for that region are displayed in resonance as a function of parts-per-million (**ppm**). Therefore, may be subject to sampling error.

Clinically important characteristic peaks are delineated in *Table 5-5*.

ILLUSTRATIVE PATTERNS

Normal brain: *See Figure 5-7*.

Tumor: *See Figure 5-7*. ↓ NAA, ↑ lactate, ↑ lipid, ↑ choline (rule of thumb: with gliomas, the higher the choline, the higher the grade up to grade 3, thereafter necrosis reduces relative choline levels and the lipid peak may be utilized).

Table 5-5   Important peaks on proton MRS

Moiety	Resonance (ppm)	Description
lipid	0.5-1.5	slightly overlaps lactate peak at TE ≈ 35
lactate	1.3	a couplet peak. Not present in normal brain. End product of anaerobic glycolysis, ∴ a marker of hypoxia. Present in: ischemia, infection, demyelinating disease, inborn errors of metabolism... At higher TE (e.g. TE = 144), the peak inverts which can help distinguish it from the lipid peak
N-acetyl aspartate (NAA)	2	a neuronal marker. Normally the tallest peak (higher than Cr or Cho). ↓ in ≈ all focal and regional brain abnormalities (CVA, tumor, MS, epilepsy, Alzheimer's disease, abscess, brain injury...)
creatine (Cr)	3*	useful primarily as a reference for choline. Higher in grey matter than white matter
choline (Cho)	3.2	marker of membrane synthesis. ↑ in neoplasms and some rare conditions of increased cell growth & in the developing brain. ★ CVA is low in choline

*   Cr has another less important peak

CVA: ↑ lactate peak predominates. Choline is characteristically low.

Abscess[17]: Reduced NAA, Cr & choline peaks, and "atypical peaks" (succinate, acetate...) from bacterial synthesis is pathognomonic for abscess (not always present). Lactate may be elevated.

Multiple sclerosis: Bland pattern. NAA slightly reduced. Lactate and lipid slightly elevated. Choline not elevated.

1. differentiating abscess from neoplasm
2. post-op enhancement vs. recurrence of tumor
3. distinguishing tumor from MS plaques: occasionally cannot be differentiated
4. in AIDS: may be able to help differentiate toxo from lymphoma from PML (PML: ↓ NAA, no significant increase in choline, lactate or lipid)
5. the promise of differentiating tumor infiltration from edema has not been borne out
6. some utility in distinguishing tumor from radiation necrosis (*see page 535*)

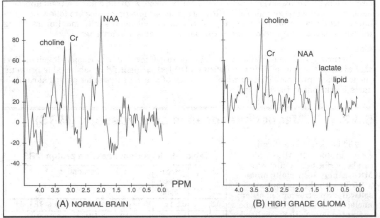

(A) NORMAL BRAIN   (B) HIGH GRADE GLIOMA

Figure 5-7 Proton MRS of (A) normal brain, and (B) high grade glioma

MULTI-VOXEL MRS

Color coded scan with selected overlay for NAA, choline... one at a time. May reduce risk of sampling error.

5.5.   Plain films

5.5.1.   Skull films

SELLA TURCICA

NORMAL ADULT DIMENSIONS ON SKULL X-RAY
    Technique: true lateral, 91 cm target to film distance, central ray 2.5 cm anterior and 1.9 cm superior to EAM. See *Figure 5-8* for illustration of the dimensions, and *Table 5-6* for normal values.
    Depth (**D**): defined as the greatest measurement from floor to diaphragma sellae.
    Length (**L**): defined as the greatest AP diameter.

Table 5-6 Normal dimensions of the sella turcica (*see Figure 5-8*)

Dimension	Max	Min	Ave
D (depth) (mm)	12	4	8.1
L (length) (mm)	16	5	10.6

ABNORMAL FINDINGS
    Pituitary adenomas tend to enlarge the sella, in contrast to craniopharyngiomas which erode the posterior clinoids. Empty sella syndrome tends to balloon the sella symmetrically, and also does not erode the clinoids.

"J" shaped sella suggests optic nerve glioma. It can also occur congenitally in Hurler's syndrome (a mucopolysaccharidosis).

MISCELLANEOUS

Water's view: x-ray tube angled up 45° (perpendicular to clivus), AKA submental vertex view.

Towne's view: x-ray tube angled down 45°, to view occiput.

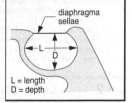
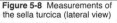

L = length
D = depth

Figure 5-8 Measurements of the sella turcica (lateral view)

BASILAR IMPRESSION

Several conditions whose names are often (erroneously) used interchangeably (exact definitions are not entirely agreed upon for all of these):

1. **platybasia**: abnormal basilar angle. Of little medical importance (used in anthropological data). May or may not be associated with basilar impression
2. **basilar impression (BI)**: upward displacement of foramen magnum margins (including occipital bone) and cervical spine (including odontoid process) into p-fossa. Some use this term for upward displacement of dens only. May be seen in:
   A. congenital conditions (BI is the most common congenital anomaly of the craniocervical junction, it is often accompanied by other anomalies[28 (p 148-9)])
      1. Down's syndrome
      2. Klippel-Feil syndrome (*see page 119*)
      3. Chiari malformation (*see page 104*)
      4. syringomyelia
   B. acquired conditions
      1. rheumatoid arthritis (in part due do incompetence of transverse ligament, see *Basilar impression in rheumatoid arthritis, page 339*)
      2. post-traumatic
3. **basilar invagination**, AKA **cranial settling**: upward indentation of skull base usually due to acquired softening of bone, often associated with atlanto-occipital fusion. Some consider this synonymous with BI. Seen in[29]:
   A. Paget's disease
   B. osteogenesis imperfecta
   C. osteomalacia
   D. rickets
   E. hyperparathyroidism

Some measurements of use (refer to *Figure 5-10*, page 141, and *Figure 5-9* below):

1. **McRae's line** ("McR" in *Figure 5-10*): drawn across foramen magnum (tip of clivus (basion) to opisthion)[30]. Should be > 19 mm (average: 35). No part of odontoid should be above this line (the most accurate for BI)

2. **Chamberlain's line** ("CL" in *Figure 5-10*)[31]: posterior hard palate to posterior margin of foramen magnum (opisthion). Less than 3 mm or half of dens should be above this line, with 6 mm being definitely pathologic. Seldom used because opisthion is often hard to see on plain film and may also be invaginated)

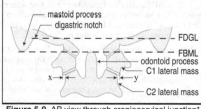

— mastoid process
— digastric notch
— FDGL
— FBML
— odontoid process
— C1 lateral mass
x→|←   →|←y
— C2 lateral mass

Figure 5-9 AP view through craniocervical junction*

3. **McGregor's baseline** ("McG" in *Figure 5-10*)[32]: posterior margin of hard palate to most caudal point of occiput. No more than 4.5 mm of dens should be above this

* FDGL = Fischgold's digastric line, FBML = Fischgold's bimastoid line, x + y = total overhang of C1 on C2 (see *Rule of Spence* page 723)

4. **Wackenheim's clivus-canal line** ("WCCL" in *Figure 5-10*): the odontoid should be tangential to or below the line that extends the course of the clivus (the clivus baseline). If the clivus is

concave or convex, this baseline is drawn to connect the basion to the base of the posterior clinoids on the clivus[33]

5. **(Fischgold's) digastric line** ("FDGL" in *Figure 5-9*): joins digastric notches. The normal distance from this line to the middle of the atlanto-occipital joint is 10 mm (decreased in BI)[34]. No part of odontoid should be above this line. More accurate than the bimastoid line (FBML

6. **Fischgold's bimastoid line** ("FBML" in *Figure 5-9*): joins tips of mastoid processes. The odontoid tip averages 2 mm above this line (range: 3 mm below to 10 mm above) and this line should cross the atlanto-occipital joint

5.5.2.   Lumbosacral (LS) spine

L4-5 is normally the lumbar disc space with the greatest vertical height. Also see *Normal LS spine measurements*, page 327.

AP view: look for defect or non visualization of the "owl's eyes" which is due to pedicle erosion which may occur with lytic tumors (common with metastatic disease).

Oblique views: look for discontinuity in neck of "Scotty dog" for defect in pars interarticularis.

5.5.3.   C-Spine

NORMAL FINDINGS

For radiographic signs of cervical spine trauma, see *Table 25-7*, page 706, and for guidelines for diagnosing clinical instability, see *Table 25-27*, page 734.

CONTOUR LINES

On a lateral C-spine x-ray, there are 4 contour lines (AKA arcuate lines). Normally each should form a smooth, gentle curve (*see Figure 5-10*):

1. posterior marginal line **(PML)**: along posterior cortical surfaces of vertebral bodies **(VB)**. Marks the anterior margin of spinal canal
2. anterior marginal line **(AML)**: along anterior cortical surfaces of VBs
3. **spinolaminar line (SLL)**: along base of spinous processes. The posterior margin of the spinal canal
4. posterior spinous line **(PSL)**: along tips of spinous processes

RELATION OF ATLAS TO OCCIPUT
See *page 719* for criteria for atlantoaxial dislocation.

RELATION OF ATLAS TO AXIS

Atlanto-dental interval (ADI)
The ADI is the distance between the anterior margin of the dens and the closest point of the anterior arch of C1 ("C1 button") on a lateral C-spine x-ray (*see Figure 5-10*). The normal maximal ADI is variously given in the range of 2 to 4 mm[18, 19]. Commonly accepted upper limits are shown in *Table 5-7*.

Atlantoaxial subluxation (AAS): Two possibilities:

1. ADI > normal: may occur with incompetence of the transverse ligament. Common in rheumatoid arthritis (*see page 338*), may also follow trauma (*see page 722*)
2. normal ADI: in the presence of an odontoid fracture (*see page 727*)

"V" shaped pre-dens space[21]: Widening of the upper space between the anterior arch of C1 and the odontoid seen on lateral C-spine flexion x-ray. It is not known if this increased mobility represents elongation or laxity of the transverse ligament and/or the posterior ligamentous complex.

Table 5-7   Normal ADI

Patient	ADI
adults	
males	≤ 3 mm
females	≤ 2.5 mm
pediatrics[20] (≤ 15 yrs)	≤ 4 mm

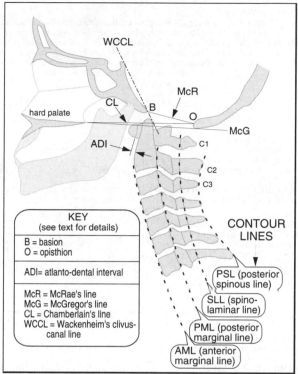

Figure 5-10 Spinal contour lines and lines used to diagnose basilar invagination
Lateral view through craniocervical junction

CANAL DIAMETER

Normal canal diameter on lateral C-spine x-ray (from spinolaminar line **(SLL)** to posterior vertebral body with 6 foot tube to film distance)[22]: **17 ± 5 mm**. In the presence of osteophytic spurs, measure from the back of the spur to the SLL.

Cervical spinal stenosis: various cutoffs for the normal minimum AP diameter have been suggested[23]. On a plain lateral C-spine x-ray this is usually measured from the posterior vertebral body (or the posterior aspect of an osteophyte) to the spinolaminar line. Some use 15 mm. Most agree that stenosis is present when the AP diameter is **< 12 mm** in an adult (*see page 334* for correlation with myelopathy).

PREVERTEBRAL SOFT TISSUE

Abnormally increased prevertebral soft tissue **(PVST)** on lateral C-spine x-ray may indicate the presence of a vertebral fracture, dislocation, or ligamentous disruption[24]. Normal values are shown in *Table 5-8*. NB: the sensitivity of these measurements is only ≈ 60% at C3 and 5% at C6[24]. Increased PVST is more likely with anterior than posterior injuries[25]. False positives may occur with basal skull/facial fractures, especially with

Table 5-8 Normal prevertebral soft tissue

Space	Level	Maximum normal width	
		Adults (mm)	Peds (mm)
retropharyngeal	C1	10	unreliable
	C2-4	5-7	
retrotracheal	C5-7	22	14

fracture of the pterygoid plates.

C-spine AP: a fracture/dislocation or ligament disruption may be diagnosed if the interspinous distance is 1.5 times that at both adjacent levels (measured from center of spinous precesses)[26]. Also look for a malalignment of spinous processes below a certain level which may be evidence of rotation due to a unilaterally locked facet.

C-spine lateral: look for "**fanning**" or "**flaring**" which is an abnormal spread of one pair of spinous processes that may also indicate ligament disruption.

PEDIATRIC C-SPINE

C1 (ATLAS) (*see Figure 5-11*)
Ossification centers[27]: usually 3
1. 1 (sometimes 2) for body (not ossified at birth; appears on x-ray during 1st yr)
2. 1 for each neural arch (appear bilaterally ≈ 7th fetal week)

Synchondroses[27]:
- synchondrosis of the spinous process: fuses by ≈ 3 yrs age
- 2 neurocentral synchondroses: fuse by ≈ age 7 yrs

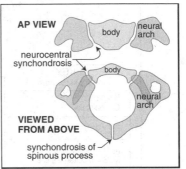

Figure 5-11 Pediatric C1 (atlas)

C2 (AXIS) (*see Figure 5-12*)
4 primary ossification centers:
- odontoid process
- vertebral body
- 2 neural arches

A secondary ossification center appears at the summit of the dens between 3-6 yrs, and fuses with dens by age 12[27].

Synchondroses: normally fuse between 3-6 years of age.

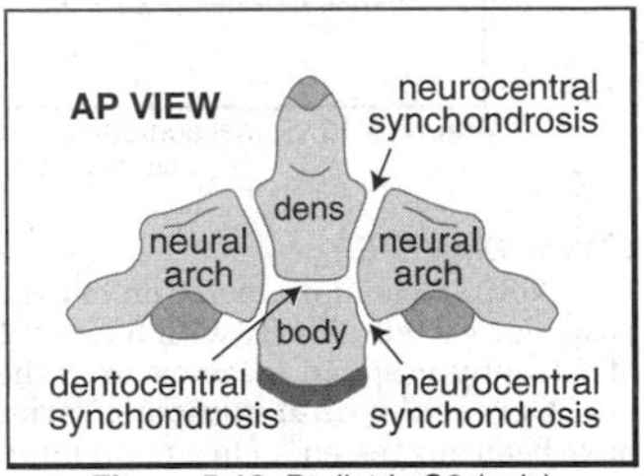

C3-7
Cervical bodies are normally wedge shaped in pediatric population (narrower anteriorly). Wedging decreases with age.

Figure 5-12 Pediatric C2 (axis)

5.6. Myelography

Lumbar myelogram
Using iohexol (Omnipaque® 140 or 180) as shown in *Table 5-1*.

Cervical myelogram with water soluble contrast via LP
Use iohexol (Omnipaque® 300 or 240) as shown in *Table 5-1*. Insert spinal needle into lumbar subarachnoid space, tilt the head of the myelogram table down with the patient's neck extended and then inject dye. If a complete cervical block is seen, have pa-

tient flex neck. If the block cannot be traversed, patient may need C1-2 puncture or MRI (first obtain a CT which may show dye above the block that cannot be appreciated on myelography alone).

Post myelographic CT

Increases sensitivity and specificity of myelography (*see page 295*). In cases of complete block on myelogram, CT will often show dye distal to the apparent site of the block.

5.7. Bone scan

Technetium-99 (^{99m}Tc) pertechnetate is a radioisotope that may be attached to various substrates for use in bone scanning. It may be used to label polyphosphate (rarely used today), diphosphonate[35] (**MDP**), or HDP (the most widely agent used currently). Bone scans with technetium-labeled compounds depends on the presence of osteoblastic activity for the deposition of tracer into the bone.

Gallium may also be used to look for more chronic osteomyelitis.

Applications for bone scans include:
1. infection
   A. osteomyelitis of the skull or spine (vertebral osteomyelitis, *see page 244*)
   B. discitis: *see page 247*
2. tumor
   A. spine metastases: *see page 518*
   B. primary bone tumors of the spine: *see page 512*
   C. skull tumors: *see page 480*
3. diseases involving abnormal bone metabolism
   A. Paget's disease: of the skull (*see page 341*) or spine (*see page 341*)
   B. hyperostosis frontalis interna: *see page 483*
4. craniosynostosis: *see page 99*
5. fractures: spine (*see page 707*) or skull
6. "low back problems": to help identify some of the above examples (*see page 293*)

5.8. References

1. Rivera E, Hardjasudarma M, Willis B K, *et al.*: Inadvertent use of ionic contrast material in myelography: Case report and management guidelines. **Neurosurgery** 36: 413-5, 1995.
2. Bohn H P, Reich L, Suljaga-Petchel K: Inadvertent intrathecal use of ionic contrast media for myelography. **AJNR** 13: 1515-9, 1992.
3. Lasser E C, Berry C C, Talner L B, *et al.*: Pretreatment with corticosteroids to alleviate reactions to intravenous contrast material. **N Engl J Med** 317: 825-9, 1987.
4. Dion J E, Gates P C, Fox A J, *et al.*: Clinical events following neuroangiography: A prospective study. **Stroke** 18: 997-1004, 1987.
5. Earnest F, Forbes G, Sandok B A, *et al.*: Complications of cerebral angiography: Prospective assessment of risk. **AJR** 142: 247-53, 1984.
6. Newton T H, Potts D G, (eds.): **Radiology of the skull and brain.** C. V. Mosby, Saint Louis, 1971.
7. Jackson E F, Ginsberg L E, Schomer D F, *et al.*: A review of MRI pulse sequences and techniques in neuroimaging. **Surg Neurol** 47: 185-99, 1997.
8. Shellock F G: **Reference manual for magnetic resonance safety.** Amirsys, Inc., Salt Lake City, Utah, 2003: pp 435-97.
9. Edelman R R, Warach S: Magnetic resonance imaging (first of two parts). **N Engl J Med** 328: 708-16, 1993.
10. Romner B, Olsson M, Ljunggren B, *et al.*: Magnetic resonance imaging and aneurysm clips: Magnetic

properties and image artifacts. **J Neurosurg** 70: 426-31, 1989.
11. Fisher M, Albers G W: Applications of diffusion-perfusion magnetic resonance imaging in acute ischemic stroke. **Neurology** 52: 1750-6, 1999.
12. Prichard J W, Grossman R I: New reasons for early use of MRI in stroke. **Neurology** 52: 1733-6, 1999 (editorial).
13. Ay H, Buonanno F S, Schaefer P W, *et al.*: Posterior leukoencephalopathy without severe hypertension: Utility of diffusion-weighted MRI. **Neurology** 51: 1369-76, 1998.
14. Schaefer P W, Buonanno F S, Gonzalez R G, *et al.*: Diffusion-weighted imaging discriminates between cytotoxic and vasogenic edema in a patient with eclampsia. **Stroke** 28: 1082-5, 1997.
15. Ay H, Buonanno F S, Rordorf G, *et al.*: Normal diffusion-weighted MRI during stroke-like deficits. **Neurology** 52: 1784-92, 1999.
16. Marks M P, Tong D C, Beaulieu C, *et al.*: Evaluation of early reperfusion and IV tPA therapy using diffusion- and perfusion-weighted MRI. **Neurology** 52: 1792-8, 1999.
17. Martinez-Perez I, Moreno A, Alonso J, *et al.*: Diagnosis of brain abscess by magnetic resonance spectroscopy. Report of two cases. **J Neurosurg** 86: 708-13, 1997.
18. Hinck V C, Hopkins C E: Measurement of the atlanto-dental interval in the adult. **Am J Roentgenol Radium Ther Nucl Med** 84: 945-51, 1960.

19. Meijers K A E, van Beusekom G T, Luyendijk W, *et al.*: Dislocation of the cervical spine with cord compression in rheumatoid arthritis. **J Bone Joint Surg** 56B: 668-80, 1974.

20. Powers B, Miller M D, Kramer R S, *et al.*: Traumatic anterior atlanto-occipital dislocation. **Neurosurgery** 4: 12-7, 1979.

21. Bohrer S P, Klein M D, Martin W: "V" shaped predens space. **Skeletal Radiol** 14: 111-6, 1985.

22. Schmidek H H, Sweet W H, (eds.): **Operative neurosurgical techniques**. 1st ed., Grune and Stratton, New York, 1982.

23. Epstein N, Epstein J A, Benjamin V, *et al.*: Traumatic myelopathy in patients with cervical spinal stenosis without fracture or dislocation: Methods of diagnosis, management, and prognosis. **Spine** 5: 489-96, 1980.

24. DeBenhe K, Havel C: Utility of prevertebral soft tissue measurements in identifying patients with cervical spine injury. **Ann Emerg Med** 24: 1119-24, 1994.

25. Miles K A, Finlay D: Is prevertebral soft tissue swelling a useful sign in injury of the cervical spine? **Injury** 19: 177-9, 1988.

26. Naidich J B, Naidich T P, Garfein C, *et al.*: The widened interspinous distance: A useful sign of anterior cervical dislocation. **Radiology** 123: 113-6, 1977.

27. Bailey D K: The normal cervical spine in infants and children. **Radiology** 59: 712-9, 1952.

28. The Cervical Spine Research Society, (ed.) **The cervical spine**. 1st ed., J.B. Lippincott, Philadelphia, 1983.

29. Jacobson G, Bleeker H H: Pseudosubluxation of the axis in children. **Am J Roentgenol** 82: 472-81, 1959.

30. McRae D L: The significance of abnormalities of the cervical spine. **AJR** 70: 23-46, 1960.

31. Chamberlain W E: Basilar impression (platybasia); bizarre developmental anomaly of occipital bone and upper cervical spine with striking and misleading neurologic manifestations. **Yale J Biol Med** 11: 487-96, 1939.

32. McGregor J: The significance of certain measurements of the skull in the diagnosis of basilar impression. **Br J Radiol** 21: 171-81, 1948.

33. VanGilder J C, Menezes A H, Dolan K D: *Radiology of the normal craniovertebral junction*. In **The craniovertebral junction and its abnormalities**. Futura Publishing, NY, 1987, Chapter 3: pp 29-68.

34. Hinck V C, Hopkins C E, Savara B S: Diagnostic criteria of basilar impression. **Radiology** 76: 579, 1961.

35. Handa J, Yamamoto I, Morita R, *et al.*: 99mTc-polyphosphate and 99mTc-diphosphonate bone scintigraphy in neurosurgical practice. **Surg Neurol** 2: 307-10, 1974.

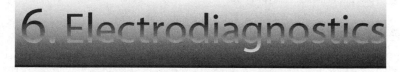

6. Electrodiagnostics

6.1.　　Electroencephalogram (EEG)

Common EEG rhythms are shown in *Table 6-1*. The primary use of EEG is in the diagnosis and management of seizure disorders. Non-convulsive use of EEG is essentially limited to monitoring for burst suppression (*see below*) (e.g. during carotid endarterectomy) or for differential diagnosis of diffuse encephalopathy, including:

Table 6-1　Common EEG rhythms

Rhythm	Symbol	Frequency
delta	Δ	0-3 Hz
theta	θ	4-7 Hz
alpha	α	8-13 Hz
beta	β	> 13 Hz

1. differentiating psychogenic unresponsiveness from organic: a normal EEG indicates either psychiatric unresponsiveness or locked-in syndrome
2. non-convulsive status epilepticus (seizures): absence or complex partial status
3. subclinical focal abnormalities: especially in patients too ill to be transported to CT. Look for e.g. PLEDs (*see below*), focal slowing...
4. specific patterns diagnostic for certain pathologies: e.g.:
   A. **periodic lateralizing epileptiform discharges (PLEDs)**: may occur with any acute focal cerebral insult (e.g. herpes simplex encephalitis **(HSE)**, abscess, tumor, embolic infarct): seen in 85% of cases of HSE (onset 2-5 d after presentation), if bilateral is ≈ diagnostic of HSE
   B. subacute sclerosing panencephalitis **(SSPE)** (pathognomonic pattern): periodic high voltage with 4-15 secs separation with accompanying body jerks, no change with painful stimulation (differential diagnosis includes PCP overdose)
   C. Creutzfeldt-Jakob disease (*see page 227*): myoclonic jerks. EEG → bilateral sharp wave 1.5-2 per second (early → slowing; later → triphasic). May resemble PLEDs, but are reactive to painful stimulation (most PLEDs are not)
   D. triphasic waves: not really specific. May be seen in hepatic encephalopathy, post-anoxia, and hyponatremia
5. objective measure of severity of encephalopathy: usually used for anoxic encephalopathy (e.g. periodic spikes with seizures indicates < 5% chance of normal neurologic outcome, with high mortality). Alpha coma, burst suppression, and electrocerebral silence are all poor prognosticators
6. differentiating hydranencephaly from severe hydrocephalus (see *Hydranencephaly*, page 180)
7. as a clinical confirmatory test in the determination of brain death (*see page 166*)

BURST SUPPRESSION
Isoelectric intervals interrupted by bursts of 8-12 Hz electrical activity that diminish to 1-4 Hz prior to electrical silence[1]. Often used as an endpoint for titrating neuroprotective drugs such as barbiturates, etomidate... (e.g. *see page 807*).

6.2.　　Evoked potentials

Clinical indications for evoked potentials **(EPs)**.
1. diagnosis: (MRI has largely replaced EPs for these 3 indications)
   A. acoustic neuroma
   B. subclinical lesions of multiple sclerosis
   C. brainstem lesions

2. intra-operative use (*see below*)

Table 6-2 Evoked potential waveforms
(note: values may differ from lab to lab)

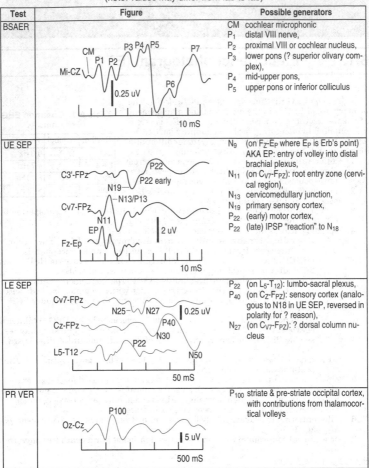

Test	Figure	Possible generators
BSAER		CM cochlear microphonic P_1 distal VIII nerve, P_2 proximal VIII or cochlear nucleus, P_3 lower pons (? superior olivary complex), P_4 mid-upper pons, P_5 upper pons or inferior colliculus
UE SEP		N_9 (on F_Z-E_P where E_P is Erb's point) AKA EP: entry of volley into distal brachial plexus, N_{11} (on C_{V7}-F_{PZ}): root entry zone (cervical region), N_{13} cervicomedullary junction, N_{19} primary sensory cortex, P_{22} (early) motor cortex, P_{22} (late) IPSP "reaction" to N_{18}
LE SEP		P_{22} (on L_5-T_{12}): lumbo-sacral plexus, P_{40} (on C_Z-F_{PZ}): sensory cortex (analogous to N18 in UE SEP, reversed in polarity for ? reason), N_{27} (on C_{V7}-F_{PZ}): ? dorsal column nucleus
PR VER		P_{100} striate & pre-striate occipital cortex, with contributions from thalamocortical volleys

INTRA-OPERATIVE EVOKED POTENTIALS

Also, *see page 3* for anesthetic requirements for intraoperative SSEP monitoring.

EPs may be used for intra-operative monitoring (e.g. monitoring hearing during resection of acoustic neuromas, or monitoring SSEPs during some spine surgery), however, their delayed nature often makes them of limited usefulness in avoiding acute intra-operative injury. A 10% increased latency of a major EP peak, or a drop in amplitude ≥ 50% is significant and should cause the surgeon to assess all variables (retractors, instruments...). Intra-operative SSEPs may be used to localize primary sensory cortex in anesthetized patients (as opposed to using brain mapping techniques in awake patients) by looking for phase reversal potentials across the central sulcus[2, 3].

EP monitoring during spine surgery

SSEPs: monitor only posterior column function, and while this correlates well with overall spinal cord function and are affected by manipulation of the spinal cord and ischemic events, they may remain unchanged with some injuries to the anterior cord.

Transcranial motor evoked potentials (TCMEPs): transcranial electrical or magnetic stimulation of motor cortex and descending motor axons with recording of motor potentials from distal spinal cord or muscle groups. Due to the large potentials, the acquisition time is shorter and feedback to the surgeon is almost immediate. However, due to patient movement from the muscle contractions, continuous recording is usually not possible (except with monitoring the response over the spinal cord). Useful for surgery involving the spinal cord (cervical or thoracic), no utility for lumbar spine surgery. In addition to general EP anesthetic requirements, neuromuscular blockade must minimized to permit ≥ 2 out of 4 twitches.

Descending evoked potentials (DEP): (formerly referred to by the misleading term as neurogenic motor evoked potentials). Rostral stimulation of the spinal cord with recording of a caudal neurogenic response from the spinal cord or peripheral nerve, or a myogenic response from a distal muscle. DEPs can be mediated primarily by sensory nerves and therefore do not represent true motor potentials. However, shown to be sensitive to spinal cord changes and may be useful when TCMEPs cannot be obtained.

ABBREVIATIONS

Abbreviations used below: **BSAER** = brain stem auditory evoked response; **UE/LE SEP** = upper/lower extremity sensory evoked potential; **PR VER** = pattern reversal visual evoked response which requires patient cooperation and visual attention as opposed to flash VER which may even be done through closed eyelids. See also references[4, 5].

Table 6-3   Normal values for evoked potentials*
(note: values may differ from lab to lab)

| Test | Parameters measured | – – Normal values – – | | Comment |
		Mean	+2.5 std dev	
BSAER	I-V peak latency	4.01 mS	**4.63 mS**	
	I-III peak latency	2.15 mS	**2.66 mS**	prolongation suggests lesion between pons and colliculus, often **acoustic neuroma**
	V absolute latency	5.7 mS	**6.27 mS**	
	III-V peak latency			prolongation suggests lesion between lower pons & midbrain, may be seen in M.S.
UE SEP	N_9-N_{18} peak latency	9.38 mS	**11.35 mS**	
LE SEP	P_{22}-P_{40} peak latency	15.62 mS	**20.82 mS**	
	P_{40} absolute latency	37.20 mS	**44.16 mS**	
PR VER	P_{100} absolute latency		**+ 3 S.D.**	
	P_{100} inter-eye difference	8-10 mS		Inter-eye difference is more sensitive with full field stimulation. Monocular defect suggests conduction defect in that optic nerve anterior to chiasm (e.g. M.S., glaucoma, compression retinal degeneration). Bilateral defect does not localize.

*   normal values in boldface are critical values used as cutoff for abnormal results

6.3.   Electromyography (EMG)

There are two portions to the EMG exam:
1. conduction measurements
2. needle exam
    A.   insertional activity
    B.   activity at rest: should be silent when needle is stationary and insertional activity has quieted

DEFINITIONS

Fibrillation potentials: following denervation of a muscle (secondary to a nerve injury), individual muscle fibers begin firing independently. Earliest onset 10 days, sometimes up to 3-4 weeks after denervation. If the nerve recovers, it may reinnervate the muscle, but with larger motor units resulting in longer duration and decreased numbers.

F-wave: nerve is stimulated, causing orthodromic and antidromic conduction. F-wave latency may be prolonged in radiculopathy (not sensitive).

SNAP: sensory nerve action potentials.

MYOTONIA
There are a number of myotonic conditions, including myotonic dystrophy. There is sustained contraction of the muscle. Classic EMG finding: "dive bomber" sound due to myotonic discharges.

LUMBAR DISC DISEASE
Also *see page 292*. SNAP may be normal, as the injury is proximal to the cell body which resides in the dorsal root ganglion (in the neural foramen). Paraspinal muscle fibrillations may occur.

Following discectomy for radiculopathy:
* motor potentials return first (if nerve injury were "complete", it would take a month to return)
* if lost, sensory potentials return last or may not return
* paraspinal potentials may no longer be useful because the muscles are cut during surgery

PLEXOPATHY
Reduction of SNAP with no paraspinal muscle fibrillations (the dorsal rami exit proximally to innervate the paraspinals, and are involved ≈ only with root lesions).

MISCELLANEOUS EMG PEARLS FOR NEUROSURGEONS
* The short head of the biceps femoris in the LE is the first muscle innervated by the peroneal division of the sciatic nerve at or just above the popliteal fossa just after the nerve splits off from the sciatic nerve. In cases e.g. of foot drop it is a good muscle to test to determine if there is a peroneal neuropathy vs. a more proximal lesion (i.e. above the popliteal fossa).
* EMG is not extremely sensitive for radiculopathy (e.g irritative radiculopathy might not be picked up), more so in the cervical region than in the lumbar region. However, when positive, it is very specific.

6.4. References

1. Donnegan J H: *The electroencephalogram*. In **Monitoring in anesthesia and critical care medicine**, Blitt C D, (ed.). Churchill Livingstone, New York, 1985: pp 323-43.
2. Gregori E M, Goldring S: Localization of function in the excision of lesions from the sensorimotor region. **J Neurosurg** 61: 1047-54, 1984.
3. Woolsey C N, Erickson T C, Gibson W E: Localization in somatic sensory and motor areas of human cerebral cortex as determined by direct recording of evoked potentials and electrical stimulation. **J Neurosurg** 51: 476-506, 1979.
4. Chiappa K H: Evoked potentials in clinical medicine (first of two parts). **N Engl J Med** 306: 1140-50, 1982.
5. Chiappa K H: Evoked potentials in clinical medicine (second of two parts). **N Engl J Med** 306: 1205-11, 1982.

7. Neurotoxicology

Also *see page 753* for plumbism (lead poisoning) from retained bullets.

7.1.   Ethanol

The acute and chronic effects of ethyl alcohol (ethanol, **EtOH**) abuse on the nervous system are protean[1], and are beyond the scope of this text (not to mention the effects of EtOH on other organ systems). Neuromuscular effects include:
1. acute intoxication: *see below*
2. effects of chronic alcohol abuse
    A. **Wernicke's encephalopathy**: *see page 151*
    B. cerebellar degeneration: due to degeneration of Purkinje cells in the cerebellar cortex, predominantly in the anterior superior vermis
    C. central pontine myelinolysis: *see page 12*
    D. stroke: increased risk of
        1. intracerebral hemorrhage: *see page 852*
        2. ischemic stroke[2]
        3. possibly aneurysmal SAH: *see page 782*
    E. peripheral neuropathy: *see page 554*
    F. skeletal myopathy
3. effects of alcohol withdrawal: usually seen in habituated drinkers with cessation or reduction of ethanol intake
    A. alcohol withdrawal syndromes: *see below*
    B. seizures: up to 33% of patients have a generalized tonic-clonic seizure 7-30 hrs after cessation of drinking (see *Alcohol withdrawal seizures*, page 261)
    C. delerium tremens (**DTs**): *see below*

ACUTE INTOXICATION

The primary effect of EtOH on the CNS is depression of neuronal excitability, impulse conduction, and neurotransmitter release due to direct effects on the cell membranes. *Table 7-1* shows the clinical effects associated with specific EtOH concentrations. **Mellanby effect**: the severity of intoxication is greater when blood alcohol levels are rising than when falling.

In most jurisdictions, individuals with blood ethanol levels ≥ 21.7 mmol/l (100 mg/dl) are defined as legally intoxicated, and a number of states have changed this to 80 mg/dl. However,

Table 7-1   Blood ethanol concentrations
(in non-alcoholic patients)

[blood EtOH]		Clinical effect
mmol/liter	mg/dl	
5.4	25	mild intoxication: altered mood, impaired cognition, incoordination
> 21.7	100	vestibular and cerebellar dysfunction: increased nystagmus, diplopia, dysarthria, ataxia
> 108.5	500	usually fatal from respiratory depression

even levels of 10.2 mmol/l (47 mg/dl) are associated with increased risk of involvement in motor vehicle accidents. Chronic alcoholism leads to increased tolerance; in habituated individuals survival with levels exceeding 1000 mg/dl has been reported.

ALCOHOL WITHDRAWAL SYNDROME

Compensation for the CNS depressant effects of EtOH occurs in chronic alcoholism. Consequently, rebound CNS hyperactivity may result from falling EtOH levels. Clinical signs of EtOH withdrawal are classified as major or minor (the degree of autonomic hyperactivity and the presence/absence of DTs differentiates these), as well as early (24-48 hrs) or late (> 48 hrs).

Signs/symptoms include: tremulousness, hyperreflexia, insomnia, N/V, autonomic hyperactivity (tachycardia, systolic HTN), agitation, myalgias, mild confusion. If EtOH withdrawal seizures occur, they tend to be early (*see page 261*). Perceptual disturbances or frank **hallucinosis** may also occur early. Hallucinosis consists of visual and/or auditory hallucinations with an otherwise clear sensorium (which distinguishes this from the hallucinations of DTs). DTs can occur 3-4 days after cessation of drinking (*see below*).

Suppressed by benzodiazepines, resumption of drinking, ß-adrenergic antagonists, or α_2-agonists.

PREVENTION OF AND TREATMENT FOR ALCOHOL WITHDRAWAL SYNDROME[3]

Mild EtOH withdrawal is managed with a quiet, supportive environment, reorientation and one-to-one contact. If symptoms progress, institute pharmacologic treatment.

Benzodiazepines

Benzodiazepines **(BDZs)** are the mainstay of treatment. They reduce autonomic hyperactivity, and may prevent seizures and/or DTs. All BDZs are effective. Initial doses are shown in *Table 7-2* and are higher than those used for treating anxiety. Symptom triggered dosing with repeated evaluation utilizing a standardized protocol (e.g. CIWA-Ar[5]) may be more efficacious than fixed-dose schedules[6]. Avoid IM administration (erratic absorption).

Adjunctive medications

Associated conditions commonly seen in patients experiencing alcohol withdrawal syndrome include dehydration, fluid and electrolyte disturbances, infection, pancreatitis, and alcoholic ketoacidosis, and should be treated accordingly.

Table 7-2 BDZ doses for EtOH withdrawal*

Drug	Dose	
	Oral	IV
chlordiazep-oxide (Librium®)	100 mg initially, then 25-50 mg PO TID-QID, gradually taper over ≈ 4 days). Additional doses may be needed for continuing agitation, up to 50 mg PO hourly[4]	–
oxazepam† (Serax®)	120 mg initially; then up to 30 mg TID-QID	–
lorazepam† (Ativan®)	4 mg initially, then 1-2 mg PO q 4 hrs	1-2 mg q 1-2 hrs
diazepam (Valium®)	20 mg PO initially, then 10 mg PO BID-QID	5-10 mg initially
midazolam (Versed®)	–	titrate drip to desired effect

*   modify as appropriate based on patient response
†   shorter half-life with fewer active metabolites

Other medications used for EtOH withdrawal itself include:
1. drugs useful for controlling HTN (caution: these agents should not be used alone because they do not prevent progression to more severe levels of withdrawal, and they may mask symptoms of withdrawal)
   A. ß-blockers: also treat most associated tachyarrhythmias
      1. atenolol (Tenormin®): reduces length of withdrawal and BDZ requirement
      2. ✖ avoid propranolol (psychotoxic reactions)
   B. α-agonists: do not use together with ß-blockers. Clonidine (*see page 5*) has been extensively studied, and can be given in patch form (takes ≈ 2 days)
2. phenobarbital: an alternative to BDZs. Long acting, and helps prophylax against seizures
3. baclofen: a small study[7] found 10 mg PO q d X 30 days resulted in rapid reduction of symptoms after the initial dose and continued abstinence
4. "supportive" medications
   A. thiamine: 100 mg IM q d x 3 d (can be given IV if needed, but there is risk of adverse reaction). Rationale: high-concentration glucose may precipitate acute Wernicke's encephalopathy in patients with thiamine deficiency
   B. folate 1 mg IM, IV or PO q d x 3 d
   C. $MgSO_4$ 1 gm x 1 on admission: helpful only if magnesium levels are low, reduces seizure risk. Be sure renal function is normal before administering
   D. vitamin B_{12} for macrocytic anemia: 100 µg IM (do not give before folate)
   E. multivitamins: of benefit *only* if patient is malnourished
5. seizures: *see page 261* for indications for treatment

A. phenytoin (Dilantin®): load with 18 mg/kg = 1200 mg/70 kg (*see page 271*)
6. ethanol drip: not widely used. 5% EtOH in D5W, start at 20 cc/hr, and titrate to a blood level of 100-150 mg/dl

DELERIUM TREMENS (DTs)

When DTs occur, they usually begin within 4 days of the onset of EtOH withdrawal, and typically persist for 1-3 days.

Signs and symptoms include: profound disorientation, agitation, tremor, insomnia, hallucinations, severe autonomic instability (tachycardia, HTN, diaphoresis, hyperthermia)[8]. Mortality is 5-10% (higher in elderly), but can be reduced with treatment (including treating associated medical problems and treatment for seizures).

Haloperidol and phenothiazines may control hallucinations, but can lower the seizure threshold. HTN and tachyarrhythmias should be treated as outline above under alcohol withdrawal syndrome.

WERNICKE'S ENCEPHALOPATHY (WE)

AKA Wernicke-Korsakoff encephalopathy. Classic triad: encephalopathy (consisting of global confusion), ophthalmoplegia, and ataxia (NB: all 3 are present in only 10-33% of cases).

Due to thiamine deficiency. Body stores of thiamine are adequate only for up to ≈ 18 days. May be seen in:
1. a certain susceptible subset of thiamine deficient alcoholics. Thiamine deficiency here is due to a combination of inadequate intake, reduced absorption, decreased hepatic storage, and impaired utilization
2. hyperemesis (as in some pregnancies)
3. starvation: including anorexia nervosa, rapid weight loss
4. gastroplication (bariatric surgery)
5. hemodialysis
6. cancers
7. AIDS
8. prolonged IV hyperalimentation

Oculomotor abnormalities occur in 96% and include: nystagmus (horizontal > vertical), lateral rectus palsy, conjugate-gaze palsies.

Gait ataxia is seen in 87%, and results from a combination of polyneuropathy, cerebellar dysfunction, and vestibular impairment.

Systemic symptoms may include: vomiting, fever.

MRI : May show high signal in T2WI and FLAIR images in the paraventricular (medial) thalamus, the floor of the 4th ventricle, and periaqueductal gray of the midbrain. These changes may resolve with treatment[9]. Atrophy of the mammillary bodies may also be seen. Normal MRI does not R/O the diagnosis.

Treatment

Wernicke's encephalopathy **(WE)** is a medical emergency. When WE is suspected, 100 mg thiamine should be given IM or IV (oral route is unreliable, *see above*) daily for 5 days. ✖ IV glucose can precipitate acute WE in thiamine deficient patients, ∴ give thiamine first.

Thiamine administration improves eye findings within hours to days; ataxia and confusion improve in days to weeks. Many patients that survive are left with horizontal nystagmus, ataxia, and 80% have **Korsakoff's syndrome** (AKA Korsakoff's psychosis), a disabling memory disturbance involving retrograde and anterograde amnesia.

7.2. Opioids

Includes heroin (which is usually injected IV, but the powder can be snorted or smoked) as well as prescription drugs. Opioids produce small pupils (miosis).

Overdose produces:
1. respiratory depression
2. pulmonary edema

3. coma
4. hypotension and bradycardia
5. seizures may occur with: propoxyphene, meperidine (Demerol®) which may also cause delerium, and the street drug combination of "T's and blues" (*see page 259*)
6. fatal overdose may occur with any agent, but is more likely with synthetic opioids such as fentanyl (Sublimaze®) among users unfamiliar with their high potency

Reversal of intoxication[10]

A test dose of naloxone (Narcan®) 0.2 mg IV avoids sudden complete reversal of all opioid effects. If no significant reaction occurs, an additional 1.8 mg (for a total dose of 2 mg) will reverse the toxicity of most opioids. If needed, the dose may be repeated q 2-3 minutes up to a total of 10 mg, although even larger doses may be needed with propoxyphene, pentazocine or buprenorphine (Buprenex®). Naloxone may precipitate narcotic withdrawal symptoms in opioid dependent patients, with anxiety or agitation, piloerection, yawning, sneezing, rhinorrhea, nausea, vomiting, diarrhea, abdominal cramps, muscle spasms... which are uncomfortable but not life threatening. Clonidine (Catapres®) may be helpful for some narcotic withdrawal symptoms.

With longer acting opioids, especially methadone (Dolophine®), repeat doses of naloxone may be obviated by the use of nalmefene (Revex®), a long-acting narcotic antagonist which is not appropriate for the initial treatment of opioid overdosage.

7.3. Cocaine

The increasing use of cocaine in its various forms (including crack) is resulting in a rise in the incidence and recognition of its deleterious effects on the CNS. Effects on other body systems (tachycardia, acute myocardial infarction, arrhythmias, rupture of ascending aorta (aortic dissection), abruptio placenta, hyperthermia, intestinal ischemia, sudden death...) are well documented elsewhere, and are not further discussed here.

Cocaine is extracted from *Erythroxylon coca* leaves (and other *Erythroxylon* species) and is thus unrelated to opioids. It blocks the re-uptake of nor-epinephrine by presynaptic adrenergic nerve terminals. It is available in 2 forms: cocaine hydrochloride (heat labile and water soluble, it is usually taken PO, IV or by nasal insufflation) and as the highly purified cocaine alkaloid (free base or crack cocaine, which is heat stable but insoluble in water and is usually smoked).

Peak toxicity occurs 60-90 minutes after ingestion (except for "body packers"), 30-60 minutes after snorting, and minutes after IV injection or smoking (freebase or crack)[10].

Acute pharmacologic effects of cocaine

Acute pharmacologic effects pertinent to the nervous system include:
1. mental status: initial CNS stimulation that first manifests as a sense of well-being and euphoria. Sometimes dysphoric agitation results, occasionally with delerium. Stimulation is followed by depression. Paranoia and toxic psychosis may occur with overdosage or chronic use. Addiction may occur
2. pupillary dilatation (mydriasis)
3. hypertension: from adrenergic stimulation

Non-pharmacologic effects related to the nervous system

1. pituitary degeneration: from chronic intranasal use
2. cerebral vasculitis: less common than with amphetamines
3. seizures: possibly related to the local anesthetic properties of cocaine
4. cerebrovascular accident (CVA, stroke)[11]
   A. intracerebral hemorrhage: see *Intracerebral hemorrhage*, *Etiologies* on page 850
   B. subarachnoid hemorrhage[12, 13]: possibly as a result of HTN in the presence of aneurysms or AVMs, however, sometimes no lesion is demonstrated on angiography[14]. May possibly be due to cerebral vasculitis
   C. ischemic stroke[15]: may result from vasoconstriction
   D. thrombotic stroke[10]
   E. TIA[16]
5. anterior spinal artery syndrome[16]
6. effects of maternal cocaine use on the fetal nervous system include[17]: microcephaly, disorders of neuronal migration, neuronal differentiation and myelination, cerebral infarction, subarachnoid and intracerebral hemorrhage, and sudden in-

fant death syndrome (SIDS) in the postnatal period

TREATMENT OF TOXICITY

Most cocaine toxicity is too short-lived to be treated. Anxiety, agitation or seizures may be treated with IV benzodiazepines (e.g. lorazepam, *see page 266*). Refractory HTN may be treated with nitroprusside (*see page 4*) or phentolamine (Regitine®, *see page 469*). IV lidocaine used to treat cardiac arrhythmias may cause seizures[10].

7.4. Amphetamines

Toxicity is similar to that of cocaine (*see above*), but longer in duration (may last up to several hours). Cerebral vasculitis may occur with prolonged abuse (*see page 63*) which may lead to cerebral infarction (*see page 774*).

Elimination of amphetamines requires adequate urine output. Antipsychotic drugs such as haloperidol (Haldol®) should not be used because of risk of seizures.

7.5. References

1. Charness M E, Simon R P, Greenberg D A: Ethanol and the nervous system. **N Engl J Med** 321: 442-54, 1989.
2. Gorelick P B: Alcohol and stroke. **Stroke** 18: 268-71, 1987.
3. Lohr R H: Treatment of alcohol withdrawal in hospitalized patients. **Mayo Clin Proc** 70: 777-82, 1995.
4. Lechtenberg R, Worner T M: Seizure risk with recurrent alcohol detoxification. **Arch Neurol** 47: 535-8, 1990.
5. Sullivan J T, Sykora K, Schneiderman J, et al.: Assessment of alcohol withdrawal: The revised clinical institute withdrawal assessment for alcohol scale (CIWA-Ar). **Br J Addict** 84: 1353-7, 1989.
6. Saitz R, Mayo-Smith M F, Roberts M S, et al.: Individualized treatment for alcohol withdrawal: A randomized double-blind controlled trial. **JAMA** 272: 519-23, 1994.
7. Addolorato G, Caputo F, Capristo E, et al.: Rapid suppression of alcohol withdrawal syndrome by baclofen. **Am J Med** 112 (3): 226-9, 2002.
8. Treatment of alcohol withdrawal. **Med Letter** 28: 75-6, 1986.
9. Watson W D, Verma A, Lenart M J, et al.: MRI in acute wernicke's encephalopathy. **Neurology** 61 (4):

527, 2003.
10. Acute reactions to drugs of abuse. **Med Letter** 38: 43-6, 1996.
11. Fessler R D, Esshaki C M, Stankewitz R C, et al.: The neurovascular complications of cocaine. **Surg Neurol** 47: 339-45, 1997.
12. Lichtenfeld P J, Rubin D B, Feldman R S: Subarachnoid hemorrhage precipitated by cocaine snorting. **Arch Neurol** 41: 223-4, 1984.
13. Oyesiku N M, Collohan A R T, Barrow D L, et al.: Cocaine-induced aneurysmal rupture: An emergent negative factor in the natural history of intracranial aneurysms? **Neurosurgery** 32: 518-26, 1993.
14. Schwartz K A, Cohen J A: Subarachnoid hemorrhage precipitated by cocaine snorting. **Arch Neurol** 41: 705, 1984 (letter).
15. Levine S R, Brust J C M, Futrell N, et al.: Cerebrovascular complications of the use of the 'crack' form of alkaloidal cocaine. **N Engl J Med** 323: 699-704, 1990.
16. Mody C K, Miller B L, McIntyre H B, et al.: Neuro logic complications of cocaine abuse. **Neurology** 38: 1189-93, 1988.
17. Volpe J J: Effect of cocaine use on the fetus. **N Engl J Med** 327: 399-407, 1992.

8. Coma

8.1. General

Consciousness has two components: arousal and content. Impairment of arousal can vary from mild (drowsiness or somnolence), to obtundation, to stupor to coma. **Coma** is the severest impairment of arousal, and is defined as the inability to obey commands, speak, or open the eyes to pain.

The Glasgow Coma Scale **(GCS)** is shown in *Table 8-1* (note: the scale is intended to assess level of consciousness and is not designed for following neurologic deficits). Some centers record a "T" next to the total score for patients whose verbal axis cannot be assessed because of intubation[2]. 90% of patients with GCS ≤ 8 and none with GCS ≥ 9 meet the above definition of coma. Thus, **GCS ≤ 8 is a** generally accepted operational definition of coma.

A scale for use in children is shown in *Table 8-2*[3].

Table 8-1 Glasgow coma* scale[1]
(recommended for age ≥ 4 yrs)

Points†	Best eye opening	Best verbal	Best motor
6	–	–	obeys
5	–	oriented	localizes pain
4	spontaneous	confused	withdraws to pain
3	to speech	inappropriate	flexion (decorticate)
2	to pain‡	incomprehensible	extensor (decerebrate)
1	none	none	none§

* technically, this is a scale of *impaired* consciousness, whereas "coma" implies unresponsiveness

† range of total points: 3 (worst) to 15 (normal)

‡ when testing eye opening to pain, use peripheral stimulus (the grimace associated with central pain may cause eye closure)

§ if no motor response, important to exclude spinal cord transection

Table 8-2 Children's coma scale* (for age < 4 yrs)

Points†	Best eye	Best verbal		Best motor
6	–	–		obeys
5	–	smiles, oriented to sound, follows objects, interacts		localizes pain
		Crying	**Interaction**	
4	spontaneous	consolable	inappropriate	withdraws to pain
3	to speech	inconsistently consolable	moaning	flexion (decorticate)
2	to pain	inconsolable	restless	extensor (decerebrate)
1	none	none	none	none

* same as adult Glasgow coma scale except for verbal response[3]

† range of total points: 3 (worst) to 15 (normal)

Coma results from one or more of the following:
- dysfunction of high brainstem (central upper pons) or midbrain
- bilateral diencephalic dysfunction
- diffuse lesions in both cerebral hemispheres (cortical or subcortical white matter)

POSTURING

The following terms are inaccurate in the implication of the location of the lesion. Decorticate posturing implies a more rostral lesion and prognosis may be better.

Decorticate posturing: Classically attributed to disinhibition by removal of corticospinal pathways above the midbrain.

Overview: abnormal flexion in UE and extension in LE.

Detail: slow flexion of arm, wrist and fingers with adduction in the UE. Extension, internal rotation, plantarflexion in LE.

Decerebrate posturing: Classically attributed to disinhibition of vestibulospinal tract (more caudal) and pontine reticular formation **(RF)** by removing inhibition of medullary RF (transection at intercollicular level, between vestibular and red nuclei).

Overview: abnormal extension in UE and LE.

Detail: opisthotonos (head and trunk extended), teeth clenched, arms extended, adducted and hyperpronated (internally rotated), wrists flexed, fingers flexed. Legs extended and internally rotated, feet plantarflexed and inverted, toes plantarflexed.

ETIOLOGIES OF COMA

TOXIC/METABOLIC CAUSES OF COMA

1. electrolyte imbalance: especially hypo- or hypernatremia, hypercalcemia, renal failure with elevated BUN & creatinine, liver failure with elevated ammonia
2. endocrine: hypoglycemia, nonketotic hyperosmolar state, DKA (diabetic ketoacidosis, AKA diabetic coma), myxedema coma, Addisonian crisis (hypoadrenalism)
3. vascular: vasculitis, DIC, hypertensive encephalopathy (*see page 64*)
4. toxic: EtOH, drug overdose (including narcotics, iatrogenic polypharmacy, barbiturates), lead intoxication, carbon monoxide (CO) poisoning, cyclosporine (causes an encephalopathy that shows white-matter changes on MRI that is often reversible with discontinuation of the drug)
5. infectious/inflammatory: meningitis, encephalitis, sepsis, lupus cerebritis, neurosarcoidosis (*see page 56*), toxic-shock syndrome
6. neoplastic: leptomeningeal carcinomatosis, rupture of neoplastic cyst
7. nutritional: Wernicke's encephalopathy, vitamin B_{12} deficiency
8. inherited metabolic disorders: porphyria, lactic acidosis
9. organ failure: uremia, hypoxemia, hepatic encephalopathy, Reye's syndrome, anoxic encephalopathy (e.g. post-resuscitation from cardiac arrest), CO_2 narcosis
10. epileptic: status epilepticus (including non-convulsive status), post-ictal state (especially with unobserved seizure)

STRUCTURAL CAUSES OF COMA

1. vascular:
   A. bilateral cortical or subcortical infarcts (e.g. with cardioembolism due to SBE, mitral stenosis, A-fib, mural thrombus...)
   B. occlusion of vessel supplying both cerebral hemispheres (e.g. severe bilateral carotid stenosis)
   C. bilateral diencephalic infarcts: well described syndrome. May be due to occlusion of a thalamo-perforator supplying both medial thalamic areas or with "top-of-the-basilar" occlusion. Initially resembles metabolic coma (including diffuse slowing on EEG), patient eventually arouses with apathy, memory loss, vertical gaze paresis
2. infectious: abscess with significant mass effect, subdural empyema, herpes simplex encephalitis
3. neoplastic: primary or metastatic
4. trauma: hemorrhagic contusions, edema, hematoma (*see below*)
5. herniation from mass effect: presumably brainstem compression causes dysfunction of reticular activating system or mass in one hemisphere causing compression of the other results in bilateral hemisphere dysfunction
6. increased intracranial pressure: reduces CBF
7. acute lateral shift of the brain: e.g. due to hematoma (subdural or epidural) (*see Table 8-3*)

Table 8-3 Effect of lateral shift on level of consciousness[4]

Amount of midline shift	Level of consciousness
0-3 mm	alert
3-4 mm	drowsy
6-8.5 mm	stuporous
8-13 mm	comatose

PSEUDOCOMA

Differential diagnosis:
1. locked-in syndrome: ventral pontine infarction
2. psychiatric: catatonia, conversion reaction
3. neuromuscular weakness: myasthenia gravis, Guillain-Barré

8.2. Approach to the comatose patient

The following covers nontraumatic coma (see *Head trauma*, page 632 for that topic). Initial evaluation: includes measures to protect brain (by providing CBF, O_2, and glucose), assesses upper brainstem (Cr. N. VIII), and rapidly identifies surgical emergencies. Keep "pseudocoma" as a possible etiology in back of mind.

APPROACH TO COMATOSE PATIENT, OUTLINE
1. cardiovascular stabilization: establish airway, check circulation (heartbeat, BP, carotid pulse), CPR if necessary
2. obtain blood for tests
   A. STAT: electrolytes (especially Na, glucose, BUN), CBC + diff, ABG
   B. others as appropriate: toxicology screen (serum & urine), calcium, ammonia, antiepileptic drug (**AED**) levels (if patient is taking AEDs)
3. administer emergency supportive medications
   A. glucose: at least 25 ml of D_{50} IVP. Due to potentially harmful effect of glucose in global ischemia, if possible check fingerstick glucose first, otherwise glucose is given without exception, unless it is known with certainty that serum glucose is normal
   B. naloxone (Narcan®): in case of narcotic overdose. 1 amp (0.4 mg) IVP
   C. flumazenil (Romazicon®): in case of benzodiazepine overdose (see page 36). Start with 0.2 mg IV over 30 seconds, wait 30 secs, then give 0.3 mg over 30 secs at 1 minute intervals up to 3 mg or until patient arouses
   D. thiamine: 50-100 mg IVP (3% of Wernicke's present with coma)
4. core neuro exam (assesses midbrain/upper pons, allows emergency measures to be instituted rapidly, more thorough evaluation possible once stabilized): → (see *Core neuro exam* below)
5. if herniation syndrome or signs of expanding p-fossa lesion with brainstem compression (see *Table 8-4*): initiate measures to lower ICP (see *ICP treatment measures*, page 655), then get a CT scan if patient begins improving, otherwise emergency surgery (see page 772). ✖ Do NOT do LP

Table 8-4 Signs of herniation syndrome or posterior fossa lesion

HERNIATION SYNDROMES	SIGNS OF P-FOSSA LESION
(also see *Herniation syndromes*, page 159)	(also see *Posterior fossa (infratentorial) tumors*, page 405)
• unilateral sensory or motor deficit • progressive obtundation→coma • unilateral 3rd nerve palsy • decorticate or decerebrate posturing (especially if unilateral)	• initial symptoms of diplopia, vertigo, bilateral limb weakness, ataxia, occipital H/A • rapid onset of deterioration/coma • bilateral motor signs at onset • miosis • absent calorics to horizontal movement, possibly with preserved vertical movements • ocular bobbing • ophthalmoplegia • multiple cranial nerve abnormalities with long tract signs • apneustic, cluster or ataxic respirations

6. if meningitis suspected (altered mental status + fever, meningeal signs...)
   A. if no indication of herniation, p-fossa mass (see *Table 8-4*), focal deficit indicating mass effect or papilledema: perform LP, start antibiotics immediately (do not wait for CSF results) (see *Meningitis*, page 212)
   B. if evidence of possible mass effect, coagulopathy or herniation, CT to R/O mass. If significant delay anticipated, consider empiric antibiotics or careful LP with small gauge needle (≤ 22 Ga.), measure opening pressure (**OP**), remove only a small amount of CSF if OP high, replace CSF if patient deteri-

orates (LP in this setting may be risky, see *Lumbar puncture*, page 615).
7. treat generalized seizures if present. If status epilepticus is suspected, treat as indicated on page 265 (obtain emergency EEG if available)
8. treat metabolic abnormalities
    A. restore acid-base balance
    B. restore electrolyte imbalance
    C. maintain body temperature
9. obtain as complete history as possible once stabilized
10. administer specific therapies

CORE NEURO EXAM (FOR COMA)

A. **respiratory** rate and pattern: the most common disorder in impaired consciousness
    1. **Cheyne-Stokes**: breathing gradually crescendos in amplitude and then trails off, followed by an expiratory pause, and then the pattern repeats. Hyperpneic phase is usually longer than apneic. Usually seen with dien-

inspiration

Cheyne-Stokes respiratory pattern

cephalic lesions or bilateral cerebral hemisphere dysfunction (non-specific), e.g. early increased ICP or metabolic abnormality. Results from an increased ventilatory response to CO_2
    2. **hyperventilation**: usually in response to hypoxemia, metabolic acidosis, aspiration, or pulmonary edema. True central neurogenic hyperventilation is rare, and usually results from dysfunction within the pons. If no other brainstem signs are present, may suggest psychiatric disorder
    3. **cluster breathing**: periods of rapid irregular breathing separated by apneic spells, may appear similar to Cheyne-Stokes, may merge with various patterns of gasping respirations. High medulla or lower pons lesion. Often an ominous sign

Cluster breathing

    4. **apneustic** (rare): a pause at full inspiration. Indicates pontine lesion, e.g. with basilar artery occlusion

Apneustic respiratory pattern

    5. **ataxic** (Biot's breathing): no pattern in rate or depth of respirations. Seen with medullary lesion. Usually preterminal

Ataxic respirations

★ B. **pupil** (size in mm) in ambient light, and in reaction to direct/consensual light
    1. equal and reactive pupils indicates toxic/metabolic cause with few exceptions (*see below*) (may have hippus). The light reflex is the most useful sign in distinguishing metabolic from structural coma
        A. the only metabolic causes of fixed/dilated pupil: glutethimide toxicity, **anoxic encephalopathy**, anticholinergics (including atropine), occasionally with botulism toxin poisoning
        B. narcotics cause small pupils (miosis) with a small range of constriction and sluggish reaction to light (in severe overdose, the pupils may be so small that a magnifying glass may be needed to see reaction)
    2. unequal (note: an afferent pupillary defect does not produce anisocoria (see *Alterations in pupillary diameter*, page 582)):
        A. fixed and dilated pupil: usually due to oculomotor palsy. Possible herniation, especially if larger pupil associated with ipsilateral 3rd nerve EOM palsy (eye deviated "down and out")
        B. possible Horner's syndrome: consider carotid occlusion/dissection
    3. bilateral pupil abnormalities
        A. pinpoint with minute reaction that can be detected with magnifying glass[5]: pontine lesion (sympathetic input is lost; parasympathetics emerge at Edinger-Westphal nucleus and are unopposed)
        B. bilateral fixed and dilated (7-10 mm): subtotal damage to medulla or imme-

diate post-anoxia or hypothermia (core temperature < 90° F (32.2° C))
  C. midposition (4-6 mm) and fixed: more extensive midbrain lesion, presumably due to interruption of sympathetics and parasympathetics
C. extraocular muscle function
  1. deviations of ocular axes at rest
     A. bilateral conjugate deviation:
        1. frontal lobe lesion (frontal center for contralateral gaze): looks toward side of destructive lesion (away from hemiparesis). Looks away from side of seizure focus (looks at jerking side), may be status epilepticus. Reflex eye movements (*see below*) are normal
        2. pontine lesion: eyes look <u>away</u> from lesion and towards hemiparesis; calorics impaired on side of lesion
        3. "wrong way gaze": medial thalamic hemorrhage. Eyes look away from lesion and towards hemiparesis (an exception to the axiom that the eyes look <u>towards</u> a destructive supratentorial lesion)[5]
        4. downward deviation: may be associated with unreactive pupils (**Parinaud's syndrome**, *see page 86*). Etiologies: thalamic or midbrain pretectal lesions, metabolic coma (especially barbiturates), may follow a seizure
     B. unilateral outward deviation on side of larger pupil (III palsy): uncal herniation
     C. unilateral inward deviation: VI (abducens) nerve
     D. <u>skew deviation</u>
        1. III or IV nerve/nucleus lesion
        2. infratentorial lesion (frequently dorsal midbrain)
  2. spontaneous eye movements
     A. "windshield wiper eyes": random roving conjugate eye movements. Non-localizing. Indicates an intact III nucleus and medial longitudinal fasciculus
     B. periodic alternating gaze, AKA "ping-pong gaze": eyes deviate side to side with frequency of ≈ 3-5 per second (pausing 2-3 secs in each direction). Usually indicates bilateral cerebral dysfunction
     C. <u>ocular bobbing</u>: repetitive rapid vertical deviation downward with slow return to neutral position. Pontine lesion (*see page 588*)
  3. internuclear ophthalmoplegia (**INO**): due to lesion in medial longitudinal fasciculus (**MLF**) (fibers crossing to contralateral III nucleus are interrupted). Eye ipsilateral to MLF lesion does not adduct on spontaneous eye movement or in response to reflex maneuvers (e.g. calorics) (*see page 585*)
  4. reflex eye movements (maneuvers to test brainstem)
     A. **oculovestibular reflex**[A], AKA **ice water calorics**: first rule-out TM perforation, then with HOB at 30°, irrigate one ear with 60-100 ml of ice water. NB: response is inhibited by neuromuscular blocking agents (**NMBA**)
        1. a comatose patient with an <u>intact</u> brainstem will have tonic conjugate eye deviation to side of cold stimulus which may be delayed up to one minute or more. There will be no fast component (nystagmus) (the cortical component) even if the brainstem is intact
           (NB: **oculocephalic reflex**[B] (doll's eyes) provides similar information as oculovestibular reflex[C], but poses a greater risk to the spinal cord if C-spine not cleared)
        2. no response: symmetrical, could be specific toxin (e.g. neuromuscular block or barbiturates), metabolic cause, brain death or possibly massive infratentorial lesion
        3. asymmetric: infratentorial lesion, especially if response inconsistent

---

A. **oculovestibular reflexes** (calorics): the anticipated response is commonly misunderstood. In a normal <u>awake</u> patient there is slow deviation towards the side of the cold stimulus with nystagmus (which is named for the rapid, cortical phase) in the *opposite* direction (hence the mnemonic "COWS" (cold-opposite, warm-same)). Nystagmus will be <u>absent</u> in the comatose patient

B. **oculocephalic reflex** ("doll's eyes" or "doll's head"): do not perform if there is any uncertainty about cervical-spine stability. In an <u>awake</u> patient, the eyes will either move with the head, or, if the movement is slow enough and the patient is fixating on an object, there will be contraversive conjugate eye movement[6] (c.f. oculovestibular reflex which does not depend on patient's level of cooperation). In a comatose patient with an intact brainstem & cranial nerves, there will also be contraversive conjugate eye movement (a positive doll's eyes response)

C. oculovestibular reflexes are absent but oculocephalic are maintained only when vestibular inputs are interrupted, e.g. streptomycin toxicity of labyrinths or bilateral acoustic neuromas

with 3rd nerve palsy (herniation). Usually maintained in toxic/metabolic coma
    4. nystagmus without tonic deviation (i.e. eyes remain in primary position) virtually diagnostic of psychogenic coma
    5. contralateral eye fails to adduct: INO (MLF lesion)
  B. **optokinetic nystagmus** presence strongly suggests psychogenic coma
D. motor: muscle tone and reflexes, response to pain, Babinski (note asymmetries)
  1. appropriate: implies corticospinal tracts and cortex intact
  2. asymmetric: supratentorial lesion (tone usually increased), unlikely in metabolic
  3. inconsistent/variable: seizures, psychiatric
  4. symmetric: metabolic (usually decreased). Asterixis, tremor, myoclonus may be present in metabolic coma
  5. hyporeflexia: consider myxedema coma, especially in patient presenting weeks after transsphenoidal surgery
  6. patterns
    A. decorticate posturing: arms flex, legs extend: large cortical or subcortical lesion
    B. decerebrate posturing: arms and legs extend: brainstem injury at or below lower midbrain
    C. arms flexed, legs flaccid: pontine tegmentum
    D. arms flaccid, legs appropriate ("man-in-the-barrel syndrome"): anoxic injury (poor prognosis)
E. **ciliospinal reflexes** (pupillary dilatation to noxious cutaneous stimuli): tests integrity of sympathetic pathways
  1. bilaterally present: metabolic
  2. unilaterally present: possible 3rd nerve lesion (herniation) if on side of larger pupil. Possible pre-existing Horner's syndrome if on side of smaller pupil
  3. bilaterally absent: usually not helpful

8.3. Herniation syndromes

Classic teaching has been that shifts in brain tissue (e.g. caused by masses or increased intracranial pressure) through rigid openings in the skull (herniation) compress other structures of the CNS producing the observed symptoms. This view has been challenged[7], with the hypothesis that herniation may be an epiphenomenon that occurs late in the process and is not actually the cause of the observations. However, herniation models still serve as useful approximations.

There are many possible herniation syndromes, the five most common are:
  1. central (transtentorial) herniation (*see page 160*) } supratentorial
  2. uncal herniation (*see page 161*) } herniation
  3. cingulate herniation: cingulate gyrus herniates under falx (AKA subfalcine herniation). Usually asymptomatic unless ACA kinks and occludes causing bi frontal infarction. Usually warns of impending transtentorial herniation
  4. upward cerebellar (*see below*) } infratentorial
  5. tonsillar herniation (*see below*) } herniation

COMA FROM SUPRATENTORIAL MASS[8]

Central and uncal herniation each causes a different form of **rostral-caudal deterioration**. Central herniation results in sequential failure of: diencephalon, midbrain, pons, medulla (*see page 160*). For uncal herniation, *see page 161*. "Classic" signs of increased ICP (HTN, bradycardia, altered respiratory pattern) usually seen with p-fossa lesions may be absent in slowly developing supratentorial masses.

Distinction between central and uncal herniation is difficult when dysfunction reaches the midbrain level or below. Predicting the location of the lesion based on the herniation syndrome is unreliable.

Clinical characteristics differentiating uncal from central herniation
  * decreased consciousness occurs early in central herniation, late in uncal
  * uncal herniation syndrome rarely gives rise to decorticate posturing

Differential diagnosis of supratentorial etiologies
1. vascular: CVA, intracerebral hemorrhage, SAH
2. inflammatory: cerebral abscess, subdural empyema, herpes simplex encephalitis
3. neoplastic: primary or metastatic
4. traumatic: epidural or subdural hematoma, depressed skull fracture

COMA FROM INFRATENTORIAL MASS

NB: it is essential to identify patients with primary posterior fossa lesions (see *Table 8-4*, page 156) as they may require emergent surgical intervention (*see page 772*).

Etiologies of infratentorial mass
1. vascular: brainstem infarction (including basilar artery occlusion), cerebellar infarction or hematoma
2. inflammatory: cerebellar abscess, central pontine myelinolysis, brainstem encephalitis
3. neoplasms: primary or metastatic
4. traumatic: epidural or subdural hematoma

HYDROCEPHALUS
Infratentorial masses can produce obstructive hydrocephalus by compressing the Sylvian aqueduct and/or 4th ventricle (*see page 404*).

UPWARD CEREBELLAR HERNIATION
Occasionally seen with p-fossa masses, may be exacerbated by ventriculostomy. Cerebellar vermis ascends above tentorium, compressing the midbrain, and possibly occluding SCAs → cerebellar infarction. May compress sylvian aqueduct → hydrocephalus.

TONSILLAR HERNIATION
Cerebellar tonsils "cone" through foramen magnum, compressing medulla → respiratory arrest. Usually rapidly fatal.

Occurs with either supra- or infra-tentorial masses or with elevated ICP. May be precipitated by LP. In many cases, there may simply be pressure on the brainstem without actual herniation[9]. There are also cases with significant cerebellar herniation through the foramen magnum with the patient remaining alert[7].

8.3.1.   Central herniation

AKA transtentorial herniation AKA tentorial herniation. Usually more chronic than uncal herniation, e.g. due to tumor, especially of frontal, parietal or occipital lobes.

The diencephalon is gradually forced through the tentorial incisura. The pituitary stalk may be sheared, resulting in diabetes insipidus. PCAs may be trapped along the open edge of the incisura, and may occlude producing cortical blindness (see *Blindness from hydrocephalus*, page 202). The brainstem suffers ischemia from compression and shearing of perforating arteries from basilar artery → hemorrhages within the brainstem (**Duret hemorrhages**).

CT or plain x-ray criteria
Downward displacement of the pineal gland may be demonstrated[10]. Perimesencephalic cisterns are compressed.

DIENCEPHALIC STAGE
Early. May be due to diffuse bilateral hemisphere dysfunction (e.g. from decreased blood flow from increased ICP) or (more likely) from bilateral diencephalic dysfuntion due to downward displacement. This stage warns of impending (irreversible) midbrain damage but is frequently reversible if the cause is treated.

Consciousness	Altered alertness is first sign; usually lethargy, agitation in some. Later: stupor → coma.
Respiration	Sighs, yawns, occasional pauses. Later: Cheyne-Stokes.
Pupils	Small (1 - 3 mm), small range of contraction.

| Oculomotor | Conjugate or slightly divergent roving eyes; if conjugate then brainstem intact. Usually positive DOLL'S EYES and conjugate ipsilateral response to cold water calorics (CWC). Impaired upgaze due to compression of superior colliculi and diencephalic pretectum (Parinaud's syndrome *see page 86*) |
| Motor | Early: appropriate response to noxious stimuli, bilateral Babinski, gegenhalten (paratonic resistance). If previously hemiparetic contralateral to lesion: may worsen. Later: motionlessness & grasp reflexes, then DECORTICATE (initially contralateral to lesion in most cases). |

MIDBRAIN - UPPER PONS STAGE

When midbrain signs fully developed (in adults), prognosis is very poor (extreme ischemia of midbrain). Fewer than 5% of cases will have a good recovery if treatment is successfully undertaken at this stage.

Respiration	Cheyne-Stokes → sustained tachypnea.
Pupils	Moderately dilated midposition (3-5 mm), fixed*.
Oculomotor	Doll's eyes & CWC impaired, may be dysconjugate. MLF lesion → **internuclear ophthalmoplegia** (when doll's or CWC elicited and dysconjugate, medially moving eye moves less than laterally moving eye).
Motor	Decorticate → bilaterally DECEREBRATE (occasionally spontaneously).

* in pontine hemorrhage pinpoint pupils appear because the loss of sympathetics leaves the parasympathetics unopposed, whereas in herniation, the parasympathetics are usually lost, too (3rd nerve injury)

LOWER PONS - UPPER MEDULLARY STAGE

Respiration	Regular, shallow and rapid (20-40/min).
Pupils	Midposition (3-5 mm), fixed.
Oculomotor	Doll's eyes and CWC unelicitable.
Motor	Flaccid. Bilateral Babinski. Occasionally LE flexion to pain.

MEDULLARY STAGE (TERMINAL STAGE)

| Respiration | Slow, irregular rate and depth, sighs/gasps. Occasionally hyperpnea alternating with apnea |
| Pupils | Dilate widely with hypoxia. |

OUTCOME AFTER CENTRAL HERNIATION

In a series of 153 patients with signs of central herniation (altered level of consciousness, anisocoria or fixed pupils, abnormal motor findings) 9% had good recovery, 18% had functional outcome, 10% were severely disabled, and 60% died[11]. Factors associated with a better result were young age (especially age ≤ 17 yrs), anisocoria with deteriorating Glasgow Coma Score and nonflaccid motor function. Factors associated with poor outcome were bilaterally fixed pupils, with only 3.5% of these patients having a functional recovery.

8.3.2. Uncal herniation

Usually occurs in rapidly expanding traumatic hematomas, frequently in the lateral middle-fossa or temporal lobe pushing medial uncus and hippocampal gyrus over edge of tentorium, entrapping third nerve and directly compressing midbrain. PCA may be occluded (as with central herniation). For CT criteria *see below*.

Impaired consciousness is NOT a reliable early sign. Earliest consistent sign: unilaterally dilating pupil. However, it is unlikely that a patient undergoing early uncal herniation would be completely neurologically intact except for anisocoria (do not dismiss confusion, agitation, etc.). Once brainstem findings appear, deterioration may be rapid (deep coma may occur within hours).

CT criteria[12]

Tentorial incisura surrounds interpeduncular and pre-pontine cisterns and brainstem. There is great interpersonal variability in the amount of space in the incisura.

Impending uncal or hippocampal herniation may be indicated by encroachment on lateral aspect of suprasellar cistern → flattening of normal pentagonal shape. Once herniation occurs CT may show: brainstem displacement and flattening, compression of contralateral cerebral peduncle, midbrain rotation with slight increase of ipsilateral subarachnoid space. Also, contralateral hydrocephalus may occur[13].

Obliteration of parasellar and interpeduncular cisterns occurs as uncus and/or hippocampus are forced through hiatus. Brainstem compression → AP elongation. Since dural structures enhance with IV contrast, this may be used to help delineate tentorial margins when necessary.

EARLY THIRD NERVE STAGE
(NOT A BRAINSTEM FINDING, DUE TO 3RD NERVE COMPRESSION)

Pupils	Unilaterally dilating pupil (may be sluggish); 85% ipsilateral to lesion[14]
Oculomotor	Doll's = normal or dysconjugate. CWC = slow ipsilateral deviation, impaired nystagmus, may be dysconjugate if external oculomotor ophthalmoplegia **(EOO)**.
Respirations	Normal.
Motor	Appropriate response to nociceptive stimulus. Contralateral Babinski.

LATE THIRD NERVE STAGE
Midbrain dysfunction occurs almost immediately after symptoms extend beyond those due to focal cerebral lesion (i.e. may skip diencephalic stage, due to lateral pressure on midbrain). Treatment delays may result in irreversible damage.

Pupils	Pupil fully dilates.
Oculomotor	Once pupil blown, then external oculomotor ophthalmoplegia (EOO).
Consciousness	Once EOO, stuporous → comatose.
Respirations	Sustained hyperventilation, rarely Cheyne-Stokes.
Motor	Usually produces contralateral weakness. However, the contralateral cerebral peduncle may be compressed against the tentorial edge causing ipsilateral hemiplegia (Kernohan's phenomenon, a false localizing sign). Then bilateral decerebration (decortication unusual).

MIDBRAIN - UPPER PONS STAGE

Pupils	Contralateral pupil fixes in midposition or full dilation. Eventually, both midposition (5-6 mm) and fixed.
Oculomotor	Impaired or absent.
Respirations	Sustained hyperpnea.
Motor	Bilateral decerebrate rigidity.

From this point onward, the uncal syndrome is indistinguishable from central herniation (*see above*).

8.4.   Hypoxic coma

Anoxic encephalopathy may be due to **anoxemic anoxia** (drop in pO_2) or **anemic anoxia** (following exsanguination or cardiac arrest). Myoclonus is commonly seen.

Pathology: lesions predominate in 3rd cortical layer (grey matter); Ammon's horn is also vulnerable. White matter is usually better preserved (due to lower O_2 requirement).

In the basal ganglia (**BG**): anoxemic anoxia severely affects globus pallidus; anemic anoxia affects the caudate nucleus and putamen. In the cerebellum: Purkinje cells, dentate nuclei, and inferior olives are affected.

Table 8-5   Patients with <u>BEST</u> chance of regaining independence*

Time of exam	Finding
< 6 hrs from onset	(pupillary light reflex present) *AND* (GCS-motor > 1) *AND* (spontaneous EOM WNL, i.e. orienting or conjugate roving)
1 day	(GCS-motor > 3) *AND* (GCS-eye improved ≥ 2 from initial)
3 days	(GCS-motor > 3) *AND* (spontaneous EOM WNL)
1 week	GCS-motor = 6
2 weeks	oculocephalic WNL

Multivariate analysis yields outcome prognosticators shown in *Table 8-5* and *Table 8-6*. NB: this analysis applies only to hypoxic-ischemic coma[15]. More recent studies confirm the poor prognosis of unreactive pupils and lack of motor response to pain[16]; if either of these findings are seen within a few hours after cardiac arrest there is an 80% risk of death or permanent vegetative state, and if present at 3 days these this rate rose to 100%.

Glucocorticoids (steroids) have been shown to have no beneficial effect on survival rate or neurological recovery rate after cardiac arrest[17].

Table 8-6   Patients with virtually NO chance of regaining independence*

Time of exam	Finding
< 6 hrs	no pupillary light reflex
1 day	(GCS-motor < 4) AND (spontaneous eye movements not orienting nor conjugate roving)
3 days	GCS-motor < 4
1 week	(GCS-motor < 6) AND (at < 6 hrs spontaneous EOM not orienting nor conjugate roving) AND (at 3 d GCS-eye < 4)
2 week	(oculocephalic not WNL) AND (at 3 d GCS-motor < 6) AND (at 3 d GCS-eye < 4) AND (at 2 wk GCS-eye not improved at least 2 points from initial)

*   abbreviations: WNL = within normal limits, GCS = Glasgow Coma Scale ("GCS-motor" refers to the motor score...); EOM = extraocular muscle;

8.5.   References

1.   Teasdale G, Jennett B: Assessment of coma and impaired consciousness: A practical scale. **Lancet** 2: 81-4, 1974.
2.   Valadka A B, Narayan R K: *Emergency room management of the head-injured patient.* In **Neurotrauma**, Narayan R K, Wilberger J E, and Povlishock J T, (eds.). McGraw-Hill, New York, 1996: pp 119-35.
3.   Hahn Y S, Chyung C, Barthel M J, *et al.*: Head injuries in children under 36 months of age: Demography and outcome. **Childs Nerv Syst** 4: 34-40, 1988.
4.   Ropper A H: Lateral displacement of the brain and level of consciousness in patients with an acute hemispheral mass. **N Engl J Med** 314: 953-8, 1986.
5.   Fisher C M: Some neuro-ophthalmological observations. **J Neurol Neurosurg Psychiatry** 30: 383-92, 1967.
6.   Buettner U W, Zee D S: Vestibular testing in comatose patients. **Arch Neurol** 46: 561-3, 1989.
7.   Fisher C M: Acute brain herniation: A revised concept. **Sem Neurology** 4: 417-21, 1984.
8.   Plum F, Posner J B: In **The diagnosis of stupor and coma**. F A Davis, Philadelphia, 3rd ed., 1980: pp 87-130.
9.   Fisher C M, Picard E H, Polak A, *et al.*: Acute hypertensive cerebellar hemorrhage: Diagnosis and surgical treatment. **J Nerv Ment Dis** 140: 38-57,

1965.
10.   Hahn F, Gurney J: C T signs of central descending transtentorial herniation. **Am J Neuroradiol** 6: 844-5, 1985.
11.   Andrews B T, Pitts L H: Functional recovery after traumatic transtentorial herniation. **Neurosurgery** 29: 227-31, 1991.
12.   Osborn A G: Diagnosis of descending transtentorial herniation by cranial CT. **Radiology** 123: 93-6, 1977.
13.   Stovring J: Descending tentorial herniation: Findings on computerized tomography. **Neuroradiology** 14: 101-5, 1977.
14.   McKissock W, Taylor J C, Bloom W H, *et al.*: Extradural hematoma: Observations on 125 cases. **Lancet** 2: 167-72, 1960.
15.   Levy D E, Caronna J J, Singer B H, *et al.*: Predicting outcome from hypoxic-ischemic coma. **JAMA** 253: 1420-6, 1985.
16.   Zandbergen E G J, de Haan R J, Stoutenbeek C P, *et al.*: Systematic review of early prediction of poor outcome in anoxic-ischemic coma. **Lancet** 352: 1808-12, 1998.
17.   Jastremski M, Sutton-Tyrell K, Vaagenes P, *et al.*: Glucocorticoid treatment does not improve neurological recovery following cardiac arrest. **JAMA** 262: 3427-30, 1989.

9. Brain death

9.1. Brain death in adults

Most states accept some form of "brain death" as a valid determination of death. The President's Commission provides the following guidelines[1]:
1. the diagnosis of death requires both cessation of function __and__ irreversibility of cessation of either cardiopulmonary system or *entire* brain (including brainstem)
2. for age < 5 years, see *Brain death in children*, page 167
3. with no "complicating conditions" listed below, there are "…no cases of brain functions returning following a 6 hr cessation, documented by clinical examination and confirmatory EEG"[A]
4. with conditions such as massive intracerebral tumor with herniation or gunshot wound to the head, it is possible to pronounce death sooner with more certainty than, e.g. with post cardiac-arrest anoxia or following a coma of unknown etiology
5. when death results from criminal assault, or there is the possibility of litigation regarding the death, extra care must be taken and legal counsel may be advisable before making the determination of brain death

BRAIN DEATH CRITERIA

Recommendations[1, 2]:

A. absence of **brainstem reflexes**:
   1. ocular examination:
      A. *fixed* pupils: no response to bright light (caution after resuscitation: *see below*), usually mid-position (4-6 mm) but may vary to dilated range[B] (9 mm) in size
      B. absent corneal reflexes[C]
      C. absent oculocephalic (doll's eyes) reflex (contraindicated if C-spine not cleared): *see page 158*
      D. absent **oculovestibular reflex** (cold water **calorics**): instill 60-100 ml ice water into one ear (do not do if TM perforated) with HOB at 30°. Brain death is excluded if any eye movement (*see page 158*). Wait at least 1 minute for response, and ≥ 5 min before testing the opposite side
   2. absent oropharyngeal reflex (gag) to stimulation of posterior pharynx
   3. no cough response to bronchial suctioning

B. **apnea test** AKA apnea challenge: no spontaneous respirations[D] after disconnection from ventilator (assesses function of medulla). Since elevating $PaCO_2$ increases ICP which could precipitate herniation and vasomotor instability, this test should be reserved for last and only used when the diagnosis of brain death is reasonably certain. Guidelines[4, 5]
   1. $PaCO_2$ should be > 60 mm Hg without respirations before apnea can be attributed to brain death (if patient does not breathe by this point, they won't breathe at a

1.	absence of brainstem reflexes
	A. fixed pupils
	B. absent corneal reflexes
	C. absent oculovestibular reflex
	D. absent oculocephalic reflex
	E. absent gag & cough reflex
2.	apnea
3.	no response to deep __central__ pain
4.	vital signs
	A. core temp > 32.2° C (90° F)
	B. SBP ≥ 90 mm Hg

A. note: EEG is __not__ mandatory, see *recommended observation periods…*, page 165
B. cervical sympathetic pathways may remain intact
C. corneal reflex: eye closing to corneal (not scleral) stimulation
D. respirations are defined as abdominal or chest excursions that produce adequate tidal volumes; if there is any question, a spirometer may be connected to the patient[3]

higher $PaCO_2$; not valid with severe COPD or CHF)
2. to prevent hypoxemia during the test (with the danger of cardiac arrhythmia or myocardial infarction):
   * precede the test with 15 minutes of ventilation with 100% O_2
   * prior to the test, adjust the ventilator to bring the $PaCO_2 \geq 40$ mm Hg (to shorten the test time and thus reduce the risk of hypoxemia)
   * during the test, have passive O_2 flow administered at 6 L/min through either a pediatric oxygen cannula or a No. 14 French tracheal suction catheter (with the side port covered with adhesive tape) passed to the estimated level of the carina
3. starting from normocapnea, the average time to reach $PaCO_2 = 60$ mm Hg is **6 minutes** (classic teaching is that $PaCO_2$ rises 3 mm Hg/min, but in actuality this varies widely, with an average 3.7 ± 2.3[4]; or 5.1 mm Hg/min if starting at normocarbia[5]). Sometimes as long as 12 minutes may be necessary
4. the test is aborted prematurely if:
   * the patient breathes: incompatible with brain death
   * significant hypotension occurs
   * if O_2 saturation drops below 80% (on pulse oximeter)
   * significant cardiac arrhythmias occur
5. if patient does not breathe, send ABG at regular intervals and at the completion of test regardless of reason for termination. If the patient does not breathe for at least 2 minutes <u>after</u> a $PaCO_2 > 60$ mm Hg is documented, then the test is valid and is compatible with brain death (if the patient is stable and ABGs results are available within a few minutes, the apnea challenge may be continued while waiting for results in case the $PaCO_2$ is < 60)
6. if $PaCO_2$ stabilizes below 60 mm Hg and the pO_2 remains adequate, try reducing the passive O_2 flow rate slightly

C. no motor function
1. no response to deep <u>central</u> pain
2. true decerebrate or decorticate posturing or seizures are incompatible with the diagnosis of brain death
3. spinal cord mediated reflex movements (including flexor plantar reflexes, flexor withdrawl, muscle stretch reflexes[6], and even abdominal and cremasteric reflexes) can be compatible with brain death, and may occasionally consist of complex movements[7], including bringing one or both arms up to the face[8], or sitting up (the "Lazarus" sign[9]) especially with hypoxemia (thought to be due to spinal cord ischemia stimulating surviving motor neurons in the upper cervical cord). If complex integrated motor movements occur, it is recommended that confirmatory testing be performed prior to pronouncement of brain death[10]

D. absence of <u>complicating conditions</u> (that could simulate brain death on exam):
1. hypothermia: core temp should be > 32.2° C (90° F). Below this temp, pupils may be fixed and dilated[11], respirations may be difficult to detect, and recovery is possible[12]
2. no evidence of remediable exogenous or endogenous intoxication, including drug or metabolic (barbiturates, benzodiazepines, meprobamate, methaqualone, trichloroethylene, paralytics, hepatic encephalopathy, hyperosmolar coma...). If there is doubt, depending on circumstances, lab tests including drug levels (serum and urine) may be sent
3. shock (SBP should be ≥ 90 mm Hg) and anoxia
4. immediately post-resuscitation: shock, anoxia, and/or (uncommonly) atropine may cause fixed and dilated pupils (for the effect of atropine, *see page 167*)
5. patients coming out of pentobarbital coma (wait until level ≈ ≤ 10 mcg/ml)
6. confirmation of brain death by use of *Clinical confirmatory tests* (EEG, angiography, CRAG, BSAER..., *see below*) is not required, but may be used as determined by judgement of attending or consulting physician

E. recommended <u>observation periods</u> during which time the patient fulfills criteria of clinical brain death before the patient may be pronounced dead:
1. in situation where <u>overwhelming</u> brain damage from an irreversible condition is well established (e.g. massive intracerebral hemorrhage), some experts will pronounce death following a single valid brain death exam in conjunction with a clinical confirmatory test
2. if an irreversible condition is well established, and clinical confirmatory tests are used: 6 hours

3. if an irreversible condition is well established and no clinical confirmatory tests are used: 12 hours
4. if diagnosis is uncertain and no clinical confirmatory tests: 12-24 hours
5. if anoxic injury is the cause of brain death: 24 hours (may be shortened if cessation of CBF is demonstrated)

CLINICAL CONFIRMATORY TESTS

CEREBRAL ANGIOGRAPHY
Criteria: absence of intracranial flow at the level of the carotid bifurcation or circle of Willis[2]). Filling of the superior sagittal sinus may occur in a delayed fashion. Interobserver validity has not been studied. Not routinely used in the diagnosis of brain death, but may be employed in difficult situations.

EEG
Can be done at bedside. Requires experienced interpreter. Does not detect brainstem activity, and electrocerebral silence (**ECS**) does not exclude the possibility of reversible coma. Thus, at least 6 hours observation is recommended in conjunction with ECS. Using ECS as a clinical confirmatory test should be done only in patients without drug intoxication, hypothermia, or shock.

Definition of **electrocerebral silence** on EEG: no electrical activity > 2 μV with the following requirements:
- recording from scalp or referential electrode pairs ≥ 10 cm apart
- 8 scalp electrodes and ear lobe reference electrodes
- inter-electrode resistance < 10,000 Ω (or impedance < 6,000 Ω) but over 100 Ω
- sensitivity of 2 μV/mm
- time constants 0.3-0.4 sec for part of recording
- no response to stimuli (pain, noise, light)
- record > 30 mins
- repeat EEG in doubtful cases
- qualified technologist and electroencephalographer with ICU EEG experience
- telephone transmission not permissible

TRANSCRANIAL DOPPLER[3]
1. small peaks in early systole without diastolic flow or reverberating flow (indicative of significantly increased ICP)
2. initial absence of doppler signals cannot be used as criteria for brain death since 10% of patients do not have temporal isonation windows

CEREBRAL RADIONUCLIDE ANGIOGRAM (CRAG)
Can be performed at the bedside with a general purpose scintillation camera with a low energy collimator. May not detect minimal blood flow to the brain, especially brainstem, therefore 6 hours observation in conjunction with CRAG is recommended unless there is a clear etiology of overwhelming brain injury (e.g. massive hemorrhage or GSW).

May be useful to confirm clinical brain death in the following settings:
1. where complicating conditions are present, e.g. hypothermia, hypotension (shock), drug intoxication
2. severe facial trauma where ocular findings may be difficult or confusing
3. in patients with severe COPD or CHF where apnea testing may not be valid
4. to shorten the observation period, especially when organ donation is a possibility

Technique
1. scintillation camera is positioned for an AP head and neck view
2. inject 20-30 mCi of 99mTc-labeled serum albumin or pertechnetate in a volume of 0.5-1.5 ml into a proximal IV port, or a central line, followed by a 30 ml NS flush
3. perform serial dynamic images at 2 second intervals for ≈ 60 seconds
4. then, obtain static images with 400,000 counts in AP and then lateral views at 5, 15 & 30 minutes after injection
5. if a study needs to be repeated because of a previous non-diagnostic study or a previous exam incompatible with brain death, a period of 12 hours should lapse

Findings

No uptake in brain parenchyma = "hollow skull phenomenon" (*see Figure 9-1*). Termination of carotid circulation at the skull base, and lack of uptake in the ACA and MCA distributions (absent "candelabra effect"). There may be delayed or faint visualization of dural venous sinuses even with brain death[13] due to connections between the extracranial circulation and the venous system.

SSEPs

Bilateral absence of N20-P22 response with median nerve stimulation.

ATROPINE

In brain death, an amp of atropine (1 mg) should not affect the heart rate due to the absence of vagal tone (it normally increase the heart rate). Although atropine in usual doses does not cause pupillary dilatation[14, 15], it is prudent to examine the pupils first to eliminate uncertainty.

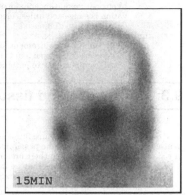

Figure 9-1 "Hollow-skull" sign on CRAG
(static AP view taken15 minutes after injection)

9.2. Brain death in children

Criteria for death: irreversible loss of cardiopulmonary or entire brain function (as in adult), but the (clinically unproven) assumption that a child's brain is more resilient results in more difficult determination of brain death. The following guidelines are proposed for patients < 5 yrs age[16]:

- these recommendations are not applicable for the premature infant
- determination of proximate cause of coma should be made to ensure absence of remediable conditions: especially toxic and metabolic disorders, sedatives, paralytics, hypothermia, hypotension (for age), and surgically treatable conditions
- criteria:
    - A. coma and apnea must coexist: including complete loss of consciousness, vocalization and volitional activity
    - B. absence of brainstem function
        1. midposition or fully dilated pupils, unresponsive to light (R/O drug effects)
        2. EOM: absence of spontaneous, doll's eyes and caloric movements of eyes
        3. absence of bulbar musculature movement: including oropharyngeal and facial muscles; absence of corneal, gag, cough, suck, and rooting reflex
        4. absence of respiratory movement (usually tested after other criteria met)
        5. flaccid tone and absence of spontaneous or induced movements (spinal myoclonus and spinal cord movements, e.g. reflex withdrawl are not included)
        6. examination results should remain consistent with brain death throughout observation period
- observation periods according to age:
    - A. in newborns born at or after term (> 38 wks): 7 days
    - B. age 7 days - 2 mos: 2 examinations and 2 EEGs 48 hrs apart (repeat exam unnecessary if cerebral radionuclide angiogram **(CRAG)** fails to visualize cerebral arteries)
    - C. age 2-12 mos: 2 examinations and 2 EEGs 24 hrs apart (repeat exam unnecessary if CRAG negative)
    - D. age > 12 mos: if irreversible condition exists, laboratory testing is not nec-

essary, and 12 hrs observation is sufficient (unclear conditions, especially hypoxic-ischemic encephalopathy, are difficult to assess, and 24 hrs observation is suggested unless electrocerebral silence on EEG or a negative CRAG confirm diagnosis)
- confirmatory tests:
  A. EEG: standard requirement for 10 cm electrode distance (*see page 167*) may be decreased in proportion to size of head
  B. CRAG: applicability to patient < 2 mos age unproven

9.3. Organ and tissue donation

State and federal laws require families of individuals satisfying criteria for brain death to be approached about the possibility of organ donation. Facts that may be conveyed to family in order to help their understanding about organ procurement:
1. any or all suitable organs may be individually specified for donation or to be excluded from consideration for donation
2. organ procurement may be done in such a way as not to interfere with an open casket funeral (i.e. disfigurement can be avoided)
3. families can receive information as to the ultimate use of any recovered organs

9.3.1. Criteria for qualification for organ donation

General exclusionary criteria for organ donation (modified[17])
1. infection
   A. untreated septicemia
   B. the following infections or conditions: AIDS, viral hepatitis, viral encephalitis, Guillain-Barré syndrome
   C. current IV drug abuse
   D. active TB
2. malignancy: brain tumors represent possible exceptions (*see below*)
3. relative exclusions: chronic untreated HTN, hypotension (desired SBP > 100 with normal CVP)
4. disease of the organs considered for donation
5. anencephalic newborns: recent consensus is that the functioning brainstem in these infants (e.g. spontaneous respirations) disqualifies them from the diagnosis of brain death (furthermore, few such organs would likely benefit others)[18]

Guidelines for inclusion (some recommendations from reference[17] **included**)
These guidelines are constantly being revised, in part due to improved results with the use of cyclosporin in recipients. In general, consultation with a transplant coordinator is recommended to determine appropriateness of donation.
1. brain death in a previously healthy individual
2. organs:
   A. **kidneys**: age > 6 mos (because of size). Normal blood pressure, BUN, serum creatinine & U/A. No SLE (because of possible lupus nephritis)
   B. **heart** and **heart/lung**: age ideally < 40 years for males and < 45 for females (above these ages, a cardiac cath is usually performed) but up to 60 yrs may be used depending on condition of heart and potential recipients). Exam by cardiologist indicating no heart disease (cardiomyopathy, valve defect, reduced ejection fraction, severe ASHD, S/P CABG). No IDDM
   C. **liver**: age > 1 mos. Normal hepatic function (normal or acceptable AST, ALT, LDH, bilirubin (direct, indirect & total) and normal clotting studies) with no history of liver disease
   D. **pancreas**: age 15 - 40 yrs. No history of diabetes. Normal serum glucose and amylase
3. tissues:
   A. corneas: age ≥ 1 yr. Neither cancer nor sepsis disqualifies (rabies and Creutzfeldt-Jakob disease are contraindications)
   B. skin: age 15-65 yrs. Excluded if cancer
   C. bone: age 15-65 yrs. Excluded if cancer
   D. bone marrow: age ≤ 50 yrs

9.3.2. Organ donation in patients with brain tumors

Among patients with a brain tumor:
1. those that are not candidates for organ donation:
    A. metastatic tumors to the brain
    B. brain tumors that have been manipulated (biopsied or excised)
    C. patients with brain tumors who have been shunted
2. those that might be candidates, but considered *high-risk* donors[A] include unmanipulated:
    A. glioblastoma multiforme
    B. anaplastic astrocytoma
    C. medulloblastoma
3. unmanipulated tumors that might not be considered high risk
    A. hemangioblastoma
    B. meningioma

Optimally, if no metastases are seen on CT (chest, abdomen and pelvis) and no mets are found at time of organ procurement, a brain biopsy would be performed after the organs are procured at the same anesthetic and the organs would not be "released" until the biopsy proves which of the above categories applies.

9.3.3. Management after brain death for organ donation

Note: once brain death occurs, cardiovascular instability eventually ensues, generally within 3-5 days, and management with pressors is usually required. Fluid and electrolyte imbalances from loss of hypothalamic regulation must be normalized. In some instances a beating-heart cadaver can be maintained for months[19].
1. consent: must be obtained from donor's legal guardian. NB: must also be obtained from medical examiner or coroner's office for all cases under their jurisdiction (in most states, death resulting from accident, within 24 hrs of hospitalization, etc.)
2. signed note in chart stating date and time patient pronounced brain dead
3. contact transplant coordinator at earliest possible time
4. wean from vasopressors if possible. Control hypotension through volume expansion whenever possible (after brain death, ADH production ceases, producing diabetes insipidus with high urine output, thus copious fluid administration is anticipated (> 250-500 ml/hr is common). Most centers prefer AVOIDING exogenous ADH (vasopressin (Pitressin®)) if possible since the risk of renal shutdown increases in brain-death
    A. start with crystalloid (D5 1/4 NS + 20 mEq KCl/L is generally a good choice since it replaces free water), replace urine cc for cc plus 100 cc/hr maintenance
    B. use colloid (FFP, albumin...) if unable to maintain BP by replacement
    C. use vasopressors if still hypotensive. Start with low dose dopamine, increase up to ≈ 10 µg/kg/min, add dobutamine if still hypotensive at this dose
    D. if UO is still > 300 ml/hr after above measures, use ADH analog (aqueous vasopressin (Pitressin®) is preferred over DDAVP to avoid renal shutdown)
5. thyroglobulin given IV converts some cells from anaerobic to aerobic metabolism which may help stave off cardiovascular collapse

LABORATORY EVALUATION [17]

General initial labs
1. serology: VDRL or RPR, HBsAg, HIV, CMV, ABO blood group, HLA tissue type
2. chemistry: electrolytes, glucose, BUN, creatinine, calcium, phosphate, liver function tests, U/A (urine analysis)
3. hematology: CBC, PT/PTT

A. high-risk organs may be considered e.g. for liver transplants in patients who are very low on the list due to age or hepatocellular cancer

4. microbiology: blood, urine and sputum cultures; sputum Gram stain

Kidney donor
1. in addition to general labs (*see above*), check BUN & creatinine ≈ q day
2. check electrolytes ≈ q 12 hrs (modify as appropriate)

Liver donor
1. in addition to general labs (*see above*), check LDH, AST, ALT, bilirubin (direct, indirect, and total)

Heart donor
1. all require an echocardiogram prior to donation

9.4.   References

1. President's Commission for the Study of Ethical Problems in Medicine: Guidelines for the determination of death. **JAMA** 246: 2184-6, 1981.
2. Quality Standards Subcommittee of the American Academy of Neurology: Practice parameters for determining brain death in adults (summary statement). **Neurology** 45: 1012-4, 1995.
3. Widjicks E F: Determining brain death in adults. **Neurology** 45: 1003-11, 1995.
4. Benzel E C, Gross C D, Hadden T A, *et al*.: The apnea test for the determination of brain death. **J Neurosurg** 71: 191-4, 1989.
5. Benzel E C, Mashburn J P, Conrad S, *et al*.: Apnea testing for the determination of brain death: A modified protocol. **J Neurosurg** 76: 1029-31, 1992.
6. Ivan L P: Spinal reflexes in cerebral death. **Neurology** 23: 650-2, 1973.
7. Turmel A, Roux A, Bojanowski M W: Spinal man after declaration of brain death. **Neurosurgery** 28: 298-302, 1991.
8. Heytens L, Verlooy J, Gheuens J, *et al*.: Lazarus sign and extensor posturing in a brain-dead patient. **J Neurosurg** 71: 449-51, 1989 (case report).
9. Ropper A H: Unusual spontaneous movements in brain-dead patients. **Neurology** 34: 1089-92, 1984.
10. Jastremski M S, Powner D, Snyder J, *et al*.: Spontaneous decerebrate movement after declaration of brain death. **Neurosurgery** 29: 479-80, 1991 (letter).
11. Treatment of hypothermia. **Med Letter** 36: 116-7, 1994.
12. Antretter H, Dapunt O E, Mueller L C: Survival after prolonged hypothermia. **N Engl J Med** 330: 219, 1994.
13. Goodman J M, Heck L L, Moore B D: Confirmation of brain death with portable isotope angiography: A review of 204 consecutive cases. **Neurosurgery** 16: 492-7, 1985.
14. Greenan J, Prasad J: Comparison of the ocular effects of atropine and glycopyrrolate with two IV induction agents. **Br J Anaesth** 57: 180-3, 1985.
15. Goetting M G, Contreras E: Systemic atropine administration during cardiac arrest does not cause fixed and dilated pupils. **Ann Emerg Med** 20: 55-7, 1991.
16. Task Force for the Determination of Brain Death in Children: Guidelines for the determination of brain death in children. **Arch Neurol** 44: 587-8, 1987.
17. Darby J M, Stein K, Grenvik A, *et al*.: Approach to management of the heartbeating "brain dead" organ donor. **JAMA** 261: 2222-8, 1989.
18. Shewmon D A, Capron A M, Peacock W J, *et al*.: The use of anencephalic infants as organ sources: A critique. **JAMA** 261: 1773-81, 1989.
19. Bernstein I M, Watson M, Simmons G M, *et al*.: Maternal brain death and prolonged fetal survival. **Obstet Gynecol** 74: 434-7, 1989.

10. CSF

10.1. General information

Cerebrospinal fluid (**CSF**) surrounds the brain and spinal cord, and may function as a shock absorber for the CNS. It may also serve an immunological function analogous to the lymphatic system[1]. It circulates within the subarachnoid space, between the arachnoid and the pial membranes.

CSF is normally a clear colorless fluid with a specific gravity of 1.007 and a pH of ≈ 7.33-7.35.

Production

80% of CSF is produced by the choroid plexuses, located in both lateral ventricles (accounts for ≈ 95% of CSF produced in the choroid plexuses) and in the 4th ventricle. Most of the rest of intracranial production occurs in the interstitial space[2]. A small amount may also be produced by the ependymal lining of the ventricles. In the spine, it is produced primarily in the dura of the nerve root sleeves. *Table 10-1* shows properties of CSF production, volumes and pressures.

Table 10-1   Normal CSF production, volumes, and pressure

Property	—— Peds ——		Adult
	Newborn	1-10 yrs	
total volume (ml)	5		150 (50% intracranial, 50% spinal)
formation rate	25 ml/d		≈ 0.3-0.35 ml/min (≈ 450-750 ml/d)
pressure* (cm of fluid)	9-12	mean: 10 normal: < 15	adult: 7-15 (> 18 usually abnormal) young adult: < 18-20

* as measured in the lumbar subarachnoid space, with the patient relaxed in the lateral decubitus position

Production rate: In the adult, CSF is produced at a rate of about 0.3 ml/min (*see Table 10-1*). In terms that are clinically relevant, this approximates 450 ml/24hrs, which means that in an adult, the CSF is "turned over" ≈ 3 times every day. The rate of formation is *independent* of the intracranial pressure[3] (except in the limiting case when ICP becomes so high that cerebral blood flow is reduced[4]).

Absorption

CSF is absorbed primarily by arachnoid villi (granulations) that extend into the dural venous sinuses. Other sites of absorption include the choroid plexuses and lymphatics. The rate of absorption is pressure dependent[5].

10.2. CSF constituents

The composition of CSF differs slightly in the ventricles where the majority of it is produced compared to the lumbar subarachnoid space.

CELLULAR COMPONENT

In normal adult CSF, there are 0-5 lymphocytes or mononuclear cells per mm^3, and no polys (PMNs) or RBCs. In the absence of RBCs, 5-10 WBCs per mm^3 is suspicious, and > 10 WBCs per mm^3 is definitely abnormal.

CSF CONSTITUENTS

Table 10-2   CSF solutes [6 (p 169), 7]
(for CEA, AFP, & hCG, see *Tumor markers*, page 500)
Data from Table 6-1 of "Cerebrospinal Fluid in Diseases of the Nervous System" by Robert A. Fishman, M.D.,
© 1980, W. B. Saunders Co., Philadelphia, PA, used with permission

Constituent	Units	CSF	Plasma	CSF:plasma ratio
osmolarity	mOsm/L	295	295	1.0
H_2O content		99%	93%	
sodium	mEq/L	138	138	1.0
potassium	mEq/L	2.8	4.5	0.6
chloride	mEq/L	119	102	1.2
calcium	mEq/L	2.1	4.8	0.4
pCO_2	mm Hg	47	41*	1.1
pH		7.33	7.41	
pO_2	mm Hg	43	104*	0.4
glucose	mg/dl	60	90	0.67
lactate	mEq/L	1.6	1.0*	1.6
pyruvate	mEq/L	0.08	0.11*	0.73
lactate:pyruvate		26	17.6*	
total protein†	mg/dl	35	7000	0.005
albumin	mg/L	155	36600	0.004
IgG	mg/L	12.3	9870	0.001

*   arterial plasma

†   Note: CSF protein is lower in ventricular fluid than in lumbar subarachnoid space

Table 10-3   Variations with age

Age group	WBC /mm³	RBC /mm³	Protein (mg/dl)	Glucose (mg/dl)	Glucose ratio (CSF:plasma)
newborn					
preemie	10	many	150	20-65	0.5-1.6
term	7-8	mod	80	30-120	0.4-2.5
infants					
1-12 mos	5-6	0	15-80		
1-2 yrs	2-3	0	15		
young child	2-3	0	20		
child 5-15 yrs	2-3	0	25		
adolescent & adult	3	0	30	40-80	0.5
senile	5	0	40*		

*   normal CSF protein rises ≈ 1 mg/dl per year of age in the adult

Table 10-4   CSF findings in various pathologic conditions (adult values)*

Condition	OP (cm H_2O)	Appearance	Cells (per mm³)	Protein (mg%)	Glucose (% serum)	Miscellaneous
normal	7-18	clear colorless	0 PMN, 0 RBC 0-5 monos	15-45	50	
acute purulent meningitis	freq ↑	turbid	few-20K (WBCs mostly PMNs)	100-1000	< 20	few cells early or if treat-ed
viral meningitis & encephalitis	nl	nl	few-350 WBCs (mostly monos)	40-100	nl	PMNs early
Guillain-Barré	nl	nl	nl	50-1000	nl	protein ↑, freq. IgG
polio	nl	nl	50-250 (monos)	40-100	nl	

Table 10-4 CSF findings in various pathologic conditions (adult values)* (continued)

Condition	OP (cm H₂O)	Appearance	Cells (per mm³)	Protein (mg%)	Glucose (% serum)	Miscellaneous
TB meningitis†	freq ↑	opalescent, yellow, fibrin clot on standing	50-500 (lymphocytes and monocytes)	60-700	20-40	PMN early, (+) AFB culture, (+) Ziel-Neelson stain
fungal meningitis	freq ↑	opalescent	30-300 (monos)	100-700	< 30	(+) India ink prep with cryptococcus
parameningeal infection	↑ if block	nl	WBCs nl or ↑ (0-800)	↑	nl	e.g. spinal epidural abscess
traumatic‡ (bloody) tap	nl	bloody; supernatant colorless	RBC:WBC ratio ≈ as in peripheral	slight ↑	nl	RBCs ↓ in successive tubes; no xanthochromia
SAH‡	↑	bloody; supernatant xanthochromic	early: ↑ RBCs / late: ↑ WBCs	50-400 / 100-800	nl or ↓	RBCs disappear in 2 wks, xanthochromia may persist for weeks
multiple sclerosis (MS)§	nl	nl	5-50 monos	nl-800	nl	usually ↑ gamma globulins (oligoclonal)

* abbreviations: OP = opening pressure; nl = normal; ↑ = increased; ↓ = decreased; freq = frequently
† the CSF findings in TB meningitis are almost pathognomonic when they occur in combination; 20-30% have acid-fast bacilli in their CSF sediment smears
‡ to differentiate traumatic tap from SAH, also see *Differentiating SAH from traumatic tap*, page 173
§ for more information on the CSF in MS, *see page 51*

TRAUMATIC TAP

Differentiating SAH from traumatic tap

For typical findings in SAH, *see page 784*. Some features helpful in differentiating SAH from TT are shown in *Table 10-5*.

Table 10-5 Features distinguishing traumatic tap from SAH

Feature	Traumatic tap (TT)	SAH
RBC count (and gross appearance of bloodiness)	declines as CSF drains (compare first tube to last tube)	usually > 100,000 RBCs/mm³, changes little as CSF drains
ratio of WBC:RBC	similar to the ratio in peripheral blood (see *Differentiating true leukocytosis from traumatic tap* above)	usually promotes a leukocytosis (elevated WBC count)
supernatant	clear	xanthochromic* (rarely in < 2 hrs, present in 70% by 6 hrs, and > 90% by 12 hrs after SAH)
clotting of fluid	usually clots if erythrocyte count > 200,000/mm³	usually does not clot
protein concentration	fresh bleeding elevates CSF protein from normal by only ≈ 1 mg per 1000 RBC	blood breakdown products elevate this more than TT (measured protein exceeds the sum of normal protein + 1 mg protein/1000 RBC)
repeat LP at higher level	usually clear	remains bloody
opening pressure	usually normal	usually elevated

* NB: other conditions can cause xanthochromia

Differentiating true leukocytosis from traumatic tap

When many RBCs and WBCs are present in the CSF due to a traumatic tap (**TT**), it may be important to tell if the WBCs are elevated or if they are present in the same ratio as in the peripheral blood. In non-anemic patients, there should be ≈ 1-2 WBCs for every 1000 RBCs (as a correction[6 (p 176)]: subtract 1 WBC for every 700 RBCs[6 (p 176)]). In the presence of anemia or peripheral leukocytosis, use **Fishman's formula**[6 (p 176)] shown in *Eq 10-1* to estimate the original WBC count in the CSF before the TT,

$$\mathrm{WBC}_{CSF\ ORIGINAL} = \mathrm{WBC}_{CSF} - \frac{\mathrm{WBC}_{BLOOD} \times \mathrm{RBC}_{CSF}}{\mathrm{RBC}_{BLOOD}} \qquad \text{Eq 10-1}$$

where $WBC_{CSF\ ORIGINAL}$ = WBC count in the CSF before the TT, WBC_{CSF} & RBC_{CSF} = WBC & RBC counts measured in the CSF, and WBC_{BLOOD} & RBC_{BLOOD} = WBC & RBC per mm^3 in the peripheral blood.

Estimating true total CSF protein content with a traumatic tap

If the hemogram and peripheral protein are normal, then have the cell count and protein content run on the <u>same tube</u>, and the correction is[6 (p 176)]:

- subtract 1 mg per 100 ml of protein for every 1000 RBC per mm^3

10.3.　Artificial CSF

A number of formulations of "artificial" CSF have been proposed over the years in order to more closely mimic the pH, osmolarity, CO_2, and membrane active ion concentration of CSF. In many instances, normal saline **(NS)** has been used in brain surgery, probably without consequence. However, renewed interest in the subject of artificial CSF has been brought about by the use of neuroendoscopy, with possible reactions to non-physiologic solutions when large volumes of fluid are exchanged, as occurs during some of these procedures. An actual reaction to NS, however, has never been proven.

In addition to simulating the constituents of CSF, it may also be well to insure a physiologic temperature of the solution[8].

Elliott's solution

AKA Solution B of Elliott and Jasper[9, 10]: an elaborate formulation that was widely used in the past.

10.4.　CSF fistula

AKA CSF leak. Two major subgroups:
1. spontaneous: rare (*see below*)
2. post-procedure or posttraumatic (more common): 67-77% of cases. Including post-transsphenoidal surgery and post skull base surgery. Subgroups:
   A. immediate
   B. delayed

CSF fistula should be suspected in patients with otorrhea or rhinorrhea after head trauma, or in patients with recurrent meningitis.

Possible routes of egress of CSF
1. mastoid air cells (especially after p-fossa surgery, e.g. for acoustic neuroma **(AN)**, *see page 435*)
2. sphenoid air cells (especially post-transsphenoidal surgery)
3. cribriform plate/ethmoidal roof (floor of frontal fossa)
4. frontal air cells
5. herniation into empty sella and then into sphenoid air sinus
6. along path of internal carotid artery
7. Rosenmüller's fossa: located just inferior to cavernous sinus, may be exposed by drilling off anterior clinoids to allow access to ophthalmic artery aneurysms
8. site of the opening of the transient lateral craniopharyngeal canal
9. percutaneously through a surgical or traumatic wound
10. petrous ridge or internal auditory canal: following temporal bone fracture or acoustic neuroma surgery (*see page 435*). Then either:
    A. **rhinorrhea**: through middle ear → eustachian tube → nasopharynx
    B. **otorrhea**: via perforated tympanic membrane → external auditory canal

TRAUMATIC FISTULA

Occur in 2-3% of all patients with head injury, 60% occur within days of trauma, 95% within 3 months[11]. 70% of cases of CSF rhinorrhea stop within 1 wk, and usually within 6 mos in the rest. Non-traumatic cases cease spontaneously in only 33%. Adult:child ratio is 10:1, rare before age 2 yrs. Anosmia is common in traumatic leaks

(78%), rare in spontaneous[12]. Most (80-85%) CSF otorrhea ceases in 5-10 days.

CSF fistula occurred in 8.9% of 101 cases of penetrating trauma, and increases the infection rate over those penetrating injuries without fistula (50% vs. 4.6%)[13]. It is reported to occur post-op in up to 30% of cases of skull-base surgery[14].

SPONTANEOUS CSF FISTULA

Nontraumatic leaks primarily occur in adults > 30 yrs. Often insidious. May be mistaken for allergic rhinitis. Unlike traumatic leaks, these tend to be intermittent, the sense of smell is usually preserved, and pneumocephalus is uncommon[15].

Sometimes associated with the following[16]
1. agenesis of the floor of the anterior fossa (cribriform plate) or middle fossa
2. empty sella syndrome: primary or post transsphenoidal surgery (see page 454)
3. increased ICP and/or hydrocephalus
4. infection of the paranasal sinuses
5. tumor: including pituitary adenomas (see page 438), meningiomas
6. a persistent remnant of the craniopharyngeal canal[17]
7. AVM[15]
8. dehiscence of the footplate of the stapes (a congenital abnormality) which can produce CSF rhinorrhea via the eustachian tube[15]

Posterior fossa
1. pediatric: usually presents with either meningitis or hearing loss
   A. preserved labyrinthine function (hearing and balance): these usually present with meningitis. 3 usual routes of fistula:
      1. facial canal: can fistulize into middle ear
      2. petromastoid canal: along path of arterial supply to mucosa of mastoid air sinuses
      3. Hyrtl's fissure (AKA tympanomeningeal fissure): links p-fossa to hypotympanum
   B. anomalies of labyrinth (hearing lost): one of several types of Mundini dysplasias, usually presenting with rounded labyrinth/cochlea that permits CSF to erode through oval or round window into auditory canal
2. adult: usually presents with conductive hearing loss with serous effusion, meningitis (often following an episode of otitis media), or cerebral abscess. Occurs most commonly through middle fossa. May be due to arachnoid granulations eroding into air sinus compartment

Spinal
Often presents with postural headache associated with neck stiffness and tenderness[18] (see page 178).

MENINGITIS IN CSF FISTULA

Incidence with posttraumatic CSF leak: 5-10%, increases as leak persists > 7 days. Meningitis is more common with spontaneous fistula. Risk may be higher in post-neurosurgical CSF fistula than in post-traumatic due to elevated ICP common in latter (forces CSF outward). If site of leak unidentified prior to attempted surgical treatment, 30% develop a recurrent leak post-op, with 5-15% of these developing meningitis before leak is stopped[19].

Meningitis may promote inflammatory changes at the site of the leak, with a resultant cessation of the leak.

Pneumococcal meningitis is the most common pathogen (83% of cases[20]), mortality is lower than in pneumococcal meningitis without underlying fistula (< 10% vs. 50%), possibly because the latter is frequently seen in elderly debilitated patients. Prognosis in children is worse[11].

EVALUATION

Determining if rhinorrhea or otorrhea is due to a CSF fistula
1. characteristics of the fluid suggesting the presence of CSF
   A. fluid is as clear as water (unless infected or admixed with blood)
   B. fluid does not cause excoriation within or outside the nose

C. patients with rhinorrhea describe the taste as salty
D. collect fluid and obtain quantitative **glucose** (urine glucose detection strips may be positive even with excess mucus). Test the fluid shortly after collection to minimize fermentation. Normal CSF glucose is > 30 mg% (usually lower with meningitis) whereas lacrimal secretions and mucus are usually < 5 mg%. A negative test is more helpful since it rules out CSF (except in hypoglycorrhachia), but there is a 45-75% chance of false positive[21 (p 1638)]
E. **ß₂-transferrin**: present in CSF, but absent in tears, saliva, nasal exudates and serum (except for newborns and patients with liver disease)[22, 23]. The only other source is the vitreous fluid of the eye. Detected by protein electrophoresis. ≈ 0.5 ml needs to be placed in a sterile container, packed in dry ice, and shipped to a lab that can perform this study
F. "**ring sign**": when a CSF leak is suspected but the fluid is blood tinged, allow the fluid to drip onto linen (sheet or pillowcase). A ring of blood with a larger concentric ring of clear fluid (so called "double ring" or halo sign) suggests the presence of CSF. An old, but unreliable, sign
2. radiographic signs of pneumocephalus on CT or skull x-ray
3. cisternogram: intrathecal injection of radionuclide tracer followed by scintigram or injection of radiopaque contrast followed by CT scan (*see below*)
4. anosmia is present in ≈ 5% of CSF leaks
5. following skull-base surgery (especially involving greater superficial petrosal nerve) there may be a **pseudo-CSF rhinorrhea** possibly due to nasal hypersecretion from imbalanced autonomic regulation of the nasal mucosa[14] ipsilateral to the surgery. Often accompanied by nasal stuffiness and absent ipsilateral lacrimation, and occasionally by facial flushing

To LOCALIZE SITE OF CSF FISTULA

90% of the time, localization does not require water-soluble contrast CT cisternography **(WS-CTC)** (*see below*).
1. CT: to R/O hydrocephalus and obstructive neoplasms. Include thin <u>coronal</u> cuts through anterior fossa all the way back to the sella turcica
   A. non-contrast (optional): to demonstrate bony anatomy
   B. with IV contrast: leak site is usually associated with abnormal enhancement of adjacent brain parenchyma (possibly from inflammation)
2. water-soluble contrast CT cisternography (procedure of choice): *see below*
3. plain skull x-ray (helpful in only 21%)
4. older tests (abandoned in favor of above):
   A. pluridirectional tomography: 53% yield, better in traumatic leaks
   B. **radionuclide cisternography (RNC)**: may be useful in leaks too slow or small to show up on WS-CTC. Various radioactive agents have been used, including: radioiodinated human serum albumin (RIHSA)[15, 24], and 500 µCi Indium[111] DPTA. Cotton pledgets are placed intranasally (anterior nasal roof, posterior nasal roof, sphenoethmoidal recess, middle meatus, and posterior floor of the nose) and are marked so that their location is known. Radiotracer is then injected intrathecally usually by lumbar puncture. Scans are performed in lateral, AP and posterior view. A protocol using In[111] DTPA is to obtain a scan shortly after injection. At 4 hours post-injection, the scan is repeated, and 0.5 ml of blood is drawn (to measure serum activity), and the pledgets are removed. The pledgets are then individually placed in a well-counter and a ratio is calculated for pledget radioactivity relative to serum. A ratio ≤ 1.3 is normal, and a ratio > 1.3 suggests leak. If no leak, the nose can be repacked and the study repeated the following morning.
   Leaks into frontal sinus will empty into nasopharynx anterior to the middle concha, unlike leaks through cribriform plate. RNC identifies the site in only 50%. May be misleading[12] with possible contamination after several hours from absorption of radioisotope into the bloodstream and accumulation in the mucosal glands of the turbinates. Patient positioning may also contaminate other pledgets
   C. intrathecal (visible) dye studies: some success with indigo carmine or fluorescein (*see page 599*) with little or no complications (✖ methylene blue is neurotoxic and should not be used, *see page 599*)
5. MRI: has little to offer in localization of CSF fistula (*see below*)

WATER-SOLUBLE CONTRAST CT CISTERNOGRAPHY

Procedure of choice. This test is performed if:

1. no site identified on plain CT (with coronals)
2. when patient is leaking clinically (the site is only sometimes identified in the absence of an active leak)
3. when multiple bony defects are identified, and it is essential to determine which site is actively leaking
4. if a bony defect seen on plain CT does not have associated changes of abnormal enhancement of adjacent brain parenchyma

Technique[25]

Use iohexol (*see page 127*, which has generally replaced metrizamide 6-7 ml of 190-220 mg/ml) injected into lumbar subarachnoid space via 22 gauge spinal needle (or 5 ml via C1-2 puncture). Patient positioned in -70° Trendelenburg **x** 3 min prone with neck gently flexed, in CT they are kept prone with head hyperextended with 5 mm coronal cuts with 3 mm overlap (use 1.5 mm cuts if necessary). May need provocative maneuvers (coronal scans prone (brow up) or in position of leak, intrathecal saline infusion (requires Harvard pump)[19]...).

Look for accumulation of contrast in air sinuses. Apparent discontinuity of bone on CT without extravassation of contrast is probably not the site of leakage (bone discontinuities may be mimicked by partial volume averaging on CT).

MRI

MRI provides little additional information for localization, but it can R/O p-fossa mass, tumor, and empty sella better than CT. Both CT and MRI can R/O hydrocephalus.

TREATMENT

Acutely after trauma, observation is justified as most cases cease spontaneously.

Prophylactic antibiotics: Controversial. There was no difference in the incidence or morbidity of meningitis between treated and untreated patients[26]. Furthermore, the risk of selecting resistant strains appears real[11] and is therefore usually avoided.

FOR PERSISTENT POSTTRAUMATIC OR POST-OP LEAKS

Non-surgical treatment

1. measures to lower ICP:
    A. bed rest: although recumbency may ameliorate symptoms, there is no other benefit from bed rest[27]
    B. avoid straining (stool softeners) and avoid blowing nose
    C. acetazolamide (250 mg PO QID) to reduce CSF production
    D. modest fluid restriction (caution post-transsphenoidal because of possible DI (*see page 16*): 1500 ml/day in adults, 75% of maintenance/day in peds
2. if leak persists (caution: first R/O obstructive hydrocephalus with CT or MRI):
    A. **LP**: q d to BID (lower pressure to near atmospheric or until H/A)
    OR
    B. continuous **lumbar drainage (CLD)**: via percutaneous catheter. Keep HOB elevated 10-15° and drip chamber at shoulder level (adjust down if leak persists). Requires ICU monitoring. If patient deteriorates with drain in place: immediately stop drainage, place patient flat in bed (or slight Trendelenburg), start 100% O_2, get CT or bedside cross-table skull x-ray (to R/O tension pneumocephalus due to drawing in of air)
3. surgical treatment in persistent cases (*see below*)

SURGICAL TREATMENT

Indications for surgical intervention

1. <u>traumatic</u> CSF leak that persists > 2 weeks in spite of non-surgical measures
2. <u>spontaneous</u> leaks and those of <u>delayed onset following trauma</u> or surgery: usually require surgery because of a high incidence of recurrence
3. leaks complicated by <u>meningitis</u>

Petrous bone

May present as otorrhea or as rhinorrhea (via the eustachian tube).

1. following posterior fossa surgery: *see page 435* for treatment following acoustic neuroma surgery
2. following mastoid fractures: may be approached via extensive mastoidectomy[15]

Leaks through cribriform plate/ethmoidal roof

Extradural approach: Generally preferred by ENT surgeons[28]. If a frontal craniotomy is being performed, an intradural approach should be used since problems may arise in dissecting the dura off of the floor of the frontal fossa, wherein the dura almost always tears and then it is difficult to know if an identified tear is the cause of the leak or if it is iatrogenic. Fluorescein dye mixed with CSF injected intrathecally may help demonstrate the leak intraoperatively (<u>CAUTION</u>: must be diluted to reduce risk of seizures, *see page 599*).

Intradural approach: Generally the procedure of choice[29]. If the fistula site is unidentified preoperatively, use a bifrontal bone flap.

General techniques of <u>intradural</u> approach:
> Post op: lumbar drain after craniotomy is controversial. Some feel CSF pressure may help enhance the seal[30]. If used, place the drip chamber at the level of shoulder for 3-5 days (for precautions, *see above*).
> Consider shunt (LP or VP) if elevated ICP or hydrocephalus is demonstrated.

Leaks into sphenoid sinus (including post-transsphenoidal surgery leak)

1. LP BID or CLD: as long as pressure > 150 mm H_2O or CSF xanthochromic
   A. if leak persists > 3 days: repack sphenoid sinus and pterygoid recesses with fat, muscle, cartilage and/or fascia lata (must reconstruct floor of sella, packing alone is inadequate). Some recommend against muscle since it putrefies and shrinks. Continue LP or CLD as above for 3-5 days post-op
   B. if leak persists > 5 days: lumboperitoneal shunt (first R/O obstructive hydrocephalus)
2. more difficult surgical approach: intracranial (intradural) approach to medial aspect of middle cranial fossa
3. consider transnasal sellar injection of fibrin glue under local anesthesia[31]

10.5.   Spontaneous intracranial hypotension

The syndrome of spontaneous intracranial hypotension is characterized by the following in the <u>absence</u> of antecedent trauma or LP (or epidural injection...)[32]:
1. orthostatic headache
2. low CSF pressure
3. diffuse pachymeningeal enhancement on cerebral MRI

In most cases, the underlying etiology is thought to be a spontaneous CSF leak from a spinal meningeal diverticulum or dural tear[18].

Clinical features

Most patients have orthostatic headache. Atypical patients have been described without H/A, or H/A that is non-positional, without pachymeningeal enhancement on MRI[33], with clinical signs of encephalopathy, cervical myelopathy, or parkinsonism[34]. Since some patients may have normal intracranial pressure, the term "CSF hypovolemia" has been suggested[35]. MRI evidence of brain descent occurred in 36%[34], and reversible pituitary enlargement with a convex superior margin[36] may also be seen. Subdural hematomas may occur as a result. Radioisotope cisternography was abnormal in 90%, and showed a leak in 40%[34].

Treatment

Treatment includes:
1. bed rest
2. analgesics
3. hydration
4. epidural blood patch **(EBP)** for appropriate cases: *see page 46*

Outcome

Complete resolution of H/A was achieved in 70%, and was higher in patients receiving EBP, and was lower in patients with multiple sites of CSF leak[34].

10.6. References

1. Binhammer R T: CSF anatomy with emphasis on relations to nasal cavity and labyrinthine fluids. **Ear Nose Throat J** 71: 292-9, 1992.
2. Sato O, Bering E A: Extraventricular formation of cerebrospinal fluid. **Brain Nerv** 19: 883-5, 1967.
3. Lorenzo A V, Page L K, Wlaters G V: Relationship between cerebrospinal fluid formation, absorption, and pressure in human hydrocephalus. **Brain** 93: 679-92, 1970.
4. Bering E A, Sato O: Hydrocephalus: Changes in formation and absorption of cerebrospinal fluid within the cerebral ventricles. **J Neurosurg** 20: 1050-63, 1963.
5. Griffith H B, Jamjoom A B: The treatment of childhood hydrocephalus by choroid plexus coagulation and artificial cerebrospinal fluid perfusion. **Br J Neurosurg** 4: 95-100, 1990.
6. Fishman R A: **Cerebrospinal fluid in diseases of the nervous system**. W. B. Saunders, Philadelphia, 1980.
7. Felgenhauer K: Protein size and cerebrospinal fluid composition. **Klin Wochenschr** 52: 1158-64, 1974.
8. Oka K, Yamamoto M, Nonaka T, et al.: The significance of artificial cerebrospinal fluid as perfusate and endoneurosurgery. **Neurosurgery** 38: 733-6, 1996.
9. Elliott K A C, Jasper H H: Physiological salt solutions for brain surgery: Studies of local pH and pial vessel reactions to buffered and unbuffered isotonic solutions. **J Neurosurg** 6: 140-52, 1949.
10. Lewis R C, Elliott K A C: Clinical uses of an artificial cerebrospinal fluid. **J Neurosurg** 7: 256-60, 1950.
11. Spetzler R F, Zabramski J M: Cerebrospinal fluid fistula. **Contemp Neurosurg** 8: 1-7, 1986.
12. Manelfe C, Cellerier P, Sobel D, et al.: CSF rhinorrhea: Evaluation with metrizamide cisternography. **AJNR** 3: 25-30, 1982.
13. Meirowsky A M, Ceveness W F, Dillon J D, et al.: CSF fistulas complicating missile wounds of the brain. **J Neurosurg** 54: 44-8, 1981.
14. Cusimano M D, Sekhar L N: Pseudo-cerebrospinal fluid rhinorrhea. **J Neurosurg** 80: 26-30, 1994.
15. Calcaterra T C: **Cerebrospinal rhinorrhea**. In Otolaryngology, English G M, (ed.). Lippincott-Raven, Philadelphia, 1992, Vol. 2, Chapter 37: pp 1-7.
16. Nutkiewicz A, DeFeo D R, Kohout R I, et al.: Cerebrospinal fluid rhinorrhea as a presentation of pituitary adenoma. **Neurosurgery** 6: 195-7, 1980.
17. Johnston W H: Cerebrospinal rhinorrhea: The study of one case and reports of twenty others collected from the literature published since nineteen hundred. **Ann Otolaryngol** 35: 1205, 1926.
18. Schievink W I, Meyer F B, Atkinson J L D, et al.: Spontaneous spinal cerebrospinal fluid leaks and intracranial hypotension. **J Neurosurg** 84: 598-605, 1996.
19. Naidich T P, Moran C J: Precise anatomic localization of atraumatic sphenoethmoidal CSF rhinorrhea by metrizamide CT cisternography. **J Neurosurg** 53: 222-8, 1980.
20. Hand W L, Sanford J P: Posttraumatic bacterial meningitis. **Ann Int Medicine** 72: 869-74, 1970.
21. Wilkins R H, Rengachary S S, (eds.): **Neurosurgery**. McGraw-Hill, New York, 1985.
22. Ryall R G, Peacock M K, Simpson D A: Usefulness of B_2-transferrin assay in the detection of cerebrospinal fluid leaks following head injury. **J Neurosurg** 77. 737-9, 1992.
23. Fransen P, Sindic C J M, Thauvoy C, et al.: Highly sensitive detection of beta-2 transferrin in rhinorrhea and otorrhea as a marker for cerebrospinal fluid (CSF) leakage. **Acta Neurochir** 109: 98-101, 1991.
24. Oberson R: Radioisotope diagnosis of rhinorrhea. **Radiol Clin Biol** 41: 28-35, 1972.
25. Ahmadi J, Weiss M H, Segall H D, et al.: Evaluation of CSF rhinorrhea by metrizamide CT cisternography. **Neurosurgery** 16: 54-60, 1985.
26. Klastersky J, Sadeghi M, Brihaye J: Antimicrobial prophylaxis in patients with rhinorrhea or otorrhea: A double blind study. **Surg Neurol** 6: 111-4, 1976.
27. Allen C, Glasziou P, Del Mar C: Bed rest: A potentially harmful treatment needing more careful evaluation. **Lancet** 354: 1229-33, 1999.
28. Calcaterra T C: Extracranial repair of cerebrospinal rhinorrhea. **Ann Otol Rhinol Laryngol** 89: 108-16, 1980.
29. Lewin W: Cerebrospinal fluid rhinorrhea in closed head injuries. **Br J Surgery** 17: 1-18, 1954.
30. Dagi T F, George E D: **Surgical management of cranial cerebrospinal fluid fistulas**. In Operative neurosurgical techniques, Schmidek H H and Sweet W H, (eds.). W.B. Saunders, Philadelphia, 3rd ed., 1995, Vol. 1: pp 117-31.
31. Fujii T, Misumi S, Onoda K, et al.: Simple management of CSF rhinorrhea after pituitary surgery. **Surg Neurol** 26: 345-8, 1986.
32. Fishman R A, Dillon W P: Dural enhancement and cerebral displacement secondary to intracranial hypotension. **Neurology** 43: 609-11, 1993.
33. Schievink W I, Tourje J: Intracranial hypotension without meningeal enhancement on magnetic resonance imaging. **J Neurosurg** 92: 475-7, 2000 (case report).
34. Chung S J, Kim J S, Lee M C: Syndrome of cerebral spinal fluid hypovolemia: Clinical and imaging features and outcome. **Neurology** 55: 1321-7, 2000.
35. Mokri B: Spontaneous cerebrospinal fluid leaks, from intracranial hypotension to cerebrospinal fluid hypovolemia: Evolution of a concept. **Mayo Clin Proc** 74: 1113-23, 1999.
36. Alvarez-Linera J, Escribano J, Benito-Leon J, et al.: Pituitary enlargement in patients with intracranial hypotension syndrome. **Neurology** 55: 1895-7, 2000.

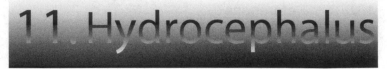
11. Hydrocephalus

11. Hydrocephalus

EPIDEMIOLOGY
Estimated prevalence: 1-1.5%.
Incidence of congenital hydrocephalus is ≈ 0.9-1.8/1000 births (reported range from 0.2 to 3.5/1000 births[1]).

FUNCTIONAL CLASSIFICATION

Two main functional subdivisions of hydrocephalus (HCP)
1. **obstructive** (AKA non-communicating): block proximal to the arachnoid granulations **(AG)**. On CT or MRI: enlargement of ventricles proximal to block (e.g. obstruction of aqueduct of Sylvius → lateral and 3rd ventricular enlargement out of proportion to the 4th ventricle, sometimes referred to as triventricular hydrocephalus)
2. **communicating** (AKA non-obstructive): CSF circulation blocked at level of AG

SPECIAL FORMS OF HYDROCEPHALUS
1. conditions that are not actually true hydrocephalus
   A. **hydrocephalus ex vacuo**: enlargement of the ventricles due to loss of cerebral tissue (cerebral atrophy), usually as a function of normal aging, but accelerated or accentuated by certain disease processes (e.g. Alzheimer's disease, Creutzfeldt-Jakob)
   B. otitic hydrocephalus: obsolete term used to describe the increased intracranial pressure seen in patients with otitis media (see see *Idiopathic intracranial hypertension*, page 493)
   C. external hydrocephalus: *see page 181*
   D. hydranencephaly: *see below*
2. normal pressure hydrocephalus **(NPH)**: *see page 199*
3. entrapped fourth ventricle: *see page 182*
4. arrested hydrocephalus: *see page 181*

HYDRANENCEPHALY
A post-neurulation defect (*see page 112*). Total or near-total absence of the cerebrum (small bands of cerebrum may be consistent with the diagnosis[2]), with intact cranial vault and meninges, the intracranial cavity being filled with CSF. There is usually progressive macrocrania, but head size may be normal (especially at birth), and, occasionally, microcephaly may occur. Facial dysmorphism is rare.
May be due to a variety of causes, the most commonly cited is bilateral ICA infarcts (which results in absence of brain tissue supplied by the anterior and middle cerebral arteries with preservation in the distribution of the PCA). May also be due to infection (congenital or neonatal herpes, toxoplasmosis, equine virus).
Less affected infants may appear normal at birth, but are often hyperirritable and retain primitive reflexes (Moro, grasp, and stepping reflex) beyond 6 mo. They rarely progress beyond spontaneous vowel production and social smiling. Seizures are common.
Progressive enlargement of CSF spaces may occur which can mimic severe ("maximal") hydrocephalus **(HCP)**. It is critical to differentiate the two since true HCP may be treated by shunting which may produce some re-expansion of the cortical mantle.

Many means to distinguish hydranencephaly and HCP have been described, and include:
1. **EEG**: shows no cortical activity in hydranencephaly (maximal HCP typically produces an abnormal EEG, but background activity will be present throughout the brain[2]) and is one of the best ways to differentiate the two
2. **CT**[2, 3], **MRI** or **ultrasound**: majority of intracranial space is occupied by CSF. Usually do not see frontal lobes or frontal horns of lateral ventricles (there may be remnants of temporal, occipital or subfrontal cortex). A structure consisting of

brainstem nodule (rounded thalamic masses, hypothalamus) and medial occipital lobes sitting on the tentorium occupies a midline position surrounded by CSF. Posterior fossa structures are grossly intact. The falx is usually intact (unlike alobar holoprosencephaly), and is not thickened, but may be displaced laterally. In HCP, some cortical mantle is usually identifiable

3. **transillumination** of the skull: a hydrocephalic head ordinarily does not transilluminate unless the patient is < 9 mos old and the cortical mantle under the light source is < 1 cm thick[4 (p 215)] or if fluid displaces the cortex inward (e.g. subdural effusions). Too nonspecific to be very helpful

4. **angiography**: in "classic" cases resulting from bilateral ICA occlusion, no flow through supraclinoid carotids and a normal posterior circulation is expected

Treatment

Shunting may be performed to control head size, but unlike the case with maximal hydrocephalus, there is no restitution of the cerebral mantle.

EXTERNAL HYDROCEPHALUS (AKA BENIGN EXTERNAL HYDROCEPHALUS)

❦ Key features
- enlarged subarachnoid spaces over the frontal poles in the first year of life
- ventricles are normal or minimally enlarged
- may be distinguished from subdural hematoma by the "cortical vein sign"
- usually resolves spontaneously by 2 years of age

Enlarged subarachnoid space (usually over the cortical sulci of the frontal poles) seen in infancy (primarily in the first year of life) usually accompanied by abnormally increasing head circumference with normal or mildly dilated ventricles[5]. There are often enlarged basal cisterns and widening of the anterior interhemispheric fissure. No other symptoms or signs should be present (although there may be slight delay only in motor milestones due to the large head). Etiology is unclear, but a defect in CSF resorption is postulated. External hydrocephalus **(EH)** may be a variant of communicating hydrocephalus[6]. No predisposing factor may be found in some cases, although EH may be associated with some craniosynostoses (especially plagiocephaly) or it may follow intraventricular hemorrhage or superior vena cava obstruction.

Differential diagnosis: EH is probably distinct from benign subdural collections (or extra-axial fluid) of infancy (*see page 678*). ★ EH must be distinguished from symptomatic chronic extra-axial fluid collections (or chronic subdural hematoma), which may be accompanied by seizures, vomiting, headache... (*see page 678*) and may be the result of child abuse. With EH, MRI or CT may demonstrate cortical veins extending from the surface of the brain to the inner table of the skull coursing through the fluid collection ("**cortical vein sign**"), whereas the collections in subdural hematomas compress the subarachnoid space which apposes the veins to the surface of the brain[8, 9].

Treatment: EH usually compensates by 12-18 mos age without shunting[10]. Recommend: follow serial ultrasound and/or CT to rule out abnormal ventricular enlargement. Emphasize to parents that this does not represent cortical atrophy. Due to increased risk for positional molding, parents may need to reposition the head while the child is sleeping[11].

A shunt may rarely be indicated when the collections are bloody (consider the possibility of child abuse) or for cosmetic reasons for severe macrocrania or frontal bossing.

"ARRESTED HYDROCEPHALUS"

The exact definition of this term is not generally agreed upon, and some use the term **compensated hydrocephalus** interchangeably. Most clinicians use these terms to refer to a situation where there is no progression or deleterious sequelae due to hydrocephalus that would require the presence of a CSF shunt. Patients and families should be advised to seek medical attention if they develop symptoms of intracranial hypertension (decompensation): headaches, vomiting, ataxia or visual symptoms[11].

Arrested hydrocephalus satisfies the following criteria in the absence of a CSF shunt:
1. near normal ventricular size
2. normal head growth curve
3. continued psychomotor development

Shunt independence

The concept of becoming independent of a shunt is not universally accepted[12]. Some feel that shunt independence occurs more commonly when the HCP is due to a block at the level of the arachnoid granulations (communicating hydrocephalus)[13], but others have shown that it can occur regardless of the etiology[14]. These patients must be followed closely as there are reports of death as late as 5 years after apparent shunt independence, sometimes without warning[13].

When to remove a disconnected or non-functioning shunt?
Note: a disconnected shunt may continue to function by CSF flow through a subcutaneous fibrous tract. Recommendations on whether or not to repair vs. remove a disconnected or non-functioning shunt:
1. when in doubt, shunt
2. indications for shunt repair (vs. removal)
   A. marginally functioning shunts
   B. the presence of any signs or symptoms of increased ICP (vomiting, upgaze palsy, sometimes H/A alone[15]...)
   C. changes in cognitive function, ↓ attention span, or emotional changes
   D. patients with aqueductal stenosis or spina bifida: most are shunt dependent
3. because of risks associated with shunt removal, surgery for this purpose alone should be performed only in the situation of a shunt infection[16]
4. patients with a nonfunctioning shunt should be followed closely with serial CTs, and possibly with serial neuropsychological evaluations

ENTRAPPED FOURTH VENTRICLE
AKA isolated fourth ventricle, as the name implies, is a 4th ventricle that neither communicates with the 3rd ventricle (through the sylvian aqueduct) nor with the basal cisterns (through the foramina of Luschka or Magendie). Usually seen with chronic shunting of the lateral ventricles, especially with post-infectious hydrocephalus (especially fungal) or in those with repeated shunt infections. Possibly as a result of adhesions forming from prolonged apposition of the ependymal lining of the aqueduct due to the diversion of CSF through the shunt. The choroid plexus of the 4th ventricle continues to produce CSF which enlarges the ventricle when there is 4th ventricular outlet obstruction or obstruction at the level of the arachnoid granulations.

Presentation may include:
1. headache
2. lower cranial nerve palsies: swallowing difficulties
3. ataxia
4. reduced level of consciousness
5. nausea/vomiting
6. may also be an incidental finding (NB: some "atypical" findings, such as reduced attention span, may be related)

Treatment
Most surgeons advocate shunting the ventricle either with a separate VP shunt, or linking into an existing shunt. Potential complications include delayed injury to the brainstem by the catheter tip as the brainstem moves into its normal position with drainage of the 4th ventricle. This may be avoided by bringing the catheter into the 4th ventricle at a slight angle through the cerebellar hemisphere.

A Torkildsen shunt (ventriculocisternal shunt) is an option for obstructive hydrocephalus if it is certain that the arachnoid granulations are functional (usually not the case with hydrocephalus of infantile onset).

An LP shunt may be considered when the 4th ventricle outlets are patent.

CT/MRI CRITERIA OF HYDROCEPHALUS
Numerous methods have been devised to attempt to quantitatively define hydrocephalus (HCP) (most date back to the early CT experience). Some are presented here for completeness. For radiologic features of *chronic* HCP, *see page 184*.

Hydrostatic hydrocephalus

Hydrostatic HCP is suggested when either[17]:
A. the size of both temporal horns (TH) is ≥ 2 mm in width (*see Figure 11-1*) (in the absence of HCP, the temporal horns should be barely visible), and the sylvian & interhemispheric fissures and cerebral sulci are not visible
OR

B. both TH are ≥ 2 mm, and the ratio

$\dfrac{FH}{ID} > 0.5$ (where FH is the largest width of the
frontal horns, and ID is the internal diameter
from inner-table to inner-table at this level) (see
Figure 11-1).

Other features suggestive of hydrostatic hydrocephalus:
1. ballooning of frontal horns of lateral ventricles ("Mickey Mouse" ventricles) and 3rd ventricle
2. periventricular low density on CT, or periventricular high intensity signal on T2WI on MRI
   suggesting **transependymal absorption** or
   migration of CSF
3. used alone, the ratio

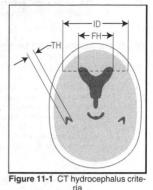

Figure 11-1 CT hydrocephalus criteria

$$\dfrac{FH}{ID} \begin{cases} < 40\% & \text{normal} \\ 40\text{-}50\% & \text{borderline} \\ > 50\% & \text{suggests hydrocephalus} \end{cases}$$

4. **Evan's ratio**: ratio of FH to maximal biparietal diameter > 30%
5. sagittal MRI may show upward bowing of the corpus callosum

ETIOLOGIES OF HYDROCEPHALUS

HCP is either due to subnormal CSF reabsorption, or rarely to CSF overproduction (as
with some choroid plexus papillomas; even
here, reabsorption is probably defective in
some as normal individuals could probably tolerate the slightly elevated CSF production rate
of these tumors). The etiologies in one series of
pediatric patients is shown in Table 11-1.
* congenital
  A. Chiari Type 2 malformation
     and/or myelomeningocele **(MM)**
     (usually occur together)

**Table 11-1 Etiologies of HCP in 170
pediatric patients with HCP[10]**

congenital (without myelomeningocele)	38%
congenital (with MM)	29%
perinatal hemorrhage	11%
trauma/subarachnoid hemorrhage	4.7%
tumor	11%
previous infection	7.6%

  B. Chiari Type 1 malformation: HCP may occur with 4th ventricle outlet ob-
     struction
  C. primary aqueductal stenosis (usually presents in infancy, rarely in adult-
     hood)
  D. secondary aqueductal gliosis: due to intrauterine infection or germinal ma-
     trix hemorrhage[19]
  E. **Dandy-Walker malformation**: atresia of foramina of Luschka & Magend-
     ie (see page 110). The incidence of this in patients with HCP is 2.4%
  F. rare X-linked inherited disorder
* acquired
  A. infectious (the most common cause of communicating HCP)
     1. post-meningitis (especially purulent and basal, including TB)
     2. cysticercosis
  B. post-hemorrhagic (2nd most common cause of communicating HCP)
     1. post-SAH (see page 783)
     2. post-intraventricular hemorrhage **(IVH)**: many will develop transient
        HCP. 20-50% of patients with large IVH develop permanent HCP
  C. secondary to masses
     1. non neoplastic: e.g. vascular malformation
     2. neoplastic: most produce obstructive HCP by blocking CSF pathways,
        especially tumors around aqueduct, e.g. medulloblastoma. A colloid
        cyst can block CSF flow at the foramen of Monro. Pituitary tumor: su-
        prasellar extension of tumor or expansion from pituitary apoplexy
  D. post-op: 20% of pediatric patients develop permanent hydrocephalus (re-
     quiring shunt) following p-fossa tumor removal. May be delayed up to 1 yr

E.   neurosarcoidosis: *see page 56*
F.   "constitutional ventriculomegaly": asymptomatic. Needs no treatment
G.   associated with spinal tumors[20]

DIFFERENTIAL DIAGNOSIS OF HYDROCEPHALUS
For etiologies of HCP, *see above*. Conditions that may mimic HCP but are not due to inadequate CSF absorption include:
1.   atrophy: sometimes referred to as "hydrocephalus ex vacuo". Does not represent altered CSF hydrodynamics, but is rather loss of brain tissue (*see page 180*)
2.   hydranencephaly: *see page 180*
3.   developmental anomalies where the ventricles appear enlarged:
     A.   agenesis of the corpus callosum: *see page 114* (may occasionally be associated with HCP, but more often merely represents expansion of the third ventricle and separation of the lateral ventricles)
     B.   septo-optic dysplasia: *see page 122*

SIGNS AND SYMPTOMS OF ACTIVE HCP

In young children
1.   cranium enlarges at a rate > facial growth
2.   irritability, poor head control, N/V
3.   fontanelle full and bulging
4.   enlargement and engorgement of scalp veins: due to reversal of flow from intracerebral sinuses due to increased intracranial pressure[21]
5.   **Macewen's sign**: cracked pot sound on percussing over dilated ventricles
6.   6th nerve (abducens) palsy: the long intracranial course is postulated to render this nerve very sensitive to pressure
7.   "setting sun sign" (upward gaze palsy): **Parinaud's syndrome** from pressure on region of suprapineal recess
8.   hyperactive reflexes
9.   irregular respirations with apneic spells
10. splaying of cranial sutures (seen on plain skull x-ray)

In older children/adults with rigid cranial vault
Symptoms of increased ICP, including: papilledema, H/A, N/V, gait changes, upgaze and/or abducens palsy. Slowly enlarging ventricles may initially be asymptomatic.

CHRONIC HCP
Features indicative of *chronic* hydrocephalus (as opposed to acute hydrocephalus):
1.   beaten copper cranium (some refer to beaten silver appearance) on plain skull x-ray[22]. By itself, does not correlate with increased ICP, however when associated with #3 and #4 below, does suggest ↑ ICP. May be seen in craniosynostosis (*see page 101* for description)
2.   3rd ventricle herniating into sella (seen on CT or MRI)
3.   erosion of sella turcica (may be due to #2 above) which sometimes produces an **empty sella**, and erosion of the dorsum sella
4.   the temporal horns may be less prominent on CT than in acute HCP
5.   **macrocrania**: by convention, OFC greater than 98th percentile[23 (pp 203)]
6.   atrophy of corpus callosum: best appreciated on sagittal MRI
7.   in infants
     A.   sutural diastasis
     B.   delayed closure of fontanelles
     C.   failure to thrive or developmental delay

OCCIPITAL-FRONTAL CIRCUMFERENCE
The occipital-frontal circumference (**OFC**) should be followed in every growing child (as part of a "well-baby" check-up, and especially in infants with documented or suspected hydrocephalus (**HCP**)). As a rule of thumb, the OFC of a normal infant should equal the distance from crown to rump[24 (rule #335)]. *See page 919* for the differential diagnosis of macrocephaly.

Normal head growth: parallels normal curves as seen on the graphs on the inside front cover, or in *Figure 11-2* and *Figure 11-3* for preemies. Any of the following may signify treatable conditions such as active HCP, subdural hematoma, or subdural effusions, and should prompt an evaluation of the intracranial contents (e.g. CT, head U/S …):

1. upward deviations (crossing curves)
2. continued head growth of more than 1.25 cm/wk
3. OFC approaching 2 standard deviations **(SD)** above normal
4. head circumference out of proportion to body length or weight, even if within normal limits for age (*see Figure 11-3*)[25]

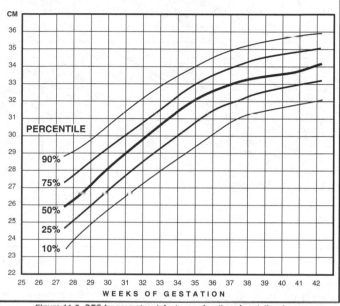

Figure 11-2 OFC for premature infants as a function of gestational age

These conditions may also be seen in the "catch-up phase" of brain growth in premature infants after they recover from their acute medical illnesses, see *Catch-up phase of brain growth* page 864). Deviations below the curves or head growth in the premature infant in the neonatal period of less than 0.5 cm/wk (excluding the first few weeks of life) may indicate microcephaly (see page 113).

Technique: measure circumference around forehead and occiput (excluding ears) three consecutive times, and use the <u>largest</u> value. OFC is then plotted on a graph of average values as a function of age[26] and followed for each individual patient. Use the graphs on the inside front cover for most children and adolescents. The graph in *Figure 11-2* shows the OFC for premature infants as a function of gestational age up to term.

The graph in *Figure 11-3* shows the relationship of head circumference, weight and length for various gestational ages.

11.1. Treatment of hydrocephalus

MEDICAL
HCP remains a surgically treated condition. Acetazolamide may be helpful for temporizing (*see below*).

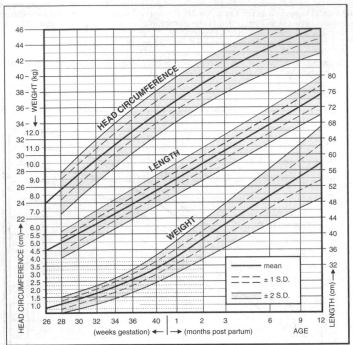

Figure 11-3 Head circumference, weight and length

(Redrawn from **Journal of Pediatrics**, "Growth Graphs for the Clinical Assessment of Infants of Varying Gestational Age", Babson S G, Benda G I, vol 89, pp 815, with permission)

Diuretic therapy

May be tried in premature infants with bloody CSF (as long as there is no evidence of active hydrocephalus) while waiting to see if there will be resumption of normal CSF absorption. However, at best this should only be considered as an adjunct to definitive treatment or as a temporizing measure.

Satisfactory control of HCP was reported in ≈ 50% of patients of age < 1 year who had stable vital signs, normal renal function and no symptoms of elevated ICP (apnea, lethargy, vomiting) using the following[27]:

- **acetazolamide** (a carbonic anhydrase inhibitor): 25 mg/kg/day PO divided TID **x** 1 day, increase 25 mg/kg/day each day until 100 mg/kg/day is reached
- simultaneously start **furosemide**: 1 mg/kg/day PO divided TID
- to counteract acidosis:
  - ◆ tricitrate (Polycitra®) 4 ml/kg/day divided QID (each ml is equivalent to 2 mEq of bicarbonate, and contains 1 mEq K^+ and 1 mEq Na^+)
  - ◆ measure serial electrolytes, and adjust dosage to maintain serum HCO_3 > 18 mEq/L
  - ◆ change to Polycitra-K® (2 mEq K^+ per ml, no Na^+) if serum potassium becomes low, or to sodium bicarbonate if serum sodium becomes low
- watch for electrolyte imbalance and acetazolamide side effects: lethargy, tachypnea, diarrhea, peristhesias (e.g. tingling in the fingertips)
- perform weekly U/S or CT scan and insert ventricular shunt if progressive ventriculomegaly occurs. Otherwise, maintain therapy for a 6 month trial, then taper dosage over 2-4 weeks. Resume 3-4 mos of treatment if progressive HCP occurs

HCP after intraventricular hemorrhage may be only transient Serial taps (ventricular or LP[28]) may temporize until resorption resumes (*see page 864*) but LPs can only be performed for <u>communicating</u> HCP. If reabsorption does not resume when the protein content of the CSF is < 100 mg/dl, then it is unlikely that spontaneous resorption will occur (i.e. a shunt will usually be necessary).

SURGICAL

Goals of therapy:

Normal sized ventricles is not the goal of therapy. Goals are optimum neurologic function and a good cosmetic result.

Options include:

1. choroid plexectomy: described by Dandy in 1918 for communicating hydrocephalus[29]. May reduce the rate but does not totally halt CSF production (only a portion of CSF is secreted by the choroid plexus, other sources include the ependymal lining of the ventricles and the dural sleeves of spinal nerve roots). Open surgery was associated with a high mortality rate (possibly due to replacement of CSF by air). Endoscopic choroid plexus coagulation was originally described in 1910 and was recently resurrected[30]
2. eliminating the obstruction: e.g. opening a stenosed sylvian aqueduct. Often higher morbidity and lower success rate than simple CSF diversion with shunts, except perhaps in the case of tumor
3. third ventriculostomy: (*see below*)
4. shunting: various shunts are described below - ventriculoperitoneal, ventriculoatrial, ventriculopleural, lumboperitoneal…

Third ventriculostomy

There has been a resurgence of interest in third ventriculostomy (**TV**) with the recent increased use of ventriculoscopic surgery (*see page 622* for technique).

Indications. TV may be used in patients with obstructive IICP. May be an option in managing shunt infection (as a means to remove all hardware without subjecting the patient to increased ICP). TV has also been proposed as an option for patients who developed subdural hematomas after shunting (the shunt is removed before the TV is performed). TV may also be indicated for slit ventricle syndrome (*see page 197*).

Contraindications: *Communicating* hydrocephalus is considered a contraindication to TV. Relative contraindications to TV would be the presence of any of the conditions associated with a low success rate (*see below*).

Complications:

1. hypothalamic injury
2. transient 3rd and 6th nerve palsies
3. uncontrollable bleeding
4. cardiac arrest[31]
5. traumatic basilar artery aneurysm[32]: possibly related to thermal injury from use of laser in performing TV

Success rate: Overall success rate is ≈ 56% (range of 60-94% for nontumoral aqueductal stenosis[32] (**AqS**)). Highest maintained patency rate is with previously untreated acquired AqS. Success rate in infants may be poor because they may not have a normally developed subarachnoid space. There is a low success rate (only ≈ 20% of TVs will remain patent) if there is pre-existing pathology including:

1. tumor
2. previous shunt
3. previous SAH
4. previous whole brain radiation (success with focal stereotactic radiosurgery is not known)
5. significant adhesions visible when perforating through the floor of the third ventricle at the time of performance of TV

11.1.1.   Shunts

See *Ventricular shunts* on page 620 for surgical insertion pointers.

SHUNT TYPE BY CATEGORY

1. ventriculoperitoneal **(VP)** shunt:
   A. most commonly used shunt in modern era
   B. lateral ventricle is the usual proximal location
2. ventriculo-atrial **(VA)** shunt ("vascular shunt"):
   A. shunts ventricles through jugular vein to superior vena cava, so-called "ven-triculo-atrial" shunt because it shunts the *cerebral ventricles* to the vascular system with the catheter tip in the region of the right *cardiac atrium*)
   B. treatment of choice when abdominal abnormalities are present (extensive abdominal surgery, peritonitis, morbid obesity, in preemies who have had NEC and may not tolerate VP shunt...)
   C. shorter length of tubing results in lower distal pressure and less siphon effect than VP shunt
3. Torkildsen shunt:
   A. shunts ventricle to cisternal space
   B. rarely used
   C. effective only in acquired obstructive HCP, as patients with congenital HCP frequently do not develop normal subarachnoid CSF pathways
4. miscellaneous: various distal projections used historically or in patients who have had significant problems with traditional shunt locations (e.g. peritonitis with VP shunt, SBE with vascular shunts):
   A. pleural space (**ventriculopleural shunt**): not a first choice, but a viable alternative if the peritoneum is not available[33]. Risk of symptomatic hydrothorax necessitating relocating distal end. Recommended only for patients > 7 yrs age
   B. gall bladder
   C. ureter or bladder: causes electrolyte imbalances due to losses through urine
5. lumboperitoneal (LP) shunt:
   A. only for communicating HCP: primarily pseudotumor cerebri or CSF fistula[34]. Useful in situations with small ventricles
   B. over age 2 yrs, percutaneous insertion with Tuohy needle is preferred
6. cyst or subdural shunt: from arachnoid cyst or subdural hygroma cavity, usually to peritoneum

Disadvantages/complications of various shunts

1. those that may occur with any shunt:
   A. obstruction: the most common cause of shunt malfunction
      ♦ proximal: ventricular catheter (the most common site)
      ♦ valve mechanism
      ♦ distal: reported incidence of 12-34%[35]. Occurs in peritoneal catheter in VP shunt (*see below*), in atrial catheter in VA shunt
   B. disconnection at a junction, or break at any point
   C. infection
   D. hardware erosion through skin, usually only in debilitated patients (especially preemies with enlarged heads and thin scalp from chronic HCP, who lay on one side of head due to elongated cranium). May also indicate silicone allergy (*see below*)
   E. seizures (ventricular shunts only): there is ≈ 5.5% risk of seizures in the first year after placement of a shunt which drops to ≈ 1.1% after the 3rd year[36] (NB: this does not mean that the shunt was the cause of all of these seizures). Seizure risk is questionably higher with frontal catheters than with parieto-occipital
   F. act as a conduit for extraneural metastases of certain tumors (e.g. medulloblastoma). This is probably a relatively low risk[37]
   G. silicone allergy[38]: rare (if it occurs at all). May resemble shunt infection with skin breakdown and fungating granulomas. CSF is initially sterile but later infections may occur. May require fabrication of a custom silicone-free device (e.g. polyurethane)
2. **VP** shunt:
   A. 17% incidence inguinal hernia (many shunts are inserted while processus vaginalis is patent)[39]
   B. need to lengthen catheter with growth: may be obviated by using long peri-

toneal catheter (*see page 621*)
- C. obstruction of peritoneal catheter:
  - ♦ may be more likely with distal slit openings ("slit valves") due to occlusion by omentum or by trapping debris from the shunt system[35]
  - ♦ by peritoneal cyst (or pseudocyst)[40]: usually associated with infection, may also be due to reaction to talc from surgical gloves. It may rarely be necessary to differentiate a CSF collection from a urine collection in patients with overdistended bladders that have ruptured (e.g. secondary to neurogenic bladder). Fluid can be aspirated percutaneously and analyzed for BUN and creatinine (which should be absent in CSF)
  - ♦ severe peritoneal adhesions: reduce surface area for CSF resorption
  - ♦ malposition of catheter tip:
    - • at time of surgery: e.g. in preperitoneal fat
    - • tubing may pull out of peritoneal cavity with growth
- D. peritonitis from shunt infection
- E. hydrocele
- F. CSF ascites
- G. tip migration
  - ♦ into scrotum[41]
  - ♦ perforation of a viscus[42]: stomach[43], bladder... More common with older spring-reinforced (Raimondi) shunt tubing
  - ♦ through the diaphragm[44]
- H. intestinal *obstruction* (as opposed to perforation): rare
- I. volvulus[45]
- J. intestinal strangulation: occurred only in patients in whom attempt was made to remove peritoneal tubing using traction on the catheter applied at the cephalad incision with subsequent breakage of the tubing leaving a residual intraabdominal segment (immediate peritoneal exploration is recommended under these circumstances)[46]
- K. overshunting: more likely than with VA shunt. Some recommend LP shunt for *communicating* hydrocephalus (*see page 196*)

3. **VA** shunt:
- A. requires repeated lengthening in growing child
- B. higher risk of infection, septicemia
- C. possible retrograde flow of blood into ventricles if valve malfunctions (rare)
- D. shunt embolus
- E. vascular complications: perforation, thrombophlebitis, pulmonary microemboli may cause pulmonary hypertension[47] (incidence ≈ 0.3%)

4. **LP** shunt:
- A. if at all possible, should not be used in growing child unless ventricular access is unavailable (e.g. due to slit ventricles) because of:
  - ♦ laminectomy in children causes scoliosis in 14%[48]
  - ♦ risk of progressive cerebellar tonsillar herniation (Chiari I malformation)[49] in up to 70% of cases[50, 51]
- B. overshunting harder to control when it occurs (a special horizontal-vertical **(H-V)** valve increases resistance when upright, *see below*)
- C. difficult access to proximal end for revision or assessment of patency (see *LP shunt evaluation*, page 622)
- D. lumbar nerve root irritation (radiculopathy)
- E. leakage of CSF around catheter
- F. pressure regulation is difficult
- G. bilateral 6th and even 7th cranial nerve dysfunction from overshunting
- H. high incidence of arachnoiditis and adhesions

MISCELLANEOUS SHUNT HARDWARE

1. tumor filter: used to prevent peritoneal or vascular seeding in tumors that may metastasize through CSF (e.g. medulloblastoma[52], PNETs, ependymoma); may eventually become occluded by tumor cells and need replacement; may be able to radiate tumor filter to "sterilize" it. The risk of "shunt mets" appears to be low[37]
2. antisiphon device: prevents siphoning effect when patient is erect
3. "horizontal-vertical valve" (H-V valve) used with LP shunts to increase the valve resistance when the patient is vertical to prevent overshunting (*see page 193*)
4. externally programmable variable pressure valves

5. on-off device: used to open or occlude shunt system by using external manipulation of shunt (e.g. Portnoy device)

SHUNT TYPE BY MANUFACTURER
Numerous shunt systems are on the market. The following describes the salient features of some commonly used shunts. Diagrams are not to scale.

X-RAY APPEARANCE OF SOME SHUNTS
The following figure depicts <u>idealized</u> x-ray appearances of some common shunts.

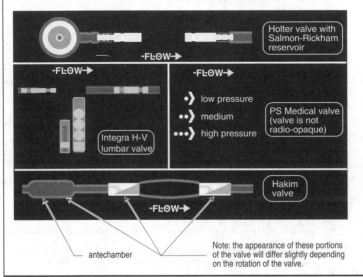

Figure 11-4 X-ray appearance of common shunts

PS MEDICAL/MEDTRONIC

Medtronic
125 Cremona Dr.
Goleta, CA 93117 USA
(800) 826-5603
www.medtronic.com

Standard contoured valve
A single one-way membrane valve design. The radio-opaque arrowhead points in the direction of flow (*see Figure 11-4*).

Pumping the valve
To pump the shunt in the "forward" direction, first occlude the inlet port (*see Figure 11-6*) with pressure from one finger on the "inlet occluder" (prevents back-

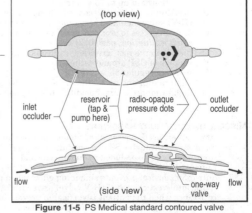

Figure 11-5 PS Medical standard contoured valve

flow into the ventricle during the next step). Then while maintaining this pressure, depress the reservoir dome with a second finger. Release both fingers, and repeat. The one-way valve regulates shunt pressure and prevents reflux of CSF during normal use and during the release phase of shunt pumping.

X-ray characteristics

The three available valve pressures are indicated by radio-opaque dots on the valve (allows x-ray identification of valve pressure): one dot = low pressure, two dots = medium, three dots = high.

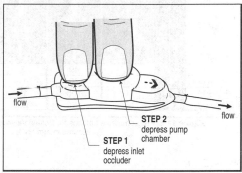

flow

STEP 2
depress pump
chamber
STEP 1
depress inlet
occluder

flow

Figure 11-6 Pumping the PS Medical valve

Strata® programmable valve

The Medtronic Strata valve is an externally adjustable valve that is programmed (using a magnet) to one of five performance level ("P/L") settings (*Figure 11-7*).

Because the valve may be inadvertently reprogrammed by external magnets, the patient must be informed to have the valve setting checked after an MRI performed for any reason.

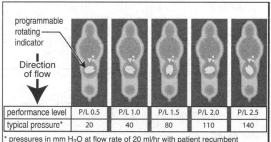

programmable rotating indicator

Direction of flow

performance level	P/L 0.5	P/L 1.0	P/L 1.5	P/L 2.0	P/L 2.5
typical pressure*	20	40	80	110	140

* pressures in mm H$_2$O at flow rate of 20 ml/hr with patient recumbent

Figure 11-7 Performance level (P/L) settings for the regular size Strata valve as seen on x-ray

SOPHYSA USA

Sophysa USA, Inc.
760 West 16th St.Bldg. N.
Costa Mesa, CA 92627 USA
(949) 548-6484
www.sophysa.com

Polaris programmable valve

The Polaris valve is an externally programmable valve that uses two attracting Samarium-Cobalt magnets to lock the pressure setting and to resist inadvertent reprogramming by environmentally encountered magnetssuch as MRI scanners, cell phones, headphones...

Available in 4 models (different pressure ranges, each identified by a unique number of radio-opaque dots), each with 5 externally adjustable positions. The x-ray appearance and corresponding pressures are shown in *Figure 11-8*.

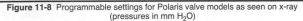

Direction of flow Model	Radiopaque dots	Position 1	Position 2	Position 3	Position 4	Position 5
SPV-140	none	10	40	80	110	140
SPV A or B	● ●	30	70	110	150	200
SPV-300	● ●	50	100	150	220	300
SPV-400	● ● ●	80	150	230	330	400

Figure 11-8 Programmable settings for Polaris valve models as seen on x-ray (pressures in mm H_2O)

NeuroCare

Distributed in U.S. by:
NeuroCare Group
8401 102nd Street
Suite 200
Pleasant Prairie, WI 53158
(800) 997-4868

Heyer-Schulte

The LPV valve is shown in *Figure 11-9*. To pump the shunt, occlude inlet port with one finger, then depress reservoir with another finger (as for

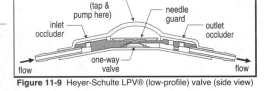

Figure 11-9 Heyer-Schulte LPV® (low-profile) valve (side view)

the PS Medical valve, *see above*). This valve may be injected in either direction by depressing the appropriate occluder while injecting into the reservoir.

Hakim shunt

Distributed by:
Integra Neurosciences
In the U.S.:
311 Enterprise Drive
Plainsboro, NJ 08536
(800) 654-2873
http://www.integra-ls.com

A dual ball-valve mechanism. To pump

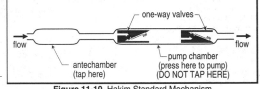

Figure 11-10 Hakim Standard Mechanism

shunt, depress the indicated portion of the valve. NB: <u>do not</u> tap here, as the silicone elastomer housing is not self-sealing. The antechamber is provided for this type of access.

INTEGRA HORIZONTAL-VERTICAL LUMBAR VALVE

May be used in lumboperitoneal shunt to increase the transmission pressure when the patient is upright to prevent overshunting. Markings used to orient the device during implantation:

1. an arrow on the inlet side of the unit indicates direction of flow
2. inlet tubing is clear
3. inlet tubing has smaller diameter than outlet tubing
4. outlet tubing is white
5. before positioning the valve and fastening it to the fascia with permanent suture, the valve should be connected to both the subarachnoid catheter (inlet) and the peritoneal catheter (outlet). The arrow on the inlet valve should point towards the patient's feet

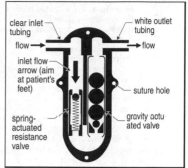

Figure 11-11 Integra H-V valve

HOLTER VALVE

Distributed by:
Codman & Shurtleff
Randolph, MA 02368
(617) 961-2300

A dual slit valve mechanism (see Figure 11-12). Usually used in combination with a Rickham or Salmon-Rickham reservoir (see Figure 11-13).

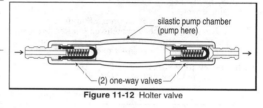

Figure 11-12 Holter valve

To pump the shunt, simply depress the indicated portion of the valve.

X-ray characteristics

The silastic tube between the two one-way valves is radiolucent (see Figure 11-4, page 190).

SALMON-RICKHAM RESERVOIR

Similar to standard Rickham reservoir except for lower profile (see Figure 11-13).

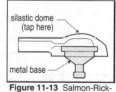

Figure 11-13 Salmon-Rickham Reservoir

11.2.   Shunt problems

Neurosurgical evaluation is usually requested for patients with a CSF shunt with variety of symptoms. Shunt "problems" usually involve one or more of the following:
1. undershunting (see below)   } accounts for most common shunt problems
2. infection (see page 214)
3. overshunting: slit ventricle syndrome, subdural hematomas... (see page 196)
4. seizures: see page 188
5. problems related to the distal catheter
   A. peritoneal: see page 188
   B. atrial: see page 189
6. skin breakdown over hardware: infection or silicone allergy (see page 188)

TAPPING A SHUNT
Indications to tap a shunt or ventricular access device (e.g. Ommaya reservoir) include:
1. to obtain CSF specimen
   A. to evaluate for shunt infection
   B. for cytology: e.g. in PNET to look for malignant cells in CSF
   C. to remove blood: e.g. in intraventricular hemorrhage
2. to evaluate shunt function
   A. measuring pressures
   B. contrast studies:
      1. proximal injection of contrast (iodinated or radio-labeled)
      2. distal injection of contrast
3. as a temporizing measure to allow function of a distally occluded shunt[53, 54]
4. to inject medication
   A. antibiotics: for shunt infection or ventriculitis
   B. chemotherapeutic (antineoplastic) agents
5. for catheters placed within tumor cyst (not a true shunt):
   A. periodic withdrawal of accumulated fluid
   B. for injection of radioactive liquid (usually phosphorous) for ablation

TECHNIQUE
(For LP shunt, see *LP shunt evaluation*, page 622).
There is a risk of introducing infection with every entry into the shunt system. With care, this may be kept to a minimum.
1. shave area
2. povidone iodine solution prep **x** 5 minutes
3. use 25 gauge butterfly needle or smaller (ideally a noncoring needle should be used): for routine taps, the needle should only be introduced into shunt components specifically designed to be tapped

To measure pressures
Steps are outlined in *Table 11-2*.

Table 11-2   Steps in tapping a shunt

Step	Information provided
1. insert needle into reservoir and look for spontaneous flow into butterfly tubing; measure pressure in manometer	• spontaneous flow indicates proximal end not completely occluded • pressure is that of ventricular system (should be < 15 cm of CSF in relaxed recumbent patient)
2. also measure the pressure with distal occluder pressed if present	• rise in pressure indicates some function of valve and distal shunt
3. if no spontaneous flow, try to aspirate CSF with syringe	• if CSF is easily aspirated, it may be that pressure seen by ventricular system is near 0 • if no CSF obtained or if difficult to aspirate, indicates proximal occlusion
4. send CSF for: C&S, protein/glucose, cell count	• checks for infection
5. fill manometer with sterile saline, & occlude proximal (inlet) occluder (with Holter valve, tap the valve itself, although this is not recommended because the hole thus created may not seal)	• measures forward transmission pressure (through valve and peritoneal catheter in presence of shunt with proximal occluder); forward pressure should be less than ventricular pressure
6. repeat measurement after injecting 3-5 ml of saline	• if peritoneal catheter is in a loculated compartment the pressure will be considerably higher after injection

INSTRUCTIONS TO PATIENTS

All patients and families of patients with hydrocephalus should be instructed regarding the following:
1. signs and symptoms of shunt malfunction or infection
2. not to pump the shunt unless instructed to do so for a specific purpose
3. prophylactic antibiotics: for the following situations (mandatory in vascular shunts, sometimes recommended in other shunts)
   A. dental procedures
   B. instrumentation of the bladder: cystoscopy, CMG, etc.

4. in a growing child: the need for periodic evaluation, including assessment of distal shunt length

UNDERSHUNTING

The shunt malfunction rate is ≈ 17% during the first year of placement in the pediatric population.

May be due to one or a number of the following:
1. blockage (occlusion)
   A. possible causes of occlusion:
      1. obstruction by choroid plexus
      2. buildup of proteinaceous accretions
      3. blood
      4. cells (inflammatory or tumor)
      5. secondary to infection
   B. site of blockage
      1. blockage of ventricular end (most common): usually by choroid plexus, may also be due to glial adhesions, intraventricular blood
      2. blockage of intermediate hardware (valves, connectors, etc., tumor filters may become obstructed by tumor cells, antisiphon devices may close due to variable overlying subcutaneous tissue pressures[55])
      3. blocked distal end (see page 189 for VP shunt)
   C. disconnection, kinking or breakage of system at any point: with age, silicone elastomers used in catheters calcify and break down, and become more rigid and fragile which may promote subcutaneous attachment[56]. Barium impregnation may accelerate this process. Tube fractures often occur near the clavicle, presumably due to the increased motion there

Signs and symptoms of undershunting
Signs and symptoms are those of active hydrocephalus, and include:
1. acute symptoms of increased intracranial pressure
   A. H/A
   B. N/V
   C. diplopia
   D. lethargy
   E. ataxia
   F. infants: apnea and/or bradycardia; irritability
   G. seizures: new onset, increase in frequency, or difficulty in control
2. acute signs of increased intracranial pressure
   A. upward gaze palsy ("setting sun sign", see Parinaud's syndrome, page 86)
   B. abducens palsy: false localizing sign
   C. field cut, or blindness (see Blindness from hydrocephalus, page 202)
   D. papilledema (rare before age 2 yrs)
   E. infants: bulging fontanelle, prominent scalp veins
3. swelling around shunt tubing: caused by CSF dissecting along shunt tract
4. chronic changes: before sutures close, OFCs crossing curves

EVALUATION OF SHUNT FOR UNDERSHUNTING
1. history and physical directed at determining presence of above signs and symptoms, also ascertain:
   A. reason for initial insertion of shunt (MM, post-meningitis, etc.)
   B. date of last revision and reason for revision
   C. presence of accessory hardware in system (e.g. antisiphon device, etc.)
   D. for children: OFC. Plot on graph of normal curves (use existing chart for that patient if available)
   E. fontanelle tension (if open): a soft pulsating fontanelle varying with respirations is normal, a tense bulging fontanelle suggests obstruction, a sunken fontanelle may be normal or may represent overshunting
   F. ability of shunt to pump and refill
      1. caution: may exacerbate obstruction, especially if shunt is occluded by ependyma due to overshunting: controversial
      2. difficult to depress: suggests distal occlusion

3. slow to refill (generally, any valve should refill in 15-30 secs): suggests proximal (ventricular) occlusion
   G. evidence of CSF dissecting along tract outside of shunt tubing
   H. in children presenting only with vomiting, especially those with cerebral palsy and feeding gastrostomy tubes, rule-out gastroesophageal reflux
2. radiographic evaluation
   A. "shunt series" (plain x-rays to visualize entire shunt: for VP shunt, AP & lateral skull + "low" CXR and/or abdominal x-ray)
      1. R/O disconnection or migration of tip by x-rays to visualize entire shunt; note: a disconnected shunt may continue to function by CSF flow through a fibrous tract; the following hardware may be radiolucent and can mimic disconnection:
         a. the central silastic part of a Holter style valve
         b. connectors ("Y" & "T" as well as straight)
         c. antisiphon devices
         d. tumor filters
      2. obtain most recent x-rays available to compare for breaks (essential for "complicated" shunts involving multiple ventricular or cyst ends or accessory hardware)
   B. in patients with open fontanelles, ultrasound is optimal method of evaluation (especially if previous U/S available)
   C. CT required if fontanelles closed, may be desirable in complicated shunt systems (e.g. cyst shunts)
   D. MRI: too costly and slow for routine shunt evaluation, shunt hardware is difficult to see. However, may be invaluable in complicated cases (may show **transependymal absorption** of CSF, loculations…)
   E. "shunt-o-gram" if it is still unclear if shunt is functioning
      1. radionuclide: *see below*
      2. x-ray: using iodinated contrast: *see below*
3. shunt tap: indications vary, generally performed if surgical exploration is considered or if infection is strongly suspected (see *Tapping a shunt*, page 194)
4. shunt exploration: sometimes even after thorough evaluation the only means to definitively prove or disprove the functioning of various shunt components is to operate and isolate and test each part of the system independently. Even when infection is not suspected, CSF and any removed hardware should be cultured.

"Shunt-o-gram"
Procedure: shave hair over reservoir & prep with Betadine. With patient supine tap the shunt by inserting a 25 gauge butterfly needle into the reservoir. Measure the pressure with a manometer. Patients with multiple ventricular catheters need to have each injected to verify its patency.

Radionuclide "shunt-o-gram" AKA radionuclide shuntography[57]: after tapping the shunt, drain 2-3 ml of CSF and send 1 ml of CSF for C&S. Inject radio-isotope (e.g. for VP shunt in an adult, use 1 mCi of ^{99m}-Tc (technecium) pertechnetate (usable range: 0.5 to 3 mCi) in 1 cc of fluid) while occluding distal flow (by compressing valve or occluding ports). Flush in isotope with remaining CSF.

Immediately image the abdomen with the gamma camera to rule out direct injection into distal tubing. Image the cranium to verify flow into ventricles (proximal patency). If spontaneous flow into abdomen is not seen after 10 minutes the patient is sat up and rescanned. If flow is not seen after 10 minutes, then the shunt is pumped. Look for diffusion of the isotope within the abdomen to rule out pseudocyst formation around catheter.

X-ray "shunt-o-gram": after tapping the shunt, drain ≈ 1 ml of CSF and send for C&S. Inject e.g. iohexol (Omnipaque 180) (*see page 127*) while occluding distal flow (by compressing valve or occluding ports).

SHUNT INFECTION

See *Shunt infection* on page 214 for evaluation and treatment.

"OVERSHUNTING"

POSSIBLE COMPLICATIONS OF OVERSHUNTING INCLUDE[58]
1. slit ventricles: including slit ventricle syndrome (*see below*)

2. intracranial hypotension: *see below*
3. subdural hematomas: *see page 198*
4. craniosynostosis and microcephaly: controversial (*see page 199*)
5. stenosis or occlusion of sylvian aqueduct

10-12% of long-term ventricular shunt patients will develop one of the above problems within 6.5 yrs of initial shunting[58]. Some experts feel that problems related to overshunting could be reduced by utilizing LP shunts for communicating hydrocephalus, and reserving ventricular shunts for obstructive HCP[58]. VP shunts may also be more likely to overdrain than VA shunts because of the longer tubing → greater siphoning effect.

INTRACRANIAL HYPOTENSION

AKA low ICP syndrome. Very rare. Symptoms similar to those of spinal H/A (postural in nature, relieved by recumbency). Although usually not associated with the following symptoms[59], they may occur[58]: N/V, lethargy, or neurologic signs (e.g. diplopia, upgaze palsy). Sometimes the symptoms resemble those of high ICP except that they are relieved when prostrate. Acute effects that may occur include[58]: tachycardia, loss of consciousness, other brain stem deficits due to a rostral shift of the intracranial contents or to low ICP.

Etiology is a siphoning effect due to the column of CSF in the shunt tube when the patient is erect[60]. Ventricles may be slit-like (as in slit ventricle syndrome (**SVS**)) or may be normal in appearance. Sometimes it is necessary to document a drop in ICP when going from supine to erect to diagnose this condition. These patients may also develop shunt occlusion and then the distinction from SVS blurs (*see below*).

With short-term symptoms, an ASD is the treatment of choice. However, patients with long-standing overshunting may not tolerate efforts to return intraventricular pressures to normal levels[58, 61].

SLIT VENTRICLES

1. asymptomatic:
   A. slit ventricles (totally collapsed lateral ventricles) may be seen on CT in 3 - 80% of patients after shunting[59, 62], most are asymptomatic
   B. these patients may occasionally present with symptoms unrelated to the shunt, e.g. true migraine
2. **slit ventricle syndrome (SVS)**: seen in < 12% of all shunted patients. Subtypes:
   A. intermittent shunt occlusion: overshunting leads to ventricular collapse (slit ventricles) which causes the ependymal lining to occlude the inlet ports of the ventricular catheter (by coaptation) producing shunt obstruction. With time, many of these patients develop low ventricular compliance[63], where even minimal dilatation results in high pressure which produces symptoms. Expansion then eventually reopens the inlet ports allowing resumption of drainage (hence the intermittent symptoms). Symptoms may resemble shunt malfunction: intermittent headaches unrelated to posture, often with N/V, drowsiness, irritability and impaired mentation. Signs may include 6th cranial nerve palsy. Incidence in shunted patients: 2-5%[59, 64]. CT or MRI scans may also show evidence of transependymal absorption of CSF
   B. total shunt malfunction (AKA normal volume hydrocephalus[63]): may occur and yet ventricles remain slit-like if the ventricles cannot expand because of subependymal gliosis, or due to the law of Laplace (which states that the pressure required to expand a large container is lower than the pressure required to expand a small container)
   C. venous hypertension with normal shunt function: may result from partial venous occlusion that occurs in some conditions (e.g. at the level of the jugular foramen in Crouzon's syndrome). Usually subsides by adulthood
3. some patients with idiopathic intracranial hypertension (pseudotumor cerebri, *see page 493*) have slit-like ventricles with consistently elevated ICP
4. intracranial hypotension: symptoms often relieved by recumbency (*see above*)

EVALUATION OF SLIT VENTRICLES

The shunt valve fills slowly if pumped when the ventricles are collapsed.

Monitoring CSF pressure: either via lumbar drain, or with a butterfly inserted into the shunt reservoir (with this method, pressure can be followed during postural changes to look for negative pressure when upright; possibly higher risk of infection with this). These patients are also monitored for pressure spikes, especially during sleep. Alternatively, these patients may be evaluated by "shunt-o-gram" (*see above*).

TREATMENT

In treating a patient with slit ventricles in imaging studies, it is important to ascertain into which of the 4 categories (*see above*) the patient falls. If the patient can be categorized, then the specific treatment listed below should be employed. Otherwise, it is probably most common to initially treat the patient empirically as intracranial hypotension, and then to move on to other methods for treatment failures.

Asymptomatic slit ventricles

Prophylactic upgrading to a higher pressure valve or insertion of an antisiphon device has largely been abandoned. However, this may be appropriate at the time of shunt revision when done for other reasons[62].

Intracranial hypotension

Postural H/A due to intracranial hypotension (true overshunting) is usually self limited, however, if symptoms persist after ≈ 3 days of bed-rest and analgesics and a trial with a tight abdominal binder, the valve should be checked for proper closing pressure. If it is low, replace with a higher pressure valve. If it is not low, an **antisiphon device (ASD)** (which, by itself, also increases the resistance of the system) alone or together with a higher pressure valve may be needed[65].

Slit ventricle syndrome

Patients with symptoms of SVS are actually suffering from intermittent *high* pressure. If total shunt malfunction is the cause, then shunt revision is indicated. For intermittent occlusion, treatment options include:
1. if symptoms occur early after shunt insertion or revision, initial expectant management may be indicated since symptoms will spontaneously resolve in many
2. revision of the proximal shunt. This may be difficult due to the small size of the ventricles. One can attempt to follow the existing tract and insert a longer or shorter length of tubing based on the pre-op imaging studies. Some advocate the placement of a second ventricular catheter, leaving the first one in place
3. patients may "respond" to either of the following interventions because the slight ventricular enlargement elevates the ependyma off of the inlet ports:
   A. valve upgrade[66] or
   B. ASD insertion[59, 65]: the procedure of choice in some opinions[58]. First described in 1973[67]
4. subtemporal decompression[68-70] sometimes with dural incision[68]. This results in dilatation of the temporal horns (evidence for elevated pressure) in most, but not all[70] cases
5. third ventriculostomy[71]: *see page 187*

Problems unrelated to shunting

For H/A consistent with migraine that are not postural, a trial with migraine-specific medications is warranted (Fiorinal®...). For treatment of idiopathic intracranial hypertension (pseudotumor cerebri), *see page 497*.

SUBDURAL HEMATOMAS

May be due to collapse of brain with tearing of bridging veins. In the pre-CT era, the incidence of subdural hematoma (**SDH**) formation following shunt insertion was probably underestimated at ≈ 1.2%. However, more recent estimates are 4-23% in adults, 2.8-5.4% in children, and is higher with normal pressure hydrocephalus (20-46%) than with "hypertensive hydrocephalus" (0.4-5%)[72, 73]. The risk of SDH is higher in the setting of longstanding hydrocephalus with a large head and little brain parenchyma (craniocerebral disproportion) with a thin cerebral mantle, as usually occurs in children with macrocephaly and large ventricles on initial evaluation. These patients have an "extremely delicate balance between subdural and intraventricular pressure"[72]. SDH can also follow shunting in elderly patients who have severe brain atrophy. The development of SDH may also be facilitated by negative pressures in the ventricles as a result of siphoning[73, 74]. There is also a low risk of epidural hematoma following CSF shunting[73].

Characteristics of the fluid: The collections may be on the same side as the shunt in 32%, on the opposite side in 21%, and bilateral in 47%[73].

At the time of discovery, the SDHs are usually subacute to chronic, and the previously large ventricles are usually collapsed. Only 1 of 19 cases showed colorless fluid[73]. In all cases tested, protein was elevated compared to CSF.

TREATMENT

Indications for treatment

Small (< 1-2 cm thick) asymptomatic collections in patients with closed cranial sutures may be followed with serial imaging. SDH were symptomatic in ≈ 40% of cases (symptoms often resemble those of shunt malfunction), and these require treatment. Treatment of SDH in children with open sutures has been advocated[73] to prevent later symptoms and/or development of macrocrania. Many authors recommend not treating asymptomatic lesions regardless of appearance[72, 75], whereas others vary their recommendations based on diverse criteria including size, appearance (chronic, acute, mixed…), etc.

Treatment techniques

A number of techniques have been described. Most involve evacuation of the SDHs by any of the usual methods (e.g. burr holes for chronic collections, craniotomy for acute collections) together with:
1. reducing the degree of shunting (i.e. to establish a lower pressure in the subdural space than in the intraventricular space, to cause the ventricles to re-expand and to prevent reaccumulation of the SDH)
    A. in shunt dependent cases
        1. replacing the valve with a higher pressure unit (upgrading the valve)
        2. increasing the pressure on a programmable pressure valve[76, 77]
        3. using a Portnoy device that can be turned off and on externally. Be sure that care providers can reliably open the device in an emergency
    B. in non-shunt dependent cases
        1. any of the methods outlined above for shunt dependent cases, or
        2. temporarily tying off the shunt[78]
    C. insertion of an anti-siphon device[67]
2. drainage of the subdural space to
    A. the cisterna magna[79]
    B. to the peritoneum with a low pressure valve (or no valve[73]). Some authors have the care-giver frequently pump the subdural valve

The goal is to achieve a delicate balance between undershunting (producing symptoms of active hydrocephalus) and overshunting (promoting the return of the SDH). Following surgery the patient should be mobilized slowly to prevent recurrence of the SDH.

CRANIOSYNOSTOSIS, MICROCEPHALY & SKULL DEFORMITIES

Also see *Craniosynostosis*, page 99. A number of skull changes have been described in infants after shunting, including[80]: thickening and inward growth of the bone of the skull base and cranial vault, decrease in size of the sella turcica, reduction in size of the cranial foramina, and craniosynostosis. The most common skull deformity was dolichocephaly from sagittal synostosis[81]. Microcephaly accounted for ≈ 6% of skull deformities after shunting (about half of these had sagittal synostosis). Some of these changes were reversible (except when complete synostosis was present) if intracranial hypertension recurred.

11.3.   Normal pressure hydrocephalus

❡ Key features
  • classic triad: dementia, gait disturbance, urinary incontinence
  • communicating hydrocephalus on CT or MRI
  • normal pressure on random LP
  • symptoms remediable with CSF shunting

First described in 1965[82], normal pressure hydrocephalus (**NPH**), AKA Hakim-Adams syndrome.
As originally described, the hydrocephalus of NPH was considered to be idiopathic.

However, in some cases an etiology can be identified:
1. post-SAH
2. post-traumatic
3. post-meningitic
4. following posterior fossa surgery
5. tumors, including carcinomatous meningitis
6. also seen in ≈ 15% of patients with Alzheimer's disease **(AD)**
7. deficiency of the arachnoid granulations
8. aqueductal stenosis may be an overlooked cause

CLINICAL
Age usually > 60 yrs. Slight male preponderance.

Clinical triad[83]
Triad is not pathognomonic, and may also be seen in vascular dementia[84].
1. gait disturbance: usually precedes other symptoms. Wide based with short, shuffling steps and unsteadiness on turning. Patients often feel like they are "glued to the floor" (so-called "magnetic gait") and may have difficulty initiating steps or turns. Absence of appendicular ataxia
2. dementia: primarily memory impairment with bradyphrenia (slowness of thought) and bradykinesia
3. urinary incontinence: usually unwitting (NB: a patient demented for any reason or with mobility impairment may have incontinence)

DIAGNOSTIC PROCEDURES
There is no test nor radiographic imaging that is pathognomonic for NPH. Numerous diagnostic criteria have been proposed for NPH to determine which patients are likely to respond to a shunt procedure in order to avoid potential complications (*see below*) and unnecessary surgery without denying surgery to those who might possibly benefit. None has proven to be of adequate reliability. Some are presented here for completeness.

LUMBAR PUNCTURE (LP)
Normal LP opening pressure **(OP)** should be < 180 mm H_2O. The response to a single LP[85] (withdrawing 15-30 ml CSF, or taking the OP down by ≈ one third) or to serial LPs may be of some predictive value. Consider ambulatory lumbar drainage (*see below*) for patients who fail to improve after a single LP. CSF should be sent for routine labs (*see page 616*).
Patients with an initial OP > 100 mm H_2O have a higher response rate to shunting.

CONTINUOUS CSF PRESSURE MONITORING
Some patients with a normal OP on LP demonstrate pressure peaks > 270 mm H_2O or recurrent B-waves[86]. These patients also tend to have a higher response rate to shunting.

AMBULATORY LUMBAR DRAINAGE[87]
Lumbar subarachnoid drain is placed with Tuohy needle, connected through a drip chamber to a closed drainage system. The drip chamber is placed at the level of the patient's ear when recumbent, or at the level of the shoulder when sitting or ambulating.
A properly functioning drain should put out ≈ 300 ml of CSF per day.
If symptoms of nerve root irritation develop during the drainage, the catheter should be withdrawn several millimeters. Daily surveillance CSF cell counts and cultures should be performed (NB: a pleocytosis of ≈ 100 cells/mm^3 is expected just with the presence of the drain).
A 5 day trial is recommended (mean time to improvement: 3 days).

CT AND MRI

Features on CT[88] and MRI[89]
1. prerequisite: communicating hydrocephalus
2. features that correlate with favorable response to shunt (these features suggest that the hydrocephalus is not due to atrophy alone[A]):

A. periventricular low density on CT or high intensity on T2WI MRI: may represent transependymal absorption of CSF. May resolve with shunting
B. compression of convexity sulci (*focal* sulcal dilation may sometimes be seen and may represent atypical reservoirs of CSF which may diminish after shunting and should not be considered as atrophy[91])
C. rounding of the frontal horns

Although some patients improve with no change in ventricles[92], clinical improvement most often accompanies reduction of ventricular size.

RADIONUCLIDE CISTERNOGRAPHY

Usefulness remains controversial. One study found that the cisternogram does not increase the diagnostic accuracy of clinical and CT criteria[93].

Technique: Lumbar subarachnoid injection of radio-isotope (e.g. 2.7 mCi of ^{99m}Tc-DTPA diluted to 1 cc with saline). Cisternograms are obtained by planar scintigraphy at 3, 6, and 24 hrs after injection (images may be obtained at 48 hrs if intraventricular activity is still seen at 24 hrs, however, an isotope other than ^{99m}Tc-DTPA must be used for such delayed images).

Conventional criteria for a normal study: Radioactivity is symmetrically distributed over the convexity 24 hrs after injection, with no intraventricular activity at any point. However, up to 41% of normals will demonstrate transient (up to 24 hrs, but not longer) activity in the ventricles[94].

Findings that may indicate a better chance for response to shunting: Of the following, only #2 is a reliable marker for NPH.
1. early scan (4-6 hrs after injection): activity in ventricles (presumed reflux from obstructed outflow). May also occur in normals (*see above*) for < 24 hrs
2. late scan (48-72 hrs): persistence of ventricular activity. Patients with this finding are most likely to improve with shunting (≈ 75% chance)
3. retained activity over convexity: these patients are less likely to improve
4. quantitative cisternography
   A. patients who clear over 50% of total intracranial radioactivity within 24 hrs are considered to have an adequate overall absorption rate, and are unlikely to improve with shunting. However others have found no correlation of clearance to shunt response
   B. one study found that if the ratio of ventricular to total intracranial activity (V/T) at 24 hours is > 32%, there would be a response to shunting, whereas V/T < 32% did not exclude the possibility of improvement[95]

MISCELLANEOUS

Cerebral blood flow (CBF) measurements: Although some studies indicate otherwise, CBF measurements show no specific findings in NPH, and are not helpful in predicting who will respond to shunting. However, increased CBF after shunting correlates with clinical improvement[96].

EEG: No specific findings on EEG in NPH.

TREATMENT

Before undertaking a surgical procedure, a dementia workup should be completed. VP shunt is the procedure of choice. Lumbar-peritoneal shunts have been used, but they tend to overshunt. In general, use a medium pressure valve[97] (closing pressure 65-90 mm H_2O) to minimize the risk of subdural hematomas (*see below*), although response rate may be higher with a low-pressure valve[98]. Gradually sit patient up over a period of several days; proceed more slowly in patients who develop low-pressure headaches. Follow patients clinically and with CT for ≈ 6-12 months.

Patients who do not improve and whose ventricles do not change should be evaluated for shunt malfunction. If not obstructed, a lower pressure valve should be tried.

A. atrophy (hydrocephalus ex vacuo), as in conditions such as Alzheimer's disease, lessens the chance of, but does not preclude, responding to a shunt (cortical atrophy is a common finding in healthy individuals of advanced age[90])

Complication rates may be as high as ≈ 35% (due to the fragility of the elderly brain)[99,100].

Potential complications include[101]:
1. subdural hematomas or hygroma (also *see page 198*): higher risk with low pressure valve and older patients who tend to have cerebral atrophy. Usually accompanied by headache, most resolve spontaneously or remain stable. Approximately one third require evacuation and tying off of shunt (temporarily or permanently). Risk may be reduced by gradual mobilization post-op
2. shunt infection
3. intraparenchymal hemorrhage in the brain
4. seizures: *see page 188*
5. delayed complications include: shunt obstruction or disconnection

OUTCOME

The most likely symptom to improve with shunting is <u>incontinence</u>, then gait disturbance, and lastly dementia. Black et al.[97] give the following markers for good candidates for improvement with shunting:

- clinical: presence of the classic triad[99] (*see page 200*). Also 77% of patients with gait disturbance as the primary symptom improved with shunting. Patients with dementia and <u>no</u> gait disturbance rarely respond to shunting
- LP: OP > 100 mm H_2O
- isotope cisternogram: typical NPH pattern. The mixed or normal pattern has no correlation with response to shunting
- continuous CSF pressure recording: pressure > 180 mm H_2O or frequent Lundberg B waves (*see page 653*)
- CT or MRI: large ventricles with flattened sulci (little atrophy)

Response is better when symptoms have been present for a shorter time.

NB: patients with suspected co-existing Alzheimer's disease **(AD)** may still improve with VP shunts, thus AD should not exclude these patients from shunting[102].

Some responders may subsequently deteriorate. Shunt malfunction and subdural collections must be ruled out before ascribing this to the natural course of the condition.

11.4. Blindness from hydrocephalus

A rare complication of hydrocephalus and/or shunt malfunction. Possible causes include:
1. occlusion of posterior cerebral arteries **(PCA)** caused by downward transtentorial herniation
2. chronic papilledema causing injury to optic nerve at the optic disc
3. dilatation of the 3rd ventricle with compression of optic chiasm

Ocular motility or visual field defects are more common with shunt malfunction than is blindness[103-106]. One series found 34 reported cases of permanent blindness in children attributed to shunt malfunction with concomitant increased ICP[107] (these authors were based in a referral center for visually impaired children, thus incidence not estimated). Another series of 100 patients with tentorial herniation (most from acute EDH and/or SDH) proven by CT; 48 patients operated; only 19 of 100 survived > 1 month (all were in operated group); 9 of 100 developed occipital lobe infarct (2 died, 3 vegetative state, remaining 4 moderate to severe disability)[108].

TYPES OF VISUAL DISTURBANCE

9 of 14 had pregeniculate (anterior visual pathway) blindness with marked optic nerve atrophy (early), and reduced pupillary light reflexes. 5 of 14 had postgeniculate (cortical) blindness with normal light responses and minimal or no optic nerve atrophy (or atrophy late). A few patients had evidence of damage in both sites.

Cortical blindness: due to lesions posterior to lateral geniculate bodies **(LGB)**, may also be seen with hypoxic injuries or trauma[109]. Occasionally associated with **Anton's syndrome** (denial of visual deficit) and with Ridoch's phenomenon (appreciation of moving objects without perception of stationary stimuli).

In patients with occipital lobe infarction

Occipital lobe infarctions **(OLI)** in PCA distribution are seen either bilaterally, or if unilateral are associated with other injuries to optic pathways posterior to LGB. The most often cited mechanism is compression of PCA resulting from brain herniating downward. Alternatively, upward cerebellar herniation (e.g. from ventricular puncture in face of a p-fossa mass) may impinge on PCA or branches with the same results[110].

OLIs are more likely with a rapid rise in ICP (doesn't allow compensatory shifts and collateral circulation to develop)[111]. Macular sparing is common.

Reported causes of OLI include: post traumatic edema, tumor, abscess, SDH, unshunted hydrocephalus, and shunt malfunction[112-114].

The occipital poles are also particularly vulnerable to diffuse hypoxia[115]; attested to by cases of cortical blindness after cardiac arrest[116]. Hypotension superimposed on compromised PCA circulation (from herniation or elevated ICP) may thus increase the risk of postgeniculate blindness[107, 111].

Both coup and contrecoup trauma may produce OLI. Unlike a PCA occlusion infarct, macular sparing is not expected in traumatic occipital lobe injury[112].

In patients with pregeniculate blindness

Elevated ICP transmits pressure to retina → bloodflow stasis, as well as mechanical trauma to optic chiasm from enlarging third ventricle (latter more commonly thought responsible for bitemporal hemianopia[103], but could, if unchecked, progress to complete visual loss). Also, if hypotension and anemia were present, consider the possibility of ischemic optic neuropathy[117-119].

These deficits are frequency unsuspected (altered mental state and the youth of many of these patients[107] makes detection difficult); an examiner must persevere to detect homonymous hemianopsias in an obtunded patient[112].

Pregeniculate blindness is less often associated with depressed sensorium than is postgeniculate (where direct compression and vascular compromise of midbrain are more likely[107]).

Cortical blindness after diffuse anoxia frequently improves (occasionally to normal); usually slowly (weeks to years quoted; several mos usually adequate)[116]. Many reports of blindness after shunt malfunction are pre-CT era, thus the presence or extent of occipital lobe infarction not ascertained. Some optimistic outcomes reported[120], however, permanent blindness or severe visual handicap are also described[112, 114]; no reliable predictor has been identified. As with infarcts elsewhere, younger patients fare better[115], but extensive calcarine infarcts on CT are probably incompatible with significant visual recovery.

11.5.   Hydrocephalus and pregnancy

Patients with CSF shunts may become pregnant, and there are at least 4 case reports of patients developing hydrocephalus during pregnancy requiring shunting[121].

With VP shunts, distal shunt problems may be higher in pregnancy. The following are management suggestions modified from Wisoff et al.[121].

Preconception management of patients with shunts

1. evaluation, including:
   A. evaluation of shunt function: preconception baseline MRI or CT. Further evaluation of shunt patency if any suspicion of malfunction. Patients with slit ventricles may have reduced compliance and may become symptomatic with very small changes in volume
   B. assessment of medications, especially anticonvulsants
2. counselling, including:
   A. genetic counselling: if the HCP is due to a neural tube defect **(NTD)**, then there is a 2-3% chance that the baby will have a NTD
   B. other recommendations include early administration of prenatal vitamins,

---

and avoiding teratogenic drugs and excessive heat (e.g. hot-tubs): see *Neural tube defects, Risk factors* on page 113.

Gravid management
1. close observation for signs of increased ICP: headache, N/V, lethargy, ataxia, seizures... Caution: these signs may mimic pre-eclampsia (which must also be ruled out). 58% of patients exhibit signs of increased ICP, which may be due to:
    A. decompensation of partial shunt malfunction
    B. shunt malfunction
    C. some show signs of increased ICP in spite of adequate shunt function, may be due to increased cerebral hydration and venous engorgement
    D. enlargement of tumor during pregnancy
    E. cerebral venous thrombosis: including dural sinus thrombosis & cortical venous thrombosis
    F. encephalopathy related to disordered autoregulation (*see page 64*)
2. patients developing symptoms of increased ICP should have CT or MRI
    A. if no change from preconception study, puncture shunt to measure ICP and culture CSF. Consider radioisotope shunt-o-gram
    B. if all studies are negative, then physiologic changes may be responsible. Treatment is bed rest, fluid restriction, and in severe cases steroids and/or diuretics. If symptoms do not abate, then early delivery is recommended as soon as fetal lung maturity can be documented (give prophylactic antibiotics for 48 hrs before delivery)
    C. if ventricles have enlarged and/or shunt malfunction is demonstrated on testing, shunt revision is performed
        1. in first two trimesters: VP shunt is preferred (do not use peritoneal trocar method after first trimester) and is tolerated well
        2. in third trimester: VA or ventriculopleural shunt is used to avoid uterine trauma or induction of labor

Intrapartum management
1. prophylactic antibiotics are recommended during labor and delivery to reduce the incidence of shunt infection. Since coliforms are the most common pathogen in L&D, Wisoff et al. recommend ampicillin 2 gm IV q 6 hrs, and gentamicin 1.5 mg/kg IV q 8 hrs in labor and **x** 48 hrs post partum[121]
2. in patients without symptoms: a vaginal delivery is performed if obstetrically feasible (lower risk of forming adhesions or infection of distal shunt). A shortened second stage is preferred since the increase in CSF pressure in this stage is probably greater than during other valsalva maneuvers[122]
3. in the patient who becomes symptomatic near term or during labor, after stabilizing the patient a C-section under general anesthesia (epidurals are contraindicated with elevated ICP) is performed with careful fluid monitoring (e.g. PA catheter) and, in severe cases, steroids and diuretics

11.6.   References

1. Lemire R J: Neural tube defects. **JAMA** 259: 558-62, 1988.
2. Sutton L N, Bruce D A, Schut L: Hydranencephaly versus maximal hydrocephalus: An important clinical distinction. **Neurosurgery** 6: 35-8, 1980.
3. Dublin A B, French B N: Diagnostic image evaluation of hydranencephaly and pictorially similar entities with emphasis on computed tomography. **Radiology** 137: 81-91, 1980.
4. Matson D D: **Neurosurgery of infancy and childhood.** 2nd ed. Charles C Thomas, Springfield, 1969.
5. Alvarez L A, Maytal J, Shinnar S: Idiopathic external hydrocephalus: Natural history and relationship to benign familial macrocephaly. **Pediatrics** 77: 901-7, 1986.
6. Barlow C F: CSF dynamics in hydrocephalus - with special attention to external hydrocephalus. **Brain Dev** 6: 119-27, 1984.
7. Chadduck W M, Chadduck J B, Boop F A: The subarachnoid spaces in craniosynostosis. **Neuro-**

surgery 30: 867-71, 1992.
8. McCluney K W, Yeakley J W, Fenstermacher J W: Subdural hygroma versus atrophy on MR brain scans: "the cortical vein sign". **AJNR** 13: 1335-9, 1992.
9. Kuzma B B, Goodman J M: Differentiating external hydrocephalus from chronic subdural hematoma. **Surg Neurol** 50: 86-8, 1998.
10. Ment L R, Duncan C C, Geehr R: Benign enlargement of the subarachnoid spaces in the infant. **J Neurosurg** 54: 504-8, 1981.
11. Sutton L N: Current management of hydrocephalus in children. **Contemp Neurosurg** 19 (21): 1-7, 1997.
12. Foltz E L, Shurtleff D B: Five-year comparative study of hydrocephalus in children with and without operation (113 cases). **J Neurosurg** 20: 1064-79, 1963.
13. Rekate H L, Nulsen F E, Mack H L, *et al.*: Establishing the diagnosis of shunt independence. **Monogr**

Neural Sci 8: 223-6, 1982.

14. Holtzer G J, De Lange S A: Shunt-independent arrest of hydrocephalus. **J Neurosurg** 39: 698-701, 1973.

15. Hemmer R: Can a shunt be removed? **Monogr Neural Sci** 8: 227-8, 1982.

16. Epstein F: Diagnosis and management of arrested hydrocephalus. **Monogr Neural Sci** 8: 105-7, 1982.

17. LeMay M, Hochberg F H: Ventricular differences between hydrostatic hydrocephalus and hydrocephalus ex vacuo by CT. **Neuroradiology** 17: 191-5, 1979.

18. Amacher A L, Wellington J: Infantile hydrocephalus: Long-term results of surgical therapy. **Childs Brain** 11: 217-29, 1984.

19. Hill A, Rozdilsky B: Congenital hydrocephalus secondary to intra-uterine germinal matrix/intraventricular hemorrhage. **Dev Med Child Neurol** 26: 509-27, 1984.

20. Kudo H, Tamaki N, Kim S, et al.: Intraspinal tumors associated with hydrocephalus. **Neurosurgery** 21: 726-31, 1987.

21. Schmidek H H, Auer L M, Kapp J P: The cerebral venous system. **Neurosurgery** 17: 663-78, 1985.

22. Tuite G F, Evanson J, Chong W K, et al.: The beaten copper cranium: A correlation between intracranial pressure, cranial radiographs, and computed tomographic scans in children with craniosynostosis. **Neurosurgery** 39: 691-9, 1996.

23. Section of Pediatric Neurosurgery of the American Association of Neurological Surgeons, (ed.) **Pediatric neurosurgery.** 1st ed., Grune and Stratton, New York, 1982.

24. Parker T: **Never trust a calm dog: And other rules of thumb.** Harper Perennial, New York, 1990.

25. Babson G G, Benda G I: **Growth graphs for the clinical assessment of infants of varying gestational age. J Pediatr** 89: 814-20, 1976.

26. Nelhaus G: Head circumference from birth to eighteen years. **Pediatrics** 41: 106-14, 1968.

27. Shinnar S, Gammon K, Bergman E W, et al.: Management of hydrocephalus in infancy: Use of acetazolamide and furosemide to avoid cerebrospinal fluid shunts. **J Pediatr** 107: 31-7, 1985.

28. Kreusser K L, Tarby T J, Kovnar E, et al.: Serial LPs for at least temporary amelioration of neonatal posthemorrhagic hydrocephalus. **Pediatrics** 75: 719-24, 1985.

29. Dandy W E: Extirpation of the choroid plexus of the lateral ventricle in communicating hydrocephalus. **Ann Surg** 68. 569-79, 1918.

30. Griffith H B, Jamjoom A B: The treatment of childhood hydrocephalus by choroid plexus coagulation and artificial cerebrospinal fluid perfusion. **Br J Neurosurg** 4: 95-100, 1990.

31. Handler M H, Abbott R, Lee M: A near-fatal complication of endoscopic third ventriculostomy: Case report. **Neurosurgery** 35: 525-8, 1994.

32. McLaughlin M R, Wahlig J B, Kaufmann A M, et al.: Traumatic basilar aneurysm after endoscopic third ventriculostomy: Case report. **Neurosurgery** 41: 1400-4, 1997.

33. Jones R F C, Currie B G, Kwok B C T: Ventriculopleural shunts for hydrocephalus: A useful alternative. **Neurosurgery** 23: 753-5, 1988.

34. James H E, Tibbs P A: Diverse clinical application of percutaneous lumboperitoneal shunts. **Neurosurgery** 8: 39-42, 1981.

35. Cozzens J W, Chandler J P: Increased risk of distal ventriculoperitoneal shunt obstruction associated with slit valves or distal slits in the peritoneal catheter. **J Neurosurg** 87: 682-6, 1997.

36. Dan N G, Wade M J: The incidence of epilepsy after ventricular shunting procedures. **J Neurosurg** 65: 19-21, 1986.

37. Berger M S, Baumeister B, Geyer J R, et al.: The risks of metastases from shunting in children with primary central nervous system tumors. **J Neurosurg** 74: 872-7, 1991.

38. Jimenez D F, Keating R, Goodrich J T: Silicone allergy in ventriculoperitoneal shunts. **Childs Nerv Syst** 10: 59-63, 1994.

39. Moazam F, Glenn J D, Kaplan B J, et al.: Inguinal hernias after ventriculoperitoneal shunt procedures in pediatric patients. **Surg Gynecol Obstet** 159: 570-2, 1984.

40. Bryant M S, Bremer A M, Tepas J J, et al.: Abdominal complications of ventriculoperitoneal shunts. **Am Surg** 54: 50-5, 1988.

41. Ram Z, Findler G, Guttman I, et al.: Ventriculoperitoneal shunt malfunction due to migration of the abdominal catheter into the scrotum. **J Pediatr Surg** 22: 1045-6, 1987.

42. Rush D S, Walsh J W: Abdominal complications of CSF-peritoneal shunts. **Monogr Neural Sci** 8: 32-4, 1982.

43. Alonso-Vanegas M, Alvarez J L, Delgado L, et al.: Gastric perforation due to ventriculo-peritoneal shunt. **Pediatr Neurosurg** 21: 192-4, 1994.

44. Lourie H, Bajwa S: Transdiaphragmatic migration of a ventriculoperitoneal catheter. **Neurosurgery** 17: 324-6, 1985.

45. Sakoda T H, Maxwell J A, Brackett C E: Intestinal volvulus secondary to a ventriculoperitoneal shunt. Case report. **J Neurosurg** 35: 95-6, 1971.

46. Couldwell W T, LeMay D R, McComb J G: Experience with use of extended length peritoneal shunt catheters. **J Neurosurg** 85: 425-7, 1996.

47. Pascual J M S, Prakash U B S: Development of pulmonary hypertension after placement of a ventriculoatrial shunt. **Mayo Clin Proc** 68: 1177-82, 1993.

48. Chumas P D, Kulkarni A V, Drake J M, et al.: Lumboperitoneal shunting: A retrospective study in the pediatric population. **Neurosurgery** 32: 376-83, 1993.

49. Welch K, Shillito J, Strand R, et al.: Chiari I "malformation": An acquired disorder? **J Neurosurg** 55: 604-9, 1982.

50. Chumas P D, Armstrong D C, Drake J M, et al.: Tonsillar herniation: The rule rather than the exception after lumboperitoneal shunting in the pediatric population. **J Neurosurg** 78: 568-73, 1993.

51. Payner T D, Prenger E, Berger T S, et al.: Acquired Chiari malformations: Incidence, diagnosis, and management. **Neurosurgery** 34: 429-34, 1994.

52. Kessler L A, Dugan P, Concannon J P: Systemic metastases of medulloblastoma promoted by shunting. **Surg Neurol** 3: 147-52, 1975.

53. Chan K H, Mann K S: Prolonged therapeutic external ventricular drainage: A prospective study. **Neurosurgery** 23: 436-8, 1988.

54. Mann K S, Yue C P, Ong G B: Percutaneous sump drainage: A palliation for oft-recurring intracranial cystic lesions. **Surg Neurol** 19: 86-90, 1983.

55. Hassan M, Higashi S, Yamashita J: Risks in using siphon-reducing devices in adult patients with normal-pressure hydrocephalus: Bench test investigations with Delta valves. **J Neurosurg** 84: 634-41, 1996.

56. Boch A-L, Hermelin É, Sainte-Rose C, et al.: Mechanical dysfunction of ventriculoperitoneal shunts caused by calcification of the silicone rubber catheter. **J Neurosurg** 88: 975-82, 1998.

57. French B N, Swanson M: Radionuclide imaging shuntography for the evaluation of shunt patency. **Monogr Neural Sci** 8: 39-42, 1982.

58. Pudenz R H, Foltz E L: Hydrocephalus: Overdrainage by ventricular shunts. A review and recommendations. **Surg Neurol** 35: 200-12, 1991.

59. McLaurin R L, Olivi A: Slit-ventricle syndrome: Review of 15 cases. **Pediat Neurosci** 13: 118-24, 1987.

60. Gruber R, Jenny P, Herzog B: Experiences with the

anti-siphon device (ASD) in shunt therapy of pediatric hydrpcephalus. **J Neurosurg** 61: 156-62, 1984.

61. Foltz E L, Blanks J P: Symptomatic low intraventricular pressure in shunted hydrocephalus. **J Neurosurg** 68: 401-8, 1988.

62. Teo C, Morris W: Slit ventricle syndrome. **Contemp Neurosurg** 21 (3): 1-4, 1999.

63. Engel M, Carmel P W, Chutorian A M: Increased intraventricular pressure without ventriculomegaly in children with shunts: "normal volume" hydrocephalus. **Neurosurgery** 5: 549-52, 1979.

64. Kiekens R, Mortier W, Pothmann R: The slit-ventricle syndrome after shunting in hydrocephalic children. **Neuropediatrics** 13: 190-4, 1982.

65. Hyde-Rowan M D, Rekate H L, Nulsen F E: Reexpansion of previously collapsed ventricles: The slit ventricle syndrome. **J Neurosurg** 56: 536-9, 1982.

66. Salmon J H: The collapsed ventricle: Management and prevention. **Surg Neurol** 9: 349-52, 1978.

67. Portnoy H D, Schult R R, Fox J L, et al.: Anti-siphon and reversible occlusion valves for shunting in hydrocephalus and preventing postshunt subdural hematoma. **J Neurosurg** 38: 729-38, 1973.

68. Epstein F J, Fleischer A S, Hochwald G M, et al.: Subtemporal craniectomy for recurrent shunt obstruction secondary to small ventricles. **J Neurosurg** 41: 29-31, 1974.

69. Holness R O, Hoffman H J, Hendrick E B: Subtemporal decompression for the slit-ventricle syndrome after shunting in hydrocephalic children. **Childs Brain** 5: 137-44, 1979.

70. Linder M, Diehl J, Sklar F H: Subtemporal decompressions for shunt-dependent ventricles: Mechanism of action. **Surg Neurol** 19: 520-3, 1983.

71. Reddy K, Fewer H D, West M, et al.: Slit ventricle syndrome with aqueduct stenosis: Third ventriculostomy as definitive treatment. **Neurosurgery** 23: 756-9, 1988.

72. Puca A, Fernandez E, Colosimo C, et al.: Hydrocephalus and macrocrania: Surgical or non-surgical treatment of postshunting subdural hematoma. **Surg Neurol** 45: 76-82, 1996.

73. Hoppe-Hirsch E, Sainte Rose C, Renier D, et al.: Pericerebral collections after shunting. **Childs Nerv Syst** 3: 97-102, 1987.

74. McCullogh D C, Fox J L: Negative intracranial pressure hydrocephalus in adults with shunts and its relationship to the production of subdural hematoma. **J Neurosurg** 40: 372-5, 1974.

75. Schut L: Comment on Puca A, et al.: Hydrocephalus and macrocrania: Surgical or non-surgical treatment of postshunting subdural hematoma. **Surg Neurol** 45: 82, 1996.

76. Dietrich U, Lumenta C, Sprick C, et al.: Subdural hematoma in a case of hydrocephalus and macrocrania: Experience with a pressure-adjustable valve. **Childs Nerv Syst** 3: 242-4, 1987.

77. Kamano S, Nakano Y, Imanishi T, et al.: Management with a programmable pressure valve of subdural hematomas caused by a ventriculoperitoneal shunt: Case report. **Surg Neurol** 35: 381-3, 1991.

78. Illingworth R D: Subdural hematoma after the treatment of chronic hydrocephalus by ventriculocaval shunts. **J Neurol Neurosurg Psychiatry** 33: 95-9, 1970.

79. Davidoff L M, Feiring E H: Subdural hematoma occurring in surgically treated hydrocephalic children with a note on a method of handling persistent accumulations. **J Neurosurg** 10: 557-63, 1963.

80. Kaufman B, Weiss M H, Young H F, et al.: Effects of prolonged cerebrospinal fluid shunting on the skull and brain. **J Neurosurg** 38: 288-97, 1973.

81. Faulhauer K, Schmitz P: Overdrainage phenomena in shunt treated hydrocephalus. **Acta Neurochir** 45: 89-101, 1978.

82. Hakim S, Adams R D: The special clinical problem of symptomatic hydrocephalus with normal CSF pressure. **J Neurol Sci** 2: 307-27, 1965.

83. Adams R D, Fisher C, Hakim S, et al.: Symptomatic occult hydrocephalus with 'normal' cerebrospinal fluid pressure. **N Engl J Med** 273: 117-26, 1965.

84. Thal L J, Grundman M, Klauber M R: Dementia: Characteristics of a referral population and factors associated with progression. **Neurology** 38: 1083-90, 1988.

85. Wood J H, Barttelt D, James A E, et al.: Normal pressure hydrocephalus: Diagnosis and patient selection for shunt surgery. **Neurology** 24: 517-26, 1974.

86. Symon L, Dorsch N W C, Stephens R J: Pressure waves in so-called low-pressure hydrocephalus. **Lancet** 2: 1291-2, 1972.

87. Haan J, Thomeer R T W M: Predictive value of temporary external lumbar drainage in normal pressure hydrocephalus. **Neurosurgery** 22: 388-91, 1988.

88. Vassilouthis J: The syndrome of normal-pressure hydrocephalus. **J Neurosurg** 61: 501-9, 1984.

89. Jack C R, Mokri B, Laws E R, et al.: MR findings in normal pressure hydrocephalus: Significance and comparison with other forms of dementia. **J Comput Assist Tomogr** 11: 923-31, 1987.

90. Schwartz M, Creasey H, Grady C L, et al.: Computed tomographic analysis of brain morphometrics in 30 healthy men, aged 21 to 81 years. **Ann Neurol** 17: 146-57, 1985.

91. Holodny A I, George A E, de Leon M J, et al.: Focal dilation and paradoxical collapse of cortical fissures and sulci in patients with normal-pressure hydrocephalus. **J Neurosurg** 89: 742-7, 1998.

92. Shenkin H A, Greenberg J O, Grossman C B: Ventricular size after shunting for idiopathic normal pressure hydrocephalus. **J Neurol Neurosurg Psychiatry** 38: 833-7, 1975.

93. Vanneste J, Augustijn P, Davies G A G, et al.: Normal-pressure hydrocephalus: Is cisternography still useful in selecting patients for a shunt? **Arch Neurol** 49: 366-70, 1992.

94. Bergstrand G, Oxenstierna G, Flyckt L, et al.: Radionuclide cisternography and computed tomography in 30 healthy volunteers. **Neuroradiology** 28: 154-60, 1986.

95. Larsson A, Moonen M, Bergh A-C, et al.: Predictive value of quantitative cisternography in normal pressure hydrocephalus. **Acta Neurol Scand** 81: 327-32, 1990.

96. Tamaki N, Kusunoki T, Wakabayashi T, et al.: Cerebral hemodynamics in normal-pressure hydrocephalus: Evaluation by 133Xe inhalation method and dynamic CT study. **J Neurosurg** 61: 510-4, 1984.

97. Black P M, Ojemann R G, Tzouras A: CSF shunts for dementia, incontinence and gait disturbance. **Clin Neurosurg** 32: 632-51, 1985.

98. McQuarrie I G, Saint-Louis L, Scherer P B: Treatment of normal-pressure hydrocephalus with low versus medium pressure cerebrospinal fluid shunts. **Neurosurgery** 15: 484-8, 1984.

99. Black P M: Idiopathic normal-pressure hydrocephalus: Results of shunting in 62 patients. **J Neurosurg** 52: 371-7, 1980.

100. Peterson R C, Mokri B, Laws E R: Surgical treatment of idiopathic hydrocephalus in elderly patients. **Neurology** 35: 307-11, 1985.

101. Udvarhelyi G B, Wood J H, James A E: Results and complications in 55 shunted patients with normal pressure hydrocephalus. **Surg Neurol** 3: 271-5, 1975.

102. Golomb J, et al.: Alzheimer's disease comorbidity in normal pressure hydrocephalus: Prevalence and shunt response. **J Neurol Neurosurg Psychiatry** 68: 778-81, 2000.

103. Humphrey P R D, Moseley I F, Russell R W R: Visual field defects in obstructive hydrocephalus. **J Neurol Neurosurg Psychiatry** 45: 591-7, 1982.

104. Calogero J A, Alexander E: Unilateral amaurosis in a hydrocephalic child with an obstructed shunt. **J Neurosurg** 34: 236-40, 1971.

105. Kojima N, Kuwamura K, Tamaki N, *et al.*: Reversible congruous homonymous hemianopia as a symptom of shunt malfunction. **Surg Neurol** 22: 253-6, 1984.

106. Black P M, Chapman P H: Transient abducens paresis after shunting for hydrocephalus. **J Neurosurg** 55: 467-9, 1981.

107. Arroyo H A, Jan J E, McCormick A Q, *et al.*: Permanent visual loss after shunt malfunction. **Neurology** 35: 25-9, 1985.

108. Sato M, Tanaka S, Kohama A, *et al.*: Occipital lobe infarction caused by tentorial herniation. **Neurosurgery** 18: 300-5, 1986.

109. Joynt R J, Honch G W, Rubin A J, *et al.*: *Occipital lobe syndromes*. In **Handbook of clinical neurology**, Frederiks J A M, (ed.). Elsevier Science Publishers, Holland, 1985, Vol. 1: pp 49-62.

110. Rinaldi I, Botton J E, Troland C E: Cortical visual disturbances following ventriculography and/or ventricular decompression. **J Neurosurg** 19: 568-576, 1962.

111. Lindenberg R, Walsh F B: Vascular compressions involving intracranial visual pathways. **Tr Am Acad Ophth Otol** 68: 677-94, 1964.

112. Hoyt W F: Vascular lesions of the visual cortex with brain herniation through the tentorial incisura. **Arch Ophthalm** 64: 44-57, 1960.

113. Barnet A B, Manson J I, Wilner E: Acute cerebral blindness in childhood. **Neurology** 20: 1147-56, 1970.

114. Keane J R: Blindness following tentorial herniation. **Ann Neurol** 8: 186-90, 1980.

115. Hoyt W F, Walsh F B: Cortical blindness with partial recovery following cerebral anoxia from cardiac arrest. **Arch Ophthalm** 60: 1061-9, 1958.

116. Weinberger H A, van der Woude R, Maier H C: Prognosis of cortical blindness following cardiac arrest in children. **JAMA** 179: 126-9, 1962.

117. Slavin M L: Ischemic optic neuropathy after cardiac arrest. **Am J Ophthalmol** 104: 435-6, 1987.

118. Sweeney P J, Breuer A C, Selhorst J B, *et al.*: Ischemic optic neuropathy: A complication of cardiopulmonary bypass surgery. **Neurology** 32: 560-2, 1982.

119. Drance S M, Morgan R W, Sweeney V P: Shock-induced optic neuropathy. A cause of nonprogressive glaucoma. **N Engl J Med** 288: 392-5, 1973.

120. Lorber J: Recovery of vision following prolonged blindness in children with hydrocephalus or following pyogenic meningitis. **Clin Pediatr** 6: 699-703, 1967.

121. Wisoff J H, Kratzert K J, Handwerker S M, *et al.*: Pregnancy in patients with cerebrospinal fluid shunts: Report of a series and review of the literature. **Neurosurgery** 29. 827-31, 1991.

122. Marx G F, Zemaitis M T, Orkin L R: CSF pressures during labor and obstetrical anesthesia. **Anesthesiology** 22: 348-54, 1981.

12. Infections

12.1. General information

12.1.1. Specific antibiotics

Some antibiotics are included herein to highlight particulars of interest to neurosurgeons.

ORAL PENICILLINS

amoxicillin + clavulanic acid (Augmentin®) — DRUG INFO

A good PO drug for superficial staph infections. Good anaerobic and anti-staphylococcal coverage. Absorption is unaffected by food. Available forms are summarized in *Table 12-1*.

***Rx* Adult**: 250 or 500 mg PO q 8 hrs or 875 mg BID (NB: use the appropriate tablet to avoid excessive clavulanate; the lower total dose of clavulanate with the 875 mg tablet may produce fewer GI side effects).
Peds: 20-40 mg/kg/d amoxicillin divided q 8 hrs.

Table 12-1   Available forms of Augmentin®

Form	Designation	Amoxicillin (mg)	Clavulanate (mg)
regular tablets	'250' tablets	250	125
	'500' tablets	500	125
	'875' tablet	875	125
chewable tablets	'125' chewables	125	31.25
	'250' chewables	250	62.5
oral suspension	'125' oral suspension	125 mg/5 ml	31.25 mg/5 ml
	'250' oral suspension	250 mg/5 ml	62.5 mg/5 ml

PARENTERAL CEPHALOSPORINS

Higher generation agents have progressively reduced activity against streptococci and penicillinase-producing *S. aureus*.

First generation cephalosporins

cefazolin (Ancef®, Kefzol®) — DRUG INFO

Good for surgical prophylaxis. Good levels in brain tissue have been documented. Poor CSF penetration (thus <u>not</u> good for meningitis). Advantage over others cephalosporins: higher serum levels (80 µg/ml) are achievable, and half life (1.8 hrs) is longer (allows q 8 hr dosing).

***Rx* Adult**: 1 gm IV q 8 hrs. **Peds**: 0-7 days → 40 mg/kg/d divided q 12 hrs; infant → 60 mg/kg/d divided q 8 hrs; child → 80 mg/kg/d divided q 6 hrs.

Third generation cephalosporins

Potency of these drugs are ≈ equivalent to aminoglycosides for: *E. coli*, klebsiella, and proteus. Only ceftazidime is adequate for <u>pseudomonas</u>. Good for "serious" infections (meningitis, endocarditis and osteomyelitis). SIDE EFFECTS: diarrhea (pseudomembranous colitis), bleeding diatheses, and may allow superinfections (enterobacter, resistant pseudomonas, enterococcus, fungus).

ceftazidime (Fortaz®) | DRUG INFO

Good for nosocomial infections. One of the <u>best</u> drugs for *Pseudomonas aeruginosa* infections (large doses tolerated well), but doesn't cover staph well. Good CNS penetration. SIDE EFFECTS: rare neutropenia with protracted administration (e.g for osteomyelitis).

Rx Adult: 1-2 gm IV/IM q 6-8 hrs (non-life threatening infections: 1 gm q 8 hrs). **Peds**: 0-4 wks → 60 mg/kg/d divided q 12 hrs; child → 150 mg/kg/d divided q 8 hrs (maximum 6 gm/d).

ceftriaxone (Rocephin®) | DRUG INFO

Good penetration into CSF. Useful for CNS infections involving GNR and for late stage Lyme disease. Long half-life allows q 12-24 hr dosing. Unlike most cephalosporins, excretion is largely dependent on liver, therefore same dosage in renal failure. May be synergistic with aminoglycosides. SIDE EFFECTS: may cause biliary sludging.

Rx Adult: 1-2 gm qd (may be given q 12 hrs for meningitis). Total daily dose < 4 gm. **Peds** (for meningitis): 75 mg/kg/d initial dose, then 100 mg/kg/d divided q 12 hrs.

MACROLIDES, VANCOMYCIN, CHLORAMPHENICOL

vancomycin (Vancocin®) | DRUG INFO

Agent of choice for *S. aureus* infections that are either methicillin resistant (if not MRSA, better results are obtained with PRSP), or that occur in patients allergic to penicillin or derivatives. Multiply resistant *S. aureus* infections may require co-treatment with rifampin. Poor for Gram negatives. Long half-life.

Rx Adult: start 1 gm IV q 8 hrs for serious infection, check levels before and after 3rd dose, and aim for peaks of 20-40 μg/ml (toxic > 50; ototoxicity and nephrotoxicity that are usually reversible occur with peaks > 200 μg/ml), and troughs of 5-10 (toxic: > 10).

PO dose for <u>pseudomembranous colitis</u>: 125 mg PO QID **x** 7-10 days (some references recommend more, but this is not necessary). **Peds**: age 0-7 days → 30 mg/kg/d divided q 12 hrs. Age > 7 days → 45 mg/kg/d divided q 8 hrs.

chloramphenicol (Chloromycetin®) | DRUG INFO

Good for: Gram (+) and Gram (−) cocci. Excellent CSF penetration (even without inflamed meninges). It is hard to find the oral form in the U.S.

Rx Adult: PO: 250-750 mg q 6 hrs (may be very difficult to find in retail pharmacies in the U.S.). IV: 50 mg/kg/d divided q 6 hrs. **Peds**: 0-7 days old → 25 mg/kg/d PO or IV q d. Infant → 50 mg/kg/d PO or IV divided q 12 hrs. Child (for meningitis) → 100 mg/kg/d IV divided q 6 hrs.

AMINOGLYCOSIDES

When given IV, only amikacin has adequate CSF penetration (and only with inflamed meninges). Not adequate monotherapy for any infection. Good adjunct for staph and GNR including sensitive pseudomonads. Poor for strep. All are oto- and nephro-toxic, however toxicities occur almost exclusively with longer use (> 8 days). More rapid kill than ß-lactams and may thus may be used initially for sepsis and then changed to a cephalosporin after ≈ 2-3 days. Increased activity in alkaline pH. Reduced activity in acidic pH, and in presence of pus and/or anaerobes (therefore may be poor for wound infections, fluoroquinolones may be better here).

Dosages based on <u>ideal</u> body weight. Obtain serum levels after 3rd dose and adjust appropriately. Dosages of all MUST be reduced in renal failure.

/ gentamicin (Garamycin®)   \ / DRUG INFO \

***Rx* Adult** (normal renal function) IV: 2 mg/kg IV loading dose then 1-1.6 mg/kg q 8 hrs maintenance, follow levels (desired peak > 4 µg/ml, trough < 2). ***Rx* Intrathecal**: 4 mg q 12-24 hrs.

/ tobramycin (Nebcin®)   \ / DRUG INFO \

The best aminoglycoside for pseudomonas (but not as good as ceftazidime).
***Rx* Adult** (normal renal function): 2 mg/kg IV loading dose then 1.6-2 mg/kg IV q 8 hrs maintenance. For age > 60, same dose q 12 hrs. Follow levels and adjust for peak 7.5-10 µg/ml, trough < 2. ***Rx* Intrathecal**: 5 mg initial dose, then 2-4 mg q 24 hrs. ***Rx* Peds**: 6-7.5 mg/kg/d divided q 6-8 hrs.

12.1.2.   Antibiotics for specific organisms

PSEUDOMONAS AERUGINOSA
Ceftazidime (Fortaz®) is the drug of choice (*see page 209*). Good CNS penetration, large doses tolerated well. Among aminoglycosides, tobramicin is the best antipseudomonal. Aminoglycosides give more rapid kill and therefore when there is a strong suspicion of pseudomonas start with ceftazidime plus tobramicin initially and then stop the tobramicin after a few days (reduces risk of aminoglycoside toxicity). Antipseudomonal penicillins are not as effective (the following are ß-lactamase susceptible): carbenicillin, ticarcillin, mezlocillin, azlocillin. Adding clavulanate to ticarcillin (Timentin®) reduces susceptibility to ß-lactamase. Adding ciprofloxacin (IV or PO) to any of the above IV medications has a synergistic effect (but is inadequate by itself for soft-tissue infections, such as wound infections).

STAPHYLOCOCCUS AUREUS
Vancomycin until it is determined that it is not MRSA, then use PRSP (e.g. nafcillin) + gentamicin (aminoglycosides give more rapid initial kill and are synergistic against staph). Stop the gentamicin after a few days (reduces risk of aminoglycoside toxicity).

For <u>oral</u> treatment of non MRSA *S. aureus* wound infections, options include 2 weeks of:
1.   Augmentin® (*see page 208*)
2.   or rifampin (600 mg PO q d) + either
   A.   trimetha/sulfa (1 DS PO BID)
   B.   or clindamycin

FUNGAL SUPERINFECTION
For fungal superinfection of the GI tract in patients on antibiotics or steroids:

/ nystatin (Mycostatin®)   \ / DRUG INFO \
   (oral suspension)

***Rx* Infants**: 1 cc (100,000 units) on each side of mouth QID.
***Rx* Adults**: if alert and swallowing mechanism is intact, 5 ml QID swish and swallow. If comatose or unable to swallow, 3 cc per NG QID and 2 cc oral swab QID.
SUPPLIED: in concentration of 100,000 units/ml.

/ fluconazole (Diflucan®)   \ / DRUG INFO \

May increase serum concentration of phenytoin, zidovudine, and oral anticoagulants, among others. Can cause liver dysfunction, which may not be reversible.
***Rx* Adults**: for oropharyngeal candidiasis, 200 mg PO the first day and then 100 mg PO qd for 2 weeks. SUPPLIED: tablets of 50, 100 or 200 mg. Powder for oral suspension which can be mixed to a volume of 35 ml of either 10 or 40 mg/ml. Also available in IV form, which is very expensive, and usually not necessary due to excellent GI absorption.

12.2. Prophylactic antibiotics

GENERAL PRINCIPLES[1]
1. antibiotics must be in tissues at time of contamination (thus, avoid "on-call" antibiotics; give 60 minutes prior to incision)
2. repeated administration vital in prolonged procedures
3. typical infecting organisms are usually predictable. Coverage for these organisms is adequate (broadening spectrum is of no value)
4. in low risk operations (e.g. carotid endarterectomy, where infections rare and seldom life-threatening) may cost more to prevent than to treat
5. prolongation of antibiotics beyond first post-op day provides no additional protection (may not be true in patients with surgical drains)
6. theoretical side effects (alteration of patient's flora, development of resistant strains in patient or hospital) have not been realized without prolonged administration of pre-op or post-op antibiotics
7. factors that increase risk of operative wound infection include:
   A. systemic factors: malnutrition, reoperation, infection at secondary site (especially UTI when GU tract manipulated), prolonged administration of antibiotics
   B. local factors: epinephrine, dehydration, hypoxia

SPECIFIC AGENTS FOR PROPHYLAXIS

1. **cephalosporins**:
   A. agents of choice where skin flora (coagulase (−) or (+) staph) are likeliest pathogens
   B. may safely be given even with history of mild, non-immediate manifestations of PCN allergy (e.g. "rashes"). Contraindicated if history of immediate or accelerated reaction (shock, bronchospasm, urticaria)
   C. **cefazolin** (Ancef®, Kefzol®):
      • effective, widely studied, therapeutic levels in brain tissue after systemic administration[2], long half-life
      • prophylactic dose: 1-2 gm (peds: 25 mg/kg up to 1 gm) IV 60 min before surgery, then q 6 hr **x** 24 hrs post-op
   D. some *S. aureus* strains are efficient in ß-lactamase degradation of cephalosporins, and cefazolin is particularly susceptible. Lower infection rates may result with cefamandole (2 gm initially, and then 1 gm q 2-3 hrs intraoperatively)[3]
   E. a semisynthetic penicillin may be more appropriate if good CSF penetration is necessary
2. **vancomycin**: alternative if cephalosporin contraindicated (incidence of anaphylactic reactions is too high for routine use). Dose (empiric): 15 mg/kg (up to 1 gm) IV pre-op, then 10 mg/kg q 8 hrs for 24 hrs post-op
3. **penicillins**: disadvantages: probably less safe, shorter half-life, may prolong bleeding times. Nafcillin is probably the best agent in this group

PROPHYLACTIC ANTIBIOTICS FOR SPECIFIC NEUROSURGICAL PROCEDURES

1. **carotid endarterectomy**: routine use not indicated (infection risk too low); when risk of infection is high, use cefazolin (as for general prophylaxis, *see above*)
2. **craniotomy**: risk of infection may be increased in prolonged or microsurgical procedures and in reoperations. No significant difference in the specific regimen used was detected in meta-analysis[4]. Options include:
   • cefazolin (*see above*)
   • clindamicin (300 mg IV) pre-op & q 4 hrs
   • vancomycin (*see above*)
   • some add gentamicin (80 mg IM) pre-op to any of these
3. **CSF shunting procedures**: efficacy has been documented when the infection

rate is unusually high for some reason (e.g. ≈ 15%). Antibiotics possibly reduce early infections, i.e. ≈ first week post-op

A. for general use
1. select one of the following:
   - cefazolin (*see above*)
   - a 1st generation cephalosporin (e.g. cephapirin (Cefadyl®) 25 mg/kg (up to 1 gm)) IVP intra-op and 6 hrs post-op
   - nafcillin 50 mg/kg (up to 2 g) IV 60 min before surgery and q 4 hrs post-op **x** 5 doses total
2. PLUS
   - intrathecal gentamicin 4 mg injected into shunt at time of placement (no longer available in U.S., but preservative-free pediatric gentamicin may be diluted appropriately and used)
B. Kaiser: suggests no antibiotics if infection rate low (< 10%). If high (> 20%) use trimethoprim (160 mg IV) plus sulfamethoxazole (800 mg IV) pre-op and q 12 hrs **x** 3 doses post-op (NB: this latter infection rate is very high, and results are thus questionable [5])
4. ICP monitors: *see page 650*
5. procedures involving incisions through **oral or pharyngeal mucosa**: gentamicin (1.7 mg/kg IV) and clindamicin (300 mg IV) pre-op & q 8 hrs post op **x** 24 hrs. Cefazolin & 3rd generation cephalosporin also effective when given over 24 hr period pre-op
6. **spinal surgery**: reduction of infection was *suggested* but was not statistically significant (low incidence would require large study)

A single blind prospective study[5] showed the incidence of post-neurosurgical operative wound infections were reduced with cefazolin (1 gm IV) plus gentamicin (80 mg IV) given one hr before incision and q 6 hrs intra-op (none post-op) with significant results in patients without foreign implants (especially craniotomies; no significant difference for spinal operations, but numbers were small). All infections were *Staph. aureus* or *epidermidis* (makes use of gentamicin questionable).

12.3.   Meningitis

Community acquired meningitis **(CAM)** is generally more fulminant than meningitis following neurosurgical procedures (the former tend to occur with more virulent organisms or impaired host defenses). Both represent medical emergencies, and should be treated immediately. Focal neurologic signs are rare in acute purulent meningitis. See *Lumbar puncture* on page 615 for a discussion about when to perform an LP.

12.3.1.   Post-neurosurgical procedure meningitis

1. usual organisms: *S. aureus*, Enterobacteriaceae, Pseudomonas sp., *pneumococci*
2. empiric antibiotics: vancomycin (to cover MRSA) + ceftazidime specifically:
   vancomycin (adult) 1 gm IV q 8 hrs: (check level before and after 3rd dose and adjust accordingly, see *Vancomycin,* page 209)
   + ceftazidime (Fortaz®) 1-2 gm IV q 8 hrs
3. for pseudomonas, add gentamicin (IV & IT)
4. if organism turns out to be non-MRSA *S. aureus*, change vancomycin to IV PRSP (e.g. nafcillin)

12.3.2.   Post craniospinal trauma meningitis (post-traumatic meningitis)

Epidemiology
Occurs in 1-20% of patients with moderate to severe head injuries[6]. Most cases occur within 2 weeks of trauma, although delayed cases have been described[7]. 75% of cases have demonstrable basal skull fracture (*see page 665*), and 58% had obvious CSF rhinorrhea.

Pathogens
As expected from above, there is a high rate of infection with organisms indigenous to the nasal cavity. The most common organisms in a series from Greece were Gram-positive cocci (*Staph. hemoliticus, S. warneri, S. cohnii, S. epidermidis*, and *Strep. pneumonia*) and Gram-negative bacilli (*E. coli, Klebsiella pneumonia, Acinetobacter anitratus*)[6].

Treatment
1. also see *CSF Fistula, Treatment* on page 177
2. antibiotics: appropriate antibiotics are selected based on CSF penetration and organism sensitivities (adapted to the pathogens common in the patient's locale; in the above series, all Gram-negative strains appeared resistant to ampicillin and third-generation cephalosporins, but were sensitive to imipenem and ciprofloxacin; Gram-positive strains were all sensitive to vancomycin). For empiric antibiotics *see page 212*
3. surgical treatment vs. "conservative treatment": controversial. Some feel that any case of posttraumatic CSF rhinorrhea should be explored[8, 9], and that cases of spontaneous cessation often represent obscuration by incarcerated brain, so-called "sham healing" with the potential for later CSF leak and/or meningitis[7]. Others support the notion that cessation (possibly with the assistance of lumbar spinal drainage) is acceptable
4. continue antibiotics for 1 week after CSF is sterilized. If rhinorrhea persists at this time, surgical repair is recommended

---

12.3.3. Recurrent meningitis

Patients with recurrent meningitis must be evaluated for the presence of abnormal communication with the intraspinal/intracranial compartment. Etiologies include dermal sinus (either spinal or cranial, *see page 118*), CSF fistula (*see page 174*), or neurenteric cyst (*see page 98*).

12.3.4. Antibiotics for specific organisms in meningitis

Route is IV unless specified otherwise.
* *S. pneumoniae*: PCN G (2nd choice: chloramphenicol)
* *N. meningitidis*: PCN G (2nd choice: chloramphenicol)
* *H. influenza*:
    A. non-penicillinase producing: ampicillin
    B. penicillinase producing: chloramphenicol
* Group B strep: ampicillin
* *L. monocytogenes*: ampicillin
* *S. aureus*
    A. initially before sensitivities known, or if MRSA or multiply resistant strains or resistant coagulase-negative *S. aureus* prevalent or suspected: vancomycin + PO rifampin + PO trimethoprim
    B. once it is known that the staph is not MRSA:
        1. infant (< 7 d): methicillin
        2. all others: nafcillin
        3. PCN allergy: vancomycin or (cefazolin via both IV + IT)
* aerobic Gram negative rods (GNR)
    A. ceftriaxone, or cefotaxime, or moxalactam (in order of preference, make alterations based on sensitivities)
    B. if aminoglycoside required, intraventricular therapy is indicated after the newborn period
* *P. aeruginosa*
    A. ceftazidime (Fortaz®) alone if not life threatening
    OR
    B. more serious infections require 2 agents (aminoglycoside gives more rapid kill, and may be used initially for 3 days and then stopped if sensitivities to ceftazidime are acceptable):
    ceftazidime + APAG + IT gentamicin 4 mg q 12 hrs (give via intraventricular route if **ventriculitis** is present)

OR
C. for overwhelming infection:
    ceftazidime + tobramicin + ticarcillin

12.4.   Shunt infection

Risk of early infection after shunt surgery: reported range is 3-20% per procedure (typically ≈ 7%).

Acceptable infection rate[10]: < 5-7% (although many published series have a rate near 20%[11], possibly due to different patient population).

Risk factors for shunt infection
Many factors have been blamed; some that seem to be better documented include:
1. young age of patient[11]: in myelomeningocele (MM) patients, waiting until the child is 2 weeks old may significantly lower the infection rate
2. length of procedure
3. open neural tube defect

Morbidity of shunt infections in children
Children with shunt infections have a increased mortality rate and risk of seizure than those without shunt infection. Those with myelomeningocele who develop ventriculitis after shunting have a lower IQ compared to those without infection[12]. Mortality ranges from 10-15%.

PATHOGENS
Over 50% of staph infections occur within 2 weeks post-shunt, 70% within 2 mos. Source is often the patient's own skin[10]. It is estimated that in ≈ 3% of operations for shunt insertion the CSF is already infected (therefore culture CSF during insertion).

Early infection
Most commonly:
1. *Staph. epidermidis* (coagulase-negative staph): 60-75% of infections (most common)
2. *S. aureus*
3. Gram-negative bacilli (GNB): 6-20% (may come from intestinal perforation)

In neonates *E. coli* and *Strep. hemoliticus* dominate.

Late infection (> 6 months after procedure)
Risk: 2.7-31% per patient (typically 6%). Almost all *S. epidermidis*. Tends to be internal type. 3.5% of patients account for 27% of infections[13].

"Late" shunt infections may be due to:
1. an indolent infection due to *Staph. epidermidis*
2. seeding of a vascular shunt during episode of septicemia (probably very rare)
3. colonization from an episode of meningitis

PRESENTATION
Non-specific syndrome: fever, N/V, lethargy, anorexia, irritability; may mimic acute abdomen. May also present as malfunction; 29% of patients presenting with shunt malfunction had positive cultures. In neonates may manifest as apneic episodes, anemia, hepatosplenomegaly, and stiff neck[14]. *S. epidermidis* infections tend to be indolent (smoldering). GNB infections usually cause more severe illness; abdominal findings more common; main clinical manifestation is fever, usually intermittent and low grade. Erythema and tenderness along shunt tubing occurs occasionally.

Shunt nephritis[15]: may occur with chronic low level infection of a ventriculovascular shunt causing immune complex deposition in renal glomeruli, characterized by proteinuria and hematuria.

Blood tests
WBC: < 10K in one fourth of shunt infections. It is > 20K in one third.
ESR: rarely normal in shunt infections.
Blood cultures: positive in less than one third of cases.
CSF: WBC is usually not > 100 cells/mm³. Gram stains may be positive ≈ 50% (yield

with *S. epidermidis* is much lower). Protein is often elevated, glucose may be low or normal. Rapid antigen tests used for community acquired meningitis are usually not helpful for the organisms that tend to cause shunt infections. CSF cultures are negative in 40% of cases (higher culture yield if CSF WBC count is > 20K).

EVALUATION OF SHUNT FOR INFECTION
1. history and physical directed at determining presence of above signs and symptoms with emphasis on
    A. history suggestive of infection at another site
        1. exposure to others with viral syndromes, including sick siblings
        2. GI source (e.g. acute gastroenteritis). Often associated with diarrhea. Diarrhea is a symptom that usually exonerates shunt infection
        3. otitis media (check tympanic membranes)
        4. tonsillitis/pharyngitis
        5. appendicitis (peritoneal inflammation may impede VP shunt outflow)
        6. URI
        7. UTI
        8. pneumonia
    B. physical exam to R/O meningismus (stiff neck, photophobia…)
2. serum WBC count with differential
3. shunt tap: should be done in cases of suspected shunt infection. Shave and prep carefully to avoid introducing infection. GNB requires different therapy and has higher morbidity than staph, thus it is desirable to identify these rare patients: > 90% of these had positive Gram-stained CSF smear (only a few Gram-positive infections have positive results). GNB have higher protein and lower glucose, and neutrophils predominate in differential (unpublished data[10])
4. CT: usually not helpful for diagnosing infection. Ependymal enhancement when it occurs is diagnostic of **ventriculitis**. CT may demonstrate shunt malfunction
5. abdominal U/S or CT: abdominal pseudocyst is suggestive of infection
6. ✖ LP: usually NOT recommended. May be hazardous in obstructive hydrocephalus **(HCP)** with a nonfunctioning shunt. Often does not yield the pathogen

TREATMENT

Antibiotics alone (without removal of shunt hardware)
Although eradication of shunt infections without removal of hardware has been reported[16 (p 595-7), 17], this has a lower success rate than with shunt removal[18], may require protracted treatment (up to 45 days in some), risks problems associated with draining infected CSF into the peritoneum (reduced CSF absorption, abdominal signs/symptoms including tenderness to full-blown peritonitis[16 (p 235)]) or vascular system (shunt nephritis (*see page 214*), sepsis…), and often requires at least partial shunt revision at some point in most cases. Treatment with antibiotics without shunt removal is therefore recommended only in cases where the patient: is terminally ill, is a poor anesthetic risk, or has slit ventricles that might be difficult to catheterize.

Removal of shunt hardware
In most instances, during the initial treatment with antibiotics the shunt is either externalized (i.e. tubing is diverted at some point distal to the ventricular catheter and connected to a closed drainage system), or sometimes the entire shunt may be removed. In the latter case, some means of CSF drainage must be provided in shunt dependent cases; either by insertion of an external ventricular drain **(EVD)**, or by intermittent ventricular taps or LPs (with communicating HCP). EVD allows easy monitoring of CSF flow, control of ICP, and repeated sampling for WBC determinations and cultures. In symptomatic patients or those with a positive CSF culture[19], any hardware removed should be cultured as only ≈ 8% are sterile in shunt infections. Skin organisms are fastidious and may take several days to grow.
If there is an abdominal pseudocyst, the fluid should be drained through the peritoneal catheter before removing it.

Empiric antibiotics
1. IV <u>vancomycin</u> used initially (penetration into CSF results in concentrations 18% that of serum).
2. PO rifampin may be added for increased coverage (10 mg/kg/day PO q 12 hrs)
3. when cultures return, change vancomycin to IV <u>nafcillin</u> unless patient is PCN allergic or cultures show MRSA (good penetration of inflamed meninges, lower toxicity than methicillin). If bactericidal activity is < 1:8, again consider adding

rifampin
4. intraventricular injection of preservative-free antibiotics may be used in addition to IV therapy, clamp EVD x 30 minutes after injection

Treatment for specific organisms
Positive cultures from shunt hardware removed at the time of shunt revision in the absence of clinical symptoms or a positive CSF culture may be due to contamination and do not require treatment[19].
1. *S. aureus* and *S. epidermidis*
   A. if sensitive (MIC ≤ 1.0 µg/ml): IT gent + (IV nafcillin, or cefazolin, or cephalothin, or cephapirin)
   B. if resistant to nafcillin (i.e. MRSA), cephalothin, or cephapirin: PO rifampin + PO trimethoprim + IV & IT vancomycin
2. Enterococcus: IV/IT ampicillin + IT gent (if intravascular shunt: add IV gent)
3. other streptococci: either antistreptococcal or above enterococcal regimen
4. aerobic GNR: base on susceptibilities; both beta-lactam & APAG IV & IT indicated
5. Corynebacterium sp. & Proprionibacterium sp. (diphtheroids)
   A. if PCN sensitive: use enterococcal regimen above
   B. if PCN resistant: IV + IT vancomycin

Intrathecal therapy
Yogev[10] cautions against <u>high</u> levels (caused neurologic effects in rabbits), he suggests striving for CSF concentrations comparable to peak blood values (e.g. 10-12 µg/ml for gent, or 25-30 µg/ml for amikacin).

Subsequent management
Once the CSF is sterile **x** 3 days, continue antibiotics an additional **10-14** days, then convert the EVD to a shunt (if an EVD was not used, it is still recommended that the shunt be replace with new hardware).

12.5.   Wound infections

12.5.1.   Laminectomy wound infection

Occurs in 0.9-5% of cases[20]. May range from superficial to severe dehiscent wound infection. The risk is increased with age, long term steroid use, obesity, and possibly DM. Intraoperative mild hypothermia (as commonly occurs in the operating room) may also increase the risk of wound infection (as demonstrated with colorectal resection[21]). Most are caused by *S. aureus*.

MANAGEMENT
1. culture the wound and/or any purulent drainage
2. start the patient empirically on vancomycin plus a third generation cephalosporin (e.g. ceftazidime)
3. modify antibiotics appropriately when culture and sensitivity results available
4. debride wound of all necrotic and devascularized tissue and any visible suture material (foreign bodies). Superficial wounds may be debrided in the office or treatment room, deep infections must be done in OR
5. shallow defects may be allowed to heal by secondary intention, and the following is one possible regimen
   A. pack the wound defect with 1/4" Iodophor® gauze
   B. dressing changes at least BID (for hospitalized patients, change q 8 hrs), remove and trim ≈ 0.5-1" of packing with each dressing change
      1. while wound is purulent, utilize 1/2 strength Betadine® wet to dry dressings
      2. when purulence subsides, switch to normal saline wet to dry
   C. antibiotics, may be useful as an adjunct to wound treatment initially, switch to oral antibiotics as early as possible, a duration of 10-14 days total is probably adequate if local wound care is being done
6. some prefer to close wound by primary intention[22], it is critical that there be no

tension on the wound for healing to occur. Some close over an irrigation system or antibiotic beads. Retention sutures may be helpful[23]

7. with large defects or when bone and/or dura becomes exposed, the use of a muscle flap (often performed by a plastic surgeon) is probably required[20]

8. CSF leakage requires exploration in the OR with watertight dural closure to prevent meningitis

12.6.   Osteomyelitis of the skull

The skull is very resistant to osteomyelitis, and hematogenous infection is rare. Most infections are due to contiguous spread (usually from an infected air sinus, occasionally from scalp abscess) or to penetrating trauma (including surgery and fetal scalp monitors[24]). With longstanding infection, edema and swelling in the area may become visible radiographically, and is called "**Pott's puffy tumor**".

Staphylococcus is the most common organism, with *S. aureus* predominating, followed by *S. epidermidis*. In neonates, *E. coli* may be the infecting organism.

Treatment

Antibiotics alone are rarely curative. Treatment is usually surgical debridement of infected skull, biting off infected bone with rongeurs until a normal snapping sound replaces the more muted sound made by rongeuring infected bone. In the case of an infected craniotomy bone flap, the flap must be removed and the edges of the skull rongeured back to healthy bone. Closure of the scalp without cranioplasty is performed.

Surgery is followed by at least 6-12 weeks of antibiotics[25], usually IV for the first 1-2 weeks, then orally for the remainder. Until MRSA is ruled out, vancomycin + a 3rd generation cephalosporin are used. Once MRSA is ruled out, vancomycin may be changed to a penicillinase resistant synthetic penicillin (e.g. nafcillin). Most treatment failures occurred in patients treated with < 4 weeks of antibiotics following surgery.

If there are no signs of infection, a cranioplasty may be performed ≈ 6 mos post-op.

12.7.   Cerebral abscess

EPIDEMIOLOGY

Approximately 1500-2500 cases per year in the U.S., with a higher incidence in developing countries. Male:female ratio is 1.5-3:1.

RISK FACTORS

Risk factors include: pulmonary abnormalities (infection, AV-fistulas..., *see below*), congenital cyanotic heart disease (*see below*), bacterial endocarditis, penetrating head trauma (*see below*) and AIDS.

VECTORS

Prior to 1980, the most common source of cerebral abscess was from contiguous spread. Now, hematogenous dissemination is the most common vector.

HEMATOGENOUS SPREAD

Abscesses arising by this means are multiple in 10-50% of cases[26]. No source can be found in up to 25% of cases. The chest is the most common origin:

- in adults: lung abscess (the most common), bronchiectasis and empyema
- in children: **congenital cyanotic heart disease (CCHD)** (estimated risk of abscess is 4-7%), especially tetralogy of Fallot. The increased Hct and low PO_2 provides an hypoxic environment suitable for abscess proliferation. Those with right-to-left (veno-atrial) shunts additionally lose the filtering effects of the lungs (the brain seems to be a preferential target for these infections over other organs). Streptococcal oral flora is frequent, and may follow dental procedures. Coexisting coagulation defects often further complicate management[27]
- pulmonary arteriovenous fistulas: ≈ 50% of these patients have **Osler-Weber-**

Rendu syndrome (AKA hereditary hemorrhagic telangectasia), and in up to 5% of these patients a cerebral abscess will eventually develop
- bacterial endocarditis: only rarely gives rise to brain abscess[28]. More likely to be associated with acute endocarditis than with subacute form
- dental abscess
- GI infections: pelvic infections may gain access to the brain via Batson's plexus

In patients with septic embolization, the risk of cerebral abscess formation is elevated in areas of previous infarction or ischemia[29].

CONTIGUOUS SPREAD
1. from purulent sinusitis: spreads by local osteomyelitis or by phlebitis of emissary veins. Virtually always singular. Rare in infants because they lack aerated paranasal and mastoid air cells. This route has become less common due to improved treatment of sinus disease
   A. middle-ear and mastoid air sinus infections → temporal lobe and cerebellar abscess. The risk of developing a cerebral abscess in an adult with active chronic otitis media is ≈ 1/10,000 per year[30] (this risk appears low, but in a 30 year-old with active chronic otitis media the lifetime risk becomes ≈ 1 in 200)
   B. nasal sinusitis → frontal lobe abscess
   C. sphenoid sinusitis: the least common location for sinusitis, but with a high incidence of intracranial complications due to venous extension to the adjacent cavernous sinus
2. odontogenic: rare. Associated with a dental procedure in the past 4 weeks in most cases[31]. May also spread hematogenously

FOLLOWING PENETRATING CRANIAL TRAUMA OR NEUROSURGICAL PROCEDURE
Post-neurosurgical: especially with traversal of an air sinus. The risk of abscess formation following civilian gunshot wounds to the brain is probably very low with the use of prophylactic antibiotics, except in cases with CSF leak not repaired surgically following traversal of an air sinus. An abscess following penetrating trauma cannot be treated by simple aspiration as with other abscesses, open surgical debridement to remove foreign matter and devitalized tissue is required. Abscess has been reported following use of intracranial pressure monitors and halo traction[32].

PATHOGENS
1. cultures from cerebral abscesses are sterile in up to 25% of cases
2. in general: Streptococcus is the most frequent organism, 33-50% are anaerobic or microaerophilic. Multiple organisms may be cultured to varying degrees, usually in only 10-30% of cases, but can approach 80-90%, and usually includes anaerobes (Bacteroides sp. common)
3. when secondary to fronto-ethmoidal sinusitis: *Strep. milleri* and *Strep. anginosus* may be seen
4. from otitis media, mastoiditis, or lung abscess: usually multiple organisms, including anaerobic strep., Bacteroides, Enterobacteriaceae (Proteus)
5. post traumatic: usually due to *S. aureus* or Enterobacteriaceae
6. Actinomyces may be associated with a dental source
7. following neurosurgical procedures: *Staph. epidermidis* and *aureus* may be seen
8. immunocompromised hosts including transplant patients (both bone marrow and solid organ) and AIDS: fungal infections are more common than otherwise would be seen. Organisms include:
   A. Toxoplasma gondii: *see page 232* and *page 233*
   B. Nocardia asteroides: *see page 223*
   C. Candida albicans
   D. Listeria monocytogenes
   E. mycobacterium
   F. *Aspergillus fumigatus* often from a primary pulmonary infection
9. infants: Gram negatives are common because IgM fraction doesn't cross placenta

PRESENTATION
Symptoms: none are specific for abscess, and many are due to edema surrounding

the lesion. Most are due to increased ICP (H/A, N/V, lethargy). Hemiparesis and seizures develop in 30-50% of cases. Papilledema is rare before 2 yrs of age.

Newborns: patent sutures and poor ability of infant brain to ward off infection → cranial enlargement. Common: seizures, meningitis, irritability, increasing OFC, and failure to thrive. Some authors say most newborns with abscess are afebrile. Tend not to do well.

EVALUATION

BLOODWORK

Peripheral WBC: may be normal or only mildly elevated in 60-70% of cases (usually > 10,000).

Blood cultures: usually negative

ESR: may be normal (especially in congenital cyanotic heart disease where polycythemia lowers the ESR).

C-reactive protein (CRP): infection anywhere in body can raise the level. Patients with brain tumor and other inflammatory condition (e.g. dental abscess) may have and elevated CRP level. Sensitivity is ≈ 90%, specificity is ≈ 77%[33].

LUMBAR PUNCTURE (LP)

The role of LP is very dubious in abscess. Although LP is abnormal in > 90%, there is no characteristic finding diagnostic of abscess. The OP is usually increased, and the WBC count and protein may be elevated. The offending organism can rarely be identified from CSF obtained by LP (unless abscess ruptures into ventricles) with positive cultures in ≈ 6-22%[34]. There is a risk of transtentorial herniation, especially with large lesions.

Σ | ✖ Due to the risk involved and the low yield of useful information, avoid LP if not already done.

IMAGING

For CT findings of various stages of abscess see below. Sensitivity approaches 100%.

Leukocyte scan with 99mTc-HMPAO (patient's own WBCs are tagged and reinjected) has close to 100% sensitivity and specificity (sensitivity will be reduced if patient is treated with steroids within 48 hrs prior to the scan)[33].

MRI spectroscopy: amino acids and acetate or lactate are diagnostic for abscess.

STAGING OF CEREBRAL ABSCESS

Table 12-2 shows the four well recognized histologic stages of cerebral abscess, and correlates this with the resistance to insertion of an aspirating needle at the time of surgery. It takes at least 2 weeks to progress through this maturation process, and steroids tend to prolong it.

CT staging

Late cerebritis (stage 2) has similar features to early capsule (stage 3) on routine con-

Table 12-2 Histologic staging of cerebral abscess

Stage	Histologic characteristics (days shown are general estimates)	Resistance to aspirating needle
1	early cerebritis: (days 1-3) early infection & inflammation, poorly demarcated from surrounding brain, toxic changes in neurons, perivascular infiltrates	intermediate resistance
2	late cerebritis: (days 4-9) reticular matrix (collagen precursor) & developing necrotic center	no resistance
3	early capsule: (days 10-13) neovascularity, necrotic center, reticular network surrounds (less well developed along side facing ventricles)	no resistance
4	late capsule: (> day 14) collagen capsule, necrotic center, gliosis around capsule	firm resistance, "pop" on entering

trast and non-contrast CT. There is some therapeutic importance in differentiating these two stages; the following aids in distinguishing[35]:
- cerebritis: tends to be more ill-defined
    A. ring-enhancement: usually appears by late cerebritis stage, usually thick
    B. further diffusion of contrast into central lumen, and/or lack of decay of enhancement on delayed scan 30-60 min after contrast infusion

- capsule:
  - A. faint rim present on pre-contrast CT (necrotic center with edematous surrounding brain cause collagen capsule to be seen)
  - B. thin ring enhancement AND delayed scans → decay of enhancement

NB: Thin ring enhancement but lack of delayed decay correlates better with cerebritis
NB: Steroids reduce degree of contrast enhancement (especially in cerebritis)

MRI staging

Table 12-3 shows MRI findings in cerebral abscess. In the cerebritis stage, the margins are ill defined.

Table 12-3 MRI findings with cerebral abscess

Stage	T1WI	T2WI
cerebritis	hypointense	hi signal
capsular	lesion center → low signal, capsule → mildly hyperintense, perilesional edema → low signal	center → iso- or hyperintense, capsule → well defined rim, perilesional edema → hi signal

TREATMENT

"There is no single best method for treating a brain abscess." Treatment usually involves surgical drainage or excision, correction of the primary source, and long-term use of antibiotics (often IV **x** 6-8 weeks followed by oral route **x** 4-8 weeks).

SURGICAL VS. PURE MEDICAL MANAGEMENT
In a patient with suspected cerebral abscess, tissue should be obtained in almost every case to confirm diagnosis and to identify pathogens (preferably before antibiotics).

MEDICAL TREATMENT
In general, surgical drainage or excision is employed in the treatment. Purely medical treatment of early abscess (cerebritis stage)[36], is controversial. NB: pathogens were cultured from well encapsulated abscesses despite adequate levels of appropriate antibiotics in 6 patients who failed medical therapy[37]. Failure may be due to poor blood supply and acidic conditions within the abscess (which may inactivate antibiotics in spite of concentrations exceeding the MIC).

Medical therapy alone is more successful if:
1. treatment begun in cerebritis stage (before complete encapsulation), even though many of these lesions subsequently go on to become encapsulated
2. small lesions: diameter of abscesses successfully treated with antibiotics alone were 0.8-2.5 cm (1.7 mean). Those that failed were 2-6 cm (4.2 mean).
   ★ **3 cm** is suggested as a cutoff[38], above this surgery should be included
3. duration of symptoms ≤ 2 wks (correlates with cerebritis stage)
4. patients show definite clinical improvement within the first week

Medical management alone considered if:
1. poor surgical candidate (NB: with local anesthesia, stereotactic biopsy can be done in almost any patient with normal blood clotting)
2. multiple abscesses, especially if small
3. abscess in critical location: e.g. dominant hemisphere or brain stem[39]
4. concomitant meningitis/ependymitis
5. hydrocephalus requiring shunt that could become infected in surgery

SURGICAL TREATMENT
Indications for initial surgical treatment include:
1. significant mass effect exerted by lesion on CT
2. difficulty in diagnosis (especially in adults)
3. proximity to ventricle: indicates likelihood of intraventricular rupture which is associated with poor outcome[27, 40]
4. evidence of significantly increased intracranial pressure
5. poor neurologic condition (patients responds only to pain, or does not even response to pain)
6. traumatic abscess associated with foreign material
7. fungal abscess
8. multiloculated abscess

9. CT scans cannot be obtained every 1-2 weeks

Surgical <u>intervention in patient being treated medically</u>:
Intervention if neurological deterioration, progression of abscess towards ventricles, or after 2 wks if the abscess is enlarged. Also considered if no decrease in size by 4 wks.

SPECIFIC MANAGEMENT
* obtain blood cultures (rarely helpful)
* initiate antibiotic therapy (preferably after biopsy specimen obtained), regardless of which mode of treatment (medical vs. surgical) is chosen (*see below*)
* LP: avoid in most cases of cerebral abscess (*see page 219*)
* anticonvulsants: used in most cases, recommended duration is 1-2 yrs

ANTIBIOTICS
1. initial antibiotics of choice (when pathogen unknown, and especially if *S. aureus* suspected), make appropriate changes as sensitivities become available. If there is no history of trauma or neurosurgical procedure, then the risk of MRSA is low:
    * <u>vancomycin</u>: covers MRSA. Adult: 1 gm IV q 12 hr. Peds: 15 mg/kg q 8 hr. Check peak & trough levels and adjust dose accordingly (*see page 209*)
    PLUS
    * a 3rd generation cephalosporin (e.g. cefotaxime (Claforan®))
    PLUS
    * one of the following
        ♦ <u>metronidazole</u> (Flagyl®). Adult: 30 mg/kg/d total usually IV (divided q 12 hrs or q 6 hrs, not to exceed 4 gm/d). Peds: 10 mg/kg IV q 8 hrs
        OR
        ♦ <u>chloramphenicol</u>. Adult: 1 gm IV q 6 hr. Peds: 15-25 mg/kg IV q 6 hr
        OR
        ♦ for post-traumatic abscess, use PO rifampin 9 mg/kg/d as 1 dose
2. if culture shows no staph (as is usual in non traumatic abscess), change nafcillin to <u>PCN G (high dose)</u>: adult: 5 M units IV q 6 hr; peds: 50,000-75,000 units/kg IV q 6 hr
3. if culture shows only strep, may use PCN G (high dose) alone
4. if cultures show staph that is <u>not</u> MRSA and the patient is not allergic to penicillin or nafcillin, substitute <u>nafcillin</u> for the vancomycin. Adult: 2 gm IV q 4 hrs. Peds: 25 mg/kg IV q 6 hrs
5. *Cryptococcus neoformans, Aspergillus sp., Candida sp.*:
    A. amphotericin B: 0.5-1 mg/kg/day. ABELCET® (amphotericin B lipid complex) 5 mg/kg/d should be used when renal function is compromised
    B. or liposomal amphotericin B: 3 mg/kg/day, increase to 15 mg/kg/d
6. in AIDS patients: *Toxoplasma gondii* is a common pathogen, and initial empiric treatment with sulfadiazine + pyrimethamine is often used (*see page 233*)

Duration of antibiotics
IV antibiotics for 6-8 wks (most commonly 6), may then D/C even if the CT abnormalities persist (neovascularity remains). NB: CT improvement may lag behind clinical improvement. Duration of treatment may be reduced if abscess and capsule entirely excised surgically. Oral antibiotics may be used following IV course. 5-20% of abscesses recur within 6 weeks of discontinuing antibiotics.

STEROIDS
Decreases likelihood of fibrous encapsulation of abscess, but may reduce penetration of antibiotics into abscess [38]. Reserved for patients with CT and clinical evidence of deterioration from marked mass effect.

CT SCAN
Repeat CT after wks #1 & #2 (more often if patient deteriorates).
Recommended follow-up: after a full course of antibiotics, CT q 2-4 wks until resolution (3.5 mos mean; range 1-11 mos). Then q 2-4 mos for 1 yr, and subsequently anytime CNS symptoms occur.

If therapy is successful, CT should show decrease in:
1. degree of ring enhancement
2. edema

---

3. mass effect
4. size of lesion: takes 1 to 4 wks (2.5 mean). 95% of lesions that will resolve with antibiotics alone decrease in size by 1 month

SURGICAL TREATMENT

Current methods consist of one of the following[41]:
1. needle aspiration: the mainstay of surgical treatment. Especially well-suited for multiple or deep lesions (*see below*)
2. surgical excision: prevents recidivism. Shortens length of time on antibiotics. Recommended in traumatic abscess to debride foreign material, and in fungal abscess because of relative antibiotic resistance (*see below*)
3. external drainage: controversial and may or may not be used
4. instillation of antibiotics directly into the abscess: has not been extremely efficacious, although it may be used as a last resort in *Aspergillus* abscesses

NEEDLE ASPIRATION

May be performed under local anesthesia if necessary. May be combined with irrigation with antibiotics or normal saline. Needs to be repeated in up to 70% of cases. May be the only surgical intervention required, but sometimes must be followed with excision (especially with multiloculated abscess). Stereotactic drainage may be ideal for deep lesions[42].

Performed through a trajectory chosen to:
1. minimize the path length through the brain
2. avoid traversing the ventricles or vital neural or vascular structures
3. avoid traversing infected structures outside the intracranial compartment (infected bone, paranasal sinuses, and scalp wounds)
4. in cases of multiples abscesses, target[26]:
    A. the largest lesion or the one causing the most symptoms
    B. once the diagnosis of abscess is confirmed
        1. any lesion $\geq$ 2.5 cm diameter
        2. lesions causing significant mass effect
        3. enlarging lesions

Cultures

Send aspirated material for the following:
1. stains
    A. Gram stain
    B. fungal stain
    C. AFB stain
2. culture
    A. routine cultures: aerobic and anaerobic
    B. fungal culture: this is not only helpful for identifying fungal infections, but since these cultures are kept for longer period and any growth that occurs will be further characterized, fastidious or indolent bacterial organisms may sometimes be identified
    C. TB culture

EXCISION

Can only be performed during the "chronic" phase (late capsule stage). Abscess is removed as any well encapsulated tumor. The length of time on antibiotics can be shortened to $\approx$ 3 days in some cases following total excision of an accessible, mature abscess (e.g. located in pole of brain). Recommended for abscesses associated with foreign body and most *Nocardia* abscesses (*see below*).

Table 12-4 Outcomes with cerebral abscess

mortality (CT era data)[26, 43]	0-10%
neurologic disability	45%
late focal or generalized seizures	27%
hemiparesis	29%

OUTCOME

In the pre-CT era, mortality ranged form 40-60%. With improvement in antibiotics, surgery, and the improved ability to diagnose and follow response with CT and/or MRI, mortality rate has been reduced to ≈ 10%, but morbidity remains high with permanent neurologic deficit or seizures in up to 50% of cases. Current outcomes are shown in *Table 12-4*. A worse prognosis is associated with poor neurologic function, intraventricular rupture of abscess, and almost 100% mortality with fungal abscesses in transplant recipients.

12.7.1. Some unusual organisms producing abscess

NOCARDIA

Nocardiosis is caused primarily by *Nocardia asteroides* (other Nocardia species such as *N. brasiliensis* are less common), a soil-born aerobic actinomycete (a bacteria, not a fungus) that is usually inoculated through the respiratory tract and produces a localized or disseminated infection. Hematogenous spread frequently results in cutaneous lesions and CNS involvement.

Nocardiosis occurs primarily in patients with chronic debilitating illnesses including:
1. neoplasms: leukemia, lymphoma…
2. conditions requiring long-term corticosteroid treatment
3. Cushing's disease
4. Paget's disease of bone
5. AIDS
6. renal or cardiac organ transplant recipients

The diagnosis is suspected in high-risk patients presenting with soft-tissue abscesses and CNS lesions. CNS involvement occurs in about one-third and includes:
1. cerebral abscess: often multiloculated
2. meningitis
3. ventriculitis in patients with CSF shunt[44]
4. epidural spinal cord compression from vertebral osteomyelitis[45]

Diagnosis: Brain biopsy may not be needed in high-risk patients with confirmed nocardia infection in other sites[44], except possibly in AIDS patients where the risk of multiple organism infections or infection plus tumor (particularly lymphoma) is considerable.

Treatment: Usually includes trimethoprim-sulfamethoxazole **(TMP-SMZ)** together with imipenem, ceftriaxone, cefuroxime or cefotaxime. Duration of treatment is at least 6 weeks, and TMP-SMZ is usually continued for many months because of the risk of relapse or hematogenous spread.

12.8. Subdural empyema

Referred to as subdural abscess prior to 1943[46]. Subdural empyema **(SDE)** is a suppurative infection that forms in the subdural space, which has no anatomic barrier to spread[47]. Antibiotic penetration into this space is poor. Distinguished from abscess which forms within brain substance, surrounded by tissue reaction with fibrin and collagen capsule formation. Hence, SDE tends to be more emergent.

SDE may be complicated by cerebral abscess (seen in 20-25% of imaging studies), cortical venous thrombosis with risk of venous infarction, or localized cerebritis.

EPIDEMIOLOGY

Less common than cerebral abscess (ratio of abscess:empyema is ≈ 5:1). Found in 32 cases in 10,000 autopsies. Male:female ratio is 3:1.

Location: 70-80% are over the convexity, 10-20% are parafalcine.

Table 12-5 Etiologies of SDE

Location	%
paranasal sinusitis (especially frontal)*	67-75
otitis (usually chronic otitis media)†	14
post surgical (neuro or ENT)	4
trauma	3
meningitis (more common in peds[49])	2
congenital heart disease	2
misc. (including pulmonary suppuration)	4
undetermined	3

* more common in adults
† no cases from otitis in a recent series[48]

ETIOLOGIES

See *Table 12-5*. Most often occurs as a result of direct extension of local infection (rarely following septicemia). Spread of the infection to the intracranial compartment may occur through the valveless diploic veins, often with associated thrombophlebitis[50].

Chronic otitis media was the leading cause of SDE in the preantibiotic era, but has now been surpassed by paranasal sinus disease especially with frontal sinus involvement[48] (may also follow mastoid sinusitis). SDE is a rare but sometimes fatal complication of cranial traction devices[48, 51]. Infection of preexisting subdural hematomas (both treated and untreated, in infants and adults) have been reported[48].

Trauma includes compound skull fractures and penetrating injuries. Other etiologies include: osteomyelitis, pneumonia, unrelated infection in diabetics.

PRESENTATION

Neurologic findings are shown in *Table 12-6*. Symptoms are due to mass effect, inflammatory involvement of the brain and meninges, and thrombophlebitis of cerebral veins and/or venous sinuses. SDE should be suspected in the presence of meningismus + unilateral hemisphere dysfunction. Marked tenderness to percussion or pressure over affected air sinuses is common[47]. Forehead or eye swelling (from emissary vein thrombosis) may occur.

Focal neurologic deficit and/or seizures usually occur late.

EVALUATION

- **CT**: IV contrast is usually helpful. CT may miss some cases (related to early generation scanners, failure to give IV contrast, poor scan quality…). If normal, repeat the CT at a later time or do an MRI if clinical suspicion persists. Findings: hypodense (but denser than CSF) crescentic or lenticular extracerebral lesion with dense enhancement of medial membrane; inward displacement of gray-white interface; ventricular distortion and effacement of basal cisterns are common findings[52]
- **MRI**: low signal on T1WI, high signal on T2WI. Pial ependymal line: a non-specific MRI finding in CNS infection
- **LP**: ✘ potentially hazardous (risk of herniation). Organisms are usually present only in cases originating from meningitis. If no meningitis: moderate sterile pleocytosis (150-600 WBC/mm^3) with PMNs predominating; glucose normal; opening pressure is usually high[47]; protein is usually elevated (range: 75-150 mg/dl)

Table 12-6 Findings on presentation with SDE*

Finding	%
fever	95
H/A	86
meningismus (nuchal rigidity…)	83
hemiparesis	80
altered mental status	76
seizures	44
sinus tenderness, swelling or inflammation	42
nausea and/or vomiting	27
homonymous hemianopsia	18
speech difficulty	17
papilledema	9

* from a review of multiple articles[48]

ORGANISMS

The causative organism varies with the specific source of the infection. SDE associated with sinusitis is often caused by aerobic and anaerobic streptococci (*see Table 12-7*). Following trauma or neurosurgical procedures, staphylococci and Gram-negative species predominate. Sterile cultures occur in up to 40%.

Table 12-7 Organisms in adult cases of SDE associated with sinusitis

aerobic streptococcus	30-50%
staphylococci	15-20%
microaerophilic and anaerobic strep	15-25%
aerobic Gram-negative rods	5-10%
other anaerobes	5-10%

TREATMENT

1. surgical drainage: indicated in most cases (nonsurgical management has been reported[53], but should only be considered with minimal neurologic involvement, limited extension and mass effect of SDE, and early favorable response to antibiotics) usually done relatively emergently
- early in the course, the pus tends to be more fluid and may be more amenable to burr hole drainage; later, loculations develop which may necessitate craniotomy
- there has been controversy over the optimal surgical treatment. Early studies indicated a better outcome with craniotomy. Recent studies show less difference
    A. critically ill patients with localized SDE may be candidates for burr-hole

drainage (usually inadequate if loculations are present). Repeat procedures may be needed, and up to 20% will later require a craniotomy
   B. craniotomy: to debride and, if possible, drain
2. antibiotics: similar to treatment for cerebral abscess
   ♦ initially: a penicillin and a third-generation cephalosporin (e.g. cefotaxime)
   ♦ metronidazole is added if there is a high suspicion of anaerobes
   ♦ for post-op SDE: substitute vancomycin for PCN (switch vancomycin to a PCN if there is no staphylococcus)
   ♦ modify antibiotics based on culture results
   ♦ duration: usually 4-6 weeks
• anticonvulsants: usually used prophylactically, mandatory if seizures occur

OUTCOME
See *Table 12-8*. Neurologic deficits were present in 55% of patients at the time of discharge[40]. Age ≥ 60 years, obtundation or coma at presentation, and SDE related to surgery or trauma carry a worse prognosis[48]. Burr-hole drainage may be associated with a worse outcome than with craniotomy, but this may have been influenced by the poorer condition of these patients. Fatal cases may have associated venous infarction of the brain.

Table 12-8 Outcome with SDE

persistent seizures	34%
residual hemiparesis	17%
mortality	10-20%

12.9.   Viral encephalitis

Encephalitides that come to the attention of the neurosurgeon usually cause imaging findings that may mimic mass lesions. Biopsy is helpful in some instances, and shunting for hydrocephalus may occasionally be needed. Those covered in this book:
1. herpes simplex encephalitis: *see below*
2. multifocal herpes varicella-zoster virus leukoencephalitis: *see page 227*
3. progressive multifocal leukoencephalopathy **(PML)**: *see page 231*

12.9.1.   Herpes simplex encephalitis

❗ Key features:
   • hemorrhagic viral encephalitis with predilection for temporal lobes
   • definitive diagnosis requires brain biopsy
   • optimal treatment: early administration of IV acyclovir

Herpes simplex encephalitis **(HSE)** AKA multifocal necrotizing encephalomyelitis, is caused by the herpes simplex virus **(HSV)** type I. It produces an acute, often (but not always) hemorrhagic, necrotizing encephalitis with edema. There is a predilection for the temporal and orbitofrontal lobes and limbic system.

Table 12-9   Adult presentation

altered consciousness	97%
fever	90%
seizures (usually focal onset)	67%
personality changes	71%
hemiparesis	33%

EPIDEMIOLOGY[54]
Estimated incidence of HSE: 1 in 750,000 to 1 million persons/yr. Equally distributed between male and females, in all races, in all ages (over 33% of cases occur in children 6 mos to 18 yrs), throughout the year.

Table 12-10   Presentation in age < 10 yrs

irritability	altered mentation
malaise	seizure
disorientation	dysphasia
hemiparesis	fever
papilledema (except in age ≤ 2 yrs)	

PRESENTATION
Patients are often confused and disoriented at onset, and progress to coma within days. Adult presentations are shown in *Table 12-9*, and for pediatrics in *Table 12-10*. Other symptoms include headache.

Diagnosis can often be made on the basis of history, CSF, and MRI. Treatment should be instituted rapidly without waiting for biopsy, before the onset of coma.

1. **CSF:** leukocytosis (mostly monos), RBCs 500-1000/mm^3, (NB: 3% have no pleocytosis), protein rises markedly as disease progresses. HSV antibodies may appear in the CSF but takes at least ≈ 14 days and is thus not useful for early diagnosis

2. **EEG:** periodic lateralizing epileptiform discharges **(PLEDs)** (triphasic high-voltage discharges every few seconds) usually from the temporal lobe. EEG may vary rapidly over few days (unusual in conditions mimicking HSE)

3. **CT:** edema predominantly localized in temporal lobes (poorer prognosis once hemorrhagic lesions visible). In one review, 38% of initial CTs were normal[55] (many were on early generation CT scanners or were done within 3 days of onset). Hemorrhages were apparent in only 12% of the initially abnormal CTs

4. **MRI:** more sensitive than CT[56], demonstrates edema as high signal on T2WI, primarily within the temporal lobe, with some extension across sylvian fissure ("transsylvian sign")[55], especially suggestive of HSE if bilateral. Differentiate from MCA infarct (which may also span sylvian fissure) by typical arterial distribution of the latter. Enhancement doesn't occur until the 2nd week

5. **technetium brain scan:** process localized to temporal lobes

6. **brain biopsy:** false negatives may occur[57]
   A. **indications:** reserved for questionable cases. May not be necessary in patients with fever, encephalopathy, compatible CSF findings, focal neuro findings (focal seizure, hemiparesis, or cranial nerve palsy), and supporting evidence of at least one of the following: focal EEG, CT, MRI or technetium brain scan abnormality
   B. should be performed within ≤ 48 hrs of starting acyclovir (otherwise false negatives may occur)
   C. anterior inferior temporal lobe is preferred site
      1. the side chosen for biopsy is the one showing maximal involvement based on clinical information (e.g. localizing seizures), EEG and/or imaging studies[58]
      2. 10 x 10 x 5 mm deep specimen obtained from anterior portion of the inferior temporal gyrus with NO COAGULATION on specimen side (cut surface with #11 blade, then cauterize pial surface on non-specimen side)
      3. 2nd specimen obtained from beneath surface specimen with fenestrated pituitary biopsy forceps
   D. virus isolation is the most specific (100%) and sensitive (96-97%) test for HSE. Other findings (less accurate): perivascular cuffing, lymphocytic infiltration, hemorrhagic necrosis, neuronophagia, intranuclear inclusions (present in 50%)
   E. if electron microscopy (EM) or immunohistofluorescence is available, 70% may be diagnosed within ≈ 3 hrs of biopsy
   F. biopsy tissue handling
      1. avoid macerating specimens for histology
      2. tissue for EM: placed in glutaraldehyde
      3. tissue for permanent histology: placed in formalin
      4. tissue for culture:
         a. handling: specimen is placed in sterile specimen container and sent directly to virology lab. If lab is closed, tissue may be:
            i. placed in regular refrigerator for up to 24 hrs
            ii. placed in –70° C freezer for indefinite time (virus remains viable for up to 5 yrs)
            iii. DO NOT place in regular freezer (destroys virus)
         b. cultures generally take at least 1 week to become positive
         c. cultures checked for 3 weeks before being declared negative
   G. biopsy results: of 432 brain biopsies meeting the above criteria, 45% had HSE, 22% had identifiable but non HSE pathology (e.g. vascular disease, other viral infection, adrenal leukodystrophy, bacterial infection...), and 33% remained without a diagnosis[59]

TREATMENT

General supportive measures: to control elevated ICP from edema, includes: elevate

HOB, mannitol, hyperventilation (dexamethasone unproven efficacy) (also see *ICP treatment measures*, page 655). Phenytoin is used for seizure prophylaxis.

Antiviral medications
Ganciclovir is gaining favor over acyclovir.

/‾‾‾‾ acyclovir (Zovirax®) ‾‾\ /‾ DRUG INFO ‾\

Rx Adult: 30 mg/kg/day, in divided q 8 hr doses in minimum volume of 100 ml IV fluid over 1 hr (caution: this fluid load may be hazardous, especially since cerebral edema is already usually problematic) for 14-21 days (some relapses have been reported after only 10 days of treatment).
Rx Children > 6 mos age: 500 mg/m^2 IV q 8 hrs **x** 10 days.
Rx Neonatal: 10 mg/kg IV q 8 hrs for 10 days.

Outcome
Six month mortality following treatment with acyclovir was influenced by:
* age (6% under age 30, 36% over age 30)
* Glasgow coma score **(GCS)** at time of treatment initiation (25% for GCS ≤ 10, 0% for GCS > 10)
* duration of disease before therapy (0% for initiating therapy within 4 days, 35% if after 4 days)

12.9.2. Multifocal varicella-zoster leukoencephalitis

Caused by the herpes varicella-zoster virus **(VZV)** which is responsible for varicella (chickenpox), herpes zoster **(HZ)** (shingles), and post-herpetic neuralgia (*see page 387*). VZV is a herpesvirus that is distinct from the *herpes simplex virus*.
Symptomatic zoster-related encephalitis occurs in < 5% of immunocompromised patients (including AIDS patients) with cutaneous zoster[60]. It typically follows cutaneous HZ by a short time (average: 9 days) although cases have been reported where many months have lapsed[61].
Manifestations include: altered level of consciousness, headache, photophobia, meningismus. Although focal neurologic deficits may occur, these are uncommon.
MRI may show multiple, discrete, round and oval lesions with minimal edema (best seen on T2WI) and minimal enhancement.
Unlike herpes simplex virus, VZV is difficult to isolate in culture. On brain biopsy, look for multiple discrete lesions within grey and white matter, with Cowdry type A intranuclear inclusion bodies in oligodendrocytes, astrocytes, and neurons, and a positive direct fluorescent antibody test directed against VZV.
There is a case report of VZV encephalitis treated with IV acyclovir[60].

12.10. Creutzfeldt-Jakob disease

❦ Key features
* an invariably fatal encephalopathy characterized by rapidly progressive dementia, ataxia and myoclonus
* death usually occurs within 1 yr of onset of symptoms
* 3 forms: 1) transmissible (possibly via prions), 2) autosomal dominant inherited, 3) sporadic
* characteristic EEG finding: bilateral sharp wave (0.5-2 per second)
* pathology: status spongiosus without inflammatory response

Creutzfeldt-Jakob disease **(CJD)** is one of 4 known rare human diseases associated with transmissible spongiform encephalopathy agents, also called prions (proteinaceous infectious particles). Although sometimes also referred to as a "slow virus", these agents contain no nucleic acids and are also resistant to processes that inactivate conventional viruses (*see Table 12-12*). Prions do not provoke an immune response.The protease-resistant protein associated with disease is designated PrP^{res} or PrP^{Sc}, and is an isoform of a naturally occurring protease-sensitive protein designated PrP^{sen} or PrP^C.

Annual incidence of CJD: 0.5-1.5 per million population[62]. Over 200 people die of CJD in the U.S. each year. CJD occurs in 3 forms: transmissible, inherited and sporadic.

Acquired prion diseases: Natural route of infection is unknown and virulence appears low, with lack of significant dissemination by respiratory, enteric, or sexual contact. There is no increased incidence in spouses (only a single conjugal pair of cases has been verified), physicians or laboratory workers. There is no evidence of transplacental transmission. The only known cases of horizontal transmission of CJD have occurred iatrogenically (*see below*). Kuru has been transmitted via handling and ingestion of infected brains in ritualistic funereal cannabalism practiced among the Fore (pronounced: "foray") linguistic group in the eastern highlands of Papua, New Guinea[63], a practice which was generally abandoned in the 1950's. Kuru is a subacute, uniformly fatal disease involving cerebellar degeneration (the word "kuru" means "to tremble" in the local language[64 (p 6)]).

Most noniatrogenically transmitted cases of CJD occur in patients > 50 yrs old, and is rare in age < 30. The incubation period can range from months to decades. The onset of symptoms following direct inoculation is usually faster (common range: 16-28 mos), but still may be much longer (up to 30 years with corneal transplant[65], and 4-21 yrs with hGH transmission).

Inherited CJD: 5-15% of cases of CJD occur in an autosomal dominant inheritance pattern with abnormalities in the amyloid gene[66] on chromosome 20 with a penetrance of 0.56[67]. Since familial CJD is dominantly inherited, analysis for the PrP gene is not indicated unless there is a history of dementia in a first degree relative.

Sporadic CJD: In ≈ 90% of cases of CJD, no infectious or familial source can be identified[66], and these cases are considered sporadic. 80% occur in persons 50-70 yrs old[62]. Sporadic cases show no abnormality in the PrP gene.

New variant CJD: Cases of atypical CJD are well-recognized. A new variant of CJD (**vCJD**) was identified in 10 cases of unusually young individuals (median age at death: 29 yrs) during 1994-95 in the United Kingdom[68], and has been strongly linked to the 1980s epidemic of bovine spongiform encephalopathy (**BSE**), dubbed "mad cow" disease by the lay press. None of the vCJD patients had periodic spikes on EEG characteristic of classic CJD, the clinical course was atypical (having prominent psychiatric symptoms and early cerebellar ataxia, somewhat similar to kuru), and brain plaques showed unusual features also reminiscent of amyloid plaques seen in kuru. A comparison of vCJD to sporadic CJD is shown in *Table 12-11*.

Table 12-11 Comparison of vCJD to sporadic CJD[62]

Characteristic	vCJD	sporadic
mean age at onset (yr)	29	60
mean duration of disease (mo)	14	5
most consistent and prominent early signs	psychiatric abnormalities, sensory symptoms	dementia, myoclonus
cerebellar signs (%)	100	40
periodic complexes on EEG (%)	0	94
pathological changes	diffuse amyloid plaques	sparse plaques in 5-10%

Table 12-12 Operating room sterilization procedures for CJD[72]

- Fully effective (recommended) procedures
  A. steam autoclaving for 1 hr at 132°C, or
  B. immersion in 1N sodium hydroxide (NaOH) for 1 hr at room temperature
- Partially effective procedures
  A. steam autoclaving at either 121° C or 132° C for 15-30 mins, or
  B. immersion in 1N NaOH for 15 mins, or lower concentrations (< 0.5N) for 1 hr at room temp, or
  C. immersion in sodium hypochlorite (household bleach) undiluted or up to 1:10 dilution (0.5%) for 1 hr[73]
- ✖ Ineffective procedures:
  boiling, UV or ionizing radiation, ethylene oxide, ethanol, formalin, beta-propiolactone, detergents, quaternary ammonium compounds, Lysol®, alcoholic iodine, acetone, potassium permanganate, routine autoclaving

Iatrogenic transmission of CJD

Described only in cases of direct contact with infected organs, tissues or surgical instruments. Has been reported with: corneal transplants[65, 69], intracerebral EEG electrodes sterilized with 70% alcohol and formaldehyde vapor after use on a CJD patient[70], operations in neurosurgical O.R.s after procedures on CJD patients, in recipients of pituitary-derived[A] human growth hormone (**hGH**)[71], and dural graft with cadaveric dura mater (Lyodura®). Recommended sterilization procedures for suspected CJD tissues and contaminated materials appear in *Table 12-12*.

Pathology

The typical form of CJD produces the classic histologic triad of neuronal loss, astrocytic proliferation, and cytoplasmic vacuoles in neurons and astrocytes (**status spongiosis**), all in the absence of an inflammatory response. There is a predilection for cerebral cortex and basal ganglia, but all parts of the CNS may be involved. In 5-10% of cases, these changes are accompanied by the deposition of amyloid plaques. Immunostaining for PrP^{res} is definitive.

Presentation

One third initially express vague feelings of fatigue, sleep disorders, or reduced appetite. Another third have neurologic symptoms including memory loss, confusion, or uncharacteristic behavior. The last third have focal signs including cerebellar ataxia, aphasia, visual deficits (including cortical blindness), or hemiparesis.

The typical course is inexorable, progression of dementia, often noticeably worse week by week, with subsequent rapid development of pyramidal tract findings (limb weakness and stiffness, pathologic reflexes), and late extrapyramidal findings (tremor, rigidity, dysarthria, bradykinesia) and myoclonus (often stimulus triggered). Clinical signs of sporadic CJD are shown in *Table 12-13*.

Supranuclear gaze palsy is an occasional finding, also usually late[67]. In early stages, CJD may resemble Alzheimer's disease (**SDAT**). 10% of cases present as ataxia without dementia or myoclonus. Cases with predominant spinal cord findings may be initially mistaken for ALS.

Myoclonus subsides in the terminal phases, and akinetic mutism ensues.

Table 12-13 Major clinical signs in sporadic CJD[62]

Sign	Freq (%)
cognitive deficits*	100
myoclonus	> 80
pyramidal tract signs	> 50
cerebellar signs	> 50
extrapyramidal signs	> 50
cortical visual deficits	> 20
abnormal extraocular movements	> 20
lower motor-neuron signs	< 20
vestibular dysfunction	< 20
seizures	< 20
sensory deficits	< 20
autonomic abnormalities	< 20

*   dementia, psychiatric and behavioral abnormalities

DIAGNOSIS

The complete "diagnostic triad" (dementia, myoclonus and periodic EEG activity) may be absent in up to 25% of cases. Diagnostic criteria have been published[74] as shown in *Table 12-14*. No patients in their series with a diagnosis other than CJD fulfilled the criteria for clinically definite CJD. The most common condition other than CJD fulfilling the criteria for clinically probable CJD was SDAT (especially difficult to distinguish in the early stages).

Table 12-14 Diagnostic criteria* of CJD[74]

•	**Pathologically confirmed** (with unequivocal spongiform changes)				
	A. clinically: requires brain biopsy (*see text*)				
	B. found at autopsy				

Clinical criteria	Mental deterioration	Myoclonus	1-2 Hz periodic EEG complexes	Any movement disorder or periodic EEG activity	Duration of illness (months)
clinically definite	+	+	+		< 12
clinically probable	+	+ OR	+		< 18
clinically possible	+			+	< 24

*   in patients with normal metabolic status and spinal fluid. If there are early cerebellar or visual symptoms and then muscular rigidity, or if another family member has died of pathologically verified CJD, then upgrade the degree of certainty to the next higher category

There is a *CSF* immunoassay for the 14-3-3 brain protein (*see below*).

Differential diagnosis

CSF examination to exclude infections such as tertiary syphilis or SSPE is recommended. Toxicity from bismuth, bromides and lithium must be ruled-out. Myoclonus is usually more prominent early in toxic/metabolic disorders than in CJD, and seizures in CJD are usually late[62].

A.   there is no longer a risk of CJD with growth hormone in the U.S. since distribution of pituitary derived hGH was halted in 1985 and current hGH is obtained from recombinant DNA technology

Diagnostic tests

- **imaging**: no characteristic CT or MR finding. These studies are frequently normal, but are essential to rule-out other conditions (e.g. herpes-simplex encephalitis, recent stroke…). Diffuse atrophy may be present, especially late. MRI may show increased intensity on T2WI in areas typically involved (basal ganglion, striatum) in up to 79% of cases (retrospectively)[75]. This is nonspecific but may help differentiate CJD from SDAT[76]
- **blood tests**: serum assays for S-100 protein are so insensitive and nonspecific[77] that it can only be used as an diagnostic adjunct
- **CSF**:
  A. routine labs: usually normal, although protein may occasionally be elevated
  B. abnormal proteins:
  1. abnormal proteins (130 & 131) have been identified in the CSF of patients with CJD[78], but the assay is technically difficult
  2. proteins 130/131 were identified as the normal neuronal protein 14-3-3, and a relatively simple immunoassay for this was developed for use on as little as 50 μl of CSF[79]. Detection of the 14-3-3 protein in the CSF has 96% sensitivity and specificity for CJD among patients with dementia. False positives may occur in other conditions involving extensive neuronal destruction including: acute CVA, herpes encephalitis, multi-infarct dementia, primary CNS lymphoma and rarely SDAT (most cases of SDAT test negative). Requires CSF (cannot be done on blood)
- **EEG**: characteristic finding of bilateral, symmetrical, periodic bi- or triphasic synchronous sharp-wave complexes, AKA **periodic spikes**, AKA pseudoperiodic sharp-wave complexes (0.5-2 per second) have ≈ 70% sensitivity and 86% specificity[80]. They resemble PLEDs (*see page 145*), but are responsive to noxious stimulus (may be absent in familial CJD[67] and in the recent UK variant (*see above*))
- **SPECT scan**: may be abnormal in vCJD even when EEG is normal[81], however the findings are not specific for vCJD
- **brain biopsy**: *see below*
- **tonsillar biopsy**: patients with variant CJD (vCJD) may have detectable levels of variant type 4 of the abnormal prion protein (PrP^Sc) in their lymphoreticular system, which may be accessed by a 1 cm wedge-biopsy of one palatine tonsil (using careful aseptic precautions)[82]

Brain biopsy

Due to lack of an effective treatment and the potential for iatrogenic infection in surgery, biopsy is reserved for cases where establishing the diagnosis is deemed important, or as part of a research study[58], or when diagnostic tests are equivocal and other potentially treatable etiologies are suspected.

Treatment and prognosis

Given the lack of demonstrated infectivity (with tissues other than brain or CSF), isolation precautions such as gowns or masks are felt to be unnecessary[62].

There is no known treatment. The disease is rapidly progressive. Median survival is 5 months, and 80% of patients with sporadic CJD die within 1 year of diagnosis[62].

12.11. Neurologic manifestations of AIDS

TYPES OF NEUROLOGIC INVOLVEMENT

40-60% of all patients with acquired immunodeficiency syndrome **(AIDS)** will develop neurologic symptoms, with one third of these presenting initially with their neurologic complaint[83, 84]. Only ≈ 5% of patients that die with AIDS have a normal brain on autopsy. One study found the CNS complications of AIDS shown in *Table 12-15*.

The most common conditions producing focal CNS lesions in AIDS[86]:
1. toxoplasmosis
2. primary CNS lymphoma
3. progressive multifocal leukoencephalopathy **(PML)**

4. cryptococcal abscess

Manifestations of CNS toxoplasmosis
1. mass lesion (toxoplasmosis abscess): the most common mass effect in AIDS patients (70-80% of cerebral mass lesions in AIDS[87]) (*see below* for CT/MRI findings)
2. meningoencephalitis
3. encephalopathy

CNS toxoplasmosis occurs late in the course of HIV infection, usually when CD4 counts are < 200 cells/mm³.

Primary CNS lymphoma (PCNSL)
Occurs in ≈ 10% of patients with AIDS[88]. PCNSL is associated with the Epstein-Barr virus (*see page 462*).

Features of PML
1. caused by a ubiquitous polyomavirus (a subgroup of papova virus, small nonenveloped viruses with a closed circular double DNA-stranded genome) called "JC virus[A]" (**JCV**). 60-80% of adults have antibodies to JCV[89]
2. frequently manifests in patients with suppressed immune systems, including
   A. AIDS: currently the most common underlying disease associated with PML
   B. prior to AIDS, the most common associated diseases were chronic lymphocytic leukemia & lymphoma
   C. allograft recipients: due to immunosuppression[90]
   D. chronic steroid therapy
   E. PML also occurs with other malignancies, and with autoimmune disorders (e.g. SLE)
3. pathologic findings: focal myelin loss (demyelination, ∴ affects white matter) with sparing of axon cylinders, surrounded by enlarged astrocytes and bizarre oligodendroglial cells with eosinophilic intranuclear inclusion bodies. EM can detect the virus. Sometimes occurs in brainstem and cerebellum
4. clinical findings: mental status changes, blindness, aphasia, progressive cranial nerve, motor, or sensory deficits and ultimately coma. Seizures are rare
5. clinical course: usually rapidly progressive to death within a few months, occasionally longer survival occurs inexplicably[91]. There is no effective treatment. Some promise initially with anti-retroviral therapy[92]
6. definitive diagnosis requires brain biopsy (sensitivity: 40-96%) although it is infrequently employed. JCV has been isolated from brain and urine. Polymerase chain reaction (PCR) of JCV DNA from CSF has been reported, and is specific but not sensitive for PML

Table 12-15 CNS complications of AIDS (320 patients[83])

Complication	%
viral syndromes	
subacute encephalitis*	17
atypical aseptic meningitis	6.5
herpes simplex encephalitis	2.8
★ progressive multifocal leukoencephalopathy (**PML**)	1.9†
viral myelitis	0.93
varicella zoster encephalitis	0.31
non-viral infections	
★ *Toxoplasma gondii*	> 32
Cryptococcus neoformans	13
Candida albicans	1.9
coccidiomycosis	0.31
Treponema pallidum	0.62
atypical *Mycobacteria*	1.9
Mycobacterium tuberculosis	0.31
Aspergillus fumigatus	0.31
bacteria (*E. coli*)	0.31
neoplasms	
★ primary CNS lymphoma	4.7
systemic lymphoma with CNS involvement	3.8
Kaposi's sarcoma (including brain mets)	0.93
CVA (stroke)	
infarct	1.6
intracerebral hemorrhage	1.2
miscellaneous/unknown	7.8

* CMV encephalitis occasionally occurs

† more recent estimate[85] of the incidence of PML in AIDS: 4%

Primary effects of AIDS infection
Neurologic involvement with infection with the Human Immunodeficiency Virus (**HIV**) (aside from opportunistic infection and tumors caused by the immunodeficient state) includes:
1. **AIDS encephalopathy**: the most common neurologic involvement, occurs in ≈ 66% of patients with AIDS involving the CNS

A. after the initials of the patient in whom it was first discovered, not to be confused with Jakob-Creutzfeldt (a prion disease) nor with Jamestown Canyon virus (also confusingly called JC virus) (a single-stranded RNA virus that occasionally causes *encephalitis* in humans)

2. AIDS dementia AKA HIV dementia complex
3. aseptic meningitis
4. cranial neuropathies: including "Bell's palsy" (occasionally bilateral)
5. AIDS related myelopathy: vacuolization of spinal cord (see *Myelopathy*, page 902)
6. peripheral neuropathies

Neurosyphilis
1. AIDS patients can develop neurosyphilis as little as 4 mos from infection[93] (unlike the 15-20 yrs usually required in non-immunocompromised patients)
2. neurosyphilis can develop in spite of what would otherwise be adequate treatment for early syphilis with benzathine PCN[93, 94]
3. the CDC recommends treating patients having symptomatic or asymptomatic neurosyphilis for at least 10 days with probenecid 500 mg PO QID plus either aqueous crystalline PCN-G, 2-4-million units IV q 4 hrs (total of 12-24-million units/d), or aqueous procaine PCN-G 2.4-million units IM q d. This 10 day regimen should be followed by benzathine PCN 2.4-million units IM q week **x** 3 weeks. Benzathine PCN is <u>NOT</u> recommended initially[95]

NEURORADIOLOGIC FINDINGS IN AIDS

A series of 200 consecutive AIDS patients[96] with neurologic symptoms followed to biopsy, autopsy, or for 2 yrs showed the following on <u>initial</u> CT:
- 81 patients (40%) had initially normal CT, only 5% of which went on to develop progression of neurologic abnormalities or developed CT abnormalities
- 75 patients (38%) showed only diffuse cerebral atrophy; 5 of these subsequently developed focal CT findings shown to be *Toxoplasma gondii* infection
- 44 patients (22%) had ≥ 1 focal lesion

See *Table 12-16* for a comparison of neuroradiologic findings in toxoplasmosis, PCNSL and PML.

CT/MRI findings in toxoplasma abscess
1. most common findings: large area (low density on CT) with mild to moderate edema, ring enhancement with IV contrast in 68% compatible with abscess (of those that did not ring enhance, many showed hypodense areas with less mass effect with slight enhancement adjacent to lesion), well circumscribed margins[97]
2. most commonly located in <u>basal ganglia</u>, are also often subcortical
3. often multiple (typically > 5 lesions[98]) and bilateral
4. usually with little to moderate mass effect[86] (in BG, may compress third ventricle and sylvian aqueduct causing obstructive hydrocephalus)
5. most patients with toxoplasmosis had evidence of cerebral atrophy

Table 12-16 Comparison of neuroradiologic lesions in AIDS*

Feature	Toxo	PCNSL	PML
Multiplicity	usually > 5	multiple but < 5	may be multiple
Enhancement	ring	homogeneous	none
Location	basal ganglia and grey-white junction	subependymal	usually limited to white matter
Mass effect	mild-moderate	mild	none-minimal
Miscellaneous	lesions surrounded by edema	may extend across corpus callosum	high signal on T2WI, low on T1WI

* abbreviations: Toxo = toxoplasmosis, PCNSL = primary CNS lymphoma, PML = progressive multifocal leukoencephalopathy

CT/MRI findings in PML (*see Table 12-16*)
Note: the appearance of PML may differ in AIDS patients from non-AIDS patients.
1. CT: diffuse areas of low density. MRI: high intensity on T2WI
2. normally involves only white matter (spares cortex), however in AIDS patients gray matter involvement has been reported
3. no enhancement (on either CT or MRI), unlike most toxoplasmosis lesions
4. no mass effect
5. no edema
6. lesions may be solitary on 36% of CTs and on 13% of MRIs
7. borders are usually more ill-defined than in toxoplasmosis[97]

CT/MRI findings in primary CNS lymphoma (PCNSL) (*see Table 12-16*)
NB: the appearance of PCNSL may differ in AIDS patients from non-AIDS patients.
1. multiple lesions with mild mass effect and edema that tend to ring-enhance on CT, or appear as areas of hypointensity surrounding central area of high intensity (target lesion) targets onT2WI MRI (unlike non-AIDS cases which tend to enhance homogeneously[99])
2. there is a greater tendency to multicentricity in AIDS patients than in the non-immunosuppressed population[100]

Imaging recommendations
MR with gadolinium is recommended as the initial screening procedure of choice for AIDS patients with CNS symptoms (lower false negative rate than CT[86]).

MANAGEMENT OF INTRACEREBRAL LESIONS

Neurosurgical consultation is often requested for biopsy in an AIDS patient with questionable lesion(s). The diagnostic dilemma is usually for low density lesions on CT, and in the United States is primarily between the following:
* toxoplasmosis: treated with pyrimethamine and sulfadiazine (*see below*)
* PML: no proven effective treatment (antiretroviral therapy may help[92])
* CNS lymphoma: usually treated with RTX (see *CNS lymphoma*, page 461)
* TB: tends to be unlikely except in Haitian population
* note: cryptococcus is more common than PML or lymphoma, but usually manifests as cryptococcal meningitis (and not as a ring enhancing lesion) (*see page 239*)

RECOMMENDATIONS
PML can usually be identified radiographically. However, radiographic imaging alone cannot reliably differentiate toxoplasmosis from lymphoma or from some other concurrent conditions (patients with toxoplasmosis may have other simultaneous diseases). Therefore, the following recommendations are made:
1. obtain baseline toxoplasmosis titers on all known AIDS patients (NB: 50% of the general population have been infected by toxo and have positive titers by age 6 years, 80-90% will be positive by middle adulthood). The chances of toxo are higher with serum antibodies > 1:16[98] (most are > 1:256)
2. multiple enhancing lesions with basal ganglion involvement in a patient whose toxo titers change from negative to positive have a high probability of being toxo
3. primary CNS lymphoma **(PCNSL)**
   A. with single lesions, lymphoma is more likely than toxo
   B. if possibility of PCNSL is strong
      1. consider LP (contraindicated in presence of mass effect)
         a. high volume LP for cytology: PCNSL can be diagnosed in ≈ 10-25% of cases using ≈ 10 ml of CSF (*see page 463* for more details)
         b. or send CSF for polymerase chain reaction **(PCR)** amplification of viral DNA of Epstein-Barr virus or JC-virus[101] (the agents responsible for AIDS-related PCNSL and PML, respectively)
      2. some recommend early biopsy[A] to identify PCNSL cases to avoid delaying RTX for 3 weeks while assessing response to antibiotics[86]
4. in patient with possible toxoplasmosis (i.e. positive toxo titers and CT findings not atypical for toxo) even if other conditions have not been excluded:
   A. empirically start: pyrimethamine (Daraprim®) (200 mg loading dose, then 75-100 mg/d), sulfadiazine (75 mg/kg PO loading dose, then 25 mg/kg q 6 hrs), folic acid (5-40 mg/d, usually 10 mg with each dose of pyrimethamine)
   B. if sulfa allergy develops (which commonly occurs), change sulfadiazine to clindamicin 400-600 mg PO or 600 mg IV q 6 hrs
   C. alternatives for complete intolerance:
      1. spiramycin (Rovamycine®) 3-4 gms/d (peds: 50-100 mg/kg/d **x** 3-4 wks)
      2. atovaquone
   D. there should be a clinical and radiographic response within 2-3 weeks[102]
   E. if response is good, reduce dosage after 6-12 weeks to 50% of the above doses and maintain for life
   F. if these drugs are continued, it should be possible to maintain control for re-

---

A. instead of biopsy, a few centers advocate empiric radiation treatment (for possible lymphoma)

mainder of patient's life (cure is not generally possible)

    G. if no response to therapy after 3 weeks (some recommend 7-10 days[103]), then consider biopsy[A]

5. perform biopsy in the following settings:

    A. in patient with negative toxo titers (note: patients occasionally have negative titers because of anergy)

    B. accessible lesion(s) atypical for toxo (i.e. non-enhancing, sparing basal ganglia, periventricular location)

    C. in the presence of extraneural infections or malignancies that may involve the CNS

    D. lesion that could be either lymphoma or toxo (e.g. single lesion, *see 3. A.*)

    E. in patients who have lesions not inconsistent with toxo but fail to respond to appropriate anti-toxo medications in the recommended time (*see above*)

    F. the role of biopsy for <u>non-enhancing</u> lesions is less well defined as the diagnosis does not influence therapy (most are PML or biopsies are non-diagnostic), it may be useful only for prognostic purposes[103]

    G. note: the risk of open biopsy in AIDS patients may be higher than non-immunocompromised patients. Stereotactic biopsy may be especially well suited, with up to 96% efficacy, fairly low morbidity (major risk: significant hemorrhage, ≈ 8% incidence) and low mortality[104, 105]

6. stereotactic biopsy guidelines:

    A. if multiple lesions are present, choose the most accessible lesion in the least eloquent brain area, or the lesion not responding to treatment

    B. biopsy the center of non-enhancing lesions, or the enhancing portion of ring-enhancing lesions

    C. recommended studies on biopsy: histology; immunoperoxidase stain for *Toxoplasma gondii*; stains for TB and fungus; culture for TB, fungi, pyogens

PROGNOSIS

Patients with CNS toxo have a median survival of 446 days, which is similar to that with PML but longer than AIDS-related PCNSL[98]. Patients with CNS lymphoma in AIDS survive on average a shorter time than similarly treated CNS lymphoma in non-immunosuppressed patients (3 months vs. 13.5 mos). Median survival is < 1 month with no treatment. CNS lymphoma in AIDS tends to occur late in the disease, and patients often die of unrelated causes (e.g. *Pneumocystis carinii* pneumonia)[103].

12.12.   Lyme disease - neurologic manifestations

Lyme disease **(LD)** is a complex multisystem disease caused by various species of Borrelia spirochetes (in North America: *Borrelia burgdorferi*) transmitted to humans by the *Ixodes scapularis* or *pacificus* ticks (the American dog tick is not involved). It was first recognized in Lyme, Connecticut in 1975, and is now the most common arthropod-borne infection in the U.S.[106].

CLINICAL FINDINGS

There are 3 clinical stages which can overlap or occur separately.

Stage 1 (early localized disease, erythema migrans and flu-like illness)

    Systemic signs of infection usually begin with a flu-like illness within days to weeks of infection, symptoms include: fever, chills, malaise, fatigue or lethargy, backache, headache, arthralgia, and myalgia. Regional or generalized lymphadenopathy may occur.

    The hallmark of LD is **erythema chronicum migrans (ECM)** (classically a "bulls-eye rash") which begins 3-30 days after the tick bite, and occurs in 60-75% of patients. ECM usually begins in the thigh, inguinal region, or axilla, and consists of an expanding macular rash with bright red borders and central clearing and induration that usually fades without scarring in 3-4 weeks. Within 30 days of the tick bite, spirochetes may be demonstrated in acellular spinal fluid.

Stage 2 (early disseminated disease)

    Several weeks to months after infection, untreated patients develop more serious organ involvement. Cardiac and neurologic involvement may occur. Manifestations include:

1. cardiac: occurs in 8%. Conduction defects (usually A-V block, generally brief and mild) and myopericarditis
2. ocular: panophthalmitis, ischemic optic atrophy, and interstitial keratitis occur rarely
3. neurologic: occurs in 10-15% of patients with stage 2 disease
   A. the clinical triad of neurologic manifestations of Lyme disease is[107]:
      • cranial neuritis (especially that mimicking Bell's palsy: Lyme disease is the most common cause of bilateral "Bell's palsy" in endemic areas)
      • meningitis
      • radiculopathy
   B. other possible neurologic involvement includes: encephalitis, myelitis, peripheral neuritis

Neurologic findings are frequently migratory, and ≈ 60% of patients have multiple neurologic findings simultaneously. In Europe, **Bannwarth's syndrome** (chronic lymphocytic meningitis, peripheral neuropathy, and radiculopathy) is the most common manifestation, and primarily affects the peripheral nervous system[108]. Neurologic symptoms usually resolve gradually.

Stage 3 (late disease)

Arthritis and chronic neurologic syndromes may occur in this stage. Arthralgias are common in stage 1, but true *arthritis* usually does not begin for months to years after infection, and is seen in ≈ 60% of cases[109]. When arthritis occurs, it may affect the knee (89%), hip (9%), shoulder (9%), ankle (7%) and/or elbow (2%)[110]. Neurologic involvement includes[111]:

1. encephalopathy[A]
2. encephalomyelitis[A]
3. peripheral neuropathy[A]
4. ataxia
5. dementia
6. sleep disorder
7. neuropsychiatric disease and fatigue syndromes

DIAGNOSIS

There is no test indicative of active infection. The spirochete is difficult to culture from infected humans. Diagnosis is easy if a history of travel to endemic areas, tick bite, and ECM are identified. *Table 12-17* shows the CDC criteria for diagnosis.

Serology

It takes 7-10 days from initial infection to develop antibodies to *B. burgdorferi*, but it takes ≈ 2-3 wks before antibodies can reliably be detected in untreated patients (antibiotics can reduce the immune response)[113]. If the first serum test is negative, it should be repeated in 4-6 weeks if the clinical suspicion of LD is strong (seroconversion from negative to positive is supportive of *B. burgdorferi* infection). False positives can occur with other borrelial and treponemal infections (e.g. syphilis, however, VDRL test will differentiate the two).

Enzyme-linked immunosorbent assay **(ELISA)** detects IgM or IgG. Antibodies to *B. burgdorferi* is the usual test method. IgM is elevated acutely, and IgG gradually rises and is elevated in almost all patients at 4-6 weeks and is usually highest in patients with arthritis[106]. Western blot may help identify false-positive ELISA results (more sensitive and specific than ELISA, however, results may vary between labs). Amplification of *B. burgdorferi* DNA by polymerase chain reaction **(PCR)** yields a more very sensitive test

Table 12-17 CDC criteria for diagnosis of Lyme disease[112]

In endemic area:
• erythema chronicum migrans **(ECM)**
• antibody titer ≥ 1:256 by IFA* and involvement of ≥ 1 organ system†
In non-endemic area:
• ECM with antibody titer ≥ 1:256
• ECM with involvement of ≥ 2 organ systems†
• antibody titer > 1:256 by IFA* and involvement of ≥ 1 organ system†

* IFA = immunofluorescence antibody
† either musculoskeletal, neurologic or cardiac

A. these conditions are chronic, and their manifestation may be subtle

that may have significant false positives, and can be positive even if the DNA is from dead organisms.

CSF

Elevated CSF IgG antibody titers to *B. burgdorferi* may occur with neurologic involvement[114]. CSF findings in late disease are usually compatible with aseptic meningitis. Oligoclonal bands and increased ratio of IgG to albumin may occur[115].

TREATMENT [111, 116, 117]

Antibiotic therapy is more effective early in the illness.

12.13. Parasitic infections of the CNS

The following is a list of some of the many parasitic infections that involve the nervous system. Those that potentially involve neurosurgical intervention have a dagger (†).
1. cysticercosis†: see *Neurocysticercosis* below
2. toxoplasmosis†: may occur as a congenital TORCH infection, or in the adult usually with AIDS (see *Neurologic manifestations of AIDS*, page 230). *Toxoplasma gondii* is an obligate intracellular protozoan that is ubiquitous but does not cause clinical infection except in immunocompromised hosts. Histologic features: necrosis containing 2-3 nm tachyzoites (cysts)
3. echinococcus†: *see page 238*
4. amebiasis†
5. schistosomiasis

† parasitic infections with a dagger are those that are more likely to involve neurosurgical attention

NEUROCYSTICERCOSIS

Cysticercosis is the most common parasitic infection involving the CNS[118]. It is caused by *Cysticercus cellulosae*, the larval stage of the pork tapeworm *Taenia solium*, which has a marked predilection for neural tissue. Cysticercosis is endemic in areas of Mexico, Eastern Europe, Asia, Central and South America, and Africa. The incidence of neurocysticercosis (encystment of larva in the brain) may reach 4% in some areas[119]. The incubation period varies between months to decades, but 83% of cases show symptoms within 7 years of exposure.

LIFE CYCLE OF T. SOLIUM

There are 3 stages to the life cycle: larva (or oncosphere), embryo and adult. *T. solium* can infect man in two different ways: as the adult worm or as the larva.

Infection with the adult worm (parasitic infection)

This type of infection results from eating undercooked infested (measly) pork. The encysted embryo is released in the small bowel and can then mature into an adult. The segmented adult worm attaches by means of four suckers and two rows of hooklets to the wall of the small intestine where it absorbs food directly through its cuticle. Man is the only known permanent host for the adult tapeworm, for which the human GI tract is the sole habitat. Proglottids (mature segments, each containing reproductive organs) produce eggs which are liberally excreted in the feces.

Infection with the larva

The disease cysticercosis occurs when animals or humans become an intermediate host for the *larval* stage by ingesting viable eggs produced by the proglottid. In the duodenum of man and pig, the shell of the ova dissolves and the thusly hatched larvae burrow through the small bowel wall to enter the lymphatics or systemic circulation and gain access to:
- brain: estimated to be involved in 60-92% of cases of cysticercosis
- skeletal muscle
- eye
- subcutaneous tissue

The most common routes of ingestion of viable eggs are:
1. food (usually vegetables) or water contaminated with eggs from human feces

2. fecal-oral autoinoculation in an individual harboring the adult form of the tapeworm due to lack of good sanitary habits or facilities
3. autoinfection by reverse peristalsis of gravid proglottids from the intestine into the stomach (a theoretical possibility that is unproven)

Once in the tissue of the intermediary host, the larva develop a cyst wall in ≈ 2 months and matures in ≈ 4 months to an embryo. Many embryos die within 5-7 yrs, these sometimes calcify. In pigs, the embryos lie dormant in the muscle, "waiting" to be eaten after which the cycle repeats.

TYPES OF NEUROLOGIC INVOLVEMENT
Involvement of the spinal cord and peripheral nerves is rare.

Two types of cysts tend to develop in the brain[120]:
1. **cysticercus cellulosae**: regular, round or oval thin-walled cyst, ranging in size from ≈ 3 to 20 mm tending to form in the parenchyma or narrow subarachnoid spaces. This cyst contains a scolex (head), is usually static, and produces only mild inflammation during the active phase
2. **cysticercus racemosus**: larger (4-12 cm), grows actively producing grape-like clusters in the basal subarachnoid spaces and produces intense inflammation. There are no larvae in these cysts. These cysts usually degenerate in 2-5 years, in which the capsule thickens and the clear cyst contents are replace by a whitish gel which undergoes calcium deposition with concomitant shrinkage of the cyst

Location of the cysts tends to fall into 1 of 4 groups:
1. meningeal: found in 27-56% of cases with neural involvement. Cysts are adherent or free-floating and are located either in:
   ♦ dorsolateral subarachnoid space: usually C. cellulosae type, causing minimal symptoms
   ♦ basal subarachnoid space: usually the expanding C. racemosus form producing arachnoiditis and fibrosis comprising a chronic meningitis with hypoglycorrhachia. Can obstruct foramina of Luschka and Magendie producing hydrocephalus, or can cause entrapment of basal cisterns → cranial neuropathies (including visual disturbance). Extremely high mortality with this form
2. parenchymal: found in 30-63%; focal or generalized seizures occurs in ≈ 50% of cases (up to 92% in some series)
3. ventricular: found in 12-18%, possibly gaining access via the choroid plexus. Pedunculated or free floating cysts occur, can block CSF flow and cause hydrocephalus with intermittent intracranial hypertension (Brun's syndrome)
4. mixed lesions: found in ≈ 23%

CLINICAL
Presentation: seizures, signs of elevated ICP, focal deficits related to the location of the cyst, and altered mental status are the most common findings. Symptoms may also be produced by the immunologic reaction to the infestation. Cranial nerve palsies can occur with basal arachnoiditis. Subcutaneous nodules may sometimes be felt.

LABORATORY EVALUATION
Mild peripheral eosinophilia can occur, but is inconsistent and thus unreliable.
CSF may be normal. Eosinophils are seen in 12-60% of cases and suggests parasitic infection. Protein may be elevated.
Stool: less than 33% of cases have *T. solium* ova in the stool.

Serology
Cysticercosis antibody titers determined by ELISA are considered significant at 1:64 in serum, and 1:8 in the CSF; checking for titers exceeding these thresholds in the serum produces a test that is more sensitive and in the CSF is more specific for cysticercosis. False negative rates are higher in cases without meningitis or with less sensitive tests. The newer enzyme-linked immunoelectrotransfer blot is ≈ 100% specific and highly sensitive[121], although sensitivity is less in cases with a solitary cyst.

RADIOGRAPHIC EVALUATION
Soft-tissue x-rays may show calcifications in subcutaneous nodules, and in thigh and shoulder muscles.
Skull x-rays show calcifications in 13-15% of cases with neurocysticercosis. May be

single or multiple. Usually circular or oval in shape.

CT
The following findings on CT have been described (modified[120, 122]):
1. ring enhancing cysts of various sizes representing living cysticerci. Little inflammatory response (edema) occurs as long as larva is alive. Characteristic finding is small (< 2.5 cm) low density cysts with eccentric punctate high density that may represent the scolex
2. low density with ring enhancement seen as an intermediate stage between living cyst and calcified remnant representing intermediate stage in granuloma formation. Resultant inflammatory reaction can cause edema, and basal arachnoiditis in cysts located in basal subarachnoid space. Often ring enhancing
3. intraparenchymal punctate calcifications (granuloma) sometimes with, but usually without surrounding enhancement, seen with dead parasites
4. hydrocephalus. Sometimes with intraventricular cysts which may be isointense with CSF on plain CT[123] and may require contrast CT ventriculography[124] or MRI to be demonstrated

TREATMENT
Steroids
May temporarily relieve symptoms, and may help decrease edema that tends to occur initially during treatment with antihelmintic drugs (e.g. dexamethasone 16 mg/d initially, subsequently tapered[120]). Steroids should probably be reserved for cases of acute deterioration during therapy[125].

Antihelmintic drugs
Corticosteroids should be used (if possible, start 2-3 d before treatment, continue during therapy). Any cysticercocidal drug may cause irreversible damage when used to treat ocular or spinal cysts, even with corticosteroid use.

Praziquantel (Biltricide®) is an antihelmintic with activity against all known species of schistosomas. Given as 50 mg/kg divided in 3 doses (same dose for pediatrics) for 15 days, there is a significant reduction in symptoms and in number of cysts seen on CT[118]. Also drug of choice for intestinal stage infestation.

Albendazole (Zentel®) 15 mg/kg per day divided in 2-3 doses, taken with a fatty meal to enhance absorption (same dose for pediatrics), given for 3 months[126, 127].

Niclosamide (Niclocide® and others) may be given orally to treat adult tapeworms in the GI tract (note: praziquantel is drug of choice). *Rx* 1 gm (2 tablets) chewed PO, repeated in 1 hour (total = 2 gm).

Intraventricular disease: There is no consensus on the efficacy of medical treatment for intraventricular cysts[128].

Surgery
Surgery may sometimes be necessary to establish the diagnosis. Stereotactic biopsy may be well suited for some cases, especially with deep lesions.

CSF diversion is necessary for patients with symptomatic hydrocephalus, although tubing may become obstructed by granulomatous inflammatory debris[129].

Surgery may be indicated for spinal cysts[119] and for intraventricular cysts which may be less responsive to medical therapy. The latter may sometimes be dealt with using stereotactic techniques and/or endoscopic instrumentation[124].

Contacts
Both patients with cysticercosis and their personal contacts should be screened for tapeworm infection since a single dose of niclosamide or praziquantel will eliminate the tapeworm[130]. Close contacts of persons with tapeworms should have screening by medical history and serologic testing for cysticercosis; if suggestive of cysticercosis a neurologic exam and CT or MRI should be done.

ECHINOCOCCOSIS
AKA **hydatid (cyst) disease**. Caused by encysted larvae of the dog tapeworm *Echinococcus granulosa* in endemic areas (Uruguay, Australia, New Zealand…). The dog is the primary definitive host of the adult worm. Intermediate hosts for the larval stage include sheep and man. Ova are excreted in dog feces and contaminate herbage eaten by sheep. After ingestion, the embryos hatch and the parasite burrows through the duodenal wall to gain hematogenous access to multiple organs (liver, lungs, heart, bone, brain).

Dogs eat these infested organs and the parasite enters the intestine where it remains. Man is infected either by eating food contaminated with ova, or by direct contact with infected dogs. CNS involvement occurs in only ≈ 3%. Produces cerebral cysts that are confined to the white matter. Primary cysts are usually solitary, secondary cysts (e.g. from embolization from cardiac cysts that rupture or from iatrogenic rupture of cerebral cysts) are usually multiple. The CT density of the cyst is similar to CSF, it does not enhance (although rim enhancement may occur if there is an inflammatory reaction), and there is little surrounding edema. It contains germinating parasitic particles called "hydatid sand" containing ≈ 400,000 scoleces/ml. The cyst enlarges slowly (rates of ≈ 1 cm per year are quoted, but this is variable and may be higher in children), and usually does not present until quite large with findings of increased ICP, seizures, or focal deficit. Patients often have eosinophilia and may have positive serologic tests for hydatid disease.

Treatment

Treatment is surgical removal of the intact cyst. Every effort must be made to avoid rupturing these cysts during removal, or else the scoleces may contaminate the adjacent tissues with possible recurrence of multiple cysts or allergic reaction. May use adjunctive medical treatment with albendazole (Zentel®) 400 mg PO BID (pediatric dose: 15 mg/kg/d) **x** 28 days, taken with a fatty meal, repeated as necessary[127].

12.14. Fungal infections of the CNS

Most are medically treated conditions that do not require neurosurgical intervention. They tend to present either with chronic meningitis or brain abscess. Some of the more common ones include
1. cryptococcosis: *see below*
   A. cryptococcoma (mucinous pseudocyst)
   B. cryptococcal meningitis
2. candidiasis: is now the most common fungal infection of the CNS, but is rarely diagnosed before autopsy. Very rare in healthy individuals
3. aspergillosis: may be associated with cerebral abscess in organ transplant patients (*see page 218*)
4. coccidiomycosis: caused by the dimorphic fungus *Coccidioides immitis*. Endemic in southwestern U.S., Mexico, and Central America. Usually presents as meningitis, with rare reports of parenchymal lesions[131]
5. mucormycosis (phycomycosis): usually occurs in diabetics (*see page 586*)

CRYPTOCOCCAL INVOLVEMENT OF THE CNS
CNS involvement is diagnosed more frequently in living patients than any other fungal disease. Occurs in healthy or immunocompromised patient.
1. cryptococcoma (mucinous pseudocyst): a parenchymal collection which occurs almost exclusively in AIDS patients. No enhancement of the lesion or the meninges. Usually 3-10 mm in diameter and are frequently located in the basal ganglia (due to spread by small perforators)
2. cryptococcal meningitis:
   A. occurs in 4-6% of patients with AIDS[132]
   B. can also occur without AIDS: *gatti* variety can infect the brain of immunocompetent hosts[133]
   C. may be associated with increased ICP (with or without hydrocephalus on CT), decreased visual acuity, and/or cranial nerve deficits
   D. late deterioration in the absence of documented infection may respond to decadron 4 mg q 6 hrs transitioned to prednisone 25 mg p.o. q d[134]

Treatment
1. antifungal agents (e.g. fluconazole, an oral triazole or amphotericin B)[135]
   A. patients with HIV require lifelong treatment
   B. non-HIV patients have a limited treatment course
2. management of intracranial hypertension **(ICHT)** (with or without hydrocephalus): controversial. Options[136]:
   A. if initial opening pressure **(OP)** on LP is WNL (< 20 cm) then a repeat LP in 2 weeks is recommended to assess culture status and to re-eval OP

B. for documented ICHT, initial management is daily LPs, draining enough CSF to reduce ICP by 50%. Daily LPs may be suspended when pressures are normal for several consecutive days
C. cases with persistent ICHT or those with visual deterioration in spite of serial LPs may be managed with:
  1. lumbar drain: temporizing. Drain to a height of ≈ 10 cm of CSF
  2. permanent shunt: neither dissemination of infection through the distal shunt nor creation of a nidus of infection refractory to medical therapy has been described[137]
    a. lumboperitoneal shunt
    b. VP or VA shunt[138, 139]

12.15. Spine infections

Spine infections may be divided into the following major categories:
1. vertebral osteomyelitis (spondylitis): *see page 243*
  A. pyogenic
  B. nonpyogenic, granulomatous
    1. tuberculous spondylitis
    2. brucellosis
    3. aspergillosis
    4. blastomycosis
    5. coccidiomycosis
    6. infection with *Candida tropicalis*
2. discitis: *see page 245*, usually associated with vertebral osteomyelitis (spondylodiscitis)
  A. spontaneous
  B. post-operative/post-procedure
3. epidural abscess (*see below*)
4. subdural empyema
5. meningitis
6. spinal cord abscess

   MRI experience suggests that patients with infectious spondylitis will develop an associated epidural abscess if untreated, and that epidural empyema is unusual in the absence of vertebral osteomyelitis[140]. Thus, the discovery of one of these conditions should prompt a search for the other.

12.15.1. Spinal epidural abscess

❢ Key features:
  • should be considered in a patient with back pain, fever, and spine tenderness
  • major risk factors: diabetes, IV drug abuse, chronic renal failure, alcoholism
  • may produce progressive myelopathy, sometimes with precipitous deterioration, therefore early surgery is recommended even if no neuro deficit
  • fever, sweats or rigors are common, but normal WBC and temperature can occur
  • classical presentation of a skin boil (furuncle) occurs in only ≈ 15%

EPIDEMIOLOGY
   Incidence: 0.2-1.2 per 10,000 hospital admissions annually[141], possibly on the rise[142]. Average age: 57.5 ± 16.6 years[143].
   Thoracic level is the most common site (≈ 50%), followed by lumbar (35%) then cervical (15%)[143]. 82% were posterior to the cord, and 18% anterior in one series[141]. SEA may span from 1 to 13 levels[144].

   Spinal epidural abscess (**SEA**) is often associated with vertebral osteomyelitis (in one series of 40 cases, osteomyelitis occurred in all cases of anterior SEA, in 85% of circumferential SEA, and no cases of posterior SEA) and intervertebral discitis.

CO-MORBID CONDITIONS
   Chronic diseases associated with compromised immunity were identified in 65% of

40 cases[145]. Associated conditions included diabetes mellitus (32%), IV drug abuse (18%), chronic renal failure (12%), alcoholism (10%), and the following in only 1 or 2 patients: cancer, recurrent UTI, Pott's disease, and positivity for HIV. Chronic steroid use and recent spinal procedure or trauma (e.g. GSW) are also risk factors[144].

CLINICAL FEATURES

Usually presents with excruciating pain localized over spine, tender to percussion. Radicular symptoms follow with subsequent distal cord findings, often beginning with bowel/bladder disturbance, abdominal distension, weakness progressing to para- and quadriplegia. Average time is 3 days from back pain to root symptoms; 4.5 days from root pain to weakness; 24 hrs from weakness to paraplegia.

Fever, sweats or rigors are common, but are not always present[144].

A furuncle may be identified in 15%.

Patients may be encephalopathic. This may range from mild to severe and may further delay diagnosis. Meningismus with a positive Kernig's sign may occur.

Patients with post-operative SEA may demonstrate surprisingly few signs or symptoms (including lack of leukocytosis, lack of fever) aside from local pain[146].

Pathophysiology of spinal cord dysfunction

Although some cord symptoms may be due to mechanical compression (including that due to vertebral body collapse), this is not always found[147]. A vascular mechanism has also been postulated, and various combinations of arterial and venous pathology have been described[141] (one autopsy series showed little arterial compromise, but did show venous compression and thrombosis, thrombophlebitis of epidural veins, and venous infarction and edema of the spinal cord[148]). Occasionally, there may be infection of the spinal cord itself, possibly by extension through the meninges.

Differential diagnosis

SEA should be considered in any patient with backache, fever, and spine tenderness[149]. Also see *Differential diagnosis, Myelopathy* on page 902.

Differential diagnosis
1. meningitis
2. acute transverse myelitis (paralysis is usually more rapid, radiographic studies are normal)
3. intervertebral disc herniation
4. spinal cord tumors
5. post-op SEA may appear similar to pseudomeningocele[146]

SOURCE SITE OF INFECTION

- hematogenous spread is the most common source (26-50% of cases) either to the epidural space or to the vertebra with extension to epidural space. Reported foci include:
    A. skin infections (most common): furuncle may be found in 15% of cases
    B. parenteral injections, especially with IV drug abuse[150]
    C. bacterial endocarditis
    D. UTI
    E. respiratory infection (including otitis media, sinusitis, or pneumonia)
    F. pharyngeal or dental abscess
- direct extension from:
    A. decubitus ulcer
    B. psoas abscess: psoas major muscle attaches to transverse processes, vertebral bodies (VB) and intervertebral discs of spinal column starting from the inferior margin of T12 VB, extending to the upper part of L5 VB
    C. penetrating trauma, including: abdominal wounds, neck wounds, GSW
    D. pharyngeal infections
    E. mediastinitis
    F. pyelonephritis with perinephric abscess
- following spinal procedures (3 of 8 of these patients had readily identified perioperative infections of periodonta, UTI, or AV-fistula[145])
    A. open procedures: especially lumbar discectomy (incidence[146] ≈ 0.67%)
    B. closed procedures: e.g. epidural catheter insertion for spinal epidural anesthesia[151-153], lumbar puncture[154]...
- a history of recent back trauma is common (in up to 30%)
- no source can be identified in up to 50% of patients in some series[155]

Operative cultures are most useful in identifying the responsible organism, these cultures may be negative (possibly more common in patients previously on antibiotics) and in these cases blood cultures may be positive. No organism may be identified in 29-50% of cases.

1. **Staph. aureus**: the most common organism (cultured in > 50%) possibly due to its propensity to form abscesses, its ubiquity, and its ability to infect normal and immunocompromised hosts (these facts help explain why many SEA arise from skin foci)
2. aerobic & anaerobic streptococcus: second most common
3. *E.coli*
4. *Pseudomonas aeruginosa*
5. *Diplococcus pneumoniae*
6. *Serratia marcescens*
7. Enterobacter
8. chronic infections:
    A. TB is the most common of these, and although it has become less widespread in the U.S. it is still responsible for 25% of cases of SEA[156], it is usually associated with vertebral osteomyelitis (Pott's disease) (see *Tuberculous vertebral osteomyelitis:*, page 245)
    B. fungal: cryptoccocis, aspergillosis, brucellosis
    C. parasitic: Echinococcus
9. multiple organisms in ≈ 10%
10. anaerobes cultured in ≈ 8%

DIAGNOSTIC TESTS

CBC: leukocytosis common in acute group (average WBC = 16,700/mm³), but usually normal in chronic (ave. WBC = 9,800/mm³)[141].

ESR elevated in most[54], usually > 30[145].

LP: performed cautiously in suspected cases at a level distant to the clinically suspected site (C1-2 puncture may be needed to do myelogram) with constant aspiration while approaching thecal sac to detect pus (danger of transmitting infection to subarachnoid space); if pus is encountered, stop advancing, send the fluid for culture, and abort the procedure. CSF protein & WBC usually elevated; glucose normal (indicative of parameningeal infection). 5 of 19 cases grew organisms identical to those in abscess.

Blood cultures: may be helpful in identifying organism in some cases.

Anergy battery: (e.g. mumps and Candida) to assess immune system.

RADIOGRAPHIC STUDIES

Plain films: Usually normal unless there is osteomyelitis of adjacent vertebral bodies (more common in infections anterior to dura). Look for lytic lesions, demineralization, and scalloping of endplates (may take 4-6 weeks after onset of infection).

MRI: Imaging study of choice. Differentiates other conditions (especially transverse myelitis or spinal cord infarction) better than myelo/CT, and doesn't require LP.

Typical findings: T1WI → hypo- or iso-intense epidural mass, vertebral osteomyelitis shows up as reduced signal in bone. T2WI → high intensity epidural mass that often enhances with gadolinium (3 patterns of enhancement: 1) dense homogeneous, 2) inhomogeneous with scattered areas of sparse or no uptake, and 3) thin peripheral enhancement[157]) but may show minimal enhancement in the acute stage when comprised primarily of pus with little granulation tissue. Vertebral osteomyelitis shows up as increased signal in bone, associated discitis produces increased signal in disc and loss of intranuclear cleft. Unenhanced MRI may miss some SEA[158], gadopentetate dimeglumine enhancement may slightly increase sensitivity[159].

Myelogram: Usually shows findings of extradural compression (e.g. "paintbrush appearance" when complete block is present). In the event of complete block, C1-2 puncture is needed to delineate upper extent (unless post-myelographic CT shows dye above the lesion). See cautions above regarding LP.

CT scan: Intraspinal gas has been described on plain CT[160]. Post-myelographic CT is more sensitive.

TREATMENT

Early surgical evacuation combined with antibiotics is the treatment of choice. Al-

though there are reports of patients managed with antibiotics alone[161-163] ± immobilization[140], rapid and irreversible deterioration has occurred even in patients treated with appropriate antibiotics who were initially neurologically intact[143, 145]. 86% of those who deteriorated were initially treated it with antibiotics alone[144]. Therefore it is recommended that nonsurgical management be reserved for the following patients (reference[161] modified[144]):
1. those with prohibitive operative risk factors
2. involvement of an extensive length of the spinal canal
3. complete paralysis for > 3 days

Surgery

Goals are establishing diagnosis and causative organism, drainage of pus and debridement of granulation tissue, and bony stabilization if necessary. Most SEA are posterior to dura and are approached with extensive laminectomy. For posteriorly located SEA and no evidence of vertebral osteomyelitis, instability will usually not follow simple laminectomy and appropriate postoperative antibiotics[155].

Specific antibiotics

If organism and source unknown, *S. aureus* most likely. Empiric antibiotics:
1. 3rd generation cephalosporin, e.g. cefotaxime (Claforan®)
PLUS
2. vancomycin: until methicillin resistant *S. aureus* **(MRSA)** can be ruled out. Once MRSA is ruled out switch to synthetic penicillin (e.g. nafcillin or oxacillin)
PLUS
3. rifampin PO

Modify antibiotics based on culture results or knowledge of source (e.g. IV drug abusers have a higher incidence of Gram-negative organisms).

Duration of treatment

For SEA, 3-4 weeks of IV antibiotics followed by 4 weeks of oral antibiotics usually suffices. 6-8 weeks of IV antibiotics are suggested if there is documented concomitant vertebral osteomyelitis[164] (although some argue that osteomyelitis is present pathologically in most cases even if not demonstrated radiographically, and therefore there should be no treatment difference between these groups[165]). Serial ESRs may also guide duration (failure to reduce suggests residual infection[142]). Immobilization for at least 6 weeks during antibiotic therapy is recommended.

OUTCOME

Fatal in 4-31% [166](the higher end of the range tends to be in older patients and in those paralyzed before surgery[145]. Patients with severe neurologic deficit rarely improve, even with surgical intervention within 6-12 hrs of onset of paralysis, although a few series have shown a chance for some recovery with treatment within 36 hrs of paralysis[149, 165]. Reversal of paralysis of caudal spinal cord segments if present for more than a few hours is rare (exception: Pott's disease has 50% return). Mortality is usually due to the original focus of infection or as a complication of residual paraplegia (e.g. pulmonary embolism).

12.15.2. Vertebral osteomyelitis

For differential diagnosis, *see Destructive lesions of the spine*, page 939. Often associated with discitis, which may be grouped together under the term *spondylodiscitis*. VO has features similar to spinal epidural abscess **(SEA)** (*see page 240*).

Vertebral body collapse and kyphotic deformity is common with possible retropulsion of necrotic bone and disc fragments against the spinal cord or cauda equina.

EPIDEMIOLOGY

Vertebral osteomyelitis **(VO)** comprises 2-4% of all cases of osteomyelitis[167]. Incidence is 1:250,000 in general population. Incidence appears to be rising. Male:female ration is 2:1. The lumbar spine is the most common site, followed by thoracic, cervical and sacrum[168].

Risk factors:
1. IV drug abuse[169]

2. diabetes mellitus: susceptible to unusual bacterial infections and even fungal osteomyelitis
3. hemodialysis: a diagnostic challenge since radiographic changes of osteomyelitis can occur even in the absence of infection (see *Destructive lesions of the spine*, page 939)
4. immunosuppression
   A. AIDS
   B. chronic corticosteroid use
   C. ethanol abuse
5. infectious endocarditis
6. following spinal surgery or invasive diagnostic or therapeutic procedures
7. may occur in elderly patients with no other identifiable risk factors[170]

Complications that my accrue:
1. spinal epidural abscess
2. subdural abscess
3. meningitis
4. bony instability
5. progressive neurologic impairment
6. unique to cervical spine involvement: pharyngeal abscess
7. unique to thoracic spine involvement: mediastinitis

CLINICAL

Signs/symptoms: localized pain (90%), fever (52%, with fever spikes and chills being rare), weight loss, paraspinal muscle spasm, radicular symptoms (50-93%) or myelopathy. VO sometimes produces few systemic effects (e.g. WBC and/or ESR may be normal). ≈ 17% of patients with VO have neurologic symptoms. The risk of paralysis may be higher in the older patient, in cervical VO (vs. thoracic or lumbar), in those with DM or rheumatoid arthritis, and in those with VO due to *S. aureus*[171]. Neurologic findings are uncommon initially, which may delay the diagnosis[172]. Sensory involvement is less common than motor and long-tract signs because compression is primarily anterior.

SOURCE OF INFECTION

Sources of spontaneous VO: UTI (the most common), respiratory tract, soft-tissues (e.g. skin boils, IV drug abuse…), dental flora, blunt trauma to the spine. In 37% of cases a source is never identified[173].

Potential routes of spread: arterial, spinal epidural venous plexus (Batson's plexus), or by direct extension (e.g. following surgery). Spontaneous spondylodiscitis in adults usually involves bone primarily, and once infection is established in the subchondral space, spread is to the adjacent disc and thence to the adjacent VB[174].

EVALUATION

Imaging

A comparison of the sensitivities and specificities of various imaging modalities is shown in *Table 12-18*.

Plain x-ray: changes take from 2-8 weeks from the onset of infection to develop. Earliest changes are loss of cortical endplate margins and loss of disc space height.

Bone scan with technetium 99m-HDP: may be positive within 1-2 days of infection. False positive increased uptake may be due to degenerative changes, recent surgery or fracture.

Table 12-18 Accuracy of various imaging modalities for vertebral osteomyelitis[175]

Modality	Sensitivity	Specificity	Accuracy
plain x-rays	82%	57%	73%
bone scan	90%	78%	86%
gallium scan	92%	100%	93%
bone scan + gallium scan	90%	100%	94%
MRI	96%	92%	94%

MRI: T1WI shows confluent low signal from the vertebral bodies and intervertebral disc space. T2WI shows increased intensity from the involved VB and disc space[175].

Laboratories

WBC: elevated in only ≈35% (rarely > 12,000), associated with poor prognosis.
ESR: elevated in almost all. Usually > 40 mm/hr. Mean: 85.
CRP: may be more sensitive than ESR, and may tend to normalize more quickly with appropriate treatment[176].

Cultures/biopsy

Culture: blood (positive in ≈ 50%), urine and any focal suppurative process. An attempt at direct culture from the involved site should be made. Ideally, cultures should be done before antibiotics are started. If feasible, percutaneous biopsy with CT or fluoroscopic guidance as required is optimal. The yield of needle biopsy cultures ranges from 60-90%. Open biopsy is more sensitive, but morbidity is higher. Cultures should include: aerobic and anaerobic, fungal and TB.

Organisms

1. as in SEA, the most common causative organism is *Staphylococcus aureus*
2. *E. coli* is a distant second
3. organisms associated with some primary infection sites[177]:
   A. IV drug abusers: *Pseudomonas aeruginosa* is common
   B. urinary tract infections: *E. coli* & *Proteus spp.* are common
   C. respiratory tract infections: *Streptococcus pneumoniae*
   D. alcohol abuse: *Klebsiella pneumoniae*
   E. endocarditis:
      1. acute endocarditis: *Staph. aureus*
      2. subacute endocarditis: *Streptococcus spp.*
4. unusual organisms include: nocardia (*see page 223*)
5. pyogenic infections are rarely polymicrobial (< 2.5%)

Tuberculous vertebral osteomyelitis:

AKA tuberculous spondylitis, AKA **Pott's disease**. More common in third world countries. Is usually symptomatic for many months. Usually affects more than one level. The most common levels involved are the lower thoracic and upper lumbar levels. Has a predilection for the vertebral body, sparing the posterior elements. Psoas abscess is common (the psoas major muscle attaches to the bodies and intervertebral discs from T12-L5). Sclerosis of the involved vertebral body may occur. Definitive diagnosis requires the identification of acid fast bacilli on culture or Gram stain of biopsy material (may be done percutaneously).

Neurologic deficit develops in 10-47% of patients[178], and may be due to medullary and radicular inflammation in most cases. The infection itself rarely extends into the spinal canal[179], however, epidural granulation tissue or fibrosis or a kyphotic bony deformity may cause cord compression[178].

The role of surgical debridement and fusion with TB is controversial, and good results may be obtained with either medical treatment or surgery. Surgery may be more appropriate when definite cord compression is documented or for complications such as abscess or sinus formation[180].

TREATMENT

90% of cases can be managed non-surgically with antibiotics and immobilization. Characteristics of potential candidates for non-surgical treatment are listed in *Table 12-19*. For details, see *Treatment*, page 242, for spinal epidural abscess. The incidence of treatment failure is increased when parenteral antibiotics are given for < 4 weeks[177]. Recommendations: IV antibiotics for at least 6 weeks (longer if ESR not normalizing) followed by 6-8 weeks of oral agents[177].

Table 12-19   Candidates for non-surgical treatment in pyogenic spontaneous spondylodiscitis[177]

• organism identified
• antibiotic sensitivity
• single disc space involvement with little VB involvement
• minimal or no neurologic deficit
• minimal or no spinal instability

12.15.3.   Discitis

An uncommon primary infection of the nucleus pulposus with secondary involvement of cartilaginous endplate and vertebral body (**VB**). May occur following a number of procedures (see *Epidemiology*, page 249) or may be "spontaneous" (the latter being more common). Often a benign, self-limited disease. Similar to vertebral osteomyelitis, except osteomyelitis primarily involves the VB and spreads secondarily to the disc space. Features and management common to spontaneous and postoperative discitis are discussed in the "general" section below, followed by sections describing characteristics unique to each (see *Spontaneous discitis*, page 248 or *Postoperative discitis* on page 249).

Many radiographic features of spondylodiscitis and tumor (metastatic and primary) are similar, but tumors rarely involve the disc space, whereas most infections begin in, or before too long, involve the disc space.

DISCITIS IN GENERAL

CLINICAL
1. symptoms:
   A. pain (the primary symptom)
      1. local pain, moderate to severe, exacerbated by virtually any motion of the spine, usually well localized to the level of involvement
      2. radiating to abdomen[181], hip, leg, scrotum, groin, or perineum
      3. radicular symptoms: in 50%[182] to 93%[183] depending on the series
   B. fever and chills (only 30-50% are febrile)
2. signs:
   A. tenderness
   B. paravertebral muscle spasm
   C. limitation of movement

RADIOGRAPHIC EVALUATION
A characteristic radiographic finding that helps distinguish infection from metastatic disease is that destruction of the disc space is highly suggestive of infection, whereas in general, <u>tumor</u> does <u>not</u> cross the disc space (see *Differentiating factors*, page 939).

PLAIN X-RAYS
Usually not helpful for early diagnosis. Sequence of changes on plain films:
* earliest changes: interspace narrowing with some demineralization of the VB. Not seen < 2-4 wks following onset of clinical symptoms, nor later than 8 wks
* sclerosis (eburnation) of adjacent cortical margins with increased density of adjacent areas of VB representing new bone formation, starting 4-12 weeks following onset of clinical symptoms
* irregularity of the adjacent vertebral endplates, with sparing of the pedicles (except for tuberculosis, which may involve the pedicles)
* in 50% of cases, the infection remains confined to the disc space, in the other 50% it spreads to adjacent VB
* a late finding is widening (ballooning) of the disc space with erosion of the VB
* circumferential bone formation may lead to exuberant spur formation between VBs 6-8 months into course of illness
* spontaneous fusion of the VB may occur

MRI
Demonstrates involvement of disc space and of VBs. MRI can R/O paravertebral or epidural spinal abscess but is poor in assessing bony fusion. As sensitive as radionuclide bone scan. Characteristic finding: decreased signal from the disc and adjacent portion of VBs on T1WI, and increased signal from these structures on T2WI. Characteristic findings may occur 3-5 days after onset of <u>symptoms</u>. MRI also rules-out other causes of post-op pain (epidural abscess, recurrent/residual disc herniation…).

The triad of gadolinium enhancement shown in *Table 12-20* is strongly suggestive of discitis (some asymptomatic patients may have some of these findings, but they rarely have all)[184].

Table 12-20 Gadolinium enhancement in discitis

Location of gadolinium enhancement	Number (out of 15 patients without discitis)	Number (out of 7 patients with discitis)
1. vertebral bone marrow	1	7
2. disc space	3	5
3. posterior annulus fibrosus	13	7

CT
May also R/O paravertebral or epidural spinal abscess, and is better for assessing bony fusion. With the addition of water soluble intrathecal contrast, also assesses the spinal canal for compromise.

Diagnostic criteria

Three basic changes on CT[185] (if all 3 are present, pathognomonic for discitis; if only the 1st 2 are present, then only 87% specific for discitis):
1. endplate fragmentation
2. paravertebral soft-tissue swelling with obliteration of fat planes
3. paravertebral abscess

SPINE POLYTOMOGRAMS

For postoperative discitis **(POD)**: performed through level of previous discectomy. Otherwise, center tomograms on painful level.

SCINTIGRAMS

Very sensitive for discitis and vertebral osteomyelitis (85% sensitivity), but may be negative in up to 85% of patients with Pott's disease. Uses either technetium-99 (abnormal as early as 7 days following onset of clinical symptoms) or gallium-67 (abnormal within 14 days). A positive scan shows focal increased uptake in adjacent endplates, and may be differentiated from osteomyelitis which will involve only one endplate. A positive scan is not specific for infection, and may also occur with neoplasms, fractures, and degenerative changes.

LABORATORY STUDIES

ESR: In non-immunocompromised patients, ESR will be elevated in almost all cases with an average of 60 mm/hr (although it can rarely occur, a normal ESR should call the diagnosis into question). Interpreting ESR may be more problematic in post-op discitis (*see page 249*). ESR may be useful to follow as an indicator of response to treatment.

C-reactive protein: *See C-reactive protein* on page 249.

WBC: Peripheral WBC is often normal, and rarely is elevated above 12,000.

PPD: Applied to help R/O Pott's disease (see *Tuberculous vertebral osteomyelitis:*, page 245), may be negative in 14% of cases[186].

Cultures: An attempt should be made to obtain direct cultures from the involved disc space. These may be obtained percutaneously with CT or other radiographic guidance (reported up to 60% positive culture rate; if available, a nucleotome provides a higher yield than e.g. Craig needle biopsy), or from intra-operative specimen (NB: surgery for open biopsy alone is usually not indicated). Staining for TB must be done in all cases.

Blood cultures may be positive in ≈ 50% of cases, and are helpful in guiding choice of antimicrobial agent when positive.

PATHOGENS

Staphylococcus aureus is the most common organism when direct cultures are obtained, followed by *S. albus* and *S. epidermidis* (*S. epidermidis* is the most common pathogen in POD). Gram negative organisms may also be found, including *E. coli* and *Proteus* species. Enteric flora in post-op discitis may due to undetected breach of the anterior longitudinal ligament with bowel perforation.

Pseudomonas aeruginosa may be more common in IV drug abusers.

H. flu is common in juvenile discitis (*see below*).

Tuberculous spondylitis (Pott's disease) may also occur.

TREATMENT

Outcome is generally good, and antibiotics together with immobilization are adequate treatment in ≈ 75% of cases. Occasionally surgery is required. Also see *Management*, page 250 under postoperative discitis for other aspects of management.

IMMOBILIZATION

Probably does not affect final outcome, but generally affords earlier pain relief, and may allow return to activity at an earlier time.

Most patients are started on strict bed rest, and are fitted for a plastic-type body jacket in which they are allowed to ambulate, and in which they remain for 6-8 weeks on the average. Alternative forms of immobilization include spica cast (provides better immobilization) and a corset-type brace.

ANTIBIOTICS
Current thinking is that most patients should receive antibiotics, guided by the results of the direct cultures when positive. In the 40-50% of cases where no organism is isolated, broad spectrum antibiotics should be used.

Two alternative treatment plans suggested:
1. treat with IV antibiotics for an arbitrary period of time, usually ≈ 4-6 weeks, followed with oral antibiotics for an additional 4-6 weeks
2. treat with IV antibiotics until the ESR normalizes, then change to PO

SURGERY
Required in only ≈ 25% of cases. Debridement may be done through the previous laminectomy site. However, if there has been significant bone loss and instability, then an anterior discectomy and fusion through a retroperitoneal approach may be required.

Surgery is reserved for:
1. situations where the diagnosis is uncertain, especially when neoplasm is a strong consideration (CT guided needle biopsy may help here)
2. decompression of neural structures, especially with associated spinal epidural abscess or compression by reactive granulation tissue. Ascending numbness, weakness, or onset of neurogenic bladder herald cauda equina syndrome
3. drainage of associated abscess, especially septated abscesses that might be recalcitrant to CT guided percutaneous needling
4. rarely, to fuse an unstable spine. Poorly endorsed in the face of active infection, especially since most go on to spontaneous fusion

Approaches
1. anterior discectomy and corpectomy removes the offending infected tissue, with strut graft using iliac crest (or, in the thoracic region, a posterolateral approach, with the strut made from the resected rib if large enough)
2. posterior laminectomy may be adequate for emergent decompression, but does not allow access to the site of pathology in cervical or thoracic regions

SPONTANEOUS DISCITIS

No recent history of surgery or instrumentation. Higher incidence of neurologic deficits and radiculopathy than with postoperative discitis (**POD**).

Two distinct types:
1. juvenile: more common; age usually < 20 yrs (*see below*)
2. adult: usually occurs in susceptible patients (diabetics, IV drug abusers)

JUVENILE DISCITIS
Age usually < 20 yrs, with a peak between 2-3 years. Probably due to the presence of primordial feeding arteries that nourish the nucleus pulposus and which involute at ≈ 20-30 yrs age. Lumbar spine is more commonly involved than thoracic or cervical. Common presentation: refusal to walk or stand progressing to refusal to sit in young children. Back pain is most common in children > 9 yrs age. Low grade fever may be present. ESR is usually 2-3 **x** normal. WBC is sometimes elevated. *H. flu* is a more commonly seen pathogen in this group.

In most cases, there is complete resolution in 9-22 weeks without recurrence in long-term follow-up studies[178 (p 365-71)]. Surgery is reserved for the rare case that progresses in spite of antibiotics, for spinal instability, or for recurrent cases.

Most authors reserve antibiotics for patients with[178 (p 365-71)]:
1. positive cultures (blood cultures or biopsy cultures)
2. elevated WBC count, constitutional symptoms, or high fever
3. poor response to rest or immobilization
4. neurologic sequelae (very rare)

Antibiotics should be given for a total of 4-6 weeks. Start with IV antibiotics, and when clinical symptoms improve convert to PO for the remainder of therapy.

POSTOPERATIVE DISCITIS

Unless otherwise specified, the following is based on a series of 27 post-op cases identified retrospectively at Duke[187].

EPIDEMIOLOGY

Incidence after lumbar discectomy[188]: 0.2-4% (realistic estimate is probably at the lower end of this range). May also occur after LP, myelogram, cervical laminectomy, lumbar sympathectomy, chemonucleolysis[189], discography (*see page 296*), fusions and other procedures. Very rare after ACDF. Risk factors include: advanced age, obesity, immunosuppression, systemic infection at the time of surgery.

PATHOPHYSIOLOGY

There is some controversy as to whether some cases of post-op discitis are not infectious[190], an autoimmune process has been implicated in some of these so-called "avascular" or "chemical" or "aseptic" discitis cases. These cases are less common than infectious ones. ESR and CRP abnormalities may be less pronounced in these patients, and biopsy of the disc space fails to grow organisms or show signs of infection (infiltrates of lymphocytes or PMNS) on microscopy[190].

In septic cases, various mechanisms for infection have been proposed: direct inoculation at the time of surgery, infection following aseptic necrosis of disc material...

CLINICAL

1. interval from operation to onset of symptoms: 3 days to 8 mos (most commonly 1-4 wks post-op, usually after an initial period of pain relief and recovery from surgery). 80% present by 3 wks
2. symptoms:
   A. moderate to (usually) severe back pain at the site of operation was the most common symptom, exacerbated by virtually any motion of the spine, often accompanied by paraspinal muscle spasms. Back pain is usually out of proportion to the findings
   B. fever (> 38° C in 9 patients; literature reports only 30-50% are febrile) and chills
   C. pain radiating to hip, leg, scrotum, groin, abdomen or perineum (true sciatica is uncommon)
3. signs: all had paravertebral muscle spasm and limited range of motion of the spine. 13 were virtually immobilized by pain. Point tenderness over infected spine occurred in 9, expressible pus in 2 (literature reports 0-8%). No new neurologic deficits were noted. Only 10-12% have associated wound infection[182]
4. lab findings:
   • ESR: 26/27 had ESR > 20 mm/hr (60 = ave.; > 40 in 17 patients; > 100 in 5 patients; the single patient < 20 was on steroids). ESR increases after uncomplicated discectomy, peaking at 2-5 days, and can fluctuate for 3-6 weeks before normalizing[191]. An elevated ESR that never decreases after surgery is a strong indicator of discitis
   • C-reactive protein (**CRP**)[191]: an acute phase protein synthesized by hepatocytes that may be a more specific indicator of post-op infection than ESR because of rapid decomposition. In the absence of discitis, CRP peaks ≈ 2-3 days post-op (to 46 ± 21 mg/L after lumbar microdiscectomy, 92 ± 47 mg/L after conventional lumbar discectomy, 70 ± 23 mg/L after anterior lumbar fusion, and 173 ± 39 mg/L after PLIF), and returns to normal values of < 10 mg/L (= 1 mg/dl) between 5-14 days post op
   • WBC: elevated > 10,000 in only 8/27 (literature: 18-30%)

RADIOGRAPHIC EVALUATION

Also, see *Radiographic evaluation*, page 246 under *Discitis in general*.

In postoperative discitis (**POD**), the average time from surgery to changes on plain x-ray is 3 mos (range: 1-8 mos). Changes are detectable earlier on polytomograms (3 wks to 2 mos). Average time from first change to spinal fusion: 2 yrs.

See *Table 12-21*. Most studies report *S. au-reus* as the most commonly identified organism, accounting for ≈ 60% of positive cultures[188], followed by other staph species. Also reported: Gram-negative organisms (including *E. coli*), *Strep viridans*, *Streptococcus species* anaerobes, TB and fungi.

Blood cultures were positive in 2 of 6 (both *S. aureus*).

For culture techniques, *see below*.

Table 12-21   Culture results
(14 patients, Craig needle biopsy)

Organism	No. of patients
Staphylococcus epidermidis	4
S. aureus	3
No growth	7

MANAGEMENT

1. admitting labs (in addition to routine): ESR, C-reactive protein, CBC, blood cultures
2. analgesics + muscle relaxants (e.g. diazepam (Valium®) 10 mg PO TID)
3. antibiotics:
   * IV antibiotics for 1-6 wks (or until ESR decreases), then PO for 1-6 mos (typically 6 weeks)
   * most start with anti-staphylococcal antibiotics (initial empiric therapy: vancomycin + PO rifampin) and a broad spectrum antibiotic (e.g. cefizox), modify based on sensitivities if positive cultures are obtained
4. activity restriction (one of the following used, usually until significant pain relief):
   * spinal immobilization with spica cast or plastic body jacket
   * strict bed rest
   * activity with corset
5. some authors recommend steroid therapy initially to assist pain relief
6. cultures: performed if radiographs suspicious, usually performed utilizing percutaneous CT-guided technique
   A. sites
      1. disc aspiration if evidence of disc space involvement
      2. needling of paraspinal mass if present
   B. send cultures for the following:
      1. stains
         a. Gram stain
         b. fungal stain
         c. AFB stain
      2. culture
         a. routine cultures: aerobic and anaerobic
         b. fungal culture: this is not only helpful for fungus, but since these cultures are kept for longer period and any growth that occurs will be further characterized, fastidious or indolent bacterial organisms may sometimes be identified
         c. TB culture
7. 3 patients in Duke series underwent anterior discectomy and fusion after unsuccessful medical therapy

OUTCOME

9 patients developed bony bridging in 12-18 mos; 10 developed bony fusion in 18-24 mos.

All patients eventually become pain free (or significantly improve). This is not the case in all series, where some report 60% were pain free at F/U, others found slight back pain in most patients, and yet others report severe chronic LBP in 75%[188]. 67-88% return to their previous work, and 12-25% received disability pension; these numbers are similar to the outcome from disc surgery in general.

No difference in outcome was found for the various activity restrictions specified, except for earlier pain relief with first two types listed above.

12.16. References

1. Kaiser A B: Antimicrobial prophylaxis in surgery. N Engl J Med 315: 1129-38, 1986.
2. Frame P T, Watanakunakorn C, McLaurin R L: Penetration of nafcillin, methicillin, and cefazolin into human brain tissue. Neurosurgery 12: 142-7, 1983.
3. Kernodle D S, Classen D C, Burke J P, et al.: Failure of cephalosporins to prevent staphylococcal aureus surgical wound infections. JAMA 263: 961-6, 1990.
4. Barker F G: Efficacy of prophylactic antibiotics for craniotomy: A meta-analysis. Neurosurgery 35: 484-92, 1994.
5. Young R F, Lawner P M: Perioperative antibiotic prophylaxis for prevention of postoperative neurosurgical infection. J Neurosurg 66: 701-5, 1987.
6. Baltas I, Tsoulfa S, Sakellariou P, et al.: Posttraumatic meningitis: Bacteriology, hydrocephalus, and outcome. Neurosurgery 35: 422-7, 1994.
7. Eljamel M S M, Foy P M: Post-traumatic CSF fistulae, the case for surgical repair. Br J Neurosurg 4: 479-83, 1990.
8. Lewin W: Cerebrospinal fluid rhinorrhea in closed head injuries. Clin Neurosurg 12: 237-52, 1966.
9. Horwitz N H, Levy C S: Comment on Baltas I, et al.: Posttraumatic meningitis: Bacteriology, hydrocephalus, and outcome. Neurosurgery 35: 426, 1994.
10. Yogev R: Cerebrospinal fluid shunt infections: A personal view. Pediatr Infect Dis 4: 113-8, 1985.
11. Ammirati M, Raimondi A: Cerebrospinal fluid shunt infections in children: A study of the relationship between the etiology of the hydrocephalus, age at the time of shunt placement, and infection. Childs Nerv Syst 3: 106-9, 1987.
12. McLone D, Czyzewski D, Raimondi A, et al.: Central nervous system infection as a limiting factor in the intelligence of children with myelomeningocele. Pediatrics 70: 338-42, 1982.
13. Amacher A L, Wellington J: Infantile hydrocephalus: Long-term results of surgical therapy. Childs Brain 11: 217-29, 1984.
14. O'Brien M, Parent A, Davis B: Management of ventricular shunt infections. Childs Brain 5: 304-9, 1979.
15. Wald S L, McLaurin R L: Shunt-associated glomerulonephritis. Neurosurgery 3: 146-50, 1978.
16. Section of Pediatric Neurosurgery of the American Association of Neurological Surgeons, (ed.) Pediatric neurosurgery. 1st ed., Grune and Stratton, New York, 1982.
17. Frame P T, McLaurin R L: Treatment of CSF shunt infections with intrashunt plus oral antibiotic therapy. J Neurosurg 60: 354-60, 1984.
18. James H E, Walsh J W, Wilson H D, et al.: Prospective randomized study of therapy in cerebrospinal fluid shunt infection. Neurosurgery 7: 459-63, 1980.
19. Steinbok P, Cochrane D D, Kestle J R W: The significance of bacteriologically positive ventriculoperitoneal shunt components in the absence of other signs of shunt infection. J Neurosurg 84: 617-23, 1996.
20. Shektman A, Granick M S, Solomon M P, et al.: Management of infected laminectomy wounds. Neurosurgery 35: 307-9, 1994.
21. Kurz A, Sessler D I, Lenhardt R: Perioperative normothermia to reduce the incidence of surgical-wound infection and shorten hospitalization. N Engl J Med 334: 1209-15, 1996.
22. Dernbach P D, Gomez H, Hahn J: Primary closure of infected spinal wounds. Neurosurgery 26: 707-9, 1990.
23. Ebersold M J: Comment on Shektman A, et al.: Primary closure of infected spinal wounds. Neurosurgery 35: 309, 1994.
24. Listinsky J L, Wood B P, Ekholm S E: Parietal osteomyelitis and epidural abscess: A delayed complication of fetal monitoring. Pediatr Radiol 16: 150-1, 1986.
25. Bullitt E, Lehman R A W: Osteomyelitis of the skull. Surg Neurol 11: 163-6, 1979.
26. Mamelak A N, Mampalam T J, Obana W G, et al.: Improved management of multiple brain abscesses: A combined surgical and medical approach. Neurosurgery 36: 76-86, 1995.
27. Takeshita M, Kagawa M, Yato S, et al.: Current treatment of brain abscess in patients with congenital cyanotic heart disease. Neurosurgery 41: 1270-9, 1997.
28. Kanter M C, Hart R G: Neurologic complications of infective endocarditis. Neurology 41: 1015-20, 1991.
29. Garvey G: Current concepts of bacterial infections of the central nervous system: Bacterial meningitis and bacterial brain abscess. J Neurosurg 59: 735-44, 1983.
30. Nunez D A, Browning G G: Risks of developing an otogenic intracranial abscess. J Laryngol Otol 104: 468-72, 1990.
31. Hollin S A, Hayashi H, Gross S W: Intracranial abscesses of odontogenic origin. Oral Surg 23: 277-93, 1967.
32. Williams F H, Nelms D K, McGaharan K M: Brain abscess: A rare complication of halo usage. Arch Phys Med Rehabil 73: 490-2, 1992.
33. Grimstad I A, Hirschberg H, Rootwelt K: 99mTc-hexamethylpropyleneamine oxime leukocyte scintigraphy and C-reactive protein levels in the differential diagnosis of brain abscesses. J Neurosurg 77: 732-6, 1992.
34. Fritz D P, Nelson P B: Brain abscess. In Central nervous system infectious diseases and therapy, Roos K L, (ed.). Marcel Dekker, New York, 1997: pp 481-98.
35. Britt R H, Enzmann D R: Clinical stages of human brain abscesses on serial CT scans after contrast infusion. J Neurosurg 59: 972-89, 1983.
36. Heineman H S, Braude A I, Osterholm J L: Intracranial suppurative disease. JAMA 218: 1542-7, 1971.
37. Black P, Graybill J R, Charache P: Penetration of brain abscess by systemically administered antibiotics. J Neurosurg 38: 705-9, 1973.
38. Rosenblum M L, Hoff J T, Norman D, et al.: Nonoperative treatment of brain abscesses in selected high-risk patients. J Neurosurg 52: 217-25, 1980.
39. Ruelle A, Zerbi D, Zuccarello M, et al.: Brain stem abscess treated successfully by medical therapy. Neurosurgery 28: 742-6, 1991.
40. Zeidman S M, Geisler F H, Olivi A: Intraventricular rupture of a purulent brain abscess: Case report. Neurosurgery 36: 189-93, 1995.
41. Stephanov S: Surgical treatment of brain abscess. Neurosurgery 22: 724-30, 1988.
42. Hollander D, Villemure J-G, Leblanc R: Thalamic abscess: A stereotactically treatable lesion. Appl Neurophysiol 50: 168-71, 1987.
43. Rosenblum M L, Hoff J T, Norman D, et al.: Decreased mortality from brain abscesses since advent of CT. J Neurosurg 49: 658-68, 1978.
44. Byrne E, Brophy B P, Pettett L V: Nocardia cerebral abscess: New concepts in diagnosis, management, and prognosis. J Neurol Neurosurg Psychiatry 42: 1038-45, 1979.

45. Awad I, Bay J W, Petersen J M: Nocardial osteomyelitis of the spine with epidural spinal cord compression - A case report. **Neurosurgery** 15: 254-6, 1984.

46. Stephanov S, Sidani A H: Intracranial subdural empyema and its management. A review of the literature with comment. **Swiss Surg** 8 (4): 159-63, 2002.

47. Kubik C S, Adams R D: Subdural empyema. **Brain** 66: 18-42, 1943.

48. Dill S R, Cobbs C G, McDonald C K: Subdural empyema: Analysis of 32 cases and review. **Clin Inf Dis** 20: 372-86, 1995.

49. Jacobson P L, Farmer T W: Subdural empyema complicating meningitis in infants: Improved prognosis. **Neurology** 31: 190-3, 1981.

50. Maniglia A J, Goodwin W J, Arnold J E, et al.: Intracranial abscess secondary to nasal, sinus, and orbital infections in adults and children. **Arch Otolaryngol Head Neck Surg** 115: 1424-9, 1989.

51. Garfin S R, Botte M J, Triggs K J, et al.: Subdural abscess associated with halo-pin traction. **J Bone Joint Surg** 70A: 1338-40, 1988.

52. Weisberg L: Subdural empyema: Clinical and computed tomographic correlations. **Arch Neurol** 43: 497-500, 1986.

53. Mauser H W, Ravijst R A P, Elderson A, et al.: Nonsurgical treatment of subdural empyema: Case report. **J Neurosurg** 63: 128-30, 1985.

54. Wilkins R H, Rengachary S S, (eds.): **Neurosurgery.** McGraw-Hill, New York, 1985.

55. Neils E W, Lukin R, Tomsick T A, et al.: Magnetic resonance imaging and computerized tomography scanning of herpes simplex encephalitis. **J Neurosurg** 67: 592-4, 1987.

56. Schroth G, Gawehn J, Thron A, et al.: The early diagnosis of herpes simplex encephalitis by MRI. **Neurology** 37: 179-83, 1987.

57. Whitley R J, Soong S-J, Dolin R, et al.: Adenosine arabinoside therapy of biopsy-proved herpes simplex encephalitis: National institute of allergy and infectious diseases collaborative antiviral study. **N Engl J Med** 297: 289-94, 1977.

58. Schlitt M J, Morawetz R B, Bonnin J M, et al.: Brain biopsy for encephalitis. **Clin Neurosurg** 33: 591-602, 1986.

59. Whitley R J, Cobbs C G, Alford C A, et al.: Diseases that mimic herpes simplex encephalitis: Diagnosis, presentation, and outcome. **JAMA** 262: 234-9, 1989.

60. Carmack M A, Twiss J, Enzmann D R, et al.: Multifocal leukoencephalitis caused by varicella-zoster virus in a child with leukemia: Successful treatment with acyclovir. **Pediatr Infect Dis J** 12: 402-6, 1993.

61. Horten B, Price R W, Jiminez D: Multifocal varicella-zoster virus leukoencephalitis temporally remote from herpes zoster. **Ann Neurol** 9: 251-66, 1981.

62. Johnson R T, Gibbs C J: Creutzfeldt-Jakob disease and related transmissible spongiform encephalopathies. **N Engl J Med** 339: 1994-2004, 1998.

63. Gajdusek D C: Unconventional viruses and the origin and disappearance of kuru. **Science** 197: 943-60, 1977.

64. Klitzman R: **The trembling mountain. A personal account of kuru, cannibals, and mad cow disease.** Plenum Trade, New York, 1998.

65. Heckmann J G, Lang C J G, Petruch F, et al.: Transmission of Creutzfeldt-Jakob disease via a corneal transplant. **J Neurol Neurosurg Psychiatry** 63: 388-90, 1997.

66. Hsiao K, Pruisner S B: Inherited human prion diseases. **Neurology** 40: 1820-7, 1990.

67. Bertoni J M, Brown P, Goldfarb L G, et al.: Familial Creutzfeldt-Jakob disease (codon 200 mutation) with supranuclear palsy. **JAMA** 268: 2413-5, 1992.

68. Will R G, Zeidler J W, Cousens S N, et al.: A new variant of Creutzfeldt-Jakob disease in the UK. **Lancet** 347: 921-5, 1996.

69. Duffy P, Wolf J, Collins G, et al.: Possible person to person transmission of Creutzfeldt-Jakob disease. **N Engl J Med** 290: 692-3, 1974.

70. Bernoulli C, Siegfried J, Baumgartner G, et al.: Danger of accidental person-to-person transmission of Creutzfeldt-Jakob disease by surgery. **Lancet** 1: 478-9, 1977.

71. Fradkin J E, Schonberger L B, Mills J L, et al.: Creutzfeldt-Jakob disease in pituitary growth hormone recipients in the United States. **JAMA** 265: 880-4, 1991.

72. Rosenberg R N, White C L, Brown P, et al.: Precautions in handling tissues, fluids and other contaminated materials from patients with documented or suspected Creutzfeldt-Jakob disease. **Ann Neurol** 12: 75-7, 1986.

73. Brown P, Gibbs C J, Amyx J L, et al.: Chemical disinfection of Creutzfeldt-Jakob virus. **N Engl J Med** 306: 1279-82, 1982.

74. Brown P, Cathala F, Castaigne P, et al.: Creutzfeldt-Jakob disease: Clinical analysis of a consecutive series of 230 neuropathologically verified cases. **Ann Neurol** 20: 597-602, 1986.

75. Finkenstaedt M, Szudra A, Zerr I, et al.: MR imaging of Creutzfeldt-Jakob disease. **Radiology** 199: 793-8, 1996.

76. Gertz H-J, Henkes H, Cervos-Navarro J: Creutzfeldt-Jakob disease: Correlation of MRI and neuropathologic findings. **Neurology** 38: 1481-2, 1988.

77. Otto M, Wiltfang J, Schutz E, et al.: Diagnosis of Creutzfeldt-Jakob disease by measurement of S100 protein in serum: Prospective case-control study. **Br Med J** 316: 577-82, 1998.

78. Harrington M G, Merril C R, Asher D M, et al.: Abnormal proteins in the cerebrospinal fluid of patients with Creutzfeldt-Jakob disease. **N Engl J Med** 315: 279-83, 1986.

79. Hsich G, Kenney K, Gibbs C J, et al.: The 14-3-3 brain protein in cerebrospinal fluid as a marker for transmissible spongiform encephalopatahies. **N Engl J Med** 335: 924-30, 1996.

80. Steinhoff B J, Räcker S, Herrendorf G, et al.: Accuracy and reliability of periodic sharp wave complexes in Creutzfeldt-Jakob disease. **Arch Neurol** 53: 162-6, 1996.

81. de Silva R, Patterson J, Hadley D, et al.: Single photon emission computed tomography in the identification of new variant Creutzfeldt-Jakob disease: Case reports. **Br Med J** 316: 593-4, 1998.

82. Hill A F, Butterworth R J, Joiner S, et al.: Investigation of variant Creutzfeldt-Jakob disease and other human prion diseases with tonsil biopsy samples. **Lancet** 353: 183-9, 1999.

83. Levy R M, Bredesen D E, Rosenblum M L: Neurological manifestations of the acquired immunodeficiency syndrome (AIDS): Experience at UCSF and review of the literature. **J Neurosurg** 62: 475-95, 1985.

84. Simpson D M, Tagliati M: Neurologic manifestations of HIV infection. **Ann Intern Med** 121: 769-85, 1994.

85. Berger J R, Kaszovitz B, Post J D, et al.: Progressive multifocal leukoencephalopathy associated with human immunodeficiency virus infection: A review of the literature with a report of sixteen cases. **Ann Intern Med** 107: 78-87, 1987.

86. Ciricillo S F, Rosenblum M L: Use of CT and MR imaging to distinguish intracranial lesions and to define the need for biopsy in AIDS patients. **J Neurosurg** 73: 720-24, 1990.

87. Chaisson R E, Griffin D E: Progressive multifocal leukoencephalopathy in AIDS. **JAMA** 364: 79-82, 1990.

88. Jean W C, Hall W A: Management of cranial and spinal infections. **Contemp Neurosurg** 20 (9): 1-10, 1998.

89. Demeter L M: *Jc, bk, and other polyomaviruses; progressive multifocal leukoencephalopathy.* In **Mandell, douglas and bennett principles and practice of infectious diseases,** Mandell G L and Bennett J E, (eds.). Churchill Livingstone, New York, 4th edition ed., 1995, Vol. 2: pp 1400-6.

90. Krupp L B, Lipton R B, Swerdlow M L, *et al.*: Progressive multifocal leukoencephalopathy: Clinical and radiographic features. **Ann Neurol** 17: 344-9, 1985.

91. Berger J R, Mucke L: Prolonged survival and partial recovery in AIDS-associated progressive multifocal leukoencephalopathy. **Neurology** 38: 1060-5, 1988.

92. Elliot B, Aromin I, Gold R, *et al.*: 2.5 year remission of AIDS-associated progressive multifocal leukoencephalopathy with combined antiretroviral therapy. **Lancet** 349: 850, 1997.

93. Johns D R, Tierney M, Felenstein D: Alterations in the natural history of neurosyphilis by concurrent infection with the human immunodeficiency virus. **N Engl J Med** 316: 1569-92, 1987.

94. Lukehart S A, Hook E W, Baker-Zander S A, *et al.*: Invasion of the central nervous system by treponema pallidum: Implications for diagnosis and treatment. **Ann Int Med** 109. 855-62, 1988.

95. Centers for Disease Control: Recommendations for diagnosing and treating syphilis in HIV-infected patients. **MMWR** 37: 600-2, 1988.

96. Levy R M, Rosenbloom S, Perrett L V: Neuroradiologic findings in AIDS: A review of 200 cases. **AJNR** 7: 833-9, 1986.

97. Jarvik J G, Hesselink J R, Kennedy C, *et al.*: Acquired immunodeficiency syndrome: Magnetic resonance patterns of brain involvement with pathologic correlation. **Arch Neurol** 45: 731-6, 1988.

98. Sadler M, Brink N S, Gazzard B G: Management of intracerebral lesions in patients with HIV: A retrospective study with discussion of diagnostic problems. **Q J Med** 91: 205 17, 1998.

99. Schwaighofer B W, Hesselink J R, Press G A, *et al.*: Primary intracranial CNS lymphoma: MR manifestations. **AJNR** 10: 725-9, 1989.

100. So Y T, Beckstead J H, Davis R L: Primary central nervous system lymphoma in acquired immune deficiency syndrome: A clinical and pathological study. **Ann Neurol** 20: 566-72, 1986.

101. Cinque P, Brytting M, Vago L, *et al.*: Epstein-Barr virus DNA in cerebrospinal fluid from patients with AIDS-related primary lymphoma of the central nervous system. **Lancet** 342: 398-401, 1991.

102. Cohn J A, Meeking M C, Cohen W, *et al.*: Evaluation of the policy of empiric treatment of suspected toxoplasma encephalitis in patients with the acquired immunodeficiency syndrome. **Am J Med** 86: 521-7, 1989.

103. Chappell E T, Guthrie B L, Orenstein J: The role of stereotactic biopsy in the management of HIV-related focal brain lesions. **Neurosurgery** 30: 825-9, 1992.

104. Levy R M, Russell E, Yungbluth M, *et al.*: The efficacy of image-guided stereotactis brain biopsy in neurologically symptomatic acquired immunodeficiency syndrome patients. **Neurosurgery** 30: 186-90, 1992.

105. Nicolato A, Gerosa M, Piovan E, *et al.*: Computerized tomography and magnetic resonance guided stereotactic brain biopsy in non-immunocompromised and AIDS patients. **Surg Neurol** 48: 267-77, 1997.

106. Nocton J J, Steere A C: Lyme disease. **Adv Int Med** 40: 69-117, 1995.

107. Pachner A R, Steere A C: The triad of neurologic manifestations of Lyme disease: Meningitis, cranial neuritis, and radiculoneuritis. **Neurology** 35: 47-53, 1985.

108. Pachner A R, Duray P, Steere: Central nervous sys-

tem manifestations of Lyme disease. **Arch Neurol** 46: 790-5, 1990.

109. Steere A C, Schoen R T, Taylor E: The clinical evolution of Lyme arthritis. **Ann Intern Med** 107: 735-31, 1987.

110. Centers for Disease Control: Lyme disease - Connecticut. **MMWR** 37: 1-3, 1988.

111. Sigal L H: Lyme disease overdiagnosis: Cause and cure. **Hosp Pract** 31: 13-5, 1996 (editorial).

112. Weinstein A, Bujak D I: *Lyme disease: A review of its clinical features.* **NY State J Med.** 1989, pp 566-71.

113. Magnarelli L A: Current status of laboratory diagnosis for Lyme disease. **Am J Med** 98 (S4A): 10-2S, 1995.

114. Wilkse B, Scheirz G, Preac-Mursic V, *et al.*: Intrathecal production of specific antibodies against borrelia burgdorferi in patients with lymphocytic meningoradiculitis (Bannwarth's syndrome). **J Infect Dis** 153: 304-14, 1986.

115. Henriksson A, Link H, Cruz M, *et al.*: Immunoglobulin abnormalities in cerebrospinal fluid and blood over the course of lymphocytic meningoradiculitis (Bannwarth's syndrome). **Ann Neurol** 20: 337-45, 1986.

116. Treatment of Lyme disease. **Med Letter** 30: 65-6, 1988.

117. Steere A C: Lyme disease. **N Engl J Med** 321: 586-96, 1989.

118. Sotelo J, Escobedo F, Rodriguez-Carbaja, *et al.*: Therapy of parenchymal brain cysticercosis with praziquantel. **N Engl J Med** 310: 1001-7, 1984.

119. Sotelo J, Guerrero V, Rubio F: Neurocysticercosis: A new classification based on active and inactive forms. **Arch Intern Med** 145: 442-5, 1985.

120. Leblanc R, Knowles K F, Melanson D, *et al.*: Neurocysticercosis: Surgical and medical management with praziquantel. **Neurosurgery** 18: 419-27, 1986.

121. Wilson M, Bryan R T, Fried J A, *et al.*: Clinical evaluation of the cysticercosis enzyme-linked immunoelectrotransfer blot in patients with neurocysticercosis. **J Infect Dis** 164: 1007-9, 1991.

122. Enzman D R: *Cysticercosis.* In **Imaging of infections and inflammations of the central nervous system: Computed tomography, ultrasound, and nuclear magnetic resonance.** Raven Press, New York, 1984: pp 103-22.

123. Madrazo I, Renteria J A G, Paredes G, *et al.*: Diagnosis of intraventricular and cisternal cysticercosis by computerized tomography with positive intra ventricular contract medium. **J Neurosurg** 55: 947-51, 1981.

124. Apuzzo M L J, Dobkin W R, Zee C-S, *et al.*: Surgical considerations in treatment of intraventricular cysticercosis: An analysis of 45 cases. **J Neurosurg** 60: 400-7, 1984.

125. Wood J H: Comment on van Dellen J R, et al.: Praziquantel (pyrazinoisoquinalone) in active cerebral cysticercosis. **Neurosurgery** 22: 95-6, 1988.

126. Sotelo J, Penagos P, Escobedo F, *et al.*: Short course of albendazole therapy for neurocysticercosis. **Arch Neurol** 45: 1130-3, 1988.

127. Drugs for parasitic infections. **Med Letter** 37: 99-108, 1995.

128. Colli B O, Carlotti C G, Machado H R, *et al.*: Treatment of patients with intraventricular cysticercosis. **Contemp Neurology** 21 (21): 1-7, 1999.

129. McCormick G F, Zee C-S, Heiden J: Cysticercosis cerebri. **Arch Neurol** 39: 534-9, 1982.

130. Centers for Disease Control: Locally acquired neurocysticercosis. **MMWR** 41: 1-4, 1992.

131. Mendel E, Milefchik E N, Ahmadi J, *et al.*: Coccidioidomycotic brain abscess: Case report. **J Neurosurg** 80: 140-2, 1994.

132. Chuck S N, Sande M A: Infections with cryptococcus neoformans in the acquired immunodeficiency syndrome. **N Engl J Med** 321: 794-9, 1989.

133. Lan S, Chang W, Lu C, et al.: Cerebral infarction in chronic meningitis: A comparison of tuberculous meningitis and cryptococcal meningitis. Q J Med 94: 247-53, 2001.

134. Lane M, McBride J, Archer J: Steroid responsive late deterioration in *cryptococcus neoformans* variety *gattii* meningitis. Neurology 63: 713-4, 2004.

135. Saag M S, Powderly W G, Cloud G A, et al.: Comparison of amphotericin B with fluconazole in the treatment of acute AIDS-associated cryptococcal meningitis. The niaid mycoses study group and the AIDS clinical trials group. N Engl J Med 326 (2): 83-9, 1992.

136. Denning D W, Armstrong R W, Lewis B H, et al.: Elevated cerebrospinal fluid pressures in patients with cryptococcal meningitis and acquired immunodeficiency syndrome. Am J Med 91 (3): 267-72, 1991.

137. Park M K, Hospenthal D R, Bennett J E: Treatment of hydrocephalus secondary to cryptococcal meningitis by use of shunting. Clin Infect Dis 28 (3): 629-33, 1999.

138. Bach M C, Tally P W, Godofsky E W: Use of cerebrospinal fluid shunts in patients having acquired immunodeficiency syndrome with cryptococcal meningitis and uncontrollable intracranial hypertension. J Neurosurg 41: 1280-3, 1997.

139. Liliang P C, Liang C L, Chang W N, et al.: Use of ventriculoperitoneal shunts to treat uncontrollable intracranial hypertension in patients who have cryptococcal meningitis without hydrocephalus. Clin Infect Dis 34 (12): E64-8, 2002.

140. Cahill D W: Infections of the spine. Contemp Neurosurg 15: 1-8, 1993.

141. Baker A S, Ojemann R G, Swartz M N, et al.: Spinal epidural abscess. N Engl J Med 293: 463-8, 1975.

142. Nussbaum E S, Rigamonti D, Standiford H, et al.: Spinal epidural abscess: A report of 40 cases and review. Surg Neurol 38: 225-31, 1992.

143. Danner R L, Hartman B J: Update of spinal epidural abscess: 35 cases and review of the literature. Rev Infect Dis 9: 265-74, 1987.

144. Curry W T, Jr., Hoh B L, Amin-Hanjani S, et al.: Spinal epidural abscess: Clinical presentation, management, and outcome. Surg Neurol 63 (4): 364-71; discussion 371, 2005.

145. Hlavin M L, Kaminski H J, Ross J S, et al.: Spinal epidural abscess: A ten-year perspective. Neurosurgery 27: 177-84, 1990.

146. Spiegelmann R, Findler G, Faibel M, et al.: Postoperative spinal epidural empyema: Clinical and computed tomography features. Spine 16: 1146-9, 1991.

147. Browder J, Meyers R: Pyogenic infections of the spinal epidural space. Surgery 10: 296-308, 1941.

148. Russell N A, Vaughan R, Morley T P: Spinal epidural infection. Can J Neurol Sci 6: 325-8, 1979.

149. Heusner A P: Nontuberculous spinal epidural infections. N Engl J Med 239: 845-54, 1948.

150. Koppel B S, Tuchman A J, Mangiardi J R, et al.: Epidural spinal infection in intravenous drug abusers. Arch Neurol 45: 1331-7, 1988.

151. Abdel-Magid R A, Kotb H I M: Spinal epidural abscess after spinal anesthesia: A favorable outcome. Neurosurgery 27: 310-1, 1990.

152. Loarie D J, Fairley H B: Epidural abscess following spinal anesthesia. Anesth Analg 57: 351-3, 1978.

153. Strong W E: Epidural abscess associated with epidural catheterization: A rare event? Report of two cases with markedly delayed presentation. Anesthesiology 74: 943-6, 1991.

154. Bergman I, Wald E R, Meyer J D, et al.: Epidural abscess and vertebral osteomyelitis following serial lumbar punctures. Pediatrics 72: 476-80, 1983.

155. Rea G L, McGregor J M, Miller C A, et al.: Surgical treatment of the spontaneous spinal epidural abscess. Surg Neurol 37: 274-9, 1992.

156. Kaufman D M, Kaplan J G, Litman N: Infectious agents in spinal epidural abscesses. Neurology 30: 844-50, 1980.

157. Post M J D, Sze G, Quencer R M, et al.: Gadolinium-enhanced MR in spinal infection. J Comput Assist Tomogr 14: 721-9, 1990.

158. Post M J D, Quencer R M, Montalvo B M, et al.: Spinal infection: Evaluation with MR imaging and intraoperative ultrasound. Radiology 169: 765-71, 1988.

159. Sandhu F S, Dillon W P: Spinal epidural abscess: Evaluation with contrast-enhanced MR imaging. AJNR 158: 1087-93, 1991.

160. Kirzner H, Oh Y K, Lee S H: Intraspinal air: A CT finding of epidural abscess. AJR 151: 1217-8, 1988.

161. Leys D, Lesoin F, Viaud C, et al.: Decreased morbidity from acute bacterial spinal epidural abscess using computed tomography and nonsurgical treatment in selected patients. Ann Neurol 17: 350-5, 1985.

162. Mampalam T J, Rosegay H, Andrews B T, et al.: Nonoperative treatment of spinal epidural infections. J Neurosurg 71: 208-10, 1989.

163. Hanigan W C, Asner N G, Elwood P W: Magnetic resonance imaging and the nonoperative treatment of spinal epidural abscess. Surg Neurol 34: 408-13, 1990.

164. Verner E F, Musher D M: Spinal epidural abscess. Med Clin North Am 69: 375-84, 1985.

165. Curling O D, Gower D J, McWhorter J M: Changing concepts in spinal epidural abscess: A report of 29 cases. Neurosurgery 27: 185-92, 1990.

166. Pereira C E, Lynch J C: Spinal epidural abscess: An analysis of 24 cases. Surg Neurol 63 Suppl 1: S26-9, 2005.

167. Schmorl G, Junghanns H: The human spine in health and disease. Grune & Stratton, New York, 1971.

168. Waldvogel F A, Vasey H: Osteomyelitis: The past decade. N Engl J Med 303: 360-70, 1980.

169. Holzman R S, Bishko R: Osteomyelitis in heroin addicts. Ann Intern Med 75: 693-6, 1971.

170. Cahill D W, Love L C, Rechtine G R: Pyogenic osteomyelitis of the spine in the elderly. J Neurosurg 74: 878-86, 1991.

171. Eismont F J, Bohlman H H, Soni P L, et al.: Pyogenic and fungal vertebral osteomyelitis with paralysis. J Bone Joint Surg 65A: 19-29, 1983.

172. Burke D R, Brant-Zawadzki M B: CT of pyogenic spine infection. Neuroradiology 27: 131-7, 1985.

173. Sapico F L, Montgomerie J Z: Pyogenic vertebral osteomyelitis: Report of nine cases and review of the literature. Rev Infect Dis 1: 754-76, 1979.

174. Skaf G S, Fehlings M G, Bouclaous C H: Medical and surgical management of pyogenic and nonpyogenic spondylodiscitis: Part I. Contemp Neurosurg 26 (19): 1-5, 2004.

175. Modic M T, Feiglin D H, Piraino D W, et al.: Vertebral osteomyelitis: Assessment using MR. Radiology 157: 157-66, 1985.

176. Rath S A, Nelf U, Schneider O, et al.: Neurosurgical management of thoracic and lumbar vertebral osteomyelitis and discitis in adults: A review of 43 consecutive surgically treated patients. Neurosurgery 38: 926-33, 1996.

177. Skaf G S, Fehlings M G, Bouclaous C H: Medical and surgical management of pyogenic and nonpyogenic spondylodiscitis: Part II. Contemp Neurosurg 26 (20): 1-5, 2004.

178. Rothman R H, Simeone F A, (eds.): The spine. 3rd ed., W.B. Saunders, Philadelphia, 1992.

179. Kinnier W S A: *Tuberculosis of the skull and spine.* In Neurology. Edward Arnold, London, 1940, Vol. 1: pp 575-83.

180. Medical Research Council Working Party on Tuberculosis of the Spine: Controlled trial of short-course regimens of chemotherapy in the ambulatory treatment of spinal tuberculosis: Results at three years of

a study in Korea. **J Bone Joint Surg** 75B: 240-8, 1993.

181. Sullivan C R, Symmonds R E: Disk infections and abdominal pain. **JAMA** 188: 655-8, 1964.
182. Malik G M, McCormick P: Management of spine and intervertebral disc space infection. **Contemp Neurosurg** 10: 1-6, 1988.
183. Kemp H B S, Jackson J W, Jeremiah J D, *et al.*: Pyogenic infections occurring primarily in intervertebral discs. **J Bone Joint Surg** 55B: 698-714, 1973.
184. Boden S D, Davis D O, Dina T S, *et al.*: Postoperative diskitis: Distinguishing early MR imaging findings from normal postoperative disk space changes. **Radiology** 184: 765-71, 1992.
185. Kopecky K K, Gilmor R L, Scott J A, *et al.*: Pitfalls of CT in diagnosis of discitis. **Neuroradiology** 27: 57-66, 1985.
186. Lifeso R M, Weaver P, Harder E H: Tuberculous spondylitis in adults. **J Bone Joint Surg** 67A: 1405-13, 1985.
187. Rawlings C E, Wilkins R H, Gallis H A, *et al.*: Postoperative intervertebral disc space infection. **Neurosurgery** 13: 371-6, 1983.
188. Iversen E, Nielsen V A H, Hansen L G: Prognosis in postoperative discitis. A retrospective study of 111 cases. **Acta Orthop Scand** 63: 305-9, 1992.
189. Deeb Z L, Schimel S, Daffner R H, *et al.*: Intervertebral disk-space infection after chymopapain injection. **AJNR** 6: 55-8, 1985.
190. Fouquet B, Goupille P, Jattiot F, *et al.*: Discitis after lumbar disc surgery. Features of "aseptic" and "septic" forms. **Spine** 17: 356-8, 1992.
191. Thelander U, Larsson S: Quantitation of C-reactive protein levels and erythrocyte sedimentation rate after spinal surgery. **Spine** 17: 400-4, 1992.

13. Seizures

13.1.   Seizure classification

Definition of a seizure: an abnormal paroxysmal cerebral neuronal discharge that results in alteration of sensation, motor function, behavior or consciousness. Seizures may be classified by type, etiology, and by epileptic syndromes.

Classification of major seizure types[1-3]

1. primary **generalized**: bilaterally symmetrical and synchronous involving both cerebral hemispheres at the onset, no local onset, consciousness lost from the start. Represents ≈ 40% of all seizures[
   A. generalized tonic-clonic **(GTC)** (nee: grand-mal seizure): generalized seizure that evolves from tonic to clonic motor activity. This is a specific type and does <u>NOT</u> include partial seizures that generalize secondarily
   B. clonic seizures: fairly symmetric, bilateral synchronous semirhythmic jerking of the UE & LE, usually with elbow flexion and knee extension
   C. tonic seizures: sudden sustained increased tone with a characteristic guttural cry or grunt as air is forced through adducted vocal cords
   D. **absence** (nee: petit-mal seizure): impaired consciousness with mild or no motor involvement (*see below*)
      1. typical absences
      2. atypical absences: more heterogeneous with more variable EEG pattern then typical absence. Seizures may last longer
   E. myoclonic seizures: shocklike body jerks (1 or more in succession) with generalized EEG discharges
   F. atonic seizures (AKA astatic seizures or "drop attacks"): sudden brief loss of tone that may cause falls
2. **partial** (nee focal seizure): implies one hemisphere involved at onset. About 57% of all seizures. A new onset of partial seizure represents a structural lesion until proven otherwise
   A. simple partial seizure (no impairment of consciousness)
      1. with motor signs (including Jacksonian)
      2. with sensory symptoms (special sensory or somatosensory)
      3. with autonomic signs or symptoms
      4. with psychic symptoms (disturbance of higher cerebral function)
   B. complex partial seizure (many used to be classified as psychomotor seizure, often attributed to temporal lobe but they can arise from any cortical area): any alteration of consciousness, usually LOC or automatisms (including lip smacking, chewing, or picking with the fingers) with autonomic aura (usually an epigastric rising sensation)
      1. simple partial onset followed by impairment of consciousness (may have premonitory **aura**)
         a. without automatisms
         b. with automatisms
      2. with impairment of consciousness at onset
         a. without automatisms (impairment of consciousness only)
         b. with automatisms
   C. partial seizure with secondary generalization
      1. simple partial evolving to generalized
      2. complex partial evolving to generalized
      3. simple partial evolving to complex partial evolving to generalized
3. unclassified epileptic seizures: ≈ 3% of all seizures

Classification by etiology (and some epileptic syndromes)
This list is not all inclusive (see reference[2, 3]).

1. **symptomatic** (AKA "secondary"): seizures of known etiology (e.g. CVA, tumor…)
   A. temporal lobe epilepsies:
      1. mesial temporal sclerosis: *see below*
2. **idiopathic** (AKA "primary"): no underlying cause. Includes:
   A. juvenile myoclonic epilepsy: *see below*
3. **cryptogenic**: seizures presumed to be symptomatic but with unknown etiology
   A. West syndrome (infantile spasms, Blitz-Nick-Salaam Krämpfe): *see below*
   B. Lennox-Gastaut syndrome: *see below*
4. special syndromes: situation-related seizures
   A. febrile seizures: *see page 264*
   B. seizures occurring only with acute metabolic or toxic event: e.g. alcohol

KEY distinctions (having therapeutic implications)

In generalized tonic-clonic seizures: primary generalized vs. partial with secondary generalization (often, local onset may not be observed).

In staring spells: absence vs. complex partial.

EPILEPSY

A disorder, not a single disease. Characterized by recurrent (2 or more), unprovoked seizures.

ABSENCE SEIZURE

Formerly called petit-mal seizure. Impaired consciousness with mild or no motor involvement (automatisms occur more commonly with bursts lasting > 7 secs). No post-ictal confusion. Aura rare. May be induced by hyperventilation x 2-3 mins. EEG shows **spike and wave** at exactly 3 per second.

UNCINATE SEIZURES

Obsolete term: "uncal fits". Seizures originating in the inferior medial temporal lobe, usually in the hippocampal region. May produce olfactory hallucinations (kakosmia or cacosmia: the perception of bad odors where none exist).

MESIAL TEMPORAL SCLEROSIS[4, 5]

The most common cause of intractable temporal lobe epilepsy. Specific pathologic basis: hippocampal sclerosis (cell loss in hippocampus on one side). Characteristics are shown in *Table 13-1*. For differential diagnosis, *see page 938*.

Adult seizures are initially responsive to medical therapy but become more varied and refractory, and may respond to seizure surgery.

JUVENILE MYOCLONIC EPILEPSY[7]

Sometimes called bilateral myoclonus. 5-10% of cases of epilepsy. An idiopathic generalized epilepsy syndrome with age-related onset consisting of 3 seizure types:
1. myoclonic jerks: predominantly after waking
2. generalized tonic-clonic seizures
3. absence

EEG → polyspike discharges. Strong family history (some studies showing linkage to the HLA region on the short arm of chromosome 6). Most responsive to depakene.

Table 13-1 Syndrome of mesial temporal-lobe epilepsy[6]

History
• higher incidence of complicated febrile seizures than in other types of epilepsy
• common family history of epilepsy
• onset in latter half of first decade of life
• auras in isolation are common
• infrequent secondarily generalized seizures
• seizures often remit for several years until adolescence or early adulthood
• seizures often become medically refractory
• common interictal behavioral disturbances (especially depression)

Clinical features of seizures
• most have aura (especially epigastric, emotional, olfactory or gustatory) x several secs
• CPS often begin with arrest & stare; oralimentary & complex automatisms are common. Posturing of contralateral arm may occur. Seizure usually lasts 1-2 mins
• postictal disorientation, recent-memory deficit, amnesia of ictus and (in dominant hemisphere) aphasia usually lasts several mins

Neurologic and laboratory features
• neuro exam: normal except memory deficit
• MRI: hippocampal atrophy and signal alteration with ipsilateral dilatation of temporal horn of lateral ventricle
• unilateral or bilateral independent anterior temporal EEG spikes with maximal amplitude in basal electrodes
• external ictal EEG activity only with CPS, usually initial or delayed focal rhythmic onset pattern of 5-7 Hz, maximal in 1 basal temporal derivation
• interictal fluorodeoxyglucose PET scan: hypometabolism in temporal lobe and possibly ipsilateral thalamus and basal ganglia
• neuropsychological testing: memory dysfunction specific to involved temporal lobe
• Wada test: amnesia with contralateral amobarbital injection (*see page 282*)

WEST SYNDROME

This term is being used less frequently as it appears not to be a homogeneous group. Classically a seizure disorder that usually appears in first year of life, and consists of recurrent, gross flexion and occasionally extension of the trunk and limbs (massive myoclonus, AKA infantile spasms, AKA salaam seizures, AKA jackknife spasms). Seizures tend to diminish with age, often abating by 5 yrs. Usually associated with mental retardation. 50% may develop complex-partial seizures, some of the rest may develop Lennox-Gastaut syndrome (*see below*). An associated brain lesion may be found in some.

EEG → the majority show either interictal **hypsarrhythmia** (huge spike/wave plus slow wave resembling muscle artifact) or modified hypsarrhythmia at some point.

Usually dramatic response of seizures and EEG findings to ACTH or corticosteroids.

LENNOX-GASTAUT SYNDROME

Rare condition that begins in childhood as atonic seizures ("drop attacks"). Often develops into tonic seizures with mental retardation. Seizures are often polymorphic, difficult to treat medically, and may occur as often as 50 per day. May also present with status epilepticus. Approximately 50% of patients have reduced seizures with valproic acid. Corpus callosotomy may reduce the number of atonic seizures.

TODD'S PARALYSIS

A post-ictal phenomena in which there is partial or total paralysis usually in areas involved in a partial seizure. More common in patients with structural lesions as the source of the seizure. The paralysis usually resolves slowly over a period of an hour or so. Thought to be due to depletion of neurons in the wake of the extensive electrical discharges of a seizure. Other similar phenomena include post-ictal aphasia and hemianopsia.

13.1.1. Factors that lower the seizure threshold

Factors that lower the seizure threshold (i.e. make it easier to provoke a seizure) in individuals with or without a prior seizure history include many items listed under *Etiologies* of *New onset seizures* (*see below*) as well as:
1. sleep deprivation
2. hyperventilation
3. photic stimulation (in some)
4. infection: systemic (febrile seizures, *see page 264*), CNS…
5. metabolic disturbances: electrolyte imbalance (especially profound hypoglycemia), pH disturbance (especially alkalosis), drugs… (*see below*)
6. head trauma: closed head injury, penetrating trauma (*see page 260*)
7. cerebral ischemia: CVA (*see below*)
8. "kindling": a concept that repeated seizures may facilitate the development of later seizures

13.2. Special types of seizures

13.2.1. New onset seizures

The age adjusted <u>incidence</u> of new onset seizures in Rochester, Minnesota was 44 per 100,000 person years[8].

Etiologies: In patients presenting with a first-time seizure, etiologies include (modified[9]):
1. following neurologic insult: either acutely (i.e. < 1 week) or remotely (> 1 week, and usually < 3 mos from insult)
    A. cerebrovascular accident (CVA, or stroke): 4.2% had a seizure within 14 days of a CVA. Risk increased with severity of stroke[10]
    B. head trauma: closed head injury, penetrating trauma (*see page 260*)
    C. CNS infection: meningitis, cerebral abscess, subdural empyema
    D. febrile seizures: *see page 264*

      E. birth asphyxia
2. underlying CNS abnormality
      A. congenital CNS abnormalities
      B. degenerative CNS disease
      C. CNS tumor: metastatic or primary
      D. hydrocephalus
      E. AVM
3. acute systemic metabolic disturbance
      A. electrolyte disorders: uremia, hyponatremia, hypoglycemia (especially profound hypoglycemia), hypercalcemia
      B. drug related, including:
          1. alcohol-withdrawal: *see page 261*
          2. cocaine toxicity: *see page 152*
          3. opioids (narcotics), principally associated with the following:
             a. propoxyphene (Darvon®)
             b. meperidine (Demerol®): may also cause delerium
             c. the street drug combination "T's and blues" (pentazocine (Talwin®) + the antihistamine tripelennamine)
          4. phenothiazine antiemetics
          5. with administration of flumazenil (Romazicon®) to treat benzodiazepine **(BDZ)** overdose (especially when BDZs are taken with other seizure lowering drugs such as tricyclic antidepressants or cocaine
          6. phencyclidine **(PCP)**: originally used as an animal tranquilizer
          7. cyclosporine: can affect Mg^{++} levels
      C. eclampsia
4. idiopathic

In 166 <u>pediatric</u> patients presenting to an emergency department with either a chief complaint of, or a discharge diagnosis of a first-time seizure[11]:
1. 110 were found to actually have either a recurrent seizure or a non-ictal event
2. of the 56 patients actually thought to have had a first-time seizure
      A. 71% were febrile seizures
      B. 21% were idiopathic
      C. 7% were "symptomatic" (hyponatremia, meningitis, drug intoxication...)

In a prospective study of 244 patients with a new-onset unprovoked seizure, only 27% had further seizures during follow-up[9, 12]. Recurrent seizures were more common in patients with a family seizure history, spike-and-waves on EEG, or a history of a CNS insult (CVA, head injury...). No patient seizure-free for 3 years had a recurrence. Following a second seizure, the risk of further seizures was high.

EVALUATION

Adults

A new-onset seizure in an <u>adult</u> in the absence of obvious cause (e.g. alcohol withdrawal) should prompt a search for an underlying basis (the onset of idiopathic seizures, i.e. epilepsy, is most common before or during adolescence). A CT or MRI (without and with enhancement) should be performed. A systemic workup should be done to identify the presence of any factors listed previously (*see above*). If all this is negative, then an MRI should be performed if not already done. If this is negative also, a repeat study (CT or MRI) should be done in ≈ 6 months and at 1 and possibly 2 years to rule-out a tumor which might not be evident on the initial study.

Pediatrics

Among pediatric patients with first-time seizures, laboratory and radiologic evaluations were often costly and not helpful[11]. A detailed history and physical exam were more helpful.

MANAGEMENT

Management of an adult with the new onset of idiopathic seizures (i.e. no abnormality found on CT or MRI, no evidence of drug withdrawal) is controversial. In one study, an EEG was performed, which if normal was followed by a sleep deprived EEG with the following observations[13]:
1. there is substantial interobserver variation in interpreting such EEGs
2. if both EEGs were normal, the 2-yr recurrence rate of seizures was 12%
3. if one or both EEGs showed epileptic discharges, the 2-yr recurrence rate was 83%

4. the presence of nonepileptic abnormalities in one or both EEGs had a 41% 2-yr recurrence rate
5. the recurrence rate with focal epileptic discharges (87%) was slightly higher than for generalized epileptic discharges (78%)

The conclusion is that EEGs thus obtained have moderate predictive value, and may be factored into the decision of whether or not to treat such seizures with AEDs.

13.2.2. Posttraumatic seizures

❡ Key points
- 2 categories: early (≤ 7 days) and late (> 7 days) after head trauma
- anticonvulsants (**AEDs**) may be used to prevent <u>early</u> posttraumatic seizures (**PTS**) in patients at high risk for seizures (*see text*)
- prophylactic AEDs do NOT reduce the frequency of late PTS
- discontinue AEDs after 1 week except for cases meeting specific criteria (*see text*)

Posttraumatic seizures (**PTS**) are often divided (arbitrarily) into: early (occurring within 1 week of injury) and late (thereafter)[14]. There may be justification for a third category: "immediate", i.e. within minutes to an hour or so.

Early PTS (≤ 7 days after head trauma)

30% incidence in severe head injury ("severe" defined as: LOC > 24 hrs, amnesia > 24 hrs, focal neuro deficit, documented contusion, or intracranial hematoma) and ≈ 1% in mild to moderate injuries. Occurs in 2.6% of children < 15 yrs age with head injury causing at least brief LOC or amnesia[15].

Early PTS may precipitate adverse events as a result of elevation of ICP, alterations in BP, changes in oxygenation, and excess neurotransmitter release[16].

Late onset PTS (> 7 days after head trauma)

Estimated incidence 10-13% within 2 yrs after "significant" head trauma (includes LOC > 2 mins, GCS < 8 on admission, epidural hematoma...) for all age groups[17, 18]. Relative risk: 3.6 times control population. Incidence in severe head injury >> moderate > mild[15].

The incidence of early PTS is higher in children than adults, but late seizures are much less frequent in children (in children who have PTS, 94.5% develop them within 24 hrs of the injury[19]). Most patients who have not had a seizure within 3 yrs of penetrating head injury will not develop seizures[20]. Risk of late PTS in children does not appear related to the occurrence of early PTS (in adults: only true for mild injuries). Risk of developing late PTS may be higher after repeated head injuries.

Penetrating trauma

The incidence of PTS is higher here with penetrating head injuries than with closed head injuries (occurs in 50% of penetrating trauma cases followed 15 yrs[21]).

TREATMENT

A prospective double blind study of patients at high risk of PTS (excluding penetrating trauma) showed a 73% reduction of risk of <u>early</u> PTS by administering 20 mg/kg loading dose of PHT within 24 hrs of injury and maintaining high therapeutic levels; but after 1 week there was no benefit in continuing the drug (based on intention to treat)[22]. Carbamazepine (Tegretol®) has also been shown to be effective in reducing the risk of early PTS, and valproic acid is currently being studied[16].

Phenytoin has adverse cognitive effects when given long-term as prophylaxis against PTS[23].

TREATMENT GUIDELINES

Based on available information (*see above*) it appears that:
1. no treatment studied effectively impedes epileptogenesis
2. in high-risk patients (*see Table 13-2*), AEDS reduces the incidence of <u>early</u> PTS
3. however, no study has shown that reducing early PTS improves outcome
4. once epilepsy has developed, continued AEDs reduces recurrence seizures

The following are therefore offered as guidelines.

Initiation of AEDs

AEDs may be considered for short term use especially if a seizure could be detrimental[A]. Early posttraumatic seizures were effectively reduced when phenytoin was used for 2 weeks following head injury with no significant increased risk of adverse effects[24].

Option: begin AEDs (usually phenytoin or carbamazepine) within 24 hrs of injury in the presence of any of the high risk criteria shown in *Table 13-2* (modified[16, 19, 22, 25]). When using PHT, load with 20 mg/kg and maintain high therapeutic levels (*see page 271*). Switch to phenobarbital if PHT not tolerated.

Table 13-2 High risk criteria for PTS

1.	acute subdural, epidural, or intracerebral hematoma
2.	open-depressed skull fracture with parenchymal injury
3.	seizure within the first 24 hrs after injury
4.	Glasgow Coma Scale score < 10
5.	penetrating brain injury
6.	history of significant alcohol abuse
7.	± cortical (hemorrhagic) contusion on CT

Discontinuation of AEDs

1. taper AEDs after 1 week of therapy except in the following:
    A. penetrating brain injury
    B. development of late PTS (i.e. a seizure > 7 days following head trauma)
    C. prior seizure history
    D. patients undergoing craniotomy[26]
2. for patients not meeting the criteria to discontinue AEDs after 1 week (*see above*):
    A. maintain ≈ 6-12 mos of therapeutic AED levels
    B. recommend EEG to rule-out presence of a seizure focus before discontinuing AEDs (predictive value) for the following:
        1. repeated seizures
        2. presence of high risk criteria shown in *Table 13-2*.

13.2.3.   Alcohol withdrawal seizures

Also, see *Alcohol withdrawal syndrome*, page 149. The withdrawal syndrome may begin hours after the EtOH peak (*see page 150* for prevention and treatment). Ethanol withdrawal seizures are classically seen in up to 33% of habituated drinkers within 7-30 hours of cessation or reduction of ethanol intake. They typically consist of 1-6 tonic-clonic generalized seizures without focality within a 6 hour period[27]. Seizures usually occur before delerium develops. They may also occur during intoxication (without withdrawal).

The seizure risk persists for 48 hrs (risk of delerium tremens (**DTs**) continues beyond that), thus a single loading dose of PHT is frequently adequate for prophylaxis. However, since most EtOH withdrawal seizures are single, brief, and self-limited, PHT has not been shown to be of benefit in uncomplicated cases and is thus usually not indicated. Chlordiazepoxide (Librium®) or other benzodiazepines administered during detoxification reduces the risk withdrawal seizures[28] (*see page 150*).

Evaluation

The following patients should have a CT scan of the brain, and should be admitted for further evaluation as well as for observation for additional seizures or for DTs:
1. those with their first EtOH withdrawal seizure
2. those with focal findings
3. those having more than 6 seizures in 6 hrs
4. those with evidence of trauma

Other causes of seizure should also be considered, e.g. a febrile patient may require an LP to R/O meningitis.

Treatment

A brief single seizure may not warrant treatment, except as outlined below. A seizure that continues beyond 3-4 minutes may be treated with diazepam or lorazepam, with further measures used as in status epilepticus (*see page 264*) if seizures persist. Loading with phenytoin (18 mg/kg = 1200 mg/70 kg, *see page 271*) and long-term treatment is indicated for:
1. a history of previous alcohol withdrawal seizures
2. recurrent seizures after admission

A. acutely, seizures may elevate ICP, and may adversely affect blood pressure and oxygen delivery, and may worsen other injuries (e.g. spinal cord injury in the setting of an unstable cervical spine)[16]

3. history of a prior seizure disorder unrelated to alcohol
4. presence of other risk factors for seizure (e.g. subdural hematoma)

13.2.4. Nonepileptic seizures

AKA pseudoseizures (although some prefer not to use this term since it may connote voluntary feigning of seizures), with the term psychogenic seizures being preferred for nonepileptic seizures (**NES**) with a psychologic etiology (psychogenic seizures are real events and may not be under voluntary control)[29].

In a major medical referral center, 20% of patients with intractable seizures have NES. Up to 50% of these may have legitimate seizures at some time as well[30]. The hazard of NES is that patients may end up needlessly taking AEDs, which in some cases may worsen NES. Possible etiologies of NES are given in *Table 13-3*. Most NES are psychogenic.

DIFFERENTIATING NES FROM EPILEPTIC SEIZURES

Distinguishing between epileptic seizures (**ES**) and NES is a common clinical dilemma. There are unusual seizures that may fool experts[31]. Some frontal lobe and temporal lobe complex partial seizures may produce bizarre behaviors that do not correspond to classic ES findings and may not produce discernible abnormalities with scalp-electrode EEG (and therefore may be misdiagnosed even with video-EEG monitoring, although this is more likely with partial seizures than with generalized). A multidisciplinary team approach may be required.

History: Attempt to document: prodromal symptoms, precipitating factors, time and environment of Sz, mode and duration of progression, ictal and postictal events, frequency and stereotypy of manifestations. Determine if patient has history of psychiatric conditions, and if they are acquainted with individuals who have ES.

Suggestive of possible NES: multiple or variable seizure types (whereas ES is usually stereotypical), fluctuating level of consciousness, denial of correlation of Sz with stress.

Table 13-3 Differential diagnosis of nonepileptic seizures[29]

1. psychologic disorders (psychogenic seizure)
A. somatoform disorders: especially conversion disorder
B. anxiety disorders: especially panic attack and posttraumatic stress disorder
C. dissociative disorders
D. psychotic disorders
E. impulse control disorders
F. attention-deficit disorders*
G. factitious disorders: including Munchausen's syndrome
2. cardiovascular disorders
A. syncope
B. cardiac arrhythmias
C. transient ischemic attacks
D. breath-holding spells*
3. migraine syndromes
A. complicated migraines*
B. basilar migraines
4. movement disorders
A. tremors
B. dyskinesias
C. tics*, spasms
D. other (including shivering)
5. parasomnias & sleep-related disorders
A. night terrors*, nightmares*, somnambulism*
B. narcolepsy, cataplexy
C. rapid eye movement behavior disorder
D. nocturnal paroxysmal dystonia
6. gastrointestinal disorders
A. episodic nausea or colic*
B. cyclic vomiting syndrome*
7. other
A. malingering
B. cognitive disorders with episodic behavioral or speech symptoms
C. medication effects or toxicity
D. daydreams*

* usually encountered in children

Psychological testing: May help. Differences occur in ES and NES on the Minnesota Multiphasic Personality Inventory (**MMPI**) scales in hypochondriasis, depression hysteria, and schizophrenia[32].

Table 13-4 contrasts some features of true seizures vs. NES, and *Table 13-5* lists some features often associated with NES, however, no characteristics are definitively diagnostic of NES since a number of them may also occur with ES.

If any two of the following are demonstrated, 96% of time this will be NES:
1. out-of-phase clonic UE movement
2. out-of-phase clonic LE movement
3. no vocalization or vocalization at start of event

Features common to both true seizures and NES: verbal unresponsiveness, rarity of automatisms and whole-body flaccidity, rarity of urinary incontinence.

Prolactin levels after seizures

Transient elevations in human serum prolactin **(HSP)** levels occur following 80% of generalized motor, 45% of complex partial, and only 15% of simple partial seizures[33]. Peak levels are reached in 15-20 minutes, and gradually return to baseline over the subsequent hour[34-36]. It has been suggested that drawing a serum prolactin level shortly after a questionable seizure may be helpful in differentiating NES (which may have elevated cortisol levels but normal HSP levels[37]).

Table 13-4 Features of ES vs. NES[30]

Feature	Epileptic seizure	NES
% males	72%	20%
clonic UE movement		
in-phase	96%	20%
out-of-phase	0	56%
clonic LE movement		
in-phase	88%	16%
out-of-phase	0	56%
vocalizations		
none	16%	56%
start of seizure	24%	44%
middle	60% "epileptic cry"	0
types	only sounds of tonic or clonic respiratory muscle contraction	moans, screams, grunts, snorts, gagging, retching, understandable statements, gasps
head turning		
unilateral	64%	16%
side-to-side	8% (slow, low amplitude)	36% (violent, high amplitude)

Repetitive seizures are associated with progressively smaller HSP elevations[38], and no rise follows absence seizures or status epilepticus (whether convulsive or absence)[39]. Greater than twofold HSP elevations consistently follow seizures that produce intense widespread high frequency mesial temporal lobe discharges; whereas such elevations do not occur in seizures not involving these limbic structures[40].

Furthermore, there may be higher baseline HSP levels in cases with right-sided interictal EEG discharges compared to those with left-sided[41], and the presence of psychopathology may affect postictal HSP elevations[42].

Therefore, the presence of HSP peaks may be strongly indicative of true seizures, but the absence may be due to a variety of complex phenomena[43]. The overall classification accuracy is ≈ 72%[36].

Table 13-5 Features often associated with NES[29]

- frequent seizures despite therapeutic AEDs
- multiple different-physician visits
- lingering prodrome or gradual ictal onset (over minutes)
- prolonged duration (> 5 mins)
- manifestations altered by distraction
- suggestible or inducible seizures
- intermittent arrhythmic and out-of-phase activity
- fluctuating intensity and severity during Sz
- side-to-side rolling, pelvic thrusting, wild movements
- bilateral motor activity with preserved consciousness
- nonphysiologic spread of neurologic signs
- absence of labored breathing or drooling after generalized convulsion
- expression of relief or indifference
- crying or whimpering
- no postictal confusion or lethargy
- disproportionate postictal mental status changes
- absence of stereotypy

13.2.5.   Febrile seizures

Definitions[44]

febrile seizure	a seizure in infants or children associated with fever with no defined cause and unaccompanied by acute neurologic illness (includes seizures during vaccination fevers)
complex febrile seizure	a convulsion that lasts longer than 15 minutes, is focal, or multiple (more than one convulsion per episode of fever)
simple febrile seizure	not complex
recurrent febrile seizure	more than one episode of fever associated with seizures

Epidemiology[44]

Febrile convulsions are the most common type of seizure. Excluding children with pre-existing neurologic or developmental abnormalities, the prevalence of febrile seizures is ≈ 2.7% (range: 2-5% in U.S. children aged 6 mos-6 yrs). The risk for developing epilepsy after a simple febrile seizure is ≈ 1%, and for a complex febrile seizure is 6% (9% for prolonged seizure, 29% for focal seizure). An underlying neurological or developmental abnormality or a family history of epilepsy increases the risk of developing epilepsy.

Treatment

In one study, the IQ in the group treated with phenobarbital was 8.4 points lower (95% confidence interval) than the placebo group, and there remained a significant difference several months after discontinuing the drug[45]. Furthermore, there was no significant reduction in seizures in the phenobarbital group. And yet, no other drug really appears well suited to treating this entity: carbamazepine and phenytoin appear ineffective, valproate may be effective but has serious risks in the < 2 yrs age group. Given the low incidence (1%) of having *afebrile* seizures (i.e. epilepsy) after a simple febrile seizure and the fact that AEDs probably do not prevent this development, there is little support for prescribing anticonvulsants in these cases. The recurrence rate of febrile seizures in children with a history of one or more febrile seizure can be reduced by administering diazepam 3.3 mg/kg PO q 8 hrs during a febrile episode (temp > 38.1 °C) and continuing until 24 hrs after the fever subsided[46].

13.3.   Status epilepticus

Definition: More than 30 minutes of (1) continuous seizure activity, or (2) multiple seizures without full recovery of consciousness between seizures[47].

Types of status epilepticus
* generalized status
  1. convulsive: generalized convulsive tonic-clonic status epilepticus **(SE)** is the most frequent type[48]. A medical emergency
  2. absence[A]
  3. secondarily generalized: accounts for ≈ 75% of generalized SE
  4. myoclonic
  5. atonic (drop attack): especially in Lennox-Gastaut syndrome (*see page 258*)
* partial status (usually related to an anatomic abnormality)
  1. simple (AKA **epilepsy partialis continuans**)
  2. complex[A]: most often from frontal lobe focus. Urgent treatment is required
  3. secondarily generalized

Epidemiology

Incidence is ≈ 100,000 cases/year in the U.S. Most cases occur in young children (among children, 73% were < 5 yrs old[49]), the next most affected group is patients over age 60 yrs. In > 50% of cases, SE is the patient's first seizure[48].

Etiologies
  1. febrile seizures: a common precipitator in young patients. 5-6% of patients pre-

---

A. in status, these may present in **twilight state**

senting with SE have a history of prior febrile seizures

2. cerebrovascular accidents: the most commonly identified cause in the elderly
3. CNS infection: in children, most are bacterial, the most common organisms were *H. influenza* and *S. pneumoniae*
4. idiopathic: accounts for ≈ one-third (in children, usually associated with fever)
5. epilepsy: is present or is subsequently diagnosed in ≈ 50% of patients presenting with SE. About 10% of adults ultimately diagnosed as having epilepsy will present in SE
6. subtherapeutic AEDs in patient with a known seizure disorder
7. electrolyte imbalance: hyponatremia (most common in children, usually due to water intoxication[49]), hypoglycemia, hypocalcemia, uremia…
8. drug intoxication (especially cocaine)
9. alcohol withdrawal
10. traumatic brain injury
11. anoxia
12. tumor

In children < 1 yr age, 75% had an acute cause: 28% were secondary to CNS infection, 30% due to electrolyte disorders, 19% associated with fever[49]. In adults, a structural lesion is more likely. In an adult, the most common cause of SE is subtherapeutic AED levels in a patient with a known seizure disorder.

Features

Most common cause is a patient with a known seizure disorder having low AED levels for any reason (non-compliance, intercurrent infection preventing PO intake of meds). One out of six patients presenting with a first time seizure will present in status epilepticus **(SE)**. In most instances, SE is a manifestation of an acute insult to the brain.

Most cases of convulsive status in adults start as partial seizures that generalize.

Morbidity and mortality from SE

Mean duration of SE in patients without neurologic sequelae is 1.5 hrs (therefore, proceed to pentobarbital anesthesia before ≈ 1 hour of SE). Recent mortality: < 10-12% (only ≈ 2% of deaths are directly attributable to SE or its complications; the rest are due to the underlying process producing the SE). Mortality in lowest amongst children (≈ 6%[49]), patients with SE related to subtherapeutic AEDs, and patients with unprovoked SE[50]. The highest mortality occurs in elderly patients and those with SE resulting from anoxia or CVA[50]. 1% of patients die during the episode itself.

Morbidity and mortality is due to[51]:
1. CNS injury from repetitive electric discharges: irreversible changes begin to appear in neurons after as little as 20 minutes of convulsive activity. Cell death is very common after 60 mins
2. systemic stress from the seizure (cardiac, respiratory, renal, metabolic)
3. CNS damage by the acute insult that provoked the SE

13.3.1. General treatment measures for status epilepticus

Treatment is directed at stabilizing the patient, stopping the seizure, and identifying the cause (determining if there is an acute insult to the brain) and if possible also treating the underlying process. Although SE is defined for seizures lasting > 30 mins, aggressive anticonvulsant therapy is indicated for any seizure lasting > 10 mins. Treatment often must be initiated prior to the availability of tests to confirm the diagnosis.

• CPR if needed
• attend airway: oral airway if feasible. O_2 by nasal cannula or bag-valve-mask. Consider intubation if respirations compromised or if seizure persists > 30 min
• IV (2 if possible: 1 for phenytoin **(PHT)** (Dilantin®), not necessary if fosphenytoin is available): start with NS
• monitor: EKG & frequent blood pressure checks
• bloodwork: electrolytes (including glucose), Mg^{++}, Ca^{++}, phenytoin level, ABG. SE due to electrolyte imbalance responds more readily to correction than to AEDs[49]
• if CNS infection is a major consideration, perform LP for CSF analysis (especially in febrile children) unless contraindicated. WBC pleocytosis up to 80 x 10⁶/L can occur following SE (benign postictal pleocytosis), and these patients should be treated with antibiotics until infection can be ruled out by negative cultures

- general meds for unknown patient:
  1. glucose:
     A. for adults: thiamine 50-100 mg IV should precede glucose bolus (in case of thiamine deficiency, e.g. in EtOH abuse). NB: can precipitate Wernicke's encephalopathy in alcoholic patients (see page 151)
     B. if fingerstick glucose can be obtained immediately and it shows hypoglycemia, or if no fingerstick glucose can be done, give 25-50 ml of D50 IV push for adults (2 ml/kg of 25% glucose for peds). Be sure blood has been sent for definitive serum glucose first
  2. naloxone (Narcan®) 0.4 mg IVP (in case of narcotics)
  3. ± bicarbonate to counter acidosis (1-2 amps depending on length of seizure)
- administer specific anticonvulsants for seizures lasting > 10 mins (see below)
- EEG monitor if possible
- if paralytics are used (e.g. to intubate), use short acting agents and be aware that muscle paralysis alone may stop visible seizure manifestations, but does not stop the electrical seizure activity in the brain, which can lead to permanent damage

13.3.2. Medications for generalized convulsive status epilepticus

Table 13-6 shows a summary of medications for status epilepticus that are outlined in further detail below (modified management scheme[47, 52-54]). Items below in boxes are considered treatment of choice. "Peds" refers to patients ≤ 16 yrs of age. Drugs should be given IV (do not use IM route). If IV access is impossible, diazepam solution (not suppository) can be given rectally.

Protocol
1. give a benzodiazepine (main side effect: respiratory depression in ≈ 12%; be prepared to intubate). Do not give if seizures have already stopped. Onset of action is rapid (1-2 mins):

Table 13-6 Summary of medications for status epilepticus in average size adult
(see text for details)

A.	lorazepam (Ativan®) 4 mg IV slowly over 2 mins, may repeat after 5 mins
B.	simultaneously load with phenytoin* • 1200 mg if not already on phenytoin • 500 mg if on phenytoin (check level)
C.	phenobarbital IV (@ < 100 mg/min) until seizures stop (up to 1400 mg) (watch BP)
D.	if seizures continue > 30 mins, intubate and begin pentobarbital (see text)

* maximum rate for phenytoin IV is 50 mg/min; for fosphenytoin it is 150 mg PE/min (see page 272)

- lorazepam (Ativan®) **0.1 mg/kg** (range: 0.02-0.12 mg/kg → 4 mg average adult dose) IV at rate < 2 mg/min, repeat if ineffective q 5 mins up to 9 mg total[55]. Peds: 0.1 mg/kg, repeat if ineffective q 2-3 mins up to 5-6 mg total. If no IV access, the same dose is given rectally

OR

- diazepam (Valium®) 0.2 mg/kg (10 mg average adult dose) IV @ 5 mg/min, repeat if ineffective q 5 mins up to 3 additional doses. Peds: 0.2-0.5 mg/kg/dose with max 5 mg if < 5 yrs, max 10 mg if ≥ 5 yrs.
  Diazepam should routinely be followed by phenytoin to prevent recurrence. Rectal dose is 0.5 mg/kg of diazepam solution up to 20 mg max, and is usually absorbed in ≈ 10 mins

OR

- in pediatric patients with frequent seizures or prophylaxis of febrile seizures and no IV access, valproic acid is well absorbed rectally, and is administered at 20 mg/kg diluted in water or vegetable oil[47]

2. simultaneously <u>load</u> with phenytoin (Dilantin®) **(PHT)** as follows (do not worry about acutely overdosing, follow dosing <u>rates</u>, monitor BP for hypotension and EKG for arrhythmias). Conventional phenytoin must be given only in NS to prevent precipitation. After giving the following loading dose, start on maintenance (see page 271)

> A. if not already on phenytoin: Adult: load with 20 mg/kg phenytoin (1400 mg for 70 kg adult) (use 15 mg/kg for elderly patients), maximum rate for phenytoin < 50 mg/min (max rate for fosphenytoin is 150 mg PE/min). Peds: 20 mg/kg, rate < 1-3 mg/kg/min

B. if on PHT and a recent level is known: a rule of thumb is giving 0.74 mg/kg to an adult raises the level by ≈ 1 µg/ml

C. if on PHT and level not known: adult: give 500 mg @ < 50 mg/min

3. proceed to each following step if seizures continue:

A. PHT additional doses of 5 mg/kg @ < 50 mg/min up to a total of 30 mg/kg

B. either[A]

> - phenobarbital: up to 20 mg/kg IV (1400 mg for 70 kg) (start infusing @ < 100 mg/min until seizures stop), takes 15-20 min to work, watch BP (a myocardial depressant).
>   Peds: 5-10 mg/kg/dose q 20-30 min to max total 30-40 mg/kg.

Phenobarbital may be preferred to PHT in patients with PHT hypersensitivity, cardiac conduction abnormality, and in neonates and young children. Maintenance phenobarbital therapy should be instituted with 24 hours of the loading dose (see page 275)

OR

- diazepam (Valium®) drip: 100 mg diazepam in 500 ml D5W @ 40 ml/min (→ level of 0.2-0.8 µg/ml). Rarely used, levels hard to check

C. prepare to initiate general anesthesia, lidocaine may be tried to temporize as shown here (usually omitted)

- lidocaine 2-3 mg/kg IVP @ 25-50 mg/min, if effective follow with drip of 50-100 mg in 250 cc D5W @ 1-2 mg/min

D. if seizures continue > 30 minutes, intubate and institute "general anesthesia" by any of the following:

> pentobarbital: load with 15 mg/kg (range: 5-20 mg/kg) IV at a rate of 25 mg/min, then place on maintenance starting at 2.5 mg/kg/hr, follow EEG and titrate while maintaining burst suppression[56, 57] (sometimes up to 3 mg/kg/hr). Monitor BP, if hypotension occurs give fluids and dopamine (see page 662 for additional measures such as PA catheter). For breakthrough seizures, give additional 50 mg pentobarbital and increase maintenance rate by 0.5 mg/kg/h

OR

benzodiazepines:
- high-dose IV lorazepam (see below)
- or midazolam (Versed®): adult: 5-10 mg bolus at < 4 mg/min, followed by 0.05-0.4 mg/kg/hr drip. Data is limited, and use should be restricted to refractory SE[54]

OR

call anesthesiologist to initiate
- general inhalation anesthesia: isoflurane (Forane®) is the preferred agent (✖ avoid enflurane (Ethrane®), see page 1). NB: this requires an anesthesia machine and usually transport to the O.R., and cannot be maintained indefinitely. Rarely, neuromuscular junction blocking agents are required (NB: paralyzing the patient and thus halting the motor activity without stopping the epileptic activity is insufficient as continued seizure activity in itself is harmful, see page 265)

OR

- propofol anesthesia: Data is limited, and use should be restricted to refractory SE[54]. May have weak intrinsic epileptogenic properties

Efficacy

Diazepam stops seizures within 3 mins in 33%, within 5 mins in 80%. PHT stops seizures in 30% after 400 mg has been given. 63% of generalized tonic-clonic SE respond to benzodiazepine + PHT. PHT is slower to control status than diazepam, but lasts longer.

Lorazepam

Not FDA approved for seizures (may still be used as "off label" indication). Among

---

A. using both phenobarbital and a benzodiazepine (e.g. diazepam) is discouraged because of increased risk of respiratory depression

benzodiazepines, lorazepam (**LZP**) is preferred (diazepam (**DZP**) redistributes rapidly in fatty tissues[58], and seizures may recur within 10-20 minutes), but causes longer sedation. LZP aborts SE in 97% of cases, vs. 68% for DZP[59]. Also, less respiratory depression than with DZP. As with all benzodiazepines:

1. respiratory depression and hypotension are exacerbated when used with other depressants (including barbiturates…)
2. effectiveness in SE is reduced by prior maintenance on other benzodiazepines (e.g. clonazepam), but is not affected by the presence of other anticonvulsants
3. tachyphylaxis may develop so that subsequent doses are less effective[60]

High-dose IV lorazepam:

LZP may also be a less toxic alternative to pentobarbital burst suppression coma[61] because, among other things, LZP does not produce systemic hypotension (this may be artifactual since in this study, burst suppression was *not* an endpoint with LZP as it is with most barbiturate protocols). It may be given as a continuous infusion or as frequent intermittent boluses. The continuous infusion protocol used by Labar[61] is shown in *Table 13-7*.

Medications to avoid in status epilepticus

1. narcotics
2. phenothiazines: including promethazine (Phenergan®)
3. neuromuscular blocking agents in the absence of AED therapy: seizures may continue and cause neurologic injury but would not be clinically evident (*see page 265*)

Table 13-7 Protocol for high-dose IV lorazepam for status epilepticus

1. used for failure to control SE with PHT level > 20 µg/ml and phenobarbital level > 40 µg/ml
2. begin IV infusion of LZP at 1 mg/hr under EEG monitoring
3. titrate up at increments of 1 mg/hr q 15 mins until ictal activity stops (rate of LZP required for seizure control varied from 0.3-9 mg/hr)
4. maintain seizure free **x** 24 hrs with LZP, keeping therapeutic levels of PHT and phenobarbital
5. then, titrate LZP down by 1 mg/hr q 1 hr as long as no seizure on EEG.
6. if SE recurs, reinstitute high dose LZP as in step *3.* above

13.3.3. Miscellaneous status epilepticus

MYOCLONIC STATUS
Treatment: valproic acid (drug of choice). Place NG, give 20 mg/kg per NG loading dose. Maintenance: 40 mg/kg/d divided (*see page 274*).
Can add lorazepam (Ativan®) or clonazepam (Klonopin®) to help with acute control.

ABSENCE STATUS EPILEPTICUS
Almost always responds to diazepam.

13.4. Antiepileptic drugs

The goal of antiepileptic drugs (**AEDs**) is seizure control (a contentious term, usually taken as reduction of seizure frequency and severity to the point to permit the patient to live a normal lifestyle without epilepsy-related limitations) with minimal or no drug toxicity. ≈ 75% of epileptics can achieve satisfactory seizure control with medical therapy[62].

13.4.1. Classification of AEDs

AEDs can be grouped as shown in *Table 13-8*.

Table 13-8 Classification of AEDs

Drug	Indications*	Page
• Barbiturates		
pentobarbital (Nembutal®)	status	
phenobarbital	status, GTC, partial Sz, febrile Sz, neonatal Sz	275
primidone (Mysoline)®		275
• Benzodiazepines		
clonazepam (Klonopin®)	Lennox-Gastaut, akinetic, myoclonic	277
clorazepate (Tranxene-SD®)	adj - partial Sz	
diazepam (Valium®)	status	266
lorazepam (Ativan®)	status	266
• GABA analogues		
gabapentin (Neurontin®)	adj - partial Sz	278
tiagabine (Gabitril®)	adj - partial Sz	280
• Hydantoins		
fosphenytoin (Cerebyx®)	status, Sz during neurosurgery, short-term replacement for oral PHT	272
phenytoin (Dilantin®)	GTC, CP, Sz during or after neurosurgery	271
• Phenyltriazenes		
lamotrigine (Lamictal®)	adj - partial Sz, adj - Lennox-Gastaut	278
• Succinimides		
ethosuximide (Zarontin®)	ABS	275
methsuximide (Celontin®)	ABS refractory to other drugs	276
• Miscellaneous		
acetazolamide (Diamox®)	centrencephalic epilepsies †	277
carbamazepine (Tegretol®, Carbatrol®)	partial Sz + complex symptomology, GTC, mixed Sz, ✘ not for absence	273
felbamate (Felbatol®)	use only with extreme caution - see text	276
levetiracetam (Keppra®)	adj - partial Sz	277
oxcarbazepine (Trileptal®)	mono or adj - partial Sz	274
topiramate (Topamax®)	adj - partial Sz or primarily GTC	279
valproate (Depakene®…)	CP (alone or with other types), ABS, adj - multiple Sz types	274
zonisamide (Zonegran®)	adj - partial Sz	

*   Indications for seizure types (does not include other uses, e.g. for chronic pain). FDA approved indications are in bold, off-label indications appear in plain text.

Abbreviations: ABS = absence, adj = adjunctive therapy, CP = complex partial, GTC = generalized tonic-clonic, PHT = phenytoin, Sz = seizure, status = status epilepticus

†   immediate release dosage form

13.4.2.   Choice of antiepileptic drug

Antiepileptic drugs (AED) for various seizure types
Boldface drugs are drug of choice (**DOC**).
1.   primary generalized
    A.   GTC (generalized tonic-clonic):
        1.   **valproic acid** (VA): if no evidence of focality some studies show fewer side effects and better control than PHT (*see page 274*)
        2.   carbamazepine: *see page 273*
        3.   **phenytoin** (PHT): *see page 271*
        4.   phenobarbital (PB): *see page 275*
        5.   primidone (PRM): *see page 275*
    B.   absence:

1. **ethosuximide**
2. **valproic acid** (VA)
3. clonazepam
4. methsuximide: *see page 276*
   C. myoclonic → benzodiazepines
   D. tonic or atonic:
      1. benzodiazepines
      2. felbamate: *see page 276*
      3. vigabatrin: *see page 279*
2. partial (simple or complex, with or without secondary generalization)[63] (VA may compare favorably with CBZ for secondarily GTC, but is less effective for complex partial seizures[64]):
   A. **carbamazepine** (CBZ)   most effective, least side effects
   B. **phenytoin** (PHT)   ↓
   C. phenobarbital (PB)   ↓
   D. primidone (PRM)   slightly less effective, more side effects
3. second line drugs for any of the above seizure types:
   A. valproate
   B. lamotrigine[A]: *see page 278*
   C. topiramate[A]: *see page 279*

13.4.3.   Anticonvulsant pharmacology[65]

GENERAL GUIDELINES

Monotherapy versus polytherapy
1. increase a given medication until seizures are controlled or side effects become intolerable (do not rely solely on therapeutic levels, which is only the range in which most patients have seizure control without side effects)
2. try monotherapy with a different drugs before resorting to two drugs together. 80% of epileptics can be controlled on monotherapy, however, failure of monotherapy indicates an 80% chance that the seizures will not be controllable pharmacologically. Only ≈ 10% benefit significantly from the addition of a second drug[64]. When > 2 AEDs are required, consider nonepileptic seizures (*see page 262*)
3. when first evaluating patients on multiple drugs, withdraw the most sedating ones first (usually barbiturates and clonazepam)

Generally, dosing intervals should be less than one half-life. Without loading dose, it takes about 5 half-lives to reach steady state.

Many AEDs affect liver function tests (**LFTs**), however, only rarely do the drugs cause enough hepatic dysfunction to warrant discontinuation. Guideline: discontinue an AED if the GGT exceeds twice normal.

SPECIFIC ANTICONVULSANTS

Table 13-9   Abbreviations

AED = antiepileptic drug; **ABS** = absence; **EC** = enteric coated; **DIV** = divided; **DOC** = drug of choice; **GTC** = generalized tonic-clonic seizure; **S/C-P** = simple or complex partial.

Pharmacokinetics: Unless otherwise specified, numbers are given for <u>oral</u> dosing form. $t_{1/2}$ = half-life; t_{PEAK} = time to peak serum level; t_{SS} = time to steady state (approximately 5 x $t_{1/2}$); $t_{D/C}$ = time to discontinue (recommended withdrawal period over which drug should be tapered); **MDF** = minimum dosing frequency. "Therapeutic level" is the average therapeutic range.

A. effective for many types of generalized seizures, but are not FDA approved for this indication

INDICATIONS
GTC, S/C-P, occasionally in ABS.

PHARMACOKINETICS
Pharmacokinetics are complicated: at low concentrations, kinetics are 1st order (elimination proportional to concentration), metabolism saturates near the therapeutic level resulting in zero-order kinetics (elimination at a constant rate). ≈ 90% of total drug is protein bound. Oral bioavailability is ≈ 90% whereas IV bioavailability is ≈ 95%; this small difference may be significant when patients are near limits of therapeutic range (due to zero-order kinetics).

$t_{1/2}$ (half-life)	t_{PEAK} (peak serum levels)	t_{SS} (steady state)	$t_{D/C}$ (discontinue)	Therapeutic level*
≈ 24 hrs (range: 9-140 hrs)†	oral suspension: 1.5-3 hrs regular capsules: 1.5-3 hrs extended release capsules: 4-12 hrs	7-21 days	4 wks	10-20 µg/ml

* therapeutic level as measured in most labs: 10-20 µg/ml (NB. it is the free PHT that is the important moiety; this is usually ≈ 1% of total PHT, thus therapeutic free PHT levels are 1-2 µg/ml; some labs are able to measure free PHT directly).

† $t_{1/2}$ for phenytoin depends on serum concentration and metabolic autoinduction

Renal failure: dosage adjustment not needed. However, serum protein binding may be altered in uremia which can obfuscate interpretation of serum phenytoin levels. *Eq 13-1* may be used to convert serum PHT concentration in a uremic patient **C (observed)**, to the expected PHT level in nonuremic patients **C (nonuremic)**.

$$C \text{ (nonuremic)} = \frac{C \text{ (observed)}}{0.1 \times \text{albumin} + 0.1}$$

Eq 13-1

ORAL DOSE
***Rx* Adult**: usual maintenance dose= 300-600 mg/d divided BID or TID (MDF = q d, for single daily dosing, either the phenytoin-sodium capsules or the extended release form should be used). Oral loading dose: 300 mg PO q 4 hrs until 17 mg/kg are given. **Peds**: oral maintenance: 4-7 mg/kg/d (MDF = BID). SUPPLIED: (oral forms): 100 mg tablets of phenytoin-sodium (sodium-salt); 30 & 100 mg Kapseals® (extended release); 50 mg chewable Infatabs® (phenytoin-acid); oral suspension 125 mg/5-ml in 8 oz (240 ml) bottles or individual 5 ml unit dose packs; pediatric suspension 30 mg/5-ml. Phenytek® 200 & 300 mg capsules.

Dosage changes
Because of zero-order kinetics, at near-therapeutic levels a small dosage change can cause large level changes. Although computer models are necessary for a high degree of accuracy, the dosing change guidelines in *Table 13-10* or the nomogram in *Figure 13-1*[66] may be used as a quick approximation.

GI absorption of phenytoin suspension or capsules may be decreased by up to 70% when given with nasogastric feedings of Osmolyte® or Isocal®[67, 68], and the suspension has been reported to have erratic absorption. Hold NG feeding for 2 hrs before and 1 hour after phenytoin dose.

Table 13-10 Guidelines for changing phenytoin dosage

Present level (mg/dl)	Change to make
< 6	100 mg/day
6-8	50 mg/day
> 8	25-30 mg/day

PARENTERAL DOSE
Phenytoin is a negative inotrope and can cause hypotension.

Conventional phenytoin may be given slow IVP or by IV drip (*see below*). The IM route should NOT be used (unreliable absorption, crystallization and sterile abscesses may develop). IV must be given slowly to reduce risk of arrhythmias and hypotension, viz. **Adult**: < 50 mg/min, **Peds**: < 1-3 mg/kg/min. The only compatible solution is NS, inject at site nearest vein to avoid precipitation.

Rx loading. Adult: 18 mg/kg slow IV. Peds: 20 mg/kg slow IV.

Rx maintenance. Adult: 200-500 mg/d (MDF = q d). Most adults have therapeutic levels on 100 mg PO TID. Peds: 4-7 mg/kg/d (MDF = BID).

Drip loading method:
Requires cardiac monitoring, and BP check q 5 minutes.
Rx Add 500 mg PHT to 50 ml NS to yield 10 mg/ml, run at 2 ml/min (20 mg/min) long enough to give 18 mg/kg (for 70 kg patient: 1200 mg over 60 mins). For more rapid administration, up to 40 mg/min may be used, or use fosphenytoin (*see below*). Decrease rate if hypotension occurs.

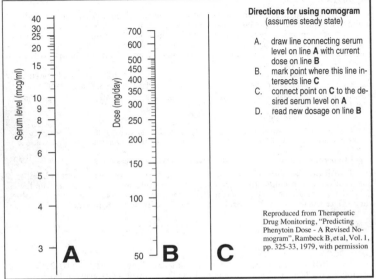

Directions for using nomogram
(assumes steady state)

A. draw line connecting serum level on line **A** with current dose on line **B**
B. mark point where this line intersects line **C**
C. connect point on **C** to the desired serum level on **A**
D. read new dosage on line **B**

Reproduced from Therapeutic Drug Monitoring, "Predicting Phenytoin Dose - A Revised Nomogram", Rambeck B, et al, Vol. 1, pp. 325-33, 1979, with permission

Figure 13-1 Nomogram for adjusting phenytoin dose

Fosphenytoin sodium injection

Fosphenytoin sodium **(FOS)** injection (Cerebyx®) is a newer formulation for administering IV phenytoin, and is indicated for short term use (≤ 5 days) when the enteral route is not usable. It is completely converted in vivo to phenytoin by organ and blood phosphatases with a conversion half-life of 10 minutes. Product labeling is given in terms of phenytoin equivalents **(PE)**. Safety in pediatric patients has not been established. Sᴜᴘ-ᴘʟɪᴇᴅ: 50 mg PE/ml in 2 & 10 ml vials (100 mg PE and 500 mg PE respectively).

Advantages of FOS (over conventional IV phenytoin):
1. less venous irritation (due to lower pH of 8.6-9 compared to 12 for phenytoin) resulting in less pain and IV extra vassa ti on
2. FOS is water soluble and therefore may be infused with dextrose or saline
3. tolerated by IM injection (IM route should not be used for status epilepticus)
4. does not come combined with propylene glycol (which can cause cardiac arrhythmias and/or hypotension itself)
5. the maximum administration rate is 3 **x** as fast (i.e. 150 mg PE/min)

SIDE EFFECTS OF PHENYTOIN

May interfere with cognitive function. May produce SLE-like syndrome, hepatic granulomas, megaloblastic anemia, cerebellar degeneration (chronic doses), hirsutism, gingival hypertrophy, hemorrhage in newborn if mother on PHT, toxic epidermal necrolysis (Stevens-Johnson variant). PHT antagonizes vitamin D → osteomalacia and rickets. Most hypersensitivity reactions occur within 2 months of initiating therapy[67]. In cases of maculopapular erythematous rash, the drug may be stopped and the patient may be rechallenged; often the rash will not recur the second time. Teratogenic (fetal hydantoin syndrome[69]).

Signs of phenytoin toxicity may develop at concentrations above 20 µg/ml (toxicity is more common at levels > 30 µg/ml) and include nystagmus (may also occur at therapeutic levels), diplopia, ataxia, asterixis, slurred speech, confusion, and CNS depression.

Drug-drug interactions: fluoxetine (Prozac®) results in elevated phenytoin levels (ave: 161% above baseline)[70]. Phenytoin may impair the efficacy of: corticosteroids, warfarin, digoxin, doxycycline, estrogens, furosemide, oral contraceptives, quinidine, rifampin, theophylline, vitamin D.

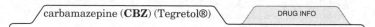

carbamazepine (**CBZ**) (Tegretol®)

INDICATIONS

Partial seizures with or without secondary generalization. Trigeminal neuralgia. An IV form for use in e.g. status epilepticus is in development.

DOSE

Rx oral route. Adult range: 600-2000 mg/d. **Peds**: 20-30 mg/kg/d. MDF = BID.

Before starting, check: CBC & platelet count (consider reticulocyte count) & serum Fe. Package insert says "recheck at frequent intervals, perhaps q week **x** 3 mos, then q month **x** 3 yrs."

Do not start CBZ (or discontinue it if patient already on CBZ) if: WBC < 4K, RBC < 3 **x** 10^6, Hct < 32%, platelets < 100K, reticulocytes < 0.3%, Fe > 150 µg%.

Start low and increment slowly: 200 mg PO q d **x** 1 wk, BID **x** 1 wk, TID **x** 1 wk. As an inpatient, dosage changes may be made every 3 days, monitoring for signs of side effects. As an outpatient, changes should be made only ≈ weekly, with levels after each change.

SUPPLIED: oral form. Scored tabs 200 mg. Chewable scored tabs 100 mg. Suspension 100 mg/5-ml. IV form: not available in the U.S. at the time of this writing. **Carbohydrate** (extended release CBZ): 200 & 300 mg tablets.

Caveats with oral forms: oral absorption is erratic, and smaller more frequent doses are preferred[71]. Oral suspension is absorbed more readily, and also ✱ should not be administered simultaneously with other liquid medicinal agents as it may result in the precipitation of a rubbery, orange mass. ✱ May aggravate hyponatremia by SIADH-like effect.

PHARMACOKINETICS

t$_{1/2}$ (half-life)	t$_{PEAK}$ (peak levels)	t$_{SS}$ (steady state)	t$_{D/C}$ (discontinue)	Therapeutic level (µg/ml)*
single dose: 20-55 hrs after chronic therapy: 10-30 hrs (adults), 8-20 hrs (peds)	4-24 hrs	up to 10 days†	4 wks	6-12

* may be misleading since the active metabolite carbamazepine-10,11-epoxide may cause toxicity and must be assayed separately

† t$_{SS}$ may subsequently fall due to autoinduction which plateaus at 4-6 wks

CBZ induces hepatic enzymes that result in increased metabolism of itself (autoinduction) as well as other drugs over a period of ≈ 3-4 weeks.

SIDE EFFECTS

✱ Drug-drug interaction: caution, propoxyphene (Darvon®), cimetidine, erythromycin and isoniazid may cause dramatic elevation of CBZ levels due to inhibition of hepatic cytochrome oxidase that degrades CBZ[72]. Side effects include:
1. drowsiness and GI upset: minimized by slow dose escalation
2. relative leukopenia in many: usually does not require discontinuing drug
3. transient diplopia
4. ataxia
5. less effect on cognitive function than PHT
6. hematological toxicity: rare. May be serious → agranulocytosis & aplastic anemia
7. Stevens-Johnson syndrome
8. SIADH
9. hepatitis (occasionally fatal) reported

oxcarbazepine (Trileptal®) DRUG INFO

Very similar efficacy profile to carbamazepine with the following differences:
1. there is no autoinduction (C-P450 is not involved in metabolism) and therefore minimal drug-drug interactions
2. no blood testing is required since:
   A. there is no liver toxicity
   B. there is no hematologic toxicity
   C. there is no need to check drug levels
3. dosing is BID
4. kinetics are linear
5. more expensive

DOSE
Rx: starting dose for pain control is 150 mg PO BID, for seizures it is 300 mg PO BID. Maximum dose 2400 mg/day total. SUPPLIED: 150, 300 & 600 mg scored tablets. 300 mg/5 ml oral suspension.

valproate DRUG INFO

Available as valproic acid (Depakene®) and divalproex sodium (Depakote®).

INDICATIONS
Effective in primary GTC. Also useful in ABS with GTC, juvenile myoclonic epilepsy, and partial seizures (not FDA approved for latter). Also FDA approved for migraine prophylaxis. Note: severe GI upset and short half life make valproic acid much less useful than Depakote® (divalproex sodium).

DOSE
Adult range: 600-3000 mg/d. **Peds** range: 15-60 mg/kg/d. MDF = q d.

Rx Start at 15 mg/kg/d, increment at 1 wk intervals by 5-10 mg/kg/d. Max recommended adult dose: 60 mg/kg/d. If daily dose > 250 mg is required, it should be divided. SUPPLIED: Oral: capsules 250 mg. Syrup 250 mg/5-ml. **Depakote®** (enteric coated) tabs: 125, 250,& 500 mg; sprinkle capsules 125 mg. IV: **Depacon®** for I.V. injection 500 mg/5 ml vial.

PHARMACOKINETICS

$t_{1/2}$ (half-life)	t_{PEAK} (peak serum levels)	t_{SS} (steady state)	$t_{D/C}$ (discontinue)	Therapeutic level (µg/ml)
8-20 hrs	(uncoated) 1-4 hrs	2-4 days	4 wks	50-100

Valproic acid **(VA)** is 90% protein bound. ASA displaces VA from serum proteins.

SIDE EFFECTS
Serious side effects are rare. <u>Pancreatitis</u> has been reported. Fatal liver failure has occurred especially if age < 2 yrs and in combination with other AEDs. <u>Teratogenic</u> (*see Contraindications* below). Drowsiness (temporary), minimal cognitive deficits, N/V (minimized with Depakote), liver dysfunction, hyperammonemia (even without liver dysfunction), weight gain, mild hair loss, tremor (dose related; similar to benign familial tremor; if severe and valproic acid is absolutely necessary, the tremor may be treated with beta blockers). May interfere with platelet function, caution with surgery on these patients.

CONTRAINDICATIONS
✖ Pregnancy: causes neural tube defects **(NTD)** in ≈ 1-2% of patients[73]. Since a correlation between peak VA levels and the risk of NTDs has been found, if VA must be used, some experts recommend changing from BID to TID dosing. ✖ Patients ≤ 2 yrs age (risk of hepatotoxicity).

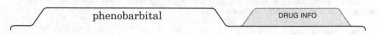

/ phenobarbital \ DRUG INFO \

INDICATIONS
Used as alternative in GTC and partial (not DOC). Had been DOC for febrile seizures, dubious benefit[45]. About as effective as PHT, but very sedating. Also used for status epilepticus (*see page 267*).

DOSE
Same dose PO, IV, or IM. MDF = q d[74, 75]. Start slowly to minimize sedation.
Rx Adult loading: 20 mg/kg slow IV (administer at rate < 100 mg/min). Maintenance: 30-250 mg/d (usually divided BID TID). **Peds** loading: 15-20 mg/kg. Maintenance: 2-6 mg/kg/d (usually divided BID). SUPPLIED: tabs 15 mg, 30 mg, 60 mg, 100 mg; elixir 20 mg/5-ml.

PHARMACOKINETICS

$t_{1/2}$ (half-life)	t_{PEAK} (peak levels)	t_{SS} (steady state)	$t_{D/C}$ (discontinue)	Therapeutic level
adult: 5 d (range: 50-160 hrs) peds: 30-70 hrs	PO & IM: 1-6 hrs	16-21 days (may take up to 30 days)	≈ 6-8 wks (reduce ≈ 25% per week)	15-30 μg/ml

Phenobarbital is a potent inducer of hepatic enzymes that metabolize other AEDs.

SIDE EFFECTS
Cognitive impairment (may be subtle and may outlast administration of the drug by at least several months[45]), thus avoid in peds; sedation; paradoxical hyperactivity (especially in peds); may cause hemorrhage in newborn if mother is on phenobarbital.

/ primidone (Mysoline®) \ DRUG INFO \

INDICATIONS
Same as phenobarbital (not DOC). NB: when used in combination therapy, low doses (50-125 mg/day) may add significant seizure control to the primary AED with few side effects.

DOSE
Rx Adult: 250-1500 mg/d. **Peds**: 15-30 mg/kg/d; MDF = BID.
Start at 125 mg/d **x** 1 wk, and inc. slowly to avoid sedation. SUPPLIED: (oral only): scored tabs 50 mg, 250 mg; suspension 250 mg/5-ml.

PHARMACOKINETICS
Metabolites include phenylethylmalonamide (PEMA) and phenobarbital. Therefore always check phenobarbital level at same time as primidone level.

$t_{1/2}$ (half-life)	t_{PEAK} (peak levels)	t_{SS} (steady state)	$t_{D/C}$ (discontinue)	Therapeutic level (μg/ml)
Primidone: 4-12 hrs derived phenobarbital: 50-160 hrs	2-5 hrs	up to 30 days	same as phenobarbital	primidone: 1-15 derived phenobarbital: 10-30

SIDE EFFECTS
Same as phenobarbital, plus: loss of libido, rare macrocytic anemia.

/ ethosuximide (Zarontin®) \ DRUG INFO \

INDICATIONS
DOC in ABS.

DOSE
Rx **Adult**: 500-1500 mg/d. **Peds**: 10-40 mg/kg/d; MDF = q d. SUPPLIED: oral only;
capsules 250 mg; syrup 250 mg/5-ml.

PHARMACOKINETICS

$t_{1/2}$ (half-life)	t_{PEAK} (peak levels)	t_{SS} (steady state)	Therapeutic level (μg/ml)
adult: 40-70 hrs peds: 20-40 hrs	1-4 hrs	adult: up to 14 days peds: up to 7 days	40-100

SIDE EFFECTS
N/V; lethargy; hiccoughs; H/A; rarely: eosinophilia, leukopenia, erythema multiforme, Stevens-Johnson syndrome, SLE-like syndrome. Toxic levels → psychotic behavior.

methsuximide (Celontin®) DRUG INFO

INDICATIONS
Indicated for absence seizures refractory to other drugs.

DOSE
Rx optimum dose must be determined by trial. Start with 300 mg PO q d, increase
by 300 mg at weekly intervals PRN to a maximum of 1200 mg/d. SUPPLIED: 150 & 300 mg
capsules.

felbamate (Felbatol®) DRUG INFO

✘ CAUTION: Due to an unacceptably high rate of aplastic anemia and hepatic failure, felbamate **(FBM)** should *not* be used except in those circumstances where the benefit clearly outweighs the risk; then, hematologic consultation is recommended by the
manufacturer. See *Side effects* below (also for drug-drug interactions).
FBM is efficacious for monotherapy and adjunctive therapy for partial seizures
(complex and secondary generalization), and reduces the frequency of atonic and GTC
seizures in Lennox-Gastaut syndrome.

PHARMACOKINETICS

$t_{1/2}$ (half-life)	t_{PEAK} (peak levels)	t_{SS} (steady state)	Therapeutic level
20-23 hrs	1-3 hrs	5-7 days	not established

DOSE
Rx: CAUTION *see above*.
Felbamate is not to be used as a
first-line drug. Patient or
guardian should sign informed
consent release. Start with
1200 mg/d divided BID, TID, or
QID, and decrease other AEDS
by one third. Increase felbamate biweekly in 600 mg increments to usual dose of 1600-

Table 13-11   Effect of felbamate on other AED levels

AED	Change in level	Recommended dos- ing change
phenytoin	↑ 30-50%	↓ 20-33%
carbamazepine	↓ 30% total ↑ 50-60% epoxide	↓ 20-33%
valproic acid	↑ 25-100%	↓ 33%

3600 mg/d (max: 45 mg/kg/d). Slow down increments and/or reduce other AEDs further
if side effects become severe. Administer at upper end of range when used as monotherapy. SUPPLIED: (oral only) 400 & 600 mg scored tablets; suspension 600 mg/5-ml.

SIDE EFFECTS
Felbamate has been associated with aplastic anemia (usually discovered after 5-30
wks of therapy) in ≈ 2-5 cases per million persons per yr, and hepatic failure (some fatal,
necessitating baseline and serial LFTs every 1-2 wks). Other side effects: insomnia, anorexia, N/V, H/A. Felbamate is a potent metabolic inhibitor, thus it is necessary to reduce

the dose of phenytoin, valproate or carbamazepine when used with felbamate[76] (*see Table 13-11*) (general rule: drop dose by one third).

levetiracetam (Keppra®) — DRUG INFO

INDICATIONS
Adjunctive therapy for partial onset Sz in adults.

DOSE
Rx start with 500 mg PO BID. Increment by 1000 mg/d q 2 weeks PRN to a maximum of 3000 mg/d.
SUPPLIED: 250, 500 & 750 mg scored film-coated tabs.

SIDE EFFECTS
Somnolence and fatigue in 15%. Dizziness in 9%.

clonazepam (Klonopin®) — DRUG INFO

A benzodiazepine derivative.

INDICATIONS
✖ Not a recommended drug for seizures (*see below*).
Used for myoclonic, atonic, and absence seizures (in absence, less effective than valproate or ethosuximide, and tolerance may develop).
NB: clonazepam usually works very well for several months, and then tends to become less effective, leaving only the sedating effects. Also, many cases have been reported of patients having seizures during withdrawal, including status epilepticus (even in patients with no history of status). Thus, may need to taper this drug over 3-6 months.

DOSE
Rx **Adult**: start at 1.5 mg/d DIV TID, increase by 0.5-1 mg q 3 d, usual dosage range is 1-12 mg/d (max 20 mg/d); MDF = q d. **Peds**: start at 0.01-0.03 mg/kg/d DIV BID or TID, increase by 0.25-0.5 mg/kg/d q 3 d; usual dosage range is 0.01-0.02 mg/kg/d; MDF = q d. SUPPLIED: oral only; scored tabs: 0.5 mg, 1 mg, 2 mg.

PHARMACOKINETICS

$t_{1/2}$ (half-life)	t_{PFAK} (peak levels)	t_{SS} (steady state)	$t_{D/C}$ (discontinue)	Therapeutic level (µg/ml)
20-60 hrs	1-3 hrs	up to 14 days	≈ 3-6 months*	0.013-0.072

* CAUTION: withdrawal seizures are common, see text above

SIDE EFFECTS
Ataxia, drowsiness, behavior changes.

zonisamide (Zonegran®) — DRUG INFO

INDICATIONS
Adjunctive therapy for partial Sz in adults.

acetazolamide (Diamox®) — DRUG INFO

The anti-epileptic effect may be either due to direct inhibition of CNS carbonic anhydrase (also reduces CSF production) or due to the slight CNS acidosis that results.

INDICATIONS
Centricephalic epilepsies (absence, nonfocal seizures). Best results are in absence

seizures; however benefit has also been observed in GTC, myoclonic jerk.

SIDE EFFECTS
Do not use in first trimester of pregnancy (may be teratogenic). The diuretic effect causes renal loss of HCO_3 which may lead to an acidotic state with long-term therapy. A sulfonamide, therefore any typical reaction to this class may occur (anaphylaxis, fever, rash, Stevens-Johnson syndrome, toxic epidermal necrolysis...). Paresthesias: medication should be discontinued.

DOSE
Rx **Adult:** 8-30 mg/kg/d in divided doses (max 1 gm/d, higher doses do not improve control). When given with another AED, the suggested starting dose is 250 mg once daily, and this is gradually increased. SUPPLIED: tablets 125, 250 mg. Diamox sequels® are sustained release 500 mg capsules. Sterile cryodessicated powder is also available in 500 mg vials for parenteral (IV) use.

gabapentin (Neurontin®) — DRUG INFO

Although developed to be a GABA agonist, it does not interact at any known GABA receptor. Efficacious for primary generalized seizures and partial seizures (with or without secondary generalization). Ineffective for absence seizures. Very low incidence of known side-effects. No known drug interactions (probably because it is renally excreted).

DOSE
Rx Adult: 300 mg PO **x** 1 day 1; 300 mg BID day 2; 300 mg TID day 3; then increase rapidly up to usual doses of ≈ 800-1800 mg per day. Doses of 1800-3600 may be needed in intractable patients. Dosage must be reduced in patients with renal insufficiency or on dialysis. SUPPLIED: 100, 300, 400 mg capsules.

PHARMACOKINETICS
Gabapentin is not metabolized, and 93% is excreted unchanged renally with plasma clearance directly proportional to creatinine clearance[77]. Does not affect hepatic microsomal enzymes, and does not affect metabolism of other AEDs. Antacids decrease bioavailablilty by ≈ 20%, therefore give gabapentin > 2 hrs after the antacid[78].

$t_{1/2}$ (half-life)	tPEAK (peak levels)	tSS (steady state)	Therapeutic level
5-7 hrs*	2-3 hrs	1-2 days	not established

* with normal renal function

SIDE EFFECTS
Somnolence, dizziness, ataxia, fatigue, nystagmus; all reduce after 2-3 weeks of drug therapy. Increased appetite. Not known to be teratogenic.

lamotrigine (Lamictal®) — DRUG INFO

Anticonvulsant effect may be due to presynaptic inhibition of glutamate release[77]. Efficacious as <u>adjunctive</u> therapy for partial seizures (with or without secondary generalization) and Lennox-Gastaut syndrome. Preliminary data suggest it may also be useful as an adjunct for refractory generalized seizures, or as monotherapy for newly diagnosed partial or generalized seizures[79]. Also FDA approved for bipolar disorder.

SIDE EFFECTS
Somnolence, dizziness, diplopia. ✖ Serious rashes requiring hospitalization and discontinuation of therapy have been reported (rash usually begins 2 weeks after initiating therapy and may be severe and potentially life-threatening, including Stevens-Johnson syndrome (more of a concern with simultaneous use of valproate), and rarely, toxic epidermal necrolysis (**TEN**)). Incidence of significant epidermal reaction may be decreased by a slow ramping-up of dosage. May increase seizure frequency in severe myoclonic epilepsy of infancy[80]. Metabolism of lamotrigine is affected by other AEDs.

DOSE

Rx Adult: In adults receiving enzyme-inducing AEDs (PHT, CBZ, or phenobarbital), start with 50 mg PO q d x 2 wks, then 50 mg BID x 2 wks, then ↑ by 100 mg/d q week until the usual maintenance dose of 200-700 mg/d (divided into 2 doses) is reached. For patients on valproic acid (**VA**) alone, the maintenance dose was 100-200 mg/d (divided into 2 doses), and VA levels drop by ≈ 25% within a few weeks of starting lamotrigine. For patients on both enzyme-inducing AEDs _and_ VA, the starting dose is 25 mg PO qod x 2 wks, then 25 mg qd x 2 wks, then ↑ by 25-50 mg/d q 1-2 wks up to a maintenance of 100-150 mg/d (divided into 2 doses). Instruct patients that rash, fever or lymphadenopathy may herald a serious reaction and that a physician should be contacted immediately. **Peds**: not indicated for use in patients < 16 yrs old due to higher incidence of potentially life-threatening rash in the pediatric population[77]. SUPPLIED: 25, 100, 150 & 200 mg tablets. 2, 5 & 25 mg chewable dispersible tablets.

PHARMACOKINETICS[79]

$t_{1/2}$ (half-life)	t_{PEAK} (peak levels)	t_{SS} (steady state)	Therapeutic level
24 hrs*	1.5-5 hrs	4-7 days	not established

* half-life is shortened to ≈ 15 hrs by PHT and CBZ, whereas valproic acid increases it to 59 hrs

vigabatrin | DRUG INFO

INDICATIONS
Effective in treating partial seizures. Less so for generalized seizures.

DOSE
Rx Adult: 1500-3000 mg/d.

topiramate (Topamax®) | DRUG INFO

May block voltage-sensitive sodium channels and enhance GABA activity at $GABA_A$ receptors and attenuate some glutamate receptors[77].

INDICATIONS[81]
As an oral adjunct to other drugs in treating refractory partial seizures.

DOSE
Rx Adult: start with 50 mg/d and increase slowly up to 200-400 mg/d[82], with no significant benefit noted at dosages > 600 mg/d[83]. SUPPLIED: 25, 100, & 200 mg tabs.

PHARMACOKINETICS
30% is metabolized in the liver, the rest is excreted unchanged in the urine.

$t_{1/2}$ (half-life)	t_{SS} (steady state)	Therapeutic level
19-25 hrs	5-7 days	not established

SIDE EFFECTS
May increase phenytoin concentration by up to 25%. Levels of topiramate are reduced by other AEDs (phenytoin, carbamazepine, valproic acid and possibly others).

Cognitive impairment (word finding difficulty, problems with concentration...), weight loss, dizziness, ataxia, diplopia, paresthesias, nervousness and confusion have been troublesome. ≈ 1.5% incidence of renal stones which usually pass spontaneously[77]

Oligohidrosis (reduced sweating) and hyperthermia, primarily in children in association with elevated environmental temperatures and/or vigorous physical activity.

A GABA uptake inhibitor, with cognitive problems of a similar frequency to that with topiramate[84].

Rx Adult: start with 4 mg/d, increase weekly by 4-8 mg to a maximum of 32-56 mg (divided BID to QID). SUPPLIED: 4, 12, 16 & 20 mg tablets.

13.4.3.1. Withdrawal of antiepileptic drugs

Most seizure recurrences develop during the first 6 months after AED withdrawal[85].

INDICATIONS FOR AED WITHDRAWAL

There is no agreement on how long a patient should be seizure-free before withdrawal of anticonvulsants, nor is there agreement on the prognostic value of EEGs and on the best time period over which to withdraw AEDs.

The following is based on a study of 92 patients with idiopathic epilepsy, who had been free of seizures for two years[86]. Generalization, e.g. to posttraumatic seizures, may not be appropriate. Taper was by 1 "unit" q 2 weeks (where a unit is defined as 200 mg for CBZ or valproic acid, or 100 mg for PHT). Follow-up: mean = 26 mos (range: 6-62).

31 patients (34%) relapsed, with the average time to relapse being 8 mos (range: 1-36). Using actuarial methods, the risk for recurrence is 5.9%/month for 3 months, then 2.7%/month for 3 months, then 0.5%/month for 3 months. Factors found to affect the likelihood of relapse include:

1. seizure type: 37% relapse rate for generalized seizures; 16% for complex or simple partial; 54% for complex partial with secondary generalization
2. number of seizures before control attained: those with ≥ 100 seizures before control had statistically significant higher relapse rate
3. the number of drugs that had to be tried before single drug therapy successfully controlled seizures: 29% if 1st drug worked, 40% if a change to a 2nd drug was needed, and 80% if a change to a 3rd drug was required
4. EEG class (*see Table 13-12*): class 4 had worst prognosis for relapse. Epileptiform discharges on EEG serves to discourage AED withdrawal[87]

Table 13-12   EEG class and seizure relapse rate

Class	– – EEG description – –		Re-lapse rate	No. of relapses/ patients at risk
	Before treatment	Before withdrawal		
1	normal	normal	34%	11/31
2	abnormal	normal	11%	4/35
3	abnormal	improved	50%	2/4
4	abnormal	unchanged	74%	14/19

In a larger randomized study[88], the most important factors identified to predict freedom from recurrent seizures were:

1. longer seizure-free period
2. use of only one AED (vs. multiple AEDs)
3. seizures other than tonic-clonic seizures

WITHDRAWAL TIMES

The recommended withdrawal times in *Table 13-13* should be used only as guidelines.

Table 13-13   Recommended AED withdrawal times

AED	Recommended withdrawal period
phenytoin, valproic acid, carbamazepine	2-4 weeks
phenobarbital	6-8 weeks (25% per week)
clonazepam	3-6 months (see CAUTION on page 277)

13.4.3.2.   Pregnancy and antiepileptic drugs

Women of childbearing potential with epilepsy should undergo counseling regarding pregnancy[89].

BIRTH CONTROL

AEDs that induce liver microsomal cytochrome P_{450} enzymes (see Table 13-14) increase the failure rate of oral contraceptives up to fourfold[90]. Patients desiring to use BCPs should employ barrier contraceptive measures until ovulation is consistently suppressed, and they should watch for breakthrough bleeding which may indicate a need for a change in the hormone dosage[85]. Non-oral hormonal contraceptives (e.g. levonorgestrel implant (Norplant®)) circumvents first pass liver degradation but should combined with a barrier method because of declining effectiveness with time.

Table 13-14 Effect of AEDs on liver cytochrome P_{450}[*]

Inducers	Noninducers
carbamazepine	valproic acid
phenobarbital	benzodiazepines
phenytoin	gabapentin
felbamate	lamotrigine
primidone	

[*] references[85, 91]

COMPLICATIONS DURING PREGNANCY

Women with epilepsy have more complications with pregnancy than mothers without epilepsy, but > 90% of pregnancies have a favorable outcome[85].

There is an increase in the number of gravid seizures in ≈ 17% (reported range: 17-30%) of epileptic women, which may be due to noncompliance or to changes of free drug levels of AEDs during pregnancy (see Table 13-15). Isolated seizures can occasionally be deleterious, but usually cause no problem. Status epilepticus poses serious risk to mother and fetus during pregnancy and should be treated aggressively.

There is also a slightly increased risk of toxemia (HTN of pregnancy) and fetal loss.

Table 13-15 Changes in free AED levels during pregnancy[92]

Drug	Change
carbamazepine	↓ 11%
phenobarbital	↓ 50%
phenytoin	↓ 31%
valproic acid	↑ 25%

BIRTH DEFECTS

The incidence of fetal malformations in offspring of patients with a known seizure disorder is ≈ 4-5%, or approximately double that of the general population[93]. The degree to which this is due to the use of AEDs vs. genetic and environmental factors is unknown. All AEDs have the potential to cause deleterious effects on the infant. Polytherapy is associated with an increased risk over monotherapy in a more than additive manner. Generally, the risk of seizures (with possible concomitant maternal and fetal hypoxia and acidosis) is felt to outweigh the teratogenic risk of most AEDs, but this must be evaluated on a case-by-case basis. Occasionally patients may be weaned off AEDs.

Specific drugs

Carbamazepine **(CBZ)** produced an increased incidence of "minor" malformations (but not of "major" malformations) in one study[94] (this study may have had methodologic problems), and may increase the incidence of neural tube defects **(NTD)**[95]. In utero exposure to phenytoin may lead to the fetal hydantoin syndrome[69, 96] and a child with an IQ lower by ≈ 10 points[97]. Phenobarbital produced the highest incidence of major malformations (9.1%) in one prospective study[98] and was also associated with most of the increase in fetal death or anomalies in another study[99]. Valproate **(VA)** causes the highest incidence of NTD (1-2%[73]), which can be detected with amniocentesis and allow an abortion if desired. TID dosing may reduce the risk of NTD (see page 274). Benzodiazepines given shortly before delivery can produce the "floppy infant syndrome"[100]. Similar effects may occur with other sedating AEDs such as phenobarbital.

Drug recommendations

A general consensus is that for most women of childbearing potential who require AEDs, that monotherapy with the lowest dose of CBZ that is effective is the method of choice if the seizure disorder is responsive to it[101]. If ineffective, then monotherapy with valproic acid (with TID dosing) is currently the recommended second choice. Folate supplementation (after confirming normal B_{12} levels, see page 904) should be used in all.

13.5. Seizure surgery

20% of patients continue to have seizures even with AEDs. Many of these patients may be candidates for surgical procedures to control their seizures[6].

INDICATIONS

Seizure disorder must be severe, medically refractory with satisfactory trials of tolerable medication for at least ≈ 1 year, and disabling to the patient. Medically **refractory** is usually considered two attempts of high-dose monotherapy with two distinct AEDs, and one attempt at polytherapy.

The three general categories of patients suitable for seizure surgery have[102]:
1. partial seizures
   A. temporal origin: the largest group of surgical candidates (especially mesial temporal epilepsy which is often medically refractory)
   B. extratemporal origin
2. secondarily generalized seizures: e.g. Lennox-Gastaut
3. unilateral, multifocal epilepsy associated with infantile hemiplegia syndrome

EVALUATION

All patients should undergo imaging study to rule out neoplasm, AVM, etc. Noninvasive techniques allow localization in the majority of cases.

NONINVASIVE TECHNIQUES

MRI
The imaging modality of choice. Extremely good for detecting hippocampal asymmetry of mesial temporal sclerosis that may produce complex partial seizures **(CPS)**[103].

CAT SCAN
A seizure focus may enhance with IV contrast shortly following a seizure. Subtle enhancement may be present on the side of the focus on interictal CT scan[104].

VIDEO-EEG MONITORING
Most centers perform pre-operative long-term inpatient video-EEG monitoring to correlate the clinically disabling seizure with appropriate electrical abnormalities and possibly to identify the seizure focus.

PET SCAN (POSITRON EMISSION TOMOGRAPHY)
Interictal PET scan using fluorine-18 deoxyglucose (^{18}FDG) shows hypometabolism lateralized to the side of temporal lobe focus in 70% of patients with medically refractory CPS (does not show actual site of origin). Useful when MRI and EEG cannot localize.

SPECT SCAN (SINGLE PHOTON EMISSION TOMOGRAPHY)
Used to demonstrate increased blood flow during a seizure to help localize site of onset. [99m] Technetium (Tc) hexamethyl-propylene-amine-oxime (HMPAO) is usually administered immediately after onset of seizure, and the scan may be obtained within several hours[105].

WADA TEST[106]
AKA intracarotid amytal test. Localizes dominant hemisphere (side of language function) and assesses ability of hemisphere without lesion to maintain memory when isolated. Usually reserved for candidates for large resections[107].

Start with angiogram (may use IV digital subtraction angiogram **(DSA)**) to assess cross flow and to R/O persistent trigeminal artery. Significant cross-flow is a relative contraindication to anesthetizing the side of dominant supply (patient goes to sleep).

Wada test may be grossly inaccurate with high flow AVM. Also, portions of hippocampus may be supplied by posterior circulation (not anesthetized by ICA injection).

EEG monitoring is usually performed during the test when it is being done for seizure surgery. Patient will show delta waves during deepest level of anesthesia.

Technique
- instruct patient as to what is expected
- catheterize ICA: usually start on side of lesion

- have patient hold contralateral arm in air, and instruct them to hold it there
- inject 100-125 mg sodium <u>amobarbital</u> (Amytal®) rapidly into internal carotid artery (effect starts almost instantaneously, begins to subside after ≈ 8 minutes (may subside in ≈ 2 minutes with AVM where flow rates are high))
- determine adequacy of injection by assessing motor function in elevated arm (should be ≈ flaccid)
- assess language skills by showing patient pictures of objects and ask them to name each one out loud and remember each one
- assess memory function by asking patient to name as many of the pictures as they can ≈ 15 minutes after test: if they have difficulty, ask them to pick out pictures from a group that contains additional ones not shown to patient
- repeat procedure on other side (use lower Amytal doses with each subsequent injection)

INVASIVE TECHNIQUES

EEG OBTAINED WITH INVASIVE ELECTRODES

Risk of infection with depth electrodes[107]: 2-10%.

Surface strip electrodes may be placed through a burr hole.

Depth electrodes may be placed stereotactically. Temporal depth electrodes may be helpful for CPS, usually to determine the laterality of the mesiotemporal source of seizure. Frontal depth electrodes are also sometimes used. 2-3% risk of intracerebral hemorrhage[107].

Subdural grid electrodes are placed with a craniotomy. These sometimes may allow sufficient mapping to permit surgery under general anesthesia without need for intraoperative mapping under local anesthesia (helpful in children or in the mentally retarded).

SURGICAL CONSIDERATIONS

Two basic types of procedure: resections and disconnections[A]:
1. resections
   A. resection of epileptic focus: higher chance of completely controlling seizures. Performed in noneloquent brain. Seizures must have focal onset (resection not encouraged if multifocal onset). Includes:
      1. anterior temporal lobectomy: *see below*
      2. amygdalo-hippocampectomy
      3. neocortical resections: especially with neuronal migration abnormalities
   B. resection of lesion in secondary epilepsy (e.g. tumor, AVM, cavernous malformation[108]...). In most cases the seizure focus is in or near the lesion, but some structural lesions are not responsible for the seizures. For seizure foci within the temporal lobe, seizure control is better when lesionectomy is accompanied by amygdalo-hippocampectomy[109]
2. disconnections: used when eloquent brain is involved, or to separate the electrical activity of the two cerebral hemispheres
   A. section of corpus callosum (callosotomy): when drop attacks are the most disabling seizure type or for multiple bilateral foci (*see below*)
   B. hemispherectomy: for unilateral seizures with widespread hemispheric lesions and profound contralateral neurologic deficit. Functional hemispherectomy isolates the abnormal side with ≈ 80% seizure control rate (similar to anatomic hemispherectomy with preservation of the basal ganglia, but with lower complication rate)
   C. multiple subpial transection[110]: for partial seizure originating in eloquent cortical areas. The cortex is transected at 5 mm intervals, thus interrupting the horizontal spread of the seizure while sparing the vertically oriented functional fibers

ANESTHETIC CONSIDERATIONS

If intraoperative electrocorticography is to be performed:

A. all of the listed procedures are for <u>refractory</u> seizures. For the definition of refractory, *see page 282*

- under local anesthesia: the only anesthetic agents that may be used are narcotics (usually fentanyl) and droperidol (the components of Innovar®)
- under general anesthesia: <u>avoid</u> benzodiazepines and barbiturates

INTRAOPERATIVE ELECTROCORTICOGRAPHY *(ECoG)*

May be performed with surface matrix that includes superior temporal gyrus and inferior frontal gyrus. Depth electrodes in the amygdala (3 cm from temporal tip) and hippocampus (5 cm from temporal tip) may also be used.

Methohexital (Brevitol®) may be given: observe for ↓ fast activity in suspected focus.

INTRAOPERATIVE CORTICAL STIMULATION

For locating motor strip, sensory cortex, or speech centers intraoperatively. Determination based on visible anatomy is unreliable. For speech center, stimulate cortex while patient names objects shown on picture cards (automatic verbalization, such as counting, is robust and may persist). Observe for effects ranging from total speech arrest to paraphasic errors.

Typical settings for a constant current generator using a bipolar electrode are shown in *Table 13-16*. If a voltage based unit is used, start at 1 volt and increase.

Table 13-16 Settings for constant current generator

Control	Setting
frequency	60 Hz
waveform	biphasic square wave
duration	2-4 mS peak-to-peak
mode	repeat
polarity	normal
current	varies between 2-16 mA

CORPUS CALLOSOTOMY

Partial or total section may be most effective for generalized major motor seizures. Of little benefit for simple or complex seizures. Benefit has been supported for:

1. frequent episodes of <u>atonic seizures</u> ("drop attacks") where loss of postural tone → falls and injuries[111] (70% reduction with callosotomy)
2. possibly for generalized seizure disorder with unilateral hemisphere damage (e.g. infantile hemiplegia syndrome); hemicortical resection may be better for this type, whereas callosotomy may promote partial seizures.
   Note: a "functional hemispherectomy" is recommended over "anatomically complete" hemispherectomy to reduce morbidity and mortality[102]
3. some patients with generalized seizures without identifiable, resectable focus

Division of the anterior two thirds of the corpus callosum **(CC)** (minimizes the risk of disconnection syndrome, *see below*) may be advantageous over complete callosotomy (controversial). Some advocate sectioning the CC with intraoperative EEG until the typical bisynchronous discharges that are usually seen become asynchronous[112]. No need to section anterior commisure. Can usually be performed via a bifrontal craniotomy utilizing a bicoronal skin incision.

May produce post-op ↓ verbalization or akinetic mutism that usually resolves in weeks. ✖ Contraindication: major behavioral and/or language deficits may occur even with partial division in patients with speech and dominant handedness located in <u>opposite</u> hemispheres ("crossed dominance"). Thus, Wada test is recommended in all left handed patients.

MRI sagittal cuts are superb for assessing extent of division of the CC[113].

DISCONNECTION SYNDROME

In a patient with a dominant left hemisphere, consists of left tactile anomia, left sided dyspraxia (may resemble hemiparesis), pseudohemianopsia, right sided anomia for smell, impaired spatial synthesis of right hand resulting in difficulty copying complex figures, decreased spontaneity of speech, incontinence.

More common with larger surgical sections of the CC. Risk is less if the anterior commisure is spared. Patients usually adapt after 2-3 months, with final function normal for most daily activities (deficits may show up on neuropsychological testing).

TEMPORAL LOBECTOMY

80% of patients with medically intractable seizures with demonstrable focus have foci in anterior temporal lobe. Most patients have neuronal loss and gliosis of mesial temporal structures. Thus, a standard resection of temporal tip (often with amygdalo-hippocampectomy) may be performed.

Limits of resection (without significant neurologic deficit)

Note that these values are generally considered safe, however, variations occur from patient to patient and only intraoperative mapping can reliably determine the location of language centers[114]. Some centers spare the superior temporal gyrus[115]. The following measurements are made along the <u>middle</u> temporal gyrus

* <u>dominant</u> temporal lobe: up to 4-5 cm may be removed. Over-resection may injure speech centers, which cannot be reliably localized visually
* <u>non-dominant</u> temporal lobe: 6-7 cm may be resected. Slight over-resection may → partial contralateral upper quadrant homonymous hemianopsia; resection of 8-9 cm → complete quadrantanopsia

Alternatively, intraoperative electrocorticography may be used to guide resection of electrically abnormal areas.

Resection should be performed in subpial plane to prevent injury to MCA branches.

AMYGDALO-HIPPOCAMPECTOMY

The amygdala lies in the roof of the anterior temporal horn of the lateral ventricle.

Two basic approaches:
1. transcortical: image guidance is very helpful
   A. Niemeyer approach[116]: 2-3 cm longitudinal cortical incision through the middle temporal gyrus centered at a point ≈ 4 cm posterior to the temporal tip
   B. approach through the anterior superior temporal gyrus
2. transylvian: approach advocated by Yasargil. More restrictive and greater risk of injury to M1 portion of MCA within sylvian fissure

Complications: vascular injury is the most significant risk.

RISKS OF SEIZURE SURGERY

Major risks are related to[117]:
1. removal of essential areas of cortex
2. injury to medullary core underlying cortical resection (projection fibers, association fibers, and/or commissural fibers): the most common deficit after temporal lobectomy is a contralateral (homonymous) superior quadrantanopsia (so-called "pie-in-the-sky" defect, due to an injury to Meyer's loop wherein the fibers for the superior visual field of the optic radiation take a slight rostral "detour" towards the temporal tip)
3. injury to vessels in area of resection → ischemic damage to areas supplied: especially sylvian branches during temporal lobectomy or ACA branches with corpus callosotomy
4. injury to nearby cranial nerves: especially third nerve during hippocampectomy where it lies medial to tentorium

PERIOPERATIVE MANAGEMENT FOR SEIZURE SURGERY

Management during evaluation:

During period when AEDs are being tapered, patient should be observed at all times (for patients not in ICU, a 24 hour-a-day sitter is required).

PRE-OP ORDERS (EPILEPTIC SURGERY)
1. taper anticonvulsants, completely D/C 1 day before surgery
2. 10 mg Decadron® PO hs before surgery, repeat PO or IV on AM of surgery
3. if seizures develop: phenobarbital 130 mg IV (@ < 100 mg/min)

POST-OP ORDERS (EPILEPTIC SURGERY)
1. for seizures in the immediate post-op period ("honeymoon seizures;"), not necessary to treat only one brief generalized seizure, otherwise load appropriately with phenytoin or phenobarbital;
2. continue 4 mg dexamethasone (Decadron®) PO q 6 hrs x <u>1 wk</u>, then taper over next week (essential to maintain for full week)

3. anticonvulsants are continued **x** 1-2 years even if no post-op seizures occur
4. before discharge:
   A. neuropsychiatric evaluation
   B. serum anticonvulsant level
   C. EEG

OUTCOME
(WITH RESECTION OF SEIZURE FOCUS)

The greatest effect of seizure surgery is <u>reduction of seizure frequency</u>[115], however, any surgical procedure may fail to have a beneficial effect.

Seizure control is usually assessed at 1,3 & 6 most post op, and then annually. A post-op MRI is usually obtained at 3 most post-op to assess extent of surgical resection. Most patients take anti-epileptic drugs (**AEDs**) for 2 years post-op, and then may be discontinued in those free of seizures.

Recurrent seizures: although late seizures may occur, 90% of seizures that recur do so within 2 years.

2 years post-op in patients maintained on AEDs: 50% are seizure-free, and 80% have over 50% reduction of seizure frequency.

For temporal lobectomies in the dominant hemisphere without intraoperative monitoring, there is a 6% risk of mild dysphasia. Significant memory deficits occur in ~ 2%.

13.6.   References

1. Commission on Classification and Terminology of the International League Against Epilepsy: Proposal for revised clinical and electroencephalographic classification of epileptic seizures. **Epilepsia** 22: 489-501, 1981.
2. Commission on Classification and Terminology of the International League Against Epilepsy: Guidelines for epidemiologic studies on epilepsy. **Epilepsia** 30: 389-99, 1989.
3. Mosewich R K, So E L: A clinical approach to the classification of seizures and epileptic syndromes. **Mayo Clin Proc** 71: 405-14, 1996.
4. French J A, Williamson P D, Thadani V M, et al.: Characteristics of medial temporal lobe epilepsy. I. Results of history and physical examination. **Ann Neurol** 34: 774-80, 1993.
5. Williamson P D, French J A, Thadani V M, et al.: Characteristics of medial temporal lobe epilepsy. II. Interictal and ictal scalp electroencephalography, neuropsychological testing, neuroimaging, surgical results, and pathology. **Ann Neurol** 34: 781-7, 1993.
6. Engel J J: Surgery for seizures. **N Engl J Med** 334: 647-52, 1996.
7. Grunewald R A, Panayiotopoulos C P: Juvenile myoclonic epilepsy: A review. **Arch Neurol** 50: 594-8, 1993.
8. Hauser W A, Annegers J F, Kurland L T: Incidence of epilepsy and unprovoked seizures in Rochester, Minnesota, 1935-1984. **Epilepsia** 34: 453-68, 1993.
9. Hauser W A, Anderson V E, Loewenson R B, et al.: Seizure recurrence after a first unprovoked seizure. **New Engl J Med** 307: 522-8, 1982.
10. Reith J, Jorgensen H S, Nakayama H, et al.: Seizures in acute stroke: Predictors and prognostic significance. The Copenhagen stroke study. **Stroke** 28: 1585-89, 1997.
11. Landfish N, Gieron-Korthals M, Weibley R E, et al.: New onset childhood seizures: Emergency department experience. **J Fla Med Assoc** 79: 697-700, 1992.
12. Hauser W A, Rich S S, Jacobs M P, et al.: Patterns of seizure occurrence and recurrence risks in patients with newly diagnosed epilepsy. **Epilepsia** 24: 516-7,

13. 1983 (abstract).
    van Donselaar C, Schimsheimer R-J, Geerts A T, et al.: Value of the electroencephalogram in adult patients with untreated idiopathic first seizures. **Arch Neurol** 49: 231-7, 1992.
14. Young B, Rapp R P, Norton J A, et al.: Failure of prophylactically administered phenytoin to prevent late posttraumatic seizures. **J Neurosurg** 58: 236-41, 1983.
15. Annegers J F, Grabow J D, Groover R V, et al.: Seizures after head trauma: A population study. **Neurology** 30: 683-9, 1980.
16. Bullock R, Chesnut R M, Clifton G, et al.: **Guidelines for the management of severe head injury**, The Brain Trauma Foundation (New York), The American Association of Neurological Surgeons (Park Ridge, Illinois), and The Joint Section of Neurotrauma and Critical Care, 1995.
17. McQueen J K, Blackwood D H R, Harris P, et al.: Low risk of late posttraumatic seizures following severe head injury. **J Neurol Neurosurg Psychiatry** 46: 899-904, 1983.
18. Young B, Rapp R P, Norton J A, et al.: Failure of prophylactically administered phenytoin to prevent early posttraumatic seizures. **J Neurosurg** 58: 231-5, 1983.
19. Hahn Y S, Fuchs S, Flannery A M, et al.: Factors influencing posttraumatic seizures in children. **Neurosurgery** 22: 864-7, 1988.
20. Weiss G H, Salazar A M, Vance S C, et al.: Predicting posttraumatic epilepsy in penetrating head injury. **Arch Neurol** 43: 771-3, 1986.
21. Temkin N R, Dikmen S S, Winn H R: Posttraumatic seizures. **Neurosurg Clin North Amer** 2: 425-35, 1991.
22. Temkin N R, Dikmen S S, Wilensky A J, et al.: A randomized, double-blind study of phenytoin for the prevention of post-traumatic seizures. **N Engl J Med** 323: 497-502, 1990.
23. Dikmen S S, Temkin N R, Miller B, et al.: Neurobehavioral effects of phenytoin prophylaxis of posttraumatic seizures. **JAMA** 265: 1271-7, 1991.
24. Haltiner A M, Newell D W, Temkin N R, et al.: Side

effects and mortality associated with use of phenytoin for early posttraumatic seizure prophylaxis. **J Neurosurg** 91: 588-92, 1999.

25. Yablon S A: Posttraumatic seizures. **Arch Phys Med Rehabil** 74: 983-1001, 1993.

26. North J B, Penhall R K, Hanieh A, *et al.*: Phenytoin and postoperative epilepsy: A double-blind study. **J Neurosurg** 58: 672-7, 1983.

27. Charness M E, Simon R P, Greenberg D A: Ethanol and the nervous system. **N Engl J Med** 321: 442-54, 1989.

28. Lechtenberg R, Worner T M: Seizure risk with recurrent alcohol detoxification. **Arch Neurol** 47: 535-8, 1990.

29. Chabolla D R, Krahn L E, So E L, *et al.*: Psychogenic nonepileptic seizures. **Mayo Clin Proc** 71: 493-500, 1996.

30. Gates J R, Ramani V, Whalen S, *et al.*: Ictal characteristics of pseudoseizures. **Arch Neurol** 42: 1183-7, 1985.

31. King D W, Gallagher B B, Marvin A J, *et al.*: Pseudoseizures: Diagnostic evaluation. **Neurology** 32: 18-23, 1982.

32. Henrichs T F, Tucker D M, Farha J, *et al.*: MMPI indices in the identification of patients evidencing pseudoseizures. **Epilepsia** 29: 184-7, 1988.

33. Wyllie E, Luders H, MacMillan J P, *et al.*: Serum prolactin levels after epileptic seizures. **Neurology** 34: 1601-4, 1984.

34. Dana-Haeri J, Trimble M R, Oxley J: Prolactin and gonadotropin changes following generalized and partial seizures. **J Neurol Neurosurg Psychiatry** 46: 331-5, 1983.

35. Prichard P B, Wannamaker B B, Sagel J, *et al.*: Serum prolactin and cortisol levels in evaluation of pseudoepileptic seizures. **Ann Neurol** 18: 87-9, 1985.

36. Laxer K D, Mullooly J P, Howell B: Prolactin changes after seizures classified by EEG monitoring. **Neurology** 35: 31-5, 1985.

37. Abbott R J, Browning M C K, Davidson D L W: Serum prolactin and cortisol concentrations after grand mal seizures. **J Neurol Neurosurg Psychiatry** 43: 163-7, 1980.

38. Jackel R A, Malkowicz D, Trivedi R, *et al.*: Reduction of prolactin response with repetitive seizures. **Epilepsia** 28: 588, 1987.

39. Tomson T, Lindbom U, Nilsson B Y, *et al.*: Serum prolactin during status epilepticus. **J Neurol Neurosurg Psychiatry** 52: 1435-7, 1989.

40. Sperling M R, Pritchard P B, Engel J, *et al.*: Prolactin in partial epilepsy: An indicator of limbic seizures. **Ann Neurol** 20: 716-22, 1986.

41. Meierkord H, Shorvon S, Lightman S, *et al.*: Comparison of the effects of frontal and temporal lobe partial seizures on prolactin levels. **Arch Neurol** 49: 225-30, 1992.

42. Dana-Haeri J, Trimble M R: Prolactin and gonadotropin changes following partial seizures in epileptic patients with and without psychopathology. **Biol Psychiatry** 19: 329-36, 1984.

43. Herzog A G: Prolactin: Quo vadis? **Arch Neurol** 49: 223-4, 1992 (editorial).

44. Verity C M, Golding J: Risk of epilepsy after febrile convulsions: A national cohort study. **BMJ** 303: 1373-6, 1991.

45. Farwell J R, Lee Y J, Hirtz D G, *et al.*: Phenobarbital for febrile seizures - effects on intelligence and on seizure recurrence. **N Engl J Med** 322: 364-9, 1990.

46. Rosman N P, Colton T, Labazzo J, *et al.*: A controlled trial of diazepam administered during febrile illnesses to prevent recurrence of febrile seizures. **N Engl J Med** 329: 79-84, 1993.

47. Working Group on Status Epilepticus: Treatment of convulsive status epilepticus. **JAMA** 270: 854-9, 1993.

48. Hauser W A: Status epilepticus: Epidemiologic considerations. **Neurology** 40 (Suppl 2): 9-13, 1990.

49. Phillips S A, Shanahan R J: Etiology and mortality of status epilepticus in children. **Arch Neurol** 46: 74-6, 1989.

50. Delorenzo R J, Pellock J M, Towne A R, *et al.*: Epidemiology of status epilepticus. **J Clin Neurophysiol** 12: 312-25, 1995.

51. Fountain N B, Lothman E W: Pathophysiology of status epilepticus. **J Clin Neurophysiol** 12: 326-42, 1995.

52. Delgado-Escueta A V, Wasterlain C, Treiman D M, *et al.*: Management of status epilepticus. **N Engl J Med** 306: 1337-40, 1982.

53. Barbosa E, Freeman J M: Status epilepticus. **Peds in Review** 4: 185-9, 1982.

54. Cascino G D: Generalized convulsive status epilepticus. **Mayo Clin Proc** 71: 787-92, 1996.

55. Levy R J, Krall R L: Treatment of status epilepticus with lorazepam. **Arch Neurol** 41: 605-11, 1984.

56. Lowenstein D H, Aminoff M J, Simon R P: Barbiturate anesthesia in the treatment of status epilepticus: Clinical experience with 14 patients. **Neurology** 38: 395-400, 1988.

57. Osorio I, Reed R C: Treatment of refractory generalized tonic-clonic status epilepticus with pentobarbital anesthesia after high-dose phenytoin. **Epilepsia** 30. 464-71, 1989.

58. Giang D, McBride M: Lorazepam versus diazepam for the treatment of status epilepticus. **Pediatr Neurol** 4: 358-61, 1988.

59. Appleton R, Sweeney A, Choonara I, *et al.*: Lorazepam versus diazepam in the acute treatment of epileptic seizures and status epilepticus. **Dev Med Child Neurol** 37: 682-8, 1995.

60. Crawford T O, Mitchell W G, Snodgrass S R: Lorazepam in childhood status epilepticus and serial seizures: Effectiveness and tachyphylaxis. **Neurology** 37: 190-5, 1987.

61. Labar D R, Auslim A, Root J: High-dose intravenous lorazepam for the treatment of refractory status epilepticus. **Neurology** 44: 1400-3, 1994.

62. Brodie M J, Dichter M A: Antiepileptic drugs. **N Engl J Med** 334: 168-75, 1996.

63. Mattson R H, Cramer J A, Collins J F, *et al.*: Comparison of carbamazepine, phenobarbital, phenytoin, and primidone in partial and secondarily generalized tonic-clonic seizures. **N Engl J Med** 313: 145-51, 1985.

64. Mattson R H, Cramer J A, Collins J F, *et al.*: A comparison of valproate with carbamazepine for the treatment of complex partial seizures and secondarily generalized tonic-clonic seizures in adults. **N Engl J Med** 327: 765-71, 1992.

65. Drugs for epilepsy. **Med Letter** 28: 91-3, 1986.

66. Rambeck B, Boenigk H E, Dunlop A, *et al.*: Predicting phenytoin dose - A revised nomogram. **Ther Drug Monit** 1: 325-33, 1979.

67. Saklad J J, Graves R H, Sharp W P: Interaction of oral phenytoin with enteral feedings. **J Parent Ent Nutr** 10: 322-3, 1986.

68. Worden J P, Wood C A, Workman C H: Phenytoin and nasogastric feedings. **Neurology** 34: 132, 1984 (letter).

69. Buehler B A, Delimont D, van Waes M, *et al.*: Prenatal prediction of risk of the fetal hydantoin syndrome. **N Engl J Med** 322: 1567-72, 1990.

70. Public Health Service: Fluoxetine-phenytoin interaction. **FDA Medical Bulletin** 24: 3-4, 1994.

71. Winkler S R, Luer M S: Antiepileptic drug review: Part 1. **Surg Neurol** 49: 449-52, 1998.

72. Oles K S, Waqar M, Penry J K: Catastrophic neurologic signs due to drug interaction: Tegretol and Darvon. **Surg Neurol** 32: 144-51, 1989.

73. Oakeshott P, Hunt G M: Valproate and spina bifida. **Br Med J** 298: 1300-1, 1989.

74. Wroblewski B A, Garvin W H: Once-daily administration of phenobarbital in adults: Clinical efficacy

and benefit. **Arch Neurol** 42: 699-700, 1985.

75. Davis A G, Mutchie K D, Thompson J A, *et al.*: Once-daily dosing with phenobarbital in children with seizure disorders. **Pediatrics** 68: 824-7, 1981.

76. Felbamate. **Med Letter** 35: 107-9, 1993.

77. Winkler S R, Luer M S: Antiepileptic drug review: Part 2. **Surg Neurol** 49: 566-8, 1998.

78. Gabapentin - A new anticonvulsant. **Med Letter** 36: 39-40, 1994.

79. Lamotrigine for epilepsy. **Med Letter** 37: 21-3, 1995.

80. Guerrini R, Dravet, C, Genton P, *et al.*: Lamotrigine and seizure aggravation in severe myoclonic epilepsy. **Epilepsia** 39: 508-12, 1998.

81. Topiramate for epilepsy. **Med Letter** 39: 51-2, 1997.

82. Faught E, Wilder B J, Ramsay R E, *et al.*: Topiramate placebo-controlled dose-ranging trial in refractory partial epilepsy using 200-, 400-, and 600-mg daily dosages. **Neurology** 46: 1684-90, 1996.

83. Privitera M, Fincham R, Penry J, *et al.*: Topiramate placebo-controlled dose-ranging trial in refractory partial epilepsy using 600-, 800-, and 1,000-mg daily dosages. **Neurology** 46: 1678-83, 1996.

84. Tiagabine for epilepsy. **Med Letter** 40: 45-6, 1998.

85. Shuster E A: Epilepsy in women. **Mayo Clin Proc** 71: 991-9, 1996.

86. Callaghan N, Garrett A, Goggin T: Withdrawal of anticonvulsant drugs in patients free of seizures for two years. **N Engl J Med** 318: 942-6, 1988.

87. Anderson T, Braathen G, Persson A, *et al.*: A comparison between one and three years of treatment in uncomplicated childhood epilepsy: A prospective study. II. The EEG as predictor of outcome after withdrawal of treatment. **Epilepsia** 38: 225-32, 1997.

88. Medical Research Council Antiepileptic Drug Withdrawal Study Group: Randomized study of antiepileptic drug withdrawal in patients in remission. **Lancet** 337 (8751): 1175-80, 1991.

89. Delgado-Escueta A, Janz D: Consensus guidelines: Preconception counseling, management, and care of the pregnant woman with epilepsy. **Neurology** 42 (Suppl 5): 149-60, 1992.

90. Mattson R H, Cramer J A, Darney P D, *et al.*: Use of oral contraceptives by women with epilepsy. **JAMA** 256: 238-40, 1986.

91. Perucca E, Hedges A, Makki K A, *et al.*: A comparative study of the relative enzyme inducing properties of anticonvulsant drugs in epileptic patients. **Br J Clin Pharmacol** 18: 401-10, 1984.

92. Yerby M S, Freil P N, McCormick K: Antiepileptic drug disposition during pregnancy. **Neurology** 42 (Suppl 5): 12-6, 1992.

93. Dias M S, Sekhar L N: Intracranial hemorrhage from aneurysms and arteriovenous malformations during pregnancy and the puerperium. **Neurosurgery** 27: 855-66, 1990.

94. Jones K L, Lacro R V, Johnson K A, *et al.*: Patterns of malformations in the children of women treated with carbamazepine during pregnancy. **N Engl J Med** 310: 1661-6, 1989.

95. Rosa F W: Spina bifida in infants of women treated with carbamazepine during pregnancy. **N Engl J Med** 324: 674-7, 1991.

96. Hanson J W, Smith D W: The fetal hydantoin syndrome. **J Pediatr** 87: 285-90, 1975.

97. Scolnik D, Nulman I, Rovet J, *et al.*: Neurodevelopment of children exposed in utero to phenytoin and carbamazepine monotherapy. **JAMA** 271: 767-70, 1994.

98. Nakane Y, Okuma T, Takahashi R, *et al.*: Multi-institutional study of the teratogenicity and fetal toxicity of antiepileptic drugs: A report of a collaborative study group in Japan. **Epilepsia** 21: 663-80, 1980.

99. Waters C H, Belai Y, Gott P S, *et al.*: Outcomes of pregnancy associated with antiepileptic drugs. **Arch Neurol** 51: 250-3, 1994.

100. Kanto J H: Use of benzodiazepines during pregnancy, labor, and lactation, with particular reference to pharmacokinetic considerations. **Drugs** 23: 354-80, 1982.

101. Saunders M: Epilepsy in women of childbearing age: If anticonvulsants cannot be avoided, use carbamazepine. **Br Med J** 199: 581, 1989.

102. National Institutes of Health Consensus Development Conference: Surgery for epilepsy. **JAMA** 264: 729-33, 1990.

103. Barkovich A J, Rowley H A, Anderman F: MR in partial epilepsy: Value of high-resolution volumetric techniques. **AJNR** 16: 339-43, 1995.

104. Oakley J, Ojemann G A, Ojemann L M, *et al.*: Identifying epileptic foci on contrast-enhanced CAT scans. **Arch Neurol** 36: 669-71, 1979.

105. Harvey A S, Hopkins I J, Bowe J M, *et al.*: Frontal lobe epilepsy: Clinical seizure characteristics and localization with ictal ^{99m}Tc-HMPAO SPECT. **Neurology** 43: 1966-80, 1993.

106. Wada J, Rasmussen T: Intracranial injection of amytal for the lateralization of cerebral speech dominance. **J Neurosurg** 17: 266-82, 1960.

107. Queenan J V, Germano I M: Advances in the neurosurgical management of adult epilepsy. **Contemp Neurosurg** 19 (16): 1-6, 1997.

108. Cohen D S, Zubay G P, Goodman R R: Seizure outcome after lesionectomy for cavernous malformations. **J Neurosurg** 83: 237-42, 1995.

109. Jooma R, Yeh H-S, Privitera M D, *et al.*: Lesionectomy versus electrophysiologically guided resection for temporal lobe tumors manifesting with complex partial seizures. **J Neurosurg** 83: 231-6, 1995.

110. Morrell F, Whisler W W, Bleck T P: Multiple subpial transection: A new approach to the surgical treatment of focal epilepsy. **J Neurosurg** 70: 231-9, 1989.

111. Gates J R, Leppik I E, Yap J, *et al.*: Corpus callosotomy: Clinical and electroencephalographic effects. **Epilepsia** 25: 308-16, 1984.

112. Marino R, Ragazzo P C: In **Epilepsy and the corpus callosum**, Reeves A G, (ed.). Plenum Press, New York, 1985: pp 281-302.

113. Bogen J E, Schultz D H, Vogel P J: Completeness of callosotomy shown by MRI in the long term. **Arch Neurol** 45: 1203-5, 1988.

114. Ojemann G A: In **Surgical treatment of the epilepsies**, Engel J, (ed.). Raven Press, New York, 1987: pp 635-9.

115. Ojemann G A: Surgical therapy for medically intractable epilepsy. **J Neurosurg** 66: 489-99, 1987.

116. Niemeyer P: *The transventricular amygdala-hippocampectomy in temporal lobe epilepsy*. In **Temporal lobe epilepsy**, Baldwin M and Bailey P, (eds.). Charles C Thomas, Springfield, 1958: pp 461-82.

117. Crandall P H: *Cortical resections*. In **Surgical treatment of the epilepsies**, Engel J, (ed.). Raven Press, New York, 1987: pp 377-404.

14. Spine

14.1.　　　Low back pain and radiculopathy

❢ Key points[1]
- low back pain is common, and in ≈ 85% of cases, no specific diagnosis can be made
- initial assessment is geared to detecting "red flags" (indicating potentially serious pathology), and in the absence of these, imaging studies and further testing of patients is usually not helpful during the first 4 weeks of low back symptoms
- relief of discomfort can be best achieved with nonprescription pain meds and/or spinal manipulation
- while activities may need to be modified, bed rest beyond 4 days may be more harmful than helpful, and patients are encouraged to return to work or their normal daily activities as soon as possible
- 89-90% of patients with low back problems will improve within 1 month even without treatment
- with or without surgery, 80% of patients with sciatica eventually recover

Low back pain (**LBP**) is extremely prevalent, and is the second most common reason for people to seek medical attention[2]. LBP accounts for ≈ 15% of all sick leave from work, and is the most common cause of disability for persons < 45 yrs age[3]. Estimates of lifetime prevalence range from 60-90%, and the annual incidence is 5%[4]. Only 1% of patients will have nerve-root symptoms, and only 1-3% have lumbar disc herniation. The prognosis for most cases of LBP is good, and improvement usually occurs with little or no medical intervention.

DEFINITIONS/CLASSIFICATIONS

radiculopathy	dysfunction of a nerve root (signs and symptoms may include: pain in the distribution of that nerve root, dermatomal sensory disturbances, weakness of muscles innervated by that nerve root, and hypoactive muscle stretch reflexes of the same muscles)
mechanical low back pain	AKA "musculoskeletal" back pain (both non-specific terms). The most common form of low back pain. May result from strain of the paraspinal muscles and/or ligaments, irritation of facet joints... Excludes anatomically identifiable causes (e.g. tumor, disc herniation...)

NOMENCLATURE FOR DISC PATHOLOGY

Historically, the terminology has been contentious and nonstandardized. Many diagnostic labels are used inconsistently (e.g. spondylosis, sprain, strain, musculoskeletal pain, myofascial pain...). A subset of nomenclature proposed by a task force[5] is shown in *Table 14-1*, which is useful primarily for consistent terminology related to radiographic reports, research....

Degenerated disc: some reports indicate that these can cause radicular pain possibly by an inflammatory mechanism[6], but this is not universally accepted.

Bulging disc: may or may not be symptomatic.

Vacuum disc: imaging findings of gas in the disc space, usually indicative of disc degeneration.

Non-Standard terms

These terms are included for completeness but are <u>not</u> recommended because they may be confusing or inaccurate[5].

Contained herniation[5]: displaced disc tissue entirely contained within an uninterrupted (but possibly distended) anulus or capsule (*see page 301* for definition of *cap-*

sule). It may be difficult to distinguish this on currently available imaging studies from an uncontained herniation which is underneath the posterior longitudinal ligament.

Ruptured disc: colloquial term usually intended to be equivalent to herniated disc.

Table 14-1 Nomenclature for lumbar disc pathology[5]

Term	Description
anular tears AKA anular fissures	separations between anular fibers, avulsions of fibers from their VB insertions, or breaks through fibers that extend radiallly, transversely, or concentrically
degeneration	desiccation, fibrosis, narrowing of the disc space, diffuse bulging of anulus beyond the disc space, extensive fissuring (i.e. numerous annular tears), mucinous degeneration of the anulus, defects and sclerosis of endplates, & osteophytes at the vertebral apophyses
degenerative disc disease	clinical syndrome of symptoms related to degenerative changes in the intervertebral disc (described above), also often considered to encompass degenerative changes *outside* the disc as well
bulging	generalized displacement of disc material (arbitrarily defined as > 50% or 180°) beyond the peripheral limits of the disc space*. Not considered a form of herniation
herniation	localized displacement of disc material (< 50% or 180°) beyond the limits of the intervertebral disc space*
	focal: < 25% of the disc circumference
	broad-based: 25-50% of the disc circumference
	protrusion: the fragment does not have a "neck" that is narrower than the fragment in any dimension
	extrusion: the fragment has a "neck" that is narrrower than the fragment in at least 1 dimension. 2 subtypes A. **sequestration**: the fragment has lost continuity with the dics of origin (AKA **free fragment**) B. **migration**: the fragment is displaced away from the site of extrusion, regardless of whether sequestered or not
	intravertebral herniation (AKA **Schmorl's node**): disc herniates in the cranio-caudal direction through the cartilaginous end-plate into the VB (*see page 313*)

* intervertebral disc space: bounded by VB endplates in the cranio-caudal dimension, and by the outer edges of the vertebral ring apophyses (exlusive of osteophytes) in the peripheral direction

Recommended classification

It is recommended[1] that acute back problems be classified into one of the 3 categories shown in *Table 14-2* based on the history and physical exam (see *Initial assessment of the patient with back pain* below).

Further evaluation, treatment, and even some information regarding prognosis can be based on this simple classification. A major goal is to detect "red flags" that may indicate potentially serious spinal or nonspinal pathology (*see page 292*).

Table 14-2 AHCPR classification of back problems

Clinical category	Description
potentially serious spinal condition	includes spinal tumor, infection, fracture, or cauda equina syndrome (*see text*)
sciatica	pain along the course of the sciatic nerve, usually resulting from nerve root compromise
nonspecific back symptoms	symptoms occurring primarily in the back that suggest neither nerve root compromise nor a serious underlying condition

NOMENCLATURE FOR SPINE PATHOLOGY OUTSIDE THE DISC

Vertebral body marrow changes:
Associated with degenerative or inflammatory changes. **Modic's classification**[7] of MRI characteristics is shown in *Table 14-3*.

Table 14-3 Modic's classification

Modic Type	Intensity changes		Description
	T1WI	T2WI	
1	↓	↑	bone marrow edema associated with acute or subacute inflammation
2	↑	iso or ↑	chronic changes: replacement of bone marrow by fat
3	↓	↓	reactive osteosclerosis

DIFFERENTIAL DIAGNOSIS

The differential diagnosis of low back pain (*see Low back pain*, page 907) overlaps with that of myelopathy. In ≈ 85% of cases of LBP no specific diagnosis can be made[8].

INITIAL ASSESSMENT OF THE PATIENT WITH BACK PAIN

Initial assessment consists of a history and physical exam focused on identifying serious underlying conditions such as: fracture, tumor, infection or cauda equina syndrome. Serious conditions presenting as low back problems are relatively rare.

HISTORY

The following information has been found to be helpful in identifying patients with serious underlying conditions such as cancer and spinal infection[1]. *Table 14-4* shows the sensitivity and specificity.

1. age
2. history of cancer (especially malignancies that are prone to skeletal metastases: prostate, breast, kidney, thyroid, lung)
3. unexplained weight loss
4. immunosuppression: from steroids, organ transplant medication, or HIV
5. prolonged use of steroids
6. duration of symptoms
7. responsiveness to previous therapy
8. pain that is worse at rest
9. history of skin infection: especially furuncle
10. history of IV drug abuse
11. UTI or other infection
12. pain radiating below the knee
13. persistent numbness or weakness in the legs
14. history of significant trauma. In a young patient: MVA, a fall from a height, or a direct blow to the back. In an older patient: minor falls, heavy lifting or even severe coughing can cause a fracture especially in the presence of osteoporosis
15. findings consistent with cauda equina syndrome (*see page 305*):
    A. bladder dysfunction (usually urinary retention, or overflow incontinence) or fecal incontinence
    B. saddle anesthesia: *see page 305*
    C. unilateral or bilateral leg weakness or pain

Table 14-4 Sensitivity and specificity of historical findings in patients with low back problems[1]

Condition	History	Sensitivity	Specificity
cancer	age ≥ 50 yrs	0.77	0.71
	previous Ca	0.31	0.98
	unexplained weight loss	0.15	0.94
	failure to improve after conservative therapy x 1 month	0.31	0.90
	any of the above	1.00	0.60
	pain > 1 month	0.50	0.81
spinal osteomyelitis	IV drug abuse, UTI, or skin infection	0.40	NA
compression fracture	age ≥ 50 yrs	0.84	0.61
	age ≥ 70yrs	0.22	0.96
	trauma	0.30	0.85
	steroid use	0.06	0.995
HLD	sciatica	0.95	0.88
spinal stenosis	pseudoclaudication	0.60	NA
	age ≥ 50 yrs	0.90*	0.70
ankylosing spondylitis	positive response to 4 out of 5 of the following	0.23	0.82
	age at onset ≤ 40 yrs	1.00	0.07
	pain not relieved when supine	0.80	0.49
	AM back stiffness	0.64	0.59
	pain ≥ 3 mos duration	0.71	0.54

* estimate

16. psychological and socioeconomic factors may influence the patient's report of symptoms (also *see page 296*), and one should inquire about:
    A. work status
    B. typical job tasks
    C. educational level
    D. pending litigation
    E. worker's compensation or disability issues
    F. failed previous treatments
    G. substance abuse
    H. depression

Less helpful than the history in identifying patients who may be harboring conditions such as cancer, but may be more helpful in detecting spinal infections.

1. spinal infection (*see page 240*): findings that suggest this as a possibility (but are also common in patients without infection)
   A. fever: common in epidural abscess and vertebral osteomyelitis, less common in discitis
   B. vertebral tenderness
   C. very limited range of spinal motion
2. findings of possible neurologic compromise: the following physical findings will identify most cases of clinically significant nerve root compromise due to L4-5 or L5-S1 HLD which comprise > 90% of cases of radiculopathy due to HLD (limiting the exam to the following might not detect the much less common upper lumbar disc herniations, which may be difficult to detect on PE, *see page 310*)
   A. dorsiflexion strength of ankle and great toe: weakness suggests L5 and some L4 dysfunction
   B. achilles reflex: diminished reflex suggests S1 root dysfunction
   C. light touch sensation of the foot:
      1. diminished over medial malleolus and medial foot: suggests L4
      2. diminished over dorsum of foot: suggests L5
      3. diminished over lateral malleolus and lateral foot: suggests S1
   D. straight leg raising (**SLR**) (also check for crossed SLR): *see page 302*

"RED FLAGS" IN THE HISTORY AND PHYSICAL EXAM FOR LOW BACK PROBLEMS

Based upon the above history and physical exam, the findings in *Table 14-5* would suggest the possibility of a serious underlying condition as the cause of the low back problem.

FURTHER EVALUATION

For over 95% of patients with acute low back problems, no further testing within the first 4 weeks of symptoms is required[1].

In the absence of any of the "red flag" conditions shown in *Table 14-5*, no further testing is recommended (even for patients suspected of having a HLD) and the treatment is similar for most patients with an acute episode of low back problems.

Simple laboratory tests including CBC and ESR are sufficiently efficacious and inexpensive that they should be obtained when there is a suspicion of back related tumor or infection.

Table 14-5 "Red flags" for patients with low back problems

Condition	Red flags
cancer or infection	1. age > 50 or < 20 yrs 2. history of cancer 3. unexplained weight loss 4. immunosuppression (*see text*) 5. UTI, IV drug abuse, fever or chills 6. back pain not improved with rest
spinal fracture	1. history of significant trauma (*see text*) 2. prolonged use of steroids 3. age > 70 yrs
cauda equina syndrome or severe neurologic compromise	1. acute onset of urinary retention or overflow incontinence 2. fecal incontinence or loss of anal sphincter tone 3. saddle anesthesia 4. global or progressive weakness in the LEs

FURTHER EVALUATION OF PATIENTS WITH LOW BACK PROBLEMS

Except for those exhibiting "red flags" (*see above*), special diagnostic tests are usually not needed during the first month of symptoms since it is not possible to predict which patients will improve (as most do) and which will not.

TESTS FOR EVIDENCE OF PHYSIOLOGIC DYSFUNCTION

EMG for low back problems: If the diagnosis of radiculopathy seems likely on clinical grounds, electrophysiologic testing is not recommended[1]. However, these tests may be useful for patients with suspicion of other conditions (e.g. neuropathy, myopathy, myelopathy...) or when the diagnosis of radiculopathy is uncertain (e.g. a HLD on MRI is not always symptomatic). Testing is highly operator dependent for accuracy.

1. needle EMG: can assess acute and chronic nerve root dysfunction, myelopathy and myopathy. Not indicated and also unreliable when symptoms present < 3-4

weeks. Overall accuracy improves with knowledge about imaging studies and clinical information[9]. Accuracy in predicting level of involvement[10] is ≈ 84%

2. H-reflex: measures sensory conduction through nerve roots. Used mostly to assess S1 radiculopathy[11]
3. SEPs: assesses sensory neurons in peripheral nerves and spinal cord. May be useful in evaluating suspected spinal stenosis or spinal myelopathy
4. nerve conduction studies (including NCVs): helps identify acute and chronic entrapment neuropathies that may mimic radiculopathy
5. ✖ not recommended for assessing acute low back problems[1]
   A. F-wave response: measures motor conduction through nerve roots, used to assess proximal neuropathies
   B. surface EMG: assesses acute and chronic recruitment patterns during static or dynamic tasks using surface (instead of needle) electrodes

Bone scan for low back problems: Description: injection of radiolabeled compounds (usually technetium-99m) that are taken up by metabolically active bone. A gamma camera is then used to localize regions of uptake. The total radiation dose is equivalent to a set of lumbar spine x-rays[1]. Contraindicated during pregnancy, and breast feeding must be suspended for a brief interval following a bone scan due to presence of radiotracer in the breast milk.

A moderately sensitive test which may be used in evaluating low back pain when spinal tumor[12], infection[13], or occult fracture is suspected from "red flags" (*see Table 14-5*) on history or examination, or results of lab tests or plain x-rays. Not very specific, but may locate occult lesions and help differentiate these conditions from degenerative changes. A positive bone scan suggesting one of these conditions usually must be confirmed by other diagnostic tests or procedures (no studies have compared bone scans to CT or MRI).

Low yield in patients with longstanding low back problems and normal plain x-rays and laboratory tests (especially ESR)[12].

Thermography for low back problems: Not recommended[1]. Did not accurately predict absence or presence of nerve root compression seen at surgery[14], and may be positive in a significant percentage of asymptomatic patients[15].

RADIOGRAPHIC EVALUATION

Diagnosing lumbar spinal stenosis or herniated intervertebral disc is usually helpful only in potential surgical candidates[16]. This includes patients with appropriate clinical syndromes who have not responded satisfactorily to adequate non-surgical treatment over a sufficient period of time, and who have no medical contraindications to surgery. Radiologic confirmation of these diagnoses usually requires CT, myelography, MRI, or some combination (*see below*). NB: myelography[17], CT[18], or MRI[19] may also show bulging or herniated lumbar discs (**HLD**) or spinal stenosis in asymptomatic patients (e.g. 24% of asymptomatic patients have herniated discs on MRI and 4% have spinal stenosis; these numbers become 36% and 21% respectively in patients 60-80 years old)[20]. Thus, these tests must be interpreted in light of clinical findings, and the anatomic level and side should correspond to the history, examination, and/or other physiologic data. Diagnostic radiology is of limited benefit as the initial evaluation in the majority of spinal disorders[21].

In the absence of red flags for serious conditions, imaging studies are not recommended in the first month of symptoms[1]. For patients who have had previous back surgery, MRI with contrast is probably the best test. Myelography (with or without CT) is invasive and has increased risk of complications, and is therefore indicated only in situations where MRI cannot be done or is inadequate, and surgery is anticipated.

Σ

Patients for whom radiographic imaging is recommended are those with:
- suspected *benign* conditions with symptoms persisting beyond 4 weeks of great enough severity to consider surgery including:
  - ◆ back related leg symptoms and clinically specific signs of nerve root compromise
  - ◆ a history of neurogenic claudication (*see page 326*) or other finding suggestive of lumbar spinal stenosis
- red flags: physical examination or other test results suggesting other serious conditions affecting the spine (e.g. cauda equina syndrome, fracture, infection, tumor, or other mass lesions or defects)

Unexpected findings occurred in only 1 in 2500 adults < 50 years age[22]. Diagnosis of surgical conditions of disc herniation and spinal stenosis cannot be made from plain films. Various congenital abnormalities of uncertain significance may be identified (e.g. spina bifida occulta), and evidence of degenerative changes (including osteophytes) are as frequent in symptomatic as in asymptomatic patients. Gonadal radiation is significant. Seldom indicated during pregnancy.

Recommendation

Not recommended for routine evaluation of patients with acute low back problems during the first month of symptoms unless a "red flag" is present (*see below*). Reserve LS x-rays for patients with a likelihood of having spinal malignancy, infection, inflammatory spondylitis, or clinically significant fracture. In these cases, plain x-rays are often just a starting point, and further study (CT, MRI…) may be indicated even if the plain x-rays are normal. "Red flags" for these conditions include the following:

1. age > 70 years, or < 20 yrs
2. systemically ill patients
3. temp > 100°F (or > 38° C)
4. history of malignancy
5. recent infection
6. patients with neurologic deficits suggesting possible cauda equina syndrome (saddle anesthesia, urinary incontinence or retention, LE weakness, *see page 305*)
7. heavy alcohol or IV drug abusers
8. diabetics
9. immunosuppressed patients (including prolonged treatment with corticosteroids)
10. recent urinary tract or spinal surgery
11. *recent* trauma: any age with significant trauma, or > 50 yrs old with mild trauma
12. unrelenting pain at rest
13. persistent pain for more than ≈ 4 weeks
14. unexplained weight loss

When spine x-rays are indicated, AP and lateral views are usually adequate[23]. Obliques and coned-down L5-S1 views more than double the radiation exposure, and add information in only 4-8% of cases[24], and can be obtained in specific instances where warranted (e.g. to diagnose spondylolysis when spondylolisthesis is found on the lateral film).

MRI

MRI has supplanted CT and myelography for diagnosing most disc herniations and also in most cases of spinal stenosis. The test of choice for patients who have had previous back surgery. Specificity and sensitivity for HLD are on the same order as CT/myelography, which is better than myelography alone[1, 25, 26].

Advantages:
1. provides information in sagittal plane (can easily evaluate cauda equina)
2. provides information regarding tissue outside of the spinal canal (e.g. extreme lateral disc herniation (*see page 311*), tumors…)
3. non-invasive and does not involve ionizing radiation

Disadvantages:
1. patients in severe pain or with claustrophobia may have difficulty holding still
2. dose not visualize bone well
3. poor for studying blood early (e.g. spinal epidural hematoma)
4. expensive (note: may be more cost effective than myelography if post-myelogram overnight hospitalization is avoided, and especially if a rare complication from myelography occurs)
5. difficult to interpret in cases of scoliosis. Myelogram/CT may be superior
6. a number of contraindications: see *Contraindications to MRI*, page 135

Findings:
In addition to demonstrating herniated lumbar disc (**HLD**) outside of the disc interspace compressing nerve root or thecal sac, MRI can demonstrate signal changes within the interspace suggestive of <u>disc degeneration</u>[27] (loss of signal intensity on T2WI, loss of disc space height).

LUMBOSACRAL CT

Not considered state of the art. If technically adequate images can be obtained (e.g.

good quality scanner, images not obscured by artifact from patient movement or obesity), CT can demonstrate most spine pathology. For HLD, sensitivity is 80-95%, and specificity is 68-88%[28, 29]. However, even some large disc herniations will be missed with plain CT. CT studies for HLD tend to be less satisfactory in the elderly. More utility with fractures.

Disc material has density (Hounsfield units) ≈ twice that of the thecal sac. Associated findings with herniated disc include:
1. loss of epidural fat (normally seen as low density in the anterolateral canal)
2. loss of normal "convexity" of thecal sac (indentation by herniated disc)

Advantages:
1. images soft tissue to a degree that may be adequate
2. excellent bony detail
3. non-invasive
4. outpatient evaluation
5. evaluates for extreme lateral disc herniation to some degree
6. evaluates paraspinal soft tissue (e.g. to rule out tumor, paraspinal abscess…)
7. advantages over MRI: faster scanning (significant in patients who have difficulty laying still for long time), less expensive, less claustrophobic, fewer contraindications (see *Contraindications to MRI*, page 135)

Disadvantages:
1. does not evaluate sagittal plane (may be partially ameliorated by eliminating skip regions and then utilizing computerized sagittal reconstructions)
2. evaluates only those levels that are scanned:
   A. higher cuts must be taken through the conus medullaris to avoid missing occasional pathology there
   B. performing cuts only through the disc spaces (a common practice) may miss pathology between the disc spaces
3. sensitivity is significantly lower than MRI or myelogram/CT

MYELOGRAPHY

With water soluble contrast, sensitivity (62-100%) and specificity (83-94%)[30-33] are similar to CT for detection of HLD. When combined with post-myelographic CT scan (myelogram/CT), the sensitivity and especially specificity increase[34]. A herniated disk in the large space between thecal sac and posterior border of vertebral bodies at L5-S1 (**insensitive space**) may not be seen on myelography (CT or MRI are usually better at detecting this).

Advantages:
1. provides information in sagittal plane (unlike plain CT)
2. evaluates cauda equina (unlike routine CT)
3. provides "functional" information about degree of stenosis (a high-degree block will allow flow of dye only after certain position changes)

Disadvantages:
1. occasionally requires overnight hospitalization
2. may miss pathology outside of the dura (including far laterally herniated disc), sensitivity is improved with post-myelographic CT
3. invasive
   A. drugs e.g. warfarin must be stopped, and sometimes converted to heparin
   B. with occasional side effects (post LP H/A, N/V, rare seizures)
4. iodine allergic patients
   A. requires iodine allergy prep
   B. may still be risky (especially in severely iodine allergic patients)

Findings:
HLD produces extradural filling defect at the level of the intervertebral disc. Massive disc herniation or severe lumbar stenosis may produce a total or near total block. In some cases of HLD, the finding may be very subtle and may consist of a cut-off of the filling (with contrast) of the nerve root sleeve (compared to normal nerve(s) on contralateral side or at other levels). Another subtle finding may be a "dual shadow" on lateral view.

BONE SCAN
See *page 293*

Injection of water-soluble contrast agent directly into the nucleus pulposus of the intervertebral disc being studied. Results of the test depend on volume of dye accepted into the disc, the pressure needed to inject the dye, the configuration of the dye (including leakage from the confines of the disc space) on radiographic imaging (plain x-rays produce the so-called "discogram", CT scan may also be utilized), and reproduction of the patient's pain on injection. Some of the basis for performing a discogram is to identify levels that may produce "discogenic pain" or "painful disc syndrome", a controversial point (see *PRACTICE PARAMETER 14-5*, page 300).

Critique:

Invasive. Interpretation is equivocal, and complications may occur (disc space infection, disc herniation, and significant radiation exposure with CT-discography). May be abnormal in asymptomatic patients[35, 36] (as any of the above tests may be) although the false positive rate may not be quite this high[37]. See *PRACTICE PARAMETER 14-9*, page 301 for recommendations.

PSYCHOSOCIAL FACTORS

Although some patients with chronic LPB (> 3 months duration) may have started off with a diagnosable condition, psychological and socioeconomic factors (such as depression, secondary gain…) may come to play a significant role in perpetuating or amplifying pain. Psychological factors, especially elevated hysteria or hypochondriasis scales on the Minnesota Multiphasic Personality Inventory **(MMPI)** were found to be a better predictor of outcome than findings on radiographic imaging in one study[9]. A screening scale of 5 factors has been proposed[38] (positive findings in any 3 suggests psychological distress):

1. pain on simulated axial loading: press on top of head
2. inconsistent performance: e.g. difficulty tolerating straight leg raising **(SLR)** while supine, but no difficulty when sitting
3. overreaction during the physical exam
4. inappropriate tenderness that is superficial or widespread } these two items may not be reliable,
5. motor or sensory abnormalities not corresponding to anatomic confines } the others are potentially reliable[39]

However, the usefulness of this information is limited, and no effective interventions have been identified to address these factors. Therefore the AHCPR panel was unable to recommend specific assessment tools or interventions[1].

TREATMENT

An initial period of nonsurgical management ("conservative" treatment, *see below*) is indicated except in the following circumstances where urgent surgery is indicated: symptoms of a cauda equina syndrome (urinary retention, saddle anesthesia…, see *Cauda equina syndrome*, page 305), progressive neurologic deficit, or profound motor weakness. A relative indication for proceeding to surgery without conservative management is severe pain that cannot be sufficiently controlled with adequate pain medication (rare).

If specific diagnoses such as herniated intervertebral lumbar disc or symptomatic lumbar stenosis are made, surgical treatment for these conditions may be considered if the patient fails to improve satisfactorily. In cases where no specific diagnosis can be made, management consists of conservative treatment and following the patient to rule out the possible development of symptoms suggestive of a more serious diagnosis that may not have initially been evident.

"CONSERVATIVE" TREATMENT

This term has regrettably come to be used for non-surgical management. With slight modification, similar approaches can be used for mechanical low back pain, as well as for acute radiculopathy from disc herniation.

Recommendations (based on AHCPR findings[1] in the absence of "red flags"[A]):

A. some key literature citations are given here, primarily those from the better studies that support the Agency for Health Care Policy and Research **(AHCPR)** panel recommendations. However, refer to Bigos et al.[1] for full analysis and list of references

1. activity modifications: no studies were found that met the panels review criteria for adequate evidence. However, the following information was felt to be useful:
   A. bed rest:
      1. the theoretical objective is to reduce symptoms by reducing pressure on the nerve roots and/or intradiscal pressures which is lowest in the supine semi-Fowler position[41], and also to reduce movements which are experienced as painful by the patient
      2. deactivation from prolonged bed rest (> 4 days) appears to be worse for patients (producing weakness, stiffness, and increased pain) than a gradual return to normal activities[42]
      3. recommendations: the majority of patients with low back problems will not require bed rest. Bed rest for 2-4 days may be an option for those with severe initial *radicular* symptoms, however, this may be no better than watchful waiting[43] and may be harmful[44]
   B. activity modification
      1. the goal is to achieve a tolerable level of discomfort while continuing sufficient physical activity to minimize disruption of daily activities
      2. risk factors: although there is not agreement on their exact role, the following were identified as having an increased incidence of low back problems. Jobs requiring heavy or repetitive lifting, total body vibration (from vehicles or industrial machinery), asymmetric postures, or postures sustained for long periods (including prolonged sitting)
      3. recommendations: temporarily limit heavy lifting, prolonged sitting, and bending or twisting of the back. Establish activity goals to help focus attention on expected return to full functional status
   C. exercise (may be part of a physical therapy program):
      1. during the 1st month of symptoms, low-stress aerobic exercise can minimize debility due to inactivity. In the first 2 weeks, utilize exercises that minimally stress the back: walking, bicycling, or swimming
      2. conditioning exercises for trunk muscles (especially back extensors, and possibly abdominal muscles) are helpful if symptoms persist (during the first 2 weeks, these exercises may aggravate symptoms)
      3. there is no evidence to support stretching of back muscles, or to recommend back-specific exercise machines over traditional exercise
      4. recommended exercise quotas that are gradually escalated results in better outcome than having patients simply stop when pain occurs[45]
2. analgesics:
   A. for the initial short-term period, acetaminophen (**APAP**) or NSAIDs (*see page 28*) may be used
   B. stronger analgesics (mostly opioids, *see page 30*) may be required for severe pain, usually severe radicular pain. For non-specific back pain, there was no earlier return to full activity than with NSAIDs or APAP[1]. Opioids should not be used > 2-3 weeks, at which time NSAIDs should be instituted
3. muscle relaxants (*see page 34*)
   A. muscle spasms have not been proven to cause pain, and the most commonly used muscle relaxants have no peripheral effect on muscle spasm
   B. probably more effective than placebo, but have not been shown to be more effective than NSAIDs
   C. potential for side effects: drowsiness (in up to 30%). Most manufacturers recommend use for < 2-3 weeks. Agents such as chlorzoxazone (Parafon Forte® and others) may be associated with risk of serious and potentially fatal hepatotoxicity[46]
4. education: (may be provided as part of a physical therapy program)
   A. explanation of the condition to the patient[47] in understandable terms, and positive reassurance that the condition will almost certainly subside[48] have been shown to be more effective than many other forms of treatment
   B. proper posture, sleeping positions, lifting techniques... should be conveyed to the patient. Formal "back school" seems to be marginally effective[49]
5. spinal manipulation therapy (**SMT**): defined as manual therapy in which loads are applied to the spine using long or short lever methods with the selected joint being taken to its end range of voluntary motion, followed by application of an impulse loading (may be part of a physical therapy program)
   A. may be helpful for patients with acute low back problems without radiculopathy when used in the first month of symptoms (efficacy after 1 month is unproven) for a period not to exceed 1 month

B. insufficient evidence to recommend SMT in the presence of radiculopathy
C. SMT should not be used in the face of severe or progressive neurologic deficit until serious conditions have been ruled out
D. ✖ reports of arterial dissection (especially vertebral artery) (*see page 883*) and CVA, myelopathy & subdural hematoma with cervical SMT and cauda equina syndrome with lumbar SMT[50-52] and the uncertainty of benefits have led to the questioning of the use of SMT[50] (especially cervical)

6. epidural injections:
   A. epidural (cortico)steroid injections **(ESI)**: there is no evidence that this is effective in treating acute radiculopathy[53]. Prospective studies yield varied results[54]. Some improvement at 3 & 6 weeks may occur (but no functional benefit, and no change in the need for surgery), with no benefit at 3 months[55]. The response in chronic back pain is poor in comparison to acute pain. ESI may be an option for short-term relief of *radicular* pain when control on oral medications is inadequate or for patients who are not surgical candidates
   B. there is no evidence to support the use of epidural injections of steroids, local anesthetics and/or opioids for LBP without radiculopathy
   C. efficacy with conditions such as lumbar spinal stenosis are conflicting [54]

PRACTICE PARAMETER 14-1 INJECTION THERAPY FOR LOW-BACK PAIN

Therapeutic recommendations

Options[40]: lumbar epidural injections or trigger point injections are not recommended for long-term relief of chronic LBP. These techniques or facet injections may be used to provide temporary relief in select patients

Diagnostic recommendations

Options[40]: **lumbar facet injections**
- may predict the response to radiofrequency facet ablation
- ✖ not recommended as a diagnostic tool to predict the response to lumbar fusion

---

✖ Not recommended by the AHCPR panel[1] for treatment of acute low back problems in the absence of "red flags" (see *Table 14-5*, page 292):

1. medications
   A. oral steroids: no difference was found at one week and 1 year after randomization to receive 1 week therapy with oral dexamethasone or placebo[56]
   B. colchicine: conflicting evidence shows either some[57] or no[58] therapeutic benefit. Side effects of N/V and diarrhea[1]
   C. antidepressant medications: most studies of these medications were for *chronic* back pain. Some methodologically flawed studies failed to show benefits when compared to placebo for chronic (not acute) LBP[59]

2. physical treatments
   A. TENS (transcutaneous electrical nerve stimulation): not statistically significantly better than placebo, and added no benefit to exercise alone[60]
   B. traction (including pelvic traction): not demonstrated to be effective[61]
   C. physical agents and modalities: including heat (including diathermy), ice, ultrasound. Benefit is insufficiently proven, however, self-administered home programs for application of heat or cold may be considered. Ultrasound and diathermy should not be used in pregnancy
   D. lumbar corsets and support belts: not proven beneficial for acute back problems. Prophylactic use has been advocated, but this is controversial[62]
   E. biofeedback: has not been studied for acute back problems. Primarily advocated for chronic LBP, where effectiveness is controversial[63]

3. injection therapy
   A. trigger point and ligamentous injections: the theory that trigger points cause or perpetuate LBP is controversial and disputed by many experts. Injections of local anesthetic are of equivocal efficacy
   B. facet joint injections: theoretical basis is that there exists a **"facet syndrome"** producing LBP which is aggravated by spine extension, with no nerve root tension signs (*see page 302*). No studies have adequately investigated injections for pain < 3 months duration. For chronic LBP, neither the agent nor the location (intrafacet or pericapsular) made a significant difference in outcomes[64, 65]
   C. epidural injections in the absence of radiculopathy: *see above*

D. acupuncture: no studies were found that evaluated the use in acute back problems. All randomized clinical trials found were for patients with *chronic* LBP, and even the best studies were felt to be mediocre and contradictory.

SURGICAL TREATMENT

Indications for surgery for herniated lumbar disc:

1. in patients with < 4-8 weeks duration of symptoms:
   A. those with "red flags" that would make them candidates for urgent treatment (e.g. cauda equina syndrome, progressive neurologic deficit...)
   B. inability to control pain with adequate pain medication (uncommon) may require earlier radiographic evaluation and consideration for surgery
2. patients with ≥ 4-8 weeks of symptoms of sciatica that are both severe and disabling and are not improving with time, with a radiographically identified abnormality that correlates with findings on the history and physical exam

---

PRACTICE PARAMETER 14-2 MRI & DISCOGRAPHY FOR PATIENT SELECTION FOR LUMBAR FUSION*

Guidelines[66]:
- MRI is recommended as the initial diagnostic test
- normal appearing discs on MRI should not be considered for discography or treatment
- lumbar discography should not be used as a stand-alone test
- if discography is used: to consider a disc level for treatment there should be a concordant pain response† & associated MRI abnormalities‡

Options[66]: discography should be reserved for equivocal MRI findings, especially at levels adjacent to unequivocally abnormal levels

---

* for recommendations on use of facet injections, see *PRACTICE PARAMETER 14-1*, page 298

† concordant pain response: pain identical or very similar to the patient's usual pain complaints (NB: discography can produce severe LBP in patients with no prior complaints[35, 36])

‡ abnormal disc morphology on MRI: loss of T2WI signal intensity, disc space collapse, modic changes, and high-intensity zones (these findings also frequently occur in asymptomatic patients[67])

Indications for fusion for chronic LBP without stenosis or spondylolisthesis:

PRACTICE PARAMETER 14-3 LUMBAR FUSION FOR LBP WITHOUT STENOSIS OR SPONDYLOLISTHESIS

Standards[68]: lumbar fusion is recommended for carefully selected patients* with disabling LBP due to one- or two-level degenerative disease without stenosis or spondylolisthesis

Options[68, 70]: intensive PT and cognitive therapy is recommended as a option for patients with LBP in whom conventional medical management has failed

---

* in the primary quoted study[69] patients had chronic LBP for ≥ 2 years and had radiologic evidence of disc degeneration at L4-L5, L5-S1, or both, and had failed best medical management

---

PRACTICE PARAMETER 14-4 CHOICE OF FUSION TECHNIQUE

Guidelines[71]: for ALIF or ALIF + instrumentation, the addition of a posterolateral fusion is not recommended*

Options[71]:
- either a posterolateral fusion or an interbody fusion (PLIF, TLIF or ALIF) are options for patients with LBP due to DDD at 1 or 2 levels
- an interbody graft is an option to improve fusion rates and functional outcome†
- ✖ the use of multiple approaches (anterior + posterior) is not recommended as a routine option for LBP without deformity

---

* the demonstrated benefit does not outweigh the additional time and blood loss involved

† caution: the improvement in fusion rate and outcome is marginal, and interbody fusion is associated with an increased complication rate, especially with combined approaches (e.g. 360° fusion)

The type of surgical procedure chosen is tailored to the specific condition identified. Examples are shown in *Table 14-6*. Discussion of some options is also provided below.

Lumbar spinal fusion

Although there is no consensus on the indications[72], lumbar spinal fusion (**LSF**) is accepted treatment for fracture/dislocation or instability resulting from tumor or infection.

For degenerative spine disease, practice parameters have been developed and are included herein.

Table 14-6 Surgical options for low back problems

Condition	Surgical treatment options
"routine" HLD	• standard discectomy and microdiscectomy are of similar efficacy • chymopapain: acceptable, but less efficacious than above. Significant risk of anaphylaxis (*see page 306*) • intradiscal procedures: nucleotome, laser disc decompression. Not recommended (*see page 306*)
foraminal or far lateral HLD	• partial or total facetectomy (*see page 312*) • extracanal approach (*see page 312*) • endoscopic techniques
lumbar spinal stenosis	• simple decompressive laminectomy • laminectomy plus fusion: may be indicated for patients with degenerative spondylolisthesis, stenosis and radiculopathy

---

PRACTICE PARAMETER 14-5 LUMBAR FUSION FOR DISC HERNIATION

Options[73]:
- lumbar fusion is <u>not</u> routinely recommended following disc excision in patients with HLD or recurrent HLD causing radiculopathy
- lumbar fusion is a potential adjunct to disc excision in cases of a HLD or recurrent HLD:
  - ♦ with evidence of preoperative lumbar spinal deformity or instability
  - ♦ in patients with chronic axial LBP associated with radiculopathy

Instrumentation as an adjunct to fusion

PRACTICE PARAMETER 14-6 PEDICLE SCREW FIXATION

Options[74]: pedicle screw fixation is recommended as a treatment option for patients with LBP treated with posterolateral fusion who are at high risk for fusion failure*

* routine use of pedicle screws is discouraged because of conflicting evidence of benefit, together with considerable evidence of increased cost and complications

The use of instrumentation increases the fusion rate[75]. Hardware used in the absence of fusion will eventually fatigue, especially in the region of the lumbar lordosis. Therefore, instrumentation must be viewed as a temporary internal stabilizing measure while awaiting the fusion process to complete.

Surgical fusion options

Early experience with midline fusions resulted in lumbar spinal stenosis as a late complication. Therefore, current fusion techniques use postero-lateral fusion, or anterior or posterior lumbar interbody fusion.

Posterior lumbar interbody fusion (PLIF): Bilateral laminectomy and aggressive discectomy followed by the placement of bone grafts into the decorticated disc space. It has been advocated to reduce the movement in an abnormal "motion segment" (defined as the area between two vertebra). Relatively contraindicated with well preserved disc-space height.

Many PLIFs when studied ≈ 1 year later show re-collapse of the disc space, which raises the question as to whether the PLIF has any benefit over simple discectomy.

Stand-alone PLIFs may be associated with progressive spondylolisthesis at that level and are usually supplemented with pedicle screws/rods. PLIF is relatively contraindicated when the disk space is very tall.

Anterior lumbar interbody fusion: Relatively contraindicated in males because of risk of retrograde ejaculation in 1-2%.

Use of bone graft extenders/substitutes as an adjunct to fusion

---
PRACTICE PARAMETER 14-7 BONE GRAFT EXTENDERS & SUBSTITUTES

Standards[76]: autologous bone or recombinant human bone morphogenetic protein (rhBMP-2) bone graft substitute is recommended in the setting of an ALIF in conjunction with a threaded titanium cage

Options[76]:
- rhBMP-2 in conjunction with hydroxyapatite and tricalcium phosphate may be substituted for autograft in some cases of posterolateral fusion
- calcium phosphate is recommended as a bone graft extender, especially when combined with autologous bone
---

Assessing surgical lumbar fusion: See *PRACTICE PARAMETER 14-8.*

PRACTICE PARAMETER 14-8 RADIOGRAPHIC ASSESSMENT OF FUSION

Standards[77]: static x-rays alone are <u>not</u> recommended

Guidelines[77]:
- in the <u>absence</u> of rigid instrumentation, lack of motion between vertebrae on lateral flexion/extension x-rays is highly suggestive of successful fusion
- ✖ technetium-99 bone scanning is <u>not</u> recommended

Options[77]: radiographic techniques, often in combination, may be used when failed lumbar fusion is suspected, including: static and flexion/extension x-rays, CT scan
---

NB: there is weak correlation between fusion and clinical outcome.

PRACTICE PARAMETER 14-9 CORRELATION BETWEEN FUSION & OUTCOME

Options[78]: the correlation between fusion and clinical outcome is not strong, and in given situation fusion status may be *unrelated* to outcome
---

CHRONIC LOW BACK PAIN

Rarely can an anatomic diagnosis be made in patients with chronic LBP ≥ 3 months duration[79]. Also, see *Psychosocial factors*, page 296. Patients with chronic pain syndromes **(CPS)** refer to their problems with affective or emotional terms with a higher frequency than those with acute pain[80]. The amount of time that a patient has been out of work due to low back problems is related to the chances of the patient getting back to work as shown in *Table 14-7.*

Table 14-7 Chances of patients going back to work

Time out of work	Chances of getting back to work
< 6 mos	50%
1 yr	20%
2 yrs	< 5%

14.2.   Intervertebral disc herniation

INTERVERTEBRAL DISC

The function of the intervertebral disc is to permit stable motion of the spine while supporting and distributing loads under movement.

ANATOMY

Anulus fibrosus (anulus may alternatively be spelled annulus, but fibrosus is the only correct spelling and is distinct from *fibrosis*)[5]: the multilaminated ligament that encompasses the periphery of the disc space. Attaches to the end-plate cartilage and ring apophyseal bone. Blends centrally with the nucleus pulposus.

Nucleus pulposus: the central portion of the disc. A remnant of the notocord.

Capsule[5]: combined fibers of the anulus fibrosus and the posterior longitudinal ligament (this term is useful because these 2 structures may not be distinguishable on imaging studies).

14.2.1.   Lumbar disc herniation

CLINICAL ASPECTS

The posterior longitudinal ligament is strongest in the midline, and the postero-lateral annulus may bear a disproportionate portion of the load. Therefore, most herniated lumbar discs **(HLD)** occur posteriorly, slightly off to one side, compressing a nerve root, characteristically causing severe radicular pain. 65% of free fragments that migrate move superiorly.

Characteristic findings on the history often include:
1. symptoms may start off with back pain, which after days or weeks gradually or sometimes suddenly yields to radicular pain often with reduction of the back pain
2. precipitating factors: various factors are often blamed, but are rarely identified[81] with certainty
3. pain relief upon flexing the knee and thigh
4. patients generally avoid excessive movements, however, remaining in any one position (sitting, standing, or lying) too long may also exacerbate the pain, sometimes necessitating position changes at intervals that range from every few minutes to 10-20 minutes. This is distinct from constant writhing in pain e.g. with ureteral obstruction
5. exacerbation with coughing, sneezing, or straining at the stool: this positive **"cough effect"** occurred in 87% in one series[82]
6. **bladder symptoms**: the incidence of voiding dysfunction is 1-18%[83 (p 966)]. Most consist of difficulty voiding, straining, or urinary retention. Reduced bladder sensation may be the earliest finding. Later it is not unusual to see "irritative" symptoms including urinary urgency, frequency (including nocturia), increased post-void residual. Less commonly enuresis, and dribbling incontinence is reported in radiculopathy[84] (note: frank urinary retention may be seen in cauda equina syndrome, *see below*). Occasionally a HLD may present only with bladder symptoms which may improve after surgery[85]. Laminectomy may improve bladder function, but this cannot be assured

PHYSICAL FINDINGS IN RADICULOPATHY

Back pain per se is usually a minor component (only 1% of patients with acute low back pain have sciatica[4]), and when it is the only presenting symptom, other causes should be sought (see *Low back pain*, page 907). Sciatica has such a high sensitivity for disc herniation, that the likelihood of a clinically significant disc herniation[86] in the absence of sciatica is ≈ 1 in 1000. Exceptions include a central disc herniation which may cause symptoms of lumbar stenosis (i.e. neurogenic claudication) or a cauda equina syndrome.

Nerve root impingement gives rise to a set of signs and symptoms present to variable degrees. Characteristic syndromes are described for the most common nerve roots involved (see *Nerve root syndromes* below).

In a series of patients referred to neurosurgical outpatient clinics for radiating leg pain, 28% had motor loss (yet only 12% listed motor weakness as a presenting complaint), 45% had sensory disturbance, and 51% had reflex changes[87].

Findings suggestive of nerve root impingement include the following. *Table 14-8* shows the sensitivity and specificity of some findings on the exam among patients with sciatica.
1. signs/symptoms of radiculopathy (see *Table 14-9*, page 304)
   A. pain radiating down LE
   B. motor weakness
   C. dermatomal sensory changes
   D. reflex changes: mental factors may influence symmetry[88]
2. positive nerve root tension sign(s): including Lasègue's sign (*see below*)
3. tenderness over the sciatic notch

Nerve root tension signs

Includes[89]:
1. **Lasègue's sign**: AKA straight leg raising **(SLR)** test. Helps differentiate sciatica from pain due to hip pathology. Test: with patient supine, raise afflicted limb by the ankle until pain is elicited[90] (should occur at < **60°**, tension in nerve increases little above this angle).

A positive test consists of leg pain or peristhesias in the distribution of pain (back pain alone does not qualify). The patient may also extend the hip (by lifting it off table) to reduce the angle. Although not part of Lasègue's sign, ankle dorsiflexion with SLR usually augments pain due to nerve root compression. SLR primarily tenses L5 and S1, L4 less so, and more proximal roots very little. Nerve-root compression produces a positive Lasègue's sign in ≈ 83% of cases[82] (more likely to be positive in patients < 30 yrs age with HLD[91]). May be positive in lumbosacral plexopathy (see page 555). Note: flexing both thighs with the knees extended ("long-sitting" or sitting knee extension) may be tolerated further than flexing the single symptomatic side alone

2. **Cram test**: with patient supine, raise the symptomatic leg with the knee slightly flexed. Then, extend the knee. Results similar to SLR

Table 14-8 Sensitivity and specificity of physical findings for HLD in patients with sciatica[1]

Test	Comment	Sensitivity	Specificity
ipsilateral SLR	positive result: pain at < 60° elevation	0.80	0.40
crossed SLR	reproduction of contralateral pain	0.25	0.90
↓ ankle jerk	HLD usually at L5-S1 (total absence increases specificity)	0.50	0.60
sensory loss	area of loss is poor in localizing level of HLD	0.50	0.50
↓ patellar reflex	suggests upper HLD	0.50	NA
WEAKNESS			
knee extension (quadriceps)	HLD usually at L3-4	< 0.01	0.99
ankle dorsiflexion (anterior tibialis)	HLD usually at L4-5	0.35	0.70
ankle plantarflexion (gastrocs)	HLD usually at L5-S1	0.06	0.95
great toe extension (EHL)	HLD at L5-S1 in 60%, at L4-5 in 30%	0.50	0.70

3. **crossed straight leg-raising** test AKA **Fajersztajn's sign**: SLR on the painless leg causes contralateral limb pain (a greater degree of elevation is usually required than the painful side). More specific but less sensitive than SLR (97% of patients undergoing surgery with this sign have confirmed HLD[92]). May correlate with a more <u>central</u> disc herniation

4. **femoral stretch test**[93], AKA **reverse straight leg raising**: patient prone, examiner's palm at popliteal fossa, knee is maximally dorsiflexed. Often positive with L2, L3, or L4 nerve root compression (e.g. in upper lumbar disc herniation), or with extreme lateral lumbar disc herniation (may also be positive in diabetic femoral neuropathy or psoas hematoma); in these situations SLR (Lasègue's sign) is frequently negative (since L5 & S1 not involved)

5. **"bowstring sign"**: once pain occurs with SLR, lower the foot to the bed by flexing knee, keeping the hip flexed. Sciatic pain ceases with this maneuver, but hip pain persists

6. **sitting knee extension** test: with patient seated and both hips and knees flexed 90°, slowly extend one knee. Stretches nerve roots as much as a moderate degree of SLR

Other signs useful in evaluation for lumbar radiculopathy

1. **FABER**: an acronym for Flexion ABduction External-Rotation, AKA FABERE test (the trailing "e" is for extension), AKA Patrick's-test. A test of hip motion. Method: the hip and knee are flexed and the lateral malleolus is placed on the contralateral knee. The ipsilateral knee is gently displaced downward towards the exam table. This stresses the hip joint and does not usually exacerbate true nerve-root compression, often markedly positive in the presence of hip joint disease (e.g. trochanteric bursitis, see page 326), sacroiliitis or mechanical low-back pain

2. **Trendelenburg sign**: examiner observes pelvis from behind while patient raises one leg while standing. Normally the pelvis remains horizontal. A positive sign occurs when the pelvis tilts down toward the side of the lifted leg indicating weakness of the contralateral thigh adductors (primarily L5 innervated)

3. **crossed adductors**: in eliciting knee jerk (**KJ**), the contralateral thigh adductors contract. In the presence of a <u>hyper</u>active ipsilateral KJ it may indicate an upper motor neuron lesion, in the presence of a <u>hypo</u>active ipsilateral KJ it may be a form of pathological spread, indicating nerve root irritability

Due to the facts listed below, a herniated lumbar disc **(HLD)** usually spares the nerve root exiting at that interspace, and impinges on the nerve exiting from the neural foramen one level <u>below</u> (e.g. a L5-S1 HLD usually causes S1 radiculopathy). This gives rise to the characteristic lumbar nerve root syndromes shown in *Table 14-9*.

Important facts in lumbar disc disease:

1. in the lumbar region, the nerve root exits <u>below</u> and in close proximity to the pedicle of its like-numbered vertebra
2. the intervertebral disc space is located well below the pedicle
3. in the modal (most common) human spine, there are 24 presacral vertebrae, however

Table 14-9   Lumbar disc syndromes

	— Lumbar disc level —		
	L3-4	**L4-5**	**L5-S1**
root usually compressed	L4	L5	S1
% of lumbar discs	3-10% (5% average)	40-45%	45-50%
reflex diminished	knee jerk* (Westphal's sign)	medial hamstring†	Achilles* (ankle jerk)
motor weakness	quadriceps femoris (knee extension)	tibialis anterior (foot drop) & EHL‡	gastrocnemius (plantarflexion), ± EHL‡
decreased sensation§	medial malleolus & medial foot	large toe web & dorsum of foot	lateral malleolus & lateral foot
pain distribution	anterior thigh	posterior LE	posterior LE, often to ankle

* **Jendrassik maneuver** may reinforce (patient pulls hands apart against each other while reflex is elicited)

† medial hamstring reflex is unreliable (not always pure L5), may also stimulate adductors when eliciting

‡ see WEAKNESS in *Table 14-8*, page 303 for breakdown

§ sensory impairment is most common in the distal extremes of the dermatome[94]

some individuals have 23 and others have 25[A]. Thus, a HLD at the ultimate disc space (usually L5-S1) most often impinges on the 25th nerve root (however, in the variant cases, it may actually impinge on the 24th or 26th root)[95]

RADIOGRAPHIC EVALUATION

See *Radiographic evaluation* on page 293 under *Low back pain*.

NONSURGICAL TREATMENT

For nonsurgical treatment, see *"Conservative" treatment*, page 296.

SURGICAL TREATMENT

INDICATIONS

In spite of multiple attempts, no one has been able to determine which patients are likely to improve on their own and which would be better served with surgery.

1. failure of non-surgical management: over 85% of patients with acute disc herniation will improve <u>without</u> surgical intervention in an average of 6 weeks[96] (70% within 4 weeks[97]). Most clinicians advocate waiting somewhere between 5-8 weeks from the onset of radiculopathy before considering surgery (assuming none of the items listed below applies)
2. **"EMERGENT SURGERY":** (i.e. before 5-8 weeks have lapsed). Indications:
   A. cauda equina syndrome **(CES)**: (*see below*)
   B. <u>progressive</u> motor deficit (e.g. foot drop): paresis of unknown duration is a doubtful indication for surgery [81, 98, 99] (no study has documented that there is less motor deficit in surgically treated patients with this finding). However, the acute development or progression of motor weakness is considered an indication for rapid surgical decompression
   C. "urgent" surgery may be indicated for patients whose pain remains intolerable in spite of adequate narcotic pain medication

---

A. variations include: 11 or 13 rib bearing vertebrae, or a lumbosacral transitional vertebrae; the terminology of a "lumbarized S1 vertebrae" or a "sacralized L5 vertebrae" is imprecise and confusing

3. ± patients who do not want to invest the time in a trial of non-surgical treatment if it is possible that they will still require surgery at the end of the trial

Cauda equina syndrome

Syndrome usually due to compression of the cauda equina. See *Table 17-70*, page 517 for features to help differentiate CES from a conus lesion.

Possible **findings** in CES:
1. sphincter disturbance:
   A. urinary retention: the most consistent finding. Sensitivity ≈ 90% (at some point in time during course)[100, 101]. Have patient empty bladder and check post-void residual. In a patient without retention, only 1 in 1000 will have a CES. Cystometrogram (when done) shows a hypotonic bladder with decreased sensation and increased capacity
   B. urinary and/or fecal incontinence[102] (some patients with urinary retention will present with overflow incontinence)
   C. anal sphincter tone: diminished in 60-80%
2. **"saddle anesthesia"**: the most common sensory deficit. Distribution: region of the anus, lower genitals, perineum, over the buttocks, posterior-superior thighs. Sensitivity ≈ 75%. Once total perineal anesthesia develops, patients tend to have permanent bladder paralysis[103]
3. significant motor weakness: usually involves more than a single nerve root (if untreated, may progress to paraplegia)
4. low back pain and/or sciatica (sciatica is usually bilateral, but may be unilateral or entirely absent, prognosis may be worse when absent or bilateral[101])
5. bilateral absence of Achilles reflex has been noted[104]
6. sexual dysfunction (usually not detected until a later time)

Etiologies of CES includes:
1. massive herniated lumbar disc: *see below*
2. tumor
   A. from compression: e g with metastatic disease to the spine with epidural extension
   B. **intravascular lymphomatosis (B-cell lymphoma)**: a circulating lymphoma without solid mass (*see page 463*). Often presents with CNS findings: CES, dementia, enhancing meninges on MRI, lymphoma cells in CSF
3. trauma
4. spinal epidural hematoma
5. free fat graft following discectomy[105]
6. ankylosing spondylitis: etiology is often obscure (*see page 344*)

CES from HLD: May be due to massive ruptured disc, usually midline, most common at L4-5, often superimposed on a preexisting condition (spinal stenosis, tethered cord...)[102].

Prevalence of CES:
1. 0.0004 in all patients with LBP[86]
2. only ≈ 1-2% of HLD that come to surgery[86]

Time course: CES tends to develop either acutely, or (less typically) slowly (prognosis is worse in the acute onset group, especially for return of bladder function, which occurred in only ≈ 50%)[100]. 3 patterns[106]:
- Group I - sudden onset of CES symptoms with no previous symptoms related to the low back
- Group II - previous history of recurrent backache and sciatica, the latest episode resulting in CES
- Group III - presentation with backache and bilateral sciatica that later develop CES

Surgical issues: A bilateral laminectomy is advised[102]. Occasionally, when it is difficult to remove a very tense midline disc, transdural removal will be necessary[104].

Timing of discectomy in CES: controversial, and the point of contention in numerous law suits. In spite of early reports emphasizing rapid decompression[104], other reports found no correlation between the time to surgery after presentation and the return of function[100, 101]. Some evidence supports the goal of performing surgery **within 48 hours** (although performing surgery within 24 hours is desirable if possible, there is no statistically significant proof that delaying up to 48 hrs is detrimental)[107, 108].

Once it is decided to treat surgically, options include:
1. trans-canal approaches
   A. standard open lumbar laminectomy and discectomy: 65-85% reported no sciatica one year post-op compared to 36% for conservative treatment[109]. Long-term results (> 1 year) were similar. 10% of patients underwent further back surgery during the first year[109]
   B. "microdiscectomy"[110, 111]: similar to standard procedure, however smaller incision is utilized. Advantages may be cosmetic, shortened hospital stay, lower blood loss. May be more difficult to retrieve some fragments[112 (p 1319), 113]. Overall efficacy is similar to standard discectomy[114]
2. intradiscal procedures (see below)
   A. chemonucleolysis: using chymopapain (see below)
   B. automated percutaneous lumbar discectomy: utilizes a nucleotome
   C. percutaneous endoscopic discectomy: see below
   D. intradiscal endothermal therapy (**IDET** or **IDTA**): see below
   E. laser disc decompression

Chemonucleolysis

Acceptable treatment, but less efficacious than routine or micro-discectomy[1]. Utilizes **chymopapain** (Chymodiactin®) injected intradiscally. Proven more effective than placebo injection[115, 116]. Typical success rates: at 1 year 85% of patients undergoing discectomy had good or excellent results compared to 44%[117] to 63%[118] for chemonucleolysis (**CNL**). Although sciatica improves in both groups, only the discectomy group had significant improvement in back pain[117]. In one study, at 6 months 56% of patients initially having CNL had undergone surgery for unrelieved symptoms[119].

Risks[120, 121]:

Risk of the significant complication of anaphylaxis (sometimes fatal) may be reduced by skin-tests for allergic sensitivity to the agent. Other complications reported include: discitis[122], neurologic injury, vascular injury, thrombophlebitis, PE, transverse myelitis[123] (very uncommon).

Intradiscal surgical procedures (ISP)

ISPs (see below for specific procedures) are among the most controversial procedures for lumbar spine surgery. The theoretical advantage is that epidural scarring is avoided, and that a smaller incision or even just a puncture site is used. This is also purported to reduce postoperative pain and hospital stay (often performed as an outpatient procedure). The conceptual problem with ISPs is that they are directed at removing disc material from the center of the disc space (which is not producing symptoms) and rely on the reduced intradiscal pressure to decompress the herniated portion of the disc from the nerve root. Only ≈ 10-15% of patients considered for surgical treatment of disc disease are candidates for an ISP. ISPs are usually done under local anesthetic in order to permit the patient to report nerve root pain to identify impingement on a nerve root by the surgical instrument or needle. Overall, ISPs are not recommended until controlled trials prove the efficacy[1].

Indications utilized by proponents of intradiscal procedures:
1. type of disc herniation: appropriate only for "contained" disc herniation (i.e. outer margin of anulus fibrosus intact)
2. appropriate level: best for L4-5 HLD. May also be used at L3-4. Difficult but often workable (utilizing angled instruments or other techniques) at L5-S1 because of the angle required and interference by iliac crest
3. not recommended in presence of severe neurologic deficit[124]

Results:

"Success" rate (≈ pain free and return to work when appropriate) reported ranges from 37-75%[125-127].

Automated percutaneous lumbar discectomy: Utilizes a nucleotome[128] to remove disc material from the center of the intervertebral disc space. Significantly less efficacious than chymopapain[127], with 1 year success rate of 37% (compared to 66% for CNL). Complications include cauda equina syndrome from improper nucleotome placement[129].

Laser disc decompression: Insertion of a needle into the disc, and introduction of a laser fiberoptic cable through the needle to allow a laser to burn a hole in the center of the disc [130, 131] (with or without endoscopic visualization).

Percutaneous endoscopic lumbar discectomy (PELD): This term refers to an essentially intradiscal procedure indicated primarily for contained disc herniations, although some small "noncontained" fragments may be treatable[132]. No large randomized study has been done to compare the technique to the accepted standard, open discectomy (with or without microscope). In one report[133], of 326 patients with L4-5 HLD, only 8 appropriate candidates for PELD (i.e. 2.4% of HLD at L3-4) were found. Of these 8, only 3 were reported as having a good result. This study is not adequate for evaluating the technique.

Intradiscal endothermal therapy (IDET) : AKA intradiscal electrothermal anuloplasty **(IDTA)**. Efficacy: 23-60% at 1 year for treating "internal disc disruption"[134] (radial fissures in the nucleus pulposus extending into the anulus fibrosus) which is purported to account for 40% of patients with chronic low back pain of unknown etiology[135].

ADJUNCTIVE TREATMENT IN LUMBAR LAMINECTOMY

Epidural steroids following discectomy

In a single-blinded non-randomized study of the use of epidural steroids (methylprednisolone acetate (Depo-Medrol®), dose not specified) irrigation of the thecal sac and nerve root following discectomy prior to wound closure found no statistically significant evidence of benefit in terms of amount of post-op analgesic medication needed, duration of hospital stay, or time to return to work[136]. However, the combination of *systemic* steroids at the start of the case (Depo-Medrol® 160 mg IM and methylprednisolone sodium succinate (Solu-Medrol®) 250 mg IV) combined with infiltration of 30 ml of 0.25% bipuvicaine (Marcaine®) into the paraspinal muscles at incision and closure, may reduce hospital stay and post-op narcotic requirements[137].

Methods to reduce scar formation

Epidural free fat graft: The use of an autogenous free fat graft in the epidural space is a fairly common practice, that is employed in an attempt to reduce post-op epidural scar formation. Opinion varies widely as to the effectiveness, some feel it is helpful, others feel it actually exacerbates scarring[138]. In some patients, no evidence of the graft will be found on reoperation years later. The fat graft can very rarely be a cause of nerve root compression[139] or cauda equina syndrome[105] within the first few days post-op, and there is a case report of compression 6 years following surgery[140].

Other measures: Other measures include the placement of barrier films or gels[141].

RISKS OF LUMBAR LAMINECTOMY

Overall risk of mortality in large series[142, 143]: 6 per 10,000 (i.e. 0.06%), most often due to septicemia, MI, or PE. Complication rates are very difficult to determine accurately[109], but the following is included as a guideline.

Common complications

(consider discussing these as part of informed consent)
1. infection:
   A. superficial wound infection: 0.9-5%[144] (risk is increased with age, long term steroids, obesity, ? DM): most are caused by *S. aureus* (see *Laminectomy wound infection*, page 216 for management)
   B. deep infection: < 1%(*see below* under *Uncommon complications*)
2. increased motor deficit: 1-8% (some transient)
3. unintended "incidental" durotomy[A]: (*see below*) incidence is 0.3-13% (risk increases to ≈ 18% in re-do operations)[145]. Possible sequelae include those listed in *Table 14-10*
   A. CSF fistula (external CSF leak): the risk of a CSF fistula requiring operative repair is ≈ 10 per 10,000[142]
   B. pseudomeningocele: 0.7-2%[145] (may appear similar radiographically to spinal epidural abscess **(SEA)**, but post-op SEA often enhances, is more irregular, and is associated with muscle edema)
4. recurrent herniated lumbar disc (same level either side): 4% (with 10 year follow-up)[146] (*see page 317*)

Uncommon complications

1. direct injury to neural structures. For large disc herniations, consider a bilateral

---

A. the term "unintended durotomy" has been recommended in preference to "dural tear" (*see below*)

exposure to reduce risk
2. injury to structures anterior to the vertebral bodies **(VB)**: injured by breaching the anterior longitudinal ligament **(ALL)** through the disc space, e.g. with pituitary rongeur. The depth of disc space penetration with instruments should be kept ≤ **3 cm**, since 5% of lumbar discs had diameters as small as 3.3 cm[147]. Asymptomatic perforations of the ALL occur in up to 12% of discectomies. Breach of the ALL risks potential injuries to:
    A. great vessels[148]: risks include potentially fatal hemorrhage, and arteriovenous fistula which may present years later. Most such injuries occur with L4-5 discectomies. Only ≈ 50% bleed into the disc space intraoperatively, the rest bleed into the retroperitoneum. Emergent laparotomy is indicated, preferably by a surgeon with vascular surgical experience, if available. Mortality rate is 37-67%
        1. aorta: the aortic bifurcation is on the left side of the lower part of the L4 VB, and so the aorta may be injured above this level
        2. below L4, the common iliac arteries may be injured
        3. veins (more common than arterial injuries)
            a. vena cava at and above L4
            b. common iliac veins below L4
    B. ureters
    C. bowel: at L5-S1 the ileum is the most likely viscus to be injured
    D. sympathetic trunk
3. rare infections:
    A. meningitis
    B. deep infection: < 1%. Including:
        1. discitis: 0.5% (*see page 245*),
        2. spinal epidural abscess **(SEA)**: 0.67% (*see page 240*)
4. cauda equina syndrome: may be caused by post-op spinal epidural hematoma (*see below*). Incidence was 0.21% in one series of 2842 lumbar discectomies[149] and 0.14% in a series of 12,000 spine operations[150]. Red flags: urinary retention, anesthesia that may be saddle or <u>bilateral</u> LE
5. complications of positioning:
    A. compression neuropathies: ulnar, peroneal nerves. Use padding over elbows and avoid pressure on posterior popliteal fossa
    B. anterior tibial compartment syndrome: due to pressure on anterior compartment of leg (reported with Andrew's frame). An orthopedic emergency that may require emergent fasciotomy
    C. pressure on the eye: corneal abrasions, damage to the anterior chamber
    D. cervical spine injuries during positioning due to relaxed muscles under anesthesia
6. post op arachnoiditis: risk factors include epidural hematoma, patients who tend to develop hypertrophic scar, post op discitis, and intrathecal injection of Pantopaque®, anesthetic agents or steroids. Surgical treatment is disappointing. Intrathecal depo-medrol may provide short-term relief (in spite of the fact that steroids are a risk factor for the development of arachnoiditis). Also *see page 315*
7. thrombophlebitis and deep-vein thrombosis with risk of pulmonary embolism **(PE)**[142]: 0.1% (see *Thromboembolism in neurosurgery*, page 25)
8. reflex sympathetic dystrophy **(RSD)**: has been reported in up to 1.2% of cases, usually after posterior decompression with fusion, often following reoperations[151] with onset 4 days to 20 weeks post-op. *See page 396* for a critique of RSD. Treatment includes some or all of: PT, sympathetic blocks, oral methylprednisolone, removal of hardware if any
9. very rare: Ogilvie's syndrome (pseudo-obstruction of the colon) has been reported as a complication of spinal surgery/trauma, spinal or epidural anesthesia, spinal metastases, and myelography[152]

Unintended durotomy
Unintentional opening of the dura during spinal surgery has an incidence of 0-14%[153].

Terminology: The terms "unintended durotomy", "incidental durotomy"[153], or even just "dural opening", have been recommended in preference to "dural tear" which may imply carelessness[145] when none was present. Dural openings have been associated with one or more alleged complications or sequelae in medical malpractice suits involving surgery on the lumbar spine.

The injury: By itself, opening the dura intentionally or otherwise is not expected to have a deleterious effect on the patient[145, 154]. In fact, dural opening is often a standard part of the operation for intradural disc herniation[155], tumors, etc.. Although not frequent, unintended durotomy is not an unusual occurrence, and alone, is not considered an act of malpractice. However, it may result from an event or events that produce more serious injuries. These events and injuries should be dealt with on their own merits.

Possible sequelae include those listed in *Table 14-10*. A CSF leak may produce "spinal headache" with its associated symptoms (*see page 46*), and if it breaches the skin it may be a risk factor for developing meningitis. Pain or sensory/motor deficits may be associated with injuries to nerve roots or herniation of nerve roots through the dural opening.

Table 14-10 Possible sequelae of dural opening

Well documented
1. CSF leak
A. contained: pseudomeningocele
B. external: CSF fistula
2. herniation of nerve roots thorough opening
3. associated nerve root contusion, laceration or injury to the cauda equina
4. CSF leak collapses the thecal sac and may increase blood loss from epidural bleeding

Less well documented
1. arachnoiditis
2. chronic pain
3. bladder, bowel and/or sexual dysfunction

Etiologies: For incidence, *see above*. Potential causes are many, and include[145]: unanticipated anatomic variations, adhesion of the dura to removed bone, slippage of an instrument, an obscured fold of dura caught in a rongeur or curette, thinning of the dura in cases of longstanding stenosis, and the possibility of a delayed CSF leak caused by perforation of the dura when it expands onto a surgically created spicule of bone[156]. The risk may be increased with anterior decompression for OPLL, with revision surgery, and with the use of high-speed drills[153].

Treatment: If the opening is recognized at the time of surgery, watertight primary closure (with or without patch graft) should be attempted with nonabsorbable suture if at all possible to prevent pseudomeningocele and/or CSF fistula. Fibrin glue may be used to supplement primary closure[153].

Although bed rest **x** 4-7 days is often advocated to reduce symptoms and facilitate healing, when watertight closure has been achieved, normal post-op mobilization is not associated with a high failure rate (bed rest is recommended if symptoms develop)[153].

In one report of 8 patients with leaks that appeared post-op, re-operation was avoided when treated by resuturing the skin under local anesthesia, followed by bed rest in slight Trendelenburg position (to reduce pressure on the leakage site), broad spectrum antibiotics and antibiotic ointment over the skin incision, and daily puncture and drainage of the subcutaneous collection[157].

Also, *see page 46* for other treatment measures for H/A associated with CSF leak.

POST-OP CARE

Post-op orders

The following are guidelines for post-operative orders for a lumbar laminectomy without intra-operative complications; variations between surgeons and institutions must be taken into consideration:
1. admit post-anesthesia recovery (PAR) unit
2. vital signs on the nursing unit: q 2° **x** 4 hrs, q 4° **x** 24°, then q 8°
3. activity: up with assist, advance as tolerated
4. nursing care
   A. I's & O's
   B. intermittent catheterization q 4-6° PRN no void
   C. *optional*: TED hose (may reduce risk of DVT) or PCB
   D. *optional (if drain used):* empty drain q 8° and PRN
5. diet: clear liquids, advance as tolerated
6. IV: D5 1/2 NS + 20 mEq KCl/l @ 75 ml/hr, D/C when tolerating PO well (after antibiotics D/C'd if prophylactic antibiotics are used)
7. meds
   A. laxative of choice (**LOC**) PRN
   B. sodium docussate (e.g. Colace®) 100 mg PO BID when tolerating PO (stool softener, does not substitute for LOC)
   C. *optional:* prophylactic antibiotics if used at your institution
   D. acetaminophen (Tylenol®) 650 mg PO or PR q 3° PRN

E. *narcotic analgesic*
F. *optional*: steroids are used by some surgeons to reduce nerve-root irritation from surgical manipulation
8. labs
A. *optional (if significant blood loss during surgery):* CBC

Post-op check
In addition to routine, the following should be checked:
❑ 1. strength of lower extremities, especially muscles relevant to nerve root, e.g. gastrocnemius for L5-S1 surgery, EHL for L4-5 surgery...
❑ 2. appearance of dressing: look for signs of excessive bleeding, CSF leak...
❑ 3. signs of **cauda equina syndrome** (*see page 305*), e.g. by post-op spinal epidural hematoma:
   A. loss of perineal sensation ("saddle anesthesia")
   B. inability to void: may not be not unusual after lumbar laminectomy, more concerning if accompanied by loss of perineal sensation
   C. pain out of the ordinary for the post-op period
   D. weakness of multiple muscle groups

Any new neurologic deficit should prompt rapid evaluation for spinal epidural hematoma[150] **(EDH)**. Delayed deficits may be due to EDH or epidural abscess. Post-op films in the recovery room can rule out graft or hardware malposition for fusions or instrumentation procedures, or changes in alignment. The diagnostic test of choice is MRI. If contraindicated or not available, CT/myelography may be indicated. An extradural defect immediately post-op suggests EDH.

OUTCOME OF SURGICAL TREATMENT
In a series of 100 patients undergoing discectomy, at 1 year post-op 73% had complete relief of leg pain and 63% had complete relief of back pain; at 5-10 years the numbers were 62% for each category[82]. At 5-10 years post-op, only 14% felt that the pain was the same or worse than pre-op (i.e. 86% felt improved), and 5% qualified as having a **failed back syndrome** (not returned to work, requiring analgesics, receiving worker's compensation, see *Failed back syndrome*, page 314).

In the only randomized study comparing standard discectomy with conservative treatment, two groups of ≈ 60 patients with a documented herniated disc that failed to improve after 14 days of rest (without strong indications for surgery, e.g. cauda equina syndrome, unbearable pain...) were randomized to surgery or continued conservative treatment (however, ≈ 25% of patients from the conservative treatment group were referred to surgery for prolonged or worsening pain). There was a significantly better outcome at 1 year follow-up in the surgical group, this was not significant at 4 years, and at 10 years neither group reported sciatica or back pain[81], provided that patients who did not improve satisfactorily after conservative treatment underwent surgery.

In patients with a diminished knee-jerk or ankle-jerk pre-op, 35% and 43% (respectively) still had reduced reflexes 1 year post-op[87]; reflexes were lost post-op in 3% and 10% respectively. The same study found that motor loss was improved in 80%, aggravated in 3%, and was newly present in 5% post-op; and that sensory loss was improved in 69% and was worsened in 15% post-op.

Recurrent disc herniation: (*see page 317*)

HERNIATED UPPER LUMBAR DISCS
(LEVELS L1-2, L2-3, & L3-4)

L4-5 & L5-S1 herniated lumbar discs **(HLD)** account for most cases of HLD (up to 98%[86]); 24% of patients with HLD at L3-4 frequently have a past history of a HLD at L4-5 or L5-S1, suggesting a generalized tendency towards disc herniation. In a series of 1,395 HLDs, there were 4 at L1-2 (0.28% incidence), 18 at L2-3 (1.3%), and 51 at L3-4 (3.6%)[158].

PRESENTATION
Typically presents with LBP, onset following trauma or strain in 51%. With progression, paresthesias and pain in the anterior thigh occur, with complaints of leg weakness (especially on ascending stairs).

Quadriceps femoris was the most common muscle involved, demonstrating weakness and sometimes atrophy.

Straight leg raising was positive in only 40%. Psoas stretch test was positive in 27%. Femoral stretch test may be positive (*see page 303*).

50% had reduced or absent knee jerk; 18% had ankle jerk abnormalities; reflex changes were more common with L3-4 HLD (81%) than L1-2 (none) or L2-3 (44%).

EXTREME LATERAL LUMBAR DISC HERNIATIONS

Definition: herniation of a disc at (**foraminal disc herniation**) or distal to (**extraforaminal lumbar disc herniation**) the facet (some authors do not consider foraminal disc herniation to be "extreme lateral"). See *Figure 14-1*.

Incidence (*see Table 14-11*): 3-10% of herniated lumbar discs (**HLD**) (series with higher numbers[159] include some HLD that are not truly *extreme* lateral).

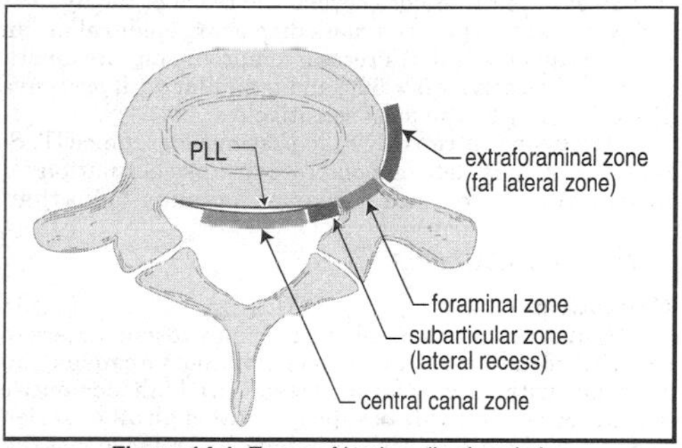

Differs from the more common (more medially located) HLD in that:

Figure 14-1 Zones of lumbar disc herniation

- the nerve root involved is usually the one exiting <u>at</u> that level (c.f. the root exiting at the level below)
- straight leg raising (**SLR**) is negative in 85-90% of cases ≥ 1 week after onset (excluding double herniations; ≈ 65% will be negative if double herniations are included); may have positive femoral stretch test (*see page 303*)
- pain is reproduced by lateral bending to the side of herniation in 75%
- myelography alone rarely diagnostic (usually requires CT[160, 161] or MRI)
- higher incidence of extruded fragments (60%)
- higher incidence of double herniations on the same side at the same level (15%)
- pain tends to be more severe than with routine HLD (may be due to fact that the dorsal root ganglion may be compressed directly)

Table 14-11 Incidence of extreme lateral HLD by level*

Disc level	No.	%
L1-2	1	1%
L2-3	11	8%
L3-4	35	24%
L4-5	82	60%
L5-S1	9	7%

* series of 138 cases[159]

Occurs most commonly at <u>L4-5</u> and next at L3-4 (*see Table 14-11*), thus L4 is the most common nerve involved and L3 is next. With a clinical picture of an upper lumbar nerve root compression (i.e. radiculopathy with negative SLR), chances are ≈ 3 to 1 that it is an extremely lateral HLD rather than an upper lumbar disc herniation.

PRESENTATION

Quadriceps weakness, reduction of patellar reflex, and diminished sensation in the L3 or L4 dermatome are the most common findings.

Differential diagnosis includes:
1. lateral recess stenosis or superior articular facet hypertrophy
2. retroperitoneal hematoma or tumor
3. diabetic neuropathy (amyotrophy): *see page 556*
4. spinal tumor
   A. benign (schwannoma or neurofibroma)
   B. malignant tumors
   C. lymphoma
5. infection
   A. localized (spinal epidural abscess)

B. psoas muscle abscess
C. granulomatous disease
6. spondylolisthesis (with pars defect)
7. compression of conjoined nerve root
8. on MRI, enlarged foraminal veins may mimic extreme lateral disc herniation

RADIOGRAPHIC DIAGNOSIS

Radiographic diagnosis may be elusive, and up to one third are initially missed[162]. However, if actively sought, many asymptomatic far-lateral disc herniations may be demonstrated on CT or MRI.

Myelography: fails to disclose the pathology even with water soluble contrast in 87% of cases due to the fact that the nerve root compression occurs distal to the nerve root sleeve (and therefore beyond the reach of the dye)[163].

CT scan[161]: reveals a mass displacing epidural fat and encroaching on the intervertebral foramen or lateral recess, compromising the emerging root. Or, may be lateral to foramen. Sensitivity is ≈ 50% and is similar with *post-myelographic* CT[163]. Post-discography CT[164] may be the most sensitive test (94%)[163].

MRI: similar sensitivity to post-myelographic CT. Sagittal views through the neural foramen may help demonstrate the disc herniation[162]. MRI may have ≈ 8% false positive rate due to presence of enlarged foraminal veins that mimic extreme lateral HLD[165].

SURGICAL TREATMENT

Foraminal discs

Usually requires mesial facetectomy to gain access to the region lateral to the dural sac without undue retraction on nerve root or cauda equina. Caution: total facetectomy combined with discectomy may result in a high incidence of instability (total facetectomy alone causes ≈ 10% rate of slippage), although other series found this risk to be lower (≈ 1 in 33[166, 167]). An alternative technique is to remove just the lateral portion of the superior articular facet below[168]. Endoscopic techniques may be well suited for herniated discs in this location[169].

Discs herniated beyond (lateral to) the foramen

Numerous approaches are used, including:
1. traditional **midline hemilaminectomy**: the ipsilateral facet must be partially or completely removed. The safest way to find the exiting nerve root is take the laminectomy of the inferior portion of the upper vertebral level (e.g. L4 for a L4-5 HLD) high enough to expose the nerve root axilla, and then follow the nerve laterally through the neural foramen by removing facet until the HLD is identified
2. **lateral approach** (i.e. extra-canal) through a paramedian incision[170]. Advantages: the facet joint is preserved (facet removal combined with discectomy may lead to instability), muscle retraction is easier. Disadvantages: unfamiliar approach for most surgeons and the nerve cannot be followed medial to lateral

DISC HERNIATIONS IN PEDIATRICS

Less than one percent of surgery for herniated lumbar disc is performed on patients between the ages of 10 and 20 yrs (one series at Mayo found 0.4% of operated HLD in patients < 17 yrs age[171]). These patients often have few neurologic findings except for a consistently positive straight leg raising test[172]. Herniated disc material in youths tends to be firm, fibrous and strongly attached to the cartilaginous end-plate unlike the degenerated material usually extruded in adult disc herniation. Plain radiographs disclosed an unusually high frequency of congenital spine anomalies (transitional vertebra, hyperlordosis, spondylolisthesis, spina bifida…). 78% did well after their first operation[171].

INTRADURAL DISC HERNIATION

Herniation of a fragment of disc into the thecal sac, or into the nerve root sleeve (the latter sometimes referred to as "intraradicular" disc herniation) has been recognized with a reported incidence of 0.04-1.1% of disc herniations[155, 173]. Although it may be suspected on the basis of pre-op myelography or MRI, the diagnosis is rarely made preoperatively[173]. Intraoperatively, it may be suggested by the impression of a tense firm mass within the nerve root sleeve or by the negative exploration of a level with obvious clinical signs and clear cut radiographic abnormalities (after verifying that the correct level is exposed).

Surgical treatment:
Although a surgical dural opening may be utilized[155], others have found this to be necessary in a minority of cases[174].

INTRAVERTEBRAL DISC HERNIATION

AKA Schmorl's node or nodule. AKA Schmor's (no "l") nodule AKA Geipel hernia[175]. Disc herniation through the cartilaginous end plate into the cancellous bone of the vertebral body (**VB**) (AKA intraspongious disc herniation). Often an incidental finding on x-ray or MRI. Clinical significance is controversial. May produce low back pain initially that lasts ≈ 3-4 months after onset. Diffuse displacement (as may be seen in osteoporosis) is sometimes referred to as a **balloon disc**[5].

Clinical findings
During the acute (symptomatic) phase, patients may exhibit LBP that is aggravated by weight bearing and movement. There may be tenderness to percussion or manual compression over the involved segment.

Radiographic findings
Plain x-ray: ≤ 33% may be seen on plain x-rays[176]. They may not be detectable acutely until sclerotic osseous bone casting develops.

MRI: the extrusion of disc material into the VB is easily appreciated on sagittal images. It has been suggested[177] that acute (symptomatic) lesions may appear differentiated from chronic (asymptomatic) lesions by the presence of MRI findings of inflammation in the bone marrow immediately surrounding the node as outlined in *Table 14-12*.

Table 14-12 MRI signal intensity in Schmorl's nodes*

Lesion	T1WI	T2WI
symptomatic (acute)	low	high
asymptomatic (chronic)	high†	low†

* signal intensity in surrounding marrow

† the same as normal marrow

Treatment
Conservative treatment is indicated, usually consisting of non-steroidal anti-inflammatory drugs (NSAIDs). Occasionally stronger pain medication and/or lumbar bracing may be required. Surgery is rarely indicated.

Outcome
With conservative treatment, symptoms generally resolve within 3-4 months of onset (as with most vertebral body fractures).

JUXTAFACET CYSTS OF THE LUMBAR SPINE

The term juxtafacet cyst (**JFC**) was originated by Kao et al.[178] and includes both **synovial cysts** (those having a synovial lining membrane) and **ganglion cysts** (those lacking synovial lining) adjacent to a spinal facet joint or arising from the ligamentum flavum. Distinction between these two types of cysts may be difficult (*see below*) and is clinically unimportant[179].

JFC occur primarily in the lumbar spine (although cysts in the cervical[180-182] and thoracic[183] spine have been described). They were first reported in 1880 by von Gruker during an autopsy[184], and were first diagnosed clinically in 1968[185]. The etiology is unknown (possibilities include: synovial fluid extrusion from the joint capsule, latent growth of a developmental rest, myxoid degeneration and cyst formation in collagenous connective tissue...), increased motion seems to have a role in many cysts, and the role of trauma in the pathogenesis is debated[181, 186] but probably plays a role in a small number (≈ 14%)[187]. JFC are relatively rare, only 3 cases were identified in a series of 1,500 spinal CT exams[188], but the frequency of diagnosis may be on the rise due to the widespread use of MRI and an increasing awareness of the condition.

Clinical
The average age was 63 years in one series[187] and 58 years in a review of 54 cases in the literature[189] (range: 33-87) with a slight female preponderance in both series. Most

occur in patients with severe spondylosis and facet joint degeneration[190], 25% had degenerative spondylolisthesis[187]. L4-5 is the most common level[187, 191]. They may be bilateral. Pain is the most common symptom, and is usually radicular. Some JFC may contribute to canal stenosis and can produce neurogenic claudication[192] (*see page 326*) or on occasion a cauda equina syndrome. Symptoms may be more intermittent in nature than with firm compressive lesions, such as HLD. A sudden exacerbation in pain may be due to hemorrhage within the cyst. Some JFC may be asymptomatic[193].

Differential diagnosis (also see *Differential diagnosis, Sciatica* on page 905). Differentiating JFC from other masses relies largely on the appearance and location. Other distinguishing features include:

1. neurofibroma: unlikely to be calcified
2. free fragment of HLD: not cystic in appearance
3. epidural or nerve root metastases: not cystic
4. dural subarachnoid root sleeve dilatation: see *Spinal meningeal cysts*, page 348
5. arachnoid cyst (from arachnoid herniation through a dural defect): not associated with facet joint, margins thinner than JFC[194]
6. perineurial cysts (Tarlov's cyst): arise in space between perineurium and endoneurium, usually on sacral roots[195], occasionally show delayed filling on myelography

Pathology

Cyst walls are composed of fibrous connective tissue of varying thickness and cellularity. There is usually no signs of infection or inflammation. There may be a synovial lining[189] (synovial cyst) or it may be absent[190] (ganglion cyst). The distinction between the two may be difficult[179], possibly owing in part to the fact that fibroblasts in ganglion cysts may form an incomplete synovial-like lining[196]. Proliferation of small venules is seen in the connective tissue. Hemosiderin staining may be present, and may or may not be associated with a history of trauma[187].

Evaluation

Identifying a JFC pre-op helps the surgeon, as the approach differs slightly from that for HLD, and the cyst might otherwise be missed or unknowingly deflated and unnecessary time wasted afterwards trying to find a compressive lesion. Or, the unwitting surgeon may misinterpret the cyst as a "transdural disc extrusion" and needlessly open the dura. Pre-op diagnoses were incorrect in 30% of operated cases of JFC[187].

Myelography: posterolateral filling defect (whereas most discs are situated anteriorly, an occasional fragment may migrate posterolaterally, whereas a JFC will always be posterolateral), often with a round extradural appearance.

CT scan: shows a low density epidural cystic lesion typically with a posterolateral juxtaarticular location. Some have calcified rim[193], and some may have gas within[197]. Erosion of bony lamina is occasionally seen[191, 198].

MRI: variable findings (may be due to differing composition of cyst fluid: serous vs. proteinaceous[199]). Unenhanced signal characteristics of non-hemorrhagic JFC are very similar to CSF. Hemorrhagic JFC are hyperintense. May be missed on sagittal imaging without contrast. Axial images may better demonstrate JFC. Gadolinium enhancement increases the sensitivity[190]. MRI usually misses bony erosion.

Treatment

Optimal treatment is not known. There is one case report of a cyst that resolved spontaneously[188]. If symptoms persist with conservative treatment, some promote cyst aspiration or facet injection with steroids[200], while most advocate surgical excision of the cyst.

Surgical treatment considerations: The cyst may be adherent to the dura. The cyst may also collapse during the surgical approach and may be missed. A JFC may serve as a marker for possible instability and should prompt an evaluation for the same. Some argue for performing a fusion since JFC may arise from instability, however, it appears that fusion is not required for a good result in many cases[200]. Therefore it is suggested that consideration for fusion be made on the basis of any instability and not merely on the basis of the presence of a JFC.

Symptomatic JFC may later develop contralateral to a surgically treated cyst[187].

FAILED BACK SYNDROME

This is a condition where there is failure to improve satisfactorily following back surgery (for herniated intervertebral disc, laminectomy for stenosis...). These patients often require analgesics and are unable to return to work. The failure rate for lumbar discectomy to provide satisfactory long-term pain relief is ≈ 8-25%[201]. Pending legal or worker's compensation claims were the most frequent deterrents to a good outcome[146].

Factors that may cause or contribute to the failed back syndrome:
1. incorrect initial diagnosis
   A. inadequate pre-op imaging
   B. clinical findings not correlated with abnormality demonstrated on imaging
   C. other causes of symptoms (sometimes in the presence of what was considered to be an appropriate lesion on imaging studies which may have been asymptomatic): e.g. trochanteric bursitis, diabetic amyotrophy...
2. continued nerve root or cauda equina compression caused by:
   A. residual disc material
   B. recurrent disc herniation at the same level: usually have pain-free interval > 6 mos post-op (see page 317)
   C. disc herniation at another level
   D. compression of nerve root by peridural **scar** (granulation) tissue (see below)
   E. pseudomeningocele
   F. epidural hematoma
   G. segmental instability: 3 patterns[202], 1) lateral rotational instability, 2) post-op spondylolisthesis, 3) post-op scoliosis
   H. lumbar spinal stenosis
      1. in patients operated for stenosis, recurrence of stenosis at the operated level (over many years)[203]
      2. development of stenosis at adjacent levels[203]
      3. development of stenosis at levels fused in the midline (the high rate of this has resulted in surgeons switching to lateral fusion)
3. permanent nerve root injury from the original disc herniation or from surgery, includes deafferentation pain which is usually constant and burning or ice cold
4. adhesive **arachnoiditis**: responsible for 6-16% of persistent symptoms in post-op patients[204] (see below)
5. discitis: usually produces exquisite back pain 2-4 weeks post-op (see page 245)
6. spondylosis
7. other causes of back pain unrelated to the original condition: paraspinal muscle spasm, myofascial syndrome... Look for trigger points, evidence of spasm
8. post-op reflex sympathetic dystrophy (**RSD**): see page 308
9. "non-anatomic factors": poor patient motivation, secondary gains, drug addiction, psychological problems... (see Psychosocial factors, page 296)

ARACHNOIDITIS (AKA ADHESIVE ARACHNOIDITIS)

Inflammatory condition of the lumbar nerve roots. Actually a misnomer, since adhesive arachnoiditis is really an inflammatory process or fibrosis that involves all three meningeal layers (pia, arachnoid, and dura). Many putative "risk factors" have been described for the development of arachnoiditis, including[205]:
1. spinal anesthesia: either due to the anesthetic agents or to detergent contaminants on the syringes used for same
2. spinal meningitis: pyogenic, syphilitic, tuberculous
3. neoplasms
4. myelographic contrast agents: less common with currently available water soluble contrast agents
5. trauma
   A. post-surgical: especially after multiple operations
   B. external trauma
6. hemorrhage
7. idiopathic

Radiographic findings in arachnoiditis

NB: Radiographic evidence of arachnoiditis may also be found in <u>asymptomatic</u> patients[205]. Arachnoiditis must be differentiated from tumor: the central adhesive type (see below) may resemble CSF seeding of tumor, and myelographic block may mimic intrathecal tumor.

Myelogram: May demonstrate complete block, or clumping of nerve roots. One of many myelographic classification systems[206] for arachnoiditis is shown in Table 14-13.

MRI: 3 patterns on MRI[207, 208]:

1. central adhesion of the nerve roots into 1 or 2 central "cords"
2. "empty thecal sac" pattern: roots adhere to meninges around periphery, only CSF signal is visible intrathecally
3. thecal sac filled with inflammatory tissue, no CSF signal. Corresponds with myelographic block and candle-dripping appearance

Arachnoiditis will usually not enhance with gadolinium as much as tumor on MRI.

PERIDURAL SCAR

Although peridural scar is frequently blamed for causing recurrent symptoms[209, 210], there has been no proof of correlation[211]. Peri-

Table 14-13 Myelographic classification of arachnoiditis

Type	Description
1	unilateral focal filling defect centered on the nerve root sleeve adjacent to disc space
2	circumferential constriction around thecal sac
3	complete obstruction with "stalactites" or "candle guttering", "candle-dripping", or "paint-brush" filling defects
4	infundibular cul-de-sac with loss of radicular striations

dural fibrosis is an inevitable sequelae to lumbar disc surgery. Even patients who are relieved of their pain following discectomy develop some scar tissue post-op[212]. Although it has been shown that if a patient has recurrent radicular pain following a lumbar discectomy there is a 70% chance that extensive peridural scar will be found on MRI[211], this study also showed that on post-op MRIs at 6 months, 43% of patients will have extensive scar, but 84% of the time this will be asymptomatic[213]. Thus, one must use clinical grounds to determine if a patient with extensive scar on MRI is in the 16% minority of patients with radicular symptoms attributable to scar[213].

For a discussion of measures to reduce peridural scarring, *see page 307.*

RADIOLOGIC EVALUATION

Patients with only persistent low back or hip pain without a strong radicular component, with a neurologic exam that is normal or unchanged from pre-op, should be treated symptomatically. Patients with signs or symptoms of recurrent radiculopathy (positive SLR is a sensitive test for nerve root compression), especially if these follow a period of apparent recovery, should undergo further evaluation.

It is critical to differentiate residual/recurrent disc herniation from scar tissue and adhesive arachnoiditis as surgical treatment has generally poor results with the latter two (see *Treatment of failed back syndrome* below).

MRI WITHOUT AND WITH IV GADOLINIUM

Diagnostic test of choice. The best exam for detecting residual or recurrent disc herniation, and to reliably differentiate disc from scar tissue. Pre-contrast studies with T1WI and T2WI yields an accuracy of ≈ 83%, comparable to IV enhanced CT[214, 215]. With the addition of gadolinium, using the protocol below yields 100% sensitivity, 71% specificity, and 89% accuracy[216]. May also detect adhesive arachnoiditis (*see above*). As scar becomes more fibrotic and calcified with time, the differential enhancement with respect to disc material attenuates and may become undetectable at some point, ≈ 1-2 years post-op[215] (some scar continues to enhance for > 20 yrs).

Recommended protocol[216]

Get pre-contrast T1WI and T2WI. Give 0.1 mmol/kg gadolinium IV. Obtain T1WI images within 10 minutes (early post-contrast). No benefit from post-contrast T2WI.

Findings on unenhanced MRI

Signal from a HLD becomes more intense as the sequence is varied from T1WI → T2WI, whereas scar tissue becomes less intense with this transition. Indirect signs (also applicable to CT):
1. mass effect: a nerve root is displaced away from disc material, whereas it may be retracted toward scar tissue by adherence to it
2. location: disc material tends to be in contiguity with the disc interspace (best seen on sagittal MRI)

Findings on enhanced MRI

On *early* (≤ 10 mins post-contrast) T1WI images: scar enhances inhomogeneously, whereas disc does not enhance at all. A nonenhancing central area surrounded by irregular enhancing material probably represents disc wrapped in scar. Venous plexus also enhances, and may be more pronounced when it is distorted by disc material, but the morphology is easily differentiated from scar tissue in these cases.

On *late* (> 30 mins post-contrast) T1WI: scar enhances homogeneously, disc had variable or no enhancement. Normal nerve roots do not enhance even on late images.

CT SCAN WITHOUT AND WITH IV (IODINATED) CONTRAST

Unenhanced CT scan density measurements are unreliable in the postoperative back[217]. Enhanced CT is only fairly good in differentiating scar (enhancing) from disc (unenhancing with possible rim enhancement). Accuracy is about equal to unenhanced MRI.

MYELOGRAPHY, WITH POST-MYELOGRAPHIC CT

Postoperative myelographic criteria alone are unreliable for distinguishing disc material from scar[205, 218]. With the addition of CT scan, neural compression is clearly demonstrated, but scar still cannot be reliably distinguished from disc.

Myelography (especially with post-myelographic CT) is very capable of demonstrating arachnoiditis[218] (*see above*).

PLAIN LS X-RAYS

Generally helpful only in cases of instability, malalignment, or spondylosis[218]. Flexion/extension views are most helpful when trying to demonstrate instability.

TREATMENT OF FAILED BACK SYNDROME

For treatment of intervertebral disc-space infection, see *Discitis*, page 245.

Symptomatic treatment

Recommended for patients who do not have radicular signs and symptoms, or for most patients demonstrated to have scar tissue or adhesive arachnoiditis on imaging. As in other cases of non-specific LBP treatment includes: short-term bed rest, analgesics (non-narcotic in most cases), anti-inflammatory medication (non-steroidal, and occasionally a short course of steroids), and physical therapy.

Surgery

Reserved for those with recurrent or residual disc herniation, segmental instability, or patients with a pseudomeningocele. Patients with post-op spinal instability should be considered for spinal fusion[202] (*see page 300*).

In most series with sufficient follow-up, success rates after reoperation are lower in patients with only epidural scar (as low as 1%) compared to those patients with disc and scar (still only ≈ 37%)[201]. An overall success rate (> 50% pain relief for > 2 yrs) of ≈ 34% was seen in one series[210], with better results in patients that were young, female, with good results following previous surgery, a small number of previous operations, employment prior to surgery, predominantly radicular (cf axial) pain, and absence of scar requiring lysis.

In addition to the absence of disc material, factors associated with poor outcome were: sensory loss involving more than one dermatome, and patients with past or pending compensation claims[201, 219].

Arachnoiditis: Surgery for carefully selected patients with arachnoiditis (those with mild radiographic involvement (Types 1 & 2 in *Table 14-13*), and < 3 previous back operations)[206] has met with moderate success (although in this series, no patient returned to work). Approximate success rate in other series[220, 221]: 50% failure, 20% able to work but with symptoms, 10-19% with no symptoms. Surgery consists of removal of extradural scar enveloping the thecal sac, removing any herniated disc fragments, and performing foraminotomies when indicated. Intradural lysis of adhesions is not indicated since no means for preventing reformation of scar has been identified[221].

RECURRENT HERNIATED LUMBAR DISC

Rates quoted in the literature range from 3-19% with the higher rates usually in series with longer follow-up[222]. In an individual series with 10 year mean F/U, the rate of recurrent disc herniation was 4% (same level, either side), one third of which occurred during the 1st year post-op (mean: 4.3 yrs)[146]. A second recurrence at the same site occurred in 1% in another series[222] with mean F/U of 4.5 yrs. In this series[222], patients presenting for a second time with disc herniation had a recurrence at the same level in 74%, but 26% had a HLD at another level. Recurrent HLD occurred at L4-5 more than twice as often as L5-S1[222].

It is often possible for a smaller amount of recurrent herniated disc to cause symptoms than in a "virgin back", due to the fact that the nerve root is often fixated by scar tissue and has little ability to deviate away from the fragment[138].

TREATMENT
Initial recommended treatment is as with a first time HLD. Nonsurgical treatment should be utilized in the absence of progressive neurologic deficit, cauda equina syndrome (CES) or intractable pain.

Surgical treatment
Disagreement occurs regarding optimal treatment. For recurrent HLD without demonstrated spinal instability, a 1992 survey showed opinion divided primarily between simple repeat discectomy (57%) vs. repeat discectomy with fusion (40%) (when instability is present, more would presumably recommend fusion).

Surgical outcome:
As with first time HLD, the outcome from surgical treatment is worse in worker's compensation cases and in patients undertaking litigation, only ≈ 40% of these patients benefit[222, 223]. A worse prognosis is also associated with: patients with < 6 mos relief after their first operation, cases where fibrosis without recurrent HLD is found at operation.

Spinal cord stimulation
One study actually showed a better response rate to spinal cord stimulation than to reoperation[224]. Since surgery for recurrent HLD carries a higher risk of dural and nerve root injury, and a lower success rate than first time operations, this may be a viable option for some patients.

14.2.2.   Cervical disc herniation

CLINICAL ASPECTS
The following facts explain the findings in herniated cervical disc (HCD):
1. in the cervical region, the nerve root exits <u>above</u> the pedicle of its like-numbered vertebra (opposite to the situation in the lumbar spine)
2. the cervical root exits through the neural foramen in close relation to the undersurface of the pedicle
3. the intervertebral disc space is located close to the inferior portion of the pedicle (unlike the lumbar region)

CERVICAL NERVE ROOT SYNDROMES (CERVICAL RADICULOPATHY)
Due to the facts listed above, a HCD usually impinges on the nerve exiting from the neural foramen <u>at</u> the level of the herniation (e.g. a C6-7 HCD usually causes a C7 radiculopathy). This gives rise to the characteristic cervical nerve root syndromes shown in Table 14-14.

Left C6 radiculopathy (e.g. from C5-6 HCD) occasionally presents with pain simulating an MI. C8 and T1 nerve root involvement may produce a partial Horner's syndrome.

Table 14-14   Cervical disc syndromes

	— Cervical disc —			
	C4-5	C5-6	C6-7	C7-T1
% of cervical discs	2%	19%	69%	10%
compressed root	C5	C6	C7	C8
reflex diminished	deltoid & pectoralis	biceps & brachioradialis	triceps	finger-jerk
motor weakness	deltoid	forearm flexion	forearm ext (wrist drop)	hand intrinsics
paresthesia & hypesthesia	shoulder	upper arm, thumb, radial forearm	fingers 2 & 3, all fingertips	fingers 4 & 5

The most common scenario for patients with herniated cervical disc is that the symptoms were present upon awakening in the morning, without identifiable trauma or stress[225].

Differential diagnosis: *see page 911.*

SIGNS USEFUL IN EVALUATING CERVICAL RADICULOPATHY

Almost all herniated cervical discs cause painful limitation of neck motion. Neck extension usually aggravates pain when cervical disc disease is present (although some patients instead exhibit pain with flexion). Some patients find relief in elevating the arm and cupping the back or the top of the head with the hand (a variation on the shoulder abduction test, *see below*). Lhermitte's sign (electrical shock-like sensation radiating down the spine) may be present.

Miscellaneous

The following tests were found to be specific, but not particularly sensitive in detecting cervical root compression[226]:

1. **Spurling's sign**[227]: radicular pain reproduced when the examiner exerts downward pressure on vertex while tilting head towards symptomatic side (sometimes adding neck extension). Causes narrowing of the intervertebral foramen and possibly increases disc bulge. Used as a "mechanical sign" analogous to SLR for lumbar disc herniation
2. **axial manual traction**: 10-15 kg of axial traction is applied to a supine patient with radicular symptoms (pull up on patient's mandible and occiput). The reduction or disappearance of radicular symptoms is a positive finding
3. **shoulder abduction test**: a sitting patient with radicular symptoms lifts their hand above their head. The reduction or disappearance of radicular symptoms is a positive finding

EVALUATION

Recommended radiologic workup in order of preference: MRI, myelogram/CT, plain CT.

MRI

Study of choice for initial evaluation for herniated cervical disc **(HCD)**. Accuracy is less than water soluble contrast myelogram/CT ($\approx$ 85-90% accuracy for MRI because of only fair to good imaging of neural foramen), but is non-invasive. For myelopathy, MRI is > 95% effective in diagnosing.

CT AND MYELOGRAM/CT

Indications: when MRI cannot be done, when resolution or image quality on MRI is inadequate, or when more bony detail is required.

Plain CT: is usually good at C5-6, is variable at C6-7 (due to artifact from patient's shoulders, depending on body habitus), and is usually poor at C7-T1.

Myelogram/CT (water soluble intrathecal contrast): invasive, may require overnight hospitalization. Accuracy is $\approx$ 98% for cervical disc disease.

TREATMENT

Over 90% of patients with acute cervical radiculopathy due to cervical disc herniation can improve without surgery[228]. The recovery period may be made more tolerable by adequate pain medication, anti-inflammatory medication (NSAIDs or short-course tapering steroids) and intermittent cervical traction (e.g. 10-15 lbs for 10-15 minutes, 2-3 **x** daily).

Surgery is indicated for those that fail to improve or those with progressive neurologic deficit while undergoing non-surgical management. A decision must be made whether to approach the disc anteriorly vs. posteriorly[225].

ACDF (ANTERIOR CERVICAL DISCECTOMY WITH FUSION)

Anterior approach is limited $\approx$ to levels C3-7.

Advantages over posterior approach:
1. safe removal of osteophytes
2. fusion of disc space affords immobility (up to 10% incidence of subluxation with extensive posterior approach)

3. only viable means of dealing with centrally herniated disc

Disadvantages over posterior approach: immobility at fused level may increase stress on adjacent disc spaces. If a fusion is performed, some surgeons prescribe a rigid collar (e.g. Philadelphia collar) for 6-12 weeks. Multiple level ACDF can devascularize the vertebral body (or bodies) between discectomies.

TECHNIQUE
To fuse or not to fuse?
Controversial. Given the absence of a randomized study, it generally depends on surgeon's preference. Arguments for fusion include maintenance of immobilization and distraction at the operated level (preventing collapse of the neural foramen). Some surgeons advocate discectomy without fusion, arguing that the amount of distraction with fusion is minimal[229], that fusion occurs in most cases, usually within 12 weeks even without a graft, and that there are risks of complications from the donor site (including pain). Fusing a level with a graft may also increase the risk of disc herniation at immediately adjacent levels.

Guidelines:
If the operation is for myelopathy with narrowing of the canal, or if the major pathology is osteophytic in nature, a fusion should strongly be considered. If the operation is for a laterally herniated "soft" disc, especially in a relatively young patient, then fusion is optional, especially with the use of the microscope and aggressive foraminotomy[230, 231].

Choice of graft material:
Autologous bone (usually from iliac crest), non-autologous bone (cadaveric) or bone substitutes (e.g. hydroxylapatite[232]). Substitutes for autologous bone eliminate problems with the donor site (*see page 321*), but may have a higher rate of absorption. There were also cases of HIV transmission from cadaveric bone grafts in 1985, however, no further cases have been reported.

POST-OP CHECK
In addition to routine, the following should be checked
❏ 1. evidence of significant post-op hematoma (wound may need to be emergently opened on floor if airway is compromised, see *Carotid endarterectomy, disruption of arteriotomy closure, management* on page 877)
      A. respiratory distress
      B. extreme difficulty swallowing
      C. tracheal deviation
❏ 2. weakness of nerve root of level operated: e.g. biceps for C5-6, triceps for C6-7
❏ 3. long tract signs (Babinski sign…) which may indicate cord compression by spinal epidural hematoma
❏ 4. in cases where bone fusion is performed: extreme swallowing difficulty may indicate anterior extrusion of bone graft impinging upon esophagus; check lateral c-spine x-ray
❏ 5. hoarseness: may indicate vocal cord paresis from recurrent laryngeal nerve injury: hold oral feeding until this can be further assessed

ACDF COMPLICATIONS
Common ones listed below, see references[233, 234]for more details.
• exposure injuries
      A. perforation of pharynx, esophagus and/or trachea: minimize by blunt retraction until longus colli separated from its attachment to vertebrae
      B. vocal cord paresis: due to injury of the recurrent laryngeal nerve (**RLN**) or vagus. Incidence: **11%** temporary, **4%** permanent paresis. Symptoms include: hoarseness, breathiness, cough, aspiration, mass sensation, dysphagia, and vocal cord fatigue[235]. Avoid sharp dissection in paratracheal muscles. Most cases probably due to prolonged retraction against trachea and not to nerve division. More common on right sided approaches where the RLN is more variable[235]
      C. vertebral artery injury: thrombosis or laceration. 0.3% incidence[234]. Risks of treating hemorrhagic complications with packing include: recurrent bleeding, AV fistula, pseudoaneurysm, and arterial thrombosis[234]. Treatment alternatives include direct repair by temporary clipping with aneurysms clips

and repair with 8-0 prolene[236] and endovascular balloon trapping
  D. carotid injury: thrombosis, occlusion, or laceration (usually by retraction)
  E. CSF fistula: usually difficult to repair directly. Place fascial graft beneath bone plug. Keep HOB elevated post op. Consider fibrin glue, lumbar drain
  F. Horner's syndrome: sympathetic plexus lies within longus coli, thus do not extend dissection far laterally into these muscles
  G. thoracic duct injury: in exposing lower cervical spine
• spinal cord or nerve root injuries
  A. spinal cord injury: especially risky in myelopathy due to narrowed canal. Minimize risk by penetrating the osteophyte at the lateral margin of interspace (increases risk to nerve root)
  B. avoid hyperextension during intubation: anesthesiologist may need to determine patient's tolerance pre-op. Consider fiberoptic guided or awake nasotracheal intubation in extreme stenosis
  C. bone graft must be shorter than interspace depth. Exercise caution in tapping graft into position
  D. rare but serious complications of C3-4 operations: sleep induced apnea[237] (possibly due to disruption of the afferent component of the central respiratory control mechanism), bradycardia & cardiorespiratory instability
• bone fusion problems
  A. failure of fusion (pseudarthrosis): incidence 2-20%. Higher with dowel technique (Cloward) than with keystone technique of Bailey & Badgley or with interbody method of Smith-Robinson (10%) or with non-fusion advocated by Hirsch. Not uniformly associated with symptoms or problems[238, 239] No treatment is required for asymptomatic pseudarthrosis
  B. anterior (kyphotic) angulation deformity: may be as high as 60% with Cloward technique (may be reduced by collar immobilization). May develop in Hirsch technique with excessive bone removal
  C. graft extrusion: 2% incidence (rarely requires re-operation unless compression of cord posteriorly, or esophagus or trachea anteriorly occurs)
  D. donor site complications: hematoma/seroma, infection, fracture of ilium, injury to lateral femoral cutaneous nerve, persistent pain due to scar, bowel perforation
• miscellaneous
  A. wound infection: incidence < 1%
  B. post-op hematoma: placing cervical collar in O.R. may delay recognition
  C. transient dysphagia and hoarseness: inevitable. Due to retraction and edema. If edema is severe, may cause tracheal obstruction
  D. adjacent level degeneration: controversial whether this represents a sequelae to altered biomechanics from surgery, or a predisposition to cervical spondylosis[240]. Many (≈ 70%) are asymptomatic[241]
  E. postoperative discomfort: sensation of lump in throat. Nagging discomfort in neck, shoulder, and interscapular regions (may last several months)
  F. reflex sympathetic dystrophy (RSD): rarely described in the literature[242], possibly due to stellate ganglion injury (see page 396)

POSTERIOR CERVICAL DECOMPRESSION

Not necessary for unilateral radiculopathy (use either ACD or keyhole laminotomy). Consists of removal of cervical lamina (laminectomy) and spinous processes in order to convert the spinal canal from a "tube" to a "trough".

Usually reserved for the following conditions:
1. multiple cervical discs or osteophytes (anterior cervical discectomy (ACD) can readily treat only 2, or possibly 3, levels) with myelopathy
2. where the disc herniation is superimposed on cervical stenosis, and the latter is more diffuse and/or more significant (see Cervical spinal stenosis, page 331)
3. in professional speakers or singers where the 5% risk of permanent voice change due to recurrent laryngeal nerve injury with ACD is unacceptable

POSTERIOR KEYHOLE LAMINOTOMY

AKA "keyhole foraminotomy".A technique to decompress only individual nerve roots (but not the spinal cord) by creating a small "keyhole" in the lamina to access the nerve root.

Indications for keyhole approach (c.f. ACD):

1. monoradiculopathy with posterolateral <u>soft</u> disc sequestration (small <u>lateral</u> osteophytic spurs may also be addressed)
2. radiculopathy in patients who are professional speakers or singers (*see above*)
3. for lower (e.g. C7, C8 or T1) or upper (e.g. C3 or C4) cervical nerve root compression, especially in a patient with a short thick neck, making an anterior approach more difficult

Outcome

A number of large series have reported good or excellent outcome in the range of 90-96%[244].

14.2.3.   Thoracic disc herniation

Account for 0.25-0.75% of all protruded discs. 80% occur between the 3rd and 5th decades. 75% are below T8, with a peak of 26% at T11-12. A history of trauma may be elicited in 25% of cases.

Most common symptoms: pain (60%), sensory changes (23%), motor changes (18%).

SURGICAL TREATMENT

Surgery for thoracic disc disease is problematic because of the difficulty of anterior approaches. The proportionately tighter space between cord and canal compared to the cervical and lumbar regions, and the watershed blood supply create a significant risk of cord injury with attempts to manipulate the cord when trying to work anteriorly to it from a posterior approach. Herniated thoracic discs are also frequently calcified.

APPROACHES

Open surgical approaches are divided into 3 basic categories (some use 4[246]):

1. posterior (midline laminectomy): primary indication is for decompression of posteriorly situated intracanalicular pathology (e.g. metastatic tumor) especially over multiple levels. There is a high failure and complication rate when used for single-level anterior pathology (e.g. midline disc herniation)
2. posterolateral
   A. lateral gutter: laminectomy plus removal of pedicle; alternatively, a transpedicular approach may be used[247]
   B. costotransversectomy (*see below*)
3. anterolateral (transthoracic)

An option to open surgery is thoracoscopic surgery.

CHOICE OF APPROACH

For anterior approaches to the thoracic spine, see sections beginning on *page 613*.

For a laterally herniated thoracic disc without myelopathy: posterolateral approach with medial facetectomy is technically simple, and has generally good results. For a central disc herniation, or when myelopathy is present: transthoracic approach has the lowest incidence of cord injury with the best operative results (*see Table 14-15*). For anterior access, unless pathology is predominantly left-sided, a right-sided thoracotomy is preferred because the heart does not impede access.

Table 14-15   Results with various approaches for thoracic spine pathology[248]

Approach	Indication	Total no.	— OUTCOME —			
			Normal	Improved	Same	Worse
laminectomy	posteriorly located tumor	129	15%	42%	11%	32%
posterolateral (transpedicular)	radicular pain with lateral disc herniation; biopsy of tumor	27	37%	45%	11%	7%
lateral (costotransversectomy)	fair for midline disc; good ipsilateral access, poor access to opposite side	43	35%	53%	12%	0
transthoracic	best for midline lesions, especially for reaching both sides of cord	12	67%	33%	0	0

COSTOTRANSVERSECTOMY

Indications: was widely used to drain tuberculous spine abscess, may be used for lateral disc herniation, biopsy of VB or pedicle, limited decompression of spinal cord from tumor. Involves resection of the transverse process and at least ≈ 4 cm of the posterior rib. A serious risk of this approach is interruption of a significant radicular artery which may compromise spinal cord blood supply (see *Spinal cord vasculature*, page 75). There is also a risk of pneumothorax which is less serious.

TRANSTHORACIC APPROACH

Indications: thoracic disc disease, burst fractures of the thoracic spine, etc.

Advantages[249]:
- excellent anterior exposure (especially advantageous for multiple levels)
- little compromise of stability (due to supporting effect of rib cage)
- low risk of mechanical cord injury

Disadvantages:
- requires thoracic surgeon (or familiarity with thoracic surgery)
- some risk of vascular cord injury (due to sacrifice of intercostal arteries)
- definitive diagnosis may not be possible if it is uncertain prior to procedure

Possible complications:
- pulmonary complications: pleural effusion, atelectasis, pneumonia, empyema, hypoventilation
- CSF-pleural fistula

14.3.   Degenerative disc/spine disease

Since structures outside of the disc are usually involved, the term degenerative spine disease (**DSD**) may be preferable to degenerative *disc* disease. Spondylosis is a non-specific term which may include degenerative spine disease. "Cervical spondylosis" is occasionally used synonymously with cervical stenosis (see *Cervical spinal stenosis*, page 331).

DSD is a progressive deterioration of the structures of the spine including:
1. disc abnormalities:
    A. the proteoglycan content of the disc nucleus decreases with age
    B. disc desiccation (loss of hydration) occurs
    C. tears develop in the disc annulus and progress to internal disruption of the lamellar architecture. Herniation of the nucleus may occur from increased nuclear pressure under mechanical loads
    D. mucoid degeneration and ingrowth of fibrous tissue ensues (disc fibrosis)
    E. subsequently disc resorption occurs
    F. there is a loss of disc space height and increased susceptibility to injury
2. facet joint abnormalities: hypertrophy and capsular laxity
3. osteophytes often form on the edges of the VB bordering the degenerated disc
4. spondylolisthesis: subluxation of one VB on another (see *Spondylolisthesis* below)
5. spondylolysis: alternative term for isthmic spondylolisthesis (*see below*), a failure of the neural arch due to a defect in the pars interarticularis which may present as spondylolisthesis. There may be a fibrous mass from the nonunion
6. hypertrophy of the ligamentum flavum

Clinical presentation:
1. the above abnormalities may produce **spinal stenosis** which can lead to neural compromise producing the following symptoms
    A. radicular symptoms (more common in cervical spine than lumbar)
    B. neurogenic claudication (lumbar) or spinal myelopathy (cervical)
2. discogenic pain (controversial) may be less prevalent in the late stages of DSD. May contribute to "musculoskeletal low back pain" but the actual pain generators here are not definitively identified

ETIOLOGY

The etiology of DSD is multifactorial and includes:
1. cumulative effects of microtrauma and macrotrauma to the spine

2. osteoporosis
3. cigarette smoking: several epidemiologic studies have shown that the incidence of back pain, sciatica and spinal degenerative disease is higher among cigarette smokers than among nonsmokers[250, 251]. Smoking also delays bone healing and increases the risk of psudoarthrosis following spinal fusion procedures, especially in the lumbar spine[250]
4. in the lumbar spine:
   A. stresses on the spine including effects of excess body weight
   B. loss of muscle tone (primarily abdominals and paraspinals) resulting in increased dependence on the bony spine for structural support

SPONDYLOLISTHESIS

Anterior subluxation of one vertebral body on another, usually L5 on S1, occasionally L4 on L5. The Meyerding[252, 253] method of grading is shown in *Table 14-16*.

Disc herniation and nerve root compression: It is rare for a herniated lumbar disc to occur at the level of the listhesis, however the disc may "roll" out as it is exposed and produce findings on MRI that have been termed a "pseudodisc". It is more common to see a herniated disc at the level above the listhesis. If the listhesis does cause nerve root compression, it tends to involve the nerve exiting below the pedicle of the anteriorly subluxed vertebra. The compression is usually due to upward displacement of the superior articular facet of the level below together with disc material, and symptoms typically resemble neurogenic claudication, although true radiculopathy may sometimes occur.

Table 14-16 Spondylolisthesis grading

Grade	Amount of subluxation
I	< 25%
II	25-50%
III	50-75%
IV	75%-complete

CLASSIFICATION OF SPONDYLOLISTHESIS

1. isthmic spondylolisthesis: AKA **spondylolysis**: a failure of the neural arch manifesting as a defect in the **pars interarticularis** (the neck of the "Scotty dog" on oblique LS-spine x-ray). May be seen in 5-20% of spine x-rays[4]. Three types:
   A. lytic: fatigue fracture of pars
   B. elongated but intact pars: possibly due to repetitive fractures and healing
   C. acute fracture of pars
2. dysplastic: congenital. Upper sacrum or arch of L5 permits the spondylolisthesis. No pars defect. Some of these may progress (no way to identify these)
3. degenerative: due to long-standing intersegmental instability. No break in the pars. Found in 5.8% of men and 9.1% of women (many of whom are asymptomatic)[4]
4. traumatic: due to fractures in other areas of the bony hook and the pars
5. pathologic: generalized or local bone disease

ISTHMIC SPONDYLOLISTHESIS (SPONDYLOLYSIS)

Presentation

Isthmic spondylolisthesis rarely produces central canal stenosis since only the anterior part of the spinal canal is shifted forward. May present with radiculopathy, the nerve exiting under the pedicle at that level is the most vulnerable. May also present with low back. Many cases may be asymptomatic.

Management[4]
1. lesions with sclerotic borders are usually well established with little chance of healing. There is virtually no risk of further slippage nor of neurologic damage in adults, thus surgery is reserved for patients with neurologic deficit or incapacitating symptoms
2. lesions without sclerosis that show increased uptake on bone scan (indicating active lesion with potential for healing) may heal in a rigid orthosis such as the **Boston brace**
3. management of symptoms:
   A. LBP only: treat with NSAIDs, PT
   B. LBP with myelopathy, radiculopathy, or neurogenic claudication: surgical treatment (*see Table 14-17* for type of surgery)

When surgery is indicated, *Table 14-17* serves as a guide to the type of procedure.

Table 14-17   Recommended treatment for spondylolisthesis

Nature of spondylolisthesis	Nature of problem	Type of procedure needed
degenerative	nerve root compression within confines of spinal canal	decompression (preserving facets)
	spinal stenosis at the level of spondylolisthesis	decompression; some advocate with intertransverse-process fusion[254]
	nerve root compression far lateral, outside confines of spinal canal	radical decompression (Gill procedure) plus fusion
traumatic	(does not matter)	decompression plus fusion

14.3.1.   Spinal stenosis

Classified as:
1. central canal stenosis: narrowing of the AP dimension of the spinal canal. The reduction in canal size may cause local neural compression and/or compromise of the blood supply to the spinal cord (cervical) or the cauda equina (lumbar)
2. foraminal stenosis: narrowing of the neural foramen
3. lateral recess stenosis (lumbar spine only): *see page 330*

Central canal stenosis
    May be congenital (as in the achondroplastic dwarf), acquired, or most commonly acquired superimposed on congenital.
    In the lumbar region, the syndrome of neurogenic claudication (*see below*) is well recognized. In the cervical region, cervical myelopathy and ataxia (from spinocerebellar tract compression) may be present. In 5%, lumbar and cervical stenoses are symptomatic simultaneously[255]. Symptomatic spinal stenosis in the thoracic region is rare[256].

14.3.1.1.   Lumbar spinal stenosis

    Unless indicated otherwise, this discussion refers primarily to central canal stenosis
⅂ Key points
- caused by hypertrophy of facets and ligamentum flavum, may be exacerbated by disc bulging or spondylolisthesis, may be superimposed on congenital narrowing
- most common at L4-5 and then at L3-4
- symptomatic stenosis produces gradually progressive back and leg pain with standing and walking that is relieved by sitting or lying (neurogenic claudication)
- symptoms differentiated from vascular claudication which is usually relieved at rest regardless of position
- usually responds to decompressive surgery; fusion may be an adjunct

    Symptomatic lumbar stenosis is most common at L4-5, then L3-4, L2-3 and lastly L5-S1[257]. It is rare at L1-2. Generally occurs in patients with congenitally shallow lumbar canal (see *Normal LS spine measurements*, page 327) with superimposed acquired degeneration in the form of some combination of facet hypertrophy, hypertrophy of the ligamentum flavum, protruding (and often calcified) intervertebral discs, and spondylolisthesis. First recognized as a distinct clinical entity producing characteristic symptoms in the 1950's and 60's[258, 259].

May be classified as[260]:
1. **stable** form of lumbar spinal stenosis: hypertrophy of facets and ligamentum flavum accompanied by disc degeneration and collapse
2. **unstable**: have the above with superimposed
    A. degenerative spondylolisthesis: (*see page 324*) the unisegmental form
    B. degenerative scoliosis: the multisegmental form

PRESENTATION

Often presents as **neurogenic claudication (NC)**, (claudicate: from Latin, *claudico*, to limp) AKA **pseudoclaudication**. To be differentiated from **vascular claudication** (AKA intermittent claudication) which results from ischemia of exercising muscles (*see Table 14-18*). NC is unilateral or bilateral buttock, hip, thigh or leg discomfort that is precipitated by standing or walking and characteristically relieved by a change in posture to sitting, squatting, or recumbency. NC is thought to arise from ischemia of lumbosacral nerve roots, as a result of increased metabolic demand from exercise together with vascular compromise of the nerve root due to pressure from surrounding structures. NC is only moderately sensitive (≈ 60%) but is highly specific for spinal stenosis[262]. Pain may not be the major complaint, instead, some patients may develop paresthesias or LE weakness with walking.

Patients with NC may de-

Table 14-18 Clinical features distinguishing neurogenic from vascular claudication[261]

Feature	Neurogenic claudication	Vascular claudication
distribution of pain	in distribution of nerve (dermatomal)	in distribution of muscle group with common vascular supply (sclerotomal)
sensory loss	dermatomal distribution	stocking distribution
inciting factors	variable amounts of exercise, also with prolonged maintenance of a given posture (65% have pain on standing at rest); coughing produces pain in 38%	reliably reproduced with fixed amount of exercise (e.g. distance ambulated) that decreases as disease progresses; rare at rest (27% have pain on standing at rest)
relief with rest	slow (often > 30 min), variable, usually positional (stooped posture or sitting often required, ★ standing and resting is usually not sufficient)	almost immediate; not dependent on posture (relief of walking induced symptoms with standing is a key differentiating feature)
claudicating distance	variable day-to-day in 62%	constant day-to-day in 88%
discomfort on lifting or bending	common (67%)	infrequent (15%)
foot pallor on elevation	none	marked
peripheral pulses	normal; or if ↓ usually reduced only unilaterally	↓ or absent; femoral bruits are common
skin temp of feet	normal	decreased

velop the **"anthropoid posture"** (exaggerated waist flexion, possibly reduces lumbar lordosis, thereby reducing inward buckling of ligamentum flavum and also distracting facet joints). They may also complain of muscle cramping, especially in the calves.

Trochanteric bursitis (TBS) and degenerative arthritis of the hip are also included in the differential diagnosis of NC[263, 264]. Although TBS may be primary, it can also be secondary to other conditions including lumbar stenosis, degenerative arthritis of the lumbar spine or knee, and leg length discrepancy. TBS produces intermittent aching pain over the lateral aspect of the hip. Although usually chronic, it occasionally may have acute or subacute onset. Pain radiates to lateral aspect of thigh in 20-40% (so called **"pseudoradiculopathy"**), but rarely extends to the posterior thigh or as far distally as the knee. There may be numbness and paresthesia-like symptoms in the upper thigh which are usually not dermatomal in distribution. Like NC, the pain may be triggered by prolonged standing, walking and climbing, but unlike NC it is also painful to lie on the affected side. Localized tenderness over the greater trochanter can be elicited in virtually all patients, with maximal tenderness at the junction of the upper thigh and greater trochanter. Pain increases with certain hip movements, especially external rotation (over half the patients have a positive Patrick-fabere test, *see page 303*), and rarely with hip flexion/extension. Treatment includes NSAIDs, local injection of glucocorticoid (usually with local anesthetic), physical therapy (with stretching and muscle strengthening exercises) and local application of ice. No controlled studies have compared these.

NEUROLOGIC EXAM

The neurologic exam is normal in ≈ 18% of cases (including normal muscle stretch reflexes and negative straight leg raising). Absent or reduced ankle jerks and diminished knee jerks is common[262]. Pain may be reproduced by lumbar <u>extension</u>.

DIFFERENTIAL DIAGNOSIS
1. vascular insufficiency (*see above*)
2. trochanteric bursitis (*see above*)
3. disc herniation (lumbar or thoracic)
4. juxtafacet cyst (*see page 313*)
5. arachnoiditis
6. intraspinal tumor
7. functional etiologies
8. diabetic neuritis: with this, the sole of the foot is usually very tender to pressure from the examiner's thumb

ASSOCIATED CONDITIONS
1. congenital:
   A. achondroplasia
   B. congenitally narrowed canal
2. acquired:
   A. spondylolisthesis
   B. acromegaly
   C. post-traumatic
   D. Paget's disease (see *Paget's disease*, page 340)
   E. ankylosing spondylitis: *see page 313*
   F. ossification of the yellow ligament **(OYL)**

DIAGNOSTIC EVALUATION

RADIOGRAPHIC EVALUATION
Comparison of modalities:

 Lumbosacral spine x-rays: may disclose spondylolisthesis. AP diameter of canal is usually narrowed (congenitally or acquired) (see *Normal LS spine measurements* below) whereas the interpediculate distance **(IPD)** may be normal[261]. Oblique films may demonstrate pars defects.

 CT scan (either routine, or following water-soluble myelography): classically shows "**trefoil**" canal (cloverleaf shaped, with 3 leaflets). CT also demonstrates AP canal diameter, hypertrophied ligaments, facet arthropathy, and bulging annulus or herniated disc. CT is poor for demonstrating spondylolisthesis although the pars defect may be seen.

 Myelogram: lateral films often show "washboard pattern" (multiple anterior defects), AP films often show "wasp-waisting" (narrowing of dye column), may also show partial or complete (especially in prone position) block. May be difficult to perform LP if stenosis is severe (poor CSF flow and difficulty avoiding nerve roots).

 MRI: demonstrates impingement on neural structures and loss of CSF signal on T2WI at severely stenotic levels. MRI is poor for visualizing bone which contributes significantly to the pathology (may be helpful for surgical planning). Good for evaluating nerve impingement due to spondylolisthesis (possibly better than myelogram/CT) and juxtafacet cysts. Asymptomatic abnormalities are demonstrated in up to 33% of asymptomatic patients 50-70 years old[257].

NORMAL LS SPINE MEASUREMENTS
 Normal dimensions of the lumbar spine are shown in *Table 14-19* for plain film and *Table 14-20* for CT.

Table 14-19 Normal AP diameter on lateral plain film
(from spinolaminar line to posterior vertebral body)[265]

average (normal)	22-25 mm
lower limits of normal	15 mm
severe lumbar stenosis	< 11 mm

Table 14-20 Normal measurements on CT[266]

AP diameter	≥ 11.5 mm
interpediculate distance (IPD)	≥ 16 mm
canal cross-sectional area	≥ 1.45 cm²
ligamentum flavum thickness[267]	≤ 4-5 mm
height of lateral recess (*see below*)	≥ 3 mm

Interpediculate distance (IPD): The transverse diameter of the spinal canal. On plain AP x-ray of lumbar spine, an IPD < 25 mm suggests stenosis. Average normal IPDs in the lumbar and lower thoracic spine appears in *Table 14-21*. An approximation for the lumbar spine is given in *Eq 14-1*.

$$IPD \ (mm) = (lumbar \ level + 12) \times 1.5 \qquad Eq \ 14-1$$

ADJUNCTS TO RADIOGRAPHIC EVALUATION

"Bicycle test": patients with NC can usually tolerate longer periods of exercise on a bicycle than patients with intermittent (vascular) claudication because the position in bicycling flexes the waist.

Ratio of ankle to brachial blood pressure (**A:B ratio**): > 1.0 is normal; mean of 0.59 in patients with intermittent claudication; 0.26 in patients with rest pain; < 0.05 indicates impending gangrene.

Vascular lab studies (e.g. Doppler) may assist in identifying vascular insufficiency.

EMG with NCV may show multiple nerve-root abnormalities bilaterally.

Table 14-21 Normal interpediculate distance (IPD) on AP LS film[268]

Level	IPD (mm)*
T10	16-22
T11	17-24
T12	19-27
L1	21-29
L2	21-30
L3	21-31
L4	21-33
L5	23-37

* 90% tolerance range for adults (target to film distance = 40 inches (102 cm))

TREATMENT

In one study of 27 unoperated patients, 19 remain unchanged, 4 improved, and 4 worsened (mean follow-up: 49 months; range: 10-103 months)[269]. NSAIDs and physical therapy are the mainstays of nonsurgical management.

Surgical decompression is undertaken when symptoms become severe in spite of medical management. The goals of surgery are pain relief, halting progression of symptoms, and possibly reversal of some existing neurologic deficit. Most authors do not consider surgery unless the symptoms have been present > 3 months, and most patients who have surgery for this have symptoms of > 1 year duration.

Surgical technique

Undercutting the superior articular facet is often necessary to decompress the nerves in the foramen (see *Lateral recess syndrome*, page 330). Treatment of moderate stenosis at adjacent levels appears warranted as these levels have been shown to have a significant likelihood of becoming symptomatic later[203].

Progression of spondylolisthesis

May occur without decompression, but is more common following surgery[270]. However, lumbar instability following decompressive laminectomy is rare (only ≈ 1% of all laminectomies for stenosis will develop progressive subluxation). Fusion is rarely required to prevent progression of subluxation with degenerative stenosis[271].

Stability (without need for instrumentation) is thought to be maintained if > 50-66% of the facets are preserved during surgery and the disc space is not violated (maintains integrity of anterior and middle column). Younger or more active patients are at higher risk of subluxing.

One approach is to obtain flexion/extension x-rays pre-op, and follow patients after decompression. Those who develop symptomatic slippage post-op are treated by fusion, possibly in conjunction with spinal instrumentation.

PRACTICE PARAMETER 14-10 FUSION IN PATIENTS WITH LUMBAR STENOSIS WITHOUT SPONDYLOLISTHESIS

Options[272]:
- in situ posterolateral fusion is not recommended following decompression in patients with lumbar stenosis in whom there is no evidence of preexisting spinal instability or likely iatrogenic instability due to facetectomy
- in situ posterolateral fusion is recommended in patients with lumbar stenosis in whom there is evidence of spinal instability
- the addition of pedicle-screw instrumentation is not recommended in conjunction with posterolateral fusion following decompression

PRACTICE PARAMETER 14-11 FUSION IN PATIENTS WITH LUMBAR STENOSIS AND SPONDYLOLISTHESIS

Guidelines[273]: posterolateral fusion is recommended for patients with stenosis and associated degenerative spondylolisthesis who require decompression

Options[273]: pedicle screw fixation as an adjunct to posterolateral fusion should be considered in patients with stenosis and spondylolisthesis in cases where there is pre-op evidence of spinal instability* or kyphosis* at the level of the spondylolisthesis or when iatrogenic instability is anticipated

* the definition of "instability" and "kyphosis" varies, and has not been standardized

Fusion may accelerate degenerative changes at adjacent levels. Some surgeons recommend fusion at levels of spoldylolisthestic stenosis[203, 260]. Patients with combined degenerative spondylolisthesis, stenosis, and radiculopathy may be reasonable candidates for fusion[1].

BRACE THERAPY

PRACTICE PARAMETER 14-12 BRACE THERAPY AS AN ADJUNCT TO OR INSTEAD OF LUMBAR FUSION

Guidelines[274]:
- short-term use (1-3 weeks) of a rigid lumbar support is recommended for treatment of LBP of relatively short duration (< 6 months)
- bracing in patients with LBP > 6 months duration is not recommended because it has not been shown to have long-term benefit

Options[274]:
- lumbar braces may reduce the number of sick days due to LBP among workers with a previous lumbar injury. Braces are not recommended for LBP in the general working population
- the use of pre-op bracing or transpedicular external fixation as tools to predict outcome for lumbar fusion is not recommended

OUTCOME

Morbidity/mortality

Risk of in-hospital mortality is 0.32%[262]. Other risks include: unintended durotomy (see page 308) (0.32%[262] to ≈ 13%[271, 275]), deep infection (5.9%), superficial infection (2.3%), and DVT (2.8%) (see also *Risks of lumbar laminectomy* on page 307).

Success of operation

No randomized study exists comparing surgery to "conservative" treatment. Patients with a postural component to their pain had much better results (96% good result) than those without a postural component (50% good results), and the relief of leg pain was much more successful than relief of back pain[276]. Surgery is most likely to reduce LE pain and improve walking tolerance[1].

Surgical failure may be divided into two groups:
1. patients with initial improvement who develop recurrent difficulties. Although short-term improvement after surgery is common, many patients progressively

---

deteriorate over time[277]. One study found a 27% recurrence of symptoms after 5 years follow-up[203] (30% due to restenosis at the operated level, 30% due to stenosis at a new level; 75% of these patients respond to further surgery). Other etiologies include: development of herniated lumbar disc, development of late instability, coexisting medical conditions

2. patients who fail to have any post-op pain relief (early treatment failures). In one series of 45 such patients[278]:
   A. the most common finding was a lack of solid clinical and radiographic indications for surgery (e.g. non-radicular LBP coupled with modest stenosis)
   B. technical factors of surgery had less influence on outcome, with the most common finding being failure to decompress the lateral recess (which requires judicious medial facet resection or undercutting the superior articular facet)
   C. other diagnoses (e.g. arachnoiditis), missed diagnosis (spinal AVM...)

Long term outcome: Literature review[262] with long-term follow-up found good or excellent outcome after surgery with a mean of 64% (range: 26-100%). A patient satisfaction survey indicated that 37% were much improved and 29% somewhat improved (total: 66%) post-op[279]. A prospective study found a success rate of 78-88% at 6 wks and 6 months, which dropped to ≈ 70% at 1 year and 5 yrs[280]. Success rates were slightly lower for lateral recess syndrome (*see below*).

LATERAL RECESS SYNDROME

A variant of lumbar stenosis[281]. The **lateral recess** is the "gutter" alongside the pedicle in which the nerve root resides just proximal to the neural foramen (*see Figure 14-2*). It is bordered anteriorly by the vertebral body, laterally by the pedicle, and posteriorly by the superior articular facet of the inferior vertebral body. Hypertrophy of this superior articular facet compresses the nerve root. L4-5 is the most commonly involved facet.

PRESENTATION

Patients develop unilateral or bilateral leg pain predominantly when walking or standing, and usually obtain relief by squatting, sitting with the waist flexed, or lying in the fetal position. Painful burning paresthesias of the lower extremities are also described. Valsalva maneuvers usually do not exacerbate the pain. The time course is usually gradually progressive over many months to years.

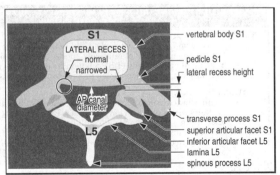

Figure 14-2 Schematic CT of L5-S1 showing the lateral recess

In comparison, a HLD usually causes increased pain on sitting, has a more abrupt onset, has pain on straight leg raising, and is worsened by Valsalva maneuvers.

The neurologic exam may be normal (including straight leg raising). Achilles reflexes may be absent.

EVALUATION

High resolution CT scan best defines the bony anatomy of the lateral recess (*see Figure 14-2* and *Table 14-22*).

MRI or water soluble contrast myelography is recommended when surgery is contemplated. Characteristic finding: flattening of nerve root as it passes beneath the hypertrophied facet joint.

Conservative treatment with lumbosacral brace may be attempted.

Surgical therapy

Indicated for unresponsive cases. Consists of laminectomy and partial (typically medial one third) facetectomy. Requires removal of the hypertrophied portion of the facet dorsal to the involved nerve root, either by undercutting, or by reducing overhanging hypertrophied facet elements until they are flush with the pedicle.

Table 14-22 Dimensions of lateral recess on CT (bone windows)

Lateral recess height	Degree of lateral recess stenosis
3-4 mm	borderline (symptomatic if other lesion co-exists, e.g. disc bulging)
< 3 mm	suggestive of lateral recess syndrome
< 2 mm	diagnostic of lateral recess syndrome

14.3.1.2. Cervical spinal stenosis

"**Cervical spondylosis**" is occasionally used synonymously with cervical spinal stenosis. However, spondylosis usually implies a more widespread degenerative condition of the cervical spine including various combinations of the following:
1. congenital spinal stenosis (the "shallow cervical canal"[282])
2. degeneration of the intervertebral disc producing a focal stenosis due to a "**cervical bar**" which is usually a combination of:
   A. osteophytic spurs ("**hard disc**" in neurosurgical jargon)
   B. and/or protrusion of intervertebral disc material ("**soft disc**")
3. hypertrophy of any of the following (which also contributes to canal stenosis):
   A. lamina
   B. dura
   C. articular facets
   D. ligaments, including
      1. ligamentum flavum: neck extension may cause an increase of infolding of the ligament from the posterior spinal canal
      2. posterior longitudinal ligament: may include ossification of the posterior longitudinal ligament (**OPLL**)[283] (see page 345). May be segmental or diffuse. Often adherent to dura
4. subluxation: due to disc and facet joint degeneration
5. altered mobility: severely spondylotic levels may be fused and are usually stable, however there is often hypermobility at certain segments
6. telescoping of the spine due to loss of height of VBs → "shingling" of laminae
7. alteration of the normal lordotic curvature[284] (NB: the amount of abnormal curvature did not correlate with the degree of myelopathy)
   A. straightening
   B. reversal of the curvature (kyphosis)
   C. exaggerated lordosis (hyperlordosis): the least common variant

Although the majority of individuals > 50 yrs old have radiologic evidence of significant degenerative disease of the cervical spine, only a small percentage will experience neurologic symptoms[285].

CLINICAL

The condition generally tends to produce three types of clinical problems[225]:
1. nerve root compression may cause radicular complaints
2. spinal cord compression may cause myelopathy. Some stereotypical syndromes are presented below (see *Cervical spondylotic myelopathy (CSM)* below)
3. pain and paresthesias in the head, neck and shoulders with little or no suggestion of radiculopathy nor abnormal physical findings. This group is the most difficult to treat, and often requires a good physician-patient relationship to decide if surgical treatment should be undertaken in an attempt to provide relief

CERVICAL SPONDYLOTIC MYELOPATHY (CSM)

Cervical spondylosis is the most common cause of myelopathy in patients > 55 yrs of age[286]. Cervical spondylotic myelopathy (CSM) develops in almost all patients with ≥

30% narrowing of the cross-sectional area of the cervical spinal canal[287] (although some patients with severe cord compression do not have myelopathy[288, 289]).

PATHOPHYSIOLOGY
Pathogenesis is controversial. Theories include the following alone or in combination:
1. direct cord compression between osteophytic bars and hypertrophy or infolding of the ligamentum flavum, especially if superimposed on congenital narrowing or cervical subluxations
2. ischemia due to compression of vascular structures (arterial deprivation and/or venous stasis)[290]
3. repeated local cord trauma by normal movements in the presence of protruded discs and/or osteophytic (spondylotic) bars (cord and root traction[291])
   A. cephalad/caudad movement with flexion extension[292]
   B. lateral traction on the cord by the dentate ligaments[293]
   C. diameter of spinal canal varies during normal flexion and extension

Pathologically[294], there is degeneration of the central grey matter at the level of compression, degeneration of the posterior columns above the lesion (particularly in the anteromedial portion), and demyelination in the lateral columns (especially the corticospinal tracts) below the lesion. Anterior spinal tracts are relatively spared. There may be atrophic changes in the ventral and dorsal roots and neurophagia of anterior horn cells.

CLINICAL
Cervical pain and mechanical signs are uncommon in cases of myelopathy. See *Table 14-23* for the frequency of symptoms in CSM in one series. In most cases the disability is mild, and the prognosis for these is good. CSM is rare in patients < 40 years of age.

Time course of symptoms
Highly variable and unpredictable. In ≈ 75% of cases of CSM, there is progression either in a stepwise fashion (in one third) or gradually progressive (two thirds)[295]. In some series, the most common pattern was that of an initial phase of deterioration followed by a stabilization that typically lasts for years and may not change thereafter[296, 297]. In these cases, the degree of disability may be established early in the course of CSM. Others disagree with such a "benign" outlook and cite that over 50% of cases continue to deteriorate with conservative treatment[285]. Sustained spontaneous improvement is probably rare[286].

Motor
Findings can be due to cord (UMN) and/or root (LMN) compression. There may be weakness and wasting of the hand muscles. Slow, stiff opening and closing of the fists may occur[299]. Clumsiness with fine motor skills (writing, buttoning buttons…) is common.
There is often proximal weakness of the lower extremities (mild to moderate iliopsoas weakness occurs in 54%) and spasticity of the LEs.

Sensory
Sensory disturbance may be minimal, and when present are often not radicular in distribution. There may be a glove-distribution sensory loss in the hands[300]. A sensory level may occur a number of levels below the area of cord compression.
LEs often exhibit loss of vibratory sense (in as many as 82%), and occasionally have reduced pin-prick sensation (9%) (almost always restricted to below the ankle). Compression of the spinocerebellar tract may cause difficulty running. Lhermitte's sign was present in only

Table 14-23 Frequency of symptoms in CSM (37 cases[298])

Finding	%
pure myelopathy	59%
myelopathy + radiculopathy	41%
reflexes	
hyperreflexia	87%
Babinski	54%
Hoffmann	13%
sensory deficits	
sensory level	41%
posterior column	39%
dermatomal arm	33%
paresthesias	21%
positive Romberg	15%
motor deficits	
arm weakness	31%
paraparesis	21%
hemiparesis	18%
quadriparesis	10%
Brown-Séquard	10%
muscle atrophy	13%
fasciculations	13%
pain	
radicular arm	41%
radicular leg	13%
cervical	8%
spasticity	54%
sphincter disturbance	49%
cervical mechanical signs	26%

2 of 37 cases. Some patients may present with a prominence of posterior column dysfunction (impaired joint position sense and 2 point discrimination)[301].

Reflexes

In 72-87%, reflexes are hyperactive at a varying distance below the level of stenosis. Clonus or Babinski's sign may also be present. **Inverted radial reflex**: flexion of the fingers in response to eliciting the brachioradialis reflex, said to be pathognomonic of CSM[302].

A hyperactive **jaw jerk** indicates upper motor neuron lesion <u>above</u> the midpons, and distinguishes long tract findings due to pathology above the foramen magnum from those below (e.g. cervical myelopathy): not helpful if absent (a normal variant).

Sphincter

Bladder sphincter symptoms are common (usually urgency), with anal sphincter disturbances being rare.

SYNDROMES

Clustering of symptoms into these 5 clinical syndromes has been described[299]:

1. transverse lesion syndrome: involvement of corticospinal and spinothalamic tracts and posterior columns, with anterior horn cells <u>segmentally</u> involved. Most frequent syndrome, possibly an "end-stage" of the disease process
2. motor system syndrome: primarily corticospinal tract and anterior horn involvement with minimal or no sensory deficit. This creates a mixture of lower motor neuron findings in the upper extremities and upper motor neuron findings (myelopathy) in the lower extremities which can mimic ALS (see below). Reflexes may be hyperactive below the area of maximal stenosis (including the upper extremities), occasionally beginning several levels below the stenosis
3. central cord syndrome: motor and sensory deficit affecting the UEs more than the LEs. This syndrome is characterized by dysfunction of the watershed areas located centrally within the cord, which may be responsible for prominence of hand symptoms[303] (results in "**numb-clumsy hands**"[304]). Lhermitte's sign may be more common in this group
4. Brown-Séquard syndrome: often with asymmetric narrowing of the canal with the side of greater narrowing producing ipsilateral corticospinal tract (upper motor neuron weakness) and posterior column dysfunction with contralateral loss of pain and temperature sensation
5. brachialgia and cord syndrome: radicular UE pain with lower motor neuron weakness, and some associated long tract involvement (motor and/or sensory)

DIFFERENTIAL DIAGNOSIS

See *Myelopathy* on page 902 for other possible causes. Some of these (e.g. spinal cord tumor, OPLL) may be demonstrated radiographically. Asymptomatic cervical spondylosis is very common, and ≈ 12% of cases of cervical myelopathy attributed to spondylosis are later found to be due to another disease process including:

1. ALS: see below
2. multiple sclerosis (**MS**): spinal cord demyelination may mimic CSM. With MS, remissions and exacerbations are common, and patients tend to be younger
3. herniated cervical disc (soft disc): patients tend to be younger than with CSM. Course is more rapid
4. subacute combined system disease: abnormal vitamin B_{12} level and possibly macrocytic anemia (see page 904)
5. (spontaneous) intracranial hypotension (see page 178)

Amyotrophic lateral sclerosis (ALS)

AKA (anterior horn) motor neuron disease (also see *Amyotrophic lateral sclerosis*, page 52). Can mimic motor system syndrome (see above). "<u>Triad</u>" of ALS: atrophic weakness of hands and forearms (early), mild LE spasticity, diffuse hyperreflexia. NB: sensory changes are conspicuously <u>absent</u>. Sphincter control is usually maintained. The development of dysarthria or hyperactive jaw-jerk may be the first clue to the presence of such a demyelinating process[305]. Lower-motor neuron (**LMN**) findings in the tongue (visible fasciculations, or positive sharp waves on EMG) or in the LEs (e.g. fasciculations and atrophy) favors the diagnosis of ALS over CSM (however, LMN findings in the LEs may occur if there is coincidental lumbar radiculopathy).

In contrast to ALS, in CSM or herniated cervical disc one usually finds neck and shoulder pain, limitation of neck movement, sensory changes, and LMN findings restrict-

---

ed to 1 or 2 spinal cord segments. Inevitably, some cases of demyelinating disease will be misdiagnosed initially as CSM until some features suggestive of the former occur.

EVALUATION

Plain x-rays
Plain cervical spine x-rays demonstrates osteophytic spurs, and malalignment if any. See *Canal diameter* on page 141 for normal dimensions and measurement techniques. Patients with CSM have an average minimal AP canal diameter of 11.8 mm[306], and values ≤ 10 mm were likely to be associated with myelopathy[307]. Patients with an AP diameter < 14 mm may be at increased risk[308], and CSM is rare in patients with a diameter > 16 mm, even with significant spurs[286].

Pavlov ratio (AKA Torg ratio[309, 310]): the ratio of the AP diameter of the spinal canal at the mid VB level to the VB at the same location. When < 0.8 is sensitive for transient neuropraxia, but since initially proposed, has been shown to have poor positive predictive value for CSM.

MRI
MRI provides information about the spinal canal, and can also show intrinsic cord abnormalities (demyelination, syringomyelia, spinal cord atrophy, edema...). Increased signal within the cord on T2WI is not uncommon, yet the exact meaning of this is controversial and it is seen in other conditions in addition to CSM[311]. It is argued whether the presence of this increased signal preoperatively correlates with more severe CSM and worse outcome[312] or not[308]. A "banana" shaped cord on axial images has a high correlation with the presence of CSM[308]. MRI also rules out other diagnostic possibilities (Chiari malformation, spinal cord tumor...). Bony structures and calcified ligaments are poorly imaged. This shortcoming and the difficulties in differentiating osteophytes from herniated discs on MRI are overcome with the addition of plain cervical spine films[313] or thin-section CT bone windows. Sagittal T2WIs tend to exaggerate the magnitude of spinal cord compression by osteophytes and/or discs, and therefore axial images and T1WIs need to be considered in the evaluation.

CT/myelogram
Plain CT scans may demonstrate a narrow canal, but do not provide adequate information regarding the discs, ligaments, spinal cord and nerve roots. Water soluble cervical myelography followed by high-resolution CT scanning provides sagittal and axial information, and delineates bony detail better than MRI[313]. Unlike MRI, does not provide information about changes within the spinal cord.

TREATMENT

NONOPERATIVE MANAGEMENT
Consists primarily of cervical bracing in an attempt to reduce motion and hence the cumulative effects of trauma on the spinal cord. The brace must be worn indefinitely and there are no well controlled studies to demonstrate the effectiveness. Outcome was acceptable in only ≈ 36% of cases (less than with surgical treatment).

SURGICAL TREATMENT

Indications
A patient presenting with myelopathy that is already established, and has been present for an unknown length of time without suggestion of progression may not derive any benefit from surgery. Indications for surgery are primarily patients with radiologic evidence of spondylotic degeneration of the cervical spine in the following settings:
1. patients with progressive myelopathy who may be neurologically stabilized with surgery (although this is controversial, see *Outcome* below)
2. patients with severe pain, i.e. the "brachialgia and cord syndrome", often have pain relief with surgical decompression
3. patients presenting early in their course (duration of symptoms < 1 yr, see *Outcome* below) fare better than those with advanced and longstanding disease. However, even patients with "end-stage" myelopathy and spinal cord atrophy occasionally respond

Choice of approach

The debate between anterior approaches (anterior cervical discectomy) and posterior approaches (decompressive cervical laminectomy) dates back to the time that both became widely practiced[225]. General sentiment is to treat anterior disease (e.g. osteophytic bar, herniated disc…) usually limited to 1 or 2 (or occasionally 3) levels with an anterior approach (utilizing anterior discectomy or vertebrectomy), and to use a posterior approach as the initial procedure in the situations outlined below. Considerations of spinal curvature may need to enter into the decision process.

NB: following a laminectomy, it may be necessary to do an anterior procedure secondarily if residual cord compression is documented on post-op MRI.

Posterior approach: situations where this would generally be the initial approach:
1. congenital cervical stenosis: where removing osteophytes still will not provide at least ≈ 12 mm of AP diameter (although removal of bars may still work)
2. disease over ≥ 3 levels (although up to 3 may occasionally be dealt with anteriorly). Sometimes with the assistance of electrodiagnostic testing, one can ascertain which 1 or 2 levels are most symptomatic and treat those anteriorly
3. primary posterior pathology (e.g. infolding of ligamentum flavum)
4. in elderly patients where (anterior) fusion over long segments and tolerance of halo bracing is not as good as in younger patients

If the patient has cervical spinal stenosis and one or perhaps two osteophytic spurs that are more prominent than any others, an option treatment would be to treat the spur(s) anteriorly, give the patient enough time to develop a solid fusion (6-8 weeks) and then do the decompressive laminectomy. If the anterior approach were to follow the laminectomy, there is a chance that the fusion will not take and a swan neck deformity might result unless fusion with instrumentation (e.g. lateral mass fixation) or bracing (e.g. halo-vest) is also utilized.

Disadvantages of the posterior approach:
1. osteophytes continue to progress following posterior decompression (when done without fusion)
2. risk of subsequent subluxation or progressive kyphotic angulation ("swan neck" deformity). Post-laminectomy multilevel instability is treated with posterior fusion (usually with lateral mass instrumentation), single level instability may be treated cautiously with anterior approach (instrumentation and/or halo may be needed to prevent kyphosis before fusion becomes solid)
3. more painful initially post-op and sometimes more prolonged rehabilitation
4. ✖ contraindicated with pre-existing swan neck deformity, and not recommended in the presence of reversal of the normal cervical lordosis (i.e. kyphotic curve) where the spinal cord won't tend to move away from the anterior compression or in the presence of ≥ 3.5 mm subluxation or > 20° rotation in the sagittal plane[308] and caution must be exercised in hyperlordosis (*see below*)

Anterior approach: Another controversy here is whether or not to use anterior cervical plates. The incidence of pseudarthrosis or graft extrusion or collapse requiring reoperation are probably lower than the incidence of complications associated with the use of plates[286].

Worsening of myelopathy has been reported in 2-5% of patients after anterior decompression[314, 315] (intraoperative SSEP monitoring may reduce this rate[315]) and C5 radiculopathy may occur (*see below*).

Posterior approach: For a decompressive cervical laminectomy, common practice dictates removal of lamina extending one or two levels beyond the stenosis above and below[316, 317]. A C3-7 laminectomy is often considered a "standard" laminectomy. An "extended laminectomy" includes C2 and sometimes C1.

Curvature considerations: an extended laminectomy has been recommended for patients with straightening of the cervical curvature[284]. In cases of hyperlordosis, posterior migration of the spinal cord following an extensive laminectomy may put increased tension on the nerve roots and blood vessels (with possible neurologic worsening), and a limited laminectomy just where the cord is compressed is recommended (see *C5 radiculopathy* below).

"Keyhole foraminotomies" or medial facetectomy with undercutting of the facets are carried out at levels involved with radiculopathy.

Position: choices are primarily: prone, lateral oblique, or sitting. The prone position has a major disadvantage of difficulty elevating the head above the heart, resulting in venous engorgement with significant operative bleeding. The sitting position has a number of inherent risks (see *Sitting position*, page 604) including cord hypoperfusion[315].

The lateral oblique position may introduce some distortion to the anatomy due to asymmetrical positioning.

The rate of post-op spinal deformity is 25-42%. Neurologic worsening has been reported in 2% in some series, higher in others. C5 radiculopathy may occur (*see below*).

To avoid significant destabilization of the cervical spine:
1. during the dissection, do not remove soft tissue overlying the facet joints (to preserve their blood supply)
2. take the laminectomy only as far lateral as the extent of the spinal canal, carefully preserving the facet joints[285] (use keyhole laminotomies where necessary)
3. avoid removing a total of one facet at any given level

OUTCOME

Even excluding cases that are later proven to have demyelinating disease, the outcome from surgery for CSM is often disappointing. Once CSM is clinically apparent, complete remission almost never occurs. The prognosis with surgery is worse with increasing severity of involvement at the time of presentation[316] and with longer duration of symptoms (48% showed clinical improvement or cure if operated within 1 yr of onset, whereas only 16% responded after 1 yr[285]). The success of surgery is also lower in patients with other degenerative diseases of the CNS (ALS, MS...).

Progression of myelopathy may be arrested by surgical decompression. This is not always borne out, and some early series[297, 318] showed similar results with conservative treatment as with laminectomy which yielded improvement in 56%, no change in 25%, and worsening in 19%. Also as discussed earlier (see *Time course of symptoms*, page 332) some cases of CSM develop most of the deficit early and then stabilize.

Some series show good results, with ≈ 64-75% patients having improvement in CSM post-op[298]. However, other authors remain less enthusiastic. Utilizing a questionnaire in 32 post-op patients operated anteriorly, 66% had relief from radicular pain, while only 33% had improvement in sensory or motor complaints[298]. In one series, half the patients had improvement in fine motor function of the hands, but the other half worsened postoperatively[319]. Spinal cord atrophy as a result of continued pressure or ischemia may be partly responsible for poor recovery. Bedridden patients with severe myelopathy rarely recover useful function.

C5 radiculopathy: Motor involvement of deltoid > biceps, without sensory involvement may follow extensive anterior or posterior decompression occurs in ≈ 3% of cases[314], and may be related to traction on the nerve root from posterior migration of the cord after decompression or to bone graft displacement.

Late deterioration: Many patients who show early improvement will develop late deterioration (7-12 yrs after reaching a plateau[308], with no radiographically apparent explanation in up to 20% of these cases[320]. In others, degeneration at levels adjacent to the operated segments may be demonstrated.

14.3.1.3.   Coincident cervical and lumbar spinal stenosis

Coincident symptomatic lumbar and cervical spinal stenosis is usually managed by first decompressing the cervical region, and later operating on the lumbar region (unless severe neurogenic claudication dominates the picture). It is also possible, in selected cases, to operate on both in a single sitting[255, 321].

14.4.   Craniocervical junction and upper cervical spine abnormalities

Abnormalities in this region are seen in a number of conditions including:
1. rheumatoid arthritis: *see page 337*
2. traumatic and post-traumatic: including odontoid fractures
3. **ankylosing spondylitis**: (*see page 343*) may result in fusion of the entire spine which spares the occipitoatlantal and/or atlantoaxial joints which can lead to instability there
4. congenital conditions:

A. Chiari malformations
B. Klippel-Feil syndrome: *see page 119*
C. Down's syndrome
D. atlantoaxial dislocation **(AAD)**
E. occipitalization of the atlas: seen in 40% of congenital AAD[322]
F. Morquio syndrome (a mucopolysaccharidosis): atlantoaxial subluxation occurs due to hypoplasia of the odontoid process and joint laxity
5. neoplasms: primary or metastatic
6. infection
7. following surgical procedures of the skull base or cervical spine: e.g. transoral resection of the odontoid

Abnormalities include:
1. basilar impression
2. atlanto-occipital dislocation
3. atlantoaxial dislocation
4. occipitalization of the atlas, or thin or deficient posterior arch of atlas[323]

TREATMENT
   Fractures of the occipital condyles, atlas or axis are usually adequately treated with external immobilization. Because traumatic occipitocervical dislocations are usually fatal, optimal treatment is not well defined. Occipitalization of the atlas may be treated by creating an "artificial atlas" from the base of the occiput and wiring to that[323].
   Indications are outlined in *Atlantoaxial fusion (C1-2 arthrodesis)* on page 623.

14.5.   Rheumatoid arthritis

   More than 85% of patients with moderate or severe rheumatoid arthritis **(RA)** have radiographic evidence of C-spine involvement[324]. For involvement in the upper C-spine, *see below*. In the subaxial C-spine, the most common pathology is subluxation.
   A grading system for neural deficit devised by Ranawat et al.[324] is shown in *Table 14-24* and has also found use in other types of spinal cord injury.

Table 14-24   Ranawat classification for spinal cord deficit

Class	Description
I	no neural deficit
II	subjective weakness + hyperreflexia + dysesthesia
III	objective weakness + long tract signs III A = ambulatory III B = quadriparetic & non ambulatory

14.5.1.   Upper cervical spine involvement

   The upper cervical spine may be involved in RA in up to 44-88% of cases[325]. Malalignment and instability result from destruction of bone and supporting ligaments by synovial proliferation. The involvement may range from mild (a few mm of asymptomatic subluxation) to severe (e.g. brain stem compression[326]).

Two common types of C-spine involvement in RA (often found together):
1. anterior **atlantoaxial subluxation**: the most common manifestation of RA in the cervical spine, found in up to 25% of patients with RA (*see below*)
2. **basilar impression (BI)**: upward translocation of the odontoid process, found in ≈ 8% of patients with RA (*see page 339*)

Less common involvement of the cervical spine in RA:
1. posterior subluxation of the atlantoaxial joint: must have either associated fracture of or near total arthritic erosion of odontoid
2. subaxial subluxations (subluxations below C2)
3. vertebral artery insufficiency secondary to changes at cranio-cervical junction[327]

Inflammatory involvement of the atlantoaxial synovial joints causes erosive changes in the odontoid process and decalcification and loosening of the insertion of the transverse ligament on the atlas. This leads to instability allowing anterior subluxation of the atlas on the axis. There are two mechanisms by which upper cervical spinal cord compression may occur: 1) by a a scissoring effect of C1 on C2, and 2) by a pannus of granulation tissue that can form around the odontoid.

Atlantoaxial subluxation (AAS) occurs in ≈ 25% of patients with RA[327]. Mean time between onset of RA symptoms to the diagnosis of AAS was 14 years (15 patients)[328].

CLINICAL

Signs and symptoms of AAS are shown in *Table 14-25*. AAS is usually slowly progressive. Mean age at onset of AAS symptoms: 57 years.

Pain is experienced locally (upper cervical and suboccipital regions, often from compression of C2 nerve root) or is referred (to mastoid, occipital, temporal, or frontal regions).

RADIOGRAPHIC EVALUATION

LATERAL C-SPINE X-RAY

Atlanto-dental interval (ADI)

The normal ADI (distance between the anterior margin of the dens and "C1-button" on lateral C-spine x-ray) in adults is < 4 mm[329, 330]. Widening of the ADI suggests possible incompetence of the transverse ligament. See *Atlanto-dental interval (ADI)* on page 140 for more details.

Table 14-25 Signs and symptoms of AAS
(15 patients with AAS[328])

Finding	%
pain	
local	67%
referred	27%
hyperreflexia	67%
spasticity	27%
paresis	27%
sensory disturbance	20%

MRI

The optimal test to evaluate the source of upper cord or medulla compression. Demonstrates location of odontoid process, extent of pannus, and effects of subluxation (may need to be performed with head flexed to evaluate this).

TREATMENT

Requires knowledge of the following information:
- natural history: AAS in most patients progresses, with a small percentage either stabilizing or fusing spontaneously. In one series[331] with 4.5 years mean follow-up, 45% of patients with 3.5-5 mm subluxation progressed to 5-8 mm, and 10% of these progressed to > 8 mm
- once myelopathy occurs, it may be irreversible
- the worse the myelopathy, the higher the risk for sudden death
- the chances of finding myelopathy are significantly increased once the subluxation reaches ≥ 9 mm[332]
- associated cranial settling further decreases the tolerance for AAS
- life expectancy of patients with RA is 10 years less than the general population[331]
- the morbidity and mortality of surgical treatment (*see below*)

When to treat?
- symptomatic patients with AAS: almost all require surgical treatment (C1-2 fusion in most cases). For management, *see below*
  A. some surgeons do not operate if the maximal dens-C1 distance is < 6 mm
- asymptomatic patients: controversial
  A. some authors feel surgical fusion is not necessary in asymptomatic patient if the dens-C1 distance is below a certain cutoff. Recommendations for this cutoff have ranged from 6 to 10 mm[333], with **8 mm** commonly cited
  B. these patients are often placed in a rigid cervical collar, e.g. while outside the home, even though it is generally acknowledged that a collar probably does not provide significant support or protection

C. NB: some cases of sudden death in previously asymptomatic RA patients may be due to AAS and may then be erroneously attributed to cardiac arrhythmias, etc., therefore all asymptomatic patients with significant instability (as defined by dens-C1 distance) should be treated surgically

Management

It is necessary to either reduce the subluxation or to decompress the upper cord before doing a C1-C2 or occipital-C1-C2 fusion.

Menezes assesses all subluxed patients for reducibility using MRI compatible Halo cervical traction as follows: start with 5 lbs, and gradually increase over a period of a week. Most cases reduce within 2-3 days. If not reduced after 7 days then it is probably not reducible. Only ≈ 20% of cases are not reducible (most of these have odontoid > 15 mm above foramen magnum).

Most require stabilization via posterior wiring and fusion, either of C1 to C2, or of occiput to C2. The latter is used when fusion is combined with decompression (posterior laminectomy of C1 with posterior enlargement of the foramen magnum). See *Atlantoaxial fusion (C1-2 arthrodesis)* on page 623.

Posterior fusion alone does not provide adequate relief if the subluxation is irreducible, or if pannus causes significant compression. In these cases, transoral odontoidectomy may be indicated. Performing the posterior stabilization and decompression first allows some patients to avoid a second operation, and permits the remainder to undergo the anterior approach without becoming destabilized. Still, some surgeons do the odontoidectomy first[333].

Reminder: the patient must be able to open the mouth greater than ≈ 25 mm in order to perform transoral odontoidectomy without splitting the mandible.

POSTERIOR FUSION

See *Atlantoaxial fusion (C1-2 arthrodesis)* on page 623 for technique. In RA, erosion and osteoporosis weakens the C1 arch, and extra care is needed to avoid fracturing it.

Morbidity and mortality

Because of the frequency of simultaneous involvement of other systems including pulmonary, cardiac, and endocrine, operative mortality ranges from 5-15%[333].

The non-fusion rate for C1-2 wiring and fusion has been reported as high as 50%[334], typical rates are lower (with 18% of patients in one series developing a fibrous union[333]). The most common site of failure of osseous fusion is the interface between the bone graft and the posterior arch of C1[335].

Post-operative care

The patient is usually mobilized almost immediately post-op in halo vest traction (some use an optional period of maintained traction before mobilization). Impaired healing in RA dictates that the Halo be worn until fusion is well established, as seen on x-ray (usually 8-12 weeks). Sonntag evaluates the patient with flexion-extension lateral C spine x-rays by disconnecting the halo ring from the vest.

BASILAR IMPRESSION IN RHEUMATOID ARTHRITIS

Erosive changes in the lateral masses of C1 → telescoping of the atlas onto the body of C2 causing ventral migration of C1 with resultant ↓ in AP diameter of the spinal canal. There is concomitant upward displacement of the dens. The posterior arch of C1 often protrudes superiorly through the foramen magnum. All of these factors lead to compression of the pons and medulla. Rheumatoid granulation tissue behind the odontoid also contributes. Vertebral artery obstruction may also play a role.

The degree of erosion of C1 correlates with

Table 14-26 Symptoms & signs of BI
(45 patients with RA[325])

Finding	%
headache	100%
progressive difficulty ambulating	80%
hyperreflexia + Babinski	80%
limb paresthesias	71%
neurogenic bladder	31%
cranial nerve dysfunction	22%
trigeminal nerve anesthesia	20%
glossopharyngeal	
vagus	
hypoglossal	
miscellaneous findings	
internuclear ophthalmoplegia	
vertigo	
diplopia	
downbeat nystagmus	
sleep apnea	
spastic quadriparesis	

the extent of odontoid invagination.

CLINICAL

See Table 14-26. Motor exam usually difficult because of severe polyarticular degeneration with pain. Sensory findings (all non-localizing): diminished vibratory, position, and light touch.

RADIOGRAPHIC EVALUATION

See *Basilar impression* on page 139 for radiographic criteria of BI.

Polytomograms: no longer available at many hospitals. Best for demonstrating bone abnormalities. Flexion-extension lateral polytomograms are optimal for determining instability.

Myelography (water soluble) with CT to follow: also good for delineating bony pathology.

MRI: optimal for demonstrating brain stem impingement, poor for showing bone.

TREATMENT

See also *Craniocervical junction and upper cervical spine abnormalities* on page 336.

CERVICAL TRACTION

May attempt with Gardner-Wells tongs. Begin with ≈ 7 lbs, and slowly increase up to 15 lbs. Some may require several weeks of traction to reduce.

SURGERY

Reducible cases: posterior occipitocervical fusion ± C1 decompressive laminectomy.

Irreducible cases: requires transoral resection of odontoid. May perform before posterior fusion (must be kept in traction while waiting for second procedure).

14.6. Paget's disease

PATHOPHYSIOLOGY

Paget's disease **(PD)** (AKA osteitis deformans) is a disorder of osteoclasts (possibly virally induced) causing increased rate of bone resorption with reactive osteoblastic overproduction of new, weaker, woven bone.

Initially there is a "hot" phase with elevated osteoclastic activity and increased intraosseous vascularity. Osteoblasts lay down a soft, nonlamellar bone. Later a "cool" phase occurs with disappearance of the vascular stroma and osteoblastic activity leaving sclerotic, radiodense, brittle bone[336] ("**ivory bone**").

Malignant degeneration

A misnomer, since the malignant changes actually occur in the reactive osteoblastic cells. About 1% (reported range: 1-14%) degenerate into sarcoma (osteogenic sarcoma, fibrous sarcoma, or chondrosarcoma)[337 (p 2642)], with the possibility of systemic (e.g. pulmonary) metastases. Malignant degeneration is much less common in the spine than in the skull or femur.

EPIDEMIOLOGY

Prevalence: ≈ 3% of population > 55 years old in the U.S. and Europe[338]. Slight male predominance. Family history of Paget's disease is found in 15-30% of cases (accuracy is poor since most are asymptomatic).

Common sites of involvement

Affinity for axial skeleton, long bones and skull. In approximate descending order of frequency: pelvis, thoracic and lumbar spine, skull, femur, tibia, fibula, and clavicles.

Only ≈ 30% of pagetic sites are symptomatic[339], the rest are discovered incidentally. The overproduction of weak bone may produce bone pain (the most common symptom), predilection for fractures and compressive syndromes (cranial nerve (*see page 918*), spinal nerve root...). Painless bowing of a long bone may be the first manifestation. A number of patients present due to pain from joint dysfunction related to PD.

NEUROSURGICAL INVOLVEMENT

PD may present to the neurosurgeon as a result of:
* back pain: usually not as a direct result of vertebral bone involvement (*see below*)
* spinal cord and/or nerve root symptoms
  ◆ compression of the spinal cord or cauda equina (relatively rare)
  ◆ spinal nerve-root compression
  ◆ vascular steal due to reactive vasodilatation adjacent to involved areas
* with skull involvement, compression of cranial nerves as they exit through bony foramina (8th nerve is most common, producing deafness or ataxia): *see page 918*
* to ascertain diagnosis in unclear bone lesions of the spine or skull

EVALUATION

1. lab work (markers may be normal in monostotic involvement):
   A. serum alkaline phosphatase: usually elevated (this enzyme is involved in bone synthesis and so may not be elevated in purely lytic Paget's disease[92] [(p 1416)]); mean 380 ± 318 IU/L (normal range: 9-44)[340]. Bone-specific alkaline phosphatase may be more sensitive and may be useful in monostotic involvement[338]
   B. calcium: usually normal (if elevated, one should R/O hyperparathyroidism)
   C. urinary hydroxyproline: found almost exclusively in cartilage. Due to the high turnover of bone, urinary hydroxyproline is often increased in PD with a mean of 280 ± 262 mg/24 hrs (normal range 18-38)[340]
2. bone scan: lights up in areas of involvement in most, but not all[340] cases
3. plain x-rays:
   A. localized enlargement of bone: a finding unique to PD (not seen in other osteoclastic diseases, such as prostatic bone mets)
   B. cortical thickening
   C. sclerotic changes
   D. osteolytic areas (in skull → osteoporosis circumscripta; in long bones → "V" shaped lesions)
   E. spinal Paget's disease often involves several contiguous levels. Pedicles and lamina are thickened, vertebral bodies are usually dense and compressed with increased width. Intervening discs are replaced by bone
4. CT: hypertrophic changes at the facet joints with coarse trabeculations

---

14.6.1. Paget's disease of the spine

PRESENTATION

The overwhelming majority of pagetic lesions are asymptomatic[92 (p 1413)] with lesions detected on radiographs or bone scan obtained for other reasons or as part of a work-up for an elevated alkaline phosphatase. Although the most common complaint in patients with Paget's disease is of back pain, this is attributable to pagetic involvement alone in only ≈ 12%[340], in the remainder it is secondary to other factors, some of which are described below.

Symptoms that may be seen:
1. symptoms from the following are slowly progressive (usually present for over 12 months; rarely < 6 mos)
   A. neural compression
      1. causes of compression
         a. due to expansion of woven bone
         b. due to osteoid tissue
         c. pagetic extension into ligamentum flavum and epidural fat[341]

2. sites of compression
   a. spinal cord (*see below*)
   b. nerve root in neural foramen
B. osteoarthritis of facet joints (Paget's disease may precipitate osteoarthritis[340])
2. symptoms from the following tend to progress more rapidly
   A. malignant (sarcomatous) change of involved bone
   B. pathologic fracture (usually gradual)
   C. neurovascular (compromise of vascular supply to nerves or spinal cord) by
      1. compression of blood vessels (arterial or venous)
      2. pagetic vascular steal (*see below*)

Spinal cord symptoms

Myelopathy or cauda equina syndrome may be due to spinal cord compression or from vascular effects (occlusion, or "steal" due to reactive vasodilatation of nearby blood vessels[92 (p 1415)]). Only ≈ 100 cases had been described as of 1981[342]. Characteristically, 3-5 adjacent vertebrae are involved[343 (p 2307)], whereas monostotic involvement is usually asymptomatic[344]. In case reports in the literature, progressive quadri- or paraparesis was the most common presentation[345]. Sensory changes are usually the first manifestation, progressing to weakness and sphincter disturbance. Pain was the only symptom in a neurologically intact patient in only 5.5%.

A rapid course (averaging 6 wks) with a sudden increase in pain is more suggestive of malignant degeneration.

TREATMENT

MEDICAL TREATMENT FOR PAGET'S DISEASE

There is no cure for Paget's disease. Medical treatment is indicated for cases that are not rapidly progressive where the diagnosis is certain, for patients who are poor surgical candidates, and pre-op if excessive bleeding cannot be tolerated. Medical therapy reverses some neurologic deficit in 50% of cases[346], but generally requires prolonged treatment (≈ 6-8 months) before improvement occurs, and may need to be continued indefinitely due to propensity for relapses. Medications used include the following.

Calcitonin derivatives

Parenteral salmon **calcitonin** (Calcimar®)[346]: reduces osteoclastic activity directly, osteoblastic hyperactivity subsides secondarily. Relapse may occur even while on calcitonin. Side effects include nausea, facial flushing, and the development of antibodies to salmon calcitonin (these patients may benefit from a more expensive synthetic human preparation (Cibacalcin®) starting at 0.5 mg SQ q d[347]).

Rx 50-100 IU (medical research council units) SQ q d **x** 1 month, then 3 injections per week for several months[338]. If used pre-op to help decrease bony vascularity, ≈ 6 months of treatment is ideal. Doses as low as ≈ 50 IU units 3 **x** per week may be used indefinitely post-op or as a sole treatment (alkaline phosphatase and urinary hydroxyproline decline by 30-50% in > half of patients in 3-6 months, but they rarely normalize).

Biphosphonates

These drugs are pyrophosphate analogues that bind to hydroxyapatite crystals and inhibit reabsorption. They also alter osteoclastic metabolism, inhibit their activity, and reduce their numbers. They are retained in bone until it is resorbed. Oral absorption of all is poor (especially in the presence of food). Bone formed during treatment is lamellar rather than woven.

Etidronate (Didronel®) (AKA EHDP): reduces normal bone mineralization (especially at doses ≥ 20 mg/kg/d) producing mineralization defects (osteomalacia) which may increase the risk of fracture but which tend to heal between courses[348]. Contraindicated in patients with renal failure, osteomalacia, or severe lytic lesions of a LE. ***Rx*** 5-10 mg/kg PO daily (average dose: 400 mg/d, or 200-300 mg/d in frail elderly patients) for 6 months, may be repeated after a 3-6 month hiatus if biochemical markers indicate relapse.

Tiludronate (Skelid®): unlike etidronate, does not appear to interfere with bone mineralization at recommended doses. Side effects: abdominal pain, diarrhea, N/V. ***Rx*** 400 mg PO qd with 6-8 ounces of plain water > 2 hrs before or after eating **x** 3 months. Available: 200 mg tablets.

Pamidronate (Aredia®): much more potent than etidronate. May cause a transient acute flu-like syndrome. Oral dosing is hindered by GI intolerance, and IV forms may be required. Mineralization defects do not occur in doses < 180 mg/course. **Rx** 90 mg/d IV **x** 3 days, or as weekly or monthly infusions.

Alendronate (Fosamax®): does not produce mineralization defects (*see page 750*).

Clodronate (Ostac®, Bonefos®): **Rx** 400-1600 mg/d PO **x** 3-6 months. 300 mg/d IV **x** 5 days.

Risedronate (Actonel®): does not interfere with bone mineralization in recommended doses[349]. **Rx**: 30 mg PO q d with 6–8 oz. of water at least 30 minutes before the first meal of the day.

Under development: ibandronate, neridronate, and others.

Plicamycin

Formerly mithramicin. A cytotoxic antibiotic that inhibits RNA synthesis with preferential toxicity for osteoclasts. Reserved for severe and extensive involvement due to dose dependent renal and hepatic impairment and possible thrombocytopenia. Not approved for treating Paget's disease in any country.

Rx 15-25 μg/kg given IV over 8-10 hours qod **x** 10 infusions.

SURGICAL TREATMENT

In general, conservative treatment of fractures in PD have a high rate of delayed union.

Surgical indications for spinal Paget's disease

1. rapid progression: indicating possible malignant change or spinal instability
2. spinal instability: severe kyphosis or compromise of canal by bone fragments from pathologic fracture. Although the collapse is usually gradual, sudden compression may occur
3. uncertain diagnosis: especially to R/O metastatic disease (osteoblastic lesions)
4. failure to improve with medications

Surgical considerations:

1. profuse bleeding is common: if significant bleeding would present an unusual problem, treat for as long as feasible pre-op with a biphosphonate or calcitonin (*see above*)
2. post-op medical treatment may be necessary to prevent recurrences[346]
3. osteogenic sarcoma
   A. surgery and chemotherapy are used, cure is less likely than in primary osteosarcoma of non-pagetic origin
   B. biopsy proven of the scalp requires en-bloc excision of scalp and tumor

Surgical outcome[345]:

In 65 patients treated with decompressive laminectomy, 55 (85%) had definite but variable degrees of improvement. Patients who had only minimal improvement were often ones with malignant changes. One patient was worse after surgery, and the operative mortality was 7 patients (10%). Survival with malignant degeneration is < 5.5 mos after admission.

14.7.   Ankylosing spondylitis

AKA Marie-Strümpell disease. One of the so-called seronegative arthropathies (ANA and serum rheumatoid factor are negative[350], unlike rheumatoid arthritis). The locus of involvement in ankylosing spondylitis (**AS**) is the entheses, (attachment points of ligaments, tendons or capsules on bones). The spine is the primary skeletal site involved, usually starting in the lumbar spine and sacroiliac joints and progressing rostrally. Non-granulomatous inflammatory changes at the entheses stimulates replacement of ligaments by bone with the ultimate result in the spine being that of osteoporotic VBs, calcified intervertebral discs (sparing the nucleus pulposus), and ossified ligaments, producing square appearing VBs with bridging syndesmophytes, the so-called "bamboo spine" or "poker spine".

Differential diagnosis:

1. early on, AS may resemble rheumatoid arthritis. However, in AS nodules do not form in joints, and rheumatoid factor is absent in the serum
2. metastatic prostate Ca in elderly male patients with sacroiliac pain and blastic changes compatible with sacroiliitis
3. Forestier's disease (*see page 347*) and DISH (*see page 346*): these overlapping con-

ditions produce exuberant bony overgrowth anterior and lateral to the disc without degeneration and ossification of the disc as in AS. Both spare the facets and SI joints, do not produce flexion deformity, and tend to occur in men > 50 yrs old (older than typical AS)[350]

4. psoriasis and Reiter's syndrome: spondylitis tends to be milder and less uniform

EPIDEMIOLOGY

Incidence is ≈ 1-3 cases per 100,000. Symptoms tend to be more pronounced in males, which has resulted in an underreporting of the condition in females and an exaggeration of the estimation of the male predominance (incidence is probably ≈ equal)[351]. Peak incidence: 17-35 yrs age. Although AS is not hereditary, first degree relatives are at increased risk.

CLINICAL

Typical initial presentation is with nonradiating low back pain, morning back stiffness, hip pain and swelling (due to large joint arthritis), exacerbated by inactivity and improved with exercise[352]. **Patrick's test** (*see page 303*) usually positive. Production of pain on compressing the pelvis with the patient in the lateral decubitus position. **Schober test** (measure distraction between skin marks on forward flexion to detect reduced mobility of the spine due to fusion[39]) is not specific for inflammatory spondylopathies[353] but may be helpful for monitoring ongoing physical therapy.

Neurosurgical involvement usually results from the following:

1. cauda equina syndrome (**CES**): etiology is frequently unclear, but is usually <u>not</u> due to stenosis or compressive lesion. In the absence of compression, surgical intervention is not indicated
2. rotatory subluxation: at occipito-atlantal and atlanto-axial joints. May occur as these are typically the last mobile segments of the spine. Incidence is much less than with rheumatoid arthritis. Lesions that might be stable in otherwise normal spines are often not stable in AS
3. myelopathy secondary to bow-stringing of the cord: laminectomy may aggravate
4. acute spinal cord injury (**SCI**): risk of SCI or CES due to fracture is increased in AS, and may occur following minimal trauma. Injuries are more common in the lower cervical spine. The rigid spine of AS when fractured acts as a long lever and is extremely unstable[354]. Delayed deterioration may be due to spinal epidural hematoma[355]
5. vertebral stress fractures: most common in the lower thoracic and upper lumbar spines, usually through the ossified intervertebral disc
6. spinal deformity
7. spinal stenosis: rare
8. basilar impression

Increased anesthetic risk in AS patients may be related to:

1. difficulty intubating due to fragile, angulated & immobile spine
2. mitral valve disease
3. myocardial conduction abnormalities
4. decreased pulmonary compliance and reduced lung volume in patients with advanced thoracic kyphoscoliosis

RADIOGRAPHIC EVALUATION

Sacroiliac joint involvement (which may be seen on AP pelvic x-rays or on oblique views through the plane of the SI joints) is one of the earliest findings, and the often symmetric osteoporosis followed by sclerosis is characteristic. "Bamboo spine" (*see above*) is also classic. Imaging of the entire spine is recommended since multiple, non-contiguous (and often unsuspected) fractures are not unusual.

MRI can rule out spinal epidural hematoma and the occasional herniated disc.

NATURAL HISTORY

Progression is slow, and patients usually remain functionally active. Thoracic kyphosis with compensatory increase in cervical and lumbar lordosis is common. The shift in center of gravity together with spine stiffness and fragility predisposes to frequent falls and further spine injuries.

Spinal cord injury: The routine of initially securing the head to a backboard with the neck in neutral position may be deleterious in the patient with kyphotic deformity related to AS[354]. AS may be suspected when the patient spontaneously holds their head in significant flexion[356], and in these cases the neck should be immobilized in that position[357]. When traction is used, the axis of traction often needs to be ventral to neutral and the use of minimal weight is recommended[354].

Subsequent treatment for SCI in AS is controversial: halo immobilization alone has been advocated by many, citing similar outcome and fewer complications. Others advocate early internal fixation because of cases of nonunion and progression of deficit while in the halo brace[354] and risk of skin breakdown under the vest due to severe kyphosis. Neurologic deficit related to cord or root compression is an indication for decompressive laminectomy and fusion[354].

Positioning for surgery may be difficult due to the immobile kyphotic spine. Anterior approaches are difficult due to extensive bridging osteophytes, and the screws for anterior plates may not hold well in the osteoporotic VBs. Posterior cervical lateral mass plating (*see page 740*) is advocated for most.

Kyphotic deformity: Severe flexion deformity may be treated by spinal osteotomy[350].

14.8. Ossification of the posterior longitudinal ligament (OPLL)

When hypertrophied or ossified, the posterior longitudinal ligament may cause myelopathy (due to direct spinal cord compression, or ischemia) and/or radiculopathy (by nerve root compression or stretching).

The age of patients with OPLL ranges from 02-01 years (mean – 53), with a slight male predominance. The prevalence increases with age. Duration of symptoms averages ~ 13 months. It is more prevalent in the Japanese population (2-3.5%)[358, 359].

PATHOPHYSIOLOGY

The pathologic basis of OPLL is unknown, but there is an increased incidence of ankylosing hyperostosis which suggests a hereditary basis.

OPLL begins with hypervascular fibrosis in the PLL which is followed by focal areas of calcification, proliferation of periosteal cartilaginous cells and finally ossification[360]. The process frequently extends into the dura. Eventually active bone marrow production may occur. The process progresses at varying rates among patients, with an average annual growth rate of 0.67 mm in the AP direction and 4.1 mm longitudinally[361].

Changes within the spinal cord involve the postero-lateral gray matter more than white matter, suggesting an ischemic basis for the neurologic involvement.

DISTRIBUTION

Average involvement: 2.7-4 levels. Frequency of involvement:
1. cervical: 70-75% of cases of OPLL. Typically begins at C3-4 and proceeds distally, often involving C4-5 and C5-6 but usually sparing C6-7
2. thoracic: 15-20% (usually upper, ~ T4-6)
3. lumbar: 10-15% (also usually upper, ~ L1-3)

PATHOLOGIC CLASSIFICATION[362]
1. segmental: confined to space behind vertebral bodies, does not cross disc spaces
2. continuous: extends from VB to VB, spanning disc space(s)
3. mixed: combines elements of both of the above with skip areas
4. other variants: includes a rare type of OPLL that is contiguous with the endplates and is confined to the disc space (involves focal hypertrophy of the PLL with punctate calcification)

EVALUATION

Plain x-rays
Often fail to demonstrate OPLL.

MRI
OPLL appears as a hypointense area and is difficult to appreciate until it reaches
≈ 5 mm thickness. On T1WI it blends in with the hypointensity of the ventral subarachnoid space; on T2WI it remains hypointense while the CSF becomes bright. Sagittal images may be very helpful in providing an overview of the extent of involvement, and T2WI may demonstrate intrinsic spinal cord abnormalities which may be associated with a worse outcome.

Myelography/CT
Myelography with post-myelographic CT (especially with 3D reconstructions) is probably best at demonstrating and accurately diagnosing OPLL.

TREATMENT

Treatment decisions
Based on clinical grade[362] as follows:
- Class I: radiographic evidence without clinical signs or symptoms. Most patients with OPLL are asymptomatic[359]. Conservative management unless severe
- Class II: patients with myelopathy or radiculopathy. Minimal or stable deficit may be followed expectantly. Significant deficit or evidence of progression warrants surgical intervention
- Class IIIA: moderate to severe myelopathy. Usually requires surgical intervention
- Class IIIB: severe to complete quadriplegia. Surgery is considered for incomplete quadriplegics showing progressive slow worsening. Rapid deterioration or complete quadriplegia, advanced age or poor medical condition are all associated with worse outcome

Technical considerations for surgery
SSEP monitoring has been recommended by some[360].
Post-operative immobilization for at least 3 months is employed with rigid collars for single level ACDF or 1-2 level corpectomies, or halo-vest traction for corpectomies > 2 levels.

Results with surgery
The incidence of pseudarthrosis after vertebral corpectomy and strut graft ranges from 5-10% and increases with the number of levels fused.
In one series there was a 10% incidence of transient worsening of neurologic function following anterior surgery[361] which may have been related to distraction.
The risk of dural tear with CSF leak following an anterior approach depends on the aggressiveness with which bone is removed from the dura, and ranges ≈ 16-25%.
Other risks of anterior approaches (e.g. esophageal injury, see *ACDF complications*, page 320) also pertain.

14.9. Ossification of the anterior longitudinal ligament (OALL)

OALL of the cervical spine and/or hypertrophic anterior cervical osteophytes may produce dramatic radiographic findings and minimal clinical symptoms. Separate from Forestier's disease (*see below*). May present with dysphagia[363].

14.10. Diffuse idiopathic skeletal hyperostosis

AKA "DISH", AKA spondylitis ossificans ligamentosa, AKA ankylosing hyperostosis, among others. A condition characterized by flowing osteophytic formation of the spine in the absence of degenerative, traumatic, or post-infectious changes. Affects Caucasians and males more commonly, and usually seen in patients in their mid 60s.
97% of cases occur in the thoracic spine, also in the lumbar spine in 90%, cervical spine in 78%, and all three segments in 70%. Sacroiliac joints are spared (unlike anky-

losing spondylitis, *see page 343*).

Usually does not produce clinical symptoms. Patients may have early morning stiffness and mild limitations of activities. May present with dysphagia or globus (a sensation of a lump in the throat, usually attributed to hysteria) due to compression of the esophagus between the osteophytes and the rigid laryngeal structures[364] (part of Forestier's disease[365]).

In cases of dysphagia, evaluation should include barium swallow to help localize the site of obstruction, and esophagoscopy to rule-out intrinsic esophageal disease. Plain x-rays and CT scan helps demonstrate the pathology. Cases that do not respond satisfactorily to dietary modifications should be considered for surgery. An anterior cervical approach, and utilization of a high-speed drill with careful protection of soft-tissue structures (esophagus, carotid sheath) without need to stabilize spine nor discectomy has been recommended[364].

14.11.   Spinal AVM

Incidence of spinal AVM (**S-AVMs**) is about 4% of primary intraspinal masses. 80% occur between age 20 and 60 years[366 (p 1850-3)]. Major classifications[367-369]:

* Type I: dural AVM. Fed by a dural artery and draining into a spinal vein via an AV shunt in the intervertebral foramen[367]. The most common type of S-AVM in the adult[370]. Generally produce symptoms of progressive myelopathy or cauda equina syndrome in middle-aged patients
* intradural AVM
  * intradural-extramedullary AVM
  * intramedullary: true AVM of the spinal cord. Fed by medullary arteries with the AV shunt contained at least partially within the spinal cord or pia. Worse prognosis than dural AVM[367]
  * Type IV: intradural perimedullary (also called arteriovenous *fistulae*). Typically occur in younger patients than Type I, and may present catastrophically with hemorrhage into the subarachnoid space[371]. These are further divided into 3 subtypes[368] shown in *Table 14-27*

Table 14-27   Merland's subclassification of Type IV (perimedullary) AV fistulas*

Sub-type	Arterial Supply	AVF	Venous Drainage
I	single (thin ASA)	single, small	slowly ascending perimedullary venous system
II	multiple (dilated ASA & PSA)	multiple, medium	
III		single, giant	giant venous ectasia, rapid metameric venous drainage

* AVF = arteriovenous fistula; ASA = anterior spinal artery; PSA = posterior spinal artery

PRESENTATION

85% present as progressive neuro deficit (back pain associated with progressive sensory loss and LE weakness over months to years). Yet, S-AVMs account for < 5% of lesions presenting as spinal cord "tumors". 10-20% of S-AVMs present as sudden onset of myelopathy usually in patients < 30 yrs age[372, 373], secondary to hemorrhage (causing SAH, hematomyelia, epidural hematoma, or watershed infarction). **Coup de poignard of Michon** = onset of SAH with sudden excruciating back pain (clinical evidence of S-AVM).

Foix-Alajouanine syndrome: acute or subacute neurologic deterioration in a patient with a S-AVM without evidence of hemorrhage. Presents as spastic → flaccid paraplegia, with ascending sensory level and loss of sphincter control. Initially thought to be due to spontaneous thrombosis of the AVM causing subacute necrotizing myelopathy[374] which would be irreversible. However, more recent evidence suggests that the myelopathy may be due to venous hypertension with secondary ischemia, and there may be improvement with treatment[375].

CLINICAL

Auscultation over spine may reveal a bruit in 2-3% of cases. Cutaneous angioma over back is present in 3-25% of cases; valsalva maneuver may enhance the redness of the angioma[373].

Selective spinal angiography is difficult and has a significant complication rate, however it is necessary for treatment planning. MRI may be able to detect spinal AVMs with greater sensitivity and safety than angiography[376]. Myelography classically shows serpiginous intradural filling defects, and should be done prone and supine (to avoid missing a dorsal AVM).

TREATMENT

Dural AVMs usually require surgery. Intradural AVMs may be amenable to interventional neuroradiologic procedures including embolization[377]. Suggested management[369] for Type IV perimedullary fistulae is shown in *Table 14-28*.

Table 14-28 Suggested management for Type IV arteriovenous fistulae[369]

Subtype	Diagnosis	Embolization	Surgery
Type I	difficult; ? reliability of MRI; tomomyelography; angiotomomyelography	difficult	easy on filum terminale; difficult on conus medullaris
Type II	easy: MRI or myelography	incomplete occlusion	on posterolateral AVFs
Type III		effective	difficult, dangerous

14.12. Spinal meningeal cysts

Spinal meningeal cysts (**SMC**): diverticula of the meningeal sac, nerve root sheath or arachnoid. May have familial tendency.

Terminology in literature is confusing. One classification system is shown in *Table 14-29*. Previously AKA Tarlov's perineural cysts, spinal arachnoid cysts, and extradural diverticula, pouches or cysts. Only congenital lesions are considered here.

- Type I SMCs above the sacrum usually have a pedicle adjacent to entrance of dorsal nerve root
- Type II SMCs: formerly called Tarlov's cysts and were differentiated from nerve root diverticula because the former were defined as communicating with subarachnoid space, and the latter not. However, intrathecal contrast CT (**ICCT**) shows both communicate. Often multiple, occur on dorsal roots anywhere, but are most prominent and symptomatic in sacrum
- Type III SMCs: may also be multiple and asymptomatic. More common along posterior subarachnoid space. Attributed to proliferation of arachnoid trabeculae

Table 14-29 Types of spinal meningeal cysts[378]

Type	Description
Type I	extradural meningeal cysts without spinal nerve root fibers
IA	"extradural meningeal/arachnoid cyst"
IB	(occult) "sacral meningocele"
Type II	extradural meningeal cysts with spinal nerve root fibers ("Tarlov's perineural cyst", "spinal nerve root diverticulum")
Type III	spinal intradural meningeal cysts ("intradural arachnoid cyst")

PRESENTATION

May be asymptomatic (i.e. incidental finding). May cause radiculopathy by pressure on adjacent nerve root (may or may not cause symptoms of nerve root from which it actually arises). Symptom complex depends on size of SMC, and proximity to spinal cord and nerve roots.

- Type I SMCs: in thoracic and cervical region, may present with acute myelopathy (spasticity and sensory level); lumbar region → LBP and radiculopathy; sacral region → sphincter disturbance
- Type II SMCs: often asymptomatic, but sacral lesions may → sciatica and/or sphincter disturbance
- Type III SMCs: may also be multiple and asymptomatic; more common along posterior subarachnoid space

EVALUATION

MRI to identify the mass, then water-soluble ICCT scan to evaluate communication of cyst with subarachnoid space.

- Type II SMCs: all 18 cases had bony erosion (demonstrated by canal widening, pedicle erosion, foraminal enlargement, or vertebral body scalloping)
- Type III SMCs: may also cause bony erosion; appear on myelogram as intradural defect, may not appear on ICCT if they communicate with subarachnoid space which causes them to blend with adjacent subarachnoid space

TREATMENT

- Type I SMCs: close ostium between cyst and subarachnoid space. Above sacrum, can usually be dissected from dura; occasionally fibrous adhesions prevent this
- Type II SMCs: no pedicle, thus either partially resect and oversew cyst wall, or excise cyst and involved nerve root. Simple aspiration is not recommended
- Type III SMCs: excise completely unless dense fibrous adhesions prevent this, in which case marsupialize cyst. Tend to recur if incompletely excised

14.13. Syringomyelia

❦ Key points
- cystic cavitation of the spinal cord (AKA syrinx)
- 70% are associated with Chiari I malformation, 10% with basilar invagination. May also be posttraumatic or associated with tumor
- symptoms: progressive neurologic deterioration over months to years, usually affecting UE first
- diameter > 5 mm + associated edema predict a more rapid deterioration
- preferred treatment is directed at correcting the causative pathophysiology

AKA **syrinx**. Cystic cavitation of the spinal cord. Rostral extension into brainstem is termed **syringobulbia**. Syrinx may be divided into specific subtypes (based on etiology, cell-type of lining, or presence/absence of communication with the central canal); terms include **hydrosyringomyelia**.

PATHOPHYSIOLOGY

Two main forms:
- **communicating syringomyelia**: primary dilatation of the central canal. Controversial if this actually occurs. Almost always associated with abnormalities of the foramen magnum, e.g. Chiari type 1 malformation (the most common form) or basilar arachnoiditis (post-infectious or idiopathic). Simple central canal dilatation with ependymal cell lining has been called **hydromyelia**.
- **noncommunicating syringomyelia**: cyst arises in cord substance and does not communicate with central canal or subarachnoid space. Etiologies include: trauma, neoplasm (mostly gliomas)

Syringomyelia is often associated with abnormalities of the foramen magnum, e.g. Chiari type 1 malformation (*see page 104*) or basilar arachnoiditis (post-infectious or idiopathic). Syrinx fluid may have the same constituency as CSF. Tumor cyst fluid is usually highly proteinaceous

Mechanism of formation
1. obstructive lesions: etiology probably lies in outlet obstruction (partial or complete) of fourth ventricle (foramina of Luschka and Magendie). Congenital conditions such as Chiari malformation type 1 or type 2, cerebellar ectopia, basilar impression (with constriction of the foramen magnum, *page 139*), Dandy-Walker syndrome, and acquired conditions such as adhesive arachnoiditis are associated with high incidence of syrinx
2. primary intraspinal pathology:
   A. intramedullary spinal cord tumors may secrete fluid, or may cause microcysts that eventually coalesce
   B. trauma: *see page 351*

14.13.1.   Non-traumatic syringomyelia

EPIDEMIOLOGY[379]
Prevalence: 8.4 cases/100,000 population. Usually presents between ages 20-50.

Associated clinical syndromes are shown in Table 14-30.

Major theories of formation of the cyst:
- hydrodynamic ("water-hammer") theory of Gardner: systolic pulsations are transmitted with each heartbeat from the intracranial cavity to the central canal. Has been essentially disproven using MRI[380]

Table 14-30   Conditions associated with syringomyelia

Condition	%*
Chiari type 1 malformation	70
basilar invagination	10
intramedullary spinal cord tumors	4

*   percent of cases of syringomyelia

- Williams' ("craniospinal dissociation") theory: maneuvers that raise CSF pressure (valsalva, coughing...) cause "hydrodissection" through the spinal cord tissue. May be more common in noncommunicating syringomyelia
- Heiss-Oldfield theory: occlusion at the foramen magnum causes CSF pulsations during cardiac systole to be transmitted through the Virchow-Robin spaces which increases the extracellular fluid which coalesce to form a syrinx[379]

CLINICAL

Presentation: highly variable. Usually progresses over months to years, with a more rapid deterioration early that gradually slows[379]. Initially, pain, weakness, atrophy and loss of pain & temperature sensation in the upper extremities is common. A myelopathy that progresses slowly over years ensues.

Characteristic syndrome
(nonspecific for intramedullary spinal cord pathology):
- sensory loss (similar to central cord syndrome) with a suspended ("cape") dissociated sensory loss (loss of pain and temperature sensation with preserved touch and joint position sense → painless ulcerations from unperceived injuries and/or burns)
- **pain**: commonly cervical and occipital. Dysesthetic pain often occurs in the distribution of the sensory loss[379]
- **weakness**: lower motor neuron weakness of the hand and arm
- painless (neurogenic) arthropathies (**Charcot's joints**) especially in the shoulder & neck due to loss of pain & temperature sensation: seen in < 5%

EVALUATION

Prior to the CT/MRI era, diagnosis relied on myelography or on autopsy.

MRI: defines anatomy in sagittal as well as axial plane. Test of choice. Cervical & thoracic spine and brain MRI (without & with contrast, to include craniocervical junction) should be obtained.

CT: low attenuation area within cord seen on either plain CT or myelogram/CT (with water soluble contrast).

Myelogram: rarely used alone (usually performed in conjunction with CT). When used alone: often normal (false negative), some → complete block at level of syrinx; iodine contrast studies may show fusiform widening of spinal cord, whereas air contrast studies may show collapse of the cord[381]. Dye may slowly leach into the cyst.

MANAGEMENT

SURGICAL TREATMENT
Options include:
1. current philosophy is to treat the underlying pathophysiology (and to use syrinx draining procedures as second choice)
   A.   posterior decompression: procedure of choice when posterior anomalies (e.g.

Chiari malformation) are present
2. shunts:
   A. disadvantages:
      1. complication rate: 16%
      2. clinical stabilization rate: 54% at 10 yrs
      3. may produce traction on spinal cord with potential for further injury
      4. prone to obstruction: 50% at 4 years
      5. does not correct underlying pathophysiology and so syrinx may recur
   B. indications: cases of diffuse arachnoiditis (e.g. following tuberculous or chemical meningitis) where the obstruction extends over many levels
   C. **K** or **T** tube drainage. Choice of distal sites includes:
      1. peritoneum[382] (difficult in cervical region)
      2. pleural cavity
      3. subarachnoid space (e.g. Heyer-Schulte-Pudenz system): requires normal CSF flow in subarachnoid space, therefore cannot use in arachnoiditis
3. percutaneous aspiration of the cyst[383] (may be used repeatedly)
4. ✖ no longer recommended:
   A. plugging the obex with muscle, teflon or other material
   B. opening the subarachnoid space & removing inferior tonsils
   C. syringostomy: usually fails to remain patent, therefore using a stent or a shunt (syringosubarachnoid or syringoperitoneal) is recommended

OUTCOME

Assessing treatment results is difficult due to rarity of the condition, variability of natural history (which may arrest spontaneously), and too short follow-up[384].

14.13.2. Posttraumatic syringomyelia

A form of noncommunicating syringomyelia. This discussion deals with cases of posttraumatic syringomyelia **(PTSx)** following penetrating injury or non-penetrating "violent" trauma to the spinal cord (injuries such as post-spinal anesthesia or following thoracic disc herniation are not included). May follow significant spinal trauma (with or without clinical spinal cord injury).

PATHOPHYSIOLOGY

Etiology appears different than that of non-posttraumatic syrinx[381]. Proposed theories are vague, and include:
1. "slosh" theory: pulsatile pressure surges of fluid in the cord following injury
2. "suck" theory: upward peaks of negative pressure (e.g. during period following Valsalva maneuver) working via a ball-valve effect
3. coalescence of microcysts[385]

EPIDEMIOLOGY

Often a late presentation following spinal cord injury, therefore incidence is higher in series with longer follow-up. Incidence increasing with increasing survival following spinal cord injury and as MRI becoming more available. Range: ≈ 0.3-3% of cord injured patients (*see Table 14-31*).

In a large number of patients followed via multicenter cooperative data bank, there were fewer cases of syrinx following cervical injuries than following thoracic injuries[387] (may be artifactual since patients with lower lesions may be more aware of ascending levels).

Table 14-31   Incidence of posttraumatic syringomyelia

Type of injury	No./risk*	Incidence
all spinal cord injury patients	30/951	3.2%
complete quadriplegics	14/177	7.9%
incomplete quadriplegics	4/181	4.5%
complete paraplegics	4/282	1.7%
incomplete paraplegics	4/181	2.2%

*   number occurring over number at risk in 951 patients followed for 11 years[386]

Latency following spinal cord injury:
- latency to symptoms: 3 mos to 34 yrs (mean 9 yrs) (earlier in complete cord lesions than incomplete: mean 7.5 vs. 9.9 yrs)
- latency to diagnosis: up to 12 yrs (mean 2.8 yrs) after onset of new symptoms

CLINICAL

The presentation of patients with PTSx is shown in *Table 14-32*. The late appearance of upper extremity symptoms in a paraplegic patient should raise a high index of suspicion of posttraumatic syringomyelia[388].

Hyperhidrosis may be the only feature of descending syringomyelia in patients with complete cord lesions[390].

EVALUATION

See *Communicating syringomyelia, Evaluation* on page 350.

One end of the cavity is often found at a site of spinal column fracture or abnormal angulation.

Table 14-32 Presentation (in 30 patients with syrinx[386])

Symptom	Initial	At time of diagnosis
pain*	57%	70%
numbness	27%	40%
increased motor deficit	23%	40%
increased spasticity	10%	23%
increased sweating (hyperhidrosis)	3%	13%
autonomic dysreflexia	3%	3%
no symptoms	7%	7%
Signs	Frequency	
ascending sensory level	93%	
depressed tendon reflexes	77%	
increased motor deficits	40%	

*   pain is often quite severe, and unrelieved with analgesics[389]

MANAGEMENT

Many authors advocate early surgical drainage of cyst as a means of reducing increased delayed deficit[391]. Some authors feel that aside from disturbing sensory symptoms, that motor loss was infrequent and therefore conservative management is indicated in most cases[392].

MEDICAL

Managed non-surgically: 31% stable, 68% progressed over yrs (longer F/U in latter).

SURGICAL

There is probably no benefit in operating on a patient with a small syrinx[386].

Surgical options:
As in *Communicating syringomyelia*, with the following differences:
- cord transection (cordectomy)[393]: an option in complete injuries only
- unlike congenital syrinx, plugging the obex is felt not to be indicated

OUTCOME

In 9 PTSx patients treated with syringosubarachnoid shunt[386]: pain relieved in all 9 (1 only slightly), motor recovery in 5/8, improved tendon reflex in 1/10. Some post-op complications in 9 patients included: 1 incomplete lesion became complete, 1 sensorimotor deterioration, transient pain in 3.

Most results are good for radicular symptoms, with dubious efficacy for autonomic symptoms or spasticity.

14.13.3.   Syringobulbia

Central cavitation of the medulla.

May present with (bilateral) peri-oral tingling and numbness, due to compression of the spinal trigeminal tracts as the fibers decussate.

14.14.   Spinal epidural hematoma

Rare. Over 200 cases of varying etiology have been reported[394], although one third of recent cases have been associated with anticoagulation therapy[395]. NSAIDs may also be a risk factor[396]. Etiologies include:
1. traumatic: including following LP or epidural anesthesia[394, 397-399] or spinal surgery[150]. Occurs predominantly in patient who is: anticoagulated[400], thrombocytopenic, or has bleeding diathesis or a vascular lesion
2. spontaneous[401]: rare. Includes hemorrhage from spinal cord AVM (*see page 347*) or from vertebral hemangioma (*see page 512*)

May occur at any level of the spine, however, thoracic is most common. Most often located posterior to spinal cord (except for hematomas following anterior cervical procedures), facilitating removal via laminectomy[395].

Presentation
The clinical picture of <u>spontaneous</u> spinal epidural hematoma is fairly consistent but nonspecific. Usually starts with severe back pain with radicular component. It may occasionally follow minor straining, and is less commonly preceded by major straining or back trauma. Spinal neurologic deficits follow, usually progressing over hours, occasionally over days. Motor weakness may go unnoticed when patients are bedridden with pain.

Treatment
Recovery without surgery is rare[396], therefore optimal treatment is immediate decompressive laminectomy in those patients who can tolerate surgery[395]. In one series, most patients who recovered underwent decompression within 72 hrs of onset of symptoms[402]. In another, decompression within 6 hours was associated with better outcome[150].

High-risk patients: for medically high-risk patients (e.g. acute MI) on anticoagulation, surgical mortality and morbidity is extremely high, and this must be considered when making the decision of whether or not to operate. In patients not operated, anticoagulants should be stopped, and reversed if possible (see *Correction of coagulopathies or reversal of anticoagulants*, page 24). Consider use of high dose methylprednisolone to minimize cord injury (see *Methylprednisolone*, page 704 under spinal cord injury). Percutaneous needle aspiration may be a consideration in high-risk patients.

14.15.   Spinal subdural hematoma

Rare. May be posttraumatic (including iatrogenic causes) or may occur spontaneously. Spinal subdural hematomas (**SSH**) that occur spontaneously or following lumbar puncture usually occur in patients with coagulopathies (primary or iatrogenic)[403].

Conservative treatment is possible in nontraumatic SSHs with minimal neurologic impairment[403].

14.16.   Coccydynia

Pain and tenderness around the coccyx. A symptom, not a diagnosis. Typically, discomfort is experienced on sitting or on rising from sitting. More common in females, possibly due to a more prominent coccyx. The condition is unusual enough in males that in the absence of trauma, strong consideration should be given to an underlying condition.

Etiologies
For differential diagnosis, see *Acute low back pain*, page 907. Better accepted etiologies include[404]:
1. local trauma (may be associated with fracture or dislocation):
   A. 25% of patients give a history of a fall

B. 12% had repetitive trauma (rowing machine, prolonged bicycle riding…)
C. 12% started with parturition
D. 5% started following a surgical procedure (half of which were in the lithotomy position)
2. idiopathic: excluding traumatic cases, no etiology can be identified in most cases
3. neoplasms
   A. chordoma
   B. giant cell tumor
   C. intradural schwannoma
   D. perineural cyst
   E. intra-osseous lipoma
   F. carcinoma of the rectum
   G. sacral hemangioma[405]
   H. pelvic metastases (e.g. from prostate cancer)
4. prostatitis

Controversial etiologies include[404, 406]:
1. local pressure over a prominent coccyx
2. referred pain:
   A. spinal disease
      1. herniated lumbosacral disc
      2. cauda equina syndrome
      3. arachnoiditis
   B. pelvic/visceral disease
      1. pelvic inflammatory disease (PID)
      2. perirectal abscess
      3. perirectal fistula
      4. pilonidal cyst
3. inflammation of the various ligaments attached to the coccyx
4. neurosis or frank hysteria

Histological evaluation of the coccyx has not helped delineate the cause, even though avascular necrosis has been suggested[407].

Evaluation

Sacrococcygeal films are often performed to rule-out a bony destructive lesion. Often, the question of a fracture may be raised, and many times cannot be definitely ruled-in or out based on this study. There may or may not be any significance of such a fracture.

Nuclear bone scans were not helpful in 50 patients with coccydynia[404].

CT scan: no consistent findings.

Treatment

Most cases resolve within ≈ 3 months of **conservative management** consisting of NSAIDs, mild analgesics, and measures to reduce pressure on the coccyx (e.g. a rubber ring ("doughnut") sitting cushion, lumbar supports to maintain sitting lumbar lordosis to shift weight from coccyx to posterior thighs)[408].

Recurrence: Occurs in ≈ 20% of conservatively treated cases, usually within the first year. Repeat therapy was often successful in providing permanent relief. More aggressive treatment may be considered for refractory cases.

Management recommendations for refractory cases[404, 408]:

1. local injection: 60% respond to corticosteroid + local anesthetic (40 mg Depo-Medrol® in 10 cc of 0.25% bipuvicaine). Recommended as initial treatment; response should be achieved by 2 injections
2. manipulation of the coccyx: usually under general anesthesia. ≈ 85% successful when combined with local injection
3. ± physiotherapy (diathermy & ultrasound): found to be of benefit only in ≈ 16%
4. caudal epidural steroid injection
5. blockade or neurolysis (with chemicals or by cryoablation[409]) of the ganglion impar (AKA ganglion of Walther, the lowest ganglion of the paired paravertebral sympathetic chain, located just anterior to the sacrococcygeal junction): some success has been described with this technique (traditionally used for intractable sympathetic perineal pain of neoplastic etiology[410])
6. neurolytic techniques directed to S4, S5 and coccygeal nerves
7. coccygectomy (surgical removal of the mobile portion of the coccyx, followed by smoothening of the residual bony prominence on the sacrum): was required in ≈ 20% of patients in one series[404], with a reported success rate of 90%. However,

many practitioners do not view this as a highly effective treatment and feel that great restraint should be used in considering this form of therapy

14.17. References

1. Bigos S, Bowyer O, Braen G, *et al.*: **Acute low back problems in adults. Clinical pratice guideline no.14. AHCPR publication no. 95-0642.** Agency for Health Care Policy and Research, Public Health Service, U.S. Department of Health and Human Services, Rockville, MD, 1994.
2. Cypress B K: Characteristics of physician visits for back symptoms: A national perspective. **Am J Public Health** 73: 389-95, 1983.
3. Cunningham L S, Kelsey J L: Epidemiology of musculoskeletal impairments and associated disability. **Am J Public Health** 74: 574-9, 1984.
4. Frymoyer J W: Back pain and sciatica. **N Engl J Med** 318: 291-300, 1988.
5. Fardon D F, Milette P C: Nomenclature and classification of lumbar disc pathology. Recommendations of the combined task forces of the North American spine society, American society of spine radiology, and American society of neuroradiology. **Spine** 26 (5): E93-E113, 2001.
6. McCarron R F, Wimpee M W, Hudkins P G, *et al.*: The inflammatory effect of nucleus pulposus: A possible element in the pathogenesis of low-back pain. **Spine** 12: 760-4, 1987.
7. Modic M T: *Degenerative disorders of the spine.* In **Magnetic resonance imaging of the spine.** Yearbook Medical, New York, 1989. pp 83-95.
8. Kelsey J L: *Idiopathic low back pain: Magnitude of the problem.* **American Academy of Orthopedic Surgeons Symposium on Idiopathic Low Back Pain.** St. Louis, C. V. Mosby Co. 1982, pp 5-8.
9. Spengler D M, Ouellette E A, Battié M, *et al.*: Elective discectomy for herniation of a lumbar disc. Additional experience with an objective method. **J Bone Joint Surg** 72A: 230-7, 1990.
10. Young A, Getty J, Jackson A, *et al.*: Variations in the pattern of muscle innervation by the L5 and S1 nerve roots. **Spine** 8: 616-24, 1983.
11. Braddon R I, Johnson E W: Standardization of H reflex and diagnostic use in S1 radiculopathy. **Arch Phys Med Rehabil** 55: 161-6, 1974.
12. Schütte H E, Park W M: The diagnostic value of bone scintigraphy in patients with low back pain. **Skeletal Radiol** 10: 1-4, 1983.
13. Whalen J L, Brown M L, McLeod R, *et al.*: Limitations of indium leukocyte imaging for the diagnosis of spine infections. **Spine** 16: 193-7, 1991.
14. Mills G H, Davies G K, Getty C J M, *et al.*: The evaluation of liquid crystal thermography in the investigation of nerve root compression due to lumbosacral lateral spinal stenosis. **Spine** 11: 427-32, 1986.
15. Harper C M, Low P A, Fealy R D, *et al.*: Utility of thermography in the diagnosis of lumbosacral radiculopathy. **Neurology** 41: 1010-4, 1991.
16. Deyo R A, Bigos S J, Maravilla K R: Diagnostic imaging procedures for the lumbar spine. **Ann Intern Med** 111: 865-7, 1989 (editorial).
17. Hitselberger W E, Witten R M: Abnormal myelograms in asymptomatic patients. **J Neurosurg** 28: 204-6, 1968.
18. Wiesel S W, Tsourmas N, Feffer H L, *et al.*: A study of computer-assisted tomography. I. The incidence of positive CAT scans in an asymptomatic group of patients. **Spine** 9: 549-51, 1984.
19. Jensen M C, Brant-Zawadzki M N, Obuchowski N, *et al.*: Magnetic resonance imaging of the lumbar spine in people without back pain. **N Engl J Med** 331: 69-73, 1994.
20. Boden S D, Davis D O, Dina T S, *et al.*: Abnormal magnetic-resonance scans of the lumbar spine in asymptomatic subjects. **J Bone Joint Surg** 72A: 403-8, 1990.
21. Spitzer W O, LeBlanc F E, Dupuis M, *et al.*: Scientific approach to the assessment and management of activity-related spinal disorders: A monograph for clinicians: Report of the Quebec task force on spinal disorders. Chapter 3: Diagnosis of the problem (the problem of diagnosis). **Spine** 12 (Suppl 7): S16-21, 1987.
22. Nachemson A L: The lumbar spine: An orthopedic challenge. **Spine** 1: 59-71, 1976.
23. World Health Organization: **A rational approach to radiodiagnostic investigations,** World Health Organization, Geneva. Technical Report Series 689, 1983.
24. Scavone J G, Latschaw R F, Rohrer G V: Use of lumbar spine films: Statistical evaluation of a university teaching hospital. **JAMA** 246: 1105-8, 1981.
25. Modic M T, Masaryk T, Boumphrey F, *et al.*: Lumbar herniated disk disease and canal stenosis: Prospective evaluation by surface coil MR, CT, and myelography. **AJR** 147: 757-65, 1986.
26. Jackson R P, Cain J E, Jacobs R, *et al.*: The neuroradiologic diagnosis of lumbar herniated nucleus pulposus: II. A comparison of computed tomography (CT), myelography, CT-myelography, and magnetic resonance imaging. **Spine** 14: 1362-7, 1989.
27. Modic M T, Pavlicek W, Weinstein M A, *et al.*: Magnetic resonance imaging of intervertebral disk disease. **Radiology** 152: 103-11, 1984.
28. Bosacco S J, Berman A T, Garbarino J L, *et al.*: A comparison of CT scanning and myelography in the diagnosis of lumbar disc herniation. **Clin Orthop** 190: 124-8, 1984.
29. Moufarrij N A, Hardy R W, Weinstein M A: Computed tomographic, myelographic, and operative findings in patients with suspected herniated lumbar discs. **Neurosurgery** 12: 184-8, 1983.
30. Aejmelaeus R, Hiltunen H, Härkönen M, *et al.*: Myelographic versus clinical diagnostics in lumbar disc disease. **Arch Orthop Trauma Surg** 103: 18-25, 1984.
31. Herron L D, Turner J: Patient selection for lumbar laminectomy and discectomy with a revised objective rating system. **Clin Orthop** 199: 145-52, 1985.
32. Kortelainen P, Puranen J, Koivisto E, *et al.*: Symptoms and signs of sciatica and their relation to the localization of the lumbar disc herniation. **Spine** 10: 88-92, 1985.
33. Hirsch C, Nachemson A: The reliability of lumbar disk surgery. **Clin Orthop** 29: 189, 1963.
34. Slebus F G, Braakman R, Schipper J, *et al.*: Noncorresponding radiological and surgical diagnoses in patients operated for sciatica. **Acta Neurochir** 94: 137-43, 1988.
35. Holt E P: The question of lumbar discography. **J Bone Joint Surg** 50A: 720-6, 1968.
36. Carragee E J, Tanner C M, Khurana S, *et al.*: The rates of false-positive lumbar discography in select patients without low back symptoms. **Spine** 25 (11): 1373-80; discussion 1381, 2000.
37. Walsh T R, Weinstein J N, Spratt K F, *et al.*: Lumbar discography in normal patients. A controlled, prospective study. **J Bone Joint Surg** 72A: 1081-8,

1990.

38. Waddell G, McCulloch J A, Kummel E, *et al.*: Non-organic physical signs in low back pain. **Spine** 5: 117-25, 1980.

39. McCombe P F, Fairbank J C T, Cockersole B C, *et al.*: Reproducibility of physical signs in low-back pain. **Spine** 14: 908-18, 1989.

40. Resnick D K, Choudhri T F, Dailey A T, *et al.*: Part 13: Injection therapies, low-back pain, and lumbar fusion. **J Neurosurg (Spine)** 2 (6): Guidelines for the performance of fusion procedures for degenerative disease of the lumbar spine: 707-15, 2005.

41. Nachemson A L: Newest knowledge of low back pain. A critical look. **Clin Orthop** 279: 8-20, 1992.

42. Deyo R A, Diehl A K, Rosenthal M: How many days of bed rest for acute low back pain? A randomized clinical trial. **N Engl J Med** 315: 1064-70, 1986.

43. Vroomen P C A J, de Krom M C T F M, Wilmink J T, *et al.*: Lack of effectiveness of bed rest for sciatica. **N Engl J Med** 340: 418-23, 1999.

44. Allen C, Glasziou P, Del Mar C: Bed rest: A potentially harmful treatment needing more careful evaluation. **Lancet** 354: 1229-33, 1999.

45. Lindström I, Ohlund C, Eek C, *et al.*: The effect of graded activity on patients with subacute low back pain: A randomized prospective clinical study with an operant-conditioning behavioral approach. **Phys Ther** 72: 279-93, 1992.

46. Chlorzoxazone hepatotoxicity. **Med Letter** 38: 46, 1996.

47. Deyo R A, Diehl A K: Patient satisfaction with medical care for low-back pain. **Spine** 11: 28-30, 1986.

48. Thomas K B: General practice consultations: Is there any point in being positive? **Br Med J** 294: 1200-2, 1987.

49. Keijsers J F E M, Bouter L M, Meertens R M: Validity and comparability of studies on the effects of back schools. **Physiother Theory Pract** 7: 177-84, 1991.

50. Di Fabio R P: Manipulation of the cervical spine: Risks and benefits. **Phys Ther** 79 (1): 50-65, 1999.

51. Ernst E: Life-threatening complications of spinal manipulation. **Stroke** 32 (3): 809-10, 2001.

52. Stevinson C, Honan W, Cooke B, *et al.*: Neurological complications of cervical spine manipulation. **J R Soc Med** 94 (3): 107-10, 2001.

53. Cuckler J M, Bernini P, Wiesel S, *et al.*: The use of epidural steroids in the treatment of lumbar radicular pain. A prospective, randomized, double-blind study. **J Bone Joint Surg** 67A: 63-6, 1985.

54. Spaccarelli K C: Lumbar and caudal epidural corticosteroid injections. **Mayo Clin Proc** 71: 169-78, 1996.

55. Carette S, Leclaire R, Marcoux S, *et al.*: Epidural corticosteroid injections for sciatica due to herniated nucleus pulposus. **N Engl J Med** 336: 1634-40, 1997.

56. Haimovic I C, Beresford H R: Dexamethasone is not superior to placebo for treating lumbosacral radicular pain. **Neurology** 36: 1593-4, 1986.

57. Meek J B, Giudice V W, McFadden J W, *et al.*: Colchicine confirmed as highly effective in disk disorders. Final results of a double-blind study. **J Neuro & Orthop Med & Surg** 6: 211-8, 1985.

58. Schnebel B E, Simmons J W: The use of oral colchicine for low-back pain. A double-blind study. **Spine** 13: 354-7, 1988.

59. Goodkin K, Gullion C M, Agras W S: A randomized, double-blind, placebo-controlled trial of trazodone hydrochloride in chronic low back pain syndrome. **J Clin Psychopharmacol** 10: 269-78, 1990.

60. Deyo R A, Walsh N E, Martin D C, *et al.*: A controlled trial of transcutaneous electrical stimulation (TENS) and exercise for chronic low back pain. **N Engl J Med** 322: 1627-34, 1990.

61. Mathews J A, Hickling J: Lumbar traction: A double-blind controlled study for sciatica. **Rheumatol Rehabil** 14: 222-5, 1975.

62. van Poppel N N M, Koes B W, van der Ploeg T, *et al.*: Lumbar supports and education for the prevention of low back pain in industry: A randomized controlled study. **JAMA** 279: 1789-94, 1998.

63. Bush C, Ditto B, Feuerstein M: A controlled evaluation of paraspinal EMG biofeedback in the treatment of chronic low back pain. **Health Psychol** 4: 307-21, 1985.

64. Carette S, Marcoux S, Truchon R, *et al.*: A controlled trial of corticosteroid injections into facet joints for chronic low back pain. **N Engl J Med** 325: 1002-7, 1991.

65. Jackson R P: The facet syndrome. Myth or reality? **Clin Orthop Rel Res** 279: 110-21, 1992.

66. Resnick D K, Choudhri T F, Dailey A T, *et al.*: Part 6: Magnetic resonance imaging and discography for patient selection for lumbar fusion. **J Neurosurg (Spine)** 2 (6): Guidelines for the performance of fusion procedures for degenerative disease of the lumbar spine: 662-9, 2005.

67. Carragee E J, Paragioudakis S J, Khurana S: 2000 volvo award winner in clinical studies: Lumbar high-intensity zone and discography in subjects without low back problems. **Spine** 25 (23): 2987-92, 2000.

68. Resnick D K, Choudhri T F, Dailey A T, *et al.*: Part 7: Intractable low-back pain without stenosis or spondylolisthesis. **J Neurosurg (Spine)** 2 (6): Guidelines for the performance of fusion procedures for degenerative disease of the lumbar spine: 670-2, 2005.

69. Fritzell P, Hagg O, Wessberg P, *et al.*: 2001 volvo award winner in clinical studies: Lumbar fusion versus nonsurgical treatment for chronic low back pain: A multicenter randomized controlled trial from the swedish lumbar spine study group. **Spine** 26 (23): 2521-32; discussion 2532-4, 2001.

70. Ivar Brox J, Sorensen R, Friis A, *et al.*: Randomized clinical trial of lumbar instrumented fusion and cognitive intervention and exercises in patients with chronic low back pain and disc degeneration. **Spine** 28 (17): 1913-21, 2003.

71. Resnick D K, Choudhri T F, Dailey A T, *et al.*: Part 11: Interbody techniques for lumbar fusion. **J Neurosurg (Spine)** 2 (6): Guidelines for the performance of fusion procedures for degenerative disease of the lumbar spine: 692-9, 2005.

72. Turner J A, Ersek M, Herron L, *et al.*: Patient outcomes after lumbar spinal fusions. **JAMA** 268: 907-11, 1992.

73. Resnick D K, Choudhri T F, Dailey A T, *et al.*: Part 8: Lumbar fusion for disc herniation and radiculopathy. **J Neurosurg (Spine)** 2 (6): Guidelines for the performance of fusion procedures for degenerative disease of the lumbar spine: 673-8, 2005.

74. Resnick D K, Choudhri T F, Dailey A T, *et al.*: Part 12: Pedicle screw fixation as an adjunct to posterolateral fusion for low-back pain. **J Neurosurg (Spine)** 2 (6): Guidelines for the performance of fusion procedures for degenerative disease of the lumbar spine: 700-6, 2005.

75. Lorenz M, Zindrick M, Schwaegler P, *et al.*: A comparison of single-level fusions with and without hardware. **Spine** 16 (Suppl 8): S455-8, 1991.

76. Resnick D K, Choudhri T F, Dailey A T, *et al.*: Part 16: Bone graft extenders and substitutes. **J Neurosurg (Spine)** 2 (6): Guidelines for the performance of fusion procedures for degenerative disease of the lumbar spine: 733-6, 2005.

77. Resnick D K, Choudhri T F, Dailey A T, *et al.*: Part 4: Radiographic assessment of fusion. **J Neurosurg (Spine)** 2 (6): Guidelines for the performance of fusion procedures for degenerative disease of the lumbar spine: 653-7, 2005.

78. Resnick D K, Choudhri T F, Dailey A T, et al.: Part 5: Correlation between radiographic and functional outcome. **J Neurosurg (Spine)** 2 (6): Guidelines for the performance of fusion procedures for degenerative disease of the lumbar spine: 658-61, 2005.

79. Gatchel R J, Mayer T G, Capra P, et al.: Quantification of lumbar function, VI: The use of psychological measures in guiding physical functional restoration. **Spine** 11: 36-42, 1986.

80. Morley S, Pallin V: Scaling the affective domain of pain: A study of the dimensionality of verbal descriptors. **Pain** 62: 39-49, 1995.

81. Weber H: Lumbar disc herniation. A controlled, prospective study with ten years of observation. **Spine** 8: 131-40, 1983.

82. Lewis P J, Weir B K A, Broad R, et al.: Long-term prospective study of lumbosacral discectomy. **J Neurosurg** 67: 49-53, 1987.

83. Wein A J: *Neuromuscular dysfunction of the lower urinary tract and its treatment*. In **Campbell's urology**, Walsh P C, Retik A B, Vaughan E D, et al., (eds.). W.B. Saunders, Philadelphia, 7th ed., 1998, Vol. 1, Chapter 29: pp 953-1006.

84. Jones D L, Moore T: The types of neuropathic bladder dysfunction associated with prolapsed lumbar intervertebral discs. **Br J Urol** 45: 39-43, 1973.

85. Ross J C, Jameson R M: Vesical dysfunction due to prolapsed disc. **Br Med J** 3: 752-4, 1971.

86. Deyo R A, Rainville J, Kent D L: What can the history and physical examination tell us about low back pain? **JAMA** 268: 760-5, 1992.

87. Blaauw G, Braakman R, Gelpke G J, et al.: Changes in radicular function following low-back surgery. **J Neurosurg** 69: 649-52, 1988.

88. Stam J, Speelman H D, van Crevel H: Tendon reflex asymmetry by voluntary mental effort in healthy subjects. **Arch Neurol** 46: 70-3, 1989.

89. Scham S M, Taylor T K F: Tension signs in lumbar disc prolapse. **Clin Orthop** 75: 195-204, 1971.

90. Dyck P: Lumbar nerve root: The enigmatic eponyms. **Spine** 9: 3-6, 1984.

91. Spangfort E V: The lumbar disc herniation. A computer-aided analysis of 2,504 operations. **Acta Orthop Scand** 142 (Suppl): 1-93, 1972.

92. Rothman R H, Simeone F A, (eds.): **The spine**. 3rd ed., W.B. Saunders, Philadelphia, 1992.

93. Estridge M N, Rouhe S A, Johnson N G: The femoral stretch test: A valuable sign in diagnosing upper lumbar disc herniations. **J Neurosurg** 57: 813-7, 1982.

94. Keegan J J: Dermatome hypalgesia associated with herniation of intervertebral disk. **Arch Neurol Psychiatry** 50: 67-83, 1943.

95. Wigh R E: Classification of the human vertebral column: Phylogenic departures and junctional anomalies. **Med Radiogr Photogr** 56: 2-11, 1980.

96. Fager C A: Observations on spontaneous recovery from intervertebral disc herniation. **Surg Neurol** 42: 282-6, 1994.

97. Weber H, Holme I, Amlie E: The natural course of acute sciatica, with nerve root symptoms in a double blind placebo controlled trial evaluating the effect of piroxicam (NSAID). **Spine** 18: 1433-8, 1993.

98. Weber H: The effect of delayed disc surgery on muscular paresis. **Acta Orthop Scand** 46: 631-42, 1975.

99. Saal J A, Saal J S: Nonoperative treatment of herniated lumbar intervertebral disc with radiculopathy: An outcome study. **Spine** 14: 431-7, 1989.

100. Kostuik J P, Harrington I, Alexander D, et al.: Cauda equina syndrome and lumbar disc herniation. **J Bone Joint Surg** 68A: 386-91, 1986.

101. O'Laoire S A, Crockard H A, Thomas D G: Prognosis for sphincter recovery after operation for cauda equina compression owing to lumbar disc prolapse. **Br Med J** 282: 1852-4, 1981.

102. Shapiro S: Cauda equina syndrome secondary to lumbar disc herniation. **Neurosurgery** 32: 743-7, 1993.

103. Scott P J: Bladder paralysis in cauda equina lesions from disc prolapse. **J Bone Joint Surg** 47B: 224-35, 1965.

104. Tay E C K, Chacha P B: Midline prolapse of a lumbar intervertebral disc with compression of the cauda equina. **J Bone Joint Surg** 61B: 43-6, 1979.

105. Prusick V D, Lint D S, Bruder J: Cauda equina syndrome as a complication of free epidural fat-grafting. **J Bone Joint Surg** 70A: 1256-8, 1988.

106. Tandon P N, Sankaran B: Cauda equina syndrome due to lumbar disc prolapse. **Indian J Orthopedics** 1: 112-9, 1967.

107. Shapiro S: Medical realities of cauda equina syndrome secondary to lumbar disc herniation. **Spine** 25: 348-51, 2000.

108. Kostuik J P: Point of view: Comment on Shapiro, S: Medical realities of cauda equina syndrome secondary to lumbar disc herniation. **Spine** 25: 351, 2000.

109. Hoffman R M, Wheeler K J, Deyo R A: Surgery for herniated lumbar discs: A literature synthesis. **J Gen Intern Med** 8 (9): 487-96, 1993.

110. Williams R W: Microlumbar discectomy: A conservative surgical approach to the virgin herniated lumbar disc. **Spine** 3: 175-82, 1978.

111. Caspar W, Campbell B, Barbier D D, et al.: The Caspar microsurgical discectomy and comparison with a conventional lumbar disc procedure. **Neurosurgery** 28: 78-87, 1991.

112. Schmidek H H, Sweet W H, (eds.): **Operative neurosurgical techniques**. 1st ed., Grune and Stratton, New York, 1982.

113. Fager C A: Lumbar discectomy: A contrary opinion. **Clin Neurosurg** 33: 419-56, 1986.

114. Tulberg T, Isacson J, Weidenhielm L: Does microscopic removal of lumbar disc herniation lead to better results than the standard procedure? Results of a one-year randomized study. **J Neurosurg** 70: 869-75, 1993.

115. Gogan W J, Fraser R D: Chymopapain. A 10-year, double-blind study. **Spine** 17: 388-94, 1992.

116. Javid M J, Nordby E J, Ford L T, et al.: Safety and efficacy of chymopapain (chymodiactin) in herniated nucleus pulposus with sciatica. Results of a randomized, double-blind study. **JAMA** 249: 2489-94, 1983.

117. Crawshaw C, Frazer A M, Merriam W F, et al.: A comparison of surgery and chemonucleolysis in the treatment of sciatica. A prospective randomized trial. **Spine** 9: 195-8, 1984.

118. van Alphen H A M, Braakman R, Bezemer P D, et al.: Chemonucleolysis versus discectomy: A randomized multicenter trial. **J Neurosurg** 70: 869-75, 1989.

119. Ejeskär A, Nachemson A, Herberts P, et al.: Surgery versus chemonucleolysis for herniated lumbar discs. A prospective study with random assignment. **Clin Orthop** 174: 236-42, 1983.

120. Bouillet R: A comparative survey of complications of surgical treatment and nucleolysis with chymopapain. **Clin Orthop** 251: 144-52, 1990.

121. Agre K, Wilson R R, Brim M, et al.: Chymodiactin postmarketing surveillance. Demographic and adverse experience data in 29,075 patients. **Spine** 9: 479-85, 1984.

122. Deeb Z L, Schimel S, Daffner R H, et al.: Intervertebral disk-space infection after chymopapain injection. **AJNR** 6: 55-8, 1985.

123. Eguro H: Transverse myelitis following chemonucleolysis: Report of a case. **J Bone Joint Surg** 65A: 1328-9, 1983.

124. Hoppenfield S: Percutaneous removal of herniated lumbar discs. 50 cases with ten-year follow-up periods. **Clin Orthop** 238: 92-7, 1989.

125. Kahanovitz N, Viola K, Goldstein T, et al.: A multicenter analysis of percutaneous discectomy. **Spine**

15: 713-5, 1990.

126. Davis G W, Onik G: Clinical experience with automated percutaneous lumbar discectomy. **Clin Orthop** 238: 98-103, 1989.

127. Revel M, Payan C, Vallee C, et al.: Automated percutaneous lumbar discectomy versus chemonucleolysis in the treatment of sciatica. **Spine** 18: 1-7, 1993.

128. Maroon J C, Onik G, Sternau L: Percutaneous automated discectomy. A new method for lumbar disc removal. Technical note. **J Neurosurg** 66: 143-6, 1987.

129. Onik G, Maroon J C, Jackson R: Cauda equina syndrome secondary to an improperly placed nucleotome probe. **Neurosurgery** 30: 412-5, 1992.

130. Yonezawa T, Onomura T, Kosaka R, et al.: The system and procedures of percutaneous intradiscal laser nucleotomy. **Spine** 15: 1175-85, 1990.

131. Choy D S J, Ascher P W, Saddekni S, et al.: Percutaneous laser disc decompression: A new therapeutic modality. **Spine** 17: 949-56, 1992.

132. Mayer H M, Brock M: Percutaneous endoscopic discectomy: Surgical technique and preliminary results compared to microsurgical discectomy. **J Neurosurg** 78: 216-25, 1993.

133. Kleinpeter G, Markowitsch M M, Bock F: Percutaneous endoscopic lumbar discectomy: Minimally invasive, but perhaps only minimally useful? **Surg Neurol** 43: 534-41, 1995.

134. Karasek M, Bogduk N: Twelve-month follow-up of a controlled trial of intradiscal thermal anuloplasty for back pain due to internal disc disruption. **Spine** 25 (20): 2601-7, 2000.

135. Schwarzer A C, Aprill C N, Derby R, et al.: The prevalence and clinical features of internal disc disruption in patients with chronic low back pain. **Spine** 20 (17): 1878-83, 1995.

136. Lavyne M H, Bilsky M H: Epidural steroids, postoperative morbidity, and recovery in patients undergoing microsurgical lumbar discectomy. **J Neurosurg** 77: 90-5, 1992.

137. Glasser R S, Knego R S, Delashaw J B, et al.: The perioperative use of corticosteroids and bupivicaine in the management of lumbar disc disease. **J Neurosurg** 78: 383-7, 1993.

138. Dunsker S B: Comment on Cobanoglu S, et al.: Complication of epidural fat graft in lumbar spine disc surgery: Case report. **Surg Neurol** 44: 481-2, 1995.

139. Cabezudo J M, Lopez A, Bacci F: Symptomatic root compression by a free fat transplant after hemilaminectomy: Case report. **J Neurosurg** 63: 633-5, 1985.

140. Cobanoglu S, Imer M, Ozylmaz F, et al.: Complication of epidural fat graft in lumbar spine disc surgery: Case report. **Surg Neurol** 44: 479-82, 1995.

141. Dunsker S, Tobler W: *A clinical study of adcon-L: A bioresorbable gel for the prevention of peridural fibrosis.* **AANS Annual Meeting.** New Orleans: 1999, pp 244-6 (abstract).

142. Ramirez L F, Thisted R: Complications and demographic characteristics of patients undergoing lumbar discectomy in community hospitals. **Neurosurgery** 25: 226-31, 1989.

143. Deyo R A, Cherkin D C, Loeser J D, et al.: Morbidity and mortality in association with operations on the lumbar spine. The influence of age, diagnosis, and procedure. **J Bone Joint Surg** 74A: 536-43, 1992.

144. Shektman A, Granick M S, Solomon M P, et al.: Management of infected laminectomy wounds. **Neurosurgery** 35: 307-9, 1994.

145. Goodkin R, Laska L L: Unintended 'incidental' durotomy during surgery of the lumbar spine: Medicolegal implications. **Surg Neurol** 43: 4-14, 1995.

146. Davis R A: A long-term outcome analysis of 984 surgically treated herniated lumbar discs. **J Neurosurg** 80: 415-21, 1994.

147. Bilsky M H, Shields C B: Complications of lumbar disc surgery. **Contemp Neurosurg** 17 (21): 1-6, 1995.

148. DeSaussure R L: Vascular injuries coincident to disc surgery. **J Neurosurg** 16: 222-39, 1959.

149. Mclaren A C, Bailey S I: Cauda equina syndrome: A complication of lumbar discectomy. **Clin Orthop** 204: 143-9, 1986.

150. Porter R W, Detwiler P W, Lawton M T, et al.: Postoperative spinal epidural hematomas: Longitudinal review of 12,000 spinal operations. **BNI Quarterly** 16: 10-7, 2000.

151. Sachs B L, Zindrick M R, Beasley R D: Reflex sympathetic dystrophy after operative procedures on the lumbar spine. **J Bone Joint Surg** 75A: 721-5, 1993.

152. Feldman R A, Karl R C: Diagnosis and treatment of Ogilvie's syndrome after lumbar spinal surgery. **J Neurosurg** 76: 1012-6, 1992.

153. Hodges S D, Humphreys C, Eck J C, et al.: Management of incidental durotomy without mandatory bed rest. **Spine** 24: 2062-4, 1999.

154. Fink L H: Unintended 'incidental' durotomy. **Surg Neurol** 45: 590, 1996 (letter).

155. Ciappetta P, Delfini R, Cantore G P: Intradural lumbar disc hernia: Description of three cases. **Neurosurgery** 8: 104-7, 1981.

156. Horwitz N H, Rizzoli H V: *Herniated intervertebral discs and spinal stenosis.* In **Postoperative complications of extracranial neurological surgery,** Horwitz N H and Rizzoli H V, (eds.). Williams and Wilkins, Baltimore, 1987: pp 1-72.

157. Waisman M, Schweppe Y: Postoperative cerebrospinal fluid leakage after lumbar spine operations. Conservative treatment. **Spine** 15: 52-3, 1991.

158. Aronson H A, Dunsmore R H: Herniated upper lumbar discs. **J Bone Joint Surg** 45: 311-7, 1963.

159. Abdullah A F, Wolber P G H, Warfield J R, et al.: Surgical management of extreme lateral lumbar disc herniations: Review of 138 cases. **Neurosurgery** 22: 648-53, 1988.

160. Godersky J C, Erickson D L, Seljeskog E L: Extreme lateral disc herniation: Diagnosis by CT scanning. **Neurosurgery** 14: 549-52, 1984.

161. Osborne D R, Heinz E R, Bullard D, et al.: Role of CT in the radiological evaluation of painful radiculopathy after negative myelography. **Neurosurgery** 14: 147-53, 1984.

162. Osborn A G, Hood R S, Sherry R G, et al.: CT/MR spectrum of far lateral and anterior lumbosacral disk herniations. **AJNR** 9: 775-8, 1988.

163. Jackson R P, Glah J J: Foraminal and extraforaminal lumbar disc herniation: Diagnosis and treatment. **Spine** 12: 577-85, 1987.

164. Angtuaco E J C, Holder J C, Boop W C, et al.: Computed tomographic discography in the evaluation of extreme lateral disc herniation. **Neurosurgery** 14: 350-2, 1984.

165. Grenier N, Greselle J-F, Douws C, et al.: MR imaging of foraminal and extraforaminal lumbar disk herniations. **J Comput Assist Tomogr** 14: 243-9, 1990.

166. Garrido E, Connaughton P N: Unilateral facetectomy approach for lateral lumbar disc herniation. **J Neurosurg** 74: 754-6, 1991.

167. Epstein N E, Epstein J A, Carras R, et al.: Far lateral lumbar disc herniations and associated structural abnormalities. An evaluation in 60 patients of the comparative value of CT, MRI, and myelo-CT in diagnosis and management. **Spine** 15: 534-9, 1990.

168. Jane J A, Haworth C S, Broaddus W C, et al.: A neurosurgical approach to far-lateral disc herniation. **J Neurosurg** 72: 143-4, 1990.

169. Ditsworth D A: Endoscopic transforaminal lumbar discectomy and reconfiguration: A posterolateral approach into the spinal canal. **Surg Neurol** 49: 588-98, 1998.

170. Maroon J C, Kopitnik T A, Schulhof L A, et al.: Di-

agnosis and microsurgical approach to far-lateral disc herniation in the lumbar spine. **J Neurosurg** 72: 378-82, 1990.

171. Ebersold M J, Quast L M, Bianco A J: Results of lumbar discectomy in the pediatric patient. **J Neurosurg** 67: 643-7, 1987.

172. Epstein J A, Epstein N E, Marc J, *et al.*: Lumbar intervertebral disk herniation in teenage children: Recognition and management of associated anomalies. **Spine** 9: 427-32, 1984.

173. Kataoka O, Nishibayashi Y, Sho T: Intradural lumbar disc herniation: Report of three cases with a review of the literature. **Spine**: 529-33, 1989.

174. Schisano G, Franco A, Nina P: Intraradicular and intradural lumbar disc herniation: Experience with nine cases. **Surg Neurol** 44: 536-43, 1995.

175. Deeg H J; Schmorl's nodule. **N Engl J Med** 298: 57, 1978 (Letter).

176. Hamanishi C, Kawabata T, Yosii T, *et al.*: Schmorl's nodes on magnetic resonance imaging. **Spine** 19: 450-3, 1994.

177. Takahashi K, Miyazaki T, Ohnari H, *et al.*: Schmorl's nodes and low-back pain. Analysis of magnetic resonance imaging findings in symptomatic and asymptomatic individuals. **Eur Spine J** 4: 56-9, 1995.

178. Kao C C, Winkler S S, Turner J H: Synovial cyst of spinal facet. Case report. **J Neurosurg** 41: 372-6, 1974.

179. Freidberg S R, Fellows T, Thomas C B, *et al.*: Experience with symptomatic epidural cysts. **Neurosurgery** 34: 989-93, 1994.

180. Cartwright M J, Nehls D G, Carrion C A, *et al.*: Synovial cyst of a cervical facet joint: Case report. **Neurosurgery** 16: 850-2, 1985.

181. Onofrio B M, Mih A D: Synovial cysts of the spine. **Neurosurgery** 22: 642-7, 1988.

182. Goffin J, Wilms G, Plets C, *et al.*: Synovial cyst at the C1-C2 junction. **Neurosurgery** 30: 914-6, 1992.

183. Lopes N M M, Aesse F F, Lopes D K: Compression of thoracic nerve root by a facet joint synovial cyst: Case report. **Surg Neurol** 38: 338-40, 1992.

184. Heary R F, Stellar S, Fobben E S: Preoperative diagnosis of an extradural cyst arising from a spinal facet joint: Case report. **Neurosurgery** 30: 415-8, 1992.

185. Kao C C, Uihlein A, Bickel W H, *et al.*: Lumbar intraspinal extradural ganglion cyst. **J Neurosurg** 29: 168-72, 1968.

186. Franck J I, King R B, Petro G R, *et al.*: A posttraumatic lumbar spinal synovial cyst. Case report. **J Neurosurg** 66: 293-6, 1987.

187. Sabo R A, Tracy P T, Weinger J M: A series of 60 juxtafacet cysts: Clinical presentation, the role of spinal instability, and treatment. **J Neurosurg** 85: 560-5, 1996.

188. Mercader J, Gomez J M, Cardenal C: Intraspinal synovial cyst: Diagnosis by CT. Follow-up and spontaneous remission. **Neuroradiology** 27: 346-8, 1985.

189. Liu S S, Williams K D, Drayer B P, *et al.*: Synovial cysts of the lumbosacral spine: Diagnosis by MR imaging. **AJNR** 10: 1239-42, 1989.

190. Silbergleit R, Gebarski S S, Brunberg J A, *et al.*: Lumbar synovial cysts: Correlation of myelographic, CT, MR, and pathologic findings. **AJNR** 11: 777-9, 1990.

191. Gorey M T, Hyman R A, Black K S, *et al.*: Lumbar synovial cysts eroding bone. **AJNR** 13: 161-3, 1992.

192. Conrad M, Pitkethly D: Bilateral synovial cysts creating spinal stenosis. **J Comput Assist Tomogr** 11: 196-7, 1987.

193. Hemminghytt S, Daniels D L, Williams M L, *et al.*: Intraspinal synovial cysts: Natural history and diagnosis by CT. **Radiology** 145: 375-6, 1982.

194. Budris D M: Intraspinal lumbar synovial cyst. **Orthopedics** 14: 618-20, 1991.

195. Tarlov I M: Spinal perineurial and meningeal cysts. **J Neurol Neurosurg Psychiatry** 33: 833-43, 1970.

196. Soren A: Pathogenesis and treatment of ganglion. **Clin Orthop** 48: 173-9, 1966.

197. Schulz E E, West W L, Hinshaw D B, *et al.*: Gas in a lumbar extradural juxtaarticular cyst: Sign of synovial origin. **Am J Radiol** 143: 875-6, 1984.

198. Munz M, Tampieri D, Robitaille Y, *et al.*: Spinal synovial cyst: Case report using magnetic resonance imaging. **Surg Neurol** 34: 431-4, 1990.

199. Martin D, Awwad E, Sundaram M: Lumbar ganglion cyst causing radiculopathy. **Orthopedics** 13: 1182-3, 1990.

200. Kurz L T, Garfin S R, Unger A S, *et al.*: Intraspinal synovial cyst causing sciatica. **J Bone Joint Surg** 67A: 865-71, 1985.

201. Law J D, Lehman R A W, Kirsch W M, *et al.*: Reoperation after lumbar intervertebral disc surgery. **J Neurosurg** 48: 259-63, 1978.

202. Markwalder T M, Battaglia M: Failed back surgery syndrome. Part 1: Analysis of the clinical presentation and results of testing procedures for instability of the lumbar spine in 171 patients. **Acta Neurochir** 123: 46-51, 1993.

203. Caputy A J, Luessenhop A J: Long-term evaluation of decompressive surgery for degenerative lumbar stenosis. **J Neurosurg** 77: 669-76, 1992.

204. Burton C V, Kirkaldy-Willis W H, Yong-Hing K, *et al.*: Causes of failure of surgery on the lumbar spine. **Clin Orthop** 157: 191-9, 1981.

205. Quencer R M, Tenner M, Rothman L: The postoperative myelogram: Radiographic evaluation of arachnoiditis and dural/arachnoidal tears. **Radiology** 123: 667-9, 1977.

206. Roca J, Moreta D, Ubierna M T, *et al.*: The results of surgical treatment of lumbar arachnoiditis. **Int Orthop** 17: 77-81, 1993.

207. Ross J S, Masaryk T J, Modic M T, *et al.*: MR imaging of lumbar arachnoiditis. **AJNR** 8: 885-92, 1987.

208. Delamarter R B, Ross J S, Masaryk T J, *et al.*: Diagnosis of lumbar arachnoiditis by magnetic resonance imaging. **Spine** 15: 304-10, 1990.

209. Martin-Ferrer S: Failure of autologous fat grafts to prevent post operative epidural fibrosis in surgery of the lumbar spine. **Neurosurgery** 24: 718-21, 1989.

210. North R B, Campbell J N, James C S, *et al.*: Failed back surgery syndrome: 5-year follow-up in 102 patients undergoing repeated operations. **Neurosurgery** 28: 685-91, 1991.

211. Ross J S, Robertson J T, Frederickson R C A, *et al.*: Association between peridural scar and recurrent radicular pain after lumbar discectomy: Magnetic resonance evaluation. **Neurosurgery** 38: 855-63, 1996.

212. Cooper P R: Comment on Ross J S, et al.: Association between peridural scar and recurrent radicular pain after lumbar discectomy. **Neurosurgery** 38: 861, 1996.

213. Sonntag V K H: Comment on Ross J S, et al.: Association between peridural scar and recurrent radicular pain after lumbar discectomy. **Neurosurgery** 38: 862, 1996.

214. Bundschuh C V, Modic M T, Ross J S, *et al.*: Epidural fibrosis and recurrent disc herniation in the lumbar spine: Assessment with magnetic resonance. **AJNR** 9: 169-78, 1988.

215. Sotiropoulos S, Chafetz N E, Lang P, *et al.*: Differentiation between postoperative scar and recurrent disk herniation: Prospective comparison of MR, CT, and contrast-enhanced CT. **AJNR** 10: 639-43, 1989.

216. Hueftle M G, Modic M T, Ross J S, *et al.*: Lumbar spine: Postoperative MR imaging with Gd-DPTA. **Radiology** 167: 817-24, 1988.

217. Braun I F, Hoffman J C, Davis P C, *et al.*: Contrast enhancement in CT differentiation between recurrent disk herniation and postoperative scar: Prospective study. **AJR** 145: 785-90, 1985.

218. Byrd S E, Cohn M L, Biggers S L, *et al*.: The radiologic evaluation of the symptomatic postoperative lumbar spine patient. **Spine** 10: 652-61, 1985.

219. Greenwood J, McGuire T H, Kimbell F: A study of the causes of failure in the herniated intervertebral disc operation. An analysis of sixty-seven reoperated cases. **J Neurosurg** 9: 15-20, 1952.

220. Jorgensen J, Hansen P H, Steenskov V, *et al*.: A clinical and radiological study of chronic lower spinal arachnoiditis. **Neuroradiology** 9: 139-44, 1975.

221. Johnston J D H, Matheny J B: Microscopic lysis of lumbar adhesive arachnoiditis. **Spine** 3: 36-9, 1978.

222. Herron L: Recurrent lumbar disc herniation: Results of repeat laminectomy and discectomy. **J Spinal Disord** 7: 161-6, 1994.

223. Waddell G, Crummel E G, Solts W N, *et al*.: Failed lumbar disc surgery and repeat surgery following industrial injuries. **J Bone Joint Surg** 61A: 201-7, 1979.

224. Bell G K, Kidd D, North R B: Cost-effectiveness analysis of spinal cord stimulation in treatment of failed back surgery syndrome. **J Pain Symptom Manage** 13 (5): 286-95, 1997.

225. Mayfield F H: Cervical spondylosis: A comparison of the anterior and posterior approaches. **Clin Neurosurg** 13: 181-8, 1966.

226. Viikari-Juntura E, Porras M, Laasonen E M: Validity of clinical tests in the diagnosis of root compression in cervical disc disease. **Spine** 14: 253-7, 1989.

227. Spurling R G, Scoville W B: Lateral rupture of the cervical intervertebral discs: A common cause of shoulder and arm pain. **Surg Gynecol Obstet** 78: 350-8, 1944.

228. Saal J, Saal Y, Yurth E: Nonoperative management of herniated cervical intervertebral disc with radiculopathy. **Spine** 21: 1877-83, 1996.

229. Murphy M A, Trimble M B, Piedmonte M R, *et al*.: Changes in the cervical foraminal area after anterior discectomy with and without a graft. **Neurosurgery** 34: 93-6, 1994.

230. Hoff J T, Wilson C B: Microsurgical approach to the anterior cervical spine and spinal cord. **Clin Neurosurg** 26: 513-28, 1979.

231. Bertalanffy H, Eggert H R: Clinical long-term results of anterior discectomy without fusion for treatment of cervical radiculopathy and myelopathy: A follow-up of 164 cases. **Acta Neurochir** 90: 127-35, 1988.

232. Senter H J, Kortyna R, Kemp W R: Anterior cervical discectomy with hydroxylapatite fusion. **Neurosurgery** 25: 39-43, 1989.

233. Tew J M, Mayfield F H: Complications of surgery of the anterior cervical spine. **Clin Neurosurg** 23: 424-34, 1976.

234. Taylor B A, Vaccaro A R, Albert T J: Complications of anterior and posterior surgical approaches in the treatment of cervical degenerative disc disease. **Semin Spine Surg** 11: 337-46, 1999.

235. Netterville J L, Koriwchak M J, Winkle M, *et al*.: Vocal fold paralysis following the anterior approach to the cervical spine. **Ann Otol Rhinol Laryngol** 105: 85-91, 1996.

236. Pfeifer B A, Freidberg S R, Jewell E R: Repair of injured vertebral artery in anterior cervical procedures. **Spine** 19: 1471-4, 1994.

237. Krieger A J, Rosomoff H L: Sleep-induced apnea. Part 2: Respiratory failure after anterior spinal surgery. **J Neurosurg** 39: 181-5, 1974.

238. DePalma A F, Cooke A J: Results of anterior interbody fusion of the cervical spine. **Clin Orthop** 60: 169-85, 1968.

239. Phillips F M, Carlson G, Emery S E, *et al*.: Anterior cervical pseudarthrosis: Natural history and treatment. **Spine** 22: 1585-9, 1997.

240. Truumees E, Herkowitz H N: Adjacent segment degeneration in the cervical spine: Incidence and management. **Semin Spine Surg** 11: 373-83, 1999.

241. Gore D R, Sepic S B: Anterior cervical fusion for degenerated or protruded discs. A review of one hundred and fifty-six patients. **Spine** 9: 667-71, 1984.

242. Hawkins R J, Bilco T, Bonutti P: Cervical spine and shoulder pain. **Clin Orthop Rel Res** 258: 142-6, 1990.

243. Aldrich F: Posterolateral microdiscectomy for cervical monoradiculopathy caused by posterolateral soft cervical disc sequestration. **J Neurosurg** 72: 370-7, 1990.

244. Zeidman S M, Ducker T B: Posterior cervical laminoforaminotomy for radiculopathy: Review of 172 cases. **Neurosurgery** 33: 356-62, 1993.

245. Collias J C, Roberts M P: *Posterior surgical approaches for cervical disc herniation and spondylotic myelopathy*. In **Operative neurosurgical techniques**, Schmidek H H and Sweet W H, (eds.). W.B. Saunders, Philadelphia, 3rd ed., 1995, Vol. 2, Chapter 146: pp 1805-16.

246. Dohn D F: Thoracic spinal cord decompression: Alternative surgical approaches and basis of choice. **Clin Neurosurg** 27: 611-23, 1980.

247. Le Roux P D, Haglund M M, Harris A B: Thoracic disc disease: Experience with the transpedicular approach in twenty consecutive patients. **Neurosurgery** 33: 58-66, 1993.

248. Arce A C, Dohrmann G J: Thoracic disc herniation. **Surg Neurol** 23: 356-61, 1985 (review).

249. Chou S N, Seljeskog E L: Alternative surgical approaches to the thoracic spine. **Clin Neurosurg** 20: 306-21, 1972.

250. Hadley M N, Reddy S V: Smoking and the human vertebral column: A review of the impact of cigarette use on vertebral bone metabolism and spinal fusion. **Neurosurgery** 41: 116-24, 1997.

251. Fogelholm R R, Alho A V: Smoking and intervertebral disc degeneration. **Med Hypotheses** 56 (4): 537-9, 2001.

252. Meyerding H W: Spondylolisthesis. **Surg Gynecol Obstet** 54: 371-7, 1932.

253. Rothman R H, Simeone F A, (eds.): **The spine**. 2nd ed., W.B. Saunders, Philadelphia, 1982.

254. Herkowitz H N, Kurz L T: Degenerative lumbar spondylolisthesis with spinal stenosis: A prospective study comparing decompression with decompression and intertransverse process arthrodesis. **J Bone Joint Surg** 73A: 802-8, 1991.

255. Epstein N E, Epstein J A, Carras R, *et al*.: Coexisting cervical and lumbar spinal stenosis: Diagnosis and management. **Neurosurgery** 15: 489-96, 1984.

256. Yamamoto I, Matsumae M, Ikeda A, *et al*.: Thoracic spinal stenosis: Experience with seven cases. **J Neurosurg** 68: 37-40, 1988.

257. Epstein N E: Symptomatic lumbar spinal stenosis. **Surg Neurol** 50: 3-10, 1998.

258. Verbiest H: A radicular syndrome from developmental narrowing of the lumbar canal. **J Bone Joint Surg** 36B: 230-7, 1954.

259. Epstein J A, Epstein B S, Lavine L: Nerve root compression associated with narrowing of the lumbar spinal canal. **J Neurol Neurosurg Psychiatry** 52: 165-76, 1962.

260. Duggal N, Sonntag V K H, Dickman C A: Fusion options and indications in the lumbosacral spine. **Contemp Neurosurg** 23 (1): 1-8, 2001.

261. Hawkes C H, Roberts G M: Neurogenic and vascular claudication. **J Neurol Sci** 38: 337-45, 1978.

262. Turner J A, Ersek M, Herron L, *et al*.: Surgery for lumbar spinal stenosis: Attempted meta-analysis of the literature. **Spine** 17: 1-8, 1992.

263. Shbeeb M I, Matteson E L: Trochanteric bursitis (greater trochanter pain syndrome). **Mayo Clin Proc** 71: 565-9, 1996.

264. Deen H G: Diagnosis and management of lumbar disk disease. **Mayo Clin Proc** 71: 283-7, 1996.

265. Ehni G: Significance of the small lumbar spinal ca-

nal. **J Neurosurg** 31: 490-4, 1969.
266. Ullrich C G, Binet E F, Sanecki M G, *et al.*: Quantitative assessment of the lumbar spinal canal by CT. **Radiology** 134: 137-43, 1980.
267. Post M J D, (ed.) **Computed tomography of the spine**. Williams and Wilkins, Baltimore, 1984.
268. Hinck V C, Clark W M, Hopkins C E: Normal interpediculate distances (minimum and maximum) in children and adult. **AJR** 97: 141-53, 1966.
269. Johnsson K E, Rosén I, Udén A: The natural course of lumbar spinal stenosis. **Acta Orthop Scand** 61 (Suppl): 24, 1990.
270. Tuite G F, Doran S E, Stern J D, *et al.*: Outcome after laminectomy for lumbar spinal stenosis. Part II: Radiographic changes and clinical correlations. **J Neurosurg** 81: 707-15, 1994.
271. Silvers H R, Lewis P J, L A H: Decompressive lumbar laminectomy for spinal stenosis. **J Neurosurg** 78: 695-701, 1993.
272. Resnick D K, Choudhri T F, Dailey A T, *et al.*: Part 10: Fusion following decompression in patients with stenosis without spondylolisthesis. **J Neurosurg (Spine)** 2 (6): Guidelines for the performance of fusion procedures for degenerative disease of the lumbar spine: 686-91, 2005.
273. Resnick D K, Choudhri T F, Dailey A T, *et al.*: Part 9: Fusion in patients with stenosis and spondylolisthesis. **J Neurosurg (Spine)** 2 (6): Guidelines for the performance of fusion procedures for degenerative disease of the lumbar spine: 679-85, 2005.
274. Resnick D K, Choudhri T F, Dailey A T, *et al.*: Part 14: Brace therapy as an adjunct to or substitute for lumbar fusion. **J Neurosurg (Spine)** 2 (6): Guidelines for the performance of fusion procedures for degenerative disease of the lumbar spine: 716-24, 2005.
275. Deburge A, Lassale B, Benoist M, *et al.*: Le traitment chirurgical des stenosis lombaires et ses resultats a propos d'une serie de 163 cas operes. **Rev Rheum Mal Osteoartic** 50: 47-54, 1983.
276. Ganz J C: Lumbar spinal stenosis: Postoperative results in terms of preoperative posture-related pain. **J Neurosurg** 72: 71-4, 1990.
277. Katz J N, Lipson S J, Larson M G, *et al.*: The outcome of decompressive laminectomy for degenerative lumbar stenosis. **J Bone Joint Surg** 73A: 809-16, 1991.
278. Deen H G, Zimmerman R S, Lyons M K, *et al.*: Analysis of early failures after lumbar decompressive laminectomy for spinal stenosis. **Mayo Clin Proc** 70: 33-6, 1995.
279. Tuite G F, Stern J D, Doran S E, *et al.*: Outcome after laminectomy for lumbar spinal stenosis. Part I: Clinical correlations. **J Neurosurg** 81: 699-706, 1994.
280. Javid M J, Hadar E J: Long-term follow-up review of patients who underwent laminectomy for lumbar stenosis: A prospective study. **J Neurosurg** 89: 1-7, 1998.
281. Ciric I, Mikhael M A, Tarkington J A, *et al.*: The lateral recess syndrome. **J Neurosurg** 53: 433-43, 1980.
282. Miller C A: Shallow cervical canal: Recognition, clinical symptoms, and treatment. **Contemp Neurosurg** 7: 1-5, 1985.
283. Nagashima C: Cervical myelopathy due to ossification of the posterior longitudinal ligament. **J Neurosurg** 37: 653-60, 1972.
284. Batzdorf U, Batzdorf A: Analysis of cervical spine curvature in patients with cervical spondylosis. **Neurosurgery** 22: 827-36, 1988.
285. Cusick J F: Pathophysiology and treatment of cervical spondylotic myelopathy. **Clin Neurosurg** 37: 661-81, 1989.
286. Cooper P R: Cervical spondylotic myelopathy. **Contemp Neurosurg** 19 (25): 1-7, 1997.
287. Yu Y L, du Boulay G H, Stevens J M, *et al.*: Com-

puted tomography in cervical spondylotic myelopathy and radiculopathy: Visualization of structures, myelographic comparison, cord measurements and clinical utility. **Neuroradiology** 28: 221-36, 1986.
288. Epstein J A, Marc J A, Hyman R A, *et al.*: Total myelography in the evaluation of lumbar disks. **Spine** 4: 121-8, 1979.
289. Houser O W, Onofrio B M, Miller G M, *et al.*: Cervical spondylotic stenosis and myelopathy: Evaluation with computed tomographic myelography. **Mayo Clin Proc** 69: 557-63, 1994.
290. Taylor A R: Vascular factors in the myelopathy associated with cervical spondylosis. **Neurology** 14: 62-8, 1964.
291. Jeffreys R V: The surgical treatment of cervical myelopathy due to spondylosis and disc degeneration. **J Neurol Neurosurg Psychiatry** 49: 353-61, 1986.
292. Adams C B T, Logue V: Studies in cervical spondylotic myelopathy: I. Movement of the cervical roots, dura and cord, and their relation to the course of the extratheca roots. **Brain** 94: 557-68, 1971.
293. Levine D N: Pathogenesis of cervical spondylotic myelopathy. **J Neurol Neurosurg Psychiatry** 62: 334-40, 1997.
294. Ogino H, Tada K, Okada K, *et al.*: Canal diameter, anteroposterior compression ratio, and spondylotic myelopathy of the cervical spine. **Spine** 8: 1-15, 1983.
295. Clarke E, Robinson P K: Cervical myelopathy: A complication of cervical spondylosis. **Brain** 79: 483-5, 1956.
296. Lees F, Aldren Turner J S: Natural history and prognosis of cervical spondylosis. **Br Med J** 2: 1607-10, 1963.
297. Nurick S: The natural history and the results of surgical treatment of the spinal cord disorder associated with cervical spondylosis. **Brain** 95: 101-8, 1972.
298. Lunsford L D, Bissonette D J, Zorub D S: Anterior surgery for cervical disc disease. Part 2: Treatment of cervical spondylotic myelopathy in 32 cases. **J Neurosurg** 53: 12-9, 1980.
299. Crandall P H, Batzdorf U: Cervical spondylotic myelopathy. **J Neurosurg** 25: 57-66, 1966.
300. Voskuhl R R, Hinton R C: Sensory impairment in the hands secondary to spondylotic compression of the cervical spinal cord. **Arch Neurol** 47: 309-11, 1990.
301. MacFadyen D J: Posterior column dysfunction in cervical spondylotic myelopathy. **Can J Neurol Sci** 11: 365-70, 1984.
302. Wiggins G C, Shaffrey C I: Laminectomy in the cervical spine: Indications, surgical techniques, and avoidance of complications. **Contemp Neurosurg** 21 (20): 1-10, 1999.
303. England J D, Hsu C Y, Vera C L, *et al.*: Spondylotic high cervical spinal cord compression presenting with hand complaints. **Surg Neurol** 25: 299-303, 1986.
304. Good D C, Couch J R, Wacasser L: "Numb, clumsy hands" and high cervical spondylosis. **Surg Neurol** 22: 285-91, 1984.
305. Campbell A M G, Phillips D G: Cervical disk lesions with neurological disorder. Differential diagnosis, treatment, and prognosis. **Br Med J** 2: 481-5, 1960.
306. Adams C B T, Logue V: Studies in cervical spondylotic myelopathy: II. The movement and contour of the spine in relation to the neural complications of cervical spondylosis. **Brain** 94: 569-86, 1971.
307. Wolf B S, Khilnani M, Malis L: The sagittal diameter of the bony cervical spinal canal and its significance in cervical spondylosis. **J of Mount Sinai Hospital** 23: 283-92, 1956.
308. Krauss W E, Ebersold M J, Quast L M: Cervical spondylotic myelopathy: Surgical indications and technique. **Contemp Neurosurg** 20 (10): 1-6, 1998.
309. Pavlov H, Torg J S, Robie B, *et al.*: Cervical spinal

stenosis: Determination with vertebral body ratio method. **Radiology** 164: 771-5, 1987.

310. Torg J S, Naranja R J, Pavlov H, *et al.*: The relationship of developmental narrowing of the cervical spinal canal to reversible and irreversible injury of the cervical spinal cord in football players. **J Bone Joint Surg** 78A: 1308-14, 1996.

311. Ratliff J, Voorhies R: Increased MRI signal intensity in association with myelopathy and cervical instability: Case report and review of the literature. **Surg Neurol** 52: 8-13, 2000.

312. Matsuda Y, Miyazaki K, Tada K, *et al.*: Increased MR signal intensity due to cervical myelopathy: Analysis of 29 surgical cases. **J Neurosurg** 74: 887-92, 1991.

313. Brown B M, Schwartz R H, Frank E, *et al.*: Preoperative evaluation of cervical radiculopathy and myelopathy by surface-coil MR imaging. **AJNR** 9: 859-66, 1988.

314. Yonenobu K, Hosono N, Iwasaki M, *et al.*: Neurologic complications of surgery for cervical compression myelopathy. **Spine** 16: 1277-82, 1991.

315. Epstein N E, Danto J, Nardi D: Evaluation of intraoperative somatosensory-evoked potential monitoring during 100 cervical operations. **Spine** 18: 737-47, 1993.

316. Epstein J, Janin Y, Carras R, *et al.*: A comparative study of the treatment of cervical spondylotic myeloradiculopathy: Experience with 50 cases treated by means of extensive laminectomy, foraminotomy, and excision of osteophytes during the past 10 years. **Acta Neurochir** 61: 89, 1982.

317. Epstein N E, Epstein J A: *Operative management of cervical spondylotic myelopathy: Technique and result of laminectomy.* In **The cervical spine**, The Cervical Spine Research Society Editorial Committee, (ed.). Lippincott-Raven, Philadelphia, 3rd ed., 1998: pp 839-48.

318. Nurick S: The pathogenesis of the spinal cord disorder associated with cervical spondylosis. **Brain** 95: 87-100, 1972.

319. Gregorius F K, Estrin T, Crandall P H: Cervical spondylotic radiculopathy and myelopathy. A long-term follow-up study. **Arch Neurol** 33: 618-25, 1976.

320. Ebersold M J, Pare M C, Quast L M: Surgical treatment for cervical spondylitic myelopathy. **J Neurosurg** 82: 745-51, 1995.

321. Dagi T F, Tarkington M A, Leech J J: Tandem lumbar and cervical spinal stenosis. **J Neurosurg** 66: 842-9, 1987.

322. Sinh G: Congenital atlanto-axial dislocation. **Neurosurg Rev** 6: 211-20, 1983.

323. Jain V K, Mittal P, Banerji D, *et al.*: Posterior occipitoaxial fusion for atlantoaxial dislocation associated with occipitalized axis. **J Neurosurg** 84: 559-64, 1996.

324. Ranawat C S, O'Leary P, Pellicci P, *et al.*: Cervical spine fusion in rheumatoid arthritis. **J Bone Joint Surg** 65A: 1003-10, 1979.

325. Menezes A H, VanGilder J C, Clark C R, *et al.*: Odontoid upward migration in rheumatoid arthritis. **J Neurosurg** 63: 500-9, 1985.

326. Smith H P, Challa V R, Alexander E: Odontoid compression of the brain stem in a patient with rheumatoid arthritis. **J Neurosurg** 53: 841-5, 1980.

327. Rana N A, Hancock D O, Taylor A R: Atlanto-axial subluxation in rheumatoid arthritis. **J Bone Joint Surg** 55B: 458-70, 1973.

328. Hildebrandt G, Agnoli A L, Zierski J: Atlanto-axial dislocation in rheumatoid arthritis: Diagnostic and therapeutic aspects. **Acta Neurochir** 84: 110-7, 1987.

329. Hinck V C, Hopkins C E: Measurement of the atlanto-dental interval in the adult. **Am J Roentgenol Radium Ther Nucl Med** 84: 945-51, 1960.

330. Meijers K A E, van Beusekom G T, Luyendijk W, *et al.*: Dislocation of the cervical spine with cord compression in rheumatoid arthritis. **J Bone Joint Surg** 56B: 668-80, 1974.

331. Smith P H, Benn R T, Sharp J: Natural history of rheumatoid cervical luxations. **Ann Rheum Dis** 31: 431-9, 1972.

332. Weissman B N W, Aliabadi P, Weinfeld M S, *et al.*: Prognostic features of atlantoaxial subluxation in rheumatoid arthritis patients. **Radiology** 144: 745-51, 1982.

333. Papadopoulos S M, Dickman C A, Sonntag V K H: Atlantoaxial stabilization in rheumatoid arthritis. **J Neurosurg** 74: 1-7, 1991.

334. Kourtopoulos H, von E C: Stabilization of the unstable upper cervical spine in rheumatoid arthritis. **Acta Neurochir** 91: 113-5, 1988.

335. Clark C R, Goetz D D, Menezes A H: Arthrodesis of the cervical spine in rheumatoid arthritis. **J Bone Joint Surg** 71A: 381-92, 1989.

336. Walpin L A, Singer F R: Paget's disease: Reversal of severe paraparesis using calcitonin. **Spine** 4: 213-9, 1979.

337. Youmans J R, (ed.) **Neurological surgery**. 3rd ed., W. B. Saunders, Philadelphia, 1990.

338. Delmas P D, Meunier P J: The management of Paget's disease of bone. **N Engl J Med** 336: 558-66, 1997.

339. Meunier P J, Salson C, Mathieu L, *et al.*: Skeletal distribution and biochemical parameters of Paget's disease. **Clin Orthop** 217: 37-44, 1987.

340. Altman R D, Brown M, Gargano F: Low back pain in Paget's disease of bone. **Clin Orthop** 217: 152-61, 1987.

341. Hadjipavlou A, Shaffer N, Lander P, *et al.*: Pagetic spinal stenosis with extradural pagetoid ossification. **Spine** 13: 128-30, 1988.

342. Douglas D L, Duckworth T, Kanis J A, *et al.*: Spinal cord dysfunction in Paget's disease of bone: Has medical treatment a vascular basis? **J Bone Joint Surg** 63B: 495-503, 1981.

343. Wilkins R H, Rengachary S S, (eds.): **Neurosurgery**. McGraw-Hill, New York, 1985.

344. Dinneen S F, Buckley T F: Spinal nerve root compression due to monostotic Paget's disease of a lumbar vertebra. **Spine** 12: 948-50, 1987.

345. Sadar E S, Walton R J, Gossman H H: Neurological dysfunction in Paget's disease of the vertebral column. **J Neurosurg** 37: 661-5, 1972.

346. Chen J-R, Rhee R S C, Wallach S, *et al.*: Neurologic disturbances in paget disease of bone: Response to calcitonin. **Neurology** 29: 448-57, 1979.

347. Human calcitonin for Paget's disease. **Med Letter** 29: 47-8, 1987.

348. Tiludronate for Paget's disease of bone. **Med Letter** 39: 65-6, 1997.

349. Risedronate for Paget's disease of bone. **Med Letter** 40: 87-8, 1998.

350. Bennett G J: Ankylosing spondylitis. **Clin Neurosurg** 37: 622-35, 1991.

351. Vender J R, McDonnell D E: Ankylosing spondylitis. **Contemp Neurosurg** 22 (25): 1-7, 2000.

352. Calin A, Porta J, Fries J F, *et al.*: Clinical history as a screening test for ankylosing spondylitis. **JAMA** 237: 2613-4, 1977.

353. Rae P S, Waddell G, Venner R M: A simple technique for measuring lumbar spinal flexion. **J R Coll Surg Edin** 29: 281-4, 1984.

354. Detwiler K N, Loftus C M, Godersky J C: Management of cervical spine injuries in patients with ankylosing spondylitis. **J Neurosurg** 72: 210-5, 1990.

355. Farhat S M, Schneider R C, Gray J M: Traumatic spinal epidural hematoma associated with cervical fractures in rheumatoid spondylitis. **J Trauma** 13: 591-9, 1973.

356. Podolsky S M, Hoffman J R, Pietrafesa C A: Neurological complications following immobilization of cervical spine fractures in a patient with ankylosing

spondylitis. **Ann Emerg Med** 12: 578-80, 1983.

357. Surin V V: Fractures of the cervical spine in patients with ankylosing spondylitis. **Acta Orthop Scand** 51: 79-84, 1980.

358. Tsuyama N: Ossification of the posterior longitudinal ligament of the spine. **Clin Orthop** 184: 71-84, 1984.

359. Nakanishi T, Mannen T, Toyokura Y: Asymptomatic ossification of the posterior longitudinal ligament of the cervical spine. **J Neurol Sci** 19: 375-81, 1973.

360. Epstein N: Diagnosis and surgical management of ossification of the posterior longitudinal ligament. **Contemp Neurosurg** 14 (22): 1-6, 1992.

361. Harsh G R, Sypert G W, Weinstein P R, *et al*.: Cervical spine stenosis secondary to ossification of the posterior longitudinal ligament. **J Neurosurg** 67: 349-57, 1987.

362. Hirabayashi K, Watanabe K, Wakano K, *et al*.: Expansive cervical laminoplasty for cervical spinal stenotic myelopathy. **Spine** 8: 693-, 1983.

363. Epstein N E, Hollingsworth R: Ossification of the cervical anterior longitudinal ligament contributing to dysphagia: Case report. **J Neurosurg** 90 (Spine 2): 261-3, 1999.

364. Burkus J K: Esophageal obstruction secondary to diffuse idiopathic skeletal hyperostosis. **Orthopedics** 11: 717-20, 1988.

365. McCafferty R R, Harrison M J, Tamas L B, *et al*.: Ossification of the anterior longitudinal ligament and Forestier's disease: An analysis of seven cases. **J Neurosurg** 83: 13-7, 1995.

366. Youmans J R, (ed.) **Neurological surgery**. 2nd ed., W. B. Saunders, Philadelphia, 1982.

367. Rosenblum B, Oldfield E H, Doppman J L, *et al*.: Spinal arteriovenous malformations: A comparison of dural arteriovenous fistulas and intradural avm's in 81 patients. **J Neurosurg** 67: 795-802, 1987.

368. Gueguen B, Merland J J, Riche M C, *et al*.: Vascular malformations of the spinal cord: Intrathecal perimedullary arteriovanous fistulas fed by medullary arteries. **Neurology** 37: 969-79, 1987.

369. Mourier K L, Gobin Y P, George B, *et al*.: Intradural perimedullary arteriovenous fistulae: Results of surgical and endovascular treatment in a series of 35 cases. **Neurosurgery** 32: 885-91, 1993.

370. Strugar J, Chyatte D: *In situ* photocoagulation of spinal dural arteriovenous malformations using the Nd:YAG laser. **J Neurosurg** 77: 571-4, 1992.

371. Bederson J B, Spetzler R F: Pathophysiology of type I spinal dural arteriovenous malformations. **BNI Quarterly** 12: 23-32, 1996.

372. Aminoff M J, Logue V: The prognosis of patients with spinal vascular malformations. **Brain** 97: 211-8, 1974.

373. Tobin W D, Layton D D: The diagnosis and natural history of spinal cord arteriovenous malformations. **Mayo Clin Proc** 51: 637-46, 1976.

374. Wirth F P, Post K D, Di Chiro G, *et al*.: Foix-Alajouanine disease. Spontaneous thrombosis of a spinal cord arteriovenous malformation: A case report. **Neurology** 20: 1114-8, 1970.

375. Criscuolo G R, Oldfield E H, Doppman J L: Reversible acute and subacute myelopathy in patients with dural arteriovenous fistulas: Foix-Alajouanine syndrome reconsidered. **J Neurosurg** 70: 354-9, 1989.

376. Barnwell S L, Dowd C F, Davis R L, *et al*.: Cryptic vascular malformations of the spinal cord: Diagnosis by magnetic resonance imaging and outcome of surgery. **J Neurosurg** 72: 403-7, 1990.

377. Anson J A, Spetzler R F: Interventional neuroradiology for spinal pathology. **Clin Neurosurg** 39: 388-417, 1991.

378. Nabors M W, Pait T G, Byrd E B, *et al*.: Updated assessment and current classification of spinal meningeal cysts. **J Neurosurg** 68: 366-77, 1988.

379. Heiss J D, Oldfield E H: Pathophysiology and treatment of syringomyelia. **Contemp Neurosurg** 25

(3): 1-8, 2003.

380. Oldfield E H, Muraszko K, Shawker T H, *et al*.: Pathophysiology of syringomyelia associated with Chiari I malformation of the cerebellar tonsils. **J Neurosurg** 80: 3-15, 1994.

381. Williams B, Terry A F, Jones F, *et al*.: Syringomyelia as a sequel to traumatic paraplegia. **Paraplegia** 19: 67-80, 1981.

382. Suzuki M, Davis C, Symon L, *et al*.: Syringoperitoneal shunt for treatment of cord cavitation. **J Neurol Neurosurg Psychiatry** 48: 620-7, 1985.

383. Booth A E, Kendall B E: Percutaneous aspiration of cystic lesions of the spinal cord. **J Neurosurg** 33: 140-4, 1970.

384. Logue V, Edwards M R: Syringomyelia and its surgical treatment. **J Neurol Neurosurg Psychiatry** 44: 273-84, 1981.

385. Kao C C, Chang L W, Bloodworth J M B: The mechanism of spinal cord cavitation following spinal cord transection: Part 2. **J Neurosurg** 46: 745-56, 1977.

386. Rossier A B, Foo D, Shillito J, *et al*.: Posttraumatic cervical syringomyelia. **Brain** 108: 439-61, 1985.

387. Vernon J D, Chir B, Silver J R, *et al*.: Posttraumatic syringomyelia. **Paraplegia** 20: 339-64, 1982.

388. Griffiths E R, McCormick C C: Posttraumatic syringomyelia (cystic myelopathy). **Paraplegia** 19: 81-8, 1981.

389. Shannon N, Symon L, Logue V, *et al*.: Clinical features, investigation and treatment of posttraumatic syringomyelia. **J Neurol Neurosurg Psychiatry** 44: 35-42, 1981.

390. Stanworth P A: The significance of hyperhidrosis in patients with posttraumatic syringomyelia. **Paraplegia** 20: 282-7, 1982.

391. Dworkin G E, Staas W E: Posttraumatic syringomyelia. **Arch Phys Med Rehabil** 66: 329-31, 1985.

392. Watson N: Ascending cystic degeneration of the cord after spinal cord injury. **Paraplegia** 19: 89-95, 1981.

393. Durward Q J, Rice G P, Ball M J, *et al*.: Selective spinal cordectomy: Clinicopathological correlation. **J Neurosurg** 56: 359-67, 1982.

394. Tekkok I H, Cataltepe K, Tahta K, *et al*.: Extradural hematoma after continuous extradural anesthesia. **Brit J Anaesth** 67: 112-5, 1991.

395. Harik S I, Raichle M E, Reis D J: Spontaneous remitting spinal epidural hematoma in a patient on anticoagulants. **N Engl J Med** 284: 1355-7, 1971.

396. Silber S H: Complete nonsurgical resolution of a spontaneous spinal epidural hematoma. **Am J Emergency Med** 14: 391-3, 1996.

397. *Neurologic complications of regional anesthesia*. In **Anesthesia for obstetrics**, Shnider S M and Levinson G, (eds.), Williams and Wilkins, Baltimore, 2nd ed., 1987: pp 319-20.

398. Sage D J: Epidurals, spinals and bleeding disorders in pregnancy: A review. **Anaesth Intens Care** 18: 319-26, 1990.

399. Gustafsson H, Rutberg H, Bengtsson M: Spinal hematoma following epidural analgesia: Report of a patient with ankylosing spondylitis and a bleeding diathesis. **Anaesthesia** 43: 220-2, 1988.

400. Dickman C A, Shedd S A, Spetzler R F, *et al*.: Spinal epidural hematoma associated with epidural anesthesia: Complications of systemic heparinization in patients receiving peripheral vascular thrombolytic therapy. 72, 1990.

401. Packer N P, Cummins B H: Spontaneous epidural hemorrhage: A surgical emergency. **Lancet** 1: 356-8, 1978.

402. Rebello M D, Dastur H M: Spinal epidural hemorrhage: A review of case reports. **Neurol India** 14: 135-45, 1966.

403. Domenicucci M, Ramieri A, Ciappetta P, *et al*.: Nontraumatic acute spinal subdural hematoma. **J Neurosurg** (Spine 1) 91: 65-73, 1999.

404. Wray C C, Easom S, Hoskinson J: Coccydynia. Etiology and treatment. **J Bone Joint Surg** 73B: 335-8, 1991.

405. Lath R, Rajshekhar V, Chacko G: Sacral hemangioma as a cause of coccydynia. **Neuroradiology** 40: 524-6, 1998.

406. Thiele G H: Coccydynia: Cause and treatment. **Dis Colon Rectum** 6: 422-35, 1963.

407. Lourie J, Young S: Avascular necrosis of the coccyx: A cause of coccydynia? Case report and histological findings in sixteen patients. **Br J Clin Pract**

39: 247-8, 1985.

408. Raj P P: *Miscelleneous pain disorders*. In **Pain medicine: A comprehensive review**, Raj P P, (ed.). C V Mosby, St. Louis, 1996, Chapter 50: pp 492-501.

409. Loev M A, Varklet V L, Wilsey B L, *et al*.: Cryoablation: A novel approach to neurolysis of the ganglion Impar. **Anesthesiology** 88: 1391-3, 1998.

410. Plancarte R, Amescua C, Patt R B, *et al*.: Superior hypogastric plexus block for pelvic cancer pain. **Anesthesiology** 73: 236-9, 1990.

15. Functional

For functional neurosurgery related to pain, see *Pain procedures*, page 390.

15.1. Brain mapping

Techniques used to identify certain areas of the brain have utility in seizure surgery as well as in treating lesions in areas of eloquent brain. Most techniques require an awake patient, with the surgery being done under local anesthesia with sedation.

Motor cortex can be localized in awake or anesthetized patients. In anesthetized patients, it is critical to reverse paralytic agents 15-30 minutes prior to applying the electrical stimulation and that a train-of-four muscle twitches can be elicited.

SSEPs may be used to locate sensory cortex in anesthetized patients (*see page 146*).

15.2. Surgical treatment of Parkinson's disease

HISTORICAL BACKGROUND

An early procedure was ligation of the anterior choroidal artery. Due to variability in distribution, destruction often extended beyond the desired confines of the pallidum and the results were too unpredictable (*see page 778*). Anterodorsal pallidotomy became an accepted procedure in the 1950's, but long-term improvement was mainly in rigidity, while tremor and bradykinesia did not improve[1]. The ventrolateral thalamus subsequently became the preferred target. Lesions there were most effective in diminishing tremor. In actuality, the tremor was often not the most debilitating symptom, particularly since it is a resting tremor at first (it may become more pervasive later), bradykinesia and rigidity were frequently more problematic. Furthermore, the procedure only reduces tremor in the contralateral half of the body, and bilateral thalamotomies were not recommended due to an unacceptably high risk of post-op dysarthria and gait disturbance. Use of thalamotomy fell off dramatically in the late 1960's with the introduction of L-dopa[2].

However, at some point most patients will experience problematic side effects and/or resistance to treatment with antiparkinsonian drugs. Tissue transplantation (e g with adrenal medullary tissue) appears to have only modest benefits (*see below*). Lesioning or stimulation techniques have therefore gained in popularity with renewed interest in the posteroventral pallidum as the target.

TISSUE TRANSPLANTATION

Tissue transplantation for Parkinson's disease is generally limited to research centers. The present status of implantation of fetal dopaminergic brain cells into Parkinson's disease patients is that it may reduce the severity of the illness and increase the effectiveness of levodopa[3]. For ethical reasons, this procedure is rarely performed in the U.S.

Other transplanted tissues include cells from the patients own adrenal medulla. After initial enthusiastic results[4], later studies failed to corroborate the dramatic outcomes, and benefits appear to be modest[5-7]. A double-blinded, randomized, placebo-controlled trial[58] of 34 subjects with severe PD noted initial improvement at 6 and 9 months, but found no efficacy 2 years after fetal mesencephalic cell transplantation. Of note: immunosuppression was only used for six months. Further research is ongoing[59].

PALLIDOTOMY[8, 9]

Pallidotomy may work by one of the following mechanisms: directly destroying portions of the internal segment of the globus pallidus (**GPi**), interrupting pallidofugal pathways, or diminishing inputs to the medial pallidum (especially from the subthalamic nucleus) (see *Pathophysiology*, page 47). Although early methodologies included stereotactic radiosurgery[10], modern techniques (excluding very select cases) rely primarily on radiofrequency or cryoprobe lesioning after confirming target location by electrical stimulation.

Electrical stimulation: Deep brain stimulation in the area of the GPi[11] and subthalamic nucleus can also relieve parkinsonian symptoms[12] without irreversibly destroying tissue.

Indications
1. patients refractory to medical therapy (including multiple agents). However, some investigators feel the response to pallidotomy might be better if done early
2. primary indication (based on an opinion survey[13]): patients with levodopa-induced dyskinesias (especially those with associated painful muscle spasms). Initial results indicate that these are very responsive to pallidotomy
3. patients primarily with rigidity or bradykinesia (unilateral or bilateral), on-off fluctuations or dystonia. Tremor may be present, but if it is the predominant symptom, then using the ventralis intermedius (**VIM**) nucleus of the thalamus as the target (for ablation (thalamotomy) or stimulation)[14] is a better procedure

Contraindications
1. patients with significant dementia: further cognitive impairment has been noted primarily in patients with cognitive deficits prior to treatment
2. patients with risk of intracerebral hemorrhage: those with coagulopathy, poorly controlled hypertension, those on anti-platelet drugs that cannot be withheld (may consider stereotactic radiosurgery lesions for these rare patients)
3. patients with ipsilateral hemianopsia: due to the risk of post-op contralateral hemianopsia from optic tract injury which would make the patient blind
4. age ≥ 85 yrs
5. patients with secondary Parkinsonism (*see page 47* for more details) i.e. not idiopathic Parkinson's disease: respond poorly, presumably due to different pathophysiology. Look for:
   A. signs of autonomic nervous system dysfunction (suggests Shy-Drager)
   B. EOM abnormalities (may occur in progressive supranuclear palsy (**PSNP**))
   C. long-tract signs
   D. cerebellar findings (as in olivo-ponto-cerebellar atrophy (**OPCA**))
   E. failure to improve with levodopa
   F. MRI: lacunar infarcts in basal ganglia (as in arteriosclerotic Parkinsonism), or tumor in region of substantia nigra
   G. PET scanning (if available): decreased striatal metabolism detected by deoxyglucose PET scan (suggests striato-nigral degeneration (**SND**))

TECHNIQUE
Antiparkinsonian medications are withheld the morning of the procedure to bring out symptoms.

RESULTS
At present, the major focus of therapy has been on improvement of *motor* symptoms. Although 97% of patients showed at least some improvement (some poor results may derive from inclusion of some patients with secondary Parkinsonism), in 17% the degree of improvement was graded as mild.

Significant reduction of levodopa induced dyskinesias occurred in 90%.Bradykinesia improved in 85%, rigidity in 75%, and tremor in 57%. Other areas of improvement include: speech, gait, posture, and reduction of on-off phenomenon and freezing. Although symptoms may be ameliorated, overall functional improvement may not be remarkable[15].

Although dosages of antiparkinsonian medication are often reduced, continued medical therapy is usually required, and no change is made for at least 2 months following pallidotomy.

Indications are that beneficial surgical effects can last ≥ 5 years, with early failures possibly due to production of too small of a lesion, and late failures possibly due to progression of the disease.

Ongoing studies are investigating longer term results, microelectrode recording, alternate lesioning targets, the role of early surgery... Until more information is available, one cannot make any statements about the optimal target, localizing method, etc.

COMPLICATIONS
Visual field deficit occurs in 2.5% due to proximity of the optic tract to the globus pallidus. Hemiparesis may occur due to the nearby passage of the internal capsule. Intracerebral hemorrhage may also occur. Dysarthria occurs in ≈ 8%, but is usually temporary. Speech difficulties and also cognitive decline may be more risky when bilateral pallidotomies are performed at the same sitting.

15.3. Spasticity

Results from lesions in upper motor neuron pathway, causing absence of inhibitory influence on alpha motor-neurons (αMN) (alpha spasticity) as well as on gamma motor neurons (intrafusal fibers) (gamma spasticity). Causes uninhibited reflex arc between αMN and Ia afferents from muscle spindles resulting in a hypertonic state of muscles with clonus, and sometimes with involuntary movements. Etiologies include: injury to cerebrum (e.g. stroke) or spinal cord (spasticity is an expected sequelae of spinal cord injury rostral to the conus medullaris), multiple sclerosis, and congenital abnormalities (e.g. cerebral palsy, spinal dysraphism).

CLINICAL
Increased resistance to passive movement, hyperactive muscle stretch reflexes, simultaneous activation of antagonistic muscle groups, may occur spontaneously or in response to minimal stimuli. Characteristic postures include scissoring of legs or hyperflexion of thighs. May be painful, or may disrupt patient's ability to sit in wheelchair, lay in bed, drive modified vehicles, sleep, etc. May also promote development of decubitus ulcers. A spastic bladder will have low capacity and will empty spontaneously.

Spasticity is often exacerbated by same type of stimuli that aggravate autonomic hyperreflexia (see *Autonomic hyperreflexia*, page 755).

The onset of spasticity following spinal cord injury may be delayed for several days to months (the latency period is attributed to "**spinal shock**", during which time there is decreased tone and reflexes)[16] (*see page 698*). Onset of spasticity following spinal shock starts with increasing flexor synergistic activity over 3-6 mos, with more gradual increases of extensor synergy which ultimately predominates in most cases.

Some "beneficial" aspects of mild spasticity:
1. maintains muscle tone and therefore bulk: provides support for patient when sitting in wheelchair, helps prevent decubitus ulcers over bony prominences
2. muscle contractions may help prevent DVTs
3. may be useful in bracing

Grading spasticity
Assessment should be performed with patient supine and relaxed. The Ashworth scale (*see Table 15-1*) is commonly used for the clinical grading of the severity of spasticity. Many attempts have been made to quantitate spasticity electrodiagnostically, the most reliable has been H-reflex measurement.

Table 15-1   Ashworth scores[17]

Ashworth score	Degree of muscle tone
1	no increase in tone (normal)
2	slight increase, a "catch" when affected part is flexed or extended
3	more marked increase, passive movements easy
4	considerable increase, passive movements difficult
5	affected part rigid in flexion or extension

TREATMENT
Depends on extent of useful function (or potential for same) present in areas at and below spasticity. Complete spinal cord injuries usually have little function, whereas patients with MS may have significant function.

1. "prevention": measures to decrease inciting stimuli (physical therapy to prevent joint damage, good skin and bladder care… see *Autonomic hyperreflexia*, page 755)
2. prolonged stretching (more than just range of motion): not only prevents joint and muscle contractures, but modulates spasticity
3. oral medications[18] (see *Surgical treatment* below for intrathecal medications): few drugs are effective without significant undesirable side effects
   A. diazepam (Valium®): activates GABA$_A$ receptors, increases pre-synaptic inhibition of αMN. Most useful in patients with complete spinal cord injuries. *Rx* start with 2 mg PO BID-TID, increase by 2 mg per day q 3 days up to a max of 20 mg TID.
   SIDE EFFECTS: may cause sedation, weakness, decreased stamina (most of which may be minimized by gradual increases in dosage). Abrupt discontinuation may cause depression, seizures, withdrawal syndrome
   B. baclofen (Lioresal®): activates GABA$_B$ receptors, causes pre-synaptic inhibition of αMN and decreases nociception. May be most useful in patients with spinal cord lesions (complete or incomplete).
   Rx start with 5 mg PO BID-TID, increase in 5 mg increments q 3 days up to max of 20 mg QID. SIDE EFFECTS: sedation, lowers seizure threshold. Must be tapered to discontinue (abrupt discontinuation may result in seizures, rebound hyper-spasticity or hallucinations).
   C. dantrolene (Dantrium®): reduces depolarization induced Ca^{++} influx into sarcoplasmic reticulum of skeletal muscle; acts on all skeletal muscle (with no preferential effect on spasmogenic reflex arc).
   Rx start with 25 mg PO q d, increase q 4-7 days to BID, TID, then QID, then by 25 mg per day up to max of ≈ 100 mg QID (may take 1 week at new steady state to see effect); SIDE EFFECTS: muscle weakness (may make ambulation impossible), sedation, idiosyncratic hepatitis (may be fatal; more common in patients on > 300 mg/d x > 2 mos) that is often preceded by anorexia, abdominal pain, N/V; D/C if no benefit is seen by ≈ 45 days; follow LFTs (SGPT or SGOT)
   D. progabide: activates both GABA$_A$ and GABA$_B$ receptors. Useful for patients with severe flexor spasms
   E. theoretical benefits may be derived from other agents, but they have not been used for some practical reason in each case [16] (e.g. phenothiazines reduce gamma spasticity, but only at high PO doses or parenterally; clonidine; Darvon; tetrahydrocannabinal…)

SURGICAL TREATMENT
Reserved for spasticity refractory to medical treatment, or where side effects of medications are intolerable. Generally either orthopedic (e.g. tendon release operations (tenotomies) of heel cord or hamstrings, iliopsoas myotomies, etc.) or neurosurgical (e.g. nerve blocks, neurectomies, myelotomy, etc.).
1. nonablative procedures
   A. intrathecal **(IT)** baclofen (*see below*)
   B. intrathecal morphine (tolerance and dependence may develop)
   C. electrical stimulation via percutaneously placed epidural electrodes[19]
2. ablative procedures, with preservation of potential for ambulation
   A. motor point block[16] (intramuscular phenol neurolysis): preserves sensation and existing voluntary function. Especially useful in patients with incomplete myelopathies; time consuming
   B. phenol nerve block: similar to motor point block, but used when spasticity more severe and complete block of muscle desired. Open phenol block used instead of percutaneous when nerve is mixed and sensory preservation is desired (also reduces post-block dysesthesias)[20]
   C. selective neurectomies[16]
      1. sciatic neurectomy (may be done with RF lesion)[21]
      2. obturator neurectomy: useful if strong hip adductor spasticity that causes scissoring and wasted energy expenditure in ambulating
      3. pudendal neurectomy: useful if excessive detrusor dyssynergy interferes with bladder retraining
   D. percutaneous radiofrequency foraminal rhizotomy: small unmyelinated sensory fibers are more sensitive to RF lesions than larger myelinated A-

alpha fibers of motor units.

Technique: start at S1 on one side, and work up to T12, then repeat on other side. At each level: verify needle position by stimulating with 0.1-0.5 V and watch for movement in appropriate myotome (tip should be extradural, avoid subarachnoid placement), ablate with 70-80° C **x** 2 mins for S1, and 70° C x 2 mins for L5 to T12 (to preserve motor function). If symptoms recur, may repeat with lesions at 90° C x 2 mins

E. myelotomies[22]
1. Bischof's myelotomy: divides anterior and posterior horns via laterally placed incision, disrupts reflex arc. No effect on α–spasticity
2. midline "T" myelotomy: interrupts reflex arc from sensory to motor units without disrupting connections from corticospinal tract to anterior motor neurons. Slightly higher risk of losing motor function. *Technique*: laminectomy from T11 to L1. Mobilize midline dorsal longitudinal vein and incise cord in midline from T12 at a depth of 3 mm to S1 at a depth of 4 mm (preserving S2-S4 maintains bladder reflex pathways. Unilateral extension up to conus medullaris reduces bladder spasticity and increases capacity before reflex emptying occurs)

F. selective dorsal rhizotomy[23, 24]: uses intraoperative EMG and electophysiological stimulation to eliminate sensory rootlets involved in "handicapping spasticity" (leaves rootlets subserving "useful spasticity" intact). Interrupts the afferent limb of pathologic reflex arc. May be temporary, but seems to persist at least ≈ 5 yrs. No effect on α–spasticity. Ambulatory children with cerebral palsy have improved gait, nonambulatory children are improved but are still not able to ambulate afterwards

G. stereotactic thalamotomy or dentatotomy: may be useful in cerebral palsy[25]. Useful for unilateral dystonia, but cannot be used for bilateral dystonia as bilateral lesions would be required which jeopardizes speech. Effective only for dystonia <u>distal</u> to shoulders or hips, and should not be used if the condition is rapidly progressive

3. ablative procedures, with <u>sacrifice</u> of potential for ambulation (in complete cord injuries, nonablative procedures are not indicated because there is no motor function to recover). Used after failure of percutaneous rhizotomy (*see above*) and "T" myelotomy (*see above*)

A. intrathecal injection of 6 ml of 10% phenol (by weight) in glycerin mixed with 4 ml of iohexol (Omnipaque® 300) (*see page 127*) for a final concentration of 6% phenol and ≈ 120 mg iodine/ml. Administered via LP at L2-3 interspace with patient in lateral decubitus position (most symptomatic side down) under fluoro until T12-S1 nerve root sleeves are filled (sparing S2-4 for bladder function). Patient is maintained in this position **x** 20-30 mins and then kept sitting upright **x** 4 hrs[26] (absolute alcohol provides more permanent blocks, but is hypobaric and more difficult to control)

B. selective anterior rhizotomy: results in flaccid paralysis with denervation atrophy of muscles

C. neurectomies, often combined with tenotomies[21]

D. intramuscular neurolysis by phenol injection[21]

E. cordectomy[27]: most drastic measure, reserved for patients who do not respond to any other measure. Results in total flaccidity with loss of benefits from mild spasticity. Converts bladder from UMN to LMN control. Works well for progressive deficit from syringomyelia and for spasticity, but poor for "phantom" leg pain[28]

F. cordotomy: rarely used

Table 15-2 Selection criteria for baclofen pump

• age 18-65 yrs (older patients treated on compassionate use basis)
• able to give informed consent
• severe, chronic spasticity (≥ 12 mos duration) due to spinal cord lesion or MS
• spasticity refractory to oral drugs (including baclofen), or unacceptable side effects
• no CSF block (e.g. on myelography)
• positive response to IT baclofen at test dose ≤ 100 μg and no response to placebo
• no implanted programmable device such as cardiac pacemaker*
• females of childbearing potential: not pregnant & using adequate contraception
• no hypersensitivity (allergy) to baclofen
• no history of stroke, impaired renal function, or severe hepatic or GI disease

* this study used a programmable IT pump

INTRATHECAL BACLOFEN[29-32]

Selection criteria used in one study[31] are shown in *Table 15-2*.

Test doses: Incremental test doses of 50, 75, and then 100 µg IT baclofen via lumbar puncture or temporary catheter were used[31], randomly alternated with placebo, with dose escalation halted if a response to active drug occurred. The following parameters were evaluated at 0.5, 1, 2, 4, 8 & 24 hrs post injection: pulse and respiratory rate, BP, hypertonia (Ashworth score, see *Table 15-1*, page 367), reflexes, spasm score, voluntary muscle movement, and adverse effects (if any, including seizures). Pump implantation was offered if there was a 2 point reduction in the Ashworth score and muscle spasm score for ≥ 4 hrs after bolus injection of active drug without intolerable side effects.

Alternatively, give 25 µg IT in the O.R., and if the patient improves, insert subcutaneous pump[18].

Table 15-3   Complications*

Complications
• mechanical problems
• pump underinfusion
• catheter problems: occlusion, kink, dislodgment, cut, break or disconnection
• wound complications
• pocket erosion
• incisional pain
• infection
• seroma (may require aspiration)
• CSF collection

*   device-related complications requiring a secondary invasive procedure

Pump systems: Available systems include Synchromed, manufactured by Medtronics, Inc., Minneapolis, MN.

Complications: Device-related complications are shown in *Table 15-3*. The frequency of most is ≈ 1%, except catheter-related problems which had a rate of ≈ 30% [31].

15.4.   Torticollis

AKA wry neck. A form of dystonia resulting in a failure to control head position (if shoulders or trunk are also involved, *dystonia* is a more proper label).

A symptom of diverse causes. Differential diagnosis includes:
1. congenital torticollis (may be the initial presentation of dystonia musculorum deformans)
2. **spasmodic torticollis**, AKA wry neck: a specific subtype of torticollis that is idiopathic by definition. The shortened sternocleidomastoid **(SCM)** muscle is usually in spasm
3. extrapyramidal lesions (including degenerative): often alleviated by lying down; EMG shows abnormal grouped activity
4. psychogenic (often mentioned, seldom verified)
5. torticollis from atlantoaxial rotatory subluxation: (*see page 721*) the elongated SCM may be in spasm (opposite of that in spasmodic torticollis)
6. neurovascular compression of the 11th nerve (*see below*)
7. hemorrhage into sternocleidomastoid muscle (with subsequent contracture)
8. infection of the cervical spine
9. cervical adenitis
10. syringomyelia
11. cerebellar tumors in children
12. bulbar palsies
13. "pseudotorticollis" may develop as an unconscious correction to reduce diplopia that occurs with imbalance of extraocular eye musculature

Non-surgical treatment of torticollis
Should be attempted first, and includes:
1. relaxation training, including biofeedback
2. thorough neuropsychiatric evaluation
3. trans-epidermal neuro-stimulation **(TENS)** to the neck

Surgical procedures
Reserved for disabling, refractory cases. Includes:
1. dorsal cord stimulation
2. local injection of botulinum toxin: may work for retrocollis, is poor for lateral torticollis (must inject posterior cervicals and both SCM, and may cause temporary pharyngeal muscle dysfunction resulting in dysphagia), and is totally ineffective for anterocollis

3. selective rhizotomy and spinal accessory nerve section

Other treatments for torticollis include
1. stereotactic electrocoagulation of Forel's H_1 field

TORTICOLLIS OF 11TH NERVE ORIGIN
1. usually a horizontal type (manifests as horizontal head movement) which may be exacerbated when supine (unlike extrapyramidal torticollis)
2. contraction of SCM is usually accompanied by activity in contralateral agonist muscles
3. may be treated surgically. Procedures include
   A. sectioning of the anastomotic branches between the 11th nerve and the upper cervical posterior root (C_1 anastomotic branch is sensory only)
   B. microvascular decompression of the 11th nerve (most cases caused by vertebral artery, but PICA compression is also described[33]). Relief takes several weeks post-op

15.5. Neurovascular compression syndromes

This section considers those syndromes due to compression of cranial nerves at the root entry zone (**REZ**) (or in the case of motor nerves, root *exit* zone) other than trigeminal neuralgia (see *Trigeminal neuralgia*, page 378 for a discussion of that entity). The REZ (AKA Obersteiner-Redlich zone) is the point where central myelin (from oligodendroglial cells) changes to peripheral myelin (from Schwann cells).
Includes: hemifacial spasm, disabling positional vertigo, some forms of torticollis of 11th nerve origin (see *Torticollis* above).

15.5.1. Hemifacial spasm

Hemifacial spasm (**HFS**) is a condition of intermittent, painless, involuntary, spasmodic contractions of muscles innervated by the facial nerve in one side of the face only. May be limited to the upper or lower half only, and excess lacrimation may be present. The condition usually begins with rare contractions of the orbicularis oculi, and slowly progresses to involve the entire half of the face and increases in frequency until the ability to see out of the affected eye is impaired. It must be distinguished from **facial myokymia** (*continuous* facial spasm) which may be a manifestation of an intrinsic brainstem glioma or of multiple sclerosis. Also in the differential diagnosis is **blepharospasm** (bilateral spasmodic closure of the orbicularis oculi muscles) which is more common in the elderly, and may be associated with organic brain syndrome. Blepharospasm is notorious for disappearing when the patient presents for medical evaluation (an effect of alerting), but may be elicited by asking patient to gently close the eyes and then rapidly open them, following which a blepharospam may occur.
HFS and **palatal myoclonus** are the only involuntary movement disorders that persist during sleep[34]. HFS may be associated with trigeminal neuralgia, geniculate neuralgia (see *Tic convulsif* page 386), or vestibular and/or cochlear[35] nerve dysfunction.
HFS is more common in women, is seen more often on the left, and usually presents after the teenages. Auditory function testing reveals abnormal acoustic middle ear reflex in almost half of patients, indicating some degree of VIII compromise[35].

ETIOLOGY
HFS is usually caused by compression of the facial nerve at the root exit zone (**REZ**) by a vessel, which is most often an artery (most commonly AICA[36] (either pre- or postmeatal[37]), but other vascular possibilities include an elongated PICA, SCA, a tortuous VA, the cochlear artery, a dolichoectatic basilar artery, AICA branches...), a vascular malformation, and rarely, veins have been implicated. In typical HFS (onset in the orbicularis oculi, and progressing downward over the face), the vessel impinges on the anterocaudal aspect of the VII/VIII nerve complex, in atypical HFS (beginning in the buccal muscles and progressing upward over the face) the compression is rostral or posterior to VII[38].

Vessels contacting the REZ of the vestibular nerve may cause vertigo, whereas tinnitus or hearing loss may result from cochlear nerve REZ compression.

Infrequently, benign tumors or a cyst in the cerebellopontine angle, multiple sclerosis, adhesions, or osseous skull deformities will be the cause of HFS.

Evidence indicates that there is not cross (ephaptic) conduction at the compressed REZ, but that the facial motonucleus is involved secondarily as a result of the REZ compression, via a phenomenon similar to kindling[39]. In addition to the spasm, a 2nd electrophysiological phenomenon associated with HFS is **synkinesis**, where stimulation of one branch of the facial nerve results in delayed discharges through another branch (average latency: 11 mSec[40]).

EVALUATION

In typical cases of HFS, the diagnostic workup is negative.

Most patients should have MRI of the posterior fossa (CT scan is less sensitive here) to R/O tumors or AVMs.

Vertebral angiography is usually not performed if imaging is normal. The neurovascular compression responsible for HFS usually cannot be identified on angiography.

TREATMENT

MEDICAL MANAGEMENT

HFS is generally a surgical condition. Early, mild cases may be managed expectantly. Carbamazepine and phenytoin are generally ineffective, unlike the situation with the causally similar condition of trigeminal neuralgia. Local injection of **botulinum toxin** (Oculinum®) may be effective in treating HFS and/or blepharospasm[41, 42].

SURGICAL MANAGEMENT

Many ablative procedures are effective for HFS (including sectioning of divisions of the facial nerve), however, this leaves the patient with some degree of facial paresis. The current procedure of choice for HFS is microvascular decompression **(MVD)** wherein the offending vessel is physically moved off of the nerve, and a sponge (e.g. Ivalon®, polyvinyl formyl alcohol foam) is interposed as a cushion. Other cushions may not prove to be as satisfactory (muscle may disappear, and Teflon felt may thin[43]).

Most often, the offending vessel approaches the nerve at a right angle, and causes grooving in the nerve. Compression must occur at the root exit zone; decompression of vessels impinging distal to this area is usually ineffective.

Operative risks of MVD (sometimes transient): facial weakness in 1-2%; hearing loss (partial or total) in 10-30% (severe in 2.8% in one series[35], 15% in another series[44]), ataxia in 1%.

Post-operatively, there may episodes of mild HFS, however they usually begin to diminish 2-3 days following MVD. Severe spasm that does not abate suggests failure to achieve adequate decompression, and reoperation should be considered.

Surgical results of MVD depends on the duration of symptoms (shorter duration has better prognosis) as well as on the age of the patient (elderly patients do less well). Complete resolution of HFS occurred in 44 (81%) of 54 patients undergoing MVD, however, 6 of these patients had relapse[44]. 5 patients (9%) had partial improvement, and 5 (9%) had no relief.

Technique of MVD

Intra-operative brainstem auditory evoked potential (BSAER)[45], or more applicable, direct VIII nerve monitoring[46] may help prevent hearing loss during MVD for 7th or 8th nerve dysfunction. Furthermore, monitoring for the disappearance of the (delayed) synkinetic response may aid in determining when adequate decompression has been achieved (generally reserved for teaching institutions)[39].

SURGICAL RESULTS

Complete resolution of spasm occurs in ≈ 85-93%[43, 47-50]. Spasm is diminished in 9%, and unchanged in 6%[50]. Of 29 patients with complete relief, 25 (86%) had immediate post-op resolution, and the remaining 4 patients took from 3 mos to 3 yrs to attain quiescence.

Recurrence
    Return of symptoms after a period of complete resolution of HFS occurs in up to 10% of patients, 86% of recurrences happen within 2 yrs of surgery, and the risk of developing recurrence after 2 yrs of post-op relief is only ≈ 1%[50].

Complications
    Ipsilateral total hearing loss occurs in ≈ 13% (range: 1.6-15%), partial hearing loss in 6%, transient facial weakness in 18%, permanent facial weakness in 6%[48], ataxia in 6%. Other complications that are minor or temporary include aseptic meningitis (AKA hemogenic meningitis) in 8.2%, hoarseness or dysphagia in 14%, CSF rhinorrhea in 0.3%, perioral herpes in 3%[51].

15.6.   Hyperhidrosis[52]

    Either essential (primary, or idiopathic) or secondary (etiologies include: hyperthyroidism, diabetes mellitus, pheochromocytoma, acromegaly, parkinsonism, CNS trauma, syringomyelia, hypothalamic tumors, menopause).
    Due to overactivity of eccrine sweat glands (found over entire body, highest concentration in palms and soles of feet). They produce a hypotonic secretion with saline as the primary constituent. These glands are under control of the sympathetic nervous system, however, the neurotransmitter is paradoxically acetycholine (i.e. they are cholinergic, unlike most sympathetic end organs which are adrenergic). Most eccrine sweat glands serve a thermoregulatory function, however, those on the palms and soles respond primarily to emotional stress.
    Essential hyperhidrosis is a generalized condition that usually manifests mostly in the palms. The incidence is unknown, although it was ≈ 1% in an Israeli study (probably high).

Treatment
Mild cases are treated medically with:
1. topical agents: astringents (potassium permanganate, tannic acid…) or antiperspirants (contact dermatitis usually limits use of these agents)
2. or systemically with anticholinergics: including atropine, probantheline bromide… (side effects of dry mouth and blurred vision usually limits use of these)
3. tap water iontophoresis: may produce keratinization of palmar epithelium

    Severe cases refractory to medical therapy may be candidates for surgical sympathectomy (see below).

15.7.   Tremor

    Thalamotomy or thalamic stimulation may be useful for tremors that are refractory to medical treatment (including parkinsonian (see page 366), essential, cerebellar and post-traumatic)[14].

15.8.   Sympathectomy

Cardiac sympathectomy
    With the advances in percutaneous coronary artery techniques, cardiovascular surgery and drugs, cardiac sympathectomy for angina pectoris has found less application. However, it may still be useful in patients who have no further treatment options. Bilateral sympathectomy from the stellate ganglion through the T7 ganglia is required. Newer thoracoscopic techniques may revive some interest in this.

Table 15-4 Indications for UE sympathectomy

• essential hyperhidrosis
• primary Raynaud's disease
• shoulder-hand syndrome
• intractable angina
• ± causalgia major (see page 389)

UPPER EXTREMITY SYMPATHECTOMY

Various pathologies that may be indications for upper extremity sympathectomy are shown in *Table 15-4*.

Removal of the only second thoracic ganglion is probably adequate, and avoids a Horner's syndrome in most. Techniques used include: anterior transthoracic, thoracic endoscopic[53], percutaneous radiofrequency, and supraclavicular. An approach via a midline posterior incision with a T3 costotransversectomy allows bilateral access[52, 54]. The risk of significant complications is ≈ 5% and include pneumothorax, intercostal neuralgia, spinal cord injury, and Horner's syndrome.

UPPER THORACIC SYMPATHECTOMY

Approaches include:
1. posterior paravertebral approach
2. axillary thoracotomy with transthoracic exposure of the sympathetic chain
3. supraclavicular, retropleural exposure
4. percutaneous radiofrequency technique[55, 56]
5. video endoscopic approach[57]

LUMBAR SYMPATHECTOMY

Primary indication is for causalgia major of the lower extremity. Preoperative lumbar sympathetic blocks may be utilized to evaluate patient for response.

Removal of the L2 and L3 sympathetic ganglion is usually adequate to remove sympathetic tone from the lower extremities (occasionally L1 and sometimes T12 are also removed for causalgia of the thigh).

The most common approach is a retroperitoneal approach through a flank incision. The patient is placed in a lateral oblique position, and the skin incision is made from the anterior superior iliac spine to the tip of the 12th rib. The peritoneum is dissected down from the muscular wall and is retracted anteriorly. The kidney and ureter are retracted anteriorly; injury to the ureter being a major risk of the operation. The sympathetic chain is identified on the lateral aspect of the vertebral bodies. The vena cava makes a right-sided approach more difficult as the aorta is easier to deal with on left-sided approaches.

15.9.   References

1. Laitinen L V, Bergenheim A T, Hariz M I: Leksell's posteroventral pallidotomy in the treatment of Parkinson's disease. **J Neurosurg** 76: 53-61, 1992.
2. Gildenberg P L: Whatever happened to stereotactic surgery? **Neurosurgery** 20: 983-7, 1987.
3. Fahn S: Fetal-tissue transplantation in Parkinson's disease. **N Engl J Med** 327: 1589-90, 1992 (editorial).
4. Madrazo I, Drucker-Colin R, Diaz V, *et al.*: Open microsurgical autograft of adrenal medulla to the right caudate nucleus in two patients with intractable Parkinson's disease. **N Engl J Med** 316: 831-4, 1987.
5. Penn R D, Goetz C G, Tanner C M, *et al.*: The adrenal medullary transplant operation for Parkinson's disease: Clinical observation in five patients. **Neurosurgery** 22: 999-1004, 1988.
6. Goetz C G, Stebbins G T, Klawans H L, *et al.*: United parkinson foundation neurotransplantation registry on adrenal medullary transplants: Presurgical, and 1- and 2-year follow-up. **Neurology** 41: 1719-22, 1991.
7. Boyer K L, Bakay R A E: The history, theory, and present status of brain transplantation. **Neurosurg Clin North Amer** 6: 113-25, 1995.
8. Iacono R P, Shima F, Lonser R R, *et al.*: The results, indications, and physiology of posteroventral palli-

dotomy for patients with Parkinson's disease. **Neurosurgery** 36: 1118-27, 1995.
9. Kondziolka D, Bonaroti E A, Lunsford L D: Pallidotomy for Parkinson's disease. **Contemp Neurosurg** 18 (6): 1-6, 1996.
10. Leksell L: Stereotactic radiosurgery. **J Neurol Neurosurg Psychiatry** 46: 797-803, 1983.
11. Iacono R P, Lonser R R, Mandybur G, *et al.*: Stimulation of the globus pallidus in Parkinson's disease. **Br J Neurosurg** 9: 505-10, 1995.
12. Limousin P, Pollack P, Benazzouz A, *et al.*: Bilateral subthalamic nucleus stimulation for severe Parkinson's disease. **Mov Disord** 10: 672-4, 1995.
13. Favre J, Taha J M, Nguyen T T, *et al.*: Pallidotomy: A survey of current practice in North America. **Neurosurgery** 39: 883-92, 1996.
14. Jankovic J, Cardoso F, Grossman R G, *et al.*: Outcome after stereotactic thalamotomy for parkinsonian, essential, and other types of tremor. **Neurosurgery** 37: 680-7, 1995.
15. Sutton J P, Couldwell W, Lew M F, *et al.*: Ventroposterior medial pallidotomy in patients with advanced Parkinson's disease. **Neurosurgery** 36: 1112-7, 1995.
16. Merritt J L: Management of spasticity in spinal cord injury. **Mayo Clin Proc** 56: 614-22, 1981.
17. Ashworth B: Preliminary trial of carisoprodal in multiple sclerosis. **Practitioner** 192: 540-2, 1964.
18. Scott B A, Pulliam M W: Management of spasticity and painful spasms in paraplegia. **Contemp Neurosurg** 9: 1-6, 1987.
19. Richardson R R, Cerullo L J, McLone D G, *et al.*: Percutaneous epidural neurostimulation in modula-

tion of paraplegic spasticity. **Acta Neurochir** 49: 235-43, 1979.

20. Garland D E, Lucie R S, Waters R L: Current use of open phenol block for adult acquired spasticity. **Clin Ortho Rel Res** 165: 217-22, 1982.

21. Herz D A, Looman J E, Tiberio A, *et al.*: The management of paralytic spasticity. **Neurosurgery** 26: 300-6, 1990.

22. Padovani R, Tognetti F, Pozzati E, *et al.*: The treatment of spasticity by means of dorsal longitudinal myelotomy and lozenge-shaped griseotomy. **Spine** 7: 103-9, 1982.

23. Privat J M, Benezech J, Frerebeau P, *et al.*: Sectorial posterior rhizotomy, a new technique of surgical treatment for spasticity. **Acta Neurochir** 35: 181-95, 1976.

24. Sindou M, Millet M F, Mortamais J, *et al.*: Results of selective posterior rhizotomy in the treatment of painful and spastic paraplegia secondary to multiple sclerosis. **Appl Neurophysiol** 45: 335-40, 1982.

25. Gornall P, Hitchcock E, Kirkland I S: Stereotaxic neurosurgery in the management of cerebral palsy. **Dev Med Child Neurol** 17: 279-86, 1975.

26. Scott B A, Weinstein Z, Chiteman R, *et al.*: Intrathecal phenol and glycerin in metrizamide for treatment of intractable spasms in paraplegia. **J Neurosurg** 63: 125-7, 1985.

27. McCarty C S: The treatment of spastic paraplegia by selective spinal cordectomy. **J Neurosurg** 11: 539-45, 1954.

28. Durward Q J, Rice G P, Ball M J, *et al.*: Selective spinal cordectomy: Clinicopathological correlation. **J Neurosurg** 56: 359-67, 1982.

29. Albright A L, Cervi A, Singletary J: Intrathecal baclofen for spasticity in cerebral palsy. **JAMA** 265: 1418-22, 1991.

30. Penn R D: Intrathecal baclofen for spasticity of spinal origin: Seven years of experience. **J Neurosurg** 77: 236-40, 1992.

31. Coffey R J, Cahill D, Steers W, *et al.*: Intrathecal baclofen for intractable spasticity of spinal origin: Results of a long-term multicenter study. **J Neurosurg** 78: 226-32, 1993.

32. Albright A L, Barron W B, Fasick P, *et al.*: Continuous intrathecal baclofen infusion for spasticity of cerebral origin. **JAMA** 270: 2475-7, 1993.

33. Shima F, Fukui M, Kitamura K, *et al.*: Diagnosis and surgical treatment of spasmodic torticollis of 11th nerve origin. **Neurosurgery** 22: 358-63, 1988.

34. Tew J M, Yeh H S: Hemifacial spasm. **Neurosurgery (Japan)** 2: 267-78, 1983.

35. Moller M B, Moller A R: Loss of auditory function in microvascular decompression for hemifacial spasm: Results in 143 consecutive cases. **J Neurosurg** 63: 17-20, 1985.

36. Yeh H S, Tew J M, Ramirez R M: Microsurgical treatment of intractable hemifacial spasm. **Neurosurgery** 9: 383-6, 1981.

37. Martin R G, Grant J L, Peace D, *et al.*: Microsurgical relationships of the anterior inferior cerebellar artery and the facial-vestibulocochlear nerve complex. **Neurosurgery** 6: 483-507, 1980.

38. Wilkins R H, Rengachary S S, (eds.): **Neurosurgery**. McGraw-Hill, New York, 1985.

39. Moller A R, Jannetta P J: Microvascular decompression in hemifacial spasm: Intraoperative electrophysiological observations. **Neurosurgery** 16: 612-8, 1985.

40. Moller A R, Jannetta P J: Hemifacial spasm: Results of electrophysiologic recording during microvascular decompression operations. **Neurology** 35: 969-74, 1985.

41. Dutton J J, Buckley E G: Botulinum toxin in the management of blepharospasm. **Arch Neurol** 43: 380-2, 1986.

42. Kennedy R H, Bartley G B, Flanagan J C, *et al.*: Treatment of blepharospasm with botulinum toxin. **Mayo Clin Proc** 64: 1085-90, 1989.

43. Rhoton A L: Comment on Payner T D and Tew J M: Recurrence of hemifacial spasm after microvascular decompression. **Neurosurgery** 38: 691, 1996.

44. Auger R G, Peipgras D G, Laws E R: Hemifacial spasm: Results of microvascular decompression of the facial nerve in 54 patients. **Mayo Clin Proc** 61: 640-4, 1986.

45. Friedman W A, Kaplan B J, Gravenstein D, *et al.*: Intraoperative brain-stem auditory evoked potentials during posterior fossa microvascular decompression. **J Neurosurg** 62: 552-7, 1985.

46. Moller A R, Jannetta P J: Monitoring auditory functions during cranial nerve microvascular decompression operations by direct recording from the eighth nerve. **J Neurosurg** 59: 493-9, 1983.

47. Jannetta P J: Neurovascular compression in cranial nerve and systemic disease. **Ann Surg** 192: 518-25, 1980.

48. Loeser J D, Chen J: Hemifacial spasm: Treatment by microsurgical facial nerve decompression. **Neurosurgery** 13: 141-6, 1983.

49. Huang C I, Chen I H, Lee L S: Microvascular decompression for hemifacial spasm: Analyses of operative findings and results in 310 patients. **Neurosurgery** 30: 53-7, 1992.

50. Payner T D, Tew J M: Recurrence of hemifacial spasm after microvascular decompression. **Neurosurgery** 38: 686-91, 1996.

51. Fukushima T: *Microvascular decompression for hemifacial spasm: Results in 2890 cases.* In **Neurovascular surgery**, Carter L P, Spetzler R F, and Hamilton M G, (eds.). McGraw-Hill, New York, 1995, Chapter 64: pp 1133-45.

52. Bay J W: Management of essential hyperhidrosis. **Contemp Neurosurg** 10: 1-5, 1988.

53. Kao M-C: Video endoscopic sympathectomy using a fiberoptic CO_2 laser to treat palmar hyperhidrosis. **Neurosurgery** 30: 131-5, 1992.

54. Dohn D F, Sava G M: Sympathectomy for vascular syndromes and hyperhidrosis of the upper extremities. **Clin Neurosurg** 25: 637-50, 1978.

55. Wilkinson H A: Percutaneous radiofrequency upper thoracic sympathectomy: A new technique. **Neurosurgery** 15: 811-4, 1984.

56. Wilkinson H A: Percutaneous radiofrequency upper thoracic sympathectomy. **Neurosurgery** 38: 715-25, 1996.

57. Lee K H, Hwang P Y K: Video endoscopic sympathectomy for palmar hyperhidrosis. **J Neurosurg** 84: 484-6, 1996.

58. Olanow C W, Goetz C G, Kordower J H, et al.: A double-blind controlled trial of bilateral fetal nigral transplantation in Parkinson's disease. **Ann Neurol** 54 (3): 403-14, 2003.

59. Snyder B J, Olanow C W: Stem cell treatment for Parkinson's disease: An update for 2005. **Curr Opin Neurol** 18 (4): 376-85, 2005.

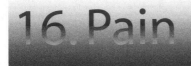

For pain medication, see *Analgesics*, page 27.

Major types of pain:
1. nociceptive
   A. somatic: well localized. Described as sharp, stabbing, aching or cramping. Results from tissue injury or inflammation, or from nerve or plexus compression. Responds to treating the underlying pathology or by interrupting the nociceptive pathway
   B. visceral: poorly localized. Poor response to primary pain medications
2. deafferentation: poorly localized. Described as crushing, tearing, tingling or numbness. Also causes burning dysesthesia numbness often with lancinating pain, and hyperpathia. Unaffected by ablative procedures
3. "sympathetically maintained" pain and the likes (e.g. causalgia): *see page 396*

16.1. Neuropathic pain syndromes

Definition: Neuropathic pain: pain caused by a lesion of the peripheral and/or central nervous system manifesting with sensory symptoms and signs[A].

Neuropathic pain syndromes **(NPS)** are typified by painful diabetic neuropathy **(PDN)** and postherpetic neuralgia **(PHN)**. Common chronic NPSs are shown in *Table 16-1*[3], divided into central or peripheral nervous system origin of the pain. The pain of PDN and PHN is typically burning and aching, and is continuous. and is characteristically refractory to medical and surgical treatment.

MEDICAL TREATMENT OF NEUROPATHIC PAIN
Treatment traditionally includes narcotic analgesics[4], and tricyclic antidepressants (*see below*). For further details and other treatment measures, *see page 555* for PDN, and *page 388* for PHN.

Tricyclic antidepressants: Use is often limited by anticholinergic and central effects and by limited pain relief[5, 6]. Possibly because serotonin potentiates the analgesic effect of endorphins and elevates pain thresholds, serotonin re-uptake blockers are more effective than norepinephrine re-uptake blockers, e.g. tranzodone (Desyrel®) blocks only serotonin. Also useful: amitriptyline (Elavil®) 75 mg daily; desipramine (Norpramin®) 10-25 mg/d; doxepin (Sinequan®) 75-150 mg/d. Some benefit may also derive from the fact that many patients with chronic pain are depressed. SIDE EFFECTS: anticholinergic effects and orthostatic hypotension, especially in the elderly.
✖ Not recommended for use in patients with is-

Table 16-1 Common neuropathic pain syndromes

Peripheral neuropathic pain
acute & chronic inflammatory demyelinating polyradiculoneuropathy (CIDP)
alcoholic polyneuropathy
chemotherapy induced polyneuropathy
complex regional pain syndrome (CRPS)
entrapment neuropathies
HIV sensory neuropathy
iatrogenic neuralgias (e.g. postthoracotomy pain)
idiopathic sensory neuropathy
neoplastic nerve compression or infiltration
nutritional-deficiency neuropathies
painful diabetic neuropathy (PDN)
phantom limb pain
postherpetic neuralgia (PHN)
postradiation plexopathy
radiculopathy
toxic exposure-related neuropathies
trigeminal neuralgia
posttraumatic neuralgias
Central neuropathic pain
cervical spondylotic myelopathy
HIV myelopathy
multiple sclerosis-related pain
Parkinson disease-related pain
postischemic myelopathy
postradiation myelopathy
poststroke pain
posttraumatic spinal cord injury pain
syringomyelia

A. Backonja[1] modified from the International Association for the Study of Pain[2]

chemic heart disease.

Gabapentin: Effective in postherpetic neuralgia **(PHN)** (*see page 388*) and painful diabetic neuropathy. Benefit also reported in pain associated with: trigeminal neuralgia, cancer[7], multiples sclerosis, HIV-related sensory neuropathy, CRPS, spinal cord injury, post-operative state[8], migraine[9] (a number of these studies may have been sponsored by the manufacturer[10]). See *page 388* for side effects, dosing & availability...

Lidocaine patch (Lidoderm®): may be effective[3]. SUPPLIED: 5% lidocaine (*see page 389*).

Tramadol (Ultram®): A centrally acting analgesic[3] (*see page 30*).

16.2. Craniofacial pain syndromes

An adapted outline appears below[11 (p 2328)]. Alternate pathways for <u>facial</u> pain include: the facial nerve (usually deep facial pain), the trigeminal motor root (portio minor), and the eighth nerve[12].

1. cephalic neuralgias
    A. trigeminal neuralgia (*see below*)
    B. glossopharyngeal neuralgia: pain usually in base of tongue and adjacent pharynx (*see page 386*)
    C. geniculate neuralgia: otalgia and deep prosopalgia (*see page 386*)
    D. **tic convulsif** (geniculate neuralgia with hemifacial spasm): *see page 386*
    E. occipital neuralgia: *see page 563*
    F. superior laryngeal neuralgia: a branch of the vagus, results primarily in laryngeal pain and occasionally pain on the auricle
    G. sphenopalatine neuralgia
    H. postherpetic neuralgia (Ramsay-Hunt syndrome): *see page 386*
    I. atypical facial pain (prosopalgia): a "wastebasket" category
2. ophthalmic pain
    A. Tolosa-Hunt syndrome: *see page 587*
    B. (Raeder's) paratrigeminal neuralgia: *see page 588*
    C. orbital pseudotumor: *see page 587*
    D. diabetic (oculomotor) neuritis
    E. optic neuritis
    F. iritis
    G. glaucoma
    H. anterior uveitis
3. otalgia (*see below*)
4. masticatory disorders
    A. dental or periodontal disease
    B. nerve injury (inferior and/or superior alveolar nerves)
    C. temporo-mandibular joint **(TMJ)** dysfunction
    D. elongated styloid process
    E. temporal & masseter myositis
5. vascular pain syndromes
    A. migraine headaches: see *Migraine*, page 45
        1. simple migraine
            a. classic
            b. common
        2. complicated migraine
            a. hemiplegic
            b. ophthalmoplegic
    B. cluster H/A (subtypes: episodic, chronic, chronic paroxysmal hemicrania)
    C. giant cell arteritis (temporal arteritis): *see page 58*
    D. toxic or metabolic vascular H/A (fever, hypercapnia, EtOH, nitrites, hypoxia, hypoglycemia, caffeine withdrawl)
    E. hypertensive H/A
    F. aneurysm or AVM (due either to mass effect or hemorrhage)
    G. basilar dolichoectasia with fifth n. compression or indentation of the pons
6. sinusitis (maximally, frontal, ethmoidal, sphenoidal)
7. neoplasia (extracranial or intracranial with referred pain or fifth n. compression)

---

8. psychogenic/idiopathic
9. tension (muscle contraction) H/A
10. post-traumatic H/A

OTALGIA

Because of redundant innervation of the region of the ear, primary otalgia may have its source in the 5th, 7th, 9th, or 10th cranial nerves or the occipital nerves[13]. As a result, sectioning of the 5th, 9th or 10th nerve or a component of the 7th (nervus intermedius, chorda tympani, geniculate ganglion) has been performed with varying results[14]. Also, microvascular decompression (**MVD**) of the corresponding nerve may also be done[15].

Work-up includes: neurotologic evaluation to rule out causes of secondary otalgia (otitis media or externa, temporal bone neoplasms…). CT or MRI should be done in any case where no cause is found.

Primary otalgia

Primary otalgia is unilateral in most ($\approx$ 80%). Trigger mechanisms are identified in slightly more than half, with cold air or water being the most common[14]. About 75% have associated aural symptoms: hearing loss, tinnitus, vertigo. Pain relief upon cocainization or nerve block of the pharyngeal tonsils suggests glossopharyngeal neuralgia (*see page 386*), however, the overlap of innervation limits the certainty.

An initial trial with medications used in trigeminal neuralgia (carbamazepine, phenytoin, baclofen…, *see page 380*) is the first line of defense. In intractable cases not responding to pharyngeal anesthesia, suboccipital exploration of the 7th (nervus intermedius) and lower cranial nerves may be indicated. If significant vascular compression is found, one may consider MVD alone. If MVD fails, or if no significant vessels are found, Rupa et al. recommend sectioning the nervus intermedius, the 9th and upper 2 fibers of 10th nerve, and a geniculate ganglionectomy (or, if glossopharyngeal neuralgia is strongly suspected, just 9th and upper 2 fibers of 10th)[14].

16.2.1. Trigeminal neuralgia

Trigeminal neuralgia (**TGN**) (AKA **tic douloureux**): paroxysmal lancinating electric-like pain lasting a few seconds, often triggered by sensory stimuli, confined to the distribution of one or more branches of the trigeminal nerve (*see Figure 16-1*) on one side of the face, with no neurologic deficit. The term "**atypical facial pain**" (**AFP**) is sometimes used to describe any other type of facial pain.

Rarely, TGN manifests as **status trigeminus**, a rapid succession of tic-like spasms triggered by seemingly any stimulus. IV carbamazepine (where available) or phenytoin may be effective for this.

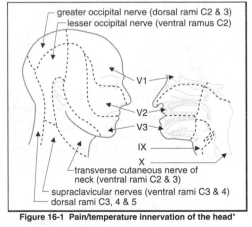

Figure 16-1 **Pain/temperature innervation of the head**[*]

EPIDEMIOLOGY

See *Table 16-2*. Annual incidence 4/100,000. There is no correlation with herpes simplex infection[16]. There is a tendency for spontaneous remission with pain free intervals of weeks or months being characteristic, regardless of treatment. 2% of patients with MS have TGN[17], whereas $\approx$ 18% of patients with bilateral trigeminal neuralgia have MS[18].

PATHOPHYSIOLOGY

Probably due to ephaptic transmission in trigeminal nerve from large-diameter partially demyelinated A fibers to thinly myelinated A-delta and C (nociceptive) fibers. Pathogenesis may be due to:

1. vascular compression of the trigeminal nerve at the root entry zone (NB: compression may be seen in up to 50% of autopsies in patients without TGN[21]):
   A. most commonly (80%) by the SCA (see *Neurovascular compression syndromes*, page 371 for more details)
   B. persistent primitive trigeminal artery[22]
   C. dolichoectatic basilar artery[23 (p 1108)]
2. posterior fossa tumor (see *Tumors and trigeminal neuralgia* below)
3. in MS, plaque within brainstem may cause TGN that is often poorly responsive to microvascular decompression

In addition to the sensory division of the trigeminal nerve, other possible pain pathways[12] include the motor branch of the 5th nerve (portio minor), or the 7th or 8th nerve.

Table 16-2	
Epidemiology[19, 20]	
age (years)	typically > 50 (average 63)
female:male	1.8:1
laterality	
right	60%
left	39%
both	1%
division involved	
V1	2%
V2	20%
V3	17%
V1 & V2	14%
V2 & V3	42%
all three	5%

EVALUATION

MRI is often used to evaluate these patients for possible intracranial tumors or MS plaques, especially in cases with atypical features.

Differential diagnosis

1. herpes zoster: pain is continuous (not paroxysmal). Characteristic vesicles and crusting usually follow pain, most often in distribution of V_1 (isolated V_1 TGN is rare). In unusual cases without vesicles differentiation may be difficult
2. dental disease
3. orbital disease
4. giant cell arteritis: tenderness over STA is common
5. intracranial tumor: primarily p-fossa, usually causes sensory deficit (*see below*)

History and physical (in addition to routine)

* history
   A. accurate description of pain localization to determine which divisions of trigeminal nerve need to be treated
   B. determine time of onset of TGN, trigger mechanisms
   C. ascertain presence and length of pain-free intervals (lack of any pain-free interval is atypical for TGN)
   D. determine duration, side-effects, dosages, and responses to medications tried
   E. inquire about history of herpetic vesicles
* physical exam: the exam should be normal in TGN, any neurologic deficit in previously unoperated patient should prompt search for structural cause, e.g. tumor (*see below*). This exam also serves as a baseline for post-op comparison
   A. assess sensation in all 3 divisions of trigeminal nerve bilaterally (include corneal reflexes)
   B. assess masseter function (bite) and pterygoid function (on opening mouth, chin deviates to weak side)
   C. assess EOM function

TUMORS AND TRIGEMINAL NEURALGIA

In > 2000 patients with facial pain seen over 10 yrs, only 16 harbored tumor (< 0.8% incidence)[24]. 3 tumors outside cranial vault included nasal carcinoma and skull base mets; all had hypalgesia and AFP. 6 middle fossa tumors included 2 meningiomas, 2 schwannomas (1 primary tumor of Gasserian ganglion), and 1 pituitary adenoma. Posterior fossa tumors are the most likely to cause symptoms that most closely resemble true TGN; of these, acoustic neuroma is most common. 2 of 7 had tumors contralateral to neuralgia (presumably due to brainstem shift). Patients with true TGN initially responded to carbamazepine, none with AFP did.

When facial pain is caused by tumor, especially with peripheral tumors, the pain is frequently atypical (usually constant), neurologic abnormalities are often present (usually sensory loss, although some are neurologically normal at first), and the age is often younger than typical TGN.

MEDICAL THERAPY FOR TRIGEMINAL NEURALGIA

carbamazepine (Tegretol®) — DRUG INFO

Complete or acceptable relief in 69% (if 600-800 mg/d are tolerated and give no relief, diagnosis of TGN is suspect[17]). SIDE EFFECTS: Drowsiness. Rash in 5-10%. Possible Stevens-Johnson syndrome. Relative leukopenia is common (usually does not require discontinuing drug). See *carbamazepine (CBZ) (Tegretol®)* on page 273 for precautions.

Rx 100 mg PO BID, increase by 200 mg/d up to maximum of 1200 mg/d divided TID.

baclofen (Lioresal®) — DRUG INFO

2nd DOC (not as effecctive as carbamazepine, but fewer side-effects). Caution: teratogenic in rats. Avoid abrupt withdrawl (can cause hallucinations and seizures). May be more effective if used in conjunction with low dose carbamazepine.

Rx Start low, 5 mg PO TID, increase q 3 d by 5 mg/dose; not to exceed 20 mg QID (80 mg/d); use smallest effective dose.

gabapentin (Neurontin®) — DRUG INFO

An anticonvulsant (*see page 278*), may act synergistically with carbamazepine and baclofen. SIDE EFFECTS: include ataxia, sedation and rash.

Rx start with 100mg po BID, titrate to 5-7mg/kg/day (3600 mg/d max).

MISCELLANEOUS DRUGS

Also possibly effective:
1. capsaicin (Zostrix®): 1 gm applied TID for several days resulted in remission of symptoms in 10 of 12 patients (4 relapsed in < 4 mos, but remained pain free for 1 yr after 2nd course)[25]
2. clonazepam (Klonopin®): works in 25% (*see page 277*)
3. lamotrigine (Lamictal®)

SURGICAL THERAPY FOR TRIGEMINAL NEURALGIA

Reserved for cases refractory to medical management, or when side effects of medications exceed risks and drawbacks of surgery.

SURGICAL OPTIONS

See review by Sweet[26] for historical perspective.
1. peripheral trigeminal nerve branch procedures to block or ablate the division involved with pain, or can be used to block the trigger[27]:
   A. means of blocking
      1. local blocks (phenol, alcohol)
      2. neurectomy of trigeminal branch involved
   B. nerve branches:
      1. V1 (ophthalmic division) at the supraorbital, supratrochlear, or infraorbital nerves
      2. V2 (maxillary division) at the foramen rotundum
      3. V3 (mandibular division) block at the foramen ovale, or neurectomy of inferior dental nerve
2. blocking the trigger: either via percutaneous rhizotomy or alcohol block
3. **percutaneous trigeminal rhizotomy (PTR)**: AKA percutaneous (stereotactic) rhizotomy **(PSR)** of trigeminal (Gasserian) ganglion (*see below*) (not truly a ster-

eotactic procedure in the current sense of the word, therefore the term *percutaneous trigeminal rhizotomy* is preferred). Objective is to selectively destroy A-delta and C fibers (nociceptive) while preserving A-alpha and beta fibers (touch). Ideally, a retrogasserian lesion (not a ganglionic lesion). May also be used to block trigger. Lesioning techniques include (*see below* for comparison of techniques):
   A. radiofrequency thermocoagulation (originated by Sweet and Wespic[28])
   B. glycerol injection into Meckel's cave[29, 30]: possibly lower incidence of sensory loss and anesthesia dolorosa than with radiofrequency lesion[31]. Water soluble contrast cisternography was recommended in original description, may not be essential[32]
   C. mechanotrauma (percutaneous microcompression (**PMC**) rhizolysis) via inflation of No. 4 Fogarty catheter balloon[33-35]
   D. injection of sterile boiling water
4. **Spiller-Frazier** subtemporal extradural approach with retrogasserian rhizotomy (rarely used today)
5. intradural retrogasserian trigeminal nerve section (sensory portion ± motor root, *see below*): may be performed during MVD if no vascular compression is identified
6. cutting descending trigeminal tract in lower medulla (99.5% success): rarely used
7. microvascular decompression (**MVD**)[36]: (*see below*) microsurgical exploration of root entry zone, usually via posterior fossa craniectomy, and displacement of vessel impinging on nerve (if such a vessel is found). Usually with the placement of a non-absorbable "insulator" (Ivalon® sponge or shredded Teflon felt - see *page 372* for relative merits of Ivalon® and Teflon felt)
8. complete section of the nerve proximal to the ganglion via a p-fossa crani
9. stereotactic radiosurgery: *see below*

SELECTION OF SURGICAL OPTION

Peripheral nerve ablation or neurectomy

Limited to pain or trigger points in territory of supraorbital/supratrochlear, infraorbital, or inferior dental nerves. Neurectomy may be a consideration especially for elderly patients who are not candidates for MVD (neurectomy may be done under local anesthesia) with pain in the forehead (to avoid anesthesia of the eye, as could occur with PTR). Disadvantages include sensory loss in the distribution of the nerve and a high rate of pain recurrence due to nerve regeneration (usually in 18-36 months) which often responds to repeat neurectomy[37]. May also be used following PTR.

Percutaneous trigeminal rhizotomy (PTR)

Patients who are poor risk for general anesthesia (elderly or those with increased risk for general anesthesia), those wishing to avoid "major" surgery, those with unresectable intracranial tumors, those with MS, patients with impaired hearing on the other side, and those with limited life expectancy (< 5 yrs) are ideal candidates for PTR[31]. For "atypical facial pain", denervating the painful region of the face benefits < 20% of patients, and worsens 20%[38]. PTR requires a patient who is able to cooperate. Recurrences are easily treated by repeat procedures. May be used to treat failures of peripheral nerve ablation.

Choice of lesion technique:
Recurrence rates and incidence of dysesthesias are comparable with the various lesioning techniques. Incidence of intraoperative hypertension is less with PMC than with radiofrequency rhizotomy (**RFR**) lesion[35] (no reports of intracerebral hemorrhage). Bradycardia occurs regularly with PMC which may not be harmful (some prophylax with atropine[39]). Paralysis of ipsilateral trigeminal motor root (e.g. pterygoids) is more common after PMC (usually temporary) than RFR, and so PMC should not be done if there is already contralateral paralysis from a previous procedure. See *page 382* for technique.

Microvascular decompression (MVD)

(For more details, *see page 385*).
Recommended for patients with inadequate medical control of pain with > 5 years anticipated survival and able to tolerate a small craniotomy[31] (surgical morbidity increases with age). Relief is often long lived, persevering 10 yrs in 70%. Incidence of facial anesthesia is much less than with PTR, and anesthesia dolorosa does not occur. Mortality: < 1%. Incidence of aseptic meningitis (AKA hemogenic meningitis): 20%. 1-10% major neurologic morbidity. Failure rate: 20-25%.
1-2% of patients with MS will have a demyelinating plaque at the root entry zone, this usually does not respond to MVD, and one should attempt a PTR.

Stereotactic radiosurgery (SRS)

Initially, this was reserved for refractory cases following multiple operations[40], now becoming more widely practiced. The least invasive procedure. Generally recommended for patients with co-morbidities, high-risk medical illness, pain refractory to prior surgical procedures, or those on anticoagulants (anticoagulation does not have to be reversed to have SRS).

Treatment plan: 4 -5 mm isocenter in the trigeminal nerve root entry zone identified on MRI. Use 70-80 Gy at the center, keeping the 80% isodose curve outside of the brainstem.

Results: Significant pain reduction after initial SRS: 80-96%[41-44], but only ≈ 65% become pain free. Median latency to pain relief: 3 months (range: 1 d-13 months)[45]. Recurrent pain occurs within three years in 10-25%. Patients with TN and multiple sclerosis are less likely to respond to SRS than those without MS. SRS can be repeated, but only after four months following the original procedure.

Favorable prognosticators: higher radiation doses, previously unoperated patient, absence of atypical pain component, normal pre-treatment sensory function[46].

Side effects: Hypesthesia occurred in 20% after initial SRS, and in 32% of those requiring repeat treatment[45] (higher rates associated with higher radiation doses[42]).

MANAGEMENT OF TREATMENT FAILURES

90% of recurrences are in distribution of previously involved divisions; 10% are in new division and may represent progression of the underlying process.

PTR may be repeated in patients who have a recurrence with some preservation of facial sensation. Attempted repeat PTR is often productive, and failures can be managed as below.

MVD may be performed in patients failing PTR, but the success rate may be reduced[47] (91% for patients undergoing MVD first, vs. 43% for those having MVD following PTR[A]). Repeat MVD may also be performed, with attention given to possible slippage of the insulating sponge, or the fact that the true offending vessel may be "artificially" moved away from the nerve secondary to the surgical positioning.

SRS can be repeated, using the same dose, with reported significant reduction in pain in 89%, and complete relief in 58%[45].

Intradural retrogasserian trigeminal nerve section

May be used as a measure of last resort in patients who have recurrent TGN following one or more PTRs in the presence of total facial anesthesia, or in patients undergoing posterior-fossa craniectomy for the purpose of MVD when no impinging vessel can be identified. In the latter case, a partial rhizotomy is performed by sectioning 2/3 of nerve, with resulting partial anesthesia. In the case of patients with facial anesthesia pre-op, consideration should be given to sectioning the motor division (portio minor) as an alternate pain pathway[12].

PERCUTANEOUS TRIGEMINAL RADIOFREQUENCY RHIZOTOMY (RFR)

Due to concerns about hemorrhage, check coagulation profile (PT/PTT, consider bleeding time), and discontinue ASA and NSAIDs, preferably 10 days pre-op. Procedure may be performed in OR with fluoro, or in angiography suite in x-ray department.

PRE-OP ORDERS (RFR)

1. NPO after MN except meds
2. continue Tegretol® & other meds PO with sips of water
3. AM of procedure: IV NS @ KVO in arm contralateral to neuralgia
4. atropine 0.4 mg IM PRN (✘ contraindications include rapid a-fib)
5. methohexital (Brevitol®) 500 mg to accompany patient to O.R. (write "do not administer")
6. non-disposable LP tray to accompany patient

TECHNIQUE (adapted[48])

NB: needle insertion and/or lesioning may cause HTN, consider monitoring BP. Use

---

A. 91% may be an unrealistically high success rate, and taking patients that fail PTR may select for a more difficult subgroup

either a straight electrode (bare 5 mm for 1 division, 7.5 mm for 2 divisions, or 10 mm for total lesions) or a curved electrode[49].

Electrode positioning
1. attach ground electrode to patients upper arm
2. prep the cheek on the involved side with Betadine
3. entry point: under methohexital (Brevitol®)[A] anesthesia (see page 36), insert electrode-needle **2.5-3 cm lateral to oral commisure**
4. trajectory:
    A. palpate the buccal mucosa with a gloved finger inside the mouth (lateral to the teeth) and with the other hand pass the electrode medial to the coronoid process of the mandible (keeping the needle deep to the oral mucosa, i.e. outside the oral cavity) initially aiming towards the plane intersecting a point **3 cm anterior to EAM** and the **medial aspect of the pupil** when the eye is directed forward. Be careful not to contaminate the field with the hand that was in the patient's mouth
    B. as insertion progresses, use fluoroscopy to direct the tip towards the intersection of the top of the petrous bone with the clivus (5-10 mm below floor of sella along clivus)
    C. upon entering foramen ovale: patient winces. Remove stylet, obtain CSF (may not occur in re-do cases), and insert electrode through needle

Intraoperative fluoroscopy may assist in localizing the needle to Meckel's cave and to R/O e.g. entry into superior orbital fissure (which can cause blindness after lesioning), or entry into foramen spinosum (middle meningeal artery). If necessary to visualize (e.g. when there is difficulty entering), the foramen ovale is optimally seen on a submental x-ray by hyperextending neck 20° and rotating head 15-20° away from side of pain[50].

Impedance measurements: from the tip of the electrode when available may help indicate location of needle tip. Impedance: CSF (or any fluid) low (≈ 40-120 Ω); connective tissue, muscle, or nerve is usually 200-300 Ω (may be up to 400 Ω); if > 400 Ω this likely indicates electrode is contacting periosteum or bone. After starting the lesion, impedance often goes down by 30 Ω transiently, and then as the lesioning continues it gradually returns to baseline or ≈ 20 Ω above it. If char develops on the electrode tip, the impedance will read higher than where it started.

Stimulation and repositioning
Once the foramen ovale is entered, the patient is allowed to wake up and is stimulated through the electrode with the following settings: frequency = 50-75 Hz, 1 mS duration, start at 0.1 V amplitude and slowly increase (usually 0.2-0.5 V is adequate, higher voltages may indicate that the needle is not near the target and that stimulation is due to far-field currents, however, in previously lesioned patients up to 4 V may sometimes be necessary). If stimulation does not reproduce pain in the distribution of the patient's TGN, then the amplitude is returned to 0, the electrode is repositioned (straight electrode: advance needle < 5 mm at a time, until the tip is in the vicinity of the clival line; curved tip electrode: advance and/or rotate) and then slowly elevate the voltage again from 0 and repeat the repositioning-stimulating process until stimulation reproduces the distribution of tic pain. If previous lesions have produced analgesia and the patient cannot feel the stimulating current, one may stimulate at 2 Hz. and watch for masseter twitch (requires preserved motor root). ✖ At no time should the needle tip extend > 8 mm beyond clival line (to avoid Cr. N. III or VI complications).

Lesioning
When stimulation produces pain in the involved distribution of the TGN, perform the first lesion under Brevitol anesthesia at 60-70° C x 90 sec. A facial flush may be noted[50]. After every lesion, perform a post-lesion assessment (see below). The goal is analgesia (but not anesthesia) in the areas of tic pain and hypalgesia in areas of trigger points. An average of three lesions are necessary at the first sitting, each ≈ 5° C higher than the previous for 90 seconds. Anesthetic may not be needed after the first lesion if moderate analgesia has been produced by previous lesions.

Post-lesion assessment
After each lesion and at completion of procedure, assess:
1. sensitivity to pinprick and light touch in all three divisions of trigeminal nerve (grading: normal, hypalgesic, analgesic, anesthetic)
2. corneal reflex bilaterally

A. some surgeons prefer propofol, however, awakening from methohexital is usually faster

3. EOM function
4. masseter muscle strength (patient clenches teeth, palpate cheeks for contraction)
5. pterygoid muscle strength (ask patient to open mouth, chin deviates towards side of pterygoid weakness)

POST-OP CARE (PTR)

Include in post-op orders:
1. ice pack to face on side of procedure for 4 hrs
2. soft diet
3. routine activity when alert
4. avoid narcotics (usually not necessary)
5. if corneal reflex impaired: natural tears 2 gtt q 2 hrs while awake to eye on affected side. Lacrilube® to eye & tape eye shut q hs

Prior to discharge from hospital, repeat post-lesion assessment (see above). Patients are then weaned off of carbamazepine as tolerated.

COMPLICATIONS[A]

1. mortality: only 17 deaths in over 22,000 procedures (includes lesser experienced neurosurgeons and patients often considered poor surgical risks)[17]
2. dysesthesias[20] (sometimes called "annoying paresthesias"): higher rate in more complete lesions
   A. minor: 9%
   B. major (requiring medical treatment): 2%
   C. **anesthesia dolorosa** (severe, constant, burning aching pain that is refractory to all treatment): 0.2-4%
3. meningitis[19]: 0.3%
4. alterations in salivation[51]: 20% (increased in 17%, decreased in 3%)

	------850 cases[49]------		315
	straight electrode (N = 700)	curved electrode (N = 150)	cases[51]
5. partial masseter weakness (usually not perceived by patient)	15-24%	7%	50%
6. oculomotor paresis (usually temporary)	2%	0	
7. reduced hearing (secondary to paresis of tensor tympani)	0	0	27%
8. **neuroparalytic keratitis** (keratitis due to fifth nerve deficit which impairs sensation)	4%	2%	0

9. intracranial hemorrhage: personal report of 7 cases (6 fatal) in > 14,000 procedures, probably due to transient HTN (SBP up to 300 torr). Consider nitroprusside (Nipride®)
10. alterations in lacrimation[51]: 20% (increased in 17%, decreased in 3%)
11. herpes simplex eruption
12. bradycardia and hypotension: 1% with RFR, up to 15% with glycerol injection
13. rare[52, 53]:
    A. carotid cavernous fistula (**CCF**): may occur with any percutaneous technique[54] (including balloon microcompression[55])
    B. temporal lobe abscess
    C. aseptic meningitis
    D. intracerebral abscess: 0.1%
    E. subarachnoid hemorrhage
    F. injury to other cranial nerves: II, III, IV & VI
    G. seizures

A. NB: some "numbness" is actually expected in most successful PTRs and occurs in 98% of cases[20], and is not considered a complication here

RESULTS (PTR)

Results of various PTR techniques compared to microvascular decompression (MVD) are shown in *Table 16-3*. Recurrence rate is higher in patients with multiple sclerosis (50% at 3 yrs mean F/U)[56].

MICROVASCULAR DECOMPRESSION (MVD) FOR TRIGEMINAL NEURALGIA
Indications:
1. patients unable to achieve adequate medical control of trigeminal neuralgia with ≥ 5 yrs anticipated survival, without significant medical or surgical risk factors[31] (although a small p-fossa exploration is usually well tolerated, surgical morbidity increases with age)

Table 16-3 Comparison of outcomes of percutaneous techniques to MVD

Parameter	Percutaneous techniques (PTR)			MVD
	RFR*	Glycerol	Balloon	
initial success rate[12, 20]	91-99%	91%	93%	85-98%
medium-term recurrence rate	19% at 6 yrs[19]	54% at 4 yrs	21% at 2 yrs	15% in 5 yrs
long-term recurrence rate	80% at 12 yrs[51] †			30% at 10 yrs
facial numbness[20]	98%	60%	72%	2%

* abbreviations: RFR = radiofrequency rhizotomy; MVD = microvascular decompression; balloon = balloon microcompression

† this author included initial failures to PTR requiring repeat procedures during same hospitalization

2. may be used in patients who do not fit the above criteria, but have intractable pain and fail PTR
3. patient with tic involving V1 for whom the risk of exposure keratitis due to corneal anesthesia would be unacceptable (e.g. already blind in contralateral eye) or patient wishing to avoid facial anesthesia for any reason
✖ patients with MS are usually not considered candidates for MVD due to low response rate

POST-OP CARE FOLLOWING MVD

Patients routinely have H/A and nausea for 2-3 days (there may be less intracranial air and less "pneumoencephalogram sickness" if the park-bench position is used instead of the sitting position). Aseptic meningitis usually responds to steroids. Some patients have continued but lessened pain for several days post-op, this usually subsides.

Include in post-op orders
1. analgesics (e.g. codeine 30-60 mg IM q 3 hrs)
2. anti-emetics (e.g. ondansetron 4 mg IV q 6 hrs)

COMPLICATIONS
1. mortality: 0.22-2% in experienced hands (> 900 procedures)[57, 58]
2. meningitis
   A. aseptic meningitis (AKA hemogenic meningitis): H/A, meningismus, mild fever, culture negative CSF, pleocytosis. Incidence: ≈ 2% (up to 20% has been reported). Usually occurs 3-7 days post-op. Responds to LP + steroids
   B. bacterial meningitis: 0.9%
3. major neurologic morbidity: 1-10% (higher rates with less experienced surgeons), including:
   A. deafness: 1%
   B. vestibular nerve dysfunction
   C. facial nerve dysfunction
4. mild facial sensory loss: 25%
5. cranial nerve palsies[59]:
   A. fourth nerve (diplopia): 4.3% (only ≈ 0.1% are permanent)
   B. facial nerve: 1.6% (most are transient)
   C. eighth nerve (hearing loss): 3%
6. postoperative hemorrhage[60]: subdural, intracerebral (1%[20]), subarachnoid
7. seizures: including status epilepticus[60]
8. infarction[60]: including posterior cerebral artery distribution, brain stem
9. pneumonia: 0.6%

---

1. success rate[A]: 75-80%;
    good but not total relief in an additional ≈ 10%
2. recurrence rate in large series is difficult to ascertain from literature; in a series
    of 40 patients followed 8.5 yrs mean[58]:
    A. major recurrence (recurrent tic not controlled by medications) rate: 31%
    B. minor recurrence (mild or controlled by medications) rate: 17%
    C. using Kaplan-Meier curve, expect 70% to be either pain free or have minor
        recurrence by 8.5 years (or ≈ 80% at 5 years)
        the risk for a major recurrence after MVD is 3.5% annually
        the risk for a minor recurrence after MVD is 1.5% annually
    D. major recurrence rate is lower for patients having major arterial cross-com-
        pression of the nerve discovered at the time of surgery (patients with venous
        compression had much higher rate)
    E. this study found no correlation between previous destructive surgery and
        major recurrence rate (in 11 patients)
    F. studies suggest that increased time from onset of symptoms or prior abla-
        tive therapies decrease the surgical success rate

16.2.2. Glossopharyngeal neuralgia

1 case for every 70 of trigeminal neuralgia[61 (p 3604-5)]. Severe, lancinating pain in distribution of glossopharyngeal and vagus nerves (throat & base of tongue most commonly
involved, radiates to ear (otalgia), occasionally to neck), occasionally with salivation and
coughing. Rarely, hypotension[62], syncope[63], cardiac arrest and convulsions may accompany. May be triggered by swallowing, talking, chewing. Trigger zones are rare.

TREATMENT

Pain may be reduced by cocainization of tonsillar pillars and fossa. Usually, the persistence and severity of pain requires surgical intervention. One may either perform microvascular decompression, or nerve division via extra- or intra-cranial approach (latter
may be required for permanent relief).

Intracranial approach: Section of preganglionic glossopharyngeal nerve (IX) and upper one third or two fibers (whichever is larger) of vagus (X). IX is readily identified at
it's dural exit zone where it is separated from X by a dural septum. The upper third of X
is usually composed of a single rootlet, or less commonly, multiple small rootlets. Initial
post-op dysphagia usually resolves. Cardiovascular complications following vagal section
have been reported, warrants close monitoring **x** 24 hrs.

16.2.3. Geniculate neuralgia

Geniculate neuralgia **(GeN)** AKA **Hunt's neuralgia** is a neuralgia affecting the facial nerve, causing paroxysmal otalgia (lancinating pain experienced deep within the
ear) radiating to the auricle, with occasional burning sensations around the ipsilateral
eye and cheek, and **prosopalgia** (pain referred to deep facial structures, including orbit,
posterior nasal and palatal regions).

Occasionally has cutaneous trigger points in the anterior EAC and tragus, and pain
may also be triggered by cold, noise, or swallowing.

GeN may be associated with herpetic infections of the geniculate ganglion (AKA
herpetic ganglionitis, AKA **Ramsay Hunt syndrome (RHS)**) in which case herpetic
lesions appear on pinna, in EAC, and possibly on TM. May include facial palsy, decreased
auditory acuity, tinnitus or vertigo. Unlike idiopathic GeN, RHS is more chronic and less
paroxysmal, tends to remit with time, usually refractory to carbamazepine.

When combined with hemifacial spasm, called **tic convulsif** (AKA convulsive tic),
usually due to neurovascular compression of both the sensory and motor roots of the facial nerve[13], most often by AICA. First described by Cushing in 1920.

Idiopathic GeN tends to be more painful than post-herpetic, and does not remit
spontaneously. Mild cases may respond to carbamazepine, sometimes in combination

---

A. rates may be lower in patients having prior destructive procedure, see *Management of treatment
    failures*, page 382

with phenytoin. Severe cases where medical treatment is not tolerated or fails may require microvascular decompression or section of the nervus intermedius (nerve of Wrisberg) (operating under local anesthesia allows verification by stimulating nerve) or geniculate ganglion.

Workup includes neuro-otologic evaluation with audiometry and ENG. Some patients may require imaging (MRI or high-resolution CT) and angio (to R/O aneurysm).

Treatment is mostly symptomatic:
* local anesthetic to EAC
* topical antibiotics for secondary infections of herpetic lesions
* pain may respond to valproate (Depakote®) 250 mg PO BID

16.3. Postherpetic neuralgia

Herpes zoster (HZ) (Greek: *zoster* - girdle) (**shingles** in lay terms): painful vesicular cutaneous eruptions caused by the herpes varicella zoster virus (**VZV**) (the etiologic agent of chickenpox, a herpesvirus distinct from herpes simplex virus). It occurs in a dermatomal distribution over one side of the thorax in ≈ 65% of cases (rarely, infections occur without vesicles, called **zoster sine herpete**). In 20% of cases it involves the trigeminal nerve (with a predilection for the ophthalmic division, called **herpes zoster ophthalmicus**). Pain usually resolves after 2-4 weeks. When the pain persists > 1 month after the vesicular eruption has healed, this pain syndrome is known as **postherpetic neuralgia (PHN)**. PHN can follow a herpes varicella infection in any site and is difficult to treat by any means (medical or surgical). It can occasionally be seen in a limb, and follows a dermatomal distribution (not a peripheral nerve distribution). PHN may remit spontaneously, but if it hasn't done so by 6 mos this is unlikely.

EPIDEMIOLOGY

Incidence of herpes zoster is ≈ 125/100,000/year in the general population, or about 850,000 cases per year in the U.S.[64]. Both sexes are equally affected. There is no seasonal variance. HZ is also more common in those with reduced immunity and in those with a coexistent malignancy (especially lympho-proliferative)[65, 66]. PHN occurs in ≈ 10% of cases of HZ[64]. Both HZ and PHN are more common in older patients (PHN is rare in age < 40 yrs, and usually occurs in age > 60) and in those with diabetes mellitus. PHN is more likely after ophthalmic HZ than after spinal segmental cases.

Table 16-4 Medical treatments for PHN*

Treatment	Efficacy
PHN treatments that appear effective	
tricyclic antidepressants	widely used(*see text*)
lidocaine patch (Lidoderm®) [67]	effective, few side effects (*see page 389*)
intrathecal steroids + lidocaine (*see text*)	appears very effective, larger studies & long-term follow-up needed
gabapentin	proven efficacy (*see text*)
oxycodone CR 10 mg PO BID[4]	proven efficacy
Treatments of questionable efficacy	
SSRIs†	may be effective
SNRIs	may be effective
tramadol	may be effective
topical capsaicin	controversial (*see text*)
iontophoresis	insufficient evidence
nonsteroidal creams	questionable
aspirin suspended in acetone, ether or chloroform	questionable
EMLA cream	questionable
Treatments that are not useful	
dextromethorphan, benzodiazepines, acyclovir, acupuncture	no benefit[68]
ketamine (NMDA receptor antagonist)	may be beneficial, but hepatotoxic
Preventative treatment	
oral antiherpetic drugs given during HZ infection	shortens length of HZ, may reduce incidence of PHN
varicella vaccination of older patients	trials of this strategy are in progress[64]

*   modified with permission from Rubin M, Relief for postherpetic neuralgia, **Neurology Alert**, 6: 33-4, 2001

†   abbreviations: oxycodone CR = controlled release (Oxycontin®); HZ = herpes zoster; PHN = postherpetic neuralgia; SNRIs = serotonin-norepinephrine reuptake inhibitor; SSRIs = selective serotonin reuptake inhibitors (e.g. Prozac®),

ETIOLOGY

It is postulated that the VZV lies dormant in the sensory ganglia (dorsal root ganglia of the spine, trigeminal (semilunar) ganglion for facial involvement) until such time that the patient's immune system is weakened and then the virus erupts. Inflammatory changes within the nerve are present early and are later replaced by fibrosis.

CLINICAL

PHN is usually described as a constant burning and aching. There may be superimposed shocks or jabs. It rarely produces throbbing or cramping pain. Pain may be spontaneous, or may be triggered by light cutaneous stimulation (allodynia) (e.g. by clothing), and may be relieved by constant pressure. The pain is present to some degree at all times with no pain-free intervals. Scars and pigmentary changes from the acute vesicular eruption are usually visible. It is not known if PHN can follow zoster sine herpete. The involved area may demonstrate hypesthesia, hypalgesia, paresthesias and dysesthesias.

MEDICAL TREATMENT

Varicella vaccination of older individuals can increase immunity to herpes zoster, but it will be several years before it can be determined if this will reduce PHN[64].

FOR HERPES ZOSTER

Treatment for the pain of the <u>acute</u> attack of herpes zoster may be accomplished with epidural or paravertebral somatic (intercostal) nerve block[69 (p 4018)].

Oral antiherpetic drugs: Also effective (they shorten the duration of pain) and also reduce the incidence of PHN. They may cause thrombotic thrombocytopenic purpura/hemolytic uremic syndrome (TTP/HUS) when used in severely immunocompromised patients at high doses. These drugs include:

Acyclovir (Zovirax®): poorly absorbed from the GI tract (15-30% bioavailability). *Rx* 800 mg PO q 4 hrs 5 times/d **x** 7 d.

Valacyclovir (Valtrex®)[70] is a prodrug of acyclovir and is more completely absorbed and should be equally as effective with fewer daily doses. *Rx* 1,000 mg PO TID starting within 72 hrs of onset of the rash **x** 7 days.

Famciclovir (Famvir®): *Rx* 500 mg PO TID **x** 7 d.

FOR POST-HERPETIC NEURALGIA

Most drugs useful for trigeminal neuralgia (*see page 380*) are less effective for PHN. Some treatment alternatives for PHN are summarized in *Table 16-4*. Details of some drugs follows. It is suggested to initiate therapy with lidocaine skin patches (*see page 389*) since this modality has the lowest potential for serious side effects[64].

Antiepileptic drugs

gabapentin (Neurontin®)　　　　　　　DRUG INFO

FDA approved only for partial seizures and postherpetic neuralgia **(PHN)**.
SIDE EFFECTS: dizziness and somnolence (usually during titration, often diminish with time). Ataxia, fatigue, peripheral edema, confusion and depression may occur.

Rx For PHN, start with 300 mg on Day 1, 300 mg BID on Day 2, and 300 mg TID on Day 3. Dose may be titrated to 1800 mg/d divided TID. To limit daytime drowsiness, patients may need to start with 100 mg at hs and increase slowly over 3-8. Although doses up to 3600 mg/day (the antiseizure dose) were studied[71] there was no significant benefit for PHN over 1800 mg/d. Lower doses are required for renal insufficiency. SUPPLIED: 100, 300 & 400 mg capsules; 600 & 800 mg scored tabs.

oxycarbazepine (Trileptal®)　　　　　　DRUG INFO

Rx 150 mg PO BID.

zonisamide (Zonegran®)　　　　　〉　DRUG INFO

Rx Initiate therapy with 100 mg PO q PM **x** 2 wks, then increase dose by 100 mg/d q 2 wks up to 400 mg/d. Bioavailability is not affected by food. Steady state is achieved within 14 days of dosage changes. **SUPPLIED:** 100 mg capsules.

Tricyclic antidepressants (TCA):
For side effects *see page 556*.

amitriptyline (Elavil®)　　　　　〉　DRUG INFO

Helpful in ≈ 66% of patients at a mean dose of 75 mg/d even without antidepressant effect[5]. **SIDE EFFECTS:** (see *Amitriptyline, side effects* page 556), minimized by starting low and slowly incrementing dose.
Rx Start with 12.5-25 mg PO q hs, and increase by the same amount q 2-5 days.

nortriptyline (Pamelor®)　　　　　〉　DRUG INFO

Fewer side effects than amitriptyline.
Rx Start with 10-20 mg PO q hs, and increase gradually.

Topical treatment:

capsaicin (Zostrix®)　　　　　〉　DRUG INFO

A vanillyl alkaloid derived from hot peppers, available without prescription for topical treatment of the pain of herpes zoster and diabetic neuropathy. Beneficial in some patients with either of these conditions (response rate at 8 weeks was 90% for PHN, 71% for diabetic neuropathy, vs. 50% with placebo in either group), although the high placebo response rate is disturbing and many authorities are skeptical[72]. Expensive. **SIDE EFFECTS:** include burning and erythema at the application site (usually subsides by 2-4 weeks).

Rx Manufacturer recommends massaging the medication into the affected area of the skin TID-QID (apply a very thin coat). Some authorities recommend q 2 hr application. Avoid contact with eyes or damaged skin. Supplied as Zostrix® (0.25% capsaicin) or Zostrix-HP® (0.75%).

lidocaine patch 5% (Lidoderm®)　　　　　〉　DRUG INFO

Often better tolerated by elderly patients than TCAs (due to pre-existing cognitive impairments, cardiac disease, or systemic illness).
Rx Apply up to 3 patches of 5% lidocaine (to cover a maximum of 420 cm^2) to intact skin q 12 hrs to cover as much of the area of greatest pain as possible[67].

Intrathecal steroids
Over 90% of patients receiving intrathecal methylprednisolone (60 mg) + 3% lidocaine (3 ml) given once per week for up to 4 weeks, reported good to excellent pain relief for up to 2 years[73]. This technique was not studied for use in PHN involving the trigeminal nerve. Further clinical trials are needed to verify the efficacy and safety[64] (potential long-term side effects include adhesive arachnoiditis).

SURGICAL TREATMENT
There is no operation that is uniformly successful in treating PHN. Numerous operations have been shown to work occasionally. Procedures that have been tried include:
1. nerve blocks: once PHN is established, nerve blocks provide only temporary relief[74]
2. cordotomy: although percutaneous cordotomy (*see page 391*) may work when the level of PHN is at least 3-4 segments below the cordotomy, this procedure is not recommended for pain of benign etiology because of possible complications and the high likelihood of pain recurrence
3. rhizotomy: including retrogasserian for facial involvement

4. neurectomies
5. sympathectomy
6. DREZ[75]: often offers good early relief, but recurrence rate is high (*see page 396*).
7. acupuncture[76]
8. TENS
9. spinal cord stimulation: *see page 395*
10. undermining the skin

16.4. Pain procedures

Medical therapy must be maximized before a patient is a candidate for a pain procedure. Usually this requires escalating the dose of oral narcotic pain medications until the point that the pain is relieved or the side effects (usually somnolence or hallucinations) are intolerable (e.g. up to 300-400 mg/day of MS Contin may sometimes be necessary).

Choice of pain procedure: *Table 16-5* shows some pain procedures that may be used for various indications. In general, nonablative procedures are exhausted before resorting to ablative procedures.

Table 16-5   Choice of pain procedures*

Unilateral pain		Bilateral or midline pain	
Head, face, neck, UE	Pain at or below C5 dermatome	Below diaphragm	Above diaphragm
stereotactic mesencephalotomy (390)	cordotomy † (391)	spinal IT narcotics (393) ↓ commissural myelotomy (392)	intraventricular narcotics (394)

*   abbreviations: IT = intrathecal, UE or LE = upper or lower extremity, numbers in parentheses = page

†   cordotomy (open or percutaneous) if pain is unresponsive to or too high for spinal IT narcotics

Types of pain procedures

For pain procedures particular to trigeminal neuralgia, *see page 380*. Techniques for other conditions include:
1. electrical stimulation
   A. deep brain stimulation[77] in periaqueductal or periventricular gray matter: *see page 395*
   B. spinal cord stimulation: *see page 395*
2. direct drug administration into the CNS:
   A. different routes: spinal (*see page 393*) epidural or intrathecal, intraventricular (*see page 394*)
   B. different agents: local anesthetics, narcotics (without motor, sensory, or sympathetic impairment seen with local anesthetics) *see page 393*
3. intracranial ablative procedures:
   A. cingulotomy: theoretically reduces the unpleasant affect of pain without eliminating the pain. Must be done bilaterally, recently with MRI. Intolerable pain usually recurs after ≈ 3 mos. 10-30% develop flattened affect
   B. medial thalamotomy: controversial. May be useful for some for nociceptive cancer pain. Performed stereotactically, *see page 396*
   C. **stereotactic mesencephalotomy**[78]: for unilateral head, neck, face and/or UE pain. Use MRI to create lesion 5 mm lateral to sylvian aqueduct at the level of the inferior colliculus. Unlike spinal cordotomy, the lesion is not near any motor tracts. Main complication is diplopia due to interference with vertical eye movement, often transient
4. spinal ablative surgical procedures
   A. cordotomy: *see below*
      1. open
      2. percutaneous
   B. cordectomy
   C. commissural myelotomy: for bilateral pain (*see page 392*)
   D. punctate midline myelotomy: for relief of visceral cancer pain
   E. dorsal root entry zone lesion: *see page 395*
   F. dorsal rhizotomy: not useful for large areas of involvement
   G. dorsal root ganglionectomy (an extraspinal procedure)
   H. sacral cordotomy: for patients with pelvic pain who have colostomy and ileostomy. A ligature is tied around the dural sac below S1 nerve roots

5. sympathectomy: possibly for causalgia major (see *Sympathectomy*, page 373 and *Complex regional pain syndrome (CRPS)* on page 396)
6. peripheral nerve procedures
   A. nerve block[79]:
      1. neurolytic: injection neurodestructive agents (e.g. phenol or absolute alcohol) on or near the target nerve
      2. nonneurolytic: using local anesthetics, sometimes in combination with corticosteroids
   B. neurectomy: (e.g. intercostal neurectomy for pain due to infiltration of chest wall by malignancy). Performed open or percutaneously with radiofrequency lesion. May sacrifice motor function with mixed nerves
   C. peripheral nerve stimulators: rarely discussed

16.4.1. Cordotomy

Interruption of the lateral spinothalamic tract fibers in the spinal cord. Cordotomy is the procedure of choice for unilateral pain below the C5 dermatomal level (≈ nipple)[A], in a terminally ill patient. Better for aching pain, poor for central pain, dysesthesias, causalgia (deafferentation pain) midline visceral pain. May be performed as an open procedure, but is more easily performed percutaneously at the C1-2 interspace (which limits the procedure to the cervical region). If there is any contralateral pain, it will tend to be magnified following the procedure and often leads to dissatisfaction with cordotomy. If there is any bladder dysfunction, it will usually be worse following cordotomy. Bilateral cervical cordotomies carries a risk of the loss of automaticity of breathing[80] (one form of sleep apnea, so-called **Ondine's curse**[81]). Therefore, if bilateral cordotomies are desired, the second should be staged after normal respiratory function and CO_2 responsiveness are verified following the first procedure, or the second stage may be done as an open procedure in the thoracic region.

Review the cross sectional spinal cord anatomy for relationships of the critical tracts (spinothalamic and corticospinal) to the dentate ligament, the anterior spinal artery, respiratory (see *Figure 3-6*, page 73), and bladder areas (see *Figure 3-15*, page 89).

PRE-OP EVALUATION

Spirometric measurement of minute volume before and after breathing a mixture of 5% CO_2 and 95% O_2 for 5 minutes. If the MV decreases, these patients are at increased risk of having sleep apnea (usually transient), no increased risk if MV increases or stays the same. Also, patients with < 50% of predicted values on PFTs are not candidates.

In patients with pulmonary cancer contralateral to the planned side of cordotomy, check that the contralateral diaphragm is functioning with fluoroscopy, otherwise if the ipsilateral diaphragm is lost due to cordotomy, the patient may be hypopneic.

PERCUTANEOUS CORDOTOMY

Indicated for unilateral pain below ≈ C4-5 in a terminally ill patient. Radiofrequency current is used to lesion the lateral spinothalamic tract.

TECHNIQUE

Patient does not need to be NPO. Usual pain medications should be given. The patient must be awake and cooperative (any movement with the needle in the cord may lacerate the cord), however one may give e.g. hydroxyzine (Vistaril®) 50 mg IM on call to procedure for relaxation.

The procedure is performed in the x-ray department with either fluoroscopic or CT guidance. For fluoroscopy, the head is placed in a Rosomoff headholder with the height adjusted to keep the mastoid process in the same horizontal plane as the acromioclavicular joint. Working on the side contralateral to the pain, local anesthetic without epinephrine is infiltrated 1 cm caudal to the mastoid tip. An 18 gauge lumbar puncture needle is inserted perfectly horizontal aiming halfway between the posterior margin of the body of C2 and the anterior portion of the C2 spinous process. Stay rostral to the C2 lamina to avoid the nerve (which is painful).

The dura will be penetrated at about the time that the tip of the needle is approxi-

---

A. occasionally pain as high up as the mandible may be treated

mately even with the midline of the odontoid process on AP fluoro. A few ml of CSF are aspirated and shaken in a syringe together with a few ml of Pantopaque®^{A}, and several ml of the mixture are injected into the subarachnoid space under lateral fluoro guidance. Some dye will layer on the anterior cord, some on the dentate ligament, and most in the posterior thecal space. The dye will only stay momentarily on the dentate ligament, thus be ready to immediately advance the needle just barely anterior to this while monitoring the tip impedance which will jump from ≈ 300-500 Ω (ohms) in the CSF to ≈ 1200-1500 Ω as the spinal cord is penetrated.

Stimulation at 100 Hz. should produce contralateral tingling at a threshold of ≤ 1 volt. No motor response should be elicited with 100 Hz. in the spinothalamic tract, and if muscle tetany occurs, lesioning must not be performed. If tingling is in the arm, lesioning will usually render from the arm and below analgesic. If tingling is in the lower extremity it will render only that limb analgesic. Stimulation at 2 Hz. should produce ipsilateral twitching of the arm or neck at ≈ 1-3 volts.

Radiofrequency lesioning is performed for 30 seconds while the patient sustains contraction of the ipsilateral hand and the voltage is gradually increased from zero. Any twitching of the hand is indication to back down on the voltage. A second lesion is performed in the same region and is usually less painful. The appropriate body area is then checked for analgesia to pinprick.

If the procedure is performed satisfactorily, an ipsilateral Horner's syndrome usually occurs.

COMPLICATIONS

For complications, see Table 16-6.

OUTCOME

In experienced hands, 94% will achieve at least significant pain relief at the time of hospital discharge. The level of analgesia falls with time. At 1 year 60% will be pain free, and at 2 years this will be only 40%.

POST-PROCEDURE MANAGEMENT

CSF leakage will cease spontaneously. Patient is kept supine for 24 hrs to prevent "spinal" (post-LP) headache. Pain medication appropriate to post-operative management is prescribed. If successful, one can rapidly stop the narcotics for the primary pain, withdrawal syndromes occur only rarely.

Table 16-6 Post-cordotomy complications

Complication	Frequency
ataxia	20%
ipsilateral paresis	5% total 3% permanent
bladder dysfunction	10% total 2% permanent
postcordotomy dysesthesia	8%
sleep induced apnea	0.3% unilateral cordotomy 3% bilateral cordotomy
death (respiratory failure)	0.3% unilateral cordotomy 1.6% bilateral cordotomy

OPEN CERVICAL CORDOTOMY (SCHWARTZ TECHNIQUE)

A relatively quick method for open cervical cordotomy[82]. Can theoretically be done under local for patients who cannot tolerate general anesthesia.

16.4.2.   Commissural myelotomy

AKA mediolongitudinal myelotomy. Interrupts pain fibers crossing in the anterior commisure on their way to the lateral spinothalamic tract.

Indications: Bilateral or midline pain, primarily below the thoracic levels (including abdomen, pelvis, perineum and lower extremities).

Technique: Outcome: 60% of patients have complete pain relief, 28% have partial, and 8% have none.

Complications: Weakness in the lower extremities occurs in ≈ 8% (usually lower motor neuron, presumably due to injury to anterior horn motor neurons). Dysesthesias occur in almost all patients, but persists > a few days in ≈ 16% (these patients also have impaired joint position sense, all of which are presumably due to posterior column injury). Bladder

---

A. Pantopaque is no longer available, and water soluble agents are less effective. A needle endoscopic technique may be able to localize the spinal cord anterior to the dentate ligaments

dysfunction is seen in ≈ 12%. Sexual dysfunction may also occur. There is a risk of injury to the anterior spinal artery (rare).

16.4.3. Punctate midline myelotomy

Indications: Pelvic and visceral pain refractory to other therapies[83].

Technique: Interruption of a midline posterior column pathway.

16.4.4. CNS narcotic administration

INTRASPINAL NARCOTICS

Spinal narcotics may be administered epidurally or intrathecally for pain relief. Satisfactory pain control can usually be achieved for pain below the neck, although for pain above the diaphragm/umbilicus some recommend intraventricular morphine[84] (*see page 394*). May also be performed on a "one-time" basis e.g. injection into epidural space following a lumbar laminectomy. Or, it may be given on a short term continuous basis, via an external epidural or intrathecal catheter. It may also be performed on an intermediate-term basis (< 60 days) with the use of a subcutaneous reservoir[85] or on a long-term basis with an implantable drug infusion pump[86] (e.g. Infusaid® or Medtronic® pump). Advantages over systemic narcotics include less sedation and/or confusion, less interference with GI motility (constipation), and possibly less N/V. The effectiveness is usually limited to ≈ 1 year and is thus not indicated for chronic benign pain. With time, increased doses are required because of the development of tolerance and/or progression of disease[87] with the concomitant development of the usual narcotic side effects.

SPINAL NARCOTICS
Must be preservative-free (for either intrathecal or epidural use). This may be prepared by a pharmacist (e.g. add enough preservative free 0.9% saline to 1 or 3 gm morphine sulfate powder to yield a total of 100 ml produces 10 or 30 mg/ml solution respectively, and then filter this through a 0.22 µm filter[88]). Alternatively, commercially available preparations include Duramorph® (available as 0.5 or 1 mg/ml) and Infumorph® (available in 20 ml ampules of 10 or 25 mg/ml), any of which may be diluted to a lower strength with preservative free diluent (normal saline). Cross tolerance to systemic narcotics does occur, and spinal narcotics are more effective in patients who have not been on continuous high dose IV opiates (patients on high-dose IV narcotics need higher initial intraspinal narcotic doses).

SIDE EFFECTS: include pruritis (often diffuse, and may be experienced most intensely in the nose), respiratory depression (the respiratory depression with spinal narcotics is usually very gradual, and is often easily detected by monitoring respiratory rate q 1 hr and taking action if the rate decreases), urinary retention, and N/V.

Trial injection
Before implanting a permanent delivery system a test injection should be performed to verify pain relief and tolerance for medication. Administered via percutaneously inserted epidural or intrathecal catheter connected to an external pump. Doses required for intrathecal catheters are usually ≈ 5-10 times lower than those for epidural catheters.

Sample post-injection orders after a one-time injection:
1. use no other narcotics for ≈ 24 hrs (with a continuous infusion additional narcotics should be withheld until the effect of the spinal narcotics has been determined)
2. 2 ampules (0.4 mg each) of naloxone (Narcan®) and syringe taped to patients bed (for the first 24 hrs after a single injection; at all times with continuous infusion)
3. head of bed elevated ≥ 10° for 24 hrs
4. record respiratory rate q1 hr for 24 hrs; if asleep and respiratory rate < 10 breaths/min, awaken patient. If unable to awaken, administer naloxone 0.4 mg IV and notify physician. Repeat naloxone 0.4 mg IV q 2 min PRN
• optional: pulse oximeter for 24 hrs
5. diphenhydramine (Benadryl®) 25 mg IV q 1 hr PRN itching
6. droperidol (Inapsine®) 0.625 mg (which is 0.25 ml of the 2.5 mg/ml standard concentration available) IV q 30-60 mins PRN nausea

7. PRN supplemental pain medication:
    A. narcotic agonist/antagonist: e.g. nalbuphine (Nubain®) 1-4 mg IV q 3 hrs
        OR
    B. ketorolac tromethamine (Toradol®) 15 mg IV or IM or 30 mg IM q 6 hrs (use
        lower dose for weight < 50 kg, age > 65 yrs, or reduced renal function)

IMPLANTABLE DRUG DELIVERY PUMPS

Although satisfactory pain control can be achieved with either epidural or intrathecal narcotics (morphine diffuses easily through the dura to the CSF where it gains access to pain receptors), epidural catheters commonly develop problems with scarring and may become less effective sooner than intrathecal catheters. Pumps should only be implanted if patients have successful pain control with test injection of spinal epidural (5-10 mg) or intrathecal (0.5-2 mg) morphine. A life expectancy of > 3 months is recommended for implantable pumps (if shorter longevity is anticipated, an external pump may be used).

One such series of commonly used implantable drug delivery pumps is manufactured by Infusaid [Infusaid, Inc., 1400 Providence Highway, Norwood, MA 02062, Phone: 1-800-451-1050]. The only needle that should be used with their devices are special 22 gauge Huber (non-coring) needles. Delivery rates increase with body temperature 10-13% per °C above 37° C, they decrease by the same amount for every °C below 37°C, and also they become inaccurate at ≤ 4 ml of reservoir fluid. These pumps should never be allowed to run until empty, as this may permanently affect accuracy and reliability of drug delivery. In addition to the pump reservoir port, most models have one or more side "bolus" ports that delivers injected fluid directly to the outlet tubing. One should not aspirate when accessing either port.

Medtronics produces a programmable pump.

Surgical insertion

Post-op pain management:

Although the pump will be infusing when the patient leaves the operating room, unless they have been on intraspinal narcotics up until the time of surgery, it will usually take several days for the drug to reach equilibrium in the CSF before the level of pain control will be adequate. This can be mitigated by a bolus infusion (3-4 mg morphine for epidural catheters, or 0.2-0.4 mg for intrathecal catheters).

Complications

Meningitis and respiratory failure are rare complications. CSF fistula and spinal H/A may occur. Disconnection or dislodgment of catheter tip may result in failure to control pain, but can usually be surgically corrected.

Outcome

Cancer pain is significantly improved in up to 90%. Success rate for neuropathic pain (e.g. postherpetic neuralgia, painful diabetic sensory neuropathy): 25-50%.

INTRAVENTRICULAR NARCOTICS

Indications

May be used for cancer pain (especially head and neck)[89] unresponsive to other methods in patients with a life expectancy < 6 mos.

Technique

An intraventricular catheter is connected to a ventricular access device. 0.5-1 mg of intrathecal morphine is injected via the VAD and usually provides ≈ 24 hrs of analgesia.

Complications

SIDE EFFECTS: common ones include dizziness, N/V. The risk of respiratory depression is minimized by using correct dosing. Complications in a series of 52 patients[89]: bacterial colonization of reservoir (4%), dislodged catheter (2%), blocked catheter (6%), postoperative meningitis (2%).

Outcome

Pain is successfully controlled in 70% at 2 mos, but thereafter the effectiveness diminishes as a result of tolerance to the narcotics.

16.4.5. Spinal cord stimulation (SCS)

Originally developed as **dorsal column stimulation (DCS)**, it has since been discovered that pain relief also occurs with ventral stimulation (without stimulation induced paresthesias seen with DCS). Pain relief in humans persists beyond the stimulation time, and is not reversed by naloxone. The exact mechanism of action is undetermined, but probably involves some combination of neurohumoral (i.e. endorphin), antidromic stimulation of a spinal pain "gate", and supraspinal center stimulation. GABA and serotonin levels have been shown to be increased with SCS. The response rate diminishes with time and by about 2 years approaches that of placebo. No blinded, randomized study has been done to determine if the procedure is effective, and until this is done, SCS will not achieve significant credibility[90]. Not helpful in cancer pain.

Indications
1. pain[91]: postlaminectomy pain syndrome (the most common indication, especially if LE pain > back pain), complex regional pain syndrome (CRPS, reflex sympathetic dystrophy), postthoracotomy pain (intercostal neuralgia), multiple sclerosis, and sometimes postherpetic neuralgia
2. functional: spastic hemiparesis, dystonia, bladder dysfunction, angina
3. ✖ generally not used for cancer pain or for patients with limited life expectancy

Technique
In order for SCS to be effective, it is necessary for the patient to feel the stimulation in the areas of pain[92]. Two techniques are used to place electrodes in the epidural space:
1. plate-like electrodes placed via hemilaminectomy
2. wire-like electrodes placed percutaneously with a Touhy needle

Following electrode placement, a trial with an external generator over several days determines if SCS is effective. The electrodes are removed unless clear improvement occurs, in which case an implantable pulse generator is placed subcutaneously.

Complications
With plate electrodes, there is a 3.5% incidence of infection which respond to electrode removal and IV antibiotics. Less common complications: electrode migration (usually seen with first few weeks), lead breakage (less common with present systems), CSF leak, radicular pain, intermittent interference with cardiac pacemakers, and weakness.

Outcome
Success rate in pain control is ≈ 50% improvement in 50% of patients in experienced hands at specialized centers where multidisciplinary approach is available[92].
Prognosticators of a poor response to SCS include: pain resulting from spinal cord injury, from lesions proximal to the ganglion (e.g. root avulsion), failed back syndrome with back pain > LE pain and multiple previous operations, psychological factors such as litigation, workers compensation, familial/marital discord or drug seeking behavior[93].

16.4.6. Deep brain stimulation

Indications
Controversial. May be considered when all other treatments have failed. Not FDA approved in the U.S., and investigational protocols have been withdrawn[94]. Deafferentation pain syndromes (anesthesia dolorosa, pain from spinal cord injury, or thalamic pain syndromes) may benefit from stimulation of sensory thalamus (ventral posteromedial **(VPM)** or ventral posterolateral **(VPL)**). Nociceptive pain syndromes are more likely to benefit from stimulation of periventricular gray matter **(PVG)** or periaqueductal gray matter **(PAG)** although PAG stimulation is rarely used because it often produces unpleasant side effects.

16.4.7. Dorsal root entry zone (DREZ) lesions

1. deafferentation pain resulting from nerve root avulsion[95-97]. This most commonly occurs in motorcycle accidents
2. spinal cord injuries **(SCI)** with pain around the lowest spared dermatome with

caudal extension of pain restricted to a few dermatomes (SCI with diffuse pain involving the entire body and limbs below the injury is less responsive)
3. post herpetic neuralgia (*see page 387*): usually good initial response, but early recurrence in ≤ few months is common, and only 25% have long-term relief of pain
4. postamputation phantom limb pain: there is some support for this in the literature, but others feel this is not a good indication[94]
5. ✖ generally not used for cancer pain

Technique: Post-op management: Bed rest for 3 days may reduce the risk of CSF leakage. Analgesics appropriate for a multilevel laminectomy are administered.

Complications: Ipsilateral weakness (related to corticospinal tract) or loss of proprioception (dorsal columns) occurs in 10% of patients, and is permanent in ≈ half (i.e. 5%).

Outcome: In pain related to brachial plexus avulsion, 80-90% long-term significant improvement can be expected. Paraplegics with pain limited to the region of injury have an 80% rate of improvement, compared to 30% for those with pain involving the entire body below the lesion.

16.4.8. Thalamotomy

Controversial & rarely used. Not a routine treatment for pain. May be useful for some nociceptive cancer pain, especially of head, neck and face. Neuropathic pain syndromes respond infrequently. The target is the medial thalamus which exhibits high-frequency bursts associated with deafferentation pain.

Pre-op preparation: CT and/or MRI is used to rule-out mass lesion and to establish target coordinates. Platelet count and coagulation studies must be within normal limits. NSAIDs should be discontinued 10 d pre-op. HTN must be avoided during surgery.

COMPLICATIONS
Mortality: < 1%. Morbidities: significant hemorrhage: 0.5%, subdural hematoma: 0.5%, hemiparesis: 1%, cognitive impairment: 20-70%. Aphasia occurs infrequently.

OUTCOME
Significant pain control occurs in ≈ 50% of those with cancer pain, but recurrence of pain is common and is seen in 60% at 6 months. Only ≈ 20% of cases of neuropathic pain respond.

16.5. Complex regional pain syndrome (CRPS)

Formerly also called causalgia (reflex sympathetic dystrophy). The term causalgia (Greek: *kausis* - burning, *algos* - pain) was introduced by Weir Mitchell in 1864. It was used to describe a rare syndrome that followed a minority of <u>partial</u> peripheral nerve injuries in the American civil war. <u>Triad</u>: burning pain, autonomic dysfunction and trophic changes.

In its severe form, **major causalgia**, was attributed to high velocity missile injuries. **Causalgia minor** denoted less severe forms, and has been described after non-penetrating trauma[98]. Shoulder-hand syndrome and Sudek's atrophy are other variant designations. In 1916, the autonomic nervous system was implicated by René Leriche, and the term **reflex sympathetic dystrophy (RSD)** later came into use[99] (but RSD may be distinct from causalgia[100]).

Post-op CRPS has been described following carpal tunnel surgery as well as surgery on the lumbar[101] (*see page 308*) and cervical spine.

At best, CRPS must be regarded as a *symptom complex*, and not as a discrete syndrome nor medical entity (see the essay by Ochoa[102]). Patients exhibiting CRPS phenomenology are not a homogeneous group, and include[103]:
1. actual CRPS (for these, Mailis proposes the term "physiogenic RSD"): a complex set of neuropathic phenomena that may occur with *or* without nerve injury
2. medical conditions distinct from CRPS but with signs and symptoms that mimic CRPS: vascular, inflammatory, neurologic...
3. the product of mere immobilization: as in severe pain avoidance behavior, or at

times psychiatric disorders
4. part of a factitious disorder with either a psychological basis (e.g. Munchausen's syndrome) or for secondary gain (financial, drug seeking...) i.e. malingering

Pathogenesis
Early theories invoked ephaptic transmission between sympathetics and afferent pain fibers. This theory is rarely cited currently. Another more recent postulate involves nor-epinephrine released at sympathetic terminals together with hypersensitivity secondary to denervation or sprouting. Many modern hypotheses do not even embrace involvement of the autonomic nervous system in all cases[99, 100, 103].

Thus, many of the alterations seen in CRPS may simply be epiphenomena rather than part of the etiopathogenetic mechanism.

CLINICAL
CRPS may be described as a phenomenology, i.e. a variable complex of signs and symptoms due to multiple etiologies included in this nonhomogeneous group[103]. No diagnostic criteria for the condition have been established, and various investigators select different factors to include or exclude patients from their studies.

Symptoms
Pain: affecting a limb, usually burning, and prominent in the hand or foot. Onset in the majority is within 24 hrs of injury (unless injury causes anesthesia, then hrs or days may intervene); however, CRPS may take days to weeks to develop. Median, ulnar and sciatic nerves are the most commonly cited involved nerves. However, it is not always possible to identify a specific nerve that has been injured. Almost any sensory stimulus worsens the pain (**allodynia** is pain induced by a nonnoxious stimulus).

Signs
The physical exam is often difficult due to pain.
Vascular changes: either vasodilator (warm and pink) or vasoconstrictor (cold, mottled blue). Trophic changes (may be partly or wholly due to immobility): dry/scaly skin, stiff joints, tapering fingers, ridged uncut nails, either long/course hair or loss of hair, sweating alterations (varies from anhidrosis to hyperhidrosis).

DIAGNOSTIC AIDS
In the absence of an agreed upon etiology or pathophysiology, there can be no basis for specific tests, and the lack of a "gold-standard" diagnostic criteria makes it impossible to verify the authenticity of any diagnostic marker. Numerous tests have been presented as aids to the diagnosis of CRPS, and essentially all have eventually been refuted. Candidates have included:
1. thermography: discredited in clinical practice
2. three phase bone scan: typical CRPS changes also occur after sympathectomy[104], which has traditionally been considered curative of CRPS
3. osteoporosis on x-ray[105], particularly periarticular demineralization: nonspecific
4. response to sympathetic block (once thought to be the sine qua non for causalgia major and minor, the response sought was relief (complete or significant) with sympathetic block of appropriate trunk (stellate for UE, lumbar for LE)): has failed to hold up once stringent placebo-controlled trials were executed
5. various autonomic tests[106]: resting sweat output, resting skin temperature, quantitative sudomotor axon reflex test

TREATMENT
In the absence of a delineated pathophysiology, treatment is judged purely by subjective impression of improvement. CRPS treatment studies have had an unusually high placebo response rate[107]. Medical therapy is usually ineffective. Proposed treatments include:
1. tricyclic antidepressants
2. 18-25% have satisfactory long-lasting relief after a series of sympathetic blocks (see *Stellate ganglion block* and *Lumbar sympathetic block* starting on *page 627*), although one report found no long-lasting benefit in any of 30 patients[108]
3. intravenous regional sympathetic block, particularly for UE CRPS: agents used include guanethidine[109] 20 mg, reserpine, bretylium..., injected IV with arterial tourniquet (sphygmomanometer cuff) inflated for 10 min. If no relief, repeat in 3-4 wks. No better than placebo in several trials[110, 111]
4. surgical sympathectomy (*see page 373*): some purport that this relieves pain in

> 90% of patients (with a few retaining some tenderness or hyperpathia). Others opine that there is no rational reason to consider sympathectomy since sympathetic blocks have been shown to be no more effective than placebo[99]

5. spinal cord stimulation: some success has been reported

16.6. References

1. Backonja M M: Defining neuropathic pain. **Anesth Analg** 97 (3): 785-90, 2003.
2. Merskey H, Bogduk N: **Classification of chronic pain: Descriptions of chronic pain syndromes and definitions of pain terms**. 2nd ed. IASP Press, Seattle, WA, 1994.
3. Dworkin R H, Backonja M, Rowbotham M C, *et al.*: Advances in neuropathic pain: Diagnosis, mechanisms, and treatment recommendations. **Arch Neurol** 60 (11): 1524-34, 2003.
4. Watson C P N, Babul N: Efficacy of oxycodone in neuropathic pain: A randomized trial in postherpetic neuralgia. **Neurology** 50: 1837-41, 1998.
5. Watson C P, Evans R J, Reed K, *et al.*: Amitriptyline versus placebo in postherpetic neuralgia. **Neurology** 32: 671-3, 1982.
6. Max M B, Lynch S A, Muir J, *et al.*: Effects of desipramine, amitriptyline, and fluoxetine on pain in diabetic neuropathy. **N Engl J Med** 326: 1250-6, 1992.
7. Bennett M I, Simpson K H: Gabapentin in the treatment of neuropathic pain. **Palliat Med** 18 (1): 5-11, 2004.
8. Dierking G, Duedahl T H, Rasmussen M L, *et al.*: Effects of gabapentin on postoperative morphine consumption and pain after abdominal hysterectomy: A randomized, double-blind trial. **Acta Anaesthesiol Scand** 48 (3): 322-7, 2004.
9. Mathew N T, Rapoport A, Saper J, *et al.*: Efficacy of gabapentin in migraine prophylaxis. **Headache** 41 (2): 119-28, 2001.
10. Gabapentin (neurontin®) for chronic pain. **Med Letter** 46: 29-31, 2004.
11. Wilkins R H, Rengachary S S, (eds.): **Neurosurgery**. McGraw-Hill, New York, 1985.
12. Keller J T, van Loveren H: Pathophysiology of the pain of trigeminal neuralgia and atypical facial pain: A neuroanatomical perspective. **Clin Neurosurg** 32: 275-93, 1985.
13. Yeh H S, Tew J M: Tic convulsif, the combination of geniculate neuralgia and hemifacial spasm relieved by vascular decompression. **Neurology** 34: 682-3, 1984.
14. Rupa V, Saunders R L, Weider D J: Geniculate neuralgia: The surgical management of primary otalgia. **J Neurosurg** 75: 505-11, 1991.
15. Young R F: Geniculate neuralgia. **J Neurosurg** 76: 888, 1992 (letter).
16. Wepsic J G: Tic douloureaux: Etiology, refined treatment. **N Engl J Med** 288: 680-1, 1973.
17. Sweet W H: The treatment of trigeminal neuralgia (tic douloureux). **N Engl J Med** 315: 174-7, 1986.
18. Brisman R: Bilateral trigeminal neuralgia. **J Neurosurg** 67: 44-8, 1987.
19. van Loveren H, Tew J M, Keller J T, *et al.*: A 10-year experience in the treatment of trigeminal neuralgia: Comparison of percutaneous stereotaxic rhizotomy and posterior fossa exploration. **J Neurosurg** 57: 757-64, 1982.
20. Taha J M, Tew J M: Comparison of surgical treatments for trigeminal neuralgia: Reevaluation of radiofrequency rhizotomy. **Neurosurgery** 38: 865-71, 1996.
21. Hardy D G, Rhoton A L: Microsurgical relationships of the superior cerebellar artery and the trigeminal

nerve. **J Neurosurg** 49: 669-78, 1978.
22. Morita A, Fukushima T, Miyazaki S, *et al.*: Tic douloureux caused by primitive trigeminal artery or its variant. **J Neurosurg** 70: 415-9, 1989.
23. Apfelbaum R I: *Trigeminal neuralgia: Vascular decompression*. In **Neurovascular surgery**, Carter L P, Spetzler R F, and Hamilton M G, (eds.). McGraw-Hill, New York, 1995, Chapter 62: pp 1107-17.
24. Bullitt E, Tew J M, Boyd J: Intracranial tumors in patients with facial pain. **J Neurosurg** 64: 865-71, 1986.
25. Fusco B M, Alessandri M: Analgesic effect of capsaicin in idiopathic trigeminal neuralgia. **Anesth Analg** 74: 375-7, 1992.
26. Sweet W H: The history of the development of treatment for trigeminal neuralgia. **Clin Neurosurg** 32: 294-318, 1985.
27. Poppen J L: **An atlas of neurosurgical techniques**. W. B. Saunders, Philadelphia, 1960.
28. Sweet W H, Wepsic J G: Controlled thermocoagulation of trigeminal ganglion and rootlets for differential destruction of pain fibers. Part I. Trigeminal neuralgia. **J Neurosurg** 40: 143-56, 1974.
29. Hakanson S: Trigeminal neuralgia treated by the injection of glycerol into the trigeminal cistern. **Neurosurgery** 9: 638-46, 1981.
30. Sweet W H, Poletti C E, Macon J B: Treatment of trigeminal neuralgia and other facial pains by the retrogasserian injection of glycerol. **Neurosurgery** 9: 647-53, 1981.
31. Lunsford L D, Apfelbaum R I: Choice of surgical therapeutic modalities for treatment of trigeminal neuralgia. **Clin Neurosurg** 32: 319-33, 1985.
32. Young R F: Glycerol rhizolysis for treatment of trigeminal neuralgia. **J Neurosurg** 69: 39-45, 1988.
33. Mullan S, Lichtor T: Percutaneous microcompression of the trigeminal ganglion for trigeminal neuralgia. **J Neurosurg** 59: 1007-12, 1983.
34. Belber C J, Rak R A: Balloon compression rhizolysis in the surgical management of trigeminal neuralgia. **Neurosurgery** 20: 908-13, 1987.
35. Lichtor T, Mullan J F: A 10-year follow-up review of percutaneous microcompression of the trigeminal ganglion. **J Neurosurg** 72: 49-54, 1990.
36. Taarnhoj P: Decompression of the posterior trigeminal root in trigeminal neuralgia. **J Neurosurg** 57: 14-7, 1982.
37. Murali R, Rovit R L: Are peripheral neurectomies of value in the treatment of trigeminal neuralgia? An analysis of new cases and cases involving previous radiofrequency Gasserian thermocoagulation. **J Neurosurg** 85: 435-7, 1996.
38. Tew J M, van Loveren H: *Percutaneous rhizotomy in the treatment of intractable facial pain (trigeminal, glossopharyngeal, and vagal nerves)*. In **Operative neurosurgical techniques**, Schmidek H H and Sweet W H, (eds.). W B Saunders, Philadelphia, 2nd ed., 1988, Vol. 2, Chapter 97: pp 1111-23.
39. Brown J A, Preul M C: Percutaneous trigeminal ganglion compression for trigeminal neuralgia. Experience in 22 cases and review of the literature. **J Neurosurg** 70: 900-4, 1989.
40. Lunsford L D: Comment on Taha J M and Tew J M: Comparison of surgical treatments for trigeminal neuralgia: Reevaluation of radiofrequency rhizoto-

41. my. **Neurosurgery** 38: 871, 1996.

41. Brisman R: Gamma knife surgery with a dose fo 75 to 76.8 gray for trigeminal neuralgia. **J Neurosurg** 100: 848-54, 2004.

42. Pollock B E, Phuong L K, Foote R L, *et al*.: High-dose trigeminal neuralgia radiosurgery associated with increased risk of trigeminal nerve dysfunction. **Neurosurgery** 49 (1): 58-62; discussion 62-4, 2001.

43. Kondziolka D, Lunsford L D, Flickinger J C: Ster-eotactic radiosurgery for the treatment of trigeminal neuralgia. **Clin J Pain** 18 (1): 42-7, 2002.

44. Massager N, Lorenzoni J, Devriendt D, *et al*.: Gam-ma knife surgery for idiopathic trigeminal neuralgia performed using a far-anterior cisternal target and a high dose of radiation. **J Neurosurg** 100 (4): 597-605, 2004.

45. Urgosik D, Liscak R, Novotny J, Jr., *et al*.: Treat-ment of essential trigeminal neuralgia with gamma knife surgery. **J Neurosurg** 102 Suppl: 29-33, 2005.

46. Maesawa S, Salame C, Flickinger J C, *et al*.: Clini-cal outcomes after stereotactic radiosurgery for idio-pathic trigeminal neuralgia. **J Neurosurg** 94 (1): 14-20, 2001.

47. Barba D, Alksne J F: Success of microvascular de-compression with and without prior surgical therapy for trigeminal neuralgia. **J Neurosurg** 60: 104-7, 1984.

48. Schmidek H H, Sweet W H, (eds.): **Operative neu-rosurgical techniques**. 1st ed., Grune and Stratton, New York, 1982.

49. Tobler W D, Tew J M, Cosman E, *et al*.: Improved outcome in the treatment of trigeminal neuralgia by percutaneous stereotactic rhizotomy with a new, curved tip electrode. **Neurosurgery** 12: 313-7, 1983.

50. Onofrio B M: Radiofrequency percutaneous Gasse-rian ganglion lesions: Results in 140 patients with trigeminal pain. **J Neurosurg** 42: 132-9, 1975.

51. Menzel J, Piotrowski W, Penzholz H: Long-term re-sults of Gasserian ganglion electrocoagulation. **J Neurosurg** 42: 140-3, 1975.

52. Wepsic J G: Complications of percutaneous surgery for pain. **Clin Neurosurg** 23: 454-64, 1976.

53. Tew J M, Keller J T: The treatment of trigeminal neuralgia by percutaneous radiofrequency tech-nique. **Clin Neurosurg** 24: 557-78, 1977.

54. Sekhar L, Heros R C, Kerber C W: Carotid-cavern-ous fistula following percutaneous retrogasserian procedures. **J Neurosurg** 51: 700-6, 1979.

55. Kuether T A, O'Neill O R, Nesbit G M, *et al*.: Direct carotid cavernous fistula after trigeminal balloon microcompression gangliolysis: Case report. **Neu-rosurgery** 39: 853-6, 1996.

56. Kondziolka D, Lunsford L D, Bissonette D J: Long-term results after glycerol rhizotomy for multiple sclerosis-related trigeminal neuralgia. **Can J Neu-rol Sci** 21: 137-40, 1994.

57. Jannetta P J: Microsurgical management of trigemi-nal neuralgia. **Arch Neurol** 42: 800, 1985.

58. Burchiel K J, Clarke H, Haglund M, *et al*.: Long-term efficacy of microvascular decompression in trigeminal neuralgia. **J Neurosurg** 69: 35-8, 1988.

59. Schmidek H H, Sweet W H, (eds.): **Operative neu-rosurgical techniques**. 2nd ed., W. B. Saunders, Philadelphia, 1988.

60. Hanakita J, Kondo A: Serious complications of mi-crovascular decompression operations for trigemi-nal neuralgia and hemifacial spasm. **Neurosurgery** 22: 348-52, 1988.

61. Youmans J R, (ed.) **Neurological surgery**. 2nd ed., W. B. Saunders, Philadelphia, 1982.

62. Weinstein R E, Herec D, Friedman J H: Hypoten-sion due to glossopharyngeal neuralgia. **Arch Neu-rol** 43: 90-2, 1986.

63. Ferrante L, Artico M, Nardacci B, *et al*.: Glossopha-ryngeal neuralgia with cardiac syncope. **Neuro-surgery** 36: 58-63, 1995.

64. Watson C P N: A new treatment for postherpetic neuralgia. **N Engl J Med** 343: 1563-5, 2000 (edito-rial).

65. Loeser J D: Herpes zoster and postherpetic neural-gia. **Pain** 25: 149-64, 1986.

66. Schimpff S, Serpick A, Stoler B, *et al*.: Varicella-zoster infection in patients with cancer. **Ann Intern Med** 76: 241-54, 1972.

67. Rowbotham M C, Davies P S, Verkempinck C, *et al*.: Lidocaine patch: Double-blind controlled trial of a new treatment method for postherpetic neural-gia. **Pain** 65: 39-44, 1996.

68. Alper B S, Lewis P R: Treatment of postherpetic neuralgia: A systematic review of the literature. **J Fam Pract** 51 (2): 121-8, 2002.

69. Youmans J R, (ed.) **Neurological surgery**. 3rd ed., W. B. Saunders, Philadelphia, 1990.

70. Valacyclovir. **Med Letter** 38. 3-4, 1996.

71. Rowbotham M C, Harden N, Stacey B, *et al*.: Gaba-pentin for the treatment of postherpetic neuralgia: A randomized controlled trial. **JAMA** 280: 1837-42, 1998.

72. Capsaicin - A topical analgesic. **Med Letter** 34: 62-3, 1992.

73. Kotani N, Kushikata T, Hashimoto H, *et al*.: Intrath-ecal methylprednisolone for intractable postherpetic neuralgia. **N Engl J Med** 343: 1514-9, 2000.

74. Dan K, Higa K, Noda B: *Nerve block for herpetic pain.* In **Advances in pain research and therapy**, Fields H, Dubner R, and Cervero F, (eds.). Raven Press, New York, 1985, Vol. 9: pp 831-8.

75. Friedman A H, Nashold B S: Dorsal root entry zone lesions for the treatment of postherpetic neuralgia. **Neurosurgery** 15: 969-70, 1984.

76. Lewith G T, Field J, Machin D: Acupuncture com-pared with placebo in post-herpetic pain. **Pain** 17: 361-8, 1983.

77. Young R F, Kroening R, Fulton W, *et al*.: Electrical stimulation of the brain in treatment of chronic pain: Experience over 5 years. **J Neurosurg** 62: 389-96, 1985.

78. Shieff C, Nashold B S: Stereotactic mesencephalot-omy. **Neurosurg Clin North Amer** 1: 825-39, 1990.

79. Marshall K A: Managing cancer pain: Basic princi-ples and invasive treatment. **Mayo Clin Proc** 71: 472-7, 1996.

80. Krieger A J, Rosomoff H L: Sleep-induced apnea. Part 1: A respiratory and autonomic dysfunction syndrome following bilateral percutaneous cervical cordotomy. **J Neurosurg** 39: 168-80, 1974.

81. Sugar O: In search of Ondine's curse. **JAMA** 240: 236-7, 1978.

82. Schwartz H G: High cervical cordotomy. **J Neuro-surg** 26: 452-5, 1967.

83. Nauta H J, Soukup V M, Fabian R H, *et al*.: Punctate midline myelotomy for the relief of visceral cancer pain. **J Neurosurg Spine** 92 (2): 125-30, 2000.

84. Lobato R D, Madrid J L, Fatela L V, *et al*.: Intraven-tricular morphine for intractable cancer pain: Ratio-nale, methods, clinical results. **Acta Anaesthesiol Scand Suppl** 85: 68-74, 1987.

85. Brazenor G A: Long term intrathecal administration of morphine: A comparison of bolus injection via reservoir with continuous infusion by implantable pump. **Neurosurgery** 21: 484-91, 1987.

86. Penn R D, Paice J A: Chronic intrathecal morphine for intractable pain. **J Neurosurg** 67: 182-6, 1987.

87. Shetter A G, Hadley M N, Wilkinson E: Administra-tion of intraspinal morphine sulfate for the treatment of intractable cancer pain. **Neurosurgery** 18: 740-7, 1986.

88. Rippe E S, Kresel J J: Preparation of morphine sul-fate solutions for intraspinal administration. **Am J Hosp Pharm** 43: 1420-1, 1986.

89. Cramond T, Stuart G: Intraventricular morphine for intractable pain of advanced cancer. **J Pain Sympt**

Manage 8: 465-73, 1993.

90. Penn R D: Comment on Spiegelmann R and Friedman W A: Spinal cord stimulation: A contemporary series. **Neurosurgery** 28: 70, 1991.

91. Kumar K, Nath R, Wyant G M: Treatment of chronic pain by epidural spinal cord stimulation. **J Neurosurg** 75: 402-7, 1991.

92. North R B, Kidd D H, Zahurak M, *et al.*: Spinal cord stimulation for chronic, intractable pain: Experience over two decades. **Neurosurgery** 32: 384-95, 1993.

93. Daniel M S, Long C, Hutcherson W L, *et al.*: Psychological factors and outcome of electrode implantation for chronic pain. **Neurosurgery** 17: 773-7, 1985.

94. Burchiel K J, Favre J: Current techniques for pain control. **Contemp Neurosurg** 19 (17): 1-6, 1997.

95. Thomas D G T, Jones S J: Dorsal root entry zone lesions (Nashold's procedure) in brachial plexus avulsion. **Neurosurgery** 15: 966-8, 1986.

96. Nashold B S: Current status of the DREZ operation: 1984. **Neurosurgery** 15: 942-4, 1984.

97. Friedman A H, Nashold B S: Dorsal root entry zone lesions for the treatment of brachial plexus avulsion injuries: A follow-up study. **Neurosurgery** 22: 369-73, 1988.

98. Sternschein M J, Myers S J, Frewin D B, *et al.*: Causalgia. **Arch Phys Med Rehabil** 56: 58-63, 1975.

99. Schott G D: An unsympathetic view of pain. **Lancet** 345: 634-6, 1995.

100. Ochoa J L, Verdugo R J: Reflex sympathetic dystrophy: A common clinical avenue for somatoform expression. **Neurol Clin** 13: 351-63, 1995.

101. Sachs B L, Zindrick M R, Beasley R D: Reflex sympathetic dystrophy after operative procedures on the lumbar spine. **J Bone Joint Surg** 75A: 721-5, 1993.

102. Ochoa J L: Reflex? Sympathetic? Dystrophy? Triple questioned again. **Mayo Clin Proc** 70: 1124-5, 1995 (editorial).

103. Mailis A: Is diabetic autonomic neuropathy protective against reflex sympathetic dystrophy? **Clin J Pain** 11: 77-81, 1995 (reply to letter).

104. Mailis A, Meindok H, Papagapiou M, *et al.*: Alterations of the three-phase bone scan after sympathectomy. **Clin J Pain** 10: 146-55, 1994.

105. Kozin F, Genant H K, Bekerman C, *et al.*: The reflex sympathetic dystrophy syndrome. **Am J Med** 60: 332-8, 1976.

106. Chelimsky T C, Low P A, Naessens J M, *et al.*: Value of autonomic testing in reflex sympathetic dystrophy. **Mayo Clin Proc** 70: 1029-40, 1995.

107. Ochoa J L: Pain mechanisms in neuropathy. **Curr Opin Neurol** 7: 407-14, 1994.

108. Dotson R, Ochoa J L, Cline M, *et al.*: A reassessment of sympathetic blocks as long term therapeutic modality for "RSD". **Pain** 5: S490, 1990.

109. Hannington-Kiff J G: Relief of Sudek's atrophy by regional intravenous guanethidine. **Lancet** 1: 1132-3, 1977.

110. Blanchard J, Ramamurthy W, Walsh N, *et al.*: Intravenous regional sympatholysis: A double-blind comparison of guanethedine, reserpine, and normal saline. **J Pain Symptom Manage** 5: 357-61, 1990.

111. Jadad A R, Carroll D, Glynn C J, *et al.*: Intravenous regional sympathetic blockade for pain relief in reflex sympathetic dystrophy: A systematic review and a randomized, double-blind crossover study. **J Pain Symptom Manage** 10: 13-20, 1995.

17. Tumor

17.1. General information

CLASSIFICATION OF CNS TUMORS

WHO classification of CNS tumors[1] (modified with adaptations from Escourolle[2])

The following is included only as a framework. Some of these tumors may be classified differently in other sections in this book. This arrow "→" denotes that the indicated cells give rise to the tumor so marked.

In summary, there are 9 categories in the WHO classification as shown in *Table 17-1* (the list that follows below adds the unofficial category "intracranial and/or intraspinal embryonal remnants").

Tumors of neuroepithelial tissue represents a significant portion of what is usually considered to be primary brain tumors. A summary of the subcategories and major tumors of this type is shown in *Table 17-2* (more details appear in the list that follows below).

A. tumors of neuroepithelial tissue
1. astrocytes[A] (see *Astrocytoma*, page 409)
   A. diffusely infiltrating astrocytomas (these tend to progress)
      1. → astrocytoma (grade II of IV[B]) (*page 411*). Variants:
         a. fibrillary
         b. gemistocytic
         c. protoplasmic
         d. mixed
      2. → anaplastic (malignant) astrocytoma (glioma grade III of IV) (*page 412*)
      3. → glioblastoma multiforme (*page 412*) **(GBM)** (glioma grade IV of IV): the most malignant astrocytoma. Variants:
         a. giant cell glioblastoma
         b. gliosarcoma
   B. more circumscribed lesions (these do <u>not</u> tend to progress to anaplastic astrocytoma and GBM)
      1. → pilocytic astrocytoma (*page 417*)
      2. → pleomorphic xanthoastrocytoma (*page 409*)

Table 17-1   9 types of CNS tumors

1.	tumors of neuroepithelial tissue
2.	tumors of cranial and spinal nerves
3.	tumors of the meninges
4.	hematopoietic neoplasms
5.	germ cell tumors
6.	cysts and tumor-like lesions
7.	tumors of the sellar region
8.	local extensions from regional tumors
9.	metastatic tumors

Table 17-2   Tumors of neuroepithelial tissue (*see text* for details)

1. astrocytic tumors
• infiltrating astrocytomas
• pilocytic astrocytomas
• pleomorphic xanthoastrocytoma
• subependymal giant cell astrocytoma
2. oligodendroglial tumors
3. ependymal tumors
4. mixed gliomas
• oligoastrocytoma
5. choroid plexus tumors
6. neuronal and mixed neuronal-glial tumors
• gangliocytoma
• ganglioglioma
• dysembryoplastic neuroepithelial tumor (DNT)
7. pineal tumors
8. embryonal tumors
• neuroblastoma
• retinoblastoma
• PNETs

A. the term **"glioma"** is occasionally used to refer to all glial tumors (e.g. "low-grade glioma" is often used when discussing low-grade tumors of any glial lineage, *see page 408*), although in its usual sense glioma (especially "high grade gliomas") refers <u>only</u> to astrocytic tumors

B. *see page 410* for details on grading astrocytomas

3. → subependymal giant cell astrocytoma (*page 504*)
2. oligodendrocytes → oligodendroglioma (*page 423*)
3. ependymocytes
    A. → ependymomas (*page 470*). Variants:
        1. cellular
        2. papillary
        3. clear cell
        4. tanycytic
    B. → anaplastic (malignant) ependymoma
    C. → myxopapillary ependymoma; occurs only in filum terminale (*page 471*)
    D. → subependymoma (*page 471*)
4. mixed gliomas
    A. oligoastrocytoma including anaplastic (malignant) oligoastrocytoma
    B. others
5. choroid plexus
    A. → choroid plexus papilloma (*page 479*)
    B. → choroid plexus carcinoma (*page 479*)
6. neuroepithelial tumors of uncertain origin
    A. astroblastoma
    B. polar spongioblastoma
    C. gliomatosis cerebri
7. neurons (and mixed neuronal-glial tumors)
    A. gangliocytoma
    B. dysplastic gangliocytoma of cerebellum (Lhermitte-Duclos)
    C. desmoplastic infantile ganglioglioma (**DIG**)
    D. dysembryoplastic neuroepithelial tumors (**DNT**) (*page 409*)
    E. gangliogliomas (*page 466*) including anaplastic (malignant) gangliogliomas
    F. central neurocytoma: *see page 425*
    G. paraganglioma of the filum terminale
    H. olfactory neuroblastoma (esthesioneuroblastoma)
        1. variant: olfactory neuroepithelioma
8. pinealocytes
    A. → pineocytomas (*page 477*) (pinealoma)
    B. → pineoblastomas (*page 477*)
    C. → mixed/transitional pineal tumors
9. embryonal tumors
    A. medulloepithelioma
    B. neuroblastoma
        1. variant: ganglioneuroblastoma
    C. retinoblastoma
    D. ependymoblastoma
    E. primitive neuroectodermal tumors (**PNET**) (*page 473*)
        1. medulloblastomas (*page 473*). Variants:
            a. desmoplastic medulloblastoma
            b. medullomyoblastoma
            c. melanotic medulloblastoma
        2. cerebral (supratentorial) and spinal PNET
B. tumors of the meninges
    1. tumors of meningothelial cells
        A. → meningiomas (*page 426*). Variants:
            1. meningothelial
            2. fibrous (fibroblastic)
            3. transitional (mixed)
            4. psammomatous
            5. angiomatous
            6. microcystic
            7. secretory
            8. clear cell
            9. chordoid
            10. lymphoplasmacyte-rich
            11. metaplastic
        B. → atypical meningioma (*page 428*)
        C. → anaplastic (malignant) meningioma (*page 428*)
    2. mesenchymal, non-meningothelial tumors
        A. benign neoplasms
            1. osteocartilaginous tumors
            2. lipoma
            3. fibrous histiocytoma
            4. others
        B. malignant neoplasms

       1. hemangiopericytoma
       2. chondrosarcoma
          a. variant: mesenchymal chondrosarcoma
       3. malignant fibrous histiocytoma
       4. rhabdomyosarcoma
       5. meningeal sarcomatosis
       6. others:
          a. e.g. primary cerebral sarcoma (rare). May result from sarcomatous change in preexisting tumor such as meningioma, glioblastoma, or oligodendroglioma

C. primary melanocytic lesions
       1. diffuse melanosis
       2. melanocytoma
       3. malignant melanoma (primary CNS) (*page 479*)
          a. variant: meningeal melanomatosis

D. tumors of uncertain histogenesis
       1. hemangioblastoma (capillary hemangioblastoma) (*page 459*)

C. tumors of cranial and spinal nerves
       1. schwannoma (neurinoma). Acoustic neuromas (*page 429*). Variants:
          A. cellular
          B. plexiform
          C. melanotic
       2. neurofibromas (*page 502*)
          A. circumscribed (solitary)
          B. plexiform
       3. malignant peripheral nerve sheath tumor (**MPNST**) (neurogenic sarcoma, anaplastic neurofibroma, "malignant schwannoma"). Variants:
          A. epithelioid
          B. MPNST with divergent mesenchymal and/or epithelial differentiation
          C. melanotic

D. lymphomas and hematopoietic neoplasms
       1. malignant lymphomas (primary CNS lymphoma) (*page 461*)
       2. plasmacytoma
       3. granulocytic sarcoma
       4. others

E. germ cell tumors
       1. germinomas (*page 477*)
       2. embryonal carcinoma
       3. yolk sac tumor (endodermal sinus tumor)
       4. choriocarcinoma
       5. teratoma (*page 477*) (from all 3 germ-cell layers)
          A. immature
          B. mature
          C. teratoma with malignant transformation
       6. mixed germ cell tumors

F. cysts and tumor-like lesions
       1. Rathke's cleft cyst (*page 457*)
       2. epidermoid cyst: AKA cholesteatomas (*page 474*)
       3. dermoid cyst (*page 474*)
       4. colloid cyst of the third ventricle (*page 457*)
       5. enterogenous cyst
       6. neuroglial cyst
       7. granular cell tumor (choristoma, pituicytoma)
       8. hypothalamic neuronal hamartoma
       9. nasal glial heterotopia
     10. plasma cell granuloma

G. tumors of the sellar region
       1. adenohypophyseal cells → pituitary adenomas (*page 438*)
       2. pituitary carcinoma
       3. craniopharyngiomas (*page 456*). Variants:
          A. adamantinomatous
          B. papillary

H. local extensions from regional tumors
       1. paraganglioma (chemodectoma)
          A. glomus jugulare tumors (*page 468*)

2. notochord → chordomas (*page 464*)
3. chondroma, chondrosarcoma
4. carcinoma
I. intracranial and/or intraspinal embryonal remnants
   1. adipose cells → lipomas (e.g. of corpus callosum, *page 114*)
J. metastatic tumors
K. unclassified tumors

17.1.1. Brain tumors - general clinical aspects

PRESENTATION

The most common presentation of brain tumors is progressive neurologic deficit (68%), usually motor weakness (45%). Headache was a presenting symptom in 54% (*see below*), and seizures in 26%. For details of presentation, see sections below for supratentorial and infratentorial tumors.

SUPRATENTORIAL TUMORS[3]
Signs and symptoms include:
1. those due to increased ICP (see *Infratentorial tumors* below):
   A. from mass effect of tumor and/or edema
   B. from blockage of CSF drainage (hydrocephalus): less common in supratentorial tumors (may occur e.g. with colloid cyst, entrapped lateral ventricle)
2. progressive focal deficits: includes weakness, dysphasia (which occurs in 37-58% of patients with left-sided brain tumors[4]): *see below*
   A. due to destruction of brain parenchyma by tumor invasion
   B. due to compression of brain parenchyma by mass and/or peritumoral edema and/or hemorrhage
   C. due to compression of cranial nerve(s)
3. headache: *see below*
4. seizures: not infrequently the first symptom of a brain tumor. Tumor should be aggressively sought in an idiopathic first time seizure in a patient > 20 years (if negative, the patient should be followed with repeat studies at later dates). Rare with posterior fossa tumors or pituitary tumors
5. mental status changes: depression, lethargy, apathy, confusion
6. symptoms suggestive of a TIA (dubbed "tumor TIA") or stroke, may be due to:
   A. occlusion of a vessel by tumor cells
   B. hemorrhage into the tumor: any tumor may hemorrhage, see *Hemorrhagic brain tumors*, page 854
   C. focal seizure
7. in the special case of pituitary tumors (see *Pituitary adenomas*, page 438):
   A. symptoms due to endocrine disturbances
   B. pituitary apoplexy: *see page 438*
   C. CSF leak

INFRATENTORIAL TUMORS
Seizures are rare (unlike supratentorial tumors, (seizures arise from irritation of cerebral cortex).
1. most posterior fossa tumors present with signs and symptoms of increased intracranial pressure (**ICP**) due to hydrocephalus (**HCP**). These include:
   A. headache: (*see below*)
   B. nausea/vomiting: due either to increased ICP from HCP, or from direct pressure on the vagal nucleus or the area postrema ("vomiting center")
   C. papilledema: estimated incidence is ≈ 50-90% (more common when the tumor impairs CSF circulation)
   D. gait disturbance/ataxia
   E. vertigo
   F. diplopia: may be due to VI nerve (abducens) palsy which may occur with increased ICP in the absence of direct compression of the nerve (*see page 586*)
2. S/S indicative of mass effect in various locations within the p-fossa

A. lesions in cerebellar <u>hemisphere</u> may cause: ataxia of the extremities, dysmetria, intention tremor
B. lesions of cerebellar <u>vermis</u> may cause: broad based gait, truncal ataxia, titubition
C. brainstem involvement usually results in multiple cranial nerve and long tract abnormalities, and should be suspected when nystagmus is present (especially rotatory or vertical)

FOCAL NEUROLOGIC DEFICITS ASSOCIATED WITH BRAIN TUMORS

In addition to nonfocal signs and symptoms (e.g. seizures, increased ICP…), as with any destructive brain lesion tumors may produce progressive deficits related to the function of the involved brain. Some characteristic "syndromes":

1. frontal lobe: abulia, dementia, personality changes. Often nonlateralizing, but apraxia, hemiparesis or dysphasia (with dominant hemisphere involvement) may occur
2. temporal lobe: auditory or olfactory hallucinations, déja vu, memory impairment. Contralateral superior quadrantanopsia may be detected on visual field testing
3. parietal lobe: contralateral motor or sensory impairment, homonymous hemianopsia. Agnosias (with dominant hemisphere involvement) and apraxias may occur (see *Clinical syndromes of parietal lobe disease*, page 87)
4. occipital lobe: contralateral visual field deficits, alexia (especially with corpus callosum involvement with infiltrating tumors)
5. posterior fossa: (*see above*) cranial nerve deficits, ataxia (truncal or appendicular)

HEADACHES WITH BRAIN TUMORS

Headache **(H/A)** may occur with or without elevated ICP. Present equally in patients with primary or metastatic tumor (≈ 50% of patients[5]). Classically described as being worse in the morning (possibly due to hypoventilation during sleep), this may actually be uncommon[5]. Often exacerbated by coughing, straining, or (in 30%) bending forward (placing head in dependent position). Associated with nausea and vomiting in 40%, may be temporarily relieved by vomiting (possibly due to hyperventilation during vomiting). These features along with the presence of a focal neurologic deficit or seizure were thought to differentiate tumor H/A from others. However, H/A in 77% of brain tumor patients were similar to tension H/A, and in 9% were migraine-like[5]. Only 8% showed the "classic" brain tumor H/A, two thirds of these patients had increased ICP.

Etiologies of tumor headache: The brain itself is not pain sensitive. H/A in the presence of brain tumor may be due to any combination of the following:

1. increased intracranial pressure **(ICP)**: which may be due to
   A. tumor mass effect
   B. hydrocephalus (obstructive or communicating)
   C. mass effect from associated edema
   D. mass effect from associated hemorrhage
2. invasion or compression of pain sensitive structures:
   A. dura
   B. blood vessels
   C. periosteum
3. secondary to difficulty with vision
   A. diplopia due to dysfunction of nerves controlling extra-ocular muscles
      1. direct compression of III, IV, or VI
      2. abducens palsy from increased ICP (*see diplopia on page 404*)
      3. internuclear ophthalmoplegia due to brainstem invasion/compression
   B. difficulty focusing: due to optic nerve dysfunction from invasion/compression
4. extreme hypertension resulting from increased ICP (part of Cushing's triad)
5. psychogenic: due to stress from loss of functional capacity (e.g. deteriorating job performance)

POSTERIOR FOSSA (INFRATENTORIAL) TUMORS

See *Posterior fossa lesions* on page 923 for differential diagnosis (includes non-neoplastic lesions as well).

In pediatric patients with a posterior fossa tumor, an MRI of the lumbar spine should be done pre-op to rule-out drop mets (post-op there may be artifact from blood).

In adults, most intraparenchymal p-fossa tumors will be metastatic, and workup for a primary should be undertaken (*see page 488*).

TREATMENT OF ASSOCIATED HYDROCEPHALUS

In cases with hydrocephalus at the time of presentation, some authors advocate initial placement of VP shunt or EVD prior to definitive surgery (waiting ≈ 2 wks before surgery) because of possibly lower operative mortality[20]. Theoretical risks of using this approach include the following:

1. placing a shunt is generally a lifelong commitment, whereas not all patients with hydrocephalus from a p-fossa tumor will require a shunt
2. possible seeding of the peritoneum with malignant tumor cells e.g. with medulloblastoma. Consider placement of tumor filter (may not be justified given the high rate of filter occlusion and the low rate of "shunt metastases"[21])
3. some shunts may become infected prior to the definitive surgery
4. definitive treatment is delayed, and the total number of hospital days may be increased
5. upward transtentorial herniation (*see page 160*) may occur if there is excessively rapid CSF drainage

Either approach (shunting followed by elective p-fossa surgery, or semi-emergent definitive p-fossa surgery) is accepted. At Children's Hospital of Philadelphia, dexamethasone is started and the surgery is performed on the next elective operating day, unless neurologic deterioration occurs necessitating emergency surgery[22].

Many surgeons place a ventriculostomy at the time of surgery. CSF is drained only after the dura is opened to help equilibrate the pressures between the infra- and supratentorial compartments. Post-op, the external ventricular drain is usually set at a low height (≈ 10 cm above the EAM) for 24 hours, and is progressively raised over the next 48 hrs and should be D/C'd by ≈ 72 hrs post-op.

FAMILIAL SYNDROMES

Several familial syndromes are associated with CNS tumors as shown in *Table 17-3*.

STEROID USE IN BRAIN TUMORS

The beneficial effect of steroids in metastatic tumors is often much more dramatic than with primary infiltrating gliomas.

Dexamethasone (Decadron®) dose for brain tumors (*see page 10* for cautions):
- for patients not previously on steroids:
  - ◆ adult: 10 mg IVP loading, then 6 mg PO/IVP q 6 hrs[7, 8]. In cases with severe vasogenic edema, doses up to 10 mg q 4 hrs may be used
  - ◆ peds: 0.5-1 mg/kg IVP loading, then 0.25-0.5 mg/kg/d PO/IVP divided q 6 hrs. NB: avoid prolonged treatment because of growth suppressant effect
- for patients already on steroids:
  - ◆ for acute deterioration, a dose of approximately double the usual dose should be tried
  - ◆ for "stress" doses, *see page 10*

Table 17-3 Familial syndromes associated with CNS tumors

Syndrome	Page	CNS tumor
von Hippel-Lindau	459	hemangioblastoma
tuberous sclerosis	504	subependymal giant cell astrocytoma
neurofibromatosis type I	502	optic glioma, astrocytoma, neurofibroma
neurofibromatosis type II	503	acoustic neuroma, meningioma, ependymoma, astrocytoma
Li-Fraumeni		astrocytoma, PNET
Turcot syndrome (BTP syndrome)[6]		glioblastoma & medulloblastoma

PROPHYLACTIC ANTICONVULSANTS IN BRAIN TUMORS

20-40% of patients with a brain tumor will have had a seizure by the time their tumor is diagnosed[9]. Antiepileptic drugs (**AEDs**) are indicated in these patients. 20-45% more will ultimately develop a seizure[9]. Although it has been studied, prophylactic AEDs does not provide substantial benefit (reduction of risk > 25% for seizure-free survival) and there are significant risks involved.

Recommendations[9]
1. prophylactic AEDs should not be used routinely in patients with newly diagnosed brain tumors (standard)
2. in patients with brain tumors undergoing craniotomy, prophylactic AEDs may be used, and if there has been no seizure, it is appropriate to taper off AEDs starting 1 week post-op (guideline)

CHEMOTHERAPY FOR BRAIN TUMORS

Some agents used for CNS tumors are shown in *Table 17-4*[10, 11].

Blood-brain barrier (BBB):
Traditionally, the BBB has been considered to be a major hindrance to the use of chemotherapy for brain tumors. In theory, the BBB effectively excludes many chemotherapeutic agents from the CNS, thereby creating a "safe haven" for some tumors, e.g. metastases. This concept has been challenged[12]. Regardless of the etiology, the response of most brain tumors to systemic chemotherapy is usually very modest, with a notable exception being a favorable response of oligodendrogliomas (*see page 424*). Considerations regarding chemotherapeutic agents in relation to the BBB include:

1. some CNS tumors may partially disrupt the BBB, especially malignant gliomas[13]
2. lipophilic agents (e.g. nitrosoureas) may cross the BBB more readily
3. selective intraarterial (e.g. intracarotid) injection[14]:

Table 17-4 Chemotherapeutic agents used for CNS tumors

Agent	Mechanism
1. nitrosoureas: carmustine (BC-NU), CCNU (lomustine) ACNU (nimustine)	DNA crosslinks, carbamoylation of amino groups
2. alkylating (methylating) agents (procarbazine, temozolomide)	DNA alkylation, interferes with protein synthesis
3. carboplatin, cisplatin	chelation via intrastrand crosslinks
4. nitrogen mustards: cyclophosphamide, isofamide, cytoxan	DNA alkylation, carbonium ion formation
5. vinca alkaloids: vincristine, vinblastine, paclitaxel	microtubule function inhibitors
6. epidophyllotoxins (ETOP-oside, VP16, teniposide, VM26)	topoisomerase II inhibitors
7. topotecan, irinotecan (CPT-11)	topoisomerase I inhibitors
8. tamoxifen	protein kinase C inhibitor
9. hydroxyurea	
10. bleomycin	
11. taxol (paxlitaxol)	
12. methotrexate	
13. cytosine, arabinoside	
14. corticosteroids: dexamethasone, prednisone	
15. fluorouracil (FU)	

produces higher local concentration of agents which increases penetration of the BBB, with lower associated systemic toxicities than would otherwise occur
4. the BBB may be iatrogenically disrupted (e.g. with mannitol) prior to administration of the agent
5. the BBB may be bypassed by intrathecal administration of agents via LP or ventricular access device (e.g. methotrexate for CNS lymphoma, *see page 464*)
6. biodegradable polymer wafers containing the agent may be directly implanted (*see page 416*)

CAT SCAN FOLLOWING SURGICAL REMOVAL OF TUMOR

To assess degree of tumor removal, a post-op brain CT without and with contrast should either be obtained within 2-3 days[15], or should be delayed at least ≈ 30 days. The non-contrast scan is important in the early post-op period to determine which areas of increased intensity are due to post-op blood and not enhancement. The contrast CT demonstrates areas of enhancement, which may represent residual tumor. After ≈ 48 hours, contrast enhancement due to post-operative inflammatory vascular changes ensues, which may be impossible to differentiate from tumor. This usually subsides by ≈ 30 days[16], but may persist for 6-8 weeks[17]. This recommendation regarding the timing of post-op CT does not apply to pituitary tumors (see *Pituitary adenomas*, page 438). The effect of steroids on contrast enhancement is controversial[18, 19], and may depend on many factors (including tumor type).

17.2. Primary brain tumors

17.2.1. Low grade gliomas

This special section is included here because the following tumors are sometimes grouped together despite the fact that they have different cell lineages.

Cell lineages considered under the heading of low-grade gliomas (**LGG**) include:
1. WHO grade II infiltrating astrocytoma (fibrillary or proto-plasmic) (*see page 411*) ⎱
2. oligodendroglia (*see page 423*) ⎰ comprise most low grade gliomas in adults
3. mixed astrocytes & oligodendroglia (oligoastrocytomas)
4. gangliogliomas (*see page 466*)
5. gangliocytomas
6. juvenile pilocytic astrocytoma (*see page 417*) ⎱ less frequent histologies
7. pleomorphic xanthoastrocytomas (*see below*) ⎰
8. dysembryoplastic neuroepithelial tumors (**DNT**) (*see below*)

Spatial definition[23, 24]
Can be used to classify LGG into 3 types (independent of histologic group).
- Type 1: solid tumor only without infiltration of brain parenchyma. Most amenable to surgical resection. Most favorable prognosis. Includes gangliogliomas, pilocytic astrocytomas, pleomorphic xanthoastrocytomas, and some protoplasmic astrocytomas (no oligodendrogliomas are in this group)
- Type 2: solid tumor associated with surrounding tumor-infiltrated brain parenchyma. Surgical resection may be possible, depending on tumor location. Often low-grade astrocytomas
- Type 3: infiltrative tumor cells without solid tumor tissue. Risk of neurologic deficit may preclude surgical resection. Usually oligodendrogliomas

Clinical
Although there are differences among the specific histological types, these tumors generally occur in young adults or children, and are often diagnosed after a history of seizures.

Neuroradiology
MRI: Most LGG are hypointense on T1WI. T2WI shows high signal changes that extend beyond the tumor volume demonstrated on other imaging sequences[24]. Only ≈ 30% enhance.
PET scans: usually shows reduced uptake of fluorodeoxyglucose compared to the rest of the brain, indicative of hypometabolism.

Diagnosis
Although imaging (and clinical) characteristics may suggest one specific tumor type, biopsy is usually required to definitively determine the diagnosis.

Treatment
Complete surgical excision is often sufficient for some of these tumors when it can be accomplished (e.g. with cystic cerebellar pilocytic astrocytomas (**PCAs**)). When this is not possible (e.g. with most hypothalamic PCAs and PCAs involving the optic nerves and chiasm), then further therapy is required, usually in the form of chemotherapy for younger children[25] (to defer the need for XRT until the patient is as old as possible).

Epidemiology

Incidence: not accurately known because the diagnosis may be missed. Estimated range: 0.8-5% of all primary brain tumors. Typically occurs in children and young adults. Most common locations: temporal or frontal. Parietal and especially occipital lobe involvement is rare. DNTs have been reported in the cerebellum, pons & basal ganglia.

Clinical

Typically associated with longstanding medically intractable seizures, usually complex partial. Symptoms usually begin before age 20.

Imaging

Cortical lesions with no surrounding edema and no midline mass effect.

CT: hypodense with distinct margins.Deformity of overlying calvaria is common.

MRI: T1WI: hypointense. T2WI: hyperintense, septations may be seen. If there is enhancement, it is usually nodular.

PET scan: hypometabolic with ^{18}Ffluorodeoxyglucose. Negative ^{11}Cmethionine uptake (unlike all other gliomas).

Pathology

A WHO Grade I glioma. Thought to arise embryologically from the secondary germinal layer (which includes subependymal layer, cerebellar external granular layer, hippocampal dentate fascia & subpial granular layer).

Multinodularity at low-power is a key feature, and the primary constituent cells are oligodendrocytes and to a lesser extent, astrocytes that are often pilocytic. Occasionally difficult to differentiate from oligodendroglioma.

Two distinct forms[28] (do not appear to have different prognoses):
1. simple form: glioneural elements consisting of axon bundles perpendicular to the cortical surface, lined with oligodendroglial-like cells that are S-100 positive and GFAP negative. Normal appearing neurons floating in a pale eosinophilic matrix are scattered between these columns (no resemblance to ganglion cells, unlike gangliogliomas)
2. complex form: glioneural elements as described above in the simple form, with glial nodules scattered throughout. The glial component may mimic a low grade fibrillary astrocytoma. Foci of cortical dysplasia occur

Outcome

Seizure control: usually improves after surgery. Degree of control seems to correlate with completeness of removal. Improvement is not as good with longer duration of intractable seizures.

Recurrence/continued growth: recurrence after complete removal, or tumor growth after partial resection is rare. Adjuvant treatment (XRT, chemotherapy...) is of no benefit. Mitoses or endothelial proliferation, seen on occasion, do not affect outcome. Malignant transformation is very rare.

PLEOMORPHIC XANTHOASTROCYTOMA *(PXA)*

In general, a compact, superficial tumor with marked cellular pleomorphism, abundant reticulin and frequent perivascular chronic inflammatory cells. Variable lipidization. Absence of vascular proliferation and necrosis[29], most but not all lack mitotic figures. Some PXAs undergo anaplastic change[30]. Often cystic with enhancing mural nodule. Usually occurs in young adults. Incomplete resections should be followed since these tumors may grow very slowly over many years before treatment is necessary, and repeat excision should be considered.

17.2.2. Astrocytoma

The most common primary intra-axial brain tumor, $\approx$ 12,000 new cases per year in the United States.

CLASSIFICATION BY CELL TYPE

The dominant cell types of astrocytomas allows their classification into one of the subdivisions shown in *Table 17-5*. The rationale for separating "ordinary" from "special" astrocytomas is based on a much different and more favorable behavior of the latter group which does not depend on grade within that group (these also tend to occur in younger patients). Current thinking has been to abandon the notion that pilocytic and microcystic cerebellar astrocytomas are the same tumor as fibrillary astrocytomas but in a different location (see *Pilocytic astrocytomas*, page 417).

Gemistocytic astrocytomas: Gemistocytes are plump cells filled with eosinophilic, hyaline cytoplasm, seen almost exclusively in gemistocytic astrocytomas and GBM. Small numbers, however, may be seen in fibrillary astrocytomas (gemistocytes should account for > 20% of tumor cells for an astrocytoma to be considered a gemistocytic astrocytoma). Gemistocytic astrocytomas are comprised primarily of these cells, but rarely occur in pure form. Often meet grade III (malignant astrocytoma) criteria.

Table 17-5 Classification of astrocytomas by cell type

"Ordinary" astrocytomas	"Special" astrocytomas
fibrillary gemistocytic protoplasmic	pilocytic microcystic cerebellar subependymal giant cell

17.2.2.1. "Ordinary" (fibrillary) astrocytomas

GRADING AND NEUROPATHOLOGY

The grading of "ordinary" astrocytomas has been historically fraught with disagreement, and a number of grading systems have been proposed over the years. The first system of Bailey and Cushing was a 3-tiered system, the Kernohan system was 4-tiered, and since then a number of 3-tiered systems have been proposed. As a result, there has been a lack of uniformity in, for example, what constitutes a glioblastoma from series to series. The current trend has been to use one of two different systems, the WHO definition or the St. Anne/Mayo system, both of which appear below.

Grading of astrocytomas remains controversial. Some special concerns:
1. sampling error: may have different degrees of malignancy in different areas
2. dedifferentiation: tumors tend to progress in malignancy over months or years (see *Dedifferentiation*, page 412)
3. histological criteria that affect prognosis include: cellularity, presence of giant cells, anaplasia, mitosis, vascular proliferation with or without endothelial proliferation, necrosis, and pseudopalisading[31]
4. in addition to histology, issues that affect clinical behavior include:
   A. patient age
   B. extent of tumor
   C. topography: tumor location, especially in relation to critical structures

NEUROPATHOLOGICAL GRADING

Kernohan system

The Kernohan system[32] divided these tumors into 4 grades (grade IV tumors are also called glioblastoma multiforme) based on the degree of presence of a number of features such as anaplasia, nuclear pleomorphism, number of mitoses... In terms of prognostication, this system distinguishes only 2 clinically different groups (grades I/II, and grades III/IV) and is less commonly used today.

Three tiered systems

There are numerous 3-tiered grading schemes, and each differs slightly. An example is shown in *Table 17-6*.

Table 17-6 A typical three tiered grading system of fibrillary astrocytic neoplasms*[33]

Characteristic	Astro-cytoma	Anaplastic astrocytoma	Glioblastoma multiforme
hypercellularity	slight	moderate	moderate to marked
pleomorphism	slight	moderate	moderate and marked
vascular proliferation	none	permitted	common (not required)
necrosis†	none	none	required (± pseudopalisading)

* to avoid confusion, grade numbers are not shown
† necrosis distinguishes anaplastic astrocytoma from glioblastoma multiforme

The World Health Organization (**WHO**) recommends a system as shown in *Table 17-7*[1], where grade I represents special types of gliomas including pilocytic astrocytomas (see *Low grade gliomas*, page 408), and the more typical astrocytic neoplasms are graded II through IV. The approximate equivalence to the Kernohan grade is also shown.

Table 17-7 Approximate equivalence of Kernohan grade (I-IV) to WHO system

Kernohan grade	WHO designation[1]	
	(I) special tumors: e.g. pilocytic astrocytomas	
I II	} (II) astrocytoma (low-grade)	
III	(III) anaplastic astrocytoma	} malignant astrocytoma
IV	(IV) glioblastoma multiforme	

The WHO criteria are shown in *Table 17-8*[1, 11].

St. Anne/Mayo grading system:
The classification system that is sometimes known as the St. Anne/Mayo (**SA/M**) system or the Daumas-Duport system[34] was devised to address histological considerations, and represents a reproducible and prognostically significant system[35]. It is restricted to "ordinary" astrocytomas, as grade has not been shown to correlate with clinical behavior in pilocytic astrocytomas.

The SA/M system assesses the presence or absence of 4 criteria (*see Table 17-9*) and then assigns a grade based on the number of criteria present (*see Table 17-10*). When the presence of any criteria is uncertain, it is considered to be absent.
The criteria tended to occur in a predictable sequence: nuclear atypia occurred in all grade 2 tumors, mitotic activity was seen in 92% of grade 3 tumors (and in none of the grade 2 tumors), necrosis and endothelial proliferation were restricted almost only to grade 4 tumors (they were seen in only 8% of grade 3 tumors).

Table 17-8 WHO classification of astrocytic tumors

Designation	Criteria
glioblastoma multiforme	highly cellular, nuclear and cellular pleomorphism, endothelial proliferation, mitotic figures, and, often, necrosis*
anaplastic astrocytoma	compared to GBM: less cellular and less pleomorphism, less mitoses and no necrosis
astrocytoma	glial tumors other than the above with little cellularity and minimal pleomorphic changes

*   although necrosis is a hallmark of GBM and is often present, it is not required for the WHO designation of GBM

Table 17-9 St. Anne/Mayo criteria

- nuclear atypia: hyperchromatasia and/or obvious variation in size and shape
- mitoses: normal or abnormal configuration
- endothelial proliferation: vascular lumina are surrounded by "piled-up" endothelial cells. Does <u>not</u> include hypervascularity
- necrosis: only when obviously present. Does <u>not</u> include pseudopalisading when seen alone

The frequencies among 287 astrocytomas were: grade 1 = 0.7%, grade 2 = 16%, grade 3 = 17.8%, and grade 4 = 65.5%.
Median survival was as follows[34]: (there were only two grade 1 patients, one survived 11 years and the other was still alive after 15 years), grade 2 = 4 years, grade 3 = 1.6 years, and grade 4 = 0.7 years (8.5 months).

**Table 17-10
St. Anne/Mayo
grade**

Grade	No. of criteria
1	0
2	1
3	2
4	3 or 4

Relative frequency of astrocytoma grades
Ratio of (glioblastoma):(anaplastic astrocytoma):(low-grade astrocytoma) is ≈ 5:3:2. Peak age incidence rises with increasing grade: 34 years for low-grade astrocytoma, 41 years for anaplastic astrocytoma, and 53 years for GBM[36].

Low-grade astrocytoma (WHO II)
These tumors tend to occur in children and young adults. Most present with seizures. There is a predilection for temporal, posterior frontal and anterior parietal lobes[37]. They demonstrate low degrees of cellularity and preservation of normal brain elements within the tumor. Calcifications are rare. Anaplasia and mitoses are absent (a single mitosis is allowed). Blood vessels may be slightly increased in number. The ultimate behavior of these tumors is usually not benign. The most important favorable prognosticator is young age. Poor prognosis is associated with findings of increased ICP, altered consciousness, personality change, significant neuro-

logic deficits[38], short duration of symptoms before diagnosis, and enhancement on imaging studies. Also *see page 408*.

Dedifferentiation: The major cause of morbidity with low-grade astrocytomas is dedifferentiation to a more malignant grade. Low grade fibrillary astrocytomas tend to undergo malignant transformation more quickly (with six-fold increased rapidity) when diagnosed after age 45 years than when diagnosed earlier[36] (*see Table 17-11*). Gemistocytic astrocytomas tend to dedifferentiate more rapidly than fibrillary astrocytomas. Once dedifferentiation occurs, median survival is 2-3 years beyond that event.

Table 17-11   Dedifferentiation rate for low grade astrocytomas

	Patients diagnosed @ age < 45 yrs	Patients diagnosed @ age ≥45 yrs
mean time to dedifferentiation	44.2 ± 17 mos	7.5 ± 5.7 mos
time to death	58 mos	14 mos

Malignant astrocytomas (WHO III & IV)
    This category encompasses anaplastic astrocytoma **(AA)** and glioblastoma multiforme **(GBM)**. Although both are "malignant", AA and GBM have distinct differences. Among 1265 patients with malignant astrocytomas, the mean age was 46 yrs for AA, and 56 yrs for GBM. Mean duration of symptoms pre-op: 5.4 mos for GBM, and 15.7 mos for AA. Malignant astrocytomas may develop from low grade astrocytomas via dedifferentiation (*see above*), however they may also arise de novo.

Glioblastoma multiforme (WHO IV)
    The most common primary brain tumor, it is also the most malignant astrocytoma.
    Histological findings associated with GBM (not all may be present, and this list does not follow any of the standard grading systems above):
• gemistocytic astrocytes
• neovascularization with endothelial proliferation
• areas of necrosis
• pseudopalisading around areas of necrosis

    Infratentorial glioblastoma multiforme **(GBM)** is rare, and often represents subarachnoid dissemination of a supratentorial GBM (used as an argument for irradiation in all patients with p-fossa GBM)[39].

MISCELLANEOUS PATHOLOGICAL FEATURES

Glial fibrillary acidic protein (GFAP) : Staining for GFAP is positive with most astrocytomas (however, may not stain positive in some poorly differentiated gliomas, and in gemistocytic astrocytomas since fibrillary astrocytes are required to be positive).

Cysts: Gliomas may have cystic central necrosis, but may also have an associated cyst even without necrosis. When fluid from these cysts is aspirated it can be differentiated from CSF by the fact that it is usually xanthochromic and often clots once removed from the body (unlike e.g. fluid from a chronic subdural). Although they may occur with malignant gliomas, cysts are more commonly associated with pilocytic astrocytomas (*see page 419*).

NEURORADIOLOGICAL GRADING AND FINDINGS
    Astrocytomas are typically located in white matter (e.g. centrum semiovale) and track through white matter tracts (*see below*). Calcifications and cysts occur in 10-20% of AA[40].

CT scan & MRI grading
    Grading gliomas by CT or MRI is imprecise[41], but may be used as a preliminary assessment (*see Table 17-12*). Neuroradiologic grading is **not** applicable to pediatric patients.
    Most low-grade gliomas do not enhance on CT or MRI (although up to 40% do[42], and may have a poorer prognosis). They are usually hypodense on CT. Most are hypointense on T1WI MRI, and show high intensity changes on T2WI

Table 17-12   Grading gliomas by CT or MRI

Kernohan grade	Radiographic features	
I	CT: low density MRI: abnormal signal	no mass effect, no enhancement
II	CT: low density MRI: abnormal signal	mass effect, no enhancement
III	complex enhancement (may not enhance)	
IV	necrosis (ring enhancement)	

that extend beyond the tumor volume. Some malignant gliomas do not enhance[41, 43]. Anaplastic astrocytomas may or may not enhance[40].

Ring-enhancement with glioblastoma multiforme (GBM): The low density center on CT represents necrosis. The enhancing ring is cellular tumor, however, tumor cells also extend as far as 15 mm beyond the ring[44].

Positron emission tomography (PET) scan
Low grade fibrillary astrocytomas appear as hypometabolic "cold" spots with fluorodeoxyglucose PET scans. Hypermetabolic "hot" spots suggest high-grade astrocytomas.

Angiographic appearance
AA's usually appear as an avascular mass. Tumor blush and AV-shunting with early draining veins are more characteristic of GBM.

SPREAD
Gliomas may spread by the following mechanisms[45] (note: < 10% of recurrent gliomas recur away from the original site[46]):
1. tracking through white matter
   A. corpus callosum **(CC)**
      1. through genu or body of CC → bilateral frontal lobe involvement (**"butterfly glioma"**)
      2. through splenium of CC → bilateral parietal lobe involvement
   B. cerebral peduncles → midbrain involvement
   C. internal capsule → encroachment of basal ganglion tumors into centrum semiovale
   D. uncinate fasciculus → simultaneous frontal and temporal lobe tumors
   E. interthalamic adhesion → bilateral thalamic gliomas
2. CSF pathways (subarachnoid seeding): 10-25% frequency of meningeal and ventricular seeding by high grade gliomas[47]
3. rarely spread systemically

MULTIPLE GLIOMAS
Multiple gliomatous masses can be seen in any one of several settings:
1. conventional glioma that has spread by one of the mechanisms previously described (*see above*)
2. **gliomatosis cerebri**: a diffuse, infiltrating astrocytoma that invades almost all of the cerebral hemispheres and brainstem. Usually low-grade[42], areas of anaplasia and glioblastoma may also occur[48] and may present as focal mass[49]. Occurs most frequently in 1st 2 decades
3. **meningeal gliomatosis**: dissemination of glioma throughout the CSF, similar to carcinomatous meningitis (*see page 491*). Occurs in up to 20% of autopsies on patients with high-grade gliomas. May present with cranial neuropathies, radiculopathies, myelopathy, dementia, and/or communicating hydrocephalus
4. multiple primary gliomas: some of the following terms are inconsistently used interchangeably: "multicentric", "multifocal", and "multiple". Reported range of occurrence is 2-20% of gliomas[50, 51] (lower end of range is probably more accurate, the higher end of the range is probably accounted for by infiltrative extension[52 (p 3117)])
   A. commonly associated with neurofibromatosis and tuberous sclerosis
   B. rarely associated with multiple sclerosis and progressive multifocal leukoencephalopathy

TREATMENT CONSIDERATIONS FOR MULTIPLE GLIOMAS
Once the diagnosis of multiple gliomatous masses has been ascertained, local therapies (e.g. surgery, interstitial radiation…) are impractical. Whole brain radiation and possibly chemotherapy are indicated.

LOW-GRADE ASTROCYTOMAS (WHO GRADE II)
Treatment options:
1. no treatment: follow serial neurologic exams and imaging studies
2. radiation
3. chemotherapy
4. combined radiation and chemotherapy
5. surgery

Analysis
No well-designed study has shown that any approach for supratentorial WHO grade II infiltrating astrocytomas in adults is clearly superior. Some treatments may simply expose the patient to the risk of treatment side effects. These tumors are slow growing, and until progression on imaging or malignant degeneration is documented, it may be no worse to not treat the patient[53]. Although this view has been challenged[54], a definitive study has yet to be performed. The following are associated with more aggressive tumors and should prompt consideration for some form of treatment:
1. extremely young patients, or patients > 50 yrs age
2. large tumors that enhance (size is one of the most important prognosticators[55])
3. short clinical history
4. evidence of progression on imaging studies

Surgery
The role of surgery in low-grade gliomas is controversial, due in part to the fact that surgery is not curative for most infiltrating hemispheric gliomas, and many of these tumors are not completely resectable. There is a trend to suggest that complete surgical removal, when possible, is associated with a better prognosis[24, 55]. However, this remains unproven.

Surgery is the principal treatment in the following situations of low-grade astrocytomas:
1. surgical biopsy or partial resection is recommended in almost all cases to establish the diagnosis since clinical and radiographic data are not definitive[37]
2. pilocytic astrocytomas
   A. cerebellar tumors occurring in children & young adults (see page 419)
   B. supratentorial pilocytic astrocytomas
3. when herniation threatens from large tumors or tumor cysts
4. tumors causing obstruction of CSF flow
5. may help in seizure control with refractory seizures
6. in an attempt to delay adjuvant therapy and its side-effects in children (especially those < 5 yrs old)[37]
7. smaller tumors are less aggressive than large ones[56] and may be better candidates for early surgery (also, see below)

The role of surgery is limited in the following situations of low-grade astrocytomas:
1. disseminated (poorly circumscribed) tumors
2. multifocal tumors
3. location in areas of eloquent brain

Technical considerations at surgery:
Since the margins of low-grade gliomas may not be readily visible at the time of surgery, adjuncts such as stereotactic and image guided techniques may be advantageous for deep tumors or in areas bordering on eloquent brain[57].
Unresolved issues: whether the extent of tumor removal influences 1) time to tumor progression, 2) incidence of malignant degeneration, and 3) period of survival. One series[58] suggested that 5-year survival improved from 50% with incomplete resection to 80% with complete resection. Some feel that early radical surgery does reduce the rate of malignant degeneration, especially when tumor volume is < 30 ml[37].

Radiation
In spite of retrospective evidence suggesting that tumor-free survival time and overall survival time after incomplete resection is prolonged by radiation[59], no well-designed study has ever been carried out[60]. A prospective dose-response trial found no difference in survival or progression-free survival between doses of 45 Gy in 5 weeks vs. 59.4 Gy in 6.6 weeks[55]. Side effects from radiation are frequent after routine whole-brain XRT and include leukoencephalopathy and cognitive impairment (see Radiation injury and necrosis, page 535).

Recommendations for XRT in low-grade gliomas (modified[60]):
1. dogmatic statements regarding XRT are unwarranted
2. in cases of gross total surgical removal, or incomplete removal in cases of pilocytic astrocytoma or cystic cerebellar astrocytoma, XRT may be withheld until tumor recurrence or progression that cannot be treated surgically is documented
3. in cases of incomplete removal of ordinary low-grade astrocytomas, post-op XRT may be considered, consisting of fractionated treatments to a maximum of **45 Gy** to the tumor bed plus surrounding margin (2 cm for enhancing, and 1 cm around hypodense zone for nonenhancing tumors) instead of whole brain XRT
4. malignant degeneration of tumor should be treated with XRT, following reoperation when appropriate

Chemotherapy
Usually reserved for tumor progression. PCV (procarbazine, CCNU, and vincristine) frequently stabilizes tumor growth. Recent evidence[61] suggests that temozolomide (Temodar®) may be effective in progressive WHO grade II astrocytomas (off label use).

MALIGNANT ASTROCYTOMAS (WHO GRADES III & IV)

Surgery
Cytoreductive surgery followed by external beam radiation (40 Gy whole-brain + 15-20 Gy to the tumor bed delivering a total of ≈ 60 Gy to the tumor) has become the standard against which other treatments are compared[62]. The extent of tumor removal and (in an inverse relationship) the volume of residual tumor on post-op imaging studies have a significant effect on time to tumor progression and median survival[63]. Alternative views suggest that surgery may be justified to reduce significant mass effect but not for reducing tumor burden[64, 65]. One must bear in mind that these tumors cannot be cured with surgery, and so the goal should be to prolong _quality_ survival; this can usually be accomplished with tumor excision for _lobar_ gliomas in patients in good neurologic condition. In _elderly_ patients (> 65 yrs age), the benefit conferred by surgery is modest (median survival of 17 weeks after biopsy + XRT, versus 30 weeks for surgery + XRT)[66].

Partial resection of a GBM carries significant risk of post-operative hemorrhage and/or edema with risk of herniation. Furthermore, the benefit of subtotal resection is dubious. Therefore, surgical excision should only be considered when the goal of gross total removal is feasible.

As a result of the above, the following are usually not candidates for surgery
1. extensive dominant lobe GBM
2. lesions with significant bilateral involvement (e.g. large butterfly gliomas)
3. elderly patients
4. patients with poor Karnofsky scores (in general, the neurologic condition on steroids is as good as it is going to get, and surgery rarely improves this)

Radiation therapy
The usual dose of XRT for malignant gliomas is 50-60 Gy. Whole brain XRT has not been shown to increase survival compared to focal XRT, and the risk of side effects is greater[67].

Brachytherapy has shown no significant benefit as an adjunct to EBRT in the initial treatment of malignant astrocytomas[68].

Chemotherapy
All agents in use have no more than a 30-40% response rate, and most have 10-20%[69]. Although not positively proven, it appears that the more complete the surgical resection, the more value the chemotherapy has[69]. When given before XRT, chemotherapy may also be useful.

Alkylating agents produce significant benefit in ≈ 10% of patients[70] (similar efficacy among all available agents: BCNU, CCNU, procarbazine...). Carmustine **(BCNU)** (BiCNU®)[71] and cisplatinum (AKA cisplatin, Platinol®) have been the primary chemotherapeutic agents used against malignant gliomas. The response may be enhanced by inhibition (via methylation) of the gene responsible for production of the DNA-repair enzyme O^6-methylguanine-DNA methyltransferase **(MGMT)**[72].

Σ | Following surgery + XRT, median survival is ≈ 9 mos, and 2-year survival is only 5-10%[73]. Meta-analysis showed an absolute increase in 1-year survival of 6% and a 2-month increase in median survival with chemotherapy. Nitrosoureas are fairly well tolerated and easy to administer. However, the quality of life during this modest increase is uncertain, making chemotherapy an option[74].

carmustine (BCNU®) | DRUG INFO

In an attempt to reduce systemic effects, intraarterial injection of carmustine has been tried[75, 76], but side effects are significant, including progressive leukoencephalopathy and visual deterioration due to retinal toxicity (attempts to offset this by selectively injecting distal to the ophthalmic artery have been disappointing). BCNU containing wafers may also be surgically implanted following tumor resection, and have been used by some following initial resection but are currently FDA approved only for *recurrent* tumor (*see below*).

The only protocol to have been fully validated by Phase 3 study[69] is maximal surgical resection when possible, followed by XRT of 60 Gy, and then BCNU at 6-week intervals of 110 mg/M².

Implantable chemotherapy:

Gliadel® wafers: carmustine (BCNU) 7.7 mg in a 200 mg prolifeprosan 20 hydrophobic polymer carrier (wafer). Following tumor removal, up to 8 wafers are applied to the resection bed at the time of surgery. The drug is released over ≈ 2-3 wks. This exposes the tumor to 113 times the concentration of BCNU that could be achieved with systemic administration[77]. In animals, only trace amounts of the drug reach the systemic circulation. FDA approved in the U.S. for implantation in *recurrent* glioblastoma multiforme.

Median survival was 28 weeks compared to 20 weeks with placebo, and 6 month survival was 64% compared to 44% with placebo[78]. In a small randomized study using implants at the time of *initial* resection, median survival increased from 40 weeks to 53 weeks[79].

No effect on blood counts occurred. The implants do increase cerebral edema, wound healing problems, and the incidence of seizures within 5 days of surgery. 8 wafers cost ≈ $12,500[80].

temozolomide (Temodar®) | DRUG INFO

An oral alkylating agent that is FDA approved for use in adults for the initial relapse of anaplastic astrocytoma and progression of disease while on a regimen containing a nitrosourea (see *Table 17-4*, page 407) and procarbazine. It has also been used (off label) for newly diagnosed GBM and AA[81] and for patients with minimal post-surgery treatment as well as for progressive low grade astrocytomas[61]. Cost: $1,300-1,500 per cycle.

Rx 150 mg/m²/d PO q d **x** 5 d. Dose for subsequent 5 day cycles every 28 days is adjusted according to nadir neutrophil and platelet counts (which occurs at day 21) during the previous cycle and the start of the next cycle (therefore check CBC on days 21 & 29).

Reoperation for recurrence

Less than 10% of recurrent gliomas recur away from the original tumor site[46]. Reoperation extends survival by an additional 36 weeks in patients with GBM, and 88 weeks in AA[82, 83] (duration of high quality survival was 10 weeks and 83 weeks respectively, and was lower with pre-op Karnofsky score < 70). In addition to Karnofsky score, significant prognosticators for response to repeat surgery include: age and time from the first operation to re-operation (shorter times → worse prognosis)[78]. Morbidity is higher with reoperation (5-18%); the infection rate is ≈ 3 **x** that for first operation, wound dehiscence is more likely.

OUTCOME

Survival with various grades of astrocytoma

In general, with "optimal treatment" the survival of the various grades of astrocytoma are approximately given in *Table 17-13* (more details may be found in other sections).

Malignant astrocytomas (WHO grades III & IV)

The following 3 statistically independent factors affect longevity:
1. patient age: consistently found to be the most significant prognosticator, with younger patients faring better. With GBM, 18 month survival is 50% for patients < 40 yrs, 20% for ages 40-60, and 10% for age > 60[84]

Table 17-13 Approximate survival for astrocytomas

Grade	Median survival
I	8-10 yrs
II	7-8 yrs
III	≈ 2-3 yrs
IV	< 1 yr

2. histological features: median survival is 36 mos for AA, and 10 mos for GBM[84] (also, *see below*)
3. performance status (e.g. Karnofsky score (KPS) *see page 899*) at presentation:
  A. with GBM, 18 month survival is 34% for KPS > 70, vs. 13% for KPS < 60[84]
  B. 5-year survival: 7.6% with KPS ≥ 70 pre-op, vs. 3.2% for KPS < 70[3]

With AA, smaller size and frontal location influence survival favorably.

Survival differences between AA and GBM:
Two large studies treated malignant gliomas by surgical resection, 60 Gy whole brain irradiation, and then various chemotherapy regimens (BCNU, procarbazine, methylprednisolone...) resulted in the survival statistics shown in *Table 17 14*.

Table 17-14   Malignant glioma life table survival statistics[33]

Tumor	– 1-yr survival –		– 2-year survival –	
	Study A	Study B	Study A	Study B
AA	60%	73%	38%	50%
GBM	36%	35%	12%	8%

STEREOTACTIC BIOPSY

Stereotactic biopsy may underestimate the occurrence of GBM by as much as 25%.
Indications for stereotactic biopsy in suspected malignant astrocytomas[85]:
1. tumors located in eloquent or inaccessible areas of brain
2. small tumors with minimal deficit
3. patients in poor medical condition precluding general anesthesia
4. to ascertain a diagnosis when one is not definitely established (including when considering a more definitive operation). Some CNS lymphomas mimic a GBM radiographically (and without immunostaining, some have also been mistaken pathologically) biopsy should be given serious consideration (to avoid operating on a lymphoma)

Technique
Yield of biopsy is highest when targets within the low density (necrotic) center and enhancing rim are chosen[44].

Outcome
In a study of 91 cases of malignant gliomas with "critical location" (i.e. deep, midline, or near eloquent brain), it was found that cytoreductive surgery may not improve survival (a limited number of patients underwent cytoreductive surgery with no obvious improvement in survival, but too few to tell if statistically significant), and that biopsy + XRT may be appropriate therapy for these non-lobar malignant tumors (*see Table 17-15*). There was no significant difference in survival between AA and GBM when the tumors were not lobar. A Karnofsky rating ≥ 70 at presentation may also portend a better prognosis (not statistically significant in this study).

Table 17-15   Survival after stereotactic Bx*
(91 patients with malignant astrocytoma[85])

Location	Tumor type	Number	Treatment	Median survival (weeks)
deep or lobar	GBM & AA	26 GBM + 4 AA	Bx only (no XRT)	≤ 11
deep	AA	6	Bx + XRT	19.4†
	GBM	22	Bx + XRT	27†
lobar	AA	17	Bx + XRT	129
	GBM	16	Bx + XRT	46.9

* abbreviations: Bx = biopsy; XRT = radiation therapy in adequate dose, defined as 50-60 Gy

† difference not statistically significant

Patients with left-sided tumors and dysphasia are at significant risk of worsening of language function following stereotactic biopsy (the risk of deterioration is low if there is no dysphasia before biopsy)[86].

17.2.2.2.   Pilocytic astrocytomas

❢ Key features
  • mean age of occurrence is lower than for typical astrocytomas
  • better prognosis than infiltrating fibrillary or diffuse astrocytomas
  • radiographic appearance: discrete appearing, contrast enhancing lesion, often cystic with mural nodule
  • pathology: compacted and loose textured astrocytes with Rosenthal fibers and/or eosinophilic granular bodies

| • danger of overgrading and overtreating if not recognized. Pathology alone may be inadequate for diagnosis; knowledge of radiographic appearance is critical

BACKGROUND AND TERMINOLOGY

Pilocytic astrocytoma (**PCA**) is the currently recommended classification of these tumors that have been referred to for many years variously as cystic cerebellar astrocytomas, juvenile pilocytic astrocytomas, optic gliomas, and hypothalamic gliomas[87 (p 77-96)]. PCAs differ markedly from infiltrating fibrillary or diffuse astrocytomas in terms of their ability to invade tissue and for malignant degeneration.

LOCATION

PCAs arise throughout the neuraxis and are more common in children and young adults:
1. **optic gliomas & hypothalamic gliomas:**
   A. PCAs arising in the optic nerve are called optic gliomas (*see page 420*)
   B. when they occur in the region of the chiasm they cannot always be distinguished clinically or radiographically from so-called hypothalamic gliomas (*see page 420*) or gliomas of the third ventricular region
2. **cerebral hemispheres:** tends to occur in older patients (i.e. young adults) than optic nerve/hypothalamic lesions. These PCAs are potentially confused with fibrillary astrocytomas possessing more malignant potential. PCAs are often distinguished by a cystic component with an enhancing mural nodule (would be atypical for a fibrillary astrocytoma), & some PCAs have dense calcifications[87]
3. **brainstem gliomas:** usually are fibrillary infiltrating type and only a small proportion are pilocytic. Those that are PCAs may comprise the majority of the prognostically favorable group described as "dorsally exophytic"[88] (*see page 420*)
4. **cerebellum:** formerly referred to as cystic cerebellar astrocytoma (*see below*)
5. **spinal cord:** PCAs may also occur here, but little information is available on these. Again, patients tend to be younger than with spinal cord fibrillary astrocytomas

PATHOLOGY

PCAs are composed of loosely knit tissue comprised of stellate astrocytes in microcystic regions containing eosinophilic granular bodies intermixed with regions of compact tissue consisting of elongated and fibrillated cells often associated with **Rosenthal fiber**[A] formation[87]. These latter two distinctive features facilitate the diagnosis. Another characteristic finding is that the tumors easily break through the pia to fill the overlying subarachnoid space. PCAs may also infiltrate into the perivascular spaces. Vascular proliferation is common. Multinucleated giant cells with peripherally located nuclei are common, especially in PCAs of the cerebellum or cerebrum. Mitotic figures may be seen, but are not as ominous as with fibrillary astrocytomas. Areas of necrosis may also be seen. In spite of well-demarcated margins grossly and on MRI, at least 64% of PCAs infiltrate the surrounding parenchyma, especially the white matter[89] (the clinical significance of this is uncertain, one study found no statistically significant decrease in survival[90]).

Differentiating from a diffuse or infiltrating fibrillary astrocytoma: Unless some of the distinctive findings described above are seen, pathology alone may not be able to differentiate. This may be especially problematic with small specimens obtained e.g. with stereotactic biopsy. Factors that suggest the diagnosis include young age, and knowledge of the radiographic appearance is often critical (*see below*).

Malignant degeneration: Malignant degeneration has been reported, often after many years. This may occur without radiation therapy (**XRT**)[91], although in most cases XRT had been administered[92].

RADIOGRAPHIC APPEARANCE

On CT or MRI, PCAs are usually well circumscribed, enhance with contrast (unlike some low-grade fibrillary astrocytomas), frequently have a cystic component with a mural nodule, and have little or no surrounding edema. Although they may occur anywhere in the CNS, they are most often periventricular.

A. Rosenthal fibers: sausage or corkscrew shaped cytoplasmic eosinophilic inclusion bodies consisting of glial filament aggregates resembling hyaline. Stain bright red on Masson trichrome smears

PILOCYTIC ASTROCYTOMA OF THE CEREBELLUM

❖ Key features
- often cystic, half of these have mural nodule
- usually presents during the second decade of life (ages 10-20 yrs)

Formerly referred to by the nonspecific and confusing term **cystic cerebellar astrocytoma**. One of the more common pediatric brain tumors (≈ 10%[93]), comprising 27-40% of pediatric p-fossa tumors[94 (p 367-74), 95 (p 3032)]. They may also occur in adults, where the mean age is lower and the post-operative survival is longer than for fibrillary astrocytomas[96].

PRESENTATION

Signs and symptoms of pilocytic astrocytoma **(PCA)** of the cerebellum are usually those of any p-fossa mass, i.e. those of hydrocephalus or cerebellar dysfunction (see *Posterior fossa (infratentorial) tumors*, page 405). Usually presents during second decade of life (ages 10-20).

PATHOLOGY

The classic "juvenile pilocytic astrocytoma" of the cerebellum is a distinctive entity with its macroscopic cystic architecture and microscopic spongy appearance[87]. For other microscopic findings, *see above*.

These tumors may be solid, but are more often cystic (hence the older term "cystic cerebellar astrocytoma"), and tend to be large at the time of diagnosis (cystic tumors: 4-5.6 cm dia; solid tumors: 2-4.8 cm dia). Cysts contain highly proteinaceous fluid (averaging ≈ 4 Hounsfield units higher density than CSF on CT[93]).

50% of cystic tumors have a mural nodule and a cyst lining of reactive, non-neoplastic cerebellar tissue or ependymal lining (non-enhancing on CT), whereas the remaining 50% lack a nodule and have a cyst wall of poorly cellular tumor[97] (enhances on CT).

Histological classification of Winston

The Winston classification system[98] is shown in *Table 17-16*. 72% of cerebellar PCAs tended to cluster with either Type A or B characteristics, 18% in his series had both, and 10% had neither.

Table 17-16 Classification of cerebellar astrocytoma

• Type A: microcysts, leptomeningeal deposits, Rosenthal fibers, foci of oligodendroglioma
• Type B: perivascular pseudorosettes, high cell density, mitosis, calcification
• common features of types A & B: hypervascularity, endothelial proliferation, parenchymal desmoplasia, pleomorphism

TREATMENT GUIDELINES

The natural history of these tumors is slow growth. Treatment of choice is surgical excision of the maximal amount of the tumor that can be removed without producing deficit. In some, invasion of brainstem or involvement of cranial nerves or blood vessels may limit resection. In tumors composed of a nodule with a true cyst, excision of the nodule is sufficient; the cyst wall is non-neoplastic and need not be removed. In tumors with a so-called "false cyst" where the cyst wall is thick and enhances (on CT or MRI), this portion must be removed also. Because of the high 5 and 10 year survival rates together with the high complication rate of radiation therapy over this time interval (see *Radiation injury and necrosis*, page 535) and the fact that many incompletely resected tumors enlarge minimally if at all over periods of 5, 10 or even 20 years, it is recommended to not radiate these patients post-op. Rather, they should be followed with serial CT or MRI and be re-operated if there is recurrence[99]. Radiation therapy is indicated for *nonresectable* recurrence (i.e. reoperation is preferred if possible) or for recurrence with malignant histology. Chemotherapy is preferable to XRT in younger patients[25].

Also, see *Posterior fossa (infratentorial) tumors*, page 405 for guidelines regarding hydrocephalus, etc.

PROGNOSIS

Children with Winston Type A cerebellar PCAs had 94% 10-yr survival, whereas those with Type B had only 29% 10-yr survival.

Tumor recurrence is relatively common, and although it has been said that they generally occur within ≈ 3 yrs of surgery[100], this is controversial and very late recurrences (violating **Collins' law**, which says that a tumor may be considered cured if it does not recur within a time period equal to the patient's age at diagnosis + 9 months) are well known[99]. Also, some tumors excised partially fail to show further growth, representing a form of cure.

About 20% of cases develop hydrocephalus requiring treatment following surgery[101]. So-called "drop metastases" are rare with PCAs.

OPTIC GLIOMA

Accounts for ≈ 2% of gliomas in adults, and 7% in children. The incidence is higher (≈ 25%) in neurofibromatosis **(NFT)** (*see page 502*).

May arise in any of the following patterns:
1. one optic nerve (without chiasmal involvement)
2. optic chiasm: less commonly involved in patients with NFT than in sporadic cases
3. multicentric in both optic nerves sparing the chiasm: almost only seen in NFT
4. may occur in conjunction with or be part of a hypothalamic glioma (*see below*)

Pathology

Most are composed of low-grade (pilocytic) astrocytes. Rarely malignant.

Presentation

<u>Painless</u> proptosis is an early sign in lesions involving one optic nerve. Chiasmal lesions produce variable and nonspecific visual defects (usually monocular) without proptosis. Large chiasmal tumors may cause hypothalamic and pituitary dysfunction, and may produce hydrocephalus by obstruction at the foramen of Monro. Gliosis of the optic nerve head may be seen on funduscopy.

Evaluation

Plain x-rays: not usually helpful, although in some cases dilatation of the optic canal can be seen in optic canal views.

CT/MRI: CT scan is excellent for imaging structures within the orbit. MRI is helpful for demonstrating chiasmal or hypothalamic involvement. On CT or MRI, involvement of the optic nerve produces contrast enhancing fusiform enlargement of the nerve usually extending > 1 cm in length.

Treatment

Tumor involving a single optic nerve, sparing the chiasm, producing proptosis and visual loss should be treated with a transcranial approach with excision of the nerve from the globe all the way back to the chiasm (a transorbital (Kronlein) approach is not appropriate since tumor may be left in the nerve stump).

Chiasmal tumors are generally not treated surgically except for biopsy (especially when it is difficult to distinguish an optic nerve glioma from a hypothalamic glioma), CSF shunting, or to remove the rare exophytic component to try and improve vision.

Further treatment: Chemotherapy[25] (especially in younger patients) or XRT is used for chiasmal tumors, for multicentric tumors, post-op if tumor is found in the chiasmal stump end of the resected nerve, and for the rare malignant tumor. Typical XRT treatment planning is for 45 Gy given in 25 fractions of 1.8 Gy.

HYPOTHALAMIC GLIOMA

Pilocytic astrocytomas of the hypothalamus and third ventricular region occur primarily in children. Radiographically, the lesion may have an intraventricular appearance. Many of these tumors have some chiasmal involvement and the distinction from optic nerve glioma cannot be made (*see above*).

May present with so-called **"diencephalic syndrome"**, a rare syndrome seen in peds, usually caused by an infiltrating glioma of the anterior hypothalamus. Classically: cachexia (loss of subcutaneous fat) associated with hyperactivity, over-alertness and an almost euphoric affect. May also see: hypoglycemia, failure to thrive, macrocephaly.

When complete resection is not possible, further treatment may be needed as outlined under optic gliomas (see *Further treatment* above).

17.2.2.3. Brainstem glioma

❡ Key features
• not a homogeneous group, MRI can differentiate malignant from benign lesions
• trend: lower grade tumors tend to occur in the upper brainstem, and higher grade tumors in the lower brainstem/medulla

| • usually presents with multiple cranial nerve palsies and long tract findings
| • most are malignant, have poor prognosis, and are not surgical candidates

Brainstem gliomas **(BSG)** tend to occur during childhood and adolescence (77% are < 20 yrs old, they comprise 1% of adult tumors[102]). They are one of the 3 most common brain tumors in pediatrics (see *Pediatric brain tumors*, page 480), comprising ≈ 10-20% of pediatric CNS tumors[88].

PRESENTATION[103]

Upper brainstem tumors tend to present with cerebellar findings and hydrocephalus, whereas lower brainstem tumors tend to present with multiple lower cranial nerve deficits and long tract findings. Due to their invasive nature, signs and symptoms usually do not occur until the tumor is fairly extensive in size.

Signs and symptoms:
1. gait disturbance
2. headache (*see page 405*)
3. nausea/vomiting
4. cranial nerve deficits: diplopia, facial asymmetry
5. distal motor weakness in 30%
6. papilledema in 50%
7. hydrocephalus in 60%, usually due to aqueductal obstruction (often late, except with periaqueductal tumors, e.g. see *Tectal gliomas* below)
8. failure to thrive (especially in age ≤ 2 yrs)

PATHOLOGY

BSG is a heterogeneous group. There may be a tendency towards lower grade tumors in the upper brainstem (76% were low-grade) versus the lower brainstem (100% of the glioblastomas were in the medulla)[104]. A cystic component is seen rarely. Calcifications are also rare. 4 growth patterns that can be identified by MRI[105] that may correlate with prognosis[106]:
1. **diffuse**: all are malignant (most are anaplastic astrocytomas, the rest are glioblastomas). On MRI these tumors extend into the adjacent region in vertical axis (e.g. medullary tumors extend into pons and/or cervical cord) with very little growth towards obex, remaining intraaxial
2. **cervicomedullary**: most (72%) are low-grade astrocytomas. The rostral extent of these tumors is limited to the spinomedullary junction. Most bulge into the obex of the 4th ventricle (some may have an actual exophytic component)
3. **focal**: extent limited to medulla (does not extend up into pons nor down into spinal cord). Most (66%) are low-grade astrocytomas
4. dorsally exophytic: may be an extension of "focal" tumors (*see above*). Many of these may actually be low grade gliomas including:
   A. pilocytic astrocytomas: *see page 417*
   B. **gangliogliomas** (*see page 466*): very rare, only 13 cases reported as of 1984. Compared to other BSGs, these patients tend to be slightly older and the medulla is involved more frequently[107]

EVALUATION

MRI

The diagnostic test of choice. MRI evaluates status of ventricles, gives optimal assessment of tumor (CT is poor in the posterior fossa) and detects exophytic component. T1WI: almost all are hypointense, homogeneous (excluding cysts). T2WI: increased signal, homogeneous (excluding cysts). Gadolinium enhancement is highly variable[105].

CT

Most do not enhance on CT, except possibly an exophytic component. If there is marked enhancement, consider other diagnoses (e.g. high grade vermian astrocytoma).

TREATMENT

SURGERY
Biopsy: should <u>not</u> be performed when the MRI shows a diffuse infiltrating brainstem lesion[108] (does not change treatment or outcome).

Treatment is usually non-surgical. Exceptions where surgery may be indicated:
1. tumors with a dorsally exophytic component[88]: *see below* these may protrude into 4th ventricle or CP angle, tend to enhance with IV contrast, tend to be lower grade
2. some success has been achieved with non-exophytic tumors that are <u>not</u> malignant astrocytomas (surgery in malignant astrocytomas is without benefit)[106] (detailed follow-up is lacking)

Dorsally exophytic tumors
These tumors are generally histologically benign (e.g. gangliogliomas) and are amenable to radical subtotal resection. Prolonged survival is possible, with a low incidence of disease progression at short-term follow-up[88].

Surgical goals in exophytic tumors include:
1. enhanced survival by subtotal removal of exophytic component[109]: broad attachment to the floor of 4th ventricle is typical and usually precludes complete excision (although some "safe entry" zones have been described[110])
2. establishing diagnosis: radiographic differentiation of exophytic brainstem gliomas tumors from other lesions (e.g. medulloblastoma, ependymoma and dermoids) may be difficult
3. tumors that demonstrate recurrent growth after resection remained histologically benign and were amenable to re-resection[88]

Complications of surgery generally consisted of exacerbation of pre-operative symptoms (ataxia, cranial nerve palsies...) which usually resolved with time.

MEDICAL
No proven chemotherapeutic regimen. Steroids are usually administered. In pediatrics, there is some indication of response to Temodar® (temozolomide).

RADIATION
Traditionally given as 45-55 Gy over a six week period, five days per week. When combined with steroids, symptomatic improvement occurs in 80% of patients.

Possible improved survival with so called **"hyperfractionation"** where multiple smaller doses per day are used.

PROGNOSIS
Most children with malignant BSG will die within 6-12 months of diagnosis. XRT may not prolong survival in patients with grade III or IV tumors. A subgroup of children have a more slowly growing tumor and may have up to 50% five-year survival. Dorsally exophytic tumors comprised of pilocytic astrocytomas may have a better prognosis.

TECTAL GLIOMAS

A topically defined diagnosis generally consisting of low-grade astrocytomas. Considered a benign subgroup of brainstem glioma. Because of location, tends to present with hydrocephalus. Focal neurologic findings are rare (diplopia, visual field deficits, nystagmus, Parinaud's syndrome, ataxia, seizures...) and are often reversible after the hydrocephalus is corrected.

Epidemiology
Comprises ≈ 6% of *surgically* treated pediatric brain tumors[111]. Presents primarily in childhood. Median age of patients becoming symptomatic = 6-14 years[111].

Pathology
Since many of these are not biopsied, meaningful statistical analysis is not possible. Pathologies identified include: WHO II diffuse astrocytoma, pilocytic astrocytomas, WHO II ependymoma, anaplastic astrocytoma, oligodendroglioma & oligoastrocytoma.

Radiographic evaluation

CT scan detects the hydrocephalus, but may miss the tumor in ≈ 50%[112]. Calcification on CT has been described in 9-25%[112, 113].

MRI is the study of choice for diagnosis and follow-up. Typically appears as a mass projecting dorsally from the quadrigeminal plate. Isointense on T1WI, iso- or hyperintense on T2WI[111, 114]. Enhancement with gadolinium occurs in 18% and is of uncertain prognostic significance.

Treatment

Due to the indolent course, open surgery is not recommended. Options include:
1. VP shunt: the standard treatment for years. Long-term results are good with a functioning shunt
2. endoscopic third ventriculostomy: may avoid the need for a shunt. Endoscopic biopsy[115] may be done at the same time through the same burr hole if it is technically feasible (requires a dilated foramen of Monro, which is often present). Long-term results unknown
3. endoscopic aqueductoplasty (with or without stenting): an option for some. Long-term results unknown

Stereotactic radiosurgery : May be offered for tumor progression (criteria are not defined; radiographic progression may not be associated with clinical deterioration[114]). Dosing should be limited to ≤ 14 Gray at the 50-70% isodose line to avoid radiation-induced side effects[116].

Prognosis

Tumor progression: described in 15-25%.

Follow-up: no accepted guidelines. Serial neurologic exams and MRIs every 6-12 months has been suggested[111].

17.2.3. Oligodendroglioma

❖ Key features
- frequently presents with seizures
- predilection for the frontal lobes
- classic histologic features of "fried egg" cytoplasm & "chicken wire" vasculature are unreliable. Calcifications are common
- grading: controversial. Recommendation: low grade and high grade
- recommended treatment: surgery for some, chemotherapy for all, XRT only for anaplastic transformation

EPIDEMIOLOGY

Oligodendroglioma **(ODG)** have long been thought to comprise only ≈ 2-4% of primary brain tumors[117, 118] or 4-8% of cerebral gliomas[118]; but recent evidence indicates these tumors have been underdiagnosed (many are misinterpreted as fibrillary astrocytomas, especially the infiltrative portion of these tumors) and ODGs may represent up to 25-33% of *glial* tumors[119, 120]. Ratio of male:female = 3:2. Primarily a tumor of adults: average age ≈ 40 years (peak be-

Table 17-17 Location of oligodendrogliomas

Location	%
supratentorial	> 90%
frontal lobes	45%
hemisphere (outside frontal lobes)	40%
within third or lateral ventricle	15%
infratentorial + spinal cord	< 10%

tween 26-46 years), but with a smaller earlier peak in childhood between 6-12 years[121]. CSF metastases reportedly occur in up to 10%, but 1% may be a more realistic estimate[117]. Spinal ODGs comprise only ≈ 2.6% of intramedullary tumors of the cord and filum.

CLINICAL

Classic presentation of ODG: a patient with seizures for many years prior to the diagnosis being made when they would present with an apoplectic event due to peri-tumoral intracerebral hemorrhage. This scenario is less common in the post CT era.

Seizures are the presenting symptoms in ≈ 50-80% of cases[117, 121]. The remainder of presenting symptoms are nonspecific for ODG, and are more often related to local mass effect and less commonly to ↑ ICP. Presenting symptoms are shown in *Table 17-18*.

Table 17-18 Presenting symptoms in 208 oligodendrogliomas[117]

Symptom	%
seizures	57%
headache	22%
mental status changes	10%
vertigo/nausea	9%

EVALUATION

Calcifications is seen in 28-60% in ODGs on plain radiographs[117], and on 90% of CTs.

PATHOLOGY

73% of tumors have microscopic calcifications[122]. Isolated tumor cells consistently penetrate largely intact parenchyma, an associated solid tumor component may or may not be present[120]. The solid portion, when present, classically demonstrates lucent perinuclear halos giving a "fried egg" appearance (actually an artifact of formalin fixation, which is not present on frozen section and may make diagnosis difficult on frozen). A "chicken-wire" vascular pattern has also been described[123]. These features are felt to be unreliable, and cells with monotonous round nuclei (often in cellular sheets) with an eccentric rim of eosinophilic cytoplasm lacking obvious cell processes are more consistent features[124].

16% of hemispheric ODGs are cystic[122] (cysts form from coalescence of microcysts from micro-hemorrhages, unlike astrocytomas which actively secrete fluid).

33-41% have a component of neoplastic astrocytic or ependymal cells (so called oligoastrocytomas or **mixed gliomas**[125] or **collision tumors**).

Most do not stain for GFAP (most ODGs contain microtubules instead of glial filaments)[126] although some do[127]. Also, in mixed gliomas, the astrocytic component may stain for GFAP.

GRADING

A work-in-progress. Historically, a number of attempts at grading ODGs have been proposed and then abandoned because of lack of prognostic significance (for a review, see reference[124]). For example, the system of Smith et al.[128] was based on 5 histopathologic features which have been shown not to be independent determinants of tumor progression (only pleomorphism has been shown to be statistically correlated with survival[124]). Necrosis does not appear to reliably predict a poor prognosis[124].

For prognostic purposes, it is suggested that ODGs be stratified into two groups: low grade and high grade[118, 124]. Although there is not uniform agreement on the means for differentiating the two, the factors shown in *Table 17-19* should be taken into account as they have been demonstrated to have prognostic significance. Using the spatial grading system for low grade gliomas (*see page 408*), no ODGs are of the Type 1 tumor (solid tumor without infiltrative component).

Table 17-19 Features associated with low-grade and high-grade oligodendrogliomas

Feature	Low grade	High grade
contrast enhancement on CT or MRI	absent	present
endothelial proliferation on histology	absent	present
pleomorphism (large variability in nuclear and cytoplasmic size and shape)	absent	present
tumor proliferation (evidenced by mitotic figures or high MIB-1 labeling index*)	absent	present
astrocytic component	absent	present

* *see page 500* for information on MIB-1 labeling

TREATMENT

Σ **Recommendation:** (*see text for details*). Chemotherapy is the primary modality (following an appropriate surgical procedure, if indicated). XRT is reserved for anaplastic transformation, if it should occur[124].

CHEMOTHERAPY

Most ODGs respond to chemotherapy, usually in < 3 mos, often with a reduction in size. The response is variable in degree and duration[129]. No pathological or clinical feature of high-grade ODGs has been identified that reliably predicts response to chemotherapy. However, allelic loss of chromosome 1p, and combined loss of chromosome arms 1p and 19q, are associated with response to chemo; and losses of both 1p and 19q were associated with longer tumor-free survival after chemo[130].

The most experience is with PCV (procarbazine 60 mg/m^2 IV, CCNU 110 mg/m^2 PO, and vincristine 1.4 mg/m^2 IV, all given on a 29 day cycle repeated every 6 weeks)[131, 132]. Also studied: temozolomide for recurrent anaplastic oligoastrocytoma showed some efficacy[133].

SURGERY

Indications for surgery:
1. ODGs with significant mass effect regardless of grade: surgery decreases the need for corticosteroids, reduces symptoms and prolongs survival[124]
2. tumors without significant mass effect:
   A. low-grade ODGs and oligoastrocytoma: surgery is recommended for resectable lesions. Gross total removal should be attempted when possible (survival is improved even more than with astrocytomas[134]), but not at the expense of neurologic function
   B. high-grade ODGs: data for improved survival is less convincing, and some studies show no advantage of gross total removal over partially resected or biopsied-only high-grade lesions[124]

POSTOPERATIVE RADIATION

Benefits of postoperative irradiation is controversial[121]. In a retrospective analysis with no set selection criteria, better survival in patients receiving > 45 Gy (1 Gy = 100 cGy) was found[135]. In another series, no difference in 5 year survival following surgery was seen with or without XRT (amount of radiation not specified)[136]. Radiation side effects of memory loss, dementia and personality changes are more common with the longer survival seen in many of these cases[137].

PROGNOSIS

Pure ODGs have a better prognosis than mixed oligoastrocytomas which are better than pure astrocytomas. An oligodendroglial component, no matter how small, confers a better prognosis.

10 year survival of 10-30% has been quoted for tumors that are completely or predominantly ODGs[135]. As a group, median survival for surgically treated lesions is given as 35 months post-op (mean 52 months)[117].

The presence of calcifications is debated as a prognosticator; in one series, calcified ODG on plain films had a longer median survival of 108 months (vs. 58 months for non-calcified)[117].

Frontal lobe ODGs survived longer than those in temporal lobes (37 months vs. 28 months postoperative survival)[117], possibly due to increased ease of radical resection with the former.

17.2.4.   Central neurocytoma

Rare. Usually considered benign, but malignant variation/behavior has been described[138]. Slow-growing well circumscribed tumor usually located in the lateral ventricles or at the septum pellucidum[139, 140]. Tends to affect young adults, usually males. Histologically, resembles oligodendrogliomas. Ultrastructure shows neuronal differentiation. Molecular oncogenesis is not known.

Usually curable by total resection[140]. Subtotal resection and histologic atypia are associated with an increased risk of recurrence, but early recurrence may occur even without malignant histologic features[138].

Variants:
1. "extraventricular neurocytomas": neurocytic neoplasms located within brain parenchyma. Not as well characterized as intraventricular type[140]
2. central liponeurocytoma: extremely rare. Classified as a glioneuronal tumor. Usually occurs in the posterior fossa of older adults[141]. Once considered a variant of medulloblastoma (called medullocytoma), has more indolent behavior[142] and characteristic morphologic features of well-differentiated neurons with the cytol-

ogy of neurocytes in addition to a population of lipidized cells resembling mature adipose tissue[142]

Treatment
1. ideal: total resection if possible
2. stereotactic radiosurgery may be effective for recurrence[143] or for incompletely removed or biopsied tumors[144]
3. chemotherapy with etoposide, cisplatin and cyclophosphamide, has been reported for recurrent progressive tumor[145]

17.2.5. Meningiomas

❗ Key features:
- slow growing, extra-axial, usually benign, arise from arachnoid (not dura)
- usually cured if completely removed, which is not always possible
- most commonly located along falx, convexity, or sphenoid bone
- often cause hyperostosis of adjacent bone
- frequently calcified. Classic histological finding: psammoma bodies

May occur anywhere that arachnoid cells are found (between brain and skull, within ventricles, and along spinal cord). Ectopic meningiomas may arise within the bone of the skull (**primary intraosseous meningiomas**)[146] and others occur in the subcutaneous tissue with no attachment to the skull. This section considers intracranial meningiomas.

Usually slow growing, circumscribed (non-infiltrating), benign lesions. Histologically malignant (incidence: ≈ 1.7% of meningiomas[147]) and/or rapidly growing varieties are also described. May be asymptomatic. Actually arise from <u>arachnoid</u> cap cells (not dura). May be multiple in up to 8% of cases[148], this finding is more common in neurofibromatosis. Occasionally forms a diffuse sheet of tumor (**meningioma en plaque**).

EPIDEMIOLOGY

As many as 3% of autopsies on patients > 60 yrs age reveals a meningioma[149]. Meningiomas account for 14.3-19% of primary intracranial neoplasms[150]. Incidence peaks at 45 years age. Female:male ratio is 1.8:1.

1.5% occur in childhood and adolescence, usually between 10-20 years age[95 (p 3263)]. 19-24% of adolescent meningiomas occur in patients with neurofibromatosis type I (von Recklinghausen's).

LOCATION

Table 17-20 lists common locations. Other locations include: CP-angle, clivus, and foramen magnum. ≈ 60-70% occur along the falx (including parasagittal), along sphenoid bone (including tuberculum sellae), or over the convexity. Childhood meningiomas are rare, 28% are intraventricular, and the posterior fossa is also a common site.

Sphenoid wing (or ridge) meningiomas
Three basic categories[152]:
1. lateral sphenoid wing (or pterional): behavior and treatment are usually similar to convexity meningioma
2. middle third (or alar)
3. medial (clinoidal): tend to encase the ICA and the MCA as well as cranial nerves in the region of the superior orbital fissure and the optic nerve. May compress brainstem. Total removal is often not possible

Parasagittal and falx meningiomas
Up to half invade the superior sagittal sinus. Grouped as:
1. anterior (ethmoidal plate to coronal suture): 33%. Most often present with H/A and mental status changes
2. middle (between coronal and lambdoidal sutures): 50%. Most often present as Jacksonian seizure and progressive monoplegia
3. posterior (lambdoidal suture to torcular Herophili): 20%. Most often present with H/A, visual symptoms, focal seizures, or mental status changes

Table 17-20 Location of adult meningiomas (series of 336 cases[151])

Location	%
parasagittal	20.8
convexity	15.2
tuberculum sellae	12.8
sphenoidal ridge	11.9
olfactory groove	9.8
falx	8
lateral ventricle	4.2
tentorial	3.6
middle fossa	3
orbital	1.2
spinal	1.2
intrasylvian	0.3
extracalvarial	0.3
multiple	0.9

Parasagittal meningiomas may originate at the level of the motor strip, and a common initial manifestation of these is a contralateral foot drop[153].

Olfactory groove meningiomas

Presentation (most reach a large size before causing symptoms) may include:
1. Foster-Kennedy syndrome: anosmia (patient is usually unaware of this), ipsilateral optic atrophy, contralateral papilledema (*see page 85*)
2. mental status changes: often with frontal lobe findings (apathy, abulia...)
3. urinary incontinence
4. posteriorly located lesions may compress the optic apparatus causing visual impairment
5. seizure

The morbidity, mortality and difficulty in achieving total removal increase significantly for tumors > 3 cm in size[154].

Tuberculum sella meningiomas

The site of origin of these tumors is only about 2 cm posterior to that of olfactory groove meningiomas[154]. These tumors are notorious for producing visual loss.

Foramen magnum meningiomas

As with any foramen magnum (**FM**) lesion, the neurologic symptoms and signs can be very confusing and often do not initially suggest a tumor in this location (*see page 492*).

In the French Cooperative Study, there were 106 FM meningiomas[155], 31% arose from the anterior lip, 56% were lateral, and 13% arose from the posterior lip of the FM. Most are intradural, but they can be extradural or a combination (the latter 2 have a lateral origin and are often invasive, which makes total removal more difficult)[156]. They may be above, below, or on both sides of the vertebral artery[156].

ASYMPTOMATIC MENINGIOMAS

Meningiomas are the most common *primary intracranial tumors*, and the routine use of CT & MRI for numerous indications has led to an increased rate of discovery of incidental (asymptomatic) meningiomas. In one series, 32% of primary brain tumors seen on imaging studies were meningiomas, and 39% of these were asymptomatic[157]. Of 63 cases followed for > 1 year with nonsurgical management, 68% showed no increase in size over an average follow-up of 36.6 mos, whereas 32% increased in size over 28 mos average follow-up[157]. Asymptomatic meningiomas with calcification seen on CT and/or hypointensity on T2WI MRI appeared to have a slower growth rate[157].

When surgery was performed, the perioperative morbidity rate was 3.5% in patients < 70 years age, and was 23% in patients > 70 years old[157] and this difference was statistically significant.

PATHOLOGY

There are a number of pathologic classification systems[1, 158, 159 (p 465)], and transitional forms between the major types exist (*see below*). More than one histological pattern may be seen in a given tumor. Most classifications include:
1. 3 main categories of "classic meningiomas"
   A. **meningotheliomatous, AKA syncytial**: the most common. Sheets of polygonal cells. Some use the term **angiomatous** for meningotheliomatous variety with closely packed blood vessels
   B. **fibrous** or **fibroblastic**: cells separated by connective tissue stroma. Consistency is more rubbery than meningotheliomatous or transitional
   C. **transitional**: intermediate between meningotheliomatous and fibrous. Cells tend to be spindle shaped, but areas of typical meningotheliomatous cells occur. Whorls, some of which are calcified (psammoma bodies)

   The following variants may be associated with any of the above 3 subtypes:
   1. **microcystic**: AKA "humid" or vacuolated meningioma. The characteristic dilated extracellular spaces are usually empty, but occasionally contain substance that stains positive for PAS (? glycoprotein) or contain fat[160]. The cysts may coalesce and form grossly or radiologically visible cysts and may resemble astrocytomas
   2. **psammomatous**: calcified meningothelial whorls (some classify these as transitional (*see above*))

3. myxomatous
4. xanthomatous: abundant cytoplasmic lipids; appear vacuolated
5. lipomatous
6. granular
7. secretory
8. chondroblastic
9. osteoblastic
10. melanotic

2. **angioblastic**: different authors use this term differently. Some also call these (meningeal) **hemangiopericytomas**. Others use the term "angioblastic" for tumors histologically similar to hemangioblastoma

3. **atypical meningioma**: this term may be applied to any of the above meningiomas possessing one or more of the following features: increased mitotic activity (1-2 mitotic figure/high-powered field), increased cellularity, focal areas of necrosis, giant cells. Cellular pleomorphism is not unusual but is not significant in and of itself. Reports suggest increasing aggressiveness with increasing atypia

4. **malignant meningiomas**: AKA anaplastic, papillary or sarcomatous. Characterized by frequent mitotic figures, cortical invasion, rapid recurrence even after apparent total removal[161], and, rarely, metastases (*see below*). Frequent mitotic figures or the presence of papillary features are strong predictors of malignancy. May be more common in younger patients. Angioblastic meningiomas show more malignant clinical characteristics than other forms[159 (p 479-83)]

Metastases

Very rarely a meningioma may metastasize outside the CNS. Most of these are angioblastic or malignant. Lung, liver, lymph nodes and heart are the most common sites.

EVALUATION

MRI

Initially thought to be poor in the detection of meningiomas, current MRI (> 0.5 tesla) will show most meningiomas on T2WI (unless it is nearly totally calcified). Gives information regarding patency of dural venous sinuses (accuracy in predicting sinus involvement is ≈ 90%[162]). "Dural tail" is a common finding[163].

CT

Appear as homogeneous, densely enhancing mass with broad base of attachment along dural border. Non-contrast Hounsfield numbers of 60-70 in a meningioma usually correlates with presence of psammomatous calcifications. There may be little cerebral edema, or it may be marked and may extend throughout the white matter of the entire hemisphere.

Intraventricular meningiomas: 50% produce extraventricular edema. On angio, these may falsely appear malignant.

Prostate cancer may mimic meningioma (prostate mets to brain are rare, but prostate frequently goes to bone, and may go to skull and can cause hyperostosis).

Angiography

Meningiomas characteristically have <u>external</u> carotid artery feeders. Exceptions: low frontal median (e.g. olfactory groove) meningiomas which feed from the ICA (ethmoidal branches of the ophthalmic artery). Suprasellar meningiomas may also be fed by large branches of the ophthalmic arteries. Parasellar meningiomas tend to feed from the ICA.

Artery of **Bernasconi & Cassinari** AKA artery of tentorium (a branch of the meningohypophyseal trunk) AKA the "Italian" artery: enlarged in lesions involving tentorium (e.g. tentorial meningiomas).

Angiography also gives information about occlusion of dural venous sinuses, especially for parasagittal/falx meningiomas. Oblique views are often best for evaluating patency of the superior sagittal sinus (**SSS**). Angiography can also help confirm diagnosis by the distinctive prolonged homogeneous tumor blush.

Plain x-rays

May show: calcifications within the tumor (in ≈ 10%), hyperostosis or blistering of the skull (including floor of frontal fossa with olfactory groove meningiomas), enlargement of vascular grooves (especially middle meningeal artery).

TREATMENT

Surgery is the treatment of choice for symptomatic meningiomas. Incidental meningiomas with no brain edema or those presenting only with seizures that are easily controlled medically may be managed expectantly with serial imaging as meningiomas tend to grow slowly, and some may "burn out" and cease growing (*see page 427*).

SURGICAL TECHNIQUE

Often very bloody. Preoperative embolization and autologous blood donation may be helpful.

Radiation therapy (XRT)

Generally regarded as ineffective as primary modality of treatment. Many prefer not to use XRT for "benign" lesions. Efficacy of XRT in preventing recurrence is controversial (*see below* under *Recurrence*); some surgeons reserve XRT for malignant (invasive), vascular, rapidly recurring ("aggressive"), or non-resectable meningiomas.

OUTCOME

5 year survival for patients with meningioma[3]: 91.3%.

RECURRENCE

The extent of surgical tumor removal is the most important factor in the prevention of recurrence. The Simpson grading system for the extent of meningioma removal is shown in *Table 17-21*. Recurrence after gross total tumor removal occurred in 11-15% of cases, but was 29% when removal is incomplete (length of follow-up not specified)[151]; 5-year recurrence rates of 37%[164]-85%[165] after partial resection are quoted. The overall recurrence rate at 20 years was 19% in one series[166], and 50% in another[165]. Malignant meningiomas have a higher recurrence rate than benign ones.

Table 17-21 Simpson grading system for removal of meningiomas[167]

Grade	Degree of removal
I	macroscopically complete removal with excision of dural attachment and abnormal bone (including sinus resection when involved)
II	macroscopically complete with endothermy coagulation (Bovie, or laser) of dural attachment
III	macroscopically complete without resection or coagulation of dural attachment or of its extradural extensions (e.g. hyperostotic bone)
IV	partial removal leaving tumor in situ
V	simple decompression (± biopsy)

Value of XRT

A retrospective series of 135 non-malignant meningiomas followed 5-15 years post-op at UCSF revealed a recurrence rate of 4% with total resection, 60% for partial resection without XRT, and 32% for partial resection with XRT[168]. Mean time to recurrence was longer in the XRT group (125 mos) than in the non-XRT group (66 mos). These results suggest that XRT may be beneficial in partially resected meningiomas. It may, however, be possible to simply follow these patients with CT or MRI without XRT.

In addition to the usual side effects of XRT (see *Radiation injury and necrosis*, page 535), there is also a case report of a malignant astrocytoma developing after XRT was used to treat a meningioma[169].

17.2.6. Acoustic neuroma

❢ Key features
- a misnomer: most are really schwannomas (not neuromas) that arise from the superior *vestibular* division of the 8th nerve (not the acoustic division)
- 3 most common early symptoms: hearing loss (insidious and progressive), tinnitus (high pitched) and dysequilibrium
- histology: benign tumors comprised of Antoni A (narrow elongated bipolar cells) and B fibers (loose reticulated)

AKA acoustic neurinomas. The term **vestibular schwannoma** has been proposed as the preferred term[170, 171] since most arise from the neurilemmal sheath of the superior division of the <u>vestibular nerve</u> at the junction of central and peripheral myelin (Obersteiner-Redlich zone, located 8-12 mm distal to brainstem, close to porus acusticus) making them schwannomas and <u>not</u> neuromas. Histologically benign. ANs arise as a result of the loss of a tumor-suppressor gene on the long arm of chromosome 22.

Epidemiology: One of the most common intracranial tumors, comprising 8-10% of tumors in most series[172]. Annual incidence is 0.78-1.15 cases per 100,000 population, resulting in ≈ 2280 new cases per year in the U.S.[173]. They typically become symptomatic after age 30. At least 95% are unilateral.

Neurofibromatosis Type 2
The incidence of acoustic neuromas (AN) is increased in neurofibromatosis (NFT), with bilateral AN being pathognomonic of neurofibromatosis Type 2 (NFT2) (central NFT, *see page 503*). Any patient < 40 yrs old with unilateral AN should also be evaluated for NFT2. Cytologically, the ANs of NFT2 are identical to sporadic cases, however in NFT2 the tumors form grape-like clusters that may infiltrate the nerve fibers (unlike most sporadic ANs which displace the eighth nerve).

CLINICAL

SYMPTOMS
Symptoms are shown in *Table 17-22*. The type of symptoms are closely correlated with tumor size. Most initially cause the triad of tinnitus, ipsilateral sensorineural hearing loss and balance difficulties. Larger tumors can cause facial numbness, weakness or twitching, and possibly brainstem symptoms. Rarely, large tumor may produce hydrocephalus. With current imaging modalities (CT and especially MRI), increasing numbers of smaller lesions are being detected.

Table 17-22 Symptoms in acoustic neuroma
(131 patients[172])

Symptom	%
hearing loss	98%
tinnitus	70%
dysequilibrium*	67%
H/A	32%
facial numbness	29%
facial weakness	10%
diplopia	10%
N/V	9%
otalgia	9%
change of taste	6%

* or vertigo

Symptoms from 8th nerve compression
Unilateral sensorineural hearing loss, tinnitus and dysequilibrium are related to pressure on the eighth nerve complex in the IAC. These are the earliest symptoms, and by the time of diagnosis, virtually all tumors have caused otologic symptoms.

Hearing loss is insidious and progressive in most (c.f. the hearing loss in Meniere's disease which fluctuates), however 10% report sudden hearing loss (see *Sudden hearing loss* below). 70% have a high frequency loss pattern, and word discrimination is usually affected (especially noticeable in telephone conversation).

The tinnitus is usually high pitched.

Sudden hearing loss: The differential diagnosis for sudden hearing loss (SHL) is extensive[174]. *Idiopathic* SHL (i.e. no identified etiology: must rule out neoplasm, infection, autoimmune, vascular and toxic causes) occurs in an estimated 10 per 100,000 population[175]. 1% of patients with SHL will be found to have an AN, and SHL may be the presenting symptom in 1-14% of patients with AN[176]. SHL with AN is presumably due to an infarction of the acoustic nerve, or acute occlusion of the cochlear artery. Treatment options for SHL include:
1. steroids: e.g. prednisone 60 mg PO q d **x** 10 d then tapered[176]
2. **✘** heparin has been shown not to be of help
3. conservative treatment: rest and salt, alcohol and tobacco restriction[177]
4. experimental: thrombolytic therapy (e.g. rt-PA) (*see page 768*)

Symptoms from 5th and 7th nerve compression
Otalgia, facial numbness and weakness, and taste changes occur as the tumor enlarges and compresses the fifth and seventh nerves. These symptoms usually do not occur until the tumor is > 2 cm. This highlights an interesting paradox: facial weakness is a rare or late occurrence, even though the 7th nerve is almost always distorted early; whereas facial numbness occurs sooner once trigeminal compression occurs (often in the presence of normal facial movement), despite the fact that the 5th nerve is farther away[178]. This may be due to the resiliency of motor nerves relative to sensory nerves.

Symptoms from compression of brainstem and other cranial nerves
Larger tumors cause brainstem compression (with ataxia, H/A, N/V, diplopia, cerebellar signs, if unchecked, coma, respiratory depression and death) and lower cranial nerve (IX, X, XII) palsies (hoarseness, dysphagia...). Obstruction of CSF circulation by larger tumors (usually > 4 cm) may produce hydrocephalus with increased ICP.

Rarely, 6th nerve involvement may cause diplopia.

SIGNS

See *Table 17-23*. VIII is the earliest cranial nerve involved. 66% of patients have no abnormal physical finding except for hearing loss. Since hearing loss is sensorineural, Weber's test will lateralize to the uninvolved side, and if there is enough preserved hearing **Rinne's test** will be positive (i.e. normal; air conduction > bone conduction). Facial nerve function may be graded clinically on the House and Brackmann scale (*see Table 17-24*).

Vestibular involvement causes nystagmus (may be central or peripheral) and abnormal electronystagmography (ENG) with caloric stimulation.

Table 17-23 Signs in 131 acoustic neuromas (excluding hearing loss)[172]

Sign	%
abnormal corneal reflex	33
nystagmus	26
facial hypoesthesia	26
facial weakness (palsy)	12
abnormal eye movement	11
papilledema	10
Babinski sign	5

DIFFERENTIAL DIAGNOSIS

See *Cerebellopontine angle (CPA) lesions* on page 922. The major differential is meningioma, or neuroma of an adjacent cranial nerve (e.g. trigeminal).

PATHOLOGY

Tumors are composed of Antoni A fibers (narrow elongated bipolar cells) and Antoni B fibers (loose reticulated).

Growth rate

Growth rate is unpredictable. Usually quoted range: ≈ **1-10 mm/yr**. However, some show no change over many years, 6% actually decrease in size[180], while some can increase in diameter up to 20 or 30 mm/yr[170, 181]. The majority of tumors (but not all[182]) will show some growth within 3 years[181].

EVALUATION

Table 17-24 Clinical grading of facial nerve function (House and Brackmann[179])

Grade	Descriptor	Detailed description
1	normal	normal facial function in all areas
2	mild dysfunction	1. gross: slight weakness noticeable on close inspection; may have very slight synkinesis 2. at rest: normal symmetry and tone 3. motion: A. forehead: slight to moderate movement B. eye: complete closure with effort C. mouth: slight asymmetry
3	moderate dysfunction	1. gross: obvious but not disfiguring asymmetry: noticeable but not severe synkinesis 2. motion: A. forehead: slight to moderate movement B. eye: complete closure with effort C. mouth: slightly weak with maximal effort
4	moderate to severe dysfunction	1. gross: obvious weakness and/or asymmetry 2. motion: A. forehead: none B. eye: incomplete closure C. mouth: asymmetry with maximum effort
5	severe dysfunction	1. gross: only barely perceptible motion 2. at rest: asymmetry 3. motion: A. forehead: none B. eye: incomplete closure
6	total paralysis	no movement

AUDIOMETRIC AND AUDIOLOGIC STUDIES

Most can be performed only if the affected ear has usable hearing. For diagnostic purposes, the expense may not be justified except in low suspicion patients, as many patients will go on to have CT or MRI regardless of audiometric findings. However, baseline studies may be helpful for later comparison (to document deterioration), or if surgery is performed to prepare for intra-operative monitoring and to compare to post-op. Also may help in treatment decision-making.

The modified **Gardener-Robertson** system for grading hearing is shown in *Table 17-25*. Mnemonic: "50/50" (Class II) is a reasonable cutoff for useful hearing (pure tone audiogram threshold ≤ 50 dB and speech discrimination score ≥ 50%). Class I patients may use the phone on that side, class II patients can localize sounds.

The American Academy of Otolaryngology-Head and Neck Surgery Foundation hearing classification system[185] is shown in *Table 17-26*.

All patients should have the following

Pure tone audiogram (PTA): May be useful as first-step screening test. Air conduction assesses the entire system, bone conduction assesses from the cochlea and proximally. PTA assesses the functionality of hearing (to help in treatment decision making) and acts as a baseline for future comparison. The single numerical score is an average of the thresholds for frequencies across the audio spectrum.

Retrocochlear lesion: VIII nerve dysfunction (typical with ANs), as opposed to a cochlear lesions (dysfunction of the hearing end-organ). <u>Progressive</u> unilateral or <u>asymmetric</u> sensorineural hearing loss of high tones occurs in > 95% of ANs[186].

Table 17-25 Gardener and Robertson modified hearing classification*

Class	Description	Pure tone audiogram† (dB)	Speech discrimination†
I	good-excellent	0-30	70-100%
II	serviceable	31-50	50-59%
III	nonserviceable	51-90	5-49%
IV	poor	91-max	1-4%
V	none	not testable	0

*   modification[183] of the Silverstein and Norrell system[184]

†   if audiogram and speech discrimination score do not qualify in the same class, use the lower class

High-frequency hearing loss is also the most common type of hearing loss with age or noise exposure, but is usually symmetrical. An unexplained hearing difference from one ear to the other of > 10-15 dB on PTA is suspicious and should be investigated further.

Speech discrimination: Maintained in conductive hearing loss, moderately impaired in cochlear hearing loss, poorest with retrocochlear lesions. A score of 4% suggests a retrocochlear lesion, as does a score that is worse than would be predicted based on PTA testing (the speech recognition threshold should be similar to PTA thresholds below 4 kHz). The median for one series of 111 AN patients was 8% with 50 patients scoring 0 (normal is 92-100%). "Rollover phenomenon": <u>decreased</u> speech discrimination of > 20% at high sound intensity, typical of retrocochlear lesions.

Additional tests that may or may not be helpful

BSAER: most common findings are prolonged I-III and I-V interpeak latencies.

Table 17-26 American Academy of Otolaryngology-Head and Neck Surgery Foundation hearing classification system

Class	Pure tone threshold (dB)*		Speech discrimination† (%)
A	≤ 30	AND	≥ 70
B	> 30 AND ≤ 50	AND	≥ 50
C	> 50	AND	5-49
D	any level		< 50

*   average of pure tone hearing thresholds by air conduction at 0.5, 1, 2 & 3 kHz

†   speech discrimination at 40 dB or maximum comfortable loudness

Including all abnormalities, < 5% false negatives, 85% specificity (distinguishes AN from labyrinthine pathology, e.g. **Meniere's disease**, which has normal interpeak latencies)[187]. Patients with cochlear hearing loss have a 25% false positive rate for AN with BSAER, and typically lose the interaural difference in peak V latency as stimulation intensity increases.

Electronystagmography (ENG): normally, 50% of the response is from each ear. It is abnormal if one side has ≤ 35% of the total. Patients with tumor arising from the inferior division of vestibular nerve may have a normal response (the horizontal semicircular canal is the dominant one, and is supplied by the superior division), also, the vestibular nerve may continue to function until almost all of the nerve fibers are affected.

Stapedial reflex & reflex decay: decay to < 50% of initial amplitude in 10 seconds is 88% specific for retrocochlear lesion.

Caloric testing: measuring the length of duration of nystagmus using ice water. A decrease of ≥ 1 min on the affected side is abnormal.

RADIOGRAPHIC EVALUATION

MRI: thin slice axial plane gadolinium enhanced MRI is the diagnostic procedure of choice with sensitivity close to 98% and almost 0% false positive rate. Characteristic findings: round or oval enhancing tumor centered on IAC. Large ANs (> 3 cm dia) may show cystic appearing areas on CT or MRI; in actuality these areas are usually solid. Adjacent blocked CSF cisterns may also give cystic appearance.

CT scan with IV contrast: second choice for imaging modality. If normal, and clinical suspicion of AN is strong, small lesions may be visualized by introducing 3-4 ml of subarachnoid air via lumbar puncture, and scanning the patient with the affected side up (to trap air in region of IAC), non-filling of the IAC is indicative of an intracanalicular mass. Even with air contrast, CT was normal in 6% in Mayo series[172]. Although many ANs enlarge the ostium of the IAC (called trumpeting) (normal diameter of the IAC is = 5-8 mm), 3-5% of ANs do not enlarge the IAC on CT; this percent may increase as patients are scanned earlier with smaller tumors. Advantage over MRI: shows bony anatomy (including mastoid air cells) which is often helpful for planning translabyrinthine approach.

TREATMENT OPTIONS

1. expectant management: follow symptoms, hearing (audiometrics) and tumor growth on serial imaging (CT or MRI q 6 mos **x** 2 yrs, then annually if stable). Intervention is performed for progression (see footnote to *Table 17-27* for details). Growth patterns observed:
   A. little or no growth: usually those contained within the IAC
   B. slow growth ≈ 2 mm/yr
   C. rapid growth: ≥ 10 mm/yr
2. radiation therapy (alone, or in conjunction with surgery)
   A. external beam radiation therapy **(EBRT)**
   B. stereotactic radiosurgery (*see page 539* for treatment details)
3. surgery: approaches include the following (*see below* for details)
   A. retrosigmoid (AKA suboccipital): may be able to spare hearing
   B. translabyrinthine (and its several variations): sacrifices hearing, may be slightly better for sparing VII
   C. extradural subtemporal (middle fossa approach): only for small lateral ANs

Selection of treatment option

In addition to the usual factors influencing the decision process with brain tumors, e.g. the patient's general medical condition, age (some use age > 65 yrs as a cutoff for surgery, but there is not universal agreement on this), etc., other factors that must be weighed include: chances of hearing preservation in those with serviceable hearing and chances of preserving VII & V nerve function (all of which are related to tumor size), demonstrated tumor growth on serial imaging, the presence of NF2, local control rates of the various treatment modalities (see *Recurrence*, page 437), and the long-term side effects of treatment in patients with these benign lesions.

The following points also figure into treatment decisions:
1. with small tumors (< 2.5 cm dia): long-term preservation of hearing and VII function is higher with MS than with SRS
2. with tumors 2.5-3 cm dia: risk of VII dysfunction is higher with MS than SRS
3. for tumors > 3 cm dia: there is ↑ risk of brainstem radiation injury following SRS
4. SRS: complication rate is reduced with lower doses[188] (but so is local control rate)

Long-term local control **(LC)** rates are likely to be lower with radiosurgery than microsurgery (*see page 437*). With small tumors (< 1.5 cm dia), long-term hearing preservation is higher with MS than SRS. **Conclusion**: surgical excision is the treatment of choice for most tumors.

Recommendations for patients *without* neurofibromatosis are shown in *Table 17-27*. Age was not a factor in surgical outcome[189]. Expectant management is an option for those cases indicated since tumor growth rate is variable and may be slow (*see page 431*). However, others argue that since

Table 17-27   Management of acoustic neuromas[180, 189]

Tumor size	Good clinical condition (ASA grade I-II)*		Poor clinical condition (ASA grade ≥ III)*
small tumor (≤ 3 cm dia)	good hearing	→ surgery†	expectant‡
	severe hearing deficit	→ expectant‡	
large tumor (> 3 cm dia)	surgery		surgery† (total or subtotal resection) with SRS§ for post-op growth

*   ASA = American Society of Anesthesiologists

†   some now consider SRS as an acceptable option (*see page 539*)

‡   **expectant management**: close observation, repeat neuro exams and serial imaging (CT or MRI q 6 mos **x** 2 yrs, then annually if stable); if symptoms progress or growth > 2 mm/year then surgery if clinical condition is good, or SRS (or possibly surgery) if poor

§   **SRS**: stereotactic radiosurgery (see *Stereotactic radiosurgery page 539* for indications), retardation of growth is observed in most cases, but long-term results are not available to fully assess therapeutic efficacy and complication rate at this time

most tumors do grow, that expectant management should be reserved only for the elderly with no symptoms from mass effect[181].

Vertigo: For patients with episodic vertigo or balance difficulties as the predominant symptom (also, see points under *Selection of treatment option* on page 433):
1. remember: patients with AN are susceptible to other causes of vertigo as well, and patients should undergo ENG and functional balance assessment
2. vertigo that is due to the AN is often self-limited, and improves in 6-8 weeks to a reasonably tolerable level with no treatment (patients may do better with so-called "vestibular rehab")
3. residual dizziness and balance disturbances are common whether stereotactic radiosurgery **(SRS)** or microsurgery **(MS)** is used, but are typically less after MS
4. after SRS: beneficial effects require a minimum of 5-6 mos, and sometimes may require up to eighteen months
5. following MS: symptoms are usually immediately worsened, but then gradually improve in most cases (except perhaps when the balance difficulties are due to brainstem compression). Symptoms are improved more rapidly than with SRS
6. **conclusion**: observation may be the best choice for ≈ 20% of patients. When treatment is desired, surgery is the best choice for most ANs producing vertigo. SRS may be the right choice for some, especially: elderly patients (> 70 yrs) with other health problems, for recurrence of AN, and for individual preference

Hydrocephalus: When hydrocephalus is present, it may require separate treatment with a CSF shunt (see *Surgical considerations*, page 435), and may possibly be done at the same time as surgery for the AN (if indicated).

SURGICAL TREATMENT

ALTERNATIVE APPROACHES[190]
* translabyrinthine: useful for tumors with primarily intracanalicular component with little CPA extension. Often preferred by neurootologists. Advantages and disadvantages are shown in *Table 17-28*
* suboccipital (posterior fossa), AKA retrosigmoid[191]: of-

Table 17-28 Merits of translabyrinthine approach

Disadvantages	Advantages
• sacrifices hearing (acceptable when hearing is already non-functional or unlikely to be spared by other approach) • limited exposure (limits maximal tumor size that can be approached) • may take longer than suboccipital approach • possibly higher rate of post-op CSF leak	• early identification of the facial nerve may result in higher preservation rate • less risk to cerebellum and lower cranial nerves • patients do not get as "ill" from blood in cisterna magna, etc. (essentially an extracranial approach)

ten preferred by neurosurgeons. Usually offers best opportunity for preservation of hearing (when possible) with possibility of preserving facial nerve, also. Disadvantages: higher morbidity than translabyrinthine; it is difficult to remove small tumors from the lateral recess of the IAC without entering the vestibule producing inner ear dysfunction, facial nerve usually presents on blind (anterior) side of tumor and is encountered late
* extradural subtemporal (middle fossa approach): limited to removal of small, laterally located intracanalicular tumors. Poor access to posterior fossa. Higher risk of VII palsy (injury at geniculate ganglion). Provides chance for preservation of hearing
* translabyrinthine approach: sacrifices hearing. Options:
   ◆ translabyrinthine-transtentorial
   ◆ translabyrinthine-suboccipital
* retromastoid

CHOICE OF APPROACH
See *Table 17-29*.
* if hearing preservation is a goal of surgery, then the translabyrinthine approach cannot be used. Note that:
1. a generous definition of functional hearing requires thresholds at least < 50 dB or speech discrimination > 50%
2. useful hearing is unlikely to be preserved post-op if:

A. pre-op speech discrimination < 75%
B. or pre-op threshold loss > 25 dB
C. or pre-op BSAER has abnormal wave morphology
D. or tumor > 2-2.5 cm diameter

- large tumors may be approached by a combined translab-suboccipital approach to debulk tumor and preserve facial nerve; a two stage approach (with 1-2 weeks in between) may improve results with very large tumors[192].

Table 17-29 Approach for AN

Tumor size	Approach*	
large (> 4 cm dia)	SO, or SO + TL combined	
medium (2-4 cm dia)	SO or TL	
small (intracanalicular) with poor hearing →	TL	
	Tumor lateral in IAC	Tumor medial in IAC
with good hearing →	MF	SO

* approach: MF = middle fossa, SO = suboccipital, TL = translabyrinthine

SURGICAL CONSIDERATIONS

The superior vestibular division of VIII is the usual origin of the tumor. The facial nerve is pushed forward by the tumor in ≈ 75% of cases (range: 50-80%), but may occasionally be pushed rostrally, less often inferiorly, and rarely posteriorly. It may be flattened to a mere ribbon on the tumor capsule surface.

Anesthesia with minimal muscle relaxants allows intra-op seventh nerve monitoring. In only ≈ 10% of large tumors is the cochlear nerve a separate band on the tumor capsule, in the remainder it is incorporated into the tumor.

Total excision of tumor is usually the goal of surgery. The only indications for planned subtotal resection is a large tumor on the side of the only ear with good hearing or those patients requiring debulking with little chance of recurrence because of limited life expectancy, especially if the facial nerve is densely adherent to the tumor[193, 194].

If hydrocephalus is present, it used to be standard practice to place a CSF shunt and wait ≈ 2 weeks before the definitive operation[190]. This is still acceptable but is less commonly done at present.

Also see references[190, 195-197].

POST-OP CARE & CARE FOR COMPLICATIONS

Cranial nerve and brainstem dysfunction

Facial nerve (VII): If eye closure is impaired due to VII dysfunction: *Rx* natural tears 2 gtts to affected eye q 2 hrs and PRN. Apply Lacrilube® to affected eye and tape it shut q hs. If there is complete VII palsy with little chance of early recovery, or if facial sensation (Vth nerve) is also impaired, tarsorrhaphy is performed within a few days.

Facial re-animation (e.g. hypoglossal-facial anastamosis) is performed after 1-2 months if VII was divided, or if no function returns after 1 year with an anatomically intact nerve.

Vestibular nerve (VIII): Vestibular dysfunction is common post-op, nausea and vomiting due to this (and also intracranial air) is common. Balance difficulties due to this clear rapidly, however, ataxia from brainstem dysfunction may have a permanent component.

Lower cranial nerves: The combination of IX, X and XII dysfunction creates swallowing difficulties and creates a risk of aspiration.

Brainstem dysfunction: Brainstem dysfunction may occur from dissection of tumor off of the brainstem. This may produce ataxia, contralateral paresthesias in the body... Although there may be improvement, once present, there is often some permanent residual.

CSF fistula

Also, see *CSF fistula*, page 174 for general information. CSF fistula may develop through the skin incision, the ear (CSF otorrhea) through a ruptured tympanic membrane, or via the eustachian tube through the nose (rhinorrhea) or down the back of the throat. Rhinorrhea may occur through any of the following routes shown in *Figure 17-1*:
1. via the apical cells to the tympanic cavity (**TC**) or eustachian tube (the most common path)
2. through the vestibule of the bony labyrinth (the posterior semicircular canal is most common area that is entered by drilling) via the oval window (which can be opened by overpacking bone wax into the labyrinth)
3. follows the perilabyrinthine cells and tracts to the mastoid antrum
4. through mastoid air cells at the craniotomy site

Most leaks are diagnosed within 1 week of surgery, although 1 presented 4 years post-op[198]. They seem to be more common with more lateral unroofing of the IAC[198]. Meningitis complicates a CSF leak in 5-25% of cases, and usually develops within days of the onset of leak[198]. Hydrocephalus may promote the development of a CSF fistula.

Treatment: 25-35% of leaks stop spontaneously (one series reported 80%)[198]. Treatment options include:
1. non-surgical:
    A. elevate HOB
    B. if leak persists: a percutaneous lumbar subarachnoid drain may be tried[199, 200], although some debate its efficacy[201], and there is a theoretical risk of drawing bacteria into the CNS
2. surgical treatment for persistent leaks:
    A. if the leak occurred because of the development of hydrocephalus, adjunctive CSF shunting is usually also necessary

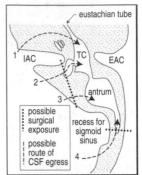

Figure 17-1 Possible routes for CSF rhinorrhea following acoustic neuroma surgery (*see text*) (right petrous bone, axial slice). Adapted from Surgical Neurology, Vol. 43, Nutik S L, Korol H W, Cerebrospinal Fluid Leak After Acoustic Neuroma Surgery, 553-7, 1995, with permission from Elsevier Science

OUTCOME & FOLLOW-UP
Complete surgical removal was reported in 97-99% of cases[202].

SURGICAL MORBIDITY AND MORTALITY
Also see *Post-op considerations for p-fossa crani's*, page 606. Estimated frequency of some complications[203]: CSF leakage in 4-27%[198] (*see above*), meningitis in 5.7%, CVA in 0.7%, subsequent requirement for CSF shunt (for hydrocephalus or to treat leak) in 6.5%. The mortality rate is ≈ 1% at specialized centers[202, 204, 205].

CRANIAL NERVE DYSFUNCTION
Table 17-30 shows statistics of VII and VIII cranial nerve preservation following suboccipital removal of ANs. For more details, *see below*.

Post-radiation cranial neuropathies generally appear 6-18 months following stereotactic radiosurgery **(SRS)**[207], and since more than half resolve within 3-6 months after the onset the recommendation is treat these with a course of corticosteroids.

Table 17-30 Cranial nerve preservation in suboccipital removal of ANs*

Size of tumor	Preserved function	
	VII nerve	VIII nerve
< 1 cm	95-100%	57%
1-2 cm	80-92%	33%
> 2 cm	50-76%	6%

* series of 135 ANs[206 (p 729)] and other sources[95 (p 3337), 202]

Facial nerve (VII)
See Table 17-24, page 431 for the House and Brackmann grading scale. Grades 1-3 are associated with acceptable function. In one surgical series, the facial nerve was preserved with all tumors ≤ 2 cm; it was preserved only in 29% of tumors > 4 cm[172]. Continuous recording of spontaneous EMG activity and responses to electrical stimulation during surgery may improve preservation of VII nerve[208, 209]. If VII is anatomically preserved, partial post-op facial weakness will usually resolve, but may take up to one year. In ≈ 13% of cases, anatomic preservation of VII is not possible.

With SRS for tumors ≤ 3 cm diameter[210]: transient VII weakness occurred in 15%, and V dysfunction (usually temporary) developed in 18%. In another series[211], 92% of cases had grade 1-2 function post op (compared to 90% for microsurgery[212]).

Vestibulo-acoustic nerve (VIII)
Patients with unilateral AN and Class I or II hearing (see *Table 17-25*, page 432) comprised ≈ 12% of cases in a large series[213]. Preservation of hearing is critically dependent on tumor size, with little chance of preservation with tumors > 1-1.5 cm diameter. Chances of preserving hearing may possibly be improved by intra-operative brainstem auditory evoked potential monitoring[214]. In centers treating large numbers of ANs, hearing *preservation* rates of 35-71% can be achieved with tumors < 1.5 cm[213, 215] (although a range of 14-48% may be more realistic[181]). Hearing may rarely be improved post-op[216].

With SRS: for tumors ≤ 3 cm diameter[210], hearing was preserved in 26% of 65 cases with pre-op pure tone threshold < 90 dB. Hearing loss has been correlated with increase in tumor size[173]. • **NB**: there is a high rate of hearing loss at 1 year.

Vestibular nerve function is rarely normal post-op. Attempts at "vestibular" sparing surgery have shown no better results than surgery not specifically addressing this issue. Most patients with unilateral loss of vestibular nerve function will learn to compensate to a significant degree with input from the contralateral side, if normal. Patients with ataxia as a result of brainstem injury from the tumor or the surgery will have more difficulties post-op. Some patients will seem to do well initially post-op with respect to vestibular nerve function, only to undergo a delayed deterioration several months post-op. These cases likely represent aberrant regeneration of the vestibular nerve fibers and may be extremely difficult to manage. Some experts advocate cutting the vestibular nerve (as for Meniere's disease, *see page 590*).

Trigeminal nerve (V)

Postoperative trigeminal nerve symptoms occur transiently in 22% and permanently in 11% following microsurgery, similar to the results of SRS[211].

Lower cranial nerves

Injuries to IX, X and XI occur infrequently following surgery on large tumors that distort the nerves and displace them inferiorly against the occipital bone.

RECURRENCE

Following microsurgery (MS)

Recurrence is highly dependent on extent of removal. However, recurrence can develop in tumors that were apparently totally removed, or when subtotal resection was performed. This can occur many years after treatment. Tumor progression rate following subtotal resection is ≈ 20%[181]. All patients should be followed with imaging (CT or MRI). In older series with up to 15 yrs follow-up, local control **(LC)** after "total resection" is ≈ 94%. More recent series with MRI follow-up indicate recurrence rates of 7-11% (3-16 yrs follow-up)[181].

Use of EBRT

EBRT may improve LC rate in incompletely resected tumors as shown in *Table 17-31* (note: with the long survival expected with benign tumors, post XRT complications may occur).

Microsurgery vs. SRS

The long-term results for SRS using the current recommended dose of 14 Gy are still not known[218]. In a non-randomized retrospective study[211] of ANs < 3 cm dia, the short-term LC rate (median 24 mos follow-up) was 97% for microsurgery vs. 94% for stereotactic radiosurgery **(SRS)**. However, for benign tumors, long-term follow-up is critical, and this study *suggests* that the long-term LC rate will be better for MS than SRS. SRS studies with long-term follow-up[219] are not directly comparable because in the cases with longest follow-up, higher radiation doses were used with a resultant higher incidence of radiation complications, and an anticipated better LC rate.

Table 17-31   Local control rates of surgery vs. surgery + EBRT for ANs[217]

Extent of surgical removal	Local control (LC)	
	Surgery	Surgery + EBRT*
gross total	60/62 (97%)	no data
near total (90-99%)	14/15 (93%)	2/2 (100%)
subtotal (< 90%)	7/13 (54%)	17/20 (85%)*
biopsy only	no data	3/3 (100%)

*   with doses < 45 Gy, LC occurred in 1 of 3 tumors radiated; with > 45 Gy LC was 94%

Initially there may be temporary enlargement of the tumor accompanied by loss of central contrast enhancement following SRS in ≈ 5% of patients[220] (with up to 2% of patients showing actual initial tumor growth), and so the need for further treatment after SRS should be postponed until there is evidence of sustained growth[221]. Surgery should be avoided during the interval from 6 to 18 months after SRS because this is time of maximum damage from the radiation[221].

Although the numbers are small, there have been indications that the rate of VII nerve injury may be higher in patients undergoing microsurgery following SRS failure[222, 223], however, this has been disputed[221]. Lastly, there is a potential for malignant transformation following SRS including **triton tumors**[224, 225] (malignant neoplasms with rhabdoid features) or the induction of skull base tumors (reported with external beam radiation[226]), as well as the risk of late arterial occlusion (the AICA lies near the surface of ANs), any of which may occur many years later.

Treatment for recurrence following microsurgery
Repeat surgery for recurrent AN is an option. One series of 23 patients[227] showed that 6 of 10 patients with moderate or normal VII function maintained at least moderate function after reoperation, 3 patients had increased ataxia, and 1 patient had a cerebellar hematoma. The use of SRS has been endorsed by some for recurrence of AN following one or more MS procedures[181]. Using SRS for recurrent ANs resulted in worsening of facial nerve function in 23% of patients with Grade I-III function before SRS (median follow-up = 43 mos), and 14% developed new trigeminal symptoms[181]. 6% of patients developed tumor progression after SRS.

HYDROCEPHALUS
May occur following treatment (MS or SRS) for AN, and may even occur years later. The increased CSF pressure may also predispose to development of a CSF fistula.

17.2.7.   Pituitary adenomas

Pituitary tumors (adenomas) arise primarily from the anterior pituitary gland (adenohypophysis) (neurohypophyseal tumors are rare) and may be classified by a number of schemes, including: by endocrine function, by light microscopy with routine histological staining methods (*see page 442*), and by electron microscopic appearance.

Microadenoma
Definition: a pituitary tumor < 1 cm diameter. Larger tumors are considered macroadenomas. Currently, 50% of pituitary tumors are < 5 mm at time of diagnosis. These may be difficult to find at the time of surgery.

DIFFERENTIAL DIAGNOSIS
See page 927 which includes non-neoplastic considerations as well.

EPIDEMIOLOGY
Pituitary tumors represent ~ 10% of intracranial tumors, although if autopsy studies are utilized the incidence is higher. They are most common in the 3rd and 4th decades of life, and equally affect both sexes. The incidence is increased in **multiple endocrine adenomatosis** or neoplasia (**MEA** or **MEN**).

CLINICAL PRESENTATION OF PITUITARY TUMORS

Pituitary tumors usually present either due to endocrinologic disturbance, or due to mass effect. Pituitary macroadenomas may produce H/A. Seizures are rarely attributable to pituitary adenomas. A small number present with pituitary apoplexy (*see below*). Rarely, invasive adenomas may present with CSF rhinorrhea[228] (*see page 442*).

Classically, pituitary tumors are divided into two groups: functional (or secreting), and non-functional (AKA endocrine-inactive, which are either non-secretory, or else secreting products such as gonadotropin that do not cause endocrinologic symptoms). The latter usually do not present until of sufficient size to cause neurologic deficits by mass effect, whereas the former frequently present earlier with symptoms caused by physiologic effects of excess hormones that they secrete[229]; this distinction is not always adhered to. Panhypopituitarism may be caused by large tumors of either variety (usually the non-functional type) as a result of compression of the pituitary.

PITUITARY APOPLEXY
⚑ Key features:
* paroxysmal H/A with endocrinologic or neurologic deficit (usually ophthalmoplegia or visual loss)
* due to expansion of a pituitary adenoma from hemorrhage or necrosis
* management: immediate administration of glucocorticoids, and transsphenoidal decompression within 7 days in most cases

Definition: Abrupt onset of headache accompanied by neurologic or endocrinologic deterioration.

Etiology: Due to sudden expansion of a mass within the sella turcica as a result of hemorrhage and/or necrosis[230, 231] or infarction within a pituitary tumor and adjacent pituitary gland. Occasionally, hemorrhage occurs into a normal pituitary gland or Rathke's cleft cyst[232].

Clinical features: Neurologic involvement includes:
1. visual disturbances: one of the most common findings. Includes:
   A. ophthalmoplegia (unilateral or bilateral): opposite the situation with a pituitary tumor, ophthalmoplegia occurs more often (78%) than visual pathway deficits (52-64%)[233]
   B. one of the typical field cuts seen in pituitary tumors (*see page 444*)
2. reduced mental status: due to ↑ ICP or hypothalamic involvement
3. cavernous sinus compression can cause venous stasis and/or pressure on any of the structures within the cavernous sinus
   A. trigeminal nerve symptoms
   B. proptosis
   C. ophthalmoplegia (Cr. N. III palsy is more common than VI)
   D. pressure on carotid artery
   E. compression of sympathetics within the cavernous sinus may produce a form of Horner's syndrome with unilateral ptosis, miosis, & anhidrosis limited to the forehead
4. when hemorrhage breaks through the tumor capsule and the arachnoid membrane into the chiasmatic cistern, signs and symptoms of SAH may be seen
   A. N/V
   B. meningismus
   C. photophobia
5. increased ICP may produce lethargy, stupor or coma
6. hypothalamic involvement may produce
   A. hypotension
   B. thermal dysautoregulation
   C. cardiac dysrhythmias
   D. respiratory pattern disturbances
   E. diabetes insipidus
   F. altered mental status: lethargy, stupor or coma
7. suprasellar expansion can produce acute hydrocephalus

Epidemiology

In Wilson's series, 3% of his patients with macroadenomas had an episode of pituitary apoplexy. In another series of 560 pituitary tumors, a high incidence of 17% was found (major attack in 7%, minor in 2%, asymptomatic in 8%)[234]. It is common for apoplexy to be the initial presentation of a pituitary tumor[235].

Evaluation

CT or MRI shows hemorrhagic mass in sella and/or suprasellar region, often distorting the anterior third ventricle.

Cerebral angiography should be considered in cases where differentiating pituitary apoplexy from aneurysmal SAH is difficult.

Management of pituitary apoplexy

Pituitary function is consistently compromised, necessitating rapid administration of corticosteroids and endocrine evaluation.

In the absence of visual deficits, prolactinomas may be treated with bromocriptine.

Rapid decompression is required for: sudden constriction of visual fields, severe and/or rapid deterioration of acuity, or neurologic deterioration due to hydrocephalus. Surgery in ≤ 7 days of pituitary apoplexy resulted in better improvement in ophthalmoplegia (100%), visual acuity (88%) and field cuts (95%) than surgery after 7 days[236]. Decompression is usually via a transsphenoidal route (transcranial approach may be advantageous in some cases). Goals of surgery:
1. to decompress the following structures if under pressure: optic apparatus, pituitary gland, cavernous sinus, third ventricle (relieving hydrocephalus)
2. obtain tissue for pathology
3. complete removal of tumor is usually not necessary
4. for hydrocephalus: ventricular drainage is generally required

---

The most common functional pituitary tumors secrete one of the following:
1. prolactin **(PRL)**: prolactinomas are the most common secretory adenoma. Causes amenorrhea-galactorrhea syndrome (AKA Forbes-Albright syndrome, AKA Ahumada-del Castillo syndrome) in females, impotence in males, and often infertility in either sex. Also causes bone loss
2. adrenocorticotropic hormone **(ACTH)**: AKA **corticotropin**. This is Cushing's *disease*. Elevated ACTH causes either:
   A. endogenous hypercortisolism (Cushing's *disease*, *see below*), or
   B. **Nelson's syndrome**: hyperpigmentation (due to melanin stimulating hormone **(MSH)** cross reactivity with ACTH). Develops in 10-30% of patients who have undergone adrenalectomy for treatment of Cushing's syndrome
3. growth hormone **(GH)**: causes acromegaly in adults (*see below*). In prepubertal children (before epiphyseal closure), it produces gigantism (very rare)

Rare pituitary adenomas secrete:
1. thyrotropin **(TSH)**: produces thyrotoxicosis
2. gonadotropins (leutinizing hormone **(LH)** and/or follicle stimulating hormone **(FSH)**): usually does not produce a clinical syndrome

Diabetes insipidus: almost never seen pre-operatively with pituitary tumors *see page 442.*

CUSHING'S SYNDROME
A constellation of findings caused by hypercortisolism. The most common cause of Cushing's syndrome **(CS)** is iatrogenic (administration of *exogenous* steroids). Possible etiologies of endogenous hypercortisolism are shown in *Table 17-32*. To determine the etiology of CS, see *Dexamethasone suppression test* on page 446.
Prevalence: 40 cases/million population. Cushing's *disease* is 9 times more common in women, whereas ectopic ACTH production is 10 times more common in males. Non-iatrogenic CS is 25% as common as acromegaly.

Table 17-32 Causes of endogenous hypercortisolism

Site of pathology	Secretion product	% of cases	ACTH levels
pituitary adenoma (Cushing's *disease*, see page 441)	ACTH	60-80%	slightly elevated*
ectopic ACTH production (tumors of lung (most common), pancreas...)	ACTH†	1-10%	very elevated
adrenal (adenoma or carcinoma)	cortisol	10-20%	low
hypothalamic or ectopic secretion of corticotropin-releasing hormone (CRH) producing hyperplasia of pituitary corticotrophs (pseudo-Cushing's state) see page 446	CRH	rare	elevated

* ACTH may be normal or slightly elevated; normal ACTH levels in the presence of hypercortisolism are considered inappropriately elevated

† cachexia often accompanies ectopic ACTH production by a malignancy

Findings in Cushing's syndrome include:
1. weight gain
   A. generalized in 50% of cases
   B. centripetal fat deposition in 50%: trunk, upper thoracic spine ("buffalo hump"), supraclavicular fat pad, neck, "dewlap tumor" (episternal fat), with round plethoric face ("moon facies") and slender extremities
2. hypertension
3. ecchymoses and purple striae, especially on flanks, breasts and lower abdomen
4. hyperglycemia: diabetes or glucose intolerance
5. amenorrhea in women, impotence in men, reduced libido in both
6. hypokalemic alkalosis
7. hyperpigmentation of skin and mucous membranes: seen only with elevated ACTH (due to MSH cross-reactivity of ACTH), i.e. Cushing's disease or ectopic ACTH production
8. atrophic, tissue-paper thin skin with easy bruising and poor wound healing
9. psychiatric: depression, emotional lability, dementia
10. osteoporosis
11. generalized muscle wasting with complaints of easy fatigability
12. elevation of other adrenal hormones: androgens may produce hirsutism and acne

Ectopic ACTH secretion:

The most common tumors are small-cell carcinoma of the lung, thymoma, carcinoid tumors, pheochromocytomas, and medullary thyroid carcinoma. Malignancies secreting ACTH are usually rapidly fatal.

Cushing's disease

Endogenous hypercortisolism due to an ACTH secreting pituitary adenoma. Over half are < 5 mm at the time of presentation which is very difficult to image with CT or MRI. Most are basophilic, some (especially the larger ones) may be chromophobic. Only ≈ 10% are large enough to produce some mass effect, which may cause enlargement of the sella, visual field deficit, cranial nerve involvement and/or hypopituitarism.

Cells contain proopiomelanocortin (**POMC**), the precursor molecule which contains amino acid sequences for ACTH, alpha-MSH, ß-lipotropin, ß-endorphin and met-en-kephalin.

ACROMEGALY

Growth hormone (**GH**) is under dual hypothalamic control via the hypophysial portal system. GH-releasing hormone (**GHRH**) stimulates pituitary secretion and synthesis of GH and induces GH gene transcription. **Somatostatin** suppresses GH release only. Somatomedin-C (AKA insulin-like growth factor-I (**IGF-I**)) is the protein secreted by the liver in response to GH that is probably responsible for most of GH's systemic effects.

Excess GH can result from pituitary adenomas, but may also occur with ectopic GH secretion by a carcinoid tumor.

In adults, elevated GH levels produces **acromegaly**[237] with findings of: skeletal overgrowth deformities (increasing hand and foot size, thickened heel pad, frontal bossing, prognathism, macroglossia), hypertension, soft tissue swelling and peripheral nerve entrapment syndromes, debilitating headache, excessive perspiration (especially palmar hyperhidrosis), oily skin, and joint pain and fatigue. 25% of acromegalics have thyromegaly with normal thyroid studies.

Patients with elevated levels of GH (including partially treated cases) have 2-3 times the expected mortality rate[238], primarily due to hypertension, diabetes, pulmonary infections, cancer, and cardiomyopathy (*see Table 17-33*). Soft-tissue swelling and nerve entrapment may be reversible with normalization of GH levels, however many disfiguring changes and health risks are permanent (*see Table 17-33*).

Elevated levels of GH in children before closure of the epiphyseal plates in the long bones produces **gigantism** instead of acromegaly.

MASS EFFECTS OF PITUITARY TUMORS

Usually (but not exclusively) seen with nonfunctioning tumors. Of functional tumors, prolactinoma is the most likely to become large enough to cause mass effect (ACTH tumor is least likely). Patients may present with headaches. Structures commonly compressed and manifestations include:

1. optic chiasm: classically resulting in bitemporal hemianopsia (noncongruous), may also cause decreasing visual acuity

Table 17-33 Risks of long-term exposure to excess growth hormone (GH)[238]

Arthropathy
• unrelated to age of onset or GH levels
• usually with longstanding acromegaly
• reversibility*:
• rapid symptomatic improvement
• bone & cartilage lesions irreversible
Peripheral neuropathy
• intermittent anesthesias, paresthesias
• sensorimotor polyneuropathy
• impaired sensation
• reversibility*:
• symptoms may improve
• onion bulbs (whorls) do not regress
Cardiovascular disease
• cardiomyopathy
• reduced LV diastolic function
• increased LV mass and arrhythmias
• fibrous hyperplasia of connective tissue
• HTN: exacerbates cardiomyopathic changes
• reversibility*: may progress even with normal GH
Respiratory disease
• upper airway obstruction: caused by soft tissue overgrowth and decreased pharyngeal muscle tone with sleep apnea in ≈ 50%
• reversibility*: generally improves
Neoplasia
• increased risk of malignancies (especially colon-Ca) & soft-tissue polyps
• reversibility*: unknown
Glucose intolerance
• occurs in 25% of acromegalics (more common with family history of DM)
• reversibility*: improves

* reversibility with normalization of GH levels

2. pituitary gland: results in varying degrees of hypopituitarism
   A. hypothyroidism: cold intolerance, myxedema, coarse hair, entrapment neuropathies (e.g. carpal tunnel syndrome)
   B. hypoadrenalism: orthostatic hypotension, easy fatigability
   C. hypogonadism: amenorrhea (women), loss of libido, infertility
   D. **diabetes insipidus**: almost never seen pre-operatively with pituitary tumors (except possibly with pituitary apoplexy, *page 438*). If DI is present, other etiologies should be sought (e.g. hypothalamic glioma, suprasellar germ cell tumor)
   E. hyperprolactinemia: PRL is under inhibitory control from the hypothalamus, and pressure on the pituitary stalk may release some inhibition (so-called "stalk-effect", *see page 445*)
3. cavernous sinus
   A. pressure on cranial nerves contained within (III, IV, V_1, V_2, VI): ptosis, facial pain, diplopia (see *Invasive pituitary adenomas* below)
   B. occlusion of the sinus: proptosis, chemosis
   C. encasement of the carotid artery by tumor: may cause slight narrowing, but complete occlusion is rare

INVASIVE PITUITARY ADENOMAS

About 5% of pituitary adenomas become locally invasive. There is evidence that the genetic make-up of these tumors may be different from more benign adenomas, even though the histology is similar. Numerous classifications systems have been devised, Wilson's system[239] (modified from Hardy[240, 241]) is shown in *Table 17-34*.

The clinical course is variable, with some tumors being more aggressive than others. Occasionally, these tumors grow to gigantic sizes (> 4 cm dia), and these are often very aggressive and follow a malignant course[242].

At times, an adenoma may push the medial wall of the cavernous sinus ahead of it without actually perforating this dural structure[243]. This is difficult to reliably identify on MRI, and the most definitive sign of cavernous sinus invasion is carotid artery encasement[244].

Table 17-34 Anatomic classification of pituitary adenoma (modified Hardy system)[239]

Extension
• Suprasellar extension
0: none
A: expanding into suprasellar cistern
B: anterior recesses of 3rd ventricle obliterated
C: floor of 3rd ventricle grossly displaced
• Parasellar extension
D*: intracranial (intradural)
E: into or beneath cavernous sinus (extradural)

Invasion/Spread
• Floor of sella intact
I: sella normal or focally expanded; tumor < 10 mm
II: sella enlarged; tumor ≥ 10 mm
• Sphenoid
III: localized perforation of sellar floor
IV: diffuse destruction of sellar floor
• Distant spread
V: spread via CSF or blood-borne

* designate: 1) anterior, 2) middle, or 3) posterior fossa

Presentation: Most of these tumors present due to compression of the optic apparatus, usually producing gradual visual deficit (sudden blindness is not unheard of). Deficits of extraocular muscles may occur with cavernous sinus invasion, and usually develop *after* visual loss. Suprasellar extension may obstruct the foramen of Monro, producing hydrocephalus. Invasion of the skull base may lead to nasal obstruction or **CSF rhinorrhea**, which occasionally may be precipitated by tumor shrinkage in response to bromocriptine[245]. Exophthalmos may occur with orbital invasion due to compromise of orbital venous drainage. Those that secrete prolactin often present with findings of hyperprolactinemia (*see page 440*) and with these, the prolactin levels are usually > 1000 ng/dl (caution: giant invasive adenomas with very high PRL production may have a falsely low PRL level, *see page 446*).

PATHOLOGICAL CLASSIFICATION OF PITUITARY TUMORS

LIGHT MICROSCOPIC APPEARANCE OF ADENOMAS

Older classification system. With newer techniques (EM, immunohistochemistry, radio-immuno assay...) many tumors previously considered nonsecretory have been found to have all the components necessary to secrete hormones. This system is of limited usefulness.

In order of decreasing frequency:
- **chromophobe**: (most common; ratio of chromophobe to acidophil is 4-20:1), originally considered "non-secretory", in actuality may produce prolactin, GH, or TSH
- **acidophil** (eosinophilic): produce prolactin, TSH, or usually <u>GH</u> → <u>gigantism</u> (in children) or <u>acromegaly</u> (in adults)
- **basophil** → gonadotropins, ß-lipotropin, or usually <u>ACTH</u> → <u>Cushing's disease</u>

CLASSIFICATION OF ADENOMAS BASED ON SECRETORY PRODUCTS
1. endocrine-active tumors: ≈ 70% of pituitary tumors produce 1 or 2 hormones that are measurable in the serum and cause defined clinical syndromes, these are classified based on their secretory product(s)
2. endocrine-inactive (nonfunctional) tumors[246]
   A. null-cell adenoma
   B. oncocytoma   } constitute the bulk of endocrine-inactive adenomas
   C. gonadotropin-secreting adenoma
   D. silent corticotropin-secreting adenoma
   E. glycoprotein-secreting adenoma

EVALUATION

Table 17-35   Summary of workup for pituitary tumors

Evaluation		Rationale	See page
• Formal visual fields		• rule out field cut from mass effect	*see below*
	• 8 A.M. cortisol*	• ↑ in hypercortisolism (Cushing's syndrome) • ↓ in hypoadrenalism (primary or secondary)	444 and 446
	• T_4, TSH	**Hypothyroidism** • T_4 ↓ & TSH ↑ in primary hypothyroidism (may produce thyrotroph hyperplasia in pituitary) • T_4 ↓ & TSH nl or ↓ in secondary hypothyroidism	445
		Hyperthyroidism (thyrotoxicosis) • T_4 ↑ & TSH ↓ in primary hyperthyroidism • T_4 ↑ & TSH ↑ in TSH-secreting adenomas	
	• prolactin	• ↑ or ↑↑ with prolactinoma • slight ↑ with stalk effect (*see page 445*)	445
	• gonadotropins (FSH, LH) and sex steroids (♀: estradiol, ♂: testosterone)	• ↓ in hypogonadotrophic hypogonadism (from mass effect causing compression of the pituitary gland) • ↑ with gonadotropin secreting adenoma	445
	• somatomedIn-C (IGF-I)	• ↑ in acromegaly • ↓ in hypopituitarism (one of the most sensitive markers)	447
	• fasting blood glucose	↓ in hypoadrenalism (primary or secondary)	444

• Radiographic studies. Either:
  • MRI without & with enhancement (test of choice)
  • *or* CT without & with enhancement (with coronal views) + cerebral angiogram
			447

(Endocrine screening spans the rows from 8 A.M. cortisol through fasting blood glucose)*

*   may be difficult to interpret, 24-hour urine free cortisol is more accurate, see text

HISTORY AND PHYSICAL
Directed to look for signs and symptoms of:
1. endocrine hyperfunction (see *Functional pituitary tumors* above)
2. endocrine deficits (due to mass effect on pituitary) (see *Mass effects of pituitary tumors*, page 441)
3. visual field deficit: bedside confrontational testing to rule-out visual field deficit (classically bitemporal hemianopsia, *see below*)
4. deficits of cranial nerves within cavernous sinus (III, IV, V_1, V_2, VI)

VISUAL FIELDS
Formal visual field testing by perimetry with a tangent screen (using the small red stimulus since desaturation of color is an early sign of chiasmal compression) or by Gold-

man or automated Humphrey perimeter (the latter requires good cooperation from the patient to be valid).

Visual field deficit patterns

Depends in part on location of chiasm with respect to sella turcica: the chiasm is located above the sella in 79%, posterior to the sella turcica (**postfixed** chiasm) in 4%; in front of the sella (pre-fixed) in 5%[247 (p 2135)]

1. compression of the optic chiasm:
   A. impinges on crossing nasal fibers producing **bitemporal hemianopsia** that obeys the vertical meridian (unlike with occipital lobe dysfunction), the classic finding associated with a pituitary tumor
   B. other reported patterns that occur rarely: monocular temporal hemianopsia
2. optic nerve compression: more likely in patients with a postfixed chiasm
   A. loss of vision in the ipsilateral eye, and if carefully sought there is usually a superior outer (temporal) quadrantanopsia in the contralateral eye[247 (p 2135)] (so-called **junctional scotoma** AKA "pie in the sky" defect) from compression of the anterior knee of Wildbrand (*see page 813*) (may also be an early finding even without a post-fixed chiasm)
   B. may produce central scotoma or monocular reduction in visual acuity
3. compression of the optic tract: may occur with a pre-fixed chiasm. Produces **homonymous hemianopsia**

ENDOCRINOLOGIC EVALUATION

BASELINE ENDOCRINE EVALUATION (modified[248])

Also, *see Table 17-35*. May give indication of tumor type, determines whether any hormones need to be replaced, serves as a baseline for comparison following treatment. Includes assessment for clinical signs and symptoms, as well as laboratory tests. Screening tests should be checked in all patients with pituitary tumors. Note: selective loss of a single pituitary hormone together with thickening of the pituitary stalk is strongly suggestive of lymphocytic hypophysitis (*see page 928*).

1. adrenal axis
   A. screening:
      1. 8 AM cortisol level: normal is 6-18 µg/100 ml. Note: AM cortisol may normally be slightly elevated. Difficult to interpret if marginal
      2. 24-hour urine free cortisol: more accurate (almost 100% sensitive and specific, false negative rare except in stress or chronic alcoholism). If not elevated several times above normal, at least 2 additional determinations should be made[249]
      3. in still questionable cases, see *Cushing's syndrome*, page 446 for the low-dose overnight DMZ suppression test and for more information
   B. further testing:
      1. **cosyntropin stimulation test**[250]: to check cortisol reserve. Draw a baseline cortisol level (fasting is not required; test can be performed at any time of day)/
         Give cosyntropin (Cortrosyn®) 1 ampoule (250 µg) IM or IV (a potent ACTH analogue), then check cortisol levels at 30 mins (optional) and at 60 mins. Normal response: peak cortisol level > 18 µg/dl with an increment > 7 µg/dl, or a peak > 20 µg/dl regardless of the increment
         a. subnormal responses indicate **adrenal insufficiency**. In primary adrenal insufficiency, pituitary ACTH secretion will be elevated. In secondary adrenal insufficiency, *chronically* reduced ACTH causes adrenal atrophy and unresponsiveness to acute exogenous ACTH stimulation
         b. a normal response rules out primary and overt secondary adrenal insufficiency, but in mild cases of reduced pituitary ACTH where adrenal atrophy has not occurred the test may be normal. In these cases further testing with metyrapone (*see page 455*) or insulin induced hypoglycemia may be indicated
      2. **insulin tolerance test**: almost always abnormal in CS. Give regular insulin 0.1 U/kg IV push, and draw blood for sugar, cortisol and GH at 0, 10, 20, 30, 45, 60, 90 and 120 mins (monitor blood sugar by fingerstick during test, and give IV glucose if patient becomes symptomatic). If fingerstick blood sugar is not < 50 by 30 minutes, give additional

regular insulin 5 U IVP
2. thyroid axis: the basis for thyroid screening is shown in *Table 17-36*

Table 17-36 Basis for thyroid screening

	T_4	TSH
Primary hypothyroidism		
• chronic primary hypothyroidism may produce secondary pituitary hyperplasia (pituitary pseudotumor) indistinguishable from adenoma on CT or MRI. Must be considered in any patient with a pituitary mass[251, 252]	↓	↑
• pathophysiology: loss of negative feedback from thyroid hormones causes increased TRH release from the hypothalamus producing secondary hyperplasia of thyrotrophic cells in the adenohypophysis (thyrotroph hyperplasia). The patient may present due to pituitary enlargement (visual symptoms, elevated PRL from stalk effect, enlarged sella on x-rays...)		
• chronic stimulation from elevated TRH may rarely produce thyrotroph adenomas		
• labs: low T_4, elevated TSH (in excess of 90-100 in patients presenting with thyrotroph hyperplasia), and the TSH response to TRH stimulation test (*see text*) will be prolonged and elevated		
Secondary hypothyroidism		
• pituitary hypothyroidism accounts for only ≈ 2-4% of all hypothyroid cases[253]	↓	↓ or nl
• ≈ 23% of patients with chromophobe adenomas develop secondary hypothyroidism if untreated (pituitary compression causes reduced TSH)		
• labs: low thyroid hormones, low or normal TSH, reduced response to TRH stimulation test		
• ✖ Caution: replacing thyroid hormone with inadequate cortisol reserves (as may occur in hypopituitarism) can precipitate adrenal crisis. Do a cosyntropin stimulation test (*see page 444*) and then replace cortisol as needed		
Primary hyperthyroidism		
• may be due to: localized hyperactive nodule, circulating antibody that stimulates the gland, or to diffuse hyperplasia (Graves' disease, AKA ophthalmic hyperthyroidism)	↑	↓
• labs: increased T_4 with subnormal TSH		
Secondary hyperthyroidism		
• TSH-secreting pituitary adenoma (rare)	↑	↑
• labs: elevated T_4 is due to elevated TSH		

A. screening: T_4 level (total or free), thyroid-stimulating hormone **(TSH)** (AKA thyrotropin). Normal values: free T_4 index is 0.8-1.5, TSH 0.4-5.5 μU/ml, total T_4 4-12 μg/100ml
B. further testing: thyrotropin-releasing hormone **(TRH)** stimulation test (indicated if T_4 is low or borderline): check baseline TSH, give 500 μg TRH IV, check TSH at 30 & 60 mins. Normal response: peak TSH twice baseline value at 30 mins. Impaired response with a low T_4 indicates pituitary deficiency. Exaggerated response suggests primary hypothyroidism

3. gonadal axis
A. screening: serum gonadotropins (FSH & LH) and sex steroids (estradiol in women, testosterone in men)
B. further testing: none dependable in differentiating pituitary from hypothalamic disorders

4. **prolactin levels**
A. should be measured in all patients with pituitary tumors, interpretation is shown in *Table 17-37*. Improvement of symptoms with surgery correlates with pre-op prolactin level **(PRL)**. If PRL is < 200 ng/ml, ≈ 80% of tumors are microadenomas, and 76% of these will have normal post-op PRL; if PRL > 200, only ≈ 20% are microadenomas.

Stalk effect: PRL is the only pituitary hormone

Table 17-37 Significance of prolactin levels*

PRL (ng/ml)	Interpretation	Possible causes
< 25	normal	
25-150	moderate elevation	• prolactinoma • "stalk effect" (*see text*) • certain drugs (e.g. phenothiazines, BCP) • primary hypothyroidism
> 150†	significant elevation	prolactinoma

* Note: ectopic sites of prolactin secretion have rarely been reported (e.g. in a teratoma[254])

† some authors recommend 200 ng/ml as the cutoff for probable prolactinomas[255]

under inhibitory regulation. Injury to the hypothalamus or pituitary stalk can cause modest elevation of PRL due to decrease in prolactin inhibitory factor **(PRIF)**. As a rule of thumb, the percent chance of an elevated PRL being due to a prolactinoma is equal to one half the PRL level. Persistent post-op PRL elevation may occur even with total tumor removal as a result of injury to stalk (usually ≤ 90 ng/ml; stalk effect doubtful if PRL > 150). Follow these patients, do not use bromocriptine

Hook effect: extremely high PRL levels may produce false negatives due to the tendency for the large numbers of PRL molecules to prevent the formation of the necessary PRL-antibody-signal complexes. Therefore, for large adenomas with a normal PRL level, have the lab perform several dilutions of the serum sample and re-run the PRL to avoid a false negative

5. growth hormone:
   A. checking a single random GH level may not be a reliable indicator and is therefore not recommended (*see page 447*)
   B. somatomedin-C (IGF-I) level (*see page 447*)
6. neurohypophysis (posterior pituitary): deficits are rare with pituitary tumors
   A. screening: check adequacy of ADH by demonstrating concentration of urine with water deprivation (see *Water deprivation test*, page 18)
   B. further testing: measurement of serum ADH in response to infusion of hypertonic saline

SPECIALIZED ENDOCRINOLOGIC TESTS

Cushing's syndrome
A. tests to determine if hypercortisolism (Cushing's syndrome, **(CS)**) is present or not, regardless of etiology if the screening 24-hr urine free cortisol (*see page 444*) is equivocal (the basis of these tests is shown in *Table 17-38*)
   1. low-dose dexamethasone **(DMZ)** suppression tests[256]:
      A. overnight low dose test: give DMZ 1 mg PO @ 11 P.M. and draw serum cortisol the next day at 8 A.M.
         1. cortisol < 5 µg/dl: Cushing's syndrome is ruled out (except for a few patients with CS who suppress at low DMZ doses, possibly due to low DMZ clearance[257])
      2. cortisol 5-10 µg/dl: indeterminate, retesting is necessary
      3. cortisol > 10 µg/dl: CS is probably present. False positives can occur in the so-called **pseudo-Cushing's state** where ectopic CRH secretion produces hyperplasia of pituitary corticotrophs that is clinically indistinguishable from pituitary ACTH producing tumors (requires further testing[257]). Seen in: 15% of obese patients, in 25% of hospitalized and chronically ill patients, in high estrogen states, in uremia, and in depression. False positives also may occur in alcoholics or patients on phenobarbital or phenytoin due increased metabolism of DMZ caused by induced hepatic microsomal degradation
   B. 2 day low dose test (used when overnight test is equivocal): give DMZ 0.5 mg PO q 6 hrs for 2 days starting at 6 A.M.; 24 hr urine collections are obtained prior to test and on the 2nd day of DMZ administration. Normal patients suppress urinary 17-hydroxycorticosteroids **(OHCS)** to less than 4 mg/24 hrs, whereas ≈ 95% of patients with CS have abnormal response (higher amounts in urine)[257]
   2. other tests include the classic low-dose DMZ suppression test: involves 4 days of urine collection[258] (not often used)
B. tests to distinguish primary Cushing's disease **(CD)** (pituitary ACTH hypersecretion) from ectopic ACTH production and adrenal tumors
   1. measure serum ACTH: low in adrenal tumors

Table 17-38 Basis for biochemical tests in Cushing's syndrome

- normally, low DMZ doses suppress ACTH release through negative feedback on hypothalamic-pituitary axis, reducing urine and serum corticosteroids
- in ≥ 98% of cases of Cushing's syndrome, suppression occurs, but at a much higher threshold
- adrenal tumors and most (85-90%) cases of ectopic ACTH production (especially bronchial Ca) will not suppress even with high dose DMZ
- ACTH response to CRH is exaggerated
- DMZ does not interfere with measurement of urinary and plasma cortisol and 17-hydroxycorticosteroids

2. abdominal CT: usually shows unilateral adrenal mass with adrenal tumors, or normal or bilateral adrenal enlargement in ACTH-dependent cases
3. high-dose dexamethasone **(DMZ)** suppression test: (NB: up to 20% of patient's with CD do not suppress with high-dose DMZ; phenytoin may also interfere with high-dose DMZ suppression[259])
4. overnight test: obtain a baseline 8 A.M. plasma cortisol level, then give DMZ 8 mg PO @ 11 P.M. and measure plasma cortisol level the next morning at 8 A.M. In 95% of CD cases plasma cortisol levels are reduced to < 50% of baseline, whereas in ectopic ACTH or adrenal tumors it will usually be unchanged
5. **metyrapone** (Metopirone®) test: performed on an inpatient basis. Give 750 mg metyrapone (suppresses cortisol synthesis) PO q 4 hrs for 6 doses. Most patients with CD will have a rise in 17-OHCS in urine of 70% above baseline, or an increase in serum 11-deoxycortisol 400-fold above baseline
6. corticotropin-releasing hormone stimulation test **(CRH)**: CD responds to exogenous CRH 0.1 μg/kg IV bolus with even further increased plasma ACTH and cortisol levels; ectopic ACTH and adrenal tumors do not[260]
7. inferior petrosal sinus sampling: may also determine likely side of a microadenoma within the pituitary (thus may be able to avoid bilateral adrenalectomy which requires lifelong gluco- and mineralo-corticoid replacement and Nelson's syndrome in 10-30%). 15% of the time this test falsely lateralizes the tumor. Look for gradient of 1.4:1 compared to peripheral to diagnose primary Cushing's disease. Mostly a research technique

Acromegaly
1. **growth hormone (GH)**: normal basal fasting level is < 5 ng/ml. In patients with acromegaly GH is > 10 ng/ml. Normal basal levels do not distinguish normal patient from GH deficiency[261]. Furthermore, due to pulsatile secretion of GH, normal patients may have sporadic peaks up to 50 ng/ml[237]. Therefore, this test is not commonly used (*see below* for somatomedin-C)
2. somatomedin-C (AKA IGF-I) level: provides an excellent integrative marker of average GH secretion. Fasting level in normals is 0.67 U/ml (range: 0.01-1.4). In acromegalics this is 6.8 U/ml (range: 2.6-21.7)[262]
3. other tests used uncommonly
   A. glucose suppression test (less precise and more expensive than measuring IGF-I, however may be more useful than IGF-I for monitoring initial response to therapy): normally, a 75 gm oral glucose load suppresses growth hormone to < 2 ng/ml (or cause a 50% reduction). This suppression is absent in acromegalics, and a few have paradoxical elevation. GH suppression may also be absent with liver disease, DM & renal failure
   B. growth-hormone releasing hormone **(GHRH)** stimulation test
   C. PRL: some GH secreting tumors also secrete PRL

RADIOGRAPHIC EVALUATION

Requires either CT or MRI. MRI has an advantage in large tumors and when evaluating for recurrence. A lateral skull x-ray may help define anatomy of sphenoid sinus in cases where transsphenoidal surgery is contemplated. ≈ 50% of pituitary tumors causing Cushing's syndrome are too small to be imaged on CT or MRI (therefore endocrinologic testing is required to prove the pituitary origin). *See page 927* for differential diagnosis of intrasellar lesions (some are indistinguishable radiographically).

Normal AP diameter of pituitary gland: female of childbearing age (≈ 13-35 yrs)[A]: ≤ 11 mm, for all others normal is ≤ 9 mm.

MRI

Imaging test of choice for pituitary tumors. Gives information about invasion of cavernous sinus, and about location and/or involvement of para-sellar carotids. MRI may fail to demonstrate tumor in 25-45% of cases of Cushing's disease[264].

Microadenoma: 75% are low signal on T1WI, and high signal on T2WI (but 25% can behave in any way, including completely opposite to above). Enhancement is time-dependent. Imaging must be done with 5 minutes of contrast administration to see a discrete microadenoma. Initially, gadolinium enhances the normal pituitary (no blood brain bar-

---

A. pituitary glands in adolescent girls may be physiologically enlarged (mean height: 8.2 ± 1.4 mm) as a result of hormonal stimulation of puberty[263]

rier) but not the pituitary tumor. After ≈ 30 minutes, the tumor enhances about the same.

Normally the neurohypophysis is high signal on T1WI (possibly due to phospholipids). Absence of this sign often correlates with diabetes insipidus.

Deviation of the pituitary stalk may also indicate the presence of a microadenoma. Normal thickness of the pituitary stalk is approximately equal to basilar artery diameter. Thickening of stalk is usually NOT adenoma, differential diagnosis here: lymphoma, lymphocytic hypophysitis (*see page 928*), granulomatous disease, hypothalamic glioma.

CT

Generally superseded by MRI. May be appropriate when MRI is contraindicated (e.g. pacemaker). When done, should include direct coronal imaging. Consider angiography to lay out parasellar carotid arteries and to R/O aneurysm as a possibility.

Calcium in pituitary usually signifies hemorrhage or infarction within tumor.

Enhancement (with IV contrast):
1. normal pituitary enhances densely (no BBB)
2. macroadenomas enhance more than normal pituitary
3. microadenomas enhance less (may just be slower). Diagnostic criteria:
   A. must have attenuation change on CT
   PLUS
   B. 2 or more of the following:
     1. focal bone erosion of sella
     2. focal superior bulge of gland
     3. displacement of stalk (this is unreliable, and may actually deviate to opposite side)

ANGIOGRAPHY

Sometimes used in cases considered for transsphenoidal surgery (e.g. as a complement to CT) to localize the parasellar carotids (note: MRI provides this information, and evaluates involvement of cavernous sinuses, usually obviating the need for angiography).

TREATMENT

See page 438 for treatment of pituitary apoplexy. *See page 452* for surgical indications.

MEDICAL TREATMENT

PROLACTINOMAS

Medical treatment is recommended in most cases with PRL > 500 (the chances of normalizing PRL surgically are very low[265]). See ★ *Indications for surgery* on page 452.

Dopamine agonists

SIDE EFFECTS:[266] (may vary with different preparations) nausea, H/A, fatigue, orthostatic hypotension with dizziness, cold induced peripheral vasodilatation, depression, nightmares and nasal congestion. Side effects are more troublesome during the first few weeks of treatment. Tolerance may be improved by bedtime dosing with food, slow dose escalation, sympathomimetics for nasal congestion, and acetaminophen 1-2 hrs before dosing to reduce H/A. Psychosis and vasospasm are rare side effects that usually necessitates discontinuation of the drug.

bromocriptine (Parlodel®)   DRUG INFO

A semi-synthetic ergot alkaloid that binds to receptors on normal and tumor lactotrophs, inhibiting synthesis and secretion of PRL and other processes regulating cell growth. Bromocriptine lowers prolactin level regardless of the whether the source is an adenoma or normal pituitary (e.g. as a result of stalk effect) to < 10% of pretreatment values in most patients. It also frequently reduces the tumor size in 6-8 weeks in 75% of patients with macroadenomas, but only as long as therapy is maintained and only for tumors that actually produce prolactin. Only ≈ 1% of prolactinomas continue to grow while the patient is on bromocriptine.

Bromocriptine can restore fertility. Continued therapy during pregnancy has been associated with a 3.3% incidence of congenital anomalies and 11% spontaneous abortion rate which is the same as for the general population. Prolactinomas may enlarge rapidly upon discontinuation of the drug. Pregnancy may also cause enlargement.

Prolonged treatment with bromocriptine may reduce the chances of surgical cure if this should be chosen at a later date. With a microadenoma, one year of bromocriptine may reduce the surgical cure rate by as much as 50%, possibly due to induced fibrosis[267]. Thus, it is suggested that if surgery is to be done that it be done in the first 6 months of bromocriptine therapy. Shrinkage of large tumors due to bromocriptine has rarely been reported to cause CSF rhinorrhea. SIDE EFFECTS: *see above*.

Rx: start with 1.25 mg (half of a 2.5 mg tablet) PO q hs (nighttime dosing reduces some side effects). Add additional 2.5 mg per day as necessary (based on PRL levels), making a dosage change every 2-4 weeks for microadenomas, or every 3-4 days for macroadenomas causing mass effect. Usual dosage is 5-7.5 mg daily (range: 2.5-15 mg) which may be given as a single dose or divided TID. Higher doses may be needed initially (e.g. for ≈ 6 mos) to bring down the PRL, and then lower doses may be able to maintain normal levels. SUPPLIED: 2.5 mg scored tabs; 5 mg capsules.

pergolide (Permax®) — DRUG INFO

A long-acting ergot alkaloid dopamine agonist that reduces PRL levels for > 24 hrs. Not FDA approved for hyperprolactinemia. Once daily dosing improves compliance. SIDE EFFECTS: *see above*.

Rx Start with 0.05 mg PO q hs, and increase by 0.025-0.05 increments (up to a maximum of ≈ 0.25 mg/d) until normal PRL levels are achieved.

cabergoline (Dostinex®) — DRUG INFO

An ergot alkaline derivative that is a selective D_2 dopamine agonist (bromocriptine (*see above*) is also a D_2 agonist but additionally affects D_1 receptors)[268]. The elimination half-life is 60-100 hrs which usually permits dosing 1-2 times weekly. Control of PRL and resumption of ovulatory cycles may be better with cabergoline[269]. SIDE EFFECTS: (*see above*) H/A and GI symptoms are reportedly less problematic than with bromocriptine.

Rx: Start with 0.25 mg PO twice weekly, and increase each dose by 0.25 mg every 4 weeks as needed to control PRL (up to a maximum of 3 mg per week). Typical dose is 0.5-1 mg twice weekly. Some combine the total dose and give it once weekly. ✖ Contraindicated in eclampsia or pre-eclampsia, uncontrolled HTN, and dosage should be reduced with severe hepatic dysfunction. SUPPLIED: 0.5 mg scored tablets.

ACROMEGALY[238]

Asymptomatic elderly patients do not require treatment since there is little evidence that intervention alters life expectancy in this group.

1. if no contraindications, surgery (usually transsphenoidal) is currently the best initial therapy (worse prognosis with macroadenomas) providing more rapid reduction in GH levels and decompression of neural structures (e.g. optic apparatus). Surgery is not recommended for elderly patients. Estimated (one-time) cost of transsphenoidal resection: $30,000 in the U.S.

2. for patients not cured[A] by surgery or with contraindications to surgery, or with recurrences after surgery or XRT, medical therapy is indicated
   A. dopamine agonists
      1. bromocriptine: (*see below*) although it benefits only a minority of patients, a first line drug since it is cheaper than pegvisomant or octreotide and is given PO
      2. other dopamine agonists: cabergoline (*see above*), pergolide (*see above*), lisuride, depo-bromocriptine (bromocriptine-LAR)
   B. pegvisomant (*see below*) should be considered for failures to above
   C. octreotide (*see below*) for those who fail to respond to the above
   D. pegvisomant or octreotide + dopamine agonist if no response to 1 drug alone (combination therapy may be more effective than either drug alone)

3. radiation for failure of medical therapy: (not recommended as initial treatment, *see page 452*)

A. the definition of "cure" with acromegaly is controversial. Many use a GH level < 3-5 ng/ml as a cutoff. Others feel that an elevated IGF-I represents lack of cure even if GH < 5. Still others require a normal IGF-I AND lack of GH rise > 2 ng/ml during an oral glucose suppression test (*see page 447*)

bromocriptine (Parlodel®) DRUG INFO

Neoplastic somatotrophs may respond fortuitously to dopamine agonists and reduce growth hormone (**GH**) secretion. Bromocriptine lowers GH levels to < 10 ng/ml in 54% of cases, to < 5 ng/ml in only ≈ 12%. Tumor shrinkage occurs in only < 20%. Higher doses are usually required than for prolactinomas. If effective, the drug may be continued but should be periodically withdrawn to assess the GH level. SIDE EFFECTS: *see page 448.* Estimated annual cost: $3,200 in the U.S.

Rx For growth hormone tumors that respond to bromocriptine, the usual dosage is 20-60 mg/d in divided doses (higher doses are unwarranted). The maximal daily dose is 100 mg. For dose escalation regimens, *see above.*

octreotide (Sandostatin®) DRUG INFO

A somatostatin analogue that is 45 times more potent than somatostatin in suppressing GH secretion but is only twice as potent in suppressing insulin secretion, has a longer half-life (≈ 2 hrs after SQ injection, compared to ≈ minutes for somatostatin), and does not result in rebound GH hypersecretion. GH levels are reduced in 71%, IGF-I levels are reduced in 93%. 50-66% have normal GH levels, 66% achieve normal IGF-I levels. Tumor volume reduces significantly in about 30% of patients. Many symptoms including H/A usually improve within the first few weeks of treatment. Annual cost to the patient: at least ≈ $7,800 in the U.S. Usually given in combination with bromocriptine.

After 50 μg SQ injection, GH secretion is suppressed within 1 hr, nadirs at 3 hrs, and remains reduced for 6-8 hrs (occasionally up to 12 hrs). SIDE EFFECTS: reduced GI motility and secretion, diarrhea, steatorrhea, flatulence, nausea, abdominal discomfort (all of these usually remit in 10 days), clinically insignificant bradycardia in 15%, cholesterol cholelithiasis (in 10-25%) or bile sludge. Asymptomatic stones require no treatment and routine ultrasonography is not required. Mild hypothyroidism or worsening of glucose intolerance may occur.

Rx: Start with 50-100 μg SQ q 8 hrs. Increase up to a maximum of 1500 μg/d (doses > 750 μg/d are rarely needed). Average dose required is 100-200 μg SQ q 8 hrs.

pegvisomant (Somavert®) DRUG INFO

A competitive GH-receptor antagonist. Treatment for ≥ 12 mos results in normal IGF-I levels in 97% of patients[270]. No change in pituitary tumor size has been observed[271]. SIDE EFFECTS: significant but reversible liver function abnormalities occur in < 1%. Serum GH increases, probably as a result of loss of negative feedback on IGF-I production.

Rx: 5-40 mg/d SQ (dose must be titrated to keep IGF-I in the normal range, to avoid GH deficiency conditions).

CUSHING'S DISEASE

Transsphenoidal surgery is the treatment of choice for most (there is no effective pituitary suppressive medication). Cure rates are ≈ 85% for microadenomas (i.e. tumors ≤ 1 cm dia), but are lower for larger tumors.

Medical therapy

For patients who fail surgical therapy or for whom surgery cannot be tolerated, medical therapy and/or radiation are utilized. Occasionally may be used for several weeks prior to planned surgery to control significant manifestations of hypercortisolism (e.g. diabetes, HTN, psychiatric disturbances…, *see page 440*).

Ketoconazole (Nizoral®)[266]: an antifungal agent that blocks adrenal steroid synthesis. The initial drug of choice. Over 75% of patients have normalization of urinary free cortisol and 17-hydroxycorticosteroid levels. SIDE EFFECTS: reversible elevations of serum hepatic transaminase (in 15%), GI discomfort, edema, skin rash. Significant hepatotoxicity occurs in 1 of 15,000 patients. Watch for evidence of adrenal insufficiency (*see page 9*).

Rx Start with 200 mg PO BID. Adjust dosage based on 24-hr urine free cortisol and 17-hydroxycorticosteroid levels. Usual maintenance doses 400-1200 mg daily in divided doses (maximum of 1600 mg daily).

Aminoglutethimide (Cytadren®)[266]: inhibits the initial enzyme in the synthesis of steroids from cholesterol. Normalizes urinary free cortisol in ≈ 50% of cases. SIDE EFFECTS: dose-dependent reversible effects include sedation, anorexia, nausea, rash and hypothyroidism (due to interference with thyroid hormone synthesis).

Rx Start with 125-250 mg PO BID. Effectiveness may diminish after several months and dose escalation may be needed. Generally do not exceed 1000 mg/d.

Metyrapone (Metopirone®): inhibits 11-ß-hydroxylase (involved in one of the final steps of cortisol synthesis) may be used alone or in combination with other drugs. Normalizes mean daily plasma cortisol in ≈ 75%. SIDE EFFECTS: lethargy, dizziness, ataxia, N/V, primary adrenal insufficiency, hirsutism and acne.

Rx Usual dose range is 750-6000 mg/d usually divided TID with meals. Initial effectiveness may diminish with time.

Mitotane (Lysodren®): related to the insecticide DDT. Inhibits several steps in glucocorticoid synthesis, and is cytotoxic to adrenocortical cells (adrenolytic agent). 75% of patients enter remission after 6-12 months of treatment, and the medication may sometimes be discontinued (however hypercortisolism may recur). SIDE EFFECTS: may be limiting, and include anorexia, lethargy, dizziness, impaired cognition, GI distress, hypercholesterolemia, adrenal insufficiency (which may necessitate supernormal doses of glucocorticoids for replacement due to induced glucocorticoid degradation).

Rx Start with 250-500 mg PO q hs, and escalate dose slowly. Usual dose range is 4-12 gm/d usually divided TID-QID. Initial effectiveness may diminish with time.

Cyproheptadine (Periactin®): a serotonin receptor antagonist that corrects the abnormalities of Cushing's disease in a small minority of patients, suggesting that some cases of "pituitary" Cushing's disease are really due to a hypothalamic disorder. Combined therapy with bromocriptine may be more effective in some patients. SIDE EFFECTS: sedation & hyperphagia with weight gain usually limit usefulness.

Rx Usual dosage range: 8-36 mg/d divided TID.

Stereotactic radiosurgery
Often normalizes serum cortisol levels. Useful for recurrence after surgery, inaccessible tumors (a.g. cavernous sinus)[272].

Adrenalectomy
Bilateral total adrenalectomy is not tolerated as well as transsphenoidal surgery. It corrects the hypercortisolism (unless there is an extra-adrenal remnant), but lifelong gluco- and mineralo-corticoid replacement are required and up to 30% develop Nelson's syndrome (*see page 440*) (incidence may be reduced by pituitary XRT). May be indicated for continued hypercortisolism after transsphenoidal surgery.

THYROTROPIN (TSH)-SECRETING ADENOMAS
Most of these tumors are large, aggressive and invasive. Cure occurs in only ≈ 40% following surgery + XRT. Normal and neoplastic anterior hypophyseal thyrotroph cells possess somatostatin receptors and most respond to octreotide (*see below*). Occasionally, beta-blockers or low-dose antithyroid drugs (e.g. Tapazole® (methimazole) ≈ 5 mg PO TID for adults) may additionally be required.

Octreotide (Sandostatin®)
Doses required are usually < than with acromegaly. TSH levels decline by > 50% in 88% of patients, and become normal in ≈ 75%. T_4 and T_3 levels decrease in almost all, with 75% becoming normal. Tumor shrinkage occurs in ≈ 33%.

Rx Start with 50-100 µg SQ q 8 hrs. Titrate to TSH, T_4 and T_3 levels.

NONFUNCTIONAL ADENOMAS
Due to poor response rates, surgery and/or XRT are usually the initial treatment of choice (*see below* for XRT).

Non-secreting adenomas
Bromocriptine has been tried with mild reductions in tumor size in only ≈ 20% of patients. The poor results are probably due to the paucity of dopaminergic receptors on cell membranes in these tumors. Octreotide reduces tumor volume in ≈ 10% of cases.

Gonadotropin-secreting tumors
Some non-functional tumors may secrete gonadotropins (FSH, LH) which do not produce a clinical syndrome. Normal and neoplastic pituitary gonadotrophs have gonadotropin-releasing hormone (**GnRH**) receptors, and may respond to long-acting GnRH agonists (by down-regulating receptors) or GnRH antagonists, but significant reductions

in tumor size does not occur.

RADIATION THERAPY

Conventional XRT usually consists of 40-50 Gy administered over 4-6 weeks.

SIDE EFFECTS:: Radiation injury to the remaining normal pituitary results in hypocortisolism, hypogonadism, or hypothyroidism in 40-50% of patients after 10 years. It may also injure the optic nerve and chiasm (possibly causing blindness), cause lethargy, memory disturbances, cranial nerve palsies, and tumor necrosis with hemorrhage and apoplexy. Cure rates but also complications are higher after proton beam therapy.

Recommendation: Radiation therapy should not be routinely used following surgical removal. Follow patient with yearly MRI. Treat recurrence with repeat operation. Consider radiation if recurrence cannot be removed and mass continues to grow.

Nonfunctional tumors

In one series of 89 nonfunctioning pituitary tumors ranging 0.5-5 cm diameter (mean = 2 cm) not totally resected because of involvement of cavernous sinus (or other inaccessible sites), half were treated with radiation therapy **(XRT)**. The recurrence rate was neither lower (and was actually higher) nor later in the XRT group[229]. However, another series of 108 pituitary macroadenomas found the recurrence rates shown in *Table 17-39* which tend to favor radiation therapy.

When used, doses of 40 or 45 Gy in 20 or 25 fractions, respectively, is recommended[274]. The oncocytic variant of null cell pituitary tumors appears to be more radioresistant than the nononcocytic undifferentiated cell adenoma[274].

Table 17-39 Recurrence rate of pituitary tumors removed transsphenoidally*

Extent of removal	Post-op XRT?	Recurrence rate
subtotal	no	50%
gross total		21%
subtotal	yes	10%
gross total		0

*   108 macroadenomas, 6 mos to 14 years follow-up[273]

Acromegaly

Not the preferred treatment. In most patients, GH levels begin to fall during the first year after XRT, and decrease gradually thereafter, reaching ≤ 10 ng/ml in 70% of patients after 10 years. It takes up to 20 years for 90% of patients to achieve GH levels < 5 ng/ml. During this latency period, patients are exposed to unacceptably high levels of GH (octreotide may be used while waiting). Patients are also still at risk for radiation side effects mentioned above. Estimated cost: $20,000.

Cushing's disease

XRT corrects hypercortisolism in 20-40%, and produces some improvement in another 40%. Improvement may not be seen for 1-2 yrs post treatment.

SURGICAL TREATMENT

★ *INDICATIONS FOR SURGERY*
1. **prolactinomas** with
    A. prolactin level **(PRL)** < 500 ng/ml in tumors that are not extensively invasive: PRL may be normalized with surgery
    B. PRL > 500 and tumor not controlled medically (≈ 18% will not respond to bromocriptine)[A]. Response should be evident by 4-6 weeks. Surgery followed by reinstitution of medical therapy may normalize PRL
2. primary **Cushing's disease**: long-term efficacy of medical therapy is inadequate
3. **acromegaly**: surgery is recommended initial treatment for most (*see page 449*)
4. macroadenomas
    A. prolactinomas: if no acute progression, these tumors may shrink dramatically on bromocriptine
    B. non-PRL tumors causing symptoms by mass effect because of large size
    C. some surgeons recommend surgery for non-PRL macroadenomas that elevate the chiasm even in the absence of endocrine abnormalities or visual

---

A.   an initial attempt at purely medical control should be made as the chances of normalizing PRL surgically with pre-op levels > 500 ng/ml are very low[265]

field deficit because of the possibility of injury to the optic apparatus

    D. *see below* for <u>invasive</u> pituitary macroadenomas

5. acute and rapid visual or other neurologic deterioration. May represent ischemia of the chiasm, or hemorrhage or infarction of the tumor (<u>pituitary apoplexy</u>). The major danger is blindness (hypopituitarism can be treated with replacement therapy). Visual loss usually require <u>emergent</u> decompression. Some surgeons feel that a transcranial approach is necessary, but transsphenoidal decompression is usually satisfactory[242, 246]

6. to obtain tissue for pathological diagnosis in questionable cases

Recommended treatment for large, invasive adenomas[242]

1. prolactinomas
    A. dopamine agonists **(DA)** (*see page 448*) unless there is unstable deficit
    B. for unstable deficit, or if the tumor does not respond to DAs: debulk the tumor transsphenoidally and then rechallenge with DA therapy

2. tumors secreting growth hormone or ACTH: an aggressive surgical approach is indicated with these tumors since the secretion product is harmful and effective medical adjuvants are lacking
    A. all patients with GH-secreting tumors should have somatostatin analog therapy before any planned surgery to improve general and cardiac risks
    B. elderly patients or tumors > 4 cm diameter: debulk tumor transsphenoidally and/or adjuvant therapy (XRT and/or medications)
    C. young age and size < 4 cm: radical surgery (may be curative)

3. nonfunctional adenomas:
    A. elderly patient: expectant management is an option, with intervention for signs of progression (radiographic or neurologic)
    B. central tumor or elderly patient with progression: transsphenoidal debulking and/or XRT (residual tumor in the region of the cavernous sinus may show little or no change over several years, and with these nonfunctional tumors, there is less harm in following them than if there is a harmful secretion product)
    C. parasellar tumor and/or young age: radical surgery (often not curative)

SURGICAL APPROACHES

1. transsphenoidal: an extra-arachnoid approach, requires no brain retraction, no external scar (aside from where a fat graft is procured). Usually the procedure of choice. Indicated for microadenomas, macroadenomas without significant extension laterally beyond the confines of the sella, patients with CSF rhinorrhea, and tumors with extension into sphenoid air sinus
    A. sublabial
    B. trans-nares

2. transcthmoidal approach[275 (p 343-50)]

3. transcranial approaches:
    A. indications: most pituitary tumors are operated by the transsphenoidal technique (*see above*), even if there is significant suprasellar extension. However, a craniotomy may be indicated for the following[246]:
        1. minimal enlargement of the sella with a large suprasellar mass, especially if the diaphragm sellae is tightly constricting the tumor (producing a "cottage loaf" tumor) and the suprasellar component is causing chiasmal compression[276 (p 124)]
        2. extrasellar extension into the middle fossa with this mass being larger than the intrasellar mass
        3. unrelated pathology may complicate a transsphenoidal approach: rare, e.g. a parasellar aneurysm
        4. unusually fibrous tumor that could not be completely removed on a previous transsphenoidal approach
        5. recurrent tumor following a previous transsphenoidal resection
    B. choices of approach
        1. subfrontal: provides access to both optic nerves. May be more difficult in patients with prefixed chiasm
        2. frontotemporal (pterional): places optic nerve and sometimes carotid artery in line of vision of tumor. There is also incomplete access to intrasellar contents. Good access for tumors with significant lateral extrasellar extension
        3. subtemporal: usually not a viable choice. Poor visualization of optic

nerve/chiasm and carotid. Does not allow total removal of intrasellar component

TRANSSPHENOIDAL SURGERY

Surgery
For pre- and post-op orders, *see below*.

Possible post-op complications
1. hormonal imbalance (including hypopituitarism)
    A. alterations in ADH: transient abnormalities are common (*see page 455* for typical post-op patterns) including DI. DI lasting > 3 mos is uncommon
    B. cortisol deficiency → hypocortisolism → Addisonian crisis if severe
    C. TSH deficiency → hypothyroidism → (rarely) myxedema coma if severe
    D. deficiency of sex hormones → hypogonadotrophic hypogonadism
2. secondary empty sella syndrome (chiasm retracts into evacuated sella → visual impairment)
3. hydrocephalus with coma[277]: may follow removal of tumors with suprasellar extension (transsphenoidally or transcranially). Consider ventriculostomy placement if hydrocephalus is present (even if not symptomatic). Possible etiologies:
    A. traction on the attached 3rd ventricle
    B. cerebral edema due to vasopressin release from manipulation of the pituitary and/or stalk
    C. tumor edema following resection
4. infection
    A. pituitary abscess[278, 279]
    B. meningitis
5. CSF rhinorrhea (fistula): 3.5% incidence[273]
6. carotid artery rupture: rare. May occur intraoperatively or in delayed fashion after surgery, often ≈ day 10 post-op (due to breakdown of fibrin around carotid, or possibly due to rupture of a pseudoaneurysm created at surgery)
7. entry into cavernous sinus with possible injury of any structure within
8. nasal septal perforation

FRONTOTEMPORAL (PTERIONAL) APPROACH
A right sided approach is usually employed (less risk to dominant hemisphere). Exceptions: when the left eye is the side of worse vision; if there is predominant left sided tumor extension; if there is other pathology on the left (e.g. aneurysm).

PERI-OPERATIVE MANAGEMENT

Pre-op orders
1. Polysporin® ointment (PSO) applied in both nostrils the night before surgery
2. antibiotics, one of the following regimens may be used:
    - chloramphenicol 500 mg IVPB at 11 PM & 6 AM
    OR
    - chloramphenicol 500 mg PO at MN & IV at 6 AM; ampicillin 1 gm PO at MN & IV at 6 AM
    OR
    - Unasyn® 1.5 gm (1 gm ampicillin + 0.5 gm sulbactam) IVPB at MN & 6 AM
3. steroids, either:
    - hydrocortisone sodium succinate (Solu-Cortef®) 50 mg IM at 11 PM & 6 AM. On call to OR: hang 1 L D₅LR + 20 mEq KCl/l + 50 mg Solu-Cortef at 75 ml/hr
    OR
    - hydrocortisone 100 mg PO at MN & IV at 6 AM
4. intra-op: continue 100 mg hydrocortisone IV q 8 hrs

Post-op orders
1. intake & output (I's & O's) q 1 hr; urine specific gravity (**SG**) q 4° and anytime urine output (**UO**) > 250 ml/hr
2. activity: BR with HOB @ 30°.
3. ice chips PRN. To avoid aspirating fat graft from sphenoid sinus, patient is not to drink through a straw and incentive spirometry is not used
4. IVF: base IV D5 1/2 NS + 20 mEq KCl/L at appropriate rate (75-100 ml/hr) PLUS: replace UO > base IV rate ml for ml with 1/2 NS.

NB: if patient receives significant fluids intra-operatively, then they may have an appropriate post-op diuresis, in which case consider replacing only ≈ 2/3 of UO > base IV rate with 1/2 NS

5. meds
   A. antibiotics: continue chloramphenicol 500 mg IVPB q 6 hr (also continue ampicillin if used pre-op), change to PO when tolerated, D/C when nasal packing removed
   B. steroids (post-op steroids are required until the adequacy of endogenous steroids is established, especially with Cushing's disease, *see below*). Either:
      • hydrocortisone 50 mg IM/IV q 6 hrs, on POD #2 change to prednisone 5 mg PO q 6 hrs x 1 day, then 5 mg PO BID, D/C on POD #6
      OR
      • hydrocortisone 50 mg IM/IV/PO BID and taper 10 mg/dose/day
   C. diabetes insipidus (DI): *see below* for typical patterns.
      Criteria: U.O. > 250 ml/hr x 1-2 hrs, and SG < 1.005 (usually < 1.003).
      If DI develops, attempt to keep up with fluid loss with IVF (*see above*); if rate is too high for IV or PO replacement (> 300 cc/hr x 4 hrs or > 500 cc/hr x 2 hrs), check urine S.G. and if < 1.005 then give a vasopressin preparation (*see below*, or see *Table 1-9*, page 18). *Caution*: danger of overtreating in case of triphasic response (*see below*), therefore use EITHER:
      • 5 U aqueous vasopressin (Pitressin®) IVP/IM/SQ q 6 hrs PRN
      OR
      • desmopressin (DDAVP®) injection SQ/IV titrated to UO. Usual adult dose: 0.5-1 ml (2-4 µg) daily in 2 divided doses
      AVOID
      ✖ avoid tannate oil suspension, because of erratic absorption and it is a long acting preparation

      THEN: when nasal packs out, either
      • intranasal DDAVP (100 µg/ml): range 0.1-0.4 ml (10-40 µg) intranasally BID (typically 0.2 ml BID)
      OR
      • clofibrate (Atromid S®) 500 mg PO QID (does not always work)
6. labs: renal profile with osmolarity q 6 hrs
7. nasal packs: remove on post-op day 3-6

Urinary output: patterns of postoperative diabetes insipidus

Manage diabetes insipidus (DI) as described above. Post-op DI generally follows one of three patterns[280] (see *Diabetes insipidus*, page 16 for details):
1. transient DI: lasts until ≈ 12-36 hrs post-op
2. "prolonged" DI: lasts months, or may be permanent
3. "triphasic response" (least common). Summary:
   ① DI → ② normalization or SIADH-like picture → ③ DI (again)

Assessment for ACTH (corticotropin) reserve[250]

If patient was not hypocortisolemic pre-op, taper and stop hydrocortisone 24-48 hrs post-op. Then, check 6 AM serum cortisol level 24 hrs after discontinuing hydrocortisone and interpret the results as shown in *Table 17-40*. If there is any question about reserve, the patient can be discharged on hydrocortisone 50 mg PO q AM and 25 mg PO q PM until adrenal reserve can be assessed.

A **metyrapone** (Metopirone®) test may be useful in cases of suspected reduced pituitary ACTH production reserve. All patients should have a cosyntropin stimulation test first to rule-out primary adrenal insufficiency (*see page 444*); ✖ do not do this test if there is primary adrenal insufficiency. Metyrapone inhibits 11-ß-hydroxylation in the adrenal cortex, reducing production of cortisol and corticosterone with concomitant increase of serum 11-deoxycortisol precursors and its 17-OHCS metabolites which appear in the urine. In response, a normal pituitary increases ACTH production. Give 2-3 grams metyrapone PO at midnight; a normal response is a serum 11-deoxycortisol level > 7 µg/dl the next morn-

Table 17-40 Interpretation of 6 AM cortisol levels

6 AM cortisol	Interpretation	Management
≥ 9 µg/dl	normal	no further tests or treatment
3-9 µg/dl	possible ACTH deficiency	place patient on hydrocortisone*
≤ 3 µg/dl	ACTH deficient	

* perform cosyntropin stimulation test (*see page 444*) 1 month post-op; D/C steroids if normal; if subnormal, then permanent replacement required

ing. CAUTION: in patients with very little reserve, the reduced cortisol may provoke adrenal insufficiency (this test is safer than the higher doses used for urinary 17-OHCS testing), ✖ do not do this test as an outpatient.

Postoperative CT scan
A study of 12 patients with macroadenomas following transsphenoidal surgery without radiation therapy demonstrated that the maximal height of the pituitary "mass" did not return to normal immediately post-op (even with total tumor removal), rather a period of 3-4 months was required[281].

> Σ The timing of the initial post-op CT or MRI to act as a baseline to rule-out future recurrence after transsphenoidal surgery may be optimal at 3-4 months post-op.

OUTCOME

FOLLOWING TRANSSPHENOIDAL SURGERY
In cases with compression of the optic apparatus, there can be significant improvements in vision following surgery[273, 282].

Biochemical outcome:
1. endocrinologic cure was attained in 25% of prolactin-secreting tumors, and in 20% of growth hormone-secreting tumors[A] (see below)
2. gross total removal was unusual in tumors with > 2 cm suprasellar extension[A]
3. the incidence of recurrence was ≈ 12%, with most recurring 4-8 years post-op[A]
4. Cushing's disease: surgical cure rates are ≈ 85% for microadenomas (i.e. tumors ≤ 1 cm dia), but are lower for larger tumors

Acromegaly
The biochemical criteria for a cure of acromegaly is a normal basal (morning) serum growth hormone level of < 5 ng/ml, and normal suppression to < 2 ng/ml after ingesting 75 gm of glucose. Somatomedin-C (IGF-I) levels should also normalize.

Transsphenoidal surgery results in biochemical cure in 85% of cases with adenomas < 10 mm diameter, no evidence of local invasion, and random GH levels < 40 ng/ml pre-op. Overall, ≈ 50% of all acromegalics undergoing transsphenoidal surgery had a biochemical cure[283]. Only 30% of macroadenomas and very few with marked suprasellar extension have surgical cure. These tumors may also recur years later.

17.2.8. Craniopharyngioma

Craniopharyngiomas (CP) tend to arise from anterior superior margin of the pituitary, and are lined with stratified squamous epithelium. Some CP may arise primarily within the third ventricle[284]. Almost all CP have solid and cystic components; fluid in the cysts varies, but usually contains cholesterol crystals. CP do not undergo malignant degeneration; but difficulty in cure makes them malignant in behavior[206 (p 905-15)]. CP are distinct from Rathke's cleft cyst, but share some similarities (see below).
Calcification: microscopically 50%. Plain x-ray: 85% in childhood, 40% in adults.

EPIDEMIOLOGY
Incidence: 2.5-4% of all brain tumors; about 50% occur in childhood (9% of Matson's series). Peak incidence: age 5-10 yrs.

ANATOMY
Arterial supply: usually small feeders from ACA and A-comm, or from ICA and P-comm (do not receive blood from PCA or BA-bifurcation unless blood supply of floor of third ventricle is parasitized).

SURGICAL TREATMENT

Pre-op endocrinologic evaluation
As for pituitary tumor (see page 444). Hypoadrenalism may be corrected rapidly, but hypothyroidism takes longer; either condition can increase surgical mortality.

A. based on a series of 108 macroadenomas[273]

Approach

Post-op

Consider all of these patients hypo-adrenal, add hydrocortisone in physiologic doses (mineralocorticoid activity) in addition to anti-edema dexamethasone taper (*see page 8*). Taper steroids slowly to avoid aseptic (chemical) meningitis.

Diabetes insipidus (**DI**): often early, may develop into a "triphasic response" (see *Urinary output: patterns of postoperative diabetes insipidus*, page 455). Best managed initially with fluid replacement. If necessary, use short acting vasopressin (prevents iatrogenic renal shutdown if a SIADH-like phase develops during vasopressin therapy).

Outcome

5-10% mortality in most series, most from hypothalamic injury (unilateral hypothalamic lesions are rarely clinically evident; bilateral injuries may produce hyperthermia and somnolence; damage to anterior osmoreceptors may → loss of thirst sensation). Five year survival is ≈ 55-85% (range from 30-93% has been reported).

RADIATION

Controversial. SIDE EFFECTS: include endocrine dysfunction, optic neuritis, dementia. Post-op XRT probably helps prevent regrowth when residual tumor is left behind[285], however, in pediatric cases it may be best to postpone XRT (to minimize deleterious effect on IQ, *see page 535*), recognizing that reoperation may be necessary for recurrence.

RECURRENCE

Most recurrences occur in < 1 year, few > 3 yrs (very delayed recurrence usually occurs in what was thought to be "total" removal). Morbidity/mortality is higher with reoperation.

17.2.9.   Rathke's cleft cyst

Rathke's cleft cyst (**RCC**) are nonneoplastic lesions that are thought to be remnants of Rathke's pouch. They are primarily intrasellar, and are found incidentally in 13-23% of necropsies[286]. The adenohypophysis arises from proliferation of the anterior wall of Rathke's pouch, and so RCC have a similar lineage to pituitary adenomas and are rarely found together[287]. RCC are often discussed in contrast to craniopharyngiomas (**CP**) (*see above*). Some features are compared in *Table 17-41*.

Table 17-41   Comparison of craniopharyngioma to Rathke's cleft cyst

Feature	Craniopharyngioma	Rathke's cleft cyst
site of origin	anterior superior margin of pituitary	pars intermedia of pituitary
cell lining	stratified squamous epithelium	single layer cuboidal epithelium
cyst contents	cholesterol crystals	resembles motor oil
surgical treatment	total removal is the goal	partial excision and drainage[288]

RCC usually appear as low-density cystic lesions on CT. One half show capsular enhancement. MRI appearance is variable[288].

17.2.10.   Colloid cyst

❢ Key features
- slow-growing benign tumor comprising < 1% of intracranial tumors
- classically occurs in the anterior 3rd ventricle, blocking foramina of Monro causing obstructive hydrocephalus involving only the lateral ventricles
- natural history: risk of sudden death has been described, but is controversial

AKA neuroepithelial cysts. Comprise 2% of gliomas, and about 0.5-1% of all intracranial tumors[289]. Usual age of diagnosis: 20-50 yrs.

PATHOGENESIS

Origin: unknown. Implicated structures include: paraphysis (evagination in roof of third ventricle, rudimentary in humans), diencephalic ependyma in the recess of the postvelar arch, ventricular neuroepithelium.

Comprised of a fibrous epithelial-lined wall filled with either mucoid or dense hyloid substance. A slow growing, benign tumor.

Most commonly found in the third ventricle in the region of the foramina of Monro, but may be seen elsewhere, e.g. in septum pellucidum[290].

PRESENTATION

Symptoms are shown in *Table 17-42*. Signs are shown in *Table 17-43*, most commonly presents either with signs of intermittent acute intracranial hypertension (classically attributed to movement of the cyst on its pedicle causing episodic obstruction of the foramina of Monro, rarely born out at operation) or with chronic hydrocephalus (from chronic obstruction). Most clinically significant cysts are > 1.5 cm in diameter.

SUDDEN DEATH

A high rate of sudden death has been reported with colloid cysts (20% in pre-CT era[291]) but is probably overestimated. The obsolete theory was that these tumors are mobile and that as a result can shift position and acutely block CSF flow with resultant herniation. Progressive obstruction from tumor growth does often produce chronic hydrocephalus, and it is possible that at some point the brain may decompensate in some cases. Changes in CSF dynamics resulting from procedures (LP, ventriculography…) may have also contributed[292]. Another proposed mechanism is disturbance of hypothalamic-mediated cardiovascular reflex control[292].

Table 17-42 Symptoms of colloid cyst at presentation*

Symptom	No.	%
headache	26	68%
gait disturbance	18	47%
disturbed mentation	14	37%
vomiting (± nausea)	14	37%
blurred vision	9	24%
incontinence	5	13%
dizziness	5	13%
tinnitus	5	13%
seizures	4	10%
acute deterioration	4	10%
diplopia	3	8%
"drop attacks"	1	
diabetes insipidus	1	
asymptomatic	1	

* 38 patients, pre-CT era[289]

DIAGNOSIS

Imaging (MRI or CT) demonstrates the tumor usually located in the anterior 3rd ventricle. Here, it often blocks both foramina of Monro causing almost pathognomonic hydrocephalus involving only the lateral ventricles (sparing the 3rd and 4th).

MRI: usually the optimal imaging technique. However, there have been cases where cysts were isointense on MRI and CT was superior[293]. MRI clearly demonstrates the location of the cyst and relation to nearby structures. Usually obviates angiogram.

CT scan: Findings are variable: most cysts are hyperdense (however, iso- and hypo-dense colloid cysts occur), and about half enhance slightly. CT is usually not quite as good as MRI, especially with isodense cysts. These tumors calcify only rarely.

✖ **LP**: contraindicated prior to placement of shunt due to risk of herniation.

Table 17-43 Signs at presentation*

Sign	No.	%
papilledema	18	47%
gait disturbance	12	32%
normal exam	10	26%
hyperreflexia	9	24%
Babinski reflex	8	21%
incoordination	5	13%
nystagmus	5	13%
tremor	4	10%
hyporeflexia	3	8%
6th nerve palsy	2	5%

* 38 patients with colloid cysts, pre-CT era[289]

TREATMENT

Optimal treatment remains controversial. Initially, shunting without treating the cyst was advocated[294]. The nature of the obstruction (both foramina of Monro) requires bilateral ventricular shunts (or, unilateral shunt with fenestration of the septum pellucidum). Presently, one form or another of direct surgical treatment is usually recommended for some or all of the following reasons:

- to prevent shunt dependency
- to reduce the possibility of tumor progression
- since the mechanism of sudden neurologic deterioration may be due to factors such as cardiovascular

instability from hypothalamic compression and not due to hydrocephalus

Surgical management options (also see *Approaches to the third ventricle*, page 610):
1. transcallosal approaches: not dependent on dilated ventricles. Higher incidence of venous infarction or forniceal injury (*see below*)
2. transcortical approach: higher incidence of post-op seizures (≈ 5%). Not feasible with normal sized ventricles (e.g. in patient with VP shunt) *see page 611*
3. stereotactic drainage: *see below*
4. ventriculoscopic removal: *see below*

TRANSCALLOSAL APPROACH

Access to the 3rd ventricle via either the foramen of Monro or by interfornicial approach. Since colloid cysts tend to occur exactly at the foramen of Monro, it is <u>rarely</u> necessary to enlarge the foramen to locate the tumor. See *Transcallosal approach to lateral or third ventricle* on page 611.

STEREOTACTIC DRAINAGE OF COLLOID CYSTS

May be useful[295], especially in patients with normal ventricles from shunting, but the contents may be too viscous[296], and the tough capsule may make blind penetration difficult. Total or even subtotal aspiration may not require further treatment in some patients; however, recurrence rate is higher than with surgical removal[297].

Early morbidity was relatively high from this procedure possibly from vascular injury or mechanical trauma; this has improved. May be more feasible with intra-operative ventriculography[298] or with a ventriculoscope[299] (some say this is the initial procedure of choice[300], with craniotomy reserved for treatment failures).

Two features that correlate with <u>unsuccessful</u> stereotactic aspiration[301]:
1. high viscosity: correlates with hyperdensity on CT (low viscosity correlated with hypo- or iso-dense CT appearance; no MRI finding correlated with viscosity)
2. deflection of the cyst from tip of aspirating needle due to small size

Stereotactic technique[302]:
1. insertion point of stereotactic needle is just anterior to right coronal suture
2. start with sharp-tipped 1.8 mm probe, and advance to 3-5 mm beyond target site (to accommodate for displacement of cyst wall)
3. use a 10 ml syringe and apply 6-8 ml of negative aspiration pressure
4. if this does not yield any material, repeat with a 2.1 mm probe
5. although complete cyst evacuation is desirable, if this cannot be accomplished an acceptable goal of aspiration is re-establishment of patency of the ventricular pathways (may be verified by injecting 1-2 cc of iohexol)

17.2.11.   Hemangioblastoma

❦ Key features
• the most common primary intra-axial tumor in the adult posterior fossa
• may occur sporadically or as part of von Hippel-Lindau disease
• may be associated with erythrocytosis (polycythemia)

Hemangioblastomas[206 (p 772-82)] (**HGB**) are histologically benign tumors. Intracranially, they occur almost exclusively in the p-fossa (the most common <u>primary</u> intra-axial p-fossa tumor in adults). Less than 100 supratentorial cases have been reported. May also occur in spinal cord (1.5-2.5% of spinal cord tumors) - *see page 509*. Relationship and/or identity with angioblastic meningiomas is controversial. Also difficult to distinguish histologically from a hypernephroma.

HGB may occur sporadically, but 20% occur as part of von Hippel-Lindau disease (*see below*). Retinal HGB and/or angiomas occur in 6% of patients with cerebellar HGBs.

VON HIPPEL-LINDAU DISEASE

A rare (1 in 36,000 live births) autosomal dominant multisystem neoplastic disorder with ≈ 90% penetrance[303] characterized by a tendency to develop retinal angiomas, hemangioblastomas (**HGB**) of the brain and spinal cord, renal cell carcinoma, pheochromocytomas, and others[304] (retinal location being 2nd most common after cerebellar) (*see Table 17-44*). The variability of von Hippel-Lindau disease (**VHL**) has lead to the suggestion of the term **hemangioblasomatosis**.

Three suggested criteria[2] for the diagnosis of VHL*:
1. one or more HGB within CNS (typically a cerebellar HGB and a retinal HGB or angioma)
2. inconstant presence of visceral lesions (usually renal and/or pancreatic tumors or cysts)
3. frequent familial incidence

* classical VHL: #1 always, #2 usually, and #3 often; other combinations represent formes frustes

HEMANGIOBLASTOMAS (IN GENERAL)

EPIDEMIOLOGY

HGB represent 1-2.5% of intracranial tumors. Comprise 7-12% of primary p-fossa tumors[305]. ≈ 85% occur in the cerebellum, 3% in spinal cord, 2-3% in medulla, and 1.5% in cerebrum[305].

Sporadic cases tend to present in the 4th decade, whereas VHL cases present earlier (peak in 3rd decade).

PRESENTATION

S/S of cerebellar HGB are usually those of any p-fossa mass (H/A, N/V, cerebellar findings... see *Posterior fossa (infratentorial) tumors*, page 405). HGB is rarely documented as a cause of apoplexy due to intracerebral hemorrhage (ICH) (lobar or cerebellar), however, some studies indicate that if cases of ICH are carefully examined, abnormal vessels consistent with HGB (and occasionally misidentified as AVM) may be found with surprising frequency (in spite of negative CT and/or angiography)[306].

Retinal HGBs tend to be located peripherally, and may hemorrhage and cause retinal detachment. Erythrocytosis may be due to erythropoietin liberated by the tumor.

PATHOLOGY

No report of malignant change. May spread thru CSF after surgery, but remain benign. No true capsule, but usually well circumscribed (narrow zone of infiltration). May be solid, or cystic with a mural nodule (70% of cerebellar lesions are cystic; nodules are very vascular, appear red, are often located near pial surface, and may be as small as 2 mm; cyst fluid is clear yellow with high protein). In cystic lesions, cyst wall is lined with non-neoplastic compressed cerebellum.

Cardinal feature: numerous capillary channels, lined by a single layer of endothelium, surrounded by reticulin fibers. Macrophages stain PAS positive.

Three types of cells:
1. endothelial
2. pericytes: surrounded by basement membrane
3. stromal: polygonal. Foamy clear cytoplasm, often lipid laden. Origin controversial

Three types of HGB recognized[307]:
1. juvenile: thin walled capillaries & dilated vessels tightly packed
2. transitional: thin walled capillaries & dilated vessels intermingled with stromal cells, some of which are lipid laden (sudanophilic)
3. clear cell: neoplasm made up almost entirely of sheets of xanthoma cells with a rich vascular stroma

EVALUATION

CT: solid lesions usually isodense with intense contrast enhancement; cystic HGBs remain low density with contrast, with the nodule enhancing.

MRI: may be preferable to CT due to the tumor's predilection for the p-fossa. May

Table 17-44 Associations with von Hippel-Lindau disease*

Common lesions	Frequency in VHL
retinal angiomatosis	
hemangioblastomas	
cerebellar (solid or cystic)	
medullary	
spinal	
pancreatic and/or renal tumors or cysts	
renal cell Ca (unilateral or bilateral)	25%
polycythemia	9-20% of intracranial HGBs

Rare lesions (pertinent to nervous system)	Frequency in VHL
supratentorial hemangioblastoma	<100 case reports
syringomyelia	
cerebellar ependymoma	
sympathetic paraganglioma	
adrenal medullary pheochromocytoma (tends to be bilateral)	10%

* see reference[206] (p 779) for more

show serpentine signal voids, especially in the periphery of the lesion. Also, peripheral hemosiderin deposits may occur from previous hemorrhages[305].

Vertebral **angiography** usually demonstrates intense vascularity (most other tumors of the p-fossa are relatively avascular); may be required in HGBs where nodule is too small to be imaged on CT/MRI. 4 patterns: 1) vascular mural nodule on side of avascular cyst, 2) vascular lesion surrounding avascular cyst, 3) solid vascular mass, & 4) multiple, separate vascular nodules.

Labs: often discloses polycythemia (no hematopoietic foci within tumor). In cases with suggestive history, labwork to rule-out catecholamine production from pheochromocytoma may be indicated (see *Endocrine studies*, page 469).

TREATMENT

Surgery
Surgical treatment may be curative in cases of sporadic HGB.

Single p-fossa lesions: cystic lesions require removal of mural nodule (otherwise, cyst will recur). Removal of cyst wall is not necessary.

Solid HGBs tend to be more difficult to remove.

Multiple lesions: if ≥ 0.8-1 cm diameter, may treat as in solitary lesion. Smaller and deeper lesions may be difficult to locate.

Radiation treatment
Effectiveness is dubious. May be useful to reduce tumor size or to retard growth, e.g. in patients who are not surgical candidates, for multiple small deep lesions, or for inoperable brainstem HGB. Does not prevent regrowth following subtotal excision.

17.2.12. CNS lymphoma

❢ Key features
  - may be primary or secondary (pathologically identical)
  - suspected with homogeneously enhancing lesion(s) in the central gray matter or corpus callosum (on MRI or CT) especially in AIDS patients
  - may present with multiple cranial-nerve palsies
  - diagnosis highly likely if tumor seen in conjunction with uveitis
  - very responsive initially to steroids (may produce "ghost tumors")

CNS involvement with lymphoma may occur secondarily from a "systemic" lymphoma, or may arise primarily in the CNS. It is controversial whether most intracranial malignant lymphomas are primary[308] or secondary[309].

SECONDARY CNS LYMPHOMA
Non CNS lymphoma is the fifth most common cause of cancer deaths in the U.S., 63% of new cases are non-Hodgkin's. Secondary CNS involvement usually occurs late in the course. Metastatic spread of systemic lymphoma to the cerebral parenchyma occurs in 1-7% of cases at autopsy[310].

PRIMARY CNS LYMPHOMA
Older names include: reticulum cell sarcoma and microglioma[311].

A rare, malignant primary CNS neoplasm comprising 0.85-2% of all primary brain tumors and 0.2-2% of malignant lymphomas[312]. May occasionally metastasize outside the CNS.

EPIDEMIOLOGY
The incidence of primary CNS lymphoma **(PCNSL)** is rising relative to other brain lesions, and will likely exceed that of low-grade astrocytomas and approach meningiomas. This is in part due to the occurrence of PCNSL in AIDS and transplant patients, but the incidence has also increased in the general population over the past 20 years[313].

Male:female ratio = 1.5:1 (based on literature review[314]).

Median age at diagnosis: 52 yrs[314] (younger among immunocompromised patients: ≈ 34 yrs).

Most common supratentorial locations: frontal lobes, then deep nucleii; periventricular also common. Infratentorially: cerebellum is the most common location.

Conditions with increased risk of primary CNS lymphomas (PCNSL)
1. collagen vascular disease
   A. systemic lupus erythematosus
   B. Sjögren's syndrome: an autoimmune connective tissue disorder
   C. rheumatoid arthritis
2. immunosuppression
   A. chronic immunosuppression in transplantation patients[315]
   B. severe-congenital immunodeficiency syndrome ("SCIDS")
   C. AIDS[316, 317]: CNS lymphoma occurs in ≈ 10% of AIDS patients, and is the first presentation in 0.6%
   D. possibly increased incidence in the elderly due to reduced competency of immune system
3. Epstein-Barr virus[318] is associated with a broad spectrum of lymphoproliferative disorders, and is detectable in ≈ 30-50% of systemic lymphomas, however, it has been associated with almost 100% of PCNSL[319], especially AIDS-related cases[320]
   (p 317)

PRESENTATION
Presentation is similar with primary or secondary CNS lymphoma: the two most common manifestations are those due to epidural spinal cord compression and those of carcinomatous meningitis (multiple cranial nerve deficits, see *Carcinomatous meningitis*, page 491). Seizures occur in up to 30% of patients[308].

Symptoms
1. presents with non-focal non-specific symptoms in over 50% of patients; at time of presentation most commonly includes:
   A. mental status changes in one third
   B. symptoms of increased ICP (H/A, N/V)
   C. generalized seizures in 9%
2. focal symptoms in 30-42% of cases:
   A. hemimotor or hemisensory symptoms
   B. partial seizures
   C. multiple cranial-nerve palsies (due to carcinomatous meningitis)
3. combination of focal and non-focal symptoms

Signs
1. non-focal in 16%:
   A. papilledema
   B. encephalopathy
   C. dementia
2. focal findings in 45% of cases:
   A. hemimotor or hemisensory deficits
   B. aphasia
   C. visual field deficits
3. combination of focal and non-focal signs

Uncommon but characteristic syndromes
1. uveocyclitis, coincident with (in 6% of cases) or preceding the diagnosis of (in 11% of cases) lymphoma
2. subacute encephalitis with subependymal infiltration
3. MS-like illness with steroid-induced remission

PATHOLOGY
Characteristic sites: corpus callosum, basal ganglia, periventricular.
The neoplastic cells are identical to those of systemic lymphomas. Most are bulky tumors that are contiguous with the ventricles or meninges.
Histologic distinguishing features: tumor cells for cuffs around blood vessels which demonstrate multiplication of basement membranes (best demonstrated with silver reticulum stain).
Frozen section distorts the cells and may lead to a misdiagnosis of malignant glioma[320 (p 320)].
Immunohistochemical stains differentiates B-cell lymphomas from T-cell lymphomas (B-cell types are more common, especially in PCNSL and in AIDS).
EM shows absence of junctional complexes (desmosomes) that are usually present in epithelial derived tumors.

Intravascular lymphomatosis[321]: Formerly: (malignant) angioendothelomatosis. A rare lymphoma with no solid mass in which malignant lymphoid cells are found in the lumen of small blood vessels in affected organs. CNS involvement is reported in most cases. Presentation is non specific: patients are often febrile, and may present with progressive multifocal cerebrovascular events (including stroke or hemorrhage), spinal cord or nerve root symptoms (including cauda equina syndrome, *see page 305*), encephalopathy or peripheral or cranial neuropathies[322]. Initial transient cerebral symptoms may mimic TIAs or seizures. The ESR is often elevated prior to initiation of steroids. Lymphoma cells may be seen in the CSF.

Painful skin nodules or plaques occur in ≈ 10% of cases, generally involving the abdomen or lower extremities, and these cases may be diagnosed with skin biopsy. Otherwise, diagnosis often requires brain biopsy (open or stereotactic), in which involved areas on imaging studies are targeted. Treatment with combination chemotherapy can result in long-term remission in some patients, but early diagnosis before permanent damage occurs is critical (diagnosis is rarely made pre-mortem).

DIAGNOSIS

On imaging (CT or MRI) 50-60% occur in one or more cerebral lobes (in grey or white matter). 25% occur in deep midline structures (septum pellucidum, basal ganglion, corpus callosum). 25% are infratentorial. 10-30% of patients have multiple lesions at the time of presentation. In contrast, systemic lymphomas that spread to the CNS tend to present with leptomeningeal involvement instead of parenchymal tumors[323].

CT: Non-AIDS-related cases tend to enhance homogeneously, whereas AIDS-related cases often have a necrotic center and appear as <u>multifocal ring-enhancing</u> lesions[324] (the wall is thicker than with an abscess).

Non-AIDS related cases: CNS lymphomas should be suspected with homogeneously enhancing lesion(s) in the central gray or corpus callosum. 75% are in contact with ependymal or meningeal surfaces (this together with dense enhancement may produce a **"pseudomeningioma pattern"**, however lymphomas lack calcifications and tend to be multiple).

60% are hyperdense to brain, only 10% are hypodense. Characteristically, > 90% of these tumors enhance; this is densely homogeneous in over 70%. As a result, when rare non-enhancing cases occur it often leads to a delay in diagnosis[325]. The appearance of enhanced PCNSL on CT has been likened to "fluffy cotton balls". There may be surrounding edema[326] and there is usually mass effect.

There is an almost diagnostic tendency of rapid partial to complete resolution on CT (and even at the time of surgery) following the administration of steroids, earning the nickname of **"ghost-cell tumor"**[327, 328] or disappearing tumor.

MRI: No pathognomonic feature. May be difficult to discern if tumor is located subependymally (signal characteristics similar to CSF); proton-weighted image may avoid this pitfall.

CSF: Should only be obtained if no mass effect. Usually abnormal, but non-specific. Most common abnormalities are elevated protein (in > 80%), and increased cell count (in 40%). Cytology is positive for lymphoma cells (pre-operatively) in only 10% (sensitivity may be higher with leptomeningeal involvement as in non-AIDS patients than with parenchymal involvement commonly seen in AIDS). Repeating up to 3 LPs may increase yield.

Angiography: Rarely helpful. 60% of cases show only an avascular mass. 30-40% show diffuse homogeneous staining or blush.

EVALUATION

All patients should be assessed (history, physical, and if appropriate, laboratory tests) for any of the conditions associated with lymphoma (*see page 462*). Since primary CNS lymphoma is very rare, any patient with CNS lymphoma should have workup for occult systemic lymphoma including:
1. careful physical exam of all lymph nodes (**LN**)
2. evaluation of perihilar and pelvic LN (CXR, CT of chest & abdomen)
3. routine blood and urine testing
4. bone marrow biopsy
5. testicular ultrasound in males
6. ophthalmologic examination (including slit-lamp evaluation of both eyes) in all
   A. for possible uveitis
   B. ≈ 28% of patients with PCNSL will also have intraocular lymphoma

TREATMENT

Surgery
Surgical decompression with partial or gross total removal does not alter patient's prognosis. The main role for surgery is for tumor biopsy, and stereotactic techniques are often well-suited for these often deep tumors[329].

Radiation therapy
The standard treatment after tissue biopsy is whole-brain radiation therapy. Doses used tend to be lower than for other primary brain tumors. ≈ 40-50 Gy total are usually given in 1.8-3 Gy daily fractions.

Chemotherapy
In non-AIDS cases, chemotherapy combined with XRT prolongs survival compared to XRT alone[330]. The addition of intraventricular (rather than just intrathecal via LP) methotrexate (**MTX**) delivered through a ventricular access device (6 doses of 12 mg twice a week, with IV leucovorin rescue) may result in even better survival[331]. In the event of an intrathecal MTX overdose (**OD**), interventions recommended[332]: ODs of up to 85 mg can be well tolerated with little sequelae; immediate LP with drainage of CSF can remove a substantial portion of the drug (removing 15 ml of CSF can eliminate ≈ 20-30% of the MTX within 2 hrs of OD). This can be followed by ventriculolumbar perfusion over several hours using 240 ml of warmed isotonic preservative-free saline entering through the ventricular reservoir and exiting through a lumbar subarachnoid catheter. For major OD of > 500 mg, add intrathecal administration of 2,000 U of carboxypeptidase G_2 (an enzyme that inactivates MTX). In cases of MTX OD, systemic toxicity should be prevented by treating with IV dexamethasone and IV (not IT) leucovorin.

PROGNOSIS
With no treatment, median survival is 1.8-3.3 months following diagnosis.
With radiation therapy[308], median survival is 10 months, with 47% 1-year median survival, and 16% 2-year median survival. 3-year survival is 8%, and 5-year survival is 3-4%. With intraventricular MTX, median time to recurrence was 41 mos[331]. Occasionally, prolonged survival may be seen[333].
About 78% of cases recur, usually ≈ 15 months after treatment (late recurrences also are seen). Of these recurrences, 93% are confined to the CNS (often at another site if the original site responded well), and 7% are elsewhere.
In AIDS-related cases, the prognosis appears worse. Although complete remission occurs in 20-50% following XRT, the median survival is only 3-5 months[334, 335], usually related to AIDS-related opportunistic infection. However, neurologic function and quality of life improve in ≈ 75%[334].

Although there are individual studies that show trends, there are no prognostic features that consistently correlate with survival.

17.2.13. Chordoma

⁑ Key features
- primary malignant tumor of the spine or clivus with high recurrence rate
- characteristic physaliphorous cells (containing intracellular mucin)
- generally slow-growing and radioresistant
- treatment of choice: wide en bloc resection, proton-beam radiation may help

Rare tumors (incidence of ≈ 0.51 cases/million) of the remnant of the primitive notochord (which normally differentiates into the nucleus pulposus of the intervertebral disks). Can arise anywhere along the neuraxis where there is remnant of notochord, however, cases tend to cluster at the two ends of the primitive notochord: 35% cranially[336] in the spheno-occipital region (clivus), and 53%[336] in the spine at the sacrococcygeal region[337]. Less commonly, they may occur in the spine above the sacrum[338]. The metastatic rate is low (5-20%)[339], but there is a high recurrence rate of 85% following surgery, and therefore aggressive RTX is usually employed post-op.

PATHOLOGY
Histologically, these tumors are considered low-grade malignancies. However, their behavior is more malignant because of the difficulty of total removal, a high recurrence rate, and the fact that they can metastasize (usually late). They are slow growing, locally

aggressive and osseodestructive. Metastases occur in about 10% of sacral tumors, usually late and after multiple resections, and most often to lung, liver and bone. Malignant transformation into fibrosarcoma or malignant fibrous histiocytoma is rare. **Physaliphorous cells** are distinctive, vacuolated cells on histology that probably represent cytoplasmic mucus vacuoles seen ultrastructurally.

RADIOGRAPHIC APPEARANCE
Usually lytic with frequent calcifications[340]. Enhances on CT with contrast[340]. Rarely, may appear as a sclerotic vertebra[341] ("ivory vertebra").

CRANIAL CHORDOMAS
Peak incidence of cranial chordomas is 50-60 years of age. These tumors are rare in patients < 30 years of age[342]. Male:female distribution is ≈ equal.

Differential diagnosis: Primarily between other cartilaginous tumors of the skull base (for differential diagnosis of other foramen magnum region tumors, *see page 924*):
1. chondrosarcomas
2. chondromas

Presentation: Usually produces cranial nerve palsies (usually oculomotor or abducens).

SACRAL CHORDOMAS
Unlike cranial chordomas, there is a male predominance[336], and these patients tend to be older. Chordomas constitute over 50% of primary bone tumors of the sacrum. May produce pain, sphincter disturbance or nerve root symptoms from local nerve root compression. It may occasionally extend cephalad into the lumbar spinal canal. It is usually confined anteriorly by the presacral fascia, and only rarely invades the wall of the rectum[343]. A firm fixed mass may be palpable between the rectum and the sacrum on rectal exam.

Evaluation
Characteristic radiographic findings: centrally located destruction of several sacral segments, with an anterior soft-tissue mass that occasionally has small calcifications. CT and MRI show the bony destruction. This is usually difficult to see on plain x-rays. MRI also shows the soft-tissue mass.

An open or CT guided percutaneous posterior biopsy can confirm the diagnosis. Transrectal biopsy should be avoided because of the potential of rectal spread[344].

Chest CT and bone scan: to R/O mets for staging purposes.

Treatment
Wide en-bloc excision with postoperative radiation is usually the best option, although this may also be only temporarily effective. Decompression is best avoided since entering the mass serves to spread tumor. Early radiation was associated with longer survival[345]. Proton radiation may offer better results than conventional XRT (*see below*).

Adverse effects of sacrectomy: If S2 nerve roots are the most caudal nerve roots spared, there is ≈ 50% chance of normal bladder and bowel control[346]. If S1 or more cephalic roots are the most caudad nerve roots spared, most will have impaired bladder control and bowel problems[346].

RADIATION THERAPY (XRT)
Best results were obtained with en bloc excision (even if marginal), sometimes combined with high-dose XRT[338, 347] (conventional XRT did not prevent recurrence when incorporated with palliative or debulking surgery[338]), but it did lengthen the interval to recurrence[347]). Higher XRT doses can be used in the sacrococcygeal region (4500-8000 rads) than in the cervical spine (4500-5500 rads) because of concerns of radiation injury to the spinal cord.

Proton beam therapy, alone[339] or combined with high-energy x-ray (photon) therapy[348, 349] may be more effective than conventional XRT alone. However, proton beam therapy requires travel to one of a very limited number of facilities with a cyclotron (in the U.S.: Boston, or Loma Linda, California) which may be difficult to arrange for what is typically ≈ 7 weeks of fractionated treatments.

17.2.14.   Ganglioglioma

❢ Key features:
- composed of two cell types: ganglion cells (neurons) and glial cells
- extremely rare (< 2% of intracranial neoplasms)
- seen primarily in the first 3 decades of life
- characterized by slow growth and a tendency to calcify

A tumor composed of two types of cells: ganglion cells (neurons) which may arise from primitive neuroblasts, and glial cells, usually astrocytic in any phase of differentiation[350].

EPIDEMIOLOGY

Location: May occur in various parts of the nervous system (cerebral hemispheres, spinal cord, brainstem, cerebellum, pineal region, thalamus, intrasellar, optic nerve, and peripheral nerve have been reported[351]). Most occur above the tentorium, primarily in or near the 3rd ventricle, in the hypothalamus or in the temporal or frontal lobes[107]. Brainstem gangliogliomas occur rarely (*see page 421*).

Incidence: Typically quoted[351] as 0.3-0.6%. One series[352] found gangliogliomas in 1.3% of all brain tumors (including mets), or 3% of *primary* brain tumors. Considering only children and young adults, incidence ranges from 1.2-7.6% of brain tumors[351].

Demographics: Occurs primarily in children and young adults (peak age of occurrence: 11 yrs).

PRESENTATION

Most common presenting symptom was seizure, or a change in a pre-existing seizure pattern. Often, the seizures are difficult to control medically.

RADIOLOGIC EVALUATION

Neuroradiologic findings are not specific for this tumor.

Plain skull x-ray: calcification was noted in 2 of 6 patients[351].

CT: all of 10 patients had a low density lesion on non-contrast CT; 8 enhanced slightly with contrast; 5 of the 10 had calcification on CT[352]. 6 of the 10 were in temporal lobe (this predilection has been noted in many but not all series), and 4 were in frontal lobe. Frequently appears cystic on CT, but still may be found to be solid at operation. Mass effect rare (suggests slow growth).

MRI: high signal on T1WI, low signal on T2WI. Calcifications appear as low signal on both[351].

Angiography: shows either an avascular or a minimally vascular mass.

PATHOLOGY

Mixture of 2 types of neoplastic cells: neuronal (ganglion) and astrocytic (glial). Very slow growing.

Two major classifications: **ganglioneuromas** (less common, more benign; predominance of neuronal component) and **gangliogliomas** (preponderance of glial cells).

Grossly: white matter mass; well-circumscribed, firm, with occasional cystic areas and calcified regions. Most dissect easily from brain, but the solid portion may show an infiltrative tendency[351].

Microscopically: ganglion cells must demonstrate nerve cell differentiation, e.g. Nissl substance and axons or dendrites. Pitfall: differentiating neoplastic neurons from neurons entrapped by an invading astrocytoma may be difficult. Also, neoplastic astrocytes may resemble neurons on light microscopy. 2 of 10 patients had areas of oligodendroglioma. One series found necrotic areas in 7 of 14 patients, minimal calcification, and Rosenthal bodies[353]. Suggested criteria for diagnosis[354]:
1. clusters of large cells potentially representing neurons (required for diagnosis)
2. no perineural clustering of glial cells around the suspected neoplastic neurons
3. fibrosis (desmoplasia)
4. calcification

Aggressive malignant changes in the glial component may dictate a poor outcome, although an "aggressive" background is not unusual and may not indicate malignancy.

TREATMENT

Recommendation is wide radical excision when possible (may be more limited in spinal cord and brainstem tumors). Close follow-up is recommended, and re-resection should be considered for recurrence. The role of XRT is unknown, and due to the deleterious effects together with the good long-term prognosis, it is not recommended initially but may be considered for recurrence[355].

PROGNOSIS

Russell and Rubenstein[356] first proposed that the grade of the astrocytic component of the tumor determines the prognosis. This has been supported by some case reports, but clinical series have not been able to correlate histology with outcome[355]. Thus, anaplasia is not significantly associated with a worse prognosis[355].

The majority of patients did well and were asymptomatic after resection. 1 patient in a series of 10 died 3 days post-op from cerebral edema.

In 58 patients, 5-year survival was 89% and 10-year survival was 84%[355]. In 9 brainstem gangliogliomas, 5-year survival was 78%.

The value of radiation therapy is not known. Consider radiation when growth is evident on follow-up CT, or when infiltration is felt to occur at time of surgery.

1 patient had degeneration to glioblastoma when a recurrence was discovered 5 years after removal (this patient received radiation therapy).

The prognosis with following subtotal resection of brainstem gangliogliomas is better than for brainstem gliomas as a group[107].

17.2.15.   Paraganglioma

AKA **chemodectoma**, AKA **glomus tumors**. *Table 17-45* shows the designation of these tumors in various sites.

These tumors arise from paraganglion cells (not chemoreceptor cells as previously thought, therefore the term *chemodectoma* is losing favor). Slow growing tumors (< 2 cm in 5 years). Histologically benign (< 10% associated

Table 17-45   Designation based on site of origin

Site	Designation
carotid bifurcation	carotid body tumors
superior vagal ganglion	glomus jugulare tumors
auricular branch of vagus	glomus tympanicum
inferior vagal (nodose) ganglion	glomus intravagale
adrenal medulla & sympathetic chain	pheochromocytoma

with lymph node involvement or distant spread). Most contain secretory granules on EM (mostly epinephrine & nor-epinephrine, and these tumors may occasionally secrete catecholamines). These tumors are not uncommonly multiple (metachronous).

CAROTID BODY TUMORS

Possibly the most common paraganglioma (pheochromocytoma may be more common). Approximately 5% are bilateral; the incidence of bilaterality increases to 26% in familial cases (these are probably autosomal dominant).

CLINICAL

Usually present as painless, slow growing mass in upper neck. Large tumors may → cranial nerve involvement (especially vagus and hypoglossal). May also cause stenosis of ICA → TIAs or stroke.

EVALUATION

1.   carotid angiogram: demonstrates predominant blood supply (usually external carotid, with possible contributions from vertebral and thyrocervical trunk). May also detect bilateral lesions. Characteristic finding: splaying of bifurcation
2.   MRI (or CT): evaluates extent, and assesses for intracranial extension

---

TREATMENT

Resection reported to carry a high complication rate, including stroke (8-20%) and cranial nerve injury (33-44%). Mortality rate is 5-13%.

GLOMUS JUGULARE TUMORS

Some authors consider glomus tumors as a category that may be subdivided into *glomus jugulare* and *glomus tympanicum* tumors. Glomus tumors are rare (0.6% of all head and neck tumors), yet the glomus tympanicum is the most common neoplasm of the middle ear. Glomus jugulare tumors **(GJT)** arise from glomus bodies, usually in the area of the jugular bulb, and track along vessels. May have finger-like extension into the jugular vein (which may embolize during resection)[357].

A very vascular tumor with main feeders from the external carotid (especially inferior tympanic branch of ascending pharyngeal artery, and branches of posterior auricular, occipital, and internal maxillary), with additional feeders from petrous portion of the ICA. Most are slow growing, although rapidly growing tumors do occur.

CLINICAL

Epidemiology

Female:male ratio is 6:1. Bilateral occurrence is almost nonexistent.

Symptoms

Patients commonly present with hearing loss and pulsatile tinnitus. Dizziness is the third most common symptoms. Ear pain may also occur.

Signs

Hearing loss may be conductive (e.g. due to obstruction of the ear canal) or sensorineural due to invasion of the labyrinth often with accompanying vertigo (the eighth nerve is the most common cranial nerve involved). Various combinations of palsies of cranial nerves IX, X, XI & XII occur (see *Jugular foramen syndromes*, page 86) with occasional VII palsy (usually from involvement within the temporal bone). Ataxia and/or hydrocephalus can occur with massive lesions that cause brainstem compression. Occasionally patients may present with symptoms due to secretory products (*see below*).

Otoscopic exam → pulsatile reddish-blue mass behind eardrum (occasionally, lamentably biopsied by ENT physician with possible ensuing massive blood loss).

PATHOLOGY

Histologically indistinguishable from carotid body tumors. May invade locally, both through temporal bone destruction and especially along pre-existing pathways (along vessels, eustachian tube, jugular vein, carotid artery). Intradural extension is rare. Malignancy may occur, but is rare. These tumors rarely metastasize.

Secretory properties

These tumors usually possess secretory granules (even the functionally inactive tumors) and may actively secrete catecholamines (similar to pheochromocytomas, occurs in only 1-4% of GJT[358]). Norepinephrine will be elevated in functionally active tumors since glomus tumors lack the methyltransferase needed to convert this to epinephrine. Alternatively, serotonin and kallikrein may be released, and may produce a carcinoid-like syndrome (bronchoconstriction, abdominal pain and explosive diarrhea, violent H/A, cutaneous flushing, hypertension, hepatomegaly and hyperglycemia)[359]. During surgical manipulation, these tumors may also release histamine and bradykinin, causing hypotension and bronchoconstriction[360].

DIFFERENTIAL DIAGNOSIS

See *Cerebellopontine angle (CPA) lesions* on page 922. The major differential is neurilemmomas (acoustic neuromas), both of which enhance on CT. A cystic component and extrinsic compression of the jugular bulb are characteristic of neurilemmomas. Angiography will differentiate difficult cases.

EVALUATION

Neurophysiologic testing
Audiometric and vestibular testing should be performed.

Imaging
1. CT or MRI used to delineate location and extent of tumor; CT is better for assessing bony involvement of the skull base
2. angiography: confirms diagnosis (helping to rule out acoustic neuroma), and ascertains patency of contralateral jugular vein in event that jugular on side of tumor must be sacrificed; jugular bulb and/or vein are usually partially or completely occluded

Endocrine studies
24 hr urine collection for: vanillylmandelic acid **(VMA),** metanephrines, and total catecholamines should be performed to assess for catecholamine secretion. In cases where elevation is found, a clonidine suppression test can be done (there will be a reduction in essential hypertension, but no change with pheochromocytoma or other tumor production).

CLASSIFICATION
A number of classification schemes have been proposed. The modified Jackson classification is shown in *Table 17-46.*

Table 17-46   Modified Jackson classification[361]

Type	Description	Intracranial extension
I	small; involves jugular bulb, middle ear & mastoid	none
II	extends under IAC	possible
III	extends into petrous apex	possible
IV	extends beyond petrous apex into clivus or infratemporal fossa	possible

TREATMENT
Surgical resection is usually simple and effective for small tumors confined to the middle ear. For larger tumors that invade and destroy bone, the relative role of surgery and/or radiation is not fully determined. With large tumors, surgery carries the risk of significant cranial nerve palsies.

MEDICAL
For tumors that actively secrete catecholamines, medical therapy is useful for palliation or as adjunctive treatment before embolization or surgery. Alpha and beta blockers given before embolization or surgery blocks possibly lethal blood pressure lability and arrhythmias. Adequate blockade takes ≈ 2-3 weeks of alpha blocker and at least 24 hours of beta blocker therapy; in emergency, 3 days of treatment may suffice.

Alpha blockers
Reduce BP by preventing peripheral vasoconstriction.
- **phenoxybenzamine** (Dibenzyline®): long acting; peak effect 1-2 hrs. Start with 10 mg PO BID and gradually increase to 40-100 mg per day divided BID
- **phentolamine** (Regitine®): short acting. Usually used IV for hypertensive crisis during surgery or embolization.
  Rx: 5 mg IV/IM (peds: 1 mg) 1-2 hrs pre-op, repeat PRN before and during surgery

Beta blockers
Reduces catecholamine induced tachycardia and arrhythmias (may also prevent hypotension that might occur if only alpha blockade is used). These drugs are not always needed, but when used ✖ NB: these drugs must not be started before starting alphablockers (to prevent hypertensive crisis and myocardial ischemia).
- **propranolol** (Inderal®): *Rx*: oral dose is 5-10 mg q 6 hrs. IV dose for use during surgery is 0.5-2 mg slow IVP
- **labetalol** (Normodyne®): may have some efficacy in blocking α_1 selective and ß non-selective (potency < propranolol), see *Hypotension (shock),* page 6

Serotonin, bradykinin, histamine release blockers
These agents may provoke bronchoconstriction that does not respond to steroids, but may respond to inhaled ß-agonists or inhaled anticholinergics. Somatostatin may be used to inhibit release of serotonin, bradykinin, or histamines. Since this drug has a

short half-life, it is preferable to give octreotide 100 μg sub-Q q 8 hrs (see page 450).

(see page 450)

RADIATION THERAPY
XRT may relieve symptoms and stop growth in spite of persistence of tumor mass. 40-45 Gy in fractions of 2 Gy has been recommended[362]. Lower doses of ≈ 35 Gy in 15 fractions of 2.35 Gy appear as effective and have fewer side effects[363]. Generally used as primary treatment only for large tumors or in patients too elderly or infirmed to undergo surgery. Some surgeons pretreat 4-6 mos pre-operatively with XRT to decrease vascularity[364] (controversial).

EMBOLIZATION
- generally reserved for large tumors with favorable blood supply (i.e. vessels that can be selectively embolized with no danger of particles passing thru to normal brain)
- post-embolization tumor swelling may compress brainstem or cerebellum
- may be used preoperatively to reduce vascularity. Performed 24-48 hours pre-op (not used prior to that, because of post-embolization edema)
- caution with actively secreting tumors which may release vasoactive substances (e.g. epinephrine) upon infarction from the embolization
- may also be used as primary treatment (± radiation) in patients who are not surgical candidates. In this case, is only palliative, as tumor will develop new blood supply
- absorbable (Gelfoam®) and non-absorbable (Ivalon®) materials have been used

SURGICAL TREATMENT
The tumor is primarily extradural, with extremely vascular surrounding dura.

Suboccipital approach may cause dangerous bleeding and usually results in incomplete resection. Team approach by a neurosurgeon in conjunction with a neuro-otologist and possibly head and neck surgeon has been advocated[275]. This approach utilizes an approach to the skull base through the neck.

ECA feeders are ligated early, followed rapidly by draining veins (to prevent systemic release of catecholamines).

Sacrifice of the jugular vein (**JV**) is tolerated if the contralateral JV is patent (often, the ipsilateral JV will already be occluded).

Complications and outcome
The most common complications are CSF fistula, facial nerve palsy, and varying degrees of dysphagia (from dysfunction of lower cranial nerves). Dysfunction of any of the cranial nerves VII thru XII can occur, and a tracheostomy should be performed if there is any doubt of lower nerve function, and a gastrostomy feeding tube may be needed temporarily or permanently. Lower cranial nerve dysfunction also predisposes to aspiration, the risk of which is also increased by impaired gastric emptying and ileus that may occur due to reduced cholecystokinin (**CCK**) levels post-op. Excessive blood loss can also occur.

Even after gross total tumor removal, recurrence rate may be as high as 33%[364, 365].

17.2.16. Ependymoma

Ependymomas arise from ependymal cells lining the cerebral ventricles and the central canal of the spinal cord. They may occur anywhere along the neuraxis.

Epidemiology:
- intracranial: comprises only ≈ 5-6% of intracranial gliomas, 69% occur in children[366], comprise 9% of pediatric brain tumors[367]
- spinal: ≈ 60% of spinal cord gliomas, 96% occur in adults[366], especially those of filum terminale (see *myxopapillary ependymoma* below)

The mean age at diagnosis is shown in *Table 17-47*.

Ependymomas have the potential to spread through the CSF through the

Table 17-47 Mean age at diagnosis[366]

Location (in 101 patients)	All patients (yrs)	Children (yrs) (age < 15 yrs)
intracranial	17.5	5
infratentorial	14.5	4.5
supratentorial	22	6.5
intraspinal	40	
intramedullary	47	
cauda region	32	

neuraxis, a process known as "seeding", resulting in so-called "drop mets" in 11%. The incidence is higher with higher grade[367]. Systemic spread occurs on rare occasion.

PATHOLOGY

World Health Organization **(WHO)** classification (for variants, *see page 402*):
1. non-anaplastic (low-grade)
   A. papillary: "classic lesion" occurring in brain or spinal cord. Can metastasize (up to 30%). Dark, small nuclei. 2 cytoplasmic patterns:
      1. differentiation along glial line: forms perivascular pseudorosettes (*see page 472*)
      2. cuboidal cells form ependymal tubules around a central blood vessel (true rosettes)
   B. **myxopapillary ependymoma**: distinctive, occurs only in filum terminale. Papillary, with microcystic vacuoles and mucosubstance (*see page 508*)
   C. subependymoma
2. anaplastic: pleomorphism, multinucleation, giant cells, mitotic figures, vascular changes and areas of necrosis (the term **ependymoblastoma** has occasionally been used for more anaplastic lesions, but this term is best reserved for a distinct, rare childhood primitive neuroectodermal tumor, *see page 474*). It is unclear if the degree of anaplasia has any effect on outcome

INTRACRANIAL EPENDYMOMAS

❡ Key features
- benign tumors, often fibrillary with epithelial appearance. Perivascular pseudorosettes may occur
- usually occur in the floor of the 4th ventricle
- potential for seeding through the neuraxis
- worse prognosis the younger the patient
- treatment: maximal resection followed by XRT

Usually well circumscribed and benign (although malignant ependymomas do occur), commonly arises in the floor of the fourth ventricle (60-70% are infratentorial, all of these occur near 4th ventricle[366], they comprise 25% of tumors in region of 4th ventricle[368] (p 2792)). Children with p-fossa ependymomas often have anaplastic tumors with a higher risk of spread through the neuraxis. Supratentorial ependymomas are often cystic. Rarely occur outside the CNS in: mediastinum, lung or ovaries. Although not as malignant histologically as medulloblastomas, ependymomas have a worse prognosis due to their propensity to invade the obex which precludes complete removal.

Subependymomas: typically occur in anterior lateral ventricles or posterior fourth ventricle, with prominent role of subependymal glial cells. Not uncommon at autopsy, rarely surgical.

CLINICAL

Symptoms

Mostly those of posterior fossa mass with increased ICP[368] (p 2795):
1. headache: 80%
2. N/V: 75%
3. ataxia or vertigo: 60%
4. seizures: only in ≈ 30% of supratentorial lesions; comprise only 1% of patients with intracranial tumors presenting with seizures

EVALUATION

CT/MRI: usually presents as a mass in the floor of fourth ventricle, often with obstructive hydrocephalus. May be difficult to distinguish from medulloblastoma **(MBS)** radiographically, the following may help:
1. calcifications are common in ependymomas, but are seen in < 10% of MBS
2. MBS: usually arises in roof of 4th ventricle (fastigium). The 4th ventricle drapes around the tumor ("**banana sign**"), c.f. ependymoma which tends to grow into 4th ventricle from floor

3. ependymomas tend to be inhomogeneous on T1WI MRI (unlike MBS)
4. the exophytic component of ependymomas tends to be high signal on T2WI MRI (with MBS this is only mildly hyperintense)

Myelogram/spinal MRI: water-soluble contrast myelography is about as sensitive as gadolinium enhanced MRI in detecting "drop mets". Myelography also provides CSF for cytology for staging.

MICROSCOPIC FEATURES

Although they are usually circumscribed with a covering layer of ependyma, they may be invasive. **Perivascular pseudorosettes** (when they occur, are diagnostic): areas of radiating processes lacking nuclei surrounding blood vessels.

TREATMENT

Surgical resection

Goal of surgery: maximal possible resection of intracranial portion without causing neurological deficits. When invasion of the floor is extensive, total excision is not possible. Postoperatively, perform LP/myelogram or MRI to look for "drop mets". 10 cc of CSF sent for cytology to quantitate (if any) number of malignant cells (may be used to follow treatment).

Lesions in fourth ventricle region are approached via midline suboccipital craniectomy.

Radiation therapy (XRT)

Ependymomas rank 2nd only to medulloblastomas in radiosensitivity. XRT is administered after surgical excision (survival is improved with post-op XRT: 50% survival time was 2 yrs longer with XRT than without[366], and 5-year survival increased from 20-40% without XRT to 40-80% with XRT[369]):
1. 45-48 Gy to tumor bed[369] (recurrence treated with additional 15-20 Gy)[368 (p 2797)]
2. spinal XRT: most radiate only if drop mets or if positive CSF cytology (however, prophylactic spinal is controversial[370])
   A. low dose XRT to entire spinal axis (median dose = 30 Gy[369])
   B. boost to any regions showing drop mets

Chemotherapy

Has little impact on newly diagnosed cases. Chemotherapy at the time of recurrence may arrest tumor progression for short periods.

OUTCOME

Operative mortality[368 (p 2797)]: 20-50% in early series; more recently: 5-8%.

Total surgical resection of primary intracranial tumor followed by craniospinal XRT as outlined above yields 41% 5-year survival. Survival tends to be worse the younger the patient (5-year survival of 20-30% in the pediatric group[367, 371], compared with up to 80% in adults). Excluding ependymoblastoma, malignant features in an ependymoma does not necessarily portend a worse prognosis[372].

The risk of recurrence is highest in patients with partial resection.

SPINAL EPENDYMOMAS

The most common spinal cord glioma below the mid-thoracic region.
See *Intramedullary spinal cord tumors* on page 508.

17.2.17.   Primitive neuroectodermal tumor (PNET)

This term has come to encompass a wide variety of previously individually named tumors which all seem to have common pathologic features suggesting origin from primitive neuroectodermal cells (although the actual cell of origin is unknown). These tumors include: medulloblastoma (the most common PNET), retinoblastoma, pineoblastoma, neuroblastoma, esthesioneuroblastoma, ependymoblastoma, and polar spongioblastoma.

These tumors may disseminate via the CSF spontaneously[373], or iatrogenically (following surgery or shunting, the latter is a rare cause of tumor dissemination[21]). Thus, all patients with PNETs require spinal axis evaluation (gadolinium enhanced MRI is about as sensitive as water-soluble myelography) and cytologic examination of CSF. Prophylactic craniospinal XRT is indicated following surgical removal. In children, cranial XRT causes intellectual impairment and growth retardation (see *Radiation injury and necrosis*, page 535) and is avoided if at all possible before 3 years of age. Extraneural metastases can also occur.

MEDULLOBLASTOMA

❦ Key features
- the most common pediatric brain malignancy and the most common PNET
- usually arises in the roof of the 4th ventricle, often producing hydrocephalus
- brainstem invasion usually limits complete surgical excision
- all patients must be evaluated for "drop mets"

Accounts for 15-20% of intracranial tumors in children[103], and is the most common malignant pediatric brain tumor[374]. Peak incidence: during 1st decade. Male:female ratio is 2:1. Usually arises in the cerebellar vermis, in the apex of the roof of the 4th ventricle (fastigium). This location predisposes to early obstructive hydrocephalus. Usual presenting symptoms: H/A, N/V, and truncal & appendicular ataxia.

Highly radiosensitive and moderately chemosensitive.

Seeding & metastases

≈ 10-35% have seeded the cranio-spinal axis at the time of diagnosis[103], and extraneural mets occur in 5% of patients[374], sometimes promoted by shunting[375] (although this is uncommon[21]).

EVALUATION

Usually appears as a solid, midline, IV-contrast-enhancing lesion on CT or MRI. Most enhance (pre-contrast may be hypo- to hyper-dense) on CT. See *Intracranial ependymomas* on page 471 for comparison of imaging characteristics. Spinal MRI with gadolinium or water-soluble contrast myelography should be done to rule-out "drop mets". Staging is done either pre-op or within 2-3 weeks of surgery.

TREATMENT

Treatment of choice: surgical debulking of as much tumor as possible (without causing neurological injury) followed by craniospinal XRT (radiation is necessary because of propensity to recur and to seed). It is better to leave a small residual on the brain-stem (these patients do fairly well) than it is to chase every last remnant off the brain-stem (neurologic deficit is more likely with this approach).

Surgical exposure of midline cerebellar medulloblastomas requires opening of the foramen magnum, usually removal of the posterior arch of C1, and occasionally the arch of C2. Tumor spread with arachnoidal thickening ("sugar coating") may occur. Invasion of or extension to the floor of the fourth ventricle (brainstem in the region of the facial colliculus) often limits excision.

XRT: optimal irradiation dose: 35-40 Gy to whole craniospinal axis + 10-15 Gy boost to tumor bed (usually posterior-fossa) and to any spinal mets seen, all fractionated over 6-7 wks. Reduce dosages by 20-25% for age < 3 yrs, or use chemotherapy instead. Lower dose radiation (25 Gy) to the neuraxis may provide acceptable control when confirmed gross total excision is achieved[376].

Chemotherapy: there is no standardized chemotherapy regimen. CCNU and vincristine are primarily used, but are usually reserved for recurrence, for poor risk patients (see *Prognosis* below), or for children < 3 yrs age.

Shunts: 30-40% of children require permanent VP shunts following p-fossa resection. The risk of shunt-related seeding has been quoted as high as 10-20%[103], but this is probably overestimated[21]. In the past, tumor filters were frequently used. They are less commonly used today because of the high incidence of obstruction.

PROGNOSIS

Poor prognosis is portended by younger age (especially if < 4 yrs), disseminated lesions, inability to perform gross-total removal, or histological differentiation along glial, ependymal, or neuronal lines. Most common site of recurrence is p-fossa.

Patients without residual tumor on post-op MRI and negative CSF results are considered **good-risk** patients with over 75% 5-year survival. Those with bulky residual tumor and dissemination in the brain, spine or CSF are **poor-risk** and have a worse prognosis, with 35-50% chance of being free of disease at 5 years[377]. Best outcome in another study: 5 and 10-yr survival of 56% & 43% respectively[374].

EPENDYMOBLASTOMA

A highly cellular embryonal form of ependymal tumor[378]. Occurs most often in age < 5 yrs. Prognosis is poor, with median post-op survival ranging from 12-20 months, and almost 100% mortality rate at 3 yrs. As with other PNETS, there is a tendency for subarachnoid seeding.

17.2.18.   Epidermoid and dermoid tumors

AKA epidermoid or dermoid *cysts*.

Comparison of dermoids and epidermoids

Both are usually developmental, benign tumors that may arise when retained ectodermal implants are trapped by two fusing ectodermal surfaces. The growth rate of these tumors is linear, like skin (rather than exponential, as with neoplastic tumors). Distinguishing features between the two tumors are shown in *Table 17-48*. They may occur in the following locations

Table 17-48   Comparison of epidermoids and dermoid

Feature	Epidermoid	Dermoid
frequency	0.5-1.5% of brain tumors	0.3% of brain tumors
lining	stratified squamous epithelium	also include dermal appendage organs (hair follicles and sebaceous glands)
contents	keratin, cellular debris, and cholesterol	same as epidermoids, plus hair and sebum
location	more common laterally (e.g. CP angle)	more commonly near midline
associated anomalies	tend to be isolated lesions	associated with other congenital anomalies in up to 50% of cases
meningitis	may have brief recurrent episodes of <u>aseptic</u> meningitis	may have repeated bouts of bacterial meningitis

1. calvaria: skull involvement occurs when ectodermal rests are included in the developing cranium (*see page 481*), epidural extension may occur with growth
2. intracranial: the most common sites include
   A. suprasellar: commonly produce bitemporal hemianopsia and optic atrophy, and only occasionally pituitary (endocrine) symptoms (including DI)
   B. sylvian fissure: may present with seizures
   C. CPA: may produce trigeminal neuralgia, especially in young patient
   D. basilar-posterior fossa: may produce lower cranial nerve findings, cerebellar dysfunction, and/or corticospinal tract abnormalities
   E. within the ventricular system: occur within the 4th ventricle more commonly than any other
3. scalp
4. within the spinal canal:
   A. most arise in the thoracic or upper lumbar spine
   B. epidermoids of the lower lumbar spine may occur iatrogenically following LP (see *Lumbar puncture*, page 615)
   C. dermoids of the spinal canal are usually associated with a dermal sinus tract (*see page 118*) and may produce recurrent bouts of spinal meningitis

EPIDERMOID CYSTS

❦ Key features
- usually arise from ectoderm trapped within or displaced into the CNS
- predilection for: CP angle, 4th ventricle, suprasellar region, spinal cord
- AKA cholesteatoma (not to be confused with cholesterol granuloma)

- grow at linear rate (unlike exponential rate of true neoplasms)
- may produce Mollaret's (aseptic) meningitis
- treatment: surgical excision; XRT has no role

AKA cholesteatoma or pearly tumor. Also *see Table 17-48* above for comparison to dermoids. Comprise 1% of intracranial tumors[379], and ≈ 7% of CPA tumors. May arise from any of the following[380]:

1. displaced dorsal midline ectodermal cell rests trapped during neural tube closure between gestational weeks 3-5
2. multipotential embryonic cell rests
3. epithelial cell rests carried to the CPA with the developing otic vesicle
4. epidermal cells displaced into CNS, e.g. by LP (see *Lumbar puncture*, page 615)

PATHOLOGY

Epidermoids are lined by stratified squamous epithelium, and contain keratin (from desquamated epithelium), cellular debris, and cholesterol[381]. Growth occurs at a linear rate like normal skin, unlike the exponential growth of true neoplasms[382]. The cyst contents may be liquid or may have a flaky consistency. They tend to spread along normal cleavage planes and surround vital structures (cranial nerves, ICA...).

Distinction from cholesterol granuloma

Epidermoid cysts have often been equated with cholesterol granulomas[383]. However, these are distinct lesions[384], the latter usually occurs following chronic inflammation. Some differences are delineated in *Table 17-49*.

Table 17-49   Characteristics of epidermoid vs. cholesterol granuloma

Feature	Epidermoid cyst	Cholesterol granuloma
origin	ectodermal remnants within CNS	chronic inflammatory cells surrounding cholesterol crystals (? from breakdown of RBC membranes)
precursor	usually congenital, occasionally acquired	chronic middle ear infection or idiopathic hemotympanum
symptoms	vary depending on location	usually involve vestibular or cochlear dysfunction
imaging	CT: low density; no enhancement; bone erosion in 33% MRI: T1WI: intensity slightly > CSF; T2WI: tumor & CSF similar hi intensity	CT: homogeneous & iso-dense; rim enhancement; extensive destruction of petrous bone MRI: increased signal on both T1WI and T2WI
gross appearance	pearly white	brown (from hemosiderin)
microscopic pathology[385]	lined with stratified squamous epithelial lining	fibroblastic proliferation, hemosiderin-laden macrophages, cholesterol clefts, giant cell reaction
ideal treatment	aggressive near-total excision	subtotal resection followed by drainage may suffice

PRESENTATION

Epidermoids may present as any mass lesion in the same location. Additionally, they may present with recurrent episodes of aseptic meningitis caused by rupture of the cyst contents. Symptoms include fever and meningeal irritation. CSF shows pleocytosis, hypoglycorrhachia, elevated protein, and negative cultures. Cholesterol crystals may be seen and can be recognized by their amorphous birefringent appearance. **Mollaret's meningitis** is a rare variant of aseptic meningitis which includes the finding of large cells in the CSF that resemble endothelial cells (which may be macrophages[386]) that may be seen in some patients with epidermoid cysts[387, 388].

EVALUATION

CT: low density, slightly greater than CSF, with no enhancement[389]. The presence of enhancement suggests the possibility of a malignant epithelial component. Bone erosion is seen in 33%.

MRI: T1WI: intensity is slightly > CSF. T2WI: tumor and CSF have similar high intensity.

TREATMENT

Caution when removing epidermoid cysts to avoid spilling contents as they are quite irritating and may cause severe chemical meningitis (Mollaret's meningitis, *see above*). Berger[380] advocates intraoperative irrigation with hydrocortisone (100 mg/L of LR) to reduce the risk of post-op communicating hydrocephalus. Peri-operative IV steroids and copious saline irrigation during surgery may provide similar results. Due to the densely adherent capsule, it is often necessary to leave remnants behind, however, if these are small this does not preclude satisfactory outcome.

In spite of adequate removal, it is not unusual to see persistent brainstem distortion on post-op imaging[384]. Post-op radiation is not indicated as the tumor is benign and XRT does not prevent recurrence[390].

17.2.19.   Pineal region tumors

Pineal region[391]: the area of the brain bounded dorsally by the splenium of the corpus callosum and the tela choroidea, ventrally by the quadrigeminal plate and midbrain tectum, rostrally by the posterior aspect of the 3rd ventricle, and caudally by the cerebellar vermis. Tumors in this region are more common in children (3-8% of pediatric brain tumors) than in adults (≤ 1%)[392]. A striking feature is the diversity of tumors that may occur in this location due to the variety of tissues and conditions normally present, as shown in *Table 17-50*. Furthermore, many tumors are of mixed cell type.

Table 17-50   Conditions giving rise to pineal region tumors

Substrate in pineal region	Tumor that may arise
pineal glandular tissue	pineocytomas and pineoblastomas
glial cells	astrocytomas (including pilocytic), oligodendrogliomas, glial cysts (AKA pineal cyst)
arachnoid cells	meningiomas, arachnoid cysts (non-neoplastic)
ependymal lining	ependymomas
sympathetic nerves	chemodectomas
rests of germ cells	germ cell tumors: choriocarcinoma, germinoma, embryonal carcinoma, endodermal sinus tumor (yolk sac tumor), and teratoma
absence of blood-brain barrier (BBB) in pineal gland	makes it a susceptible site for hematogenous metastases
remnants of ectoderm	epidermoid or dermoid cysts

Germ cell tumors **(GCT)**, ependymomas and pineal cell tumors metastasize easily through the CSF ("drop metastases").

PINEAL CYSTS *(PC)*

Usually an incidental finding (i.e. not symptomatic), seen on ≈ 4% of MRIs[393] or on 25-40% of autopsies[394] (many are microscopic). May escape detection on CT because the cyst fluid density is similar to CSF. The most common ones are intra-pineal glial-lined cysts with diameter < 1 cm. They have been regarded as benign, but the natural history is not known with certainty[395]. Etiology is obscure, they are usually benign, nonneoplastic, and may be due to ischemic glial degeneration or due to sequestration of the pineal diverticulum. They may contain clear, slightly xanthochromic, or hemorrhagic fluid. If asymptomatic, they may be followed on serial MRIs. Rarely, they may enlarge, and like other pineal region masses, may become symptomatic by causing hydrocephalus by aqueductal compression[396], gaze paresis[397] including Parinaud's syndrome, or hypothalamic symptoms.

May be difficult to detect on CT. On MRI T1WI show round or ovoid abnormality in region of pineal recess, signal varies with protein content (isointense or slightly hyperintense). T2WI occasionally show increased intensity[395]. Gadolinium occasionally enhances the cyst wall with a maximum thickness of 2 mm; irregularities of the wall with nodular enhancement suggests the lesion is not benign.

Positional H/As have been attributed to PCs, the theory is that the cyst could intermittently compress the vein of Galen and/or sylvian aqueduct[398]. This remains unproven since asymptomatic compression of the vein of Galen and the quadrigeminal plate has been demonstrated on MRI[399].

Epidermoid-dermoid cysts may also occur in the pineal region, and are larger and have different signal characteristics on MRI.

Management

Asymptomatic PCs < 2 cm diameter with typical appearance should be followed clinically and with annual imaging studies. Surgery to relieve symptoms or to obtain a diagnosis is suggested for symptomatic lesions or for ones that show changes on MRI.

Surgery options for patients with hydrocephalus:
1.   CSF shunt: may not relieve gaze disturbance

2. excision: relieves symptoms and establishes diagnosis. Low morbidity
3. stereotactic or endoscopic aspiration: may not get enough tissue for diagnosis
4. endoscopic third ventriculostomy: useful only for typical PC as it does not obtain tissue. A few cases of regression of pineal cysts after treatment have been reported[400]

PINEAL REGION NEOPLASMS

Pineal cell tumors

A pineocytoma is a well differentiated neoplasm arising from pineal epithelium. Pineoblastoma is a malignant tumor that is considered a primitive neuroectodermal tumor **(PNET)**. Both can metastasize through the CSF, and both are radiosensitive.

Germ cell tumors

Occur in the midline (suprasellar and pineal region) when they arise in the CNS. In the pineal region, these tumors occur predominantly in males. In females, GCTs are more common in the suprasellar region[401]. Aside from benign teratomas, all intracranial GCTs are malignant and may metastasize via CSF and systemically.

1. germinomas: malignant tumors of primitive germ cells that occur in the gonads (called testicular seminomas in males, dysgerminomas in females) or in the CNS. Survival with these is much better than with nongerminomatous tumors
2. nongerminomas include:
   A. embryonal carcinoma
   B. choriocarcinoma
   C. teratoma

Tumor markers

GCTs characteristically (but not always) give rise to tumor markers (ßhCG and AFP) in the CSF (see *Tumor markers used clinically*, page 500). Elevated CSF ßhCG is classically associated with choriocarcinomas, but also occurs with ≈ 10% of germinomas (which are more common). AFP is elevated with endodermal sinus tumors, embryonal carcinoma and occasionally with teratomas. When positive, these markers can be followed serially to assess treatment and to look for recurrence (they should be checked in serum and CSF). NB: these markers alone are not usually sufficient for making a definitive diagnosis of a pineal region tumor since many of these tumors are mixed cell type.

PEDIATRIC

A breakdown of pediatric pineal region tumors in one series is shown in *Table 17-51* (series A).

In 36 patients < 18 yrs age, 17 distinct histological tumor types were identified: 11 germinomas (the most common tumor), 7 astrocytomas, and the remaining 18 had 15 different tumors[402].

ADULT

GCTs and pineal cell tumors occur primarily in childhood and young adults. Thus, over the age of 40, a pineal region tumor is more likely to be a meningioma or a glioma. Series B in *Table 17-51* includes both adult and pediatric patients.

Table 17-51 Pineal region tumors

Tumor	Series A* (%)	Series B† (%)
germinoma	30	27
astrocytoma	19	26
pineocytoma	6	12
malignant teratoma	6	
unidentified germ-cell tumor	6	
choriocarcinoma	3	1.1
malignant teratoma/embryonal cell tumor	3	1.6
glioblastoma	3	
teratoma	3	4.3
germinoma/ectodermal sinus tumor	3	
dermoid	3	
embryonal cell tumor	3	
pineoblastoma	3	12
pineocytoma/pineoblastoma	3	
endodermal sinus tumor	3	
glial cyst (pineal cyst)[403]	3	2.7
arachnoid cyst	3	
metastases		2.7
meningioma		2.7
ependymoma		4.3
oligodendrogliomas		0.54
ganglioglioneuroma		2.7
lymphoma		2.7

* 36 children ≤ 18 yrs[402]

† 370 tumors in patients 3-73 yrs old[392]

CLINICAL

Almost all patients have hydrocephalus by the time of presentation, causing typical signs and symptoms of headache, vomiting, lethargy, memory disturbance, abnormally increasing head circumference in infants, and seizures. Parinaud's syndrome (or the syndrome of the sylvian aqueduct) may be present (*see page 86*). Precocious puberty may occur only in boys with choriocarcinomas or germinomas with syncytiotrophoblastic cells due to leutinizing hormone-like effects of ßhCG secreted in the CSF.

Drop metastases from CSF seeding can produce radiculopathy and/or myelopathy.

TREATMENT

The optimal management strategy for pineal region tumors has yet to be determined.

Hydrocephalus

Patients presenting acutely due to hydrocephalus may be best treated with external ventricular drainage (**EVD**). This permits control over the amount of CSF drained, prevents peritoneal seeding with tumor (a rare event[21]), and may avoid having a permanent shunt placed in the significant number of patients who will not need one after tumor removal (although ≈ 90% of patients with a pineal GCT require a shunt). Ventricular access (via EVD or Frazier burr hole) in the post-op period is important in the event of acute hydrocephalus.

Stereotactic procedures

May be used to ascertain diagnosis (biopsy), or to treat symptomatic pineal region cysts[404, 405]. Caution is advised since the pineal region has numerous vessels (vein of Galen, basal veins of Rosenthal, internal cerebral veins, posterior medial choroidal artery)[406] which may be displaced from their normal position. The complication rate of stereotactic biopsy is: ≈ 1.3% mortality, ≈ 7% morbidity, and 1 case of seeding in 370 patients, and the diagnostic rate is ≈ 94%[392]. A shortcoming of stereotactic biopsy is that it may fail to disclose the histologic heterogeneity of some tumors.

One study found that the trajectory correlated with complications, and they recommended a low frontal approach below the internal cerebral veins[407]. However, the correlation of trajectory and complications was not born out in another study[392], and they found that the complication rate was higher in firm tumors (pineocytomas, teratomas, and astrocytomas) and they recommend an open approach when the tumor appears difficult to penetrate on the first attempt at biopsy.

Stereotactic radiosurgery may be appropriate for treatment of some lesions.

Radiation treatment

Controversial. Germinomas are very sensitive to radiation (and chemotherapy), and are probably best treated with these modalities and followed. If a pineal region tumor enhances uniformly and has the classic appearance of a germinoma on MRI, some surgeons will give a test dose of 5 Gy, and if the tumor shrinks down the diagnosis of germinoma is virtually certain and XRT may be continued without surgery. Others feel that this needlessly exposes patients with benign or radioresistant tumors to XRT, and they prefer a tissue diagnosis (e.g. by stereotactic biopsy)[392]. "Trial XRT" should be avoided in tumors suspected of being teratomas or epidermoid cyst on MRI.

XRT is also utilized post-op for other malignant tumors. For highly malignant tumors or if there is evidence of CSF seeding, craniospinal XRT with a boost to the tumor bed is appropriate.

If possible, XRT is best avoided in the young child (*see page 535*). Chemotherapy may be used for the child < 3 yrs age until the child is older when XRT better tolerated[401].

Surgical treatment of the tumor

Indications: controversial. Some authors feel that most tumors (except germinomas, which are best treated with XRT) are amenable to open resection[408]. Others feel that resection should be limited to ≈ 25% of tumors which are[392]:
1. radioresistant (e.g. malignant nongerminoma GCTs): 35-50% of pineal region tumors (larger numbers occur in series not limited to pediatric patients)
2. benign (e.g. meningioma, teratomas...)
3. well encapsulated
4. NB: malignant germ cell tumors should be <u>without</u> evidence of metastases (those with metastases do not benefit from surgery on the primary tumor)

Approaches include (the choice is aided by the pre-op MRI):
1. infratentorial supracerebellar: cannot be used if MRI show that the angle of the tentorium is too steep. May be done in the sitting position (risk of air embolism,

---

see page 605) or in the Concorde position (*see page 604*)
2. occipital transtentorial: wide view. Risk of injury to visual cortex. Recommended for lesions centered at or superior to the tentorial edge or located above the vein of Galen. The occipital lobe is retracted laterally, and the tentorium is incised 1 cm lateral to the straight sinus
3. transventricular: indicated for large, eccentric lesions with ventricular dilatation. Usually via a cortical incision in the posterior portion of the superior temporal gyrus. Risks: visual defect, seizures, and on dominant side language dysfunction
4. lateral paramedian infratentorial
5. transcallosal: largely abandoned except for tumors extending into corpus callosum and third ventricle

Important surgical considerations:
    The base of the pineal gland is the posterior wall of the 3rd ventricle. The splenium of the corpus callosum lies above, and the thalamus surrounds both sides. The pineal projects posteriorly and inferiorly into the quadrigeminal cistern. The deep cerebral veins are a major obstacle to operations in this region.

Surgical outcome:
    Mortality rate: 5-10%[392]. Postoperative complications include: new visual field deficits, epidural fluid collection, infection, and cerebellar ataxia.

17.2.20. Choroid plexus tumors

Account for 0.4-1% of all intracranial tumors. Although they may occur at any age, 70% of patients are < 2 yrs old[409]. Some tumors occur in neonates, supporting the hypothesis that some of these are congenital[410].
    In adults these tumors are usually infratentorial, whereas in children they occur in the lateral ventricle[410] (a reverse from the situation for most other tumors). See *Intraventricular lesions* on page 934 for differential diagnosis.
    Most are histologically benign (**choroid plexus papilloma**), although malignant tumors (**choroid plexus carcinoma**) also occur. The tumors sometimes grow rapidly.

Presentation
    Most present with symptoms of increased ICP from hydrocephalus (H/A, N/V, craniomegaly), others may present with seizures, subarachnoid hemorrhage (with meningismus), or focal neurologic deficit (hemiparesis, sensory deficits, cerebellar signs, or cranial nerve palsies of III, IV and VI).
    Hydrocephalus may result from overproduction of CSF, although total removal of these tumors does not always cure the hydrocephalus (this occurs most often in patients with high CSF protein, hemorrhage from tumor or surgery, or ependymitis).

Treatment
    There is no role for chemotherapy or radiation for benign lesions.

Surgical treatment:
    Benign lesions may be cured surgically with total removal, and even the malignant tumors respond well to surgery. The operation may be difficult due to fragility of the tumor and bleeding from the choroidal arteries. However, persistence with a second and sometimes even third operation is recommended as 5-year survival rate of 84% can be achieved[410]. Post-operative subdural collections after transcortical tumor excision may occur, and may result from a persistent ventriculosubdural fistula, which may require subdural-peritoneal shunting[409].

17.2.21. Miscellaneous primary brain tumors

PRIMARY CNS MELANOMA
    Probably arises from melanocytes in the leptomeninges. May spread through CSF pathways. May occasionally metastasize outside the CNS to produce systemic metastases[411].
    The peak age for this tumor is in the 4th decade (compared to the 7th decade for primary cutaneous melanoma)[412].

17.3.   Pediatric brain tumors

Among all childhood cancers, brain tumors are the second
only to leukemias in incidence (20%), and are the most common
solid pediatric tumor[374], comprising 40-50% of all tumors[103]. Annual incidence: 2-5 cases per 100,000.

Types of tumors
The common pediatric brain tumors are gliomas (cerebellum, brain stem, and optic nerve), pineal tumors, craniopharyngiomas, teratomas, granulomas, and primitive neuroectodermal
tumors (**PNETs**, primarily medulloblastoma).

Meningiomas: 1.5% of meningiomas occur in childhood and
adolescence (usually between 10-20 years), comprising 0.4-4.6%
of intracranial tumors[95 (p 3263)] (see *Meningiomas* on page 426).

**Table 17-52 Loca-
tion of pediatric
brain tumors by age**

| Age | % Infrat-
entorial |
|---|---|
| 0-6 mos | 27% |
| 6-12 mos | 53% |
| 12-24 mos | 74% |
| 2-16 yrs | 42% |

Infratentorial vs. supratentorial
It has traditionally been taught that
most pediatric brain tumors (≈ 60%) are
infratentorial, and that these are
≈ equally divided among brain stem gliomas, cerebellar astrocytomas, and
medulloblastomas. In reality, the ratio of
supratentorial to infratentorial tumors is
dependent on the specific age group studied, as illustrated in *Table 17-52*. *Table
17-53* shows the breakdown for pooled
data from 1350 pediatric brain tumors.

Astrocytomas are the most common
supratentorial tumor in pediatrics as in
adulthood.

**Table 17-53   Incidence of
pediatric brain tumors***

Tumor type	Page	% of total
infratentorial tumors		54%
cerebellar astrocytomas	419	15%
medulloblastomas	473	14%
brain stem gliomas	420	12%
ependymomas[367]	470	9%
supratentorial benign astrocytomas	417	13%

* data from 1350 pediatric brain tumors[94 (p 368)]

INTRACRANIAL NEOPLASMS DURING THE FIRST YEAR OF LIFE
Brain tumors presenting during the first year of life is a different subset of tumors
than those presenting later in childhood. In a busy neurosurgical unit in a children's hospital, they represented ≈ 8% of children admitted with brain tumors, an average of only
≈ 3 admissions per year[413].

90% of brain tumors in neonates are of neuroectodermal origin, teratoma being the
most common. Some of these tumors may be congenital[414]. Other supratentorial tumors
include: astrocytoma, choroid plexus tumors, ependymomas, and craniopharyngiomas.
Posterior fossa tumors include medulloblastoma and cerebellar astrocytoma.

Many of these tumors escape diagnosis until they are very large in size due to the
elasticity of the infant skull, the adaptability of the developing nervous system to compensate for deficits, and the difficulty in examining a patient with limited neurologic rep-
ertoire and inability to cooperate. The most common presenting manifestations are
vomiting, arrest or regression of psychomotor development, macrocrania, poor feed-
ing/failure to thrive. They may also present with seizures.

17.4.   Skull tumors

See *Skull lesions* on page 930 for differential diagnosis and evaluation (including
non-neoplastic lesions). Considering only tumors, the differential diagnosis includes:
1. benign tumors
    A. osteoma: *see below*
    B. hemangioma: *see below*
    C. dermoid and epidermoid tumors: *see below*
    D. chondroma: occur mainly in conjunction with the basal synchondroses
    E. meningioma

F. aneurysmal bone cyst
2. malignant tumors: malignancy is suggested by a single large or multiple (> 6) small osteolytic lesions with margins that are ragged, undermined and lacking sclerosis[415]
   A. bone metastases to the skull. Common ones include:
      1. prostate
      2. breast
      3. lung
      4. kidney
      5. thyroid
      6. lymphoma
      7. multiple myeloma/plasmacytoma: *see page 514*
   B. chondrosarcoma
   C. osteogenic sarcoma
   D. fibrosarcoma

17.4.1.   Osteoma

Osteomas are the most common primary bone tumor of the calvaria. They are benign, slow-growing lesions, that occur commonly in the cranial vault, mastoid and paranasal air sinuses, and the mandible. Lesions within air sinuses may present as recurrent sinusitis. More common in females. Triad of Gardner's syndrome: multiple cranial osteomas (of calvaria, sinuses, and mandible), colonic polyposis, and soft-tissue tumors.

See *Localized increased density or hyperostosis of the calvaria* on page 932 for differential diagnosis.

Pathology

Consists of osteoid tissue within osteoblastic tissue, surrounded by reactive bone. Difficult to distinguish from fibrous dysplasia.

Radiographic evaluation

Skull x-ray: well demarcated, homogeneous dense projection. May arise from the inner or outer table. May be compact or spongy. Unlike meningiomas, diplöe are preserved and vascular channels are not increased.

Osteomas are "hot" on nuclear bone scan.

Treatment

Asymptomatic lesions may simply be followed. Surgery may be considered for cosmetic reasons, or if pressure on adjacent tissues produces discomfort. Lesions involving only the outer table may be removed leaving the inner table intact.

17.4.2.   Hemangioma

Comprise ≈ 7% of skull tumors[415]. These benign tumors commonly occur in the skull (discussed here) and spine (*see page 512*). Two types: cavernous (most common) and capillary (rare).

Radiographic evaluation

Skull x-ray: characteristically shows a circular lucency with honeycomb or trabecular pattern (seen in ≈ 50% of cases) or radial trabeculations producing a sunburst pattern (seen in ≈ 11% of cases)[415]. Sclerotic margins are evident in only ≈ 33%.

CT: hypodense lesion with sclerotic spaced trabeculations. Nonenhancing.

Bone scan: typically hot.

Treatment

Accessible lesions may be cured by en bloc excision or curettage. The gross appearance is of a hard, blue-domed mass beneath the pericranium. Radiation may be considered for inaccessible tumors.

17.4.3.   Epidermoid and dermoid tumors of the skull

See also *page 474* for epidermoids and dermoids in general. Skull involvement occurs when ectodermal rests are included in the developing skull. Usually midline. Arise within the diplöe and expand both inner and outer tables. Identical clinically and radiologically, dermoids contain skin appendages (dermal elements). These benign lesions may involve underlying dural venous structures or brain. They may become infected.

Radiographic evaluation
* **skull x-ray**: these osteolytic lesions have well-defined, sclerotic margins
* some imaging is required to evaluate possible intracranial involvement
    ♦ **CT**: the lesions are hypodense (keratin contains fats), and non-enhancing
    ♦ **MRI**: they are low intensity on T1WI and high signal on T2WI

Treatment
    Treatment is surgical. Bone margins are curetted. Search must be made for a tract leading to the intracranial cavity which must be followed if found. Preparation for dural sinus repair must be made for lesions overlying the sagittal sinus (including torcular Herophili). Radiation and chemotherapy are not indicated.

17.4.4.   Eosinophilic granuloma

    A generally benign local disease of bone with mononuclear cells and eosinophils, most commonly found in the skull (43-80%). May also be seen in femur (14.5%), mandible, ribs, pelvis, and the spine (vertebra plana, *see page 506*). Classified as the mildest form of **histiocytosis X** which also includes multifocal eosinophilic granuloma (Hand-Schüller-Christian disease) and Letterer-Siwe syndrome (a fulminant, malignant lymphoma of infancy)[416].

CLINICAL
    Generally a condition of youth, 70% of patients are < 20 yrs age. In a series of 26 patients[416], age range was 18 mos-49 yrs (mean: 16 yrs).
    Most common presenting symptom: tender, enlarging skull mass (> 90%). May be asymptomatic and incidentally discovered on skull x-ray obtained for other reasons. Blood tests were normal in all except 1 who had eosinophilia of 23%.
    Parietal bone was the most common site (42%), frontal bone next (31%)[416] (some series show frontal bone was the most common).

EVALUATION

Skull x-rays
    Classic radiographic finding: round or oval non-sclerotic punched out skull lesion with sharply defined margins, involving both inner and outer tables (the disease begins in diploic space), often with beveled edges. A central bone density is occasionally noted (rare, but diagnostic). No abnormal vascularity of adjacent bone. No periosteal reaction. Differentiate from hemangioma by absence of sunburst appearance.

CT scan
    Characteristic appearance of a soft tissue mass within area of bony destruction having a central density[417]. Differentiate from epidermoid which has dense surrounding sclerosis.

PATHOLOGY
    Gross: pinkish gray to purple lesion extending out of bone and involving pericranium. Dural involvement occurs in only 1 of 26 patients, but with no dural penetration.
    Microscopic: numerous histiocytes, eosinophils, and multinucleated cells in a reticulin fiber network. No evidence that this is a result of an infection.

TREATMENT
    Tendency toward spontaneous regression, however, most single lesions are treated by curettage. Multiple lesions are usually associated with extracalvarial bony involvement and are often treated with chemotherapy and/or low dose radiation therapy.

OUTCOME
    After a mean 8 years follow-up, 8 patients (31%) developed additional lesions, 5 of these were ≤ 3 yrs age (all of 5 patients < 3 yrs age)[416] (may suggest a form of Letterer-Siwe, thus young patients should be followed closely). Recurrences were local in one case, and in others involved other bones (including the skull, femur, lumbar spine) or brain (in-

cluding the hypothalamus, presenting with diabetes insipidus and growth delay).

17.4.5. Non-neoplastic skull lesions

Includes:
1. osteopetrosis (*see page 918*)
2. Paget's disease of the skull (*see page 340*)
3. hyperostosis frontalis interna (*see below*)
4. fibrous dysplasia

HYPEROSTOSIS FRONTALIS INTERNA

See page 932 for differential diagnosis. Hyperostosis frontalis interna (**HFI**) is a benign irregular nodular thickening of the inner table of the frontal bone that is almost always bilateral. The midline is spared at the insertion of the falx. Unilateral cases have been reported[418], and in these cases one must R/O other etiologies such as meningioma, calcified epidural hematoma, osteoma, fibrous dysplasia, an epidural fibrous tumor[419], or Paget's disease.

The incidence of HFI in the general population is ≈ 1.4-5%[418]. HFI is more common in women (female:male ratio may be as high as 9:1) with an incidence of 15-72% in elderly women. A number of possible associated conditions have been described (most are unproven), the majority of which are metabolic, earning it the alias of **metabolic craniopathy**. Associated conditions include:
1. Morgagni's syndrome (AKA Morgagni-Stewart-Morel syndrome): headache, obesity, virilism and neuropsychiatric disorders (including mental retardation)
2. endocrinologic abnormalities
   A. acromegaly[420] (elevated growth hormone levels)
   B. hyperprolactinemia[420]
3. metabolic abnormalities
   A. hyperphosphatasemia
   B. obesity
4. diffuse idiopathic skeletal hyperostosis (**DISH**)

CLINICAL

HFI may present without symptoms as an incidental finding on radiographic evaluation for other reasons. Many signs and symptoms have been attributed to HFI including: hypertension, seizures, headache, cranial nerve deficits, dementia, irritability, depression, hysteria, fatigability and mental dullness. The incidence of headache may be statistically higher in patients with HFI than in the general population[421].

EVALUATION

Blood tests to R/O some of the above noted conditions may be indicated in appropriate cases: check growth hormone, prolactin, phosphate, alkaline phosphatase (to R/O Paget's disease).

Plain skull x-ray shows thickening of the frontal bone with characteristic sparing of the midline. Spread to parietal and occipital bone occasionally occurs.

CT demonstrates the lesion which usually causes 5-10 mm of bone thickening, but as much as 4 cm has been reported.

Bone scan: usually shows moderate uptake in HFI (generally not as intense as with bone mets). Also, indium-111 leukocyte scan (commonly used to detect occult infection) will show accumulation in HFI (a false positive)[422, 423].

TREATMENT

Little has been written about treatment of cases where symptoms are suspected to be due to HFI. In one report, removal of the thickened bone was accomplished without evidence of dural adhesions, and with improvement in the presenting hysteria[418].

FIBROUS DYSPLASIA

Usually a benign condition in which normal bone is replaced by fibrous connective tissue (malignant transformation occurs in < 1%). Does not appear to be heritable. Most lesions occur in the ribs or craniofacial bones, especially the maxilla. May occur:

1. monostotic: most common
2. polyostotic: 25% with this form have > 50% of the skeleton involved with associated fractures and skeletal deformities
3. as part of McCune-Albright syndrome (endocrine dysfunction, café au lait spots which tend to occur on one side of the midline and tend to be more jagged than those seen in neurofibromatosis (*see page 502*), fibrous dysplasia, and precocious puberty primarily in females) and its variants

Clinical

Clinical manifestations of the fibrous dysplasia **(FD)** lesions include:
1. incidental finding (i.e. asymptomatic)
2. local pain
3. local swelling (rarely marked distortion resembling aneurysmal bone cyst may occur) or deformity
4. may predispose to pathologic fractures when they occur in long bones
5. cranial nerve involvement: including loss of hearing when the temporal bone is involved as a result of obliteration of the external auditory canal
6. seizures
7. serum alkaline phosphatase is elevated in about 33%, calcium levels are normal
8. darkened hair pigmentation overlying skull lesions
9. spontaneous scalp hemorrhages
10. rarely associated with Cushing's syndrome, acromegaly

3 forms of the FD lesions:
1. cystic (the lesions are not actually cysts in the strict sense): widening of the diplöe usually with thinning of the outer table and little involvement of the inner table. Typically occurs high in calvaria
2. sclerotic: usually involves skull base (especially sphenoid bone) and facial bones
3. mixed: appearance is similar to cystic type with patches of increased density within the lucent lesions

Ground glass appearance on x-rays is due to the thin spicules of woven bone.

Treatment

There is no cure for FD. Local procedures (mostly orthopedic) are used for deformities or bone pain that is refractory to other treatment. Neurosurgical involvement may be required for skull lesions producing refractory pain or neurologic symptoms. Calvarial lesions may be treated with curettage and cranioplasty. Calcitonin may be used for widespread lesions with bone pain and/or high serum alkaline phosphatase levels.

17.5.   Cerebral metastases

METASTASES TO THE BRAIN

Cerebral metastases are the most common brain tumor seen clinically, comprising slightly more than half of brain tumors (if one considers only imaging studies, they comprise ≈ 30%). In the U.S., the annual incidence of new cases of metastases is > 100,000, compared to 17,000 for primary brain tumors. 15-30% of patients with cancer **(Ca)** develop cerebral mets[424]. In patients with no Ca history, a cerebral met was the presenting symptom in 15%; of these, 43-60% will have an abnormal chest x-ray **(CXR)**[425, 426] (showing either a bronchogenic primary or other mets to lung).

In 9% of cases, a cerebral met is the only detectable site of spread. Cerebral mets occur in only 6% of pediatric cases.

The route of metastatic spread to the brain is usually hematogenous, although local extension can also occur.

Solitary mets:
1. CT: at the time of neurologic diagnosis, 50% are solitary on CT[427, 428] (*see page 487*)
2. MRI: if the same patients have an MRI, < 30% will be solitary[429]
3. on autopsy: mets are solitary in one third of patients with brain mets, and 1-3% of solitary mets occur in the brain stem[430]

Increasing incidence of cerebral mets: May be due to a number of factors:
1. increasing length of survival of cancer patients[431] as a result of improvements in treatment of systemic cancer
2. enhanced ability to diagnose CNS tumors due to availability of CT and/or MRI

3. many chemotherapeutic agents used systemically do not cross the blood-brain barrier **(BBB)** well, providing a "haven" for tumor growth there
4. some chemotherapeutic agents may transiently weaken the BBB and allow CNS seeding with tumor

METASTASES OF PRIMARY CNS TUMORS

Spread via CSF pathways

Tumors that may spread via CSF pathways include the following (when these tumors spread to the spinal cord, they are often called "drop mets"):
1. high grade gliomas (10-25%) (*see page 413*)
2. primitive neuroectodermal tumors **(PNET)**, especially medulloblastoma (*see page 472*)
3. ependymoma (11%) (*see page 470*)
4. pineal region tumors
   A. germ cell tumors (*see page 476*)
   B. pineocytoma and pineoblastoma (*see page 477*)
5. rarely:
   A. oligodendrogliomas (≈ 1%) (*see page 423*)
   B. hemangioblastomas (*see page 460*)
   C. primary CNS melanoma (*see page 479*)

Extraneural spread

Although most CNS tumors do not spread systemically, there is some potential for extraneural spread with the following tumors:
1. medulloblastoma (cerebellar-PNET): the most common primary responsible for extraneural spread. May spread to lung, bone marrow, lymph nodes, abdomen
2. meningioma: rarely goes to heart or lungs
3. malignant astrocytomas rarely metastasize systemically
4. ependymomas
5. pineoblastomas
6. meningeal sarcomas
7. choroid plexus tumors
8. tumors that spread through CSF pathways (*see above*) may spread via a CSF shunt (e.g. to peritoneum with VP shunt or hematogenously with a VA shunt), however, this risk is probably quite small[21]

PRIMARY CANCERS IN PATIENTS WITH CEREBRAL METASTASES

In over 2,700 adults with a primary cancer undergoing autopsy at Sloan-Kettering, the sources of cerebral metastases are shown in *Table 17-54*. Sources of brain metastases in pediatrics is shown in *Table 17-55*.

In adults, lung and breast Ca together account for > 50% of cerebral mets.

LOCATION OF CEREBRAL METS

Intracranial metastases may be either parenchymal (≈ 75%) or may involve the leptomeninges in a carcinomatous meningitis (*see page 491*). 80% of solitary metastases are located in the cerebral hemispheres.

The highest incidence of parenchymal mets is posterior to the Sylvian fissure near the junction of temporal, parietal, and occipital lobes (presumably due to embolic spread to terminal MCA branches)[433]. Many tend to arise at the gray/white-matter interface.

The cerebellum is a common site of intracranial mets, and is the location in 16% of cases of solitary brain mets. It is the most common p-fossa tumor in adults, thus "a solitary lesion in the posterior fossa of an adult is considered a metastasis until proven otherwise". Spread to the posterior fossa may be via the spinal epidural venous plexus (Bat-

Table 17-54 Sources of cerebral mets in adults

Primary	%
lung Ca	44%
breast	10%
kidney (renal cell)*	7%
GI	6%
melanoma†	3%
undetermined	10%

* a rare tumor that metastasizes frequently to brain (in 20-25% of cases)

† 16% in older series[432]

Table 17-55 Sources of cerebral mets in peds

neuroblastoma
rhabdomyosarcoma
Wilm's tumor

son's plexus) and the vertebral veins.

SPECIFIC TYPES OF CEREBRAL METS
The autopsy incidence of cerebral mets for various types of primary cancers at Sloan-Kettering Cancer Center is shown in *Table 17-56*.

LUNG CANCER
The lungs are the most common source of cerebral mets, and these are usually multiple. The lung primary may be so small as to render it occult.

Necropsy demonstrates cerebral mets in up to 50% of patients with small-cell lung Ca (**SCLC**) and non-squamous, non-small-cell lung Ca[434].

Small cell lung cancer (SCLC)
AKA "oat cell" Ca, neuroendocrine tumor. 95% arise in proximal airways, usually in mainstem or lobar bronchi. Typically younger (27-66 years) than other lung Ca. Strongly associated with cigarette smoking. Median survival: 6-10 months. Staged in 1 of 2 categories:
> **limited**: confined to an area of the chest that can be encompassed by a single radiation port
> **extensive**: metastasis outside the thorax or intrathoracic disease that cannot be contained in a single radiation port

Radiosensitive. Although SCLC comprises only ≈ 20% of primary lung cancers, it is more likely to produce cerebral mets than other bronchogenic cell types (brain mets are found in 80% of patients who survive 2 yrs after diagnosis of SCLC)[431]. Therefore prophylactic brain XRT is used even in patients without brain mets.

Treatment of primary: usually not resected; treated with XRT + chemotherapy.

Non-small cell lung cancer (NSCLC)
Includes: large cell, squamous cell, adenocarcinoma, bronchoalveolar. Retrospective analysis of patients with NSCLC completely resected from lung found a 6.8% first recurrence rate in the brain[434]. Staged with typical TNM system. Treatment of primary: grades I, II, IIIA (i.e. no distal mets, excluding single brain met): resection; higher grades receive XRT + chemotherapy.

Staging studies for known lung primary
1. PET scan: can detect small malignancies. Useful in NSCLC to determine elegibility of resection of primary; not useful in initial evaluation of SCLC
2. chest CT: usually includes adrenals and liver (thus abdomen and pelvis CT not necessary)
3. bone scan
4. brain: CT or MRI

When metastatic lung cancer is the suspected source of a newly diagnosed brain lesion, the lung lesion should be biopsied (if technically feasible) to rule out SCLC before obtaining tissue from the cerebral mass.

MELANOMA
Once cerebral mets of melanoma are detected, median survival is 113 days, and the mets contributed to the death in 94% of cases[435]. A small group with survival > 3 yrs had a single surgically treated met in the absence of other visceral lesions. Metastatic melanoma almost never responds to chemotherapy and is poorly responsive to radiation. NB: there is also a rare primary CNS melanoma.

Metastatic melanoma classically causes pial/arachnoid involvement. May be hyperdense to brain on unenhanced CT. Enhancement is less constant than for other mets (e.g. bronchogenic).

The primary site cannot be identified in up to ≈ 14% of cases[436] (extremely difficult

Table 17-56 Autopsy incidence of cerebral mets for given primary cancers

Primary	% with cerebral mets
lung	21%
breast	9%
melanoma	40%
lymphoma	1%
Hodgkin's	0
non-Hodgkin's	2%
GI	3%
colon	5%
gastric	0
pancreatic	2%
GU	11%
kidney (renal)	21%
prostate*	0
testes	46%
cervix	5%
ovary	5%
osteosarcoma	10%
neuroblastoma	5%
head and neck	6%

* uncommon, but does occur

to locate primary sites include: intraocular, GI mucosa).

RENAL-CELL CARCINOMA
Usually associated with spread to lungs, lymph nodes, liver, bone, adrenals, and contralateral kidney before invading the CNS (thus, this tumor rarely presents as isolated cerebral metastases). Look for hematuria, abdominal pain, and/or abdominal mass on palpation or CT.

CLINICAL PRESENTATION

As with most brain tumors, signs and symptoms are usually slowly progressive compared to those from vascular events (ischemic or hemorrhagic infarcts) which tend to be sudden in onset and slowly resolve, or electrical events (seizures) which tend to be sudden in onset and rapidly resolve. There are no findings that would allow differentiation of a metastatic tumor from a primary neoplasm on clinical grounds.

Signs and symptoms include:
1. those due to increased ICP from mass effect and/or blockage of CSF drainage (hydrocephalus):
   A. headache (**H/A**): the most common presenting symptom, occurs in ≈ 50%
   B. nausea/vomiting
2. focal deficits:
   A. due to compression of brain parenchyma by mass and/or peritumoral edema (e.g. monoparesis without sensory disturbance)
   B. due to compression of cranial nerve
3. seizures: occur only in ≈ 15% of cases
4. mental status changes: depression, lethargy, apathy, confusion
5. symptoms suggestive of a TIA (dubbed "tumor TIA") or stroke, may be due to:
   A. occlusion of a vessel by tumor cells
   B. hemorrhage into the tumor, especially common with metastatic melanoma, choriocarcinoma, and renal cell carcinoma[437] (see *Hemorrhagic brain tumors*, page 854). May also occur due to decreased platelet count

EVALUATION

IMAGING STUDIES (CT OR MRI)
Metastases usually appear as "non-complicated" masses on CT (i.e. round, well circumscribed), often arising at the gray/white junction. Characteristically, profound white matter edema ("fingers of edema") reach deep into brain from the tumor, usually more pronounced than that seen with primary (infiltrating) brain tumors. When multiple lesions are present (on CT or MRI of brains with multiple mets) Chamber's rule applies: "Whoever counts the most mets is right." Mets usually enhance, and must be considered in the differential diagnosis of a ring-enhancing lesion.

Solitary supratentorial lesion on CT[425]
* brain mets from solid tumors are solitary on CT in 50-65% of cases
* with negative Ca history, negative CXR and negative IVP (presumably, this would also apply if a chest/abdominal/pelvic CT was negative): 7% of solitary lesions are mets, 87% are primary brain tumors, and 6% are nonneoplastic. Yield of further workup to find primary is low (recommendation: follow serial CXRs)
* with history of treated Ca: 93% of solitary lesions are mets

MRI
More sensitive than CT, especially in the p-fossa (including brain stem). Detects multiple mets in ≈ 20% of single mets on CT[424]. Multiple projections may also assist in surgical planning.

LUMBAR PUNCTURE
May be indicated once mass lesion has been ruled out. May be most useful in diagnosing carcinomatous meningitis (*see Carcinomatous meningitis*, page 491).

METASTATIC WORKUP

Prior to obtaining tissue from brain lesion: When metastatic disease is suspected based on imaging or on surgical tissue, a search for a primary site and assessment for other lesions may be considered and should include:

1. CXR: to rule out lung primary or other mets to lung
2. CT of the chest (more sensitive that CXR), abdomen and pelvis: to rule out renal or GI primary (second choice: IVP) or liver mets
3. test stool for occult blood
4. radionuclide bone scan: for patients with bone pain or for tumors that tend to produce osseous metastases (especially: prostate, breast, kidney, thyroid & lung)
5. mammogram in women
6. PET scan: can detect small malignancies

Once pathology of brain lesion is available:
Small cell carcinoma metastatic to the brain is most likely from the lung (positive for **neuroendocrine** stains (*see page 500*)).

MANAGEMENT

With optimal treatment, median survival of patients with cerebral mets is still only ≈ 26-32 weeks, therefore management is mostly palliative (also see *Outcome*, page 490 for comparison of various treatments).

Confirming the diagnosis
Caution: 11% of patients with abnormalities on brain CT or MRI with a history of cancer (within past 5 yrs) do not have cerebral metastases[438]. Differential diagnoses include: glioblastoma multiforme, low grade astrocytoma, abscess, and nonspecific inflammatory reaction. If non-surgical treatment (e.g. chemotherapy or RTX) is being contemplated, strong consideration should be given to confirming the diagnosis by biopsy.

Management decisions
Table 17-57 shows a summary of management suggestions (details appear in following sections).

Also, surgical excision is indicated for patients with renal cell Ca or melanoma in whom chemotherapy with interleukin-2 **(IL-2)** is being considered since this drug produces significant cerebral edema if there are any cerebral mets from these primary.

MEDICAL MANAGEMENT
Initial treatment:
1. anticonvulsants: e.g. phenytoin. Generally not needed for posterior fossa lesions
2. corticosteroids: many symptoms are due to peritumoral edema (which is primarily vasogenic), and respond to steroids within 24-48 hrs. This improvement is not permanent, and prolonged steroid administration may produce side effects (see *Possible deleterious side effects of steroids*, page 10).
Rx typical dose for a patient with significant symptoms who is not already on steroids: dexamethasone (Decadron®) 10-20 mg IV, followed by 6 mg IV q 6

Table 17-57 Management suggestions for cerebral metastases*

Clinical situation	Management
unknown primary or unconfirmed diagnosis	stereotactic biopsy for ≈ all patients if surgical excision is not a consideration
uncontrolled widespread systemic cancer & obviously short life expectancy and/or poor performance status (Karnofsky ≤ 70)	(biopsy as indicated above) + WBRT or no treatment
Stable systemic disease & good performance status	
solitary met — symptomatic, large, or accessible lesion	surgical excision + WBRT
asymptomatic, small, or inaccessible lesion	WBRT ± SRS boost
multiple mets — single large lesion that is life threatening or producing mass effect	surgery for the large lesion + WBRT for the rest
≤ 3 lesions: symptomatic & can all be removed	surgery + WBRT or SRS + WBRT
≤ 3 lesions: cannot all be removed	WBRT or SRS + WBRT
> 3 lesions: with no mass effect requiring surgery	WBRT

* adapted[439]. Abbreviations: WBRT = whole brain radiation therapy, SRS = stereotactic radiosurgery

hrs for 2-3 days, after which it is converted to ≈ 4 mg PO QID. Once symptoms are controlled, this is tapered to ≈ 2-4 mg PO TID as long as symptoms do not worsen
3. H₂ antagonists (e.g. ranitidine 150 mg PO q 12 hrs)

CHEMOTHERAPY

Limitations of chemotherapy in the brain are discussed on *page 407*. If multiple lesions of known small cell Ca are detected on cerebral imaging, treatment of choice is radiation plus chemotherapy.

RADIATION THERAPY

Caution: not all brain lesions in cancer patients are mets (*see above*).

In patients not considered for surgery, steroids and radiation usually help H/A, and in ≈ 50% of cases symptoms improve or completely resolve[440]. This does not result in local control for the majority of these patients and they frequently succumb from progressive brain disease.

The usual dose is **30 Gy in 10 fractions given over 2 weeks**. With this dose, 11% of 1-yr survivors and 50% of 2-yr survivors develop severe dementia.

Tumors that are considered "radiosensitive" to whole brain radiation therapy (**WBRT**) are shown in *Table 17-58*. Other metastases, e.g. large cell Ca of the lung and malignant melanoma are considered "radioresistant".

Table 17-58 "Radiosensitive" metastases[438]
• small-cell lung Ca
• germ-cell tumors
• lymphoma
• leukemia
• multiple myeloma

Prophylactic cranial irradiation

Prophylactic cranial irradiation after resection of small cell lung carcinoma (**SCLC**) reduces relapses in brain, but does not affect survival[441].

Post-op radiation therapy

WBRT is usually recommended following craniotomy for metastatic disease[119], especially with SCLC where "micro-metastases" are presumed to be present throughout brain^A.

Optimal dose is controversial. Early reports recommended 30-39 Gy over 2-2.5 weeks (3 Gy fractions) with or without surgery[443]. This is acceptable in patients not expected to live long enough to get long-term radiation effects. Recent recommendations are for smaller daily fractions of 1.8-2.0 Gy to reduce neurotoxicity[444]. These low doses are also associated with a higher rate of recurrent brain metastases[445]. Since 50 Gy are needed to achieve > 90% control of micrometastases, some use **45-50 Gy WBRT**, plus a boost to the tumor bed to bring the total treatment up to 55 Gy, all with low **fractions of 1.80-2.0 Gy**[446].

Stereotactic radiosurgery

Inconsistent in its ability to reduce tumor size. *See page 491*.

SURGICAL MANAGEMENT

SOLITARY LESIONS

Indications favoring surgical excision of a solitary lesion:
1. primary disease quiescent
2. lesion accessible
3. lesion is symptomatic or life-threatening
4. primary tumor known to be relatively radioresistant (excision is rarely indicated for untreated brain metastases from SCLC because of its radiosensitivity)
5. for recurrent SCLC following XRT
6. diagnosis unknown: alternatively consider biopsy, e.g. stereotactic biopsy

Surgical resection in patients with progressive systemic disease and/or significant neurologic deficit is probably unjustified[447]. Also, in newly diagnosed cancer patients, craniotomy may delay systemic treatment for weeks and the ramifications of this need

---

A. some centers do not routinely administer post-op WBRT (except for very radiosensitive tumors such as SCLC) but instead follow patients with serial imaging studies and administer XRT only when metastases are documented

to be considered.

MULTIPLE LESIONS

Patients with multiple metastases generally have much worse survival than those with solitary lesions[444]. Multiple metastases are usually treated with XRT without surgery. However, if total excision of all mets is feasible, then even multiple mets may be removed with survival similar to those having a single met removed[448] (also *see Table 17-57* for summary). If only incomplete excision is possible (i.e. cannot remove all mets, or portions of 1 or more must be left behind) then there is no improvement in survival with surgery, and XRT alone is recommended. The mortality of removing > 1 met at a single sitting is not statistically significantly higher than removing a single met.

Situations where surgery may be indicated for multiple mets[449]:
1. one particular and accessible lesion is clearly symptomatic and/or life threatening (life-threatening lesions include p-fossa and large temporal lobe lesions). This is palliative treatment to reduce the symptom/threat from that particular lesion
2. multiple lesions that can all be completely removed (*see above*)
3. no diagnosis (e.g. no identifiable primary): consider stereotactic biopsy

STEREOTACTIC BIOPSY

Considered for:
1. lesions not appropriate for surgery. Includes cases with no definite diagnosis and:
   A. deep lesions
   B. multiple small lesions
2. patients not candidates for surgical resection
   A. poor medical condition
   B. poor neurologic condition
   C. active or widespread systemic disease
3. to ascertain a diagnosis
   A. when another diagnosis is possible: e.g. no other sites of metastases, long interval between primary cancer and detection of brain mets…
   B. especially if nonsurgical treatment modalities are planned (*see above*)

OUTCOME

Table 17-59 lists factors associated with better survival regardless of treatment. Also, the prognosis gets worse as the number of mets increases[439]. Median survival even with best treatment in some studies is only ≈ 6 months.

Natural history

By the time that neurologic findings develop, median survival among untreated patients is ≈ 1 month[450].

Steroids

Using steroids alone (to control edema) doubles survival[451] to 2 mos[A].

Table 17-59 Factors associated with better prognosis (with any treatment)

- Karnofsky score* > 70 (*see page 899*)
- age < 60 yrs
- metastases to brain only (no systemic mets)
- absent or controlled primary disease
- > 1 yr since diagnosis of primary
- the fewer the number of brain mets
- female gender

* the Karnofsky score is probably the most important predictor; those with a score of 100 had median survival > 150 weeks

Whole brain radiation therapy (WBRT)

WBRT + steroids increases survival to 3-6 mos[448]. 50% of deaths are due to progression of intracranial disease.

Surgery ± WBRT

Recurrence of tumor was significantly less frequent and more delayed with the use of post-op WBRT[442]. Length of survival was unchanged with supplemental use of WBRT. There is also an additional loss of cognitive function in many cases, and patients are rarely independent after WBRT.

In 33 patients treated with surgical resection of single mets and post-op WBRT[453]: median survival was 8 months; with 44% 1-yr survival. If no evidence of systemic Ca, 1-yr survival is 81%. If systemic Ca is present (active or inactive), 1-yr survival is 20%. Patients with solitary mets and no evidence of active systemic tumor have the best

---

A. NB: this is based largely on pre-CT era data, and the tumors were therefore probably larger than in current studies[452]

prognosis[440, 447]. With total removal, no recurrence nor new parenchymal mets occurred within 6 months, and the major cause of death was progression of Ca outside the CNS. A randomized trial verified the improved longevity and quality of survival of patients with solitary mets undergoing surgical excision plus WBRT vs. WBRT alone (40 weeks vs. 15 weeks median survival)[438]. The surgical mortality was 4% (≈ same as 30-day mortality in the RTX-only group). More patients treated with WBRT alone die of their brain mets than those who underwent surgery. Following total removal and post-op WBRT, 22% of patients will have recurrent brain tumor at 1 year[444]. This is better than surgery without XRT (with reported failure rates of 46%[444] and 85%[445]).

Stereotactic radiosurgery (SRS)
Also, see page 542. There has not been a randomized study to compare surgery to SRS. Retrospective studies suggest that SRS may be comparable to surgery[454]. However, a prospective (non-randomized, retrospectively matched) study[455] found a median survival of 7.5 mos with SRS vs. 16.4 mos with surgery, and a higher mortality from cerebral disease in the SRS group (with the mortality due to the SRS treated lesions and not new lesions). A local control rate of ≈ 88% has been reported, with one study also recommending WBRT following the SRS for better regional control[456].

Actuarial control rates at 1 year following SRS + WBRT were 75-80% and appear to be similar to surgery + WBRT[439]. However, SRS was unreliable in reducing tumor size.

Multiple mets
Patients with multiple mets that were totally removed have a survival that is similar to those having single mets surgically removed[448] (see above).

17.6.   Carcinomatous meningitis

Carcinomatous meningitis (CM) AKA (lepto)meningeal carcinomatosis (LMC). Found in up to 8% of patients autopsied with systemic Ca. Up to 48% may present with CM before the presence of systemic Ca is known. Most common primaries: breast, lung, then melanoma[206 (p 610-2)]. Always include lymphomatous meningitis in the differential diagnosis (see CNS lymphoma, page 461).

CLINICAL
Simultaneous onset of findings in multiple levels of neuraxis. Multiple cranial nerve findings are frequent (in up to 94%, most common: VII, III, V & VI), usually progressive. Most frequent symptoms: H/A, mental status changes, lethargy, seizure, ataxia. Non-obstructive hydrocephalus is also common. Painful radiculopathies can occur with "drop mets".

DIAGNOSIS

Lumbar puncture
Perform only after mass lesion has been ruled out with cranial CT or MRI. Although the initial LP may be normal, CSF is eventually abnormal in > 95%.

CSF should be sent for:
1. cytology to look for malignant cells (requires ≈ 10 ml for adequate evaluation for CM). Repeat if negative (45% positive on first study, 81% eventually positive after up to 6 LPs). May need to pass CSF through a millipore filter
2. bacterial and fungal cultures (including unusual organisms, e.g. cryptococcus)
3. tumor markers: carcinoembryonic antigen, alpha-fetoprotein
4. protein/glucose: elevated protein is the most common abnormality. Glucose may be as low as ≈ 40 mg% in about a third of patients

MRI
Contrast enhanced MRI is more sensitive in showing meningeal enhancement[457].

CT
May show (mild) ventricular dilatation, enhancement of basal cisterns. Sulcal enhancement may also occur with involvement of the convexities.

Myelography
Spinal seeding ("drop mets") will produce filling defects on myelography.

Untreated: < 2 months. With radiation therapy + chemotherapy: median survival is 5.8 mos (range 1-29). Chemotherapy may be given intrathecally. About half of patients die of CNS involvement, and half die of systemic disease.

17.7.   Foramen magnum tumors

DIFFERENTIAL DIAGNOSIS

See *Foramen magnum lesions* on page 924 for <u>nonneoplastic</u> lesions. Most foramen magnum **(FM)** region tumors are extra-axial. This includes:
1.   meningioma: the anterior lip of the foramen magnum is the second most common site of origin of posterior fossa meningiomas. Meningiomas comprise 38-46% of FM tumors[155, 156] (*see page 427*) and most are intradural
2.   chordoma
3.   neurilemmoma
4.   epidermoid
5.   chondroma
6.   chondrosarcoma
7.   metastases
8.   exophytic component of a brainstem tumor

PRESENTATION

In the pre-imaging era (i.e. before CT & MRI) these lesions were often diagnosed relatively late due to the unusual associated clinical syndromes and the rarity of visualizing this region on myelography.

CLINICAL FINDINGS

Symptoms:
1.   sensory
    A.   craniocervical pain: usually an early symptom, commonly in neck and occiput. Aching in nature. ↑ with head movement
    B.   sensory findings: usually occur later. Numbness and tingling of the fingers
2.   motor
    A.   spastic weakness of the extremities: weakness usually starts in the ipsilateral UE, then the ipsilateral LE, then contralateral LE, and finally contralateral UE ("rotating paralysis")

Signs:
1.   sensory
    A.   dissociated sensory loss: loss of pain and temperature contralateral to lesion with preservation of tactile sensation
    B.   loss of position and vibratory sense, greater in the upper than the lower extremities
2.   motor
    A.   spastic weakness of the extremities
    B.   atrophy of the intrinsic hand muscles: a lower motor nerve finding
    C.   cerebellar findings may rarely be present with extensive intracranial extension
3.   long tract findings
    A.   brisk muscle stretch reflexes (hyperreflexia, spasticity)
    B.   loss of abdominal cutaneous reflexes
    C.   neurogenic bladder: usually a very late finding
4.   ipsilateral Horner's syndrome: due to compression of cervical sympathetics
5.   nystagmus: classically downbeat (*see page 580*), but other types can occur

It had been postulated that long tract findings were due to direct compression at the cervicomedullary junction, and that lower motor nerve findings in the upper extremities were due to central necrosis of the grey matter as a result of compression of arterial blood supply. Anatomic study suggests that it is actually <u>venous</u> infarction at lower cervical levels (C8-T1) that is responsible for the lower motor neuron findings.

Surgical approaches:
1. transoral approach: *see page 613* for technique
   A. disadvantage: cannot reach to > 1 cm to either side of midline
   B. almost exclusively for extradural lesions (although some intra-axial lesions have been approached, the experience is extremely limited)
2. extreme lateral transcondylar approach
   A. disadvantage: lack of familiarity of most neurosurgeons with this approach
   B. advantage: excellent exposure of anterior foramen magnum with proximal control of vertebral artery
3. lateral posterior fossa approach: see *Posterior fossa (suboccipital) craniectomy*, page 604 for technique
   A. disadvantage: cannot reach midline or contralateral component, however, some tumor in these regions may be pulled into the field as the tumor is debulked

17.8. Idiopathic intracranial hypertension

❦ Key features
• papilledema and symptomatic ICP elevation > 20 cm, in the absence of intracranial mass or infection
• more common in obese females of childbearing age than general population
• imaging studies (CT or routine MRI) of brain are normal (allowed exception: slit-like ventricles). CSF is normal except for increased pressure
• usually self-limited, recurrence is common, chronic in some patients
• a preventable cause of (often permanent) blindness from optic atrophy
• risk of blindness is not reliably correlated to duration of symptoms, papilledema, H/A, Snellen visual acuity, or number of recurrences
• for patients failing medical management (weight loss, Diamox…)
   ◆ optic nerve sheath fenestration is best for visual loss without H/A
   ◆ CSF shunting is better for H/A than ONSF

Idiopathic intracranial hypertension (**IIH**), AKA **pseudotumor cerebri**, AKA **benign intracranial hypertension**, (plus numerous other obsolete terms[458]) is a heterogeneous group of conditions characterized by increased intracranial pressure with no evidence of intracranial mass, hydrocephalus, infection (e.g. chronic fungal meningitis), or hypertensive encephalopathy. Some, but not all, authors exclude patients with intracranial hypertension in the presence of dural sinus thrombosis. IIH is thus a diagnosis of exclusion. There is a juvenile and an adult form.

EPIDEMIOLOGY
1. female:male ratio reported ranges from 2:1 to 8:1 (in juvenile form)
2. obesity is reported in 11-90% of cases, and is not as prevalent in men[459]
3. incidence among obese women of childbearing years[460, 461]: 19-21/100,000, (whereas incidence in general population[458]: 1-2/100,000)
4. peak incidence in 3rd decade (range: 1-55 years). 37% of cases are in children, 90% of these are age 5-15 years. Very rare in infancy
5. frequently self limited (recurrence rate: 9-43%)
6. severe visual deficits develop in 4-12%, unrelated to duration of symptoms, degree of papilledema, headache, visual obscuration, and number of recurrences[462]. Perimetry is the best means to detect and follow visual loss

PATHOGENESIS
Not fully understood. Increased cerebral edema & brain water content, increased venous pressure & cerebral blood volume, and reduced CSF absorption have all been demonstrated. Theories that also explain the high prevalence in obese females:
1. mechanical theory: obesity → ↑ intraabdominal pressure → ↑ central venous pressure → ↓ CSF resorption → ↑ ICP[A]
2. hormonal theory: adipocytes convert androstenedione → estrone → ↑ CSF production

EVALUATION RECOMMENDATIONS

Most tests are intended to rule out conditions that may mimic IIH.

1. cerebral imaging: cerebral CT or MRI (*see below*) scan without and with contrast
2. LP:
   A. measure opening pressure **(OP)** with patient in lateral decubitus position
   B. CSF analysis to rule-out infection (e.g. fungus, TB or Lyme disease), inflammation (e.g. sarcoidosis, SLE) or neoplasm (e.g. carcinomatous meningitis)
      1. protein/glucose
      2. cell count
      3. routine & fungal cultures
      4. cytology if suspicion of carcinomatous meningitis
3. routine labs: CBC, electrolytes, PT/PTT
4. W/U for sarcoidosis or SLE if other findings suggestive (e.g. cutaneous nodules, hypercoagulable state...)
5. neuro-ophthalmologic evaluation is recommended. Includes: visual field testing using quantitative perimetry, with evaluation of size of blind spot, slit-lamp examination ± fundus photographs
6. check BP to R/O malignant HTN → hypertensive encephalopathy (*see page 497*)

Diagnostic criteria

Modified Dandy's criteria are shown in *Table 17-60*.

More specifically, four diagnostic criteria[464]:

1. CSF pressure: > 20 cm H_2O (pressures > 40 are not uncommon)[A]. Some recommend that the pressure should be > 25 to exclude normals[465]
2. CSF composition: normal glucose and cell count. Protein is normal, or in ≈ two thirds of cases it is low (< 20 mg%)
3. symptoms & signs are those of elevated ICP alone, i.e. papilledema & H/A, with no focal findings (with the allowed exception of abducens nerve palsy which may be due to increased ICP, *see page 586*)
4. normal radiologic studies of the brain (CT or MRI) with the allowed exceptions of:
   A. the occasionally seen slit ventricles (the incidence may be no higher in IIH than in age-matched controls[466]) or empty sella
   B. infantile form may have generous ventricles and large fluid spaces over brain
   C. intra-orbital abnormalities may be seen: *see below*

Table 17-60 Modified Dandy's criteria for IIH

- signs & symptoms of increased ICP
- no localizing signs other than Cr. N VI palsy* in an otherwise awake and alert patient
- increased CSF pressure without chemical or cytological abnormalities
- normal to small ventricles and no intracranial mass

* may result from ↑ ICP (*see page 586*)

CT

Usually adequate to R/O intracranial mass as a possible cause of intracranial hypertension, but may miss cases of dural sinus thrombosis. MRI & MRV are preferred.

MRI

Intracranial abnormalities are usually absent or minimal (slit ventricles, empty sella in 30-70%). However, intraorbital findings may be more substantial and include[467]:

1. flattening of the posterior sclera: occurs in 80%
2. enhancement of the prelaminar optic nerve: in 50%
3. distention of the perioptic subarachnoid space: in 45%
4. vertical tortuosity of the orbital optic nerve: in 40%
5. intraocular protrusion of the prelaminar optic nerve: in 30%

Venography

Conventional venography or MRV (MR venography) to rule-out dural sinus or venous thrombosis.

A. however, other studies have indicated that elevated venous pressure may actually be an epiphenomenon to a primary increase in ICP[463]

A. diurnal variations in CSF pressure may occasionally cause a falsely low (i.e normal) reading. In these cases, if clinical suspicion is high, an LP at a different time of day may be required

- symptoms
  - A. classic (major) symptoms
    1. H/A (the most common symptom): 94-99%. Typically retro-ocular and pulsatile. May ↑ with eye movement. Severity does not correlate with degree of CSF pressure elevation. Occasionally worse in A.M.
    2. nausea: 32% (actual vomiting is less common)
    3. visual loss (see *Visual loss in IIH* below):
        a. transient visual obscuration (**TVO**)
        b. permanent afferent visual pathway injury
    4. diplopia (more common in adult, usually due to VI nerve palsy): 30%
  - B. minor symptoms[469]
    1. neck stiffness: 30-50%
    2. tinnitus[A]: up to 60%. Usually pulse synchronous. Described as rushing noise. May be unilateral (in these, may be reduced by ipsilateral jugular vein compression + ipsilateral head rotation)
    3. ataxia: 4-11%
    4. acral paresthesias: 25%
    5. retrobulbar eye pain on eye movements
    6. arthralgia[A]: 11-18%
    7. dizziness: 32%
    8. fatigue
    9. reduced olfactory acuity
- signs (generally restricted to visual system)
  - A. papilledema:
    1. present in almost ≈ 100%
    2. idiopathic intracranial hypertension without papilledema (**IIH-WOP**)[470]. a variant of IIH. Visual loss tends not to occur
    3. usually bilateral, occasionally unilateral[471]
    4. may be mild (subtle nerve fiber elevation)
  - B. abducens nerve (Cr. N. VI) palsy: 20% (a false localizing sign, *see page 586*). The esotropia ranges from < 5 prism diopters dysconjugate angle in primary gaze to > 50[467]
  - C. changes in visual acuity: relatively insensitive assessment of visual function
  - D. enlarged blind spot (66%) and concentric constriction of peripheral fields (blindness is very rare at presentation)
  - E. visual field defect: 9%. Early changes: peripheral fields & nasal quadrant
  - F. infantile form may have only enlarging OFC, frequently self limited, usually requires only follow-up without specific treatment
  - G. conspicuous absence of altered level of consciousness in spite of high ICP

 Worsening of any of the above symptoms with postural changes that increase ICP (bending over, Valsalva maneuver…) is characteristic in idiopathic intracranial hypertension.

Visual loss in IIH

Quoted range of occurrence in IIH: 48-68% (lower numbers generally come from population based samples). A prospective study found changes by Goldman perimetry in 96% of 50 patients[472]. The only other factor associated with worsening vision is recent weight gain.

Pathomechanics: Increased ICP is transmitted along optic nerve sheath → circumferential compression of the retinal ganglion cell axons at the level of the lamina cribrosa[467].

Manifestations:
1. **transient visual obscurations (TVO)**: graying or blacking out of vision. Lasts ≈ 1 second. Uni- or bi-lateral. Typically occur with eye movement, bending over or Valsalva maneuver. Directly proportional to severity of papilledema. Frequency of TVOs parallels ICP elevation, but does not correlate with permanent visual loss

---

A. the causal relationship with IIH has been demonstrated by resolution of these symptoms with reduction of CSF pressure

2. visual loss in IIH may occur early or late, may be sudden or gradually progressive, and is not reliably correlated to duration of symptoms, papilledema, H/A, Snellen visual acuity, or number of recurrences. It may escape detection until profound. Early: usually constriction of fields and loss of color (∴ perimetry is the best test for following vision in IIH). Later: central vision is affected. Findings include: concentric constrictions, enlargement of the blind spot, inferior nasal defects, arcuate defects, cecocentral scotomas...

ASSOCIATED CONDITIONS

By definition, IIH is idiopathic. However, often what is considered "IIH" may actually be secondary to some other condition (e.g. thrombosis of the transverse sinus, see below). Many conditions that are cited as being associated with IIH may be coincidental. Four criteria shown in Table 17-61 have been suggested to establish a cause-effect relationship[468].

Table 17-61   Criteria for causality of IIH by another condition[468]

A.	meets Dandy's criteria (Table 17-60, page 494)
B.	the condition should be proven to increase ICP
C.	treatment of the condition should improve the IIH
D.	properly controlled studies should show an association between the condition and IIH

Digre[473] has proposed a scale (see Table 17-62) to rank the likelihood of association between various conditions and IIH based on the number of the criteria in Table 17-61 that are met.

Other conditions not included in this list that meet minimal criteria but are unconfirmed in case-control studies[458] include:
1. other drugs: isotretinoin (Accutane®), trimethoprim-sulfamethoxazole, cimetidine, tamoxifen
2. systemic lupus erythematosus (**SLE**)

Conditions that may be related by virtue of increased pressure in the dural sinuses (see below) (some have called this "secondary IIH" which is an oxymoron):
1. otitis media with petrosal extension (so-called otitic hydrocephalus)
2. radical neck surgery with resection of the jugular vein
3. hypercoagulable states

VENOUS HYPERTENSION & SINOVENOUS ABNORMALITIES

Venous hypertension has often been proposed as a unifying underlying cause of IIH. Abnormalities of the dural sinuses, including thrombosis, stenosis[474], obstruction, or elevated pressure have been demonstrated. While these findings may underlie a significant number of

Table 17-62   Conditions that may be associated with IIH[473]

Proven association Meets 4 criteria from Table 17-61
• obesity
Likely association Meets 3 criteria from Table 17-61
• drugs: keprone, lindane
• hypervitaminosis A
Probable association Meets 2 criteria from Table 17-61
• steroid withdrawal*
• thyroid replacement in children
• ketoprofen & indomethacin in Bartter syndrome
• hypoparathyroidism
• Addison's disease*
• uremia
• iron deficiency anemia
• drugs: tetracycline, nalidixic acid, Danazol, lithium, amiodarone, phenytoin, nitrofurantoin, cirpofloxacin, nitroglycerin
Possible association Meets 1 criterion from Table 17-61
• menstrual irregularity
• oral contraceptive use†
• Cushing's syndrome
• Vitamin A deficiency
• minor head trauma
• Behçet syndrome
Unlikely association Meets none of the criteria in Table 17-61
• hyperthyroidism
• steroid use
• immunization
Unsupported association
• pregnancy
• menarche

*   may respond to steroids

†   may be associated with dural sinus thrombosis, see text

cases, they may in actuality be epiphenomena (e.g. venous hypertension may be due to compression of the transverse sinuses by elevated intracranial pressure[463]), and it is unlikely that such abnormalities will explain all cases.

DIFFERENTIAL DIAGNOSIS
1. true mass lesions: tumor, cerebral abscess, subdural hematomas, rarely gliomatosis cerebri may be undetectable on CT and will be misdiagnosed as IIH

2. cranial venous outflow impairment (some authors consider these as IIH)[475]
   A. dural sinus thrombosis (*see above* and *page 888*)
   B. congestive heart failure
   C. superior vena cava syndrome
   D. unilateral or bilateral jugular vein or sigmoid sinus[476] obstruction
   E. hyperviscosity syndromes
   F. Masson's vegetant intravascular hemangioendothelioma[477]: an uncommon, usually benign lesion that may rarely involve the neuraxis (including intracranial occurrence)
3. Chiari I malformation (**CIM**): may produce findings similar to IIH. 6% of IIH patients have significant tonsillar ectopia, and ≈ 5% of patient with CIM have papilledema[467]
4. infection (CSF will be abnormal in most of these): encephalitis, arachnoiditis, meningitis (especially basal meningitis or granulomatous infections, e.g. syphilitic meningitis, chronic cryptococcal meningitis), chronic brucellosis
5. inflammatory conditions: e.g. neurosarcoidosis (*see page 56*), SLE
6. vasculitis: e.g. Behçet's syndrome
7. metabolic conditions: e.g. lead poisoning
8. pseudopapilledema (anomalous elevation of the optic nerve head) associated with hyperopia and drusen. Retinal venous pulsations are usually present. Especially deceptive when a patient with migraines has pseudopapilledema: treat the H/A
9. malignant hypertension: may produce H/A & bilateral optic disc edema which can be indistinguishable from papilledema. May also produce hypertensive encephalopathy (*see page 64*). Check BP in all IIH suspects
10. meningeal carcinomatosis
11. Guillain-Barré syndrome: CSF protein is usually elevated (*see page 53*)
12. following head trauma

TREATMENT AND MANAGEMENT

NATURAL HISTORY

Spontaneous resolution is common, sometimes within months, but usually after ≈ 1 year. Papilledema persists in ≈ 15%. Permanent visual loss occurs in 2-24%. Persistent H/A may occur in some. Recurs in ≈ 10% after initial resolution[467].

INTERVENTIONS

Studies are often difficult to interpret especially since spontaneous remission is common.
1. all patients must have repeated thorough ophthalmologic exams (*see above*)
2. stop possible offending drugs
3. weight loss: a weight loss of 6% usually results in complete resolution of papilledema[478]. However, resolution may be too slow for acutely threatened vision. Weight loss is also associated with reduction of other health risks of obesity. Symptoms recur if the weight is regained
   A. dieting: [479]rarely accomplished or sustained
   B. bariatric surgery: gastric bypass, laparoscopic banding...
4. treatment of asymptomatic IIH patients is controversial as there is no reliable predictor for visual loss. Close follow up with serial formal visual field evaluation is necessary. Intervention is recommended in unreliable patients, or whenever visual fields deteriorate. It is possible to lose vision without H/A or papilledema
5. most cases remit by 6-15 weeks, however relapse is common
6. medical treatment
   A. fluid and salt restriction
   B. diuretics (slows CSF production)
      1. carbonic anhydrase (**CA**) inhibitors:
         a. acetazolamide (Diamox®): **Rx** start at 125-250 mg PO q 8-12 hrs, or long acting Diamox Sequels® 500 mg PO BID. Increase by 250 mg/day until symptoms improve, side effects occur, or 2 gm/day reached. SIDE EFFECTS: (in high doses): acral paresthesias, nausea, metabolic acidosis, altered taste, renal calculi, drowsiness. Rare: Stevens-Johnson syndrome, toxic epidermal necrolysis, agranulocytosis. ✖ Contraindicated with allergy to sulfa or a history of renal calculi
         b. methazolamide (Neptazane®): better tolerated but less effec-

tive. *Rx* 50-100 mg PO BID-TID. SIDE EFFECTS: similar to acetazolamide

    c.   topiramate (Topamax®): anticonvulsant with secondary inhibi-
tion of CA. *Rx* 200 mg PO BID. SIDE EFFECTS: Similar to acetazolamide, but can be used in sulfa allergic patients

  2. furosemide (Lasix®)

    a.   start: 160 mg per day in adults, adjust per symptoms and eye
exam (not to CSF pressure)

    b.   if ineffective, double (320 mg/day)

    c.   monitor K⁺ levels and supplement as needed

  C. if ineffective, add steroids (options: dexamethasone (Decadron®) 12 mg/day,
prednisone 40-60 mg/day, or methylprednisolone 250 mg IV q 6 hrs). May ↑
CSF resorption in cases of inflammation or venous thrombosis. Can be used
as temporizing agents for patients awaiting surgery. A reduction in symptoms should occur by 2 weeks, after which time the steroid should be tapered over 2 weeks. Long-term use is not recommended due to, among other
things, associated weight gain

  7. surgical therapy[206] [(p 250-3)] only for cases refractory to above, or where visual loss is
progressive or is severe initially or unreliable patient:

    A. serial LPs until remission (25% remit after 1st LP[480]): remove up to 30 ml to
halve OP, perform qod until OP < 20 cm H₂0, then decrease to q wk (no patient who had remission by 2nd LP had OP > 350 on 1st LP). Use a large
gauge needle (e.g. 18 Ga) which may help promote a post-LP CSF leak into
subcutaneous tissues. LPs may be difficult in obese patients. Revisions may
be required in up to 50%. SIDE EFFECTS: include sciatica from nerve root irritation, acquired cerebellar tonsillar herniation (*see page 189*), spinal H/A
(from intracranial hypotension)

    B. shunts

      1. lumbar shunt: usually lumboperitoneal. May be difficult in obese pa-
tient. May need a horizontal-vertical valve (*see page 189*) to prevent
H/A from intracranial hypotension. Alternative: lumbopleural shunt

      2. other shunts may be used, especially when arachnoiditis precludes
use of lumbar subarachnoid space, e.g.:

        • VP shunt: often difficult since the ventricles are frequently
small or slit-like[481]. Stereotactic techniques may make this more
technically feasible

        • cisterna magna shunt: may shunt to vascular system

    C. optic nerve sheath fenestration: *see below*

    D. obsolete treatment (presented for historical interest): subtemporal (advo-
cated by Dandy) or suboccipital decompression. Usually bilateral silver-dol-
lar size craniectomies under temporalis muscle to floor of middle fossa, open
dura, cover brain with absorbable sponge, close fascia and muscle watertight, anticonvulsants were started due to risk of post-op seizures

  8. interventional procedures: venous sinus stenting may be considered for refractory
cases[482]

  9. patients should be followed at least two years (with repeat imaging, e.g. MRI) to
R/O occult tumor

Optic nerve sheath fenestration (ONSF)[483-485]

    Generally better for protection of vision and reversal of papilledema than for other
symptoms (e.g. H/A). Performed via medial or less commonly a lateral orbitotomy or
transconjunctival medial approach. May reverse or stabilize visual deterioration[486] and
sometimes (but not always) lowers ICP (by continued CSF filtration) and may protect the
contralateral eye (if not, contralateral ONSF must be performed). Has succeeded in cases
where visual loss progressed after LP shunting[487], possibly due to poor communication
between orbital and intracranial subarachnoid spaces. SIDE EFFECTS: potential adverse include: pupillary dysfunction, peripapillary hemorrhage, chemosis, chorioretinal
scarring[488], diplopia (usually self-limited) from medial rectus disruption. Repeat fenestration is needed in 0-6%[467].

MANAGEMENT RECOMMENDATIONS FOR SPECIFIC SITUATIONS
Weight loss should be attempted in all.

  1. IIH patients with H/A and no visual loss: medical therapy to control ↑ ICP and
H/A. ONSF not recommended. Shunting is an option if medical management fails

  2. IIH with visual loss without H/A:

A. mild visual loss: acetazolamide 500-1500 mg/d, follow-up q 2 weeks
B. moderate visual loss: acetazolamide 2000-3000 mg/d, follow-up q week
C. severe visual loss that doesn't respond to acetazolamide, or optic disc at risk:
1. methylprednisolone 250 mg IV q 6 hrs + acetazolamide 1000 mg PO BID
2. if no improvement: ONSF. Consider shunt if ICP > 300 mm H_2O
3. IIH with visual loss AND H/A: for patients with surgical indications, either surgical procedure is appropriate. Shunting may relieve both problems simultaneously. ONSF may be more reliable to relieve the visual problems (the failure rate may be lower than the shunt malfunction rate) but is not as good for the H/A
4. IIHWOP: symptomatic treatment for H/A, diuretics
5. IIH in children and adolescents:
A. may be seen with withdrawal of steroids used for asthma
B. search for and correction of underlying etiology (offending drugs listed above, hypercalcemia, cancer…)
C. acetazolamide has been used with success
6. IIH in pregnancy:
A. women who first present with IIH during pregnancy: resolution of IIH following delivery is common
B. women who become pregnant during therapy:
1. 1st trimester: observation, limitation of weight gain, serial LPs.
✖ Acetazolamide should be avoided because of teratogenicity
2. 2nd & 3rd trimester: acetazolamide has been used safely, but involvement of high-risk obstetrician specialist is advised
7. pseudopapilledema (associated with drusen, etc., in the absence of IIH): no interventions[467]. Reassurance and H/A management are employed

17.9. Empty sella syndrome

Empty sella syndrome (ESS) can be "primary" or "secondary".

Primary empty sella syndrome

Herniation of the arachnoid membrane into the sella turcica[489] which can act as a mass, probably as a result of repeated CSF pulsation. The sella can become enlarged (see *Sella turcica*, page 138 for normal dimensions) and the pituitary gland may become compressed against the floor.

Most of these patients are obese women. The frequency of intrasellar arachnoid herniation is higher in patients with pituitary tumors and in those with increased intracranial pressure for any reason (including idiopathic intracranial hypertension, *see page 493*) than in the general population.

These patients usually present with symptoms that do not suggest an intrasellar abnormality including: headache (the most common symptom), dizziness, seizures… Occasionally patients may develop CSF rhinorrhea, deterioration of vision (acuity or field deficit resulting from kinking of optic chiasm due to herniation into the sella), or amenorrhea-galactorrhea syndrome.

Clinically evident endocrine disturbances are rare with primary ESS, however up to 30% have abnormal pituitary function tests, most commonly reduced growth hormone secretion following stimulation. Mild elevation of prolactin (PRL) and reduction of ADH may occur, probably from compression of the stalk. These patients show a normal PRL rise with TRH stimulation (whereas patients with prolactinomas do not).

Surgical treatment is usually not indicated, except in the case of CSF rhinorrhea. In this setting, it is necessary to determine if there is increased ICP, and if so, if there is an identifiable cause. Simple shunting for hydrocephalus runs the risk of producing tension pneumocephalus from air drawn in through the former leak site. This may necessitate transsphenoidal repair with simultaneous external lumbar drainage, to be converted to a permanent shunt shortly thereafter.

Secondary empty sella syndrome[490]

Occurs following successful transsphenoidal removal of a pituitary tumor. Often presents with visual deterioration due to herniation of the optic chiasm into the surgically evacuated sella.

17.10. Tumor markers

TUMOR MARKERS USED HISTOLOGICALLY IN NEUROSURGERY

GLIAL FIBRILLARY ACIDIC PROTEIN (GFAP)

Polypeptide, MW = 49,000 Daltons. Although the presence of GFAP usually indicates astroglial origin, it may occasionally be seen in oligodendrogliomas, ependymomas, and choroid plexus papillomas[159 p (30-1)]. GFAP is only rarely found outside the CNS (in nonmyelinated Schwann cells, epithelium of the lens, hepatic Kupffer cells...). Thus, the presence of GFAP in a tumor found in the CNS is usually taken as good evidence for glial origin of the tumor. GFAP also occurs in normal brain parenchyma.

S-100 PROTEIN

A low molecular weight (21,000 Daltons) calcium-binding protein. Used on tissue microscopy for pathology. May participate in regulation of microtubule assembly. In CNS tumors, the distribution is similar to GFAP, but it is not as specific as GFAP (may be found in other cell types such as stellate cells of the adenohypophysis, chondrocytes)[159 p (34-5)], melanomas. In the peripheral nervous system, it is localized in Schwann cells. May be helpful in distinguishing Schwann cells from perineurial cells.

Clinically has been measured in serum (see below).

CYTOKERATIN (HIGH & LOW MOLECULAR WEIGHT)

Stains epithelial cells. Most primary brain tumors do not stain positive. Supports the diagnosis of carcinoma. Therefore, may help distinguish metastatic tumors (that stain positive) from primary CNS tumors.

MIB-1 (AKA MONOCLONAL MOUSE ANTI-HUMAN KI-67 ANTIBODY)

Immunohistochemical stain for cells leaving the G_0/G_1-phase and entering the S-phase (performing DNA synthesis). A high MIB-1 labeling index denotes high mitotic activity which often correlates with degree of malignancy. Most often used in lymphomas and breast cancer. Also used in astrocytomas where a MIB-1 ≥ 7-9% suggests an anaplastic tumor, while MIB-1 < 5% favors a low-grade tumor.

NEUROENDOCRINE STAINS

Includes:
1. chromagranin: stains for neural crest derivatives, viz. pituitary adenomas, paragangliomas, neuroendocrine tumors
2. synaptophysin: stains neuronal and pineal tumors, PNET & medulloblastomas
3. neuron specific enolase (NSE): very sensitive but not specific for neuroendocrine

Metastases that are positive for neuroendocrine stains include: small cell carcinoma of the lung, malignant pheochromocytoma, Merkel cell tumor. Metastatic small cell tumors to the brain staining positive for neuroendocrine stains are almost all due to lung.

STAINING PATTERNS[491]

An individual tumor may lack a marker that is typically representative of its type. Therefore, a positive stain is more significant than a negative stain. General staining patterns are shown in Table 10-63.

TUMOR MARKERS USED CLINICALLY

HUMAN CHORIONIC GONADOTROPIN (hCG)

A glycoprotein, MW = 45,000. Secreted by placental trophoblastic epithelium. Beta chain (ß-hCG) is normally present only in the fetus or in gravid or postpartum females, otherwise it indicates disease. Classically associated with choriocarcinoma (uterine or testicular), also found in patients with embryonal cell tumors, teratocarcinoma of testis, and others.

CSF ß-hCG is 0.5-2% of serum ß-hCG in non-CNS tumors. Higher levels are diagnostic of cerebral mets from uterine or testicular choriocarcinoma, or primary choriocarcinoma or embryonal cell carcinoma of pineal (*see page 476*) or suprasellar region.

Table 10-63 Immunohistochemical staining patterns
for nervous system tumor masses of epithelioid cells*

Neoplasm	Immunohistochemical stain response† ‡					
	GFAP	CAM5.2	EMA	S-100	CgA	Syn
oligodendroglioma	+		−		−	
ependymoma				+		−
choroid plexus papilloma						+
chordoma		+				
craniopharyngioma	−		+	−	−	−
carcinoma						
pituitary adenoma					+	+
paraganglioma		−				
meningioma		+				
melanoma				+	−	−
hemangioblastoma		−	−			

* modified from McKeever, P E, Immunohistochemistry of the Nervous System, in Dobbs, D J Diagnostic Immunohistochemistry, Churchill Livingstone, NY, © 2002

† abbreviations: GFAP = glial fibrillary acidic protein, EMA = epithelial membrane antigen, CAM5.2 = cytokeratin CAM5.2, CgA = chromogranin A, syn = synaptophysin

‡ a "+" or a "−" sign indicates presence or absence of the stain respectively; a darkened entries indicate that the stain is not decisive for that particular tumor

ALPHA-FETOPROTEIN

Alpha-fetoprotein (**AFP**) is a normal fetal glycoprotein (MW = 70,000) initially produced by the yolk sac, and later by the fetal liver. It is found in the fetal circulation throughout gestation, and drops rapidly during the first few weeks of life, reaching normal adult levels by age 1 yr. It is detectable only in trace amounts in normal adult males or nonpregnant females. It is present in amniotic fluid in normal pregnancies, and is detectable in maternal serum starting at ≈ 12-14 weeks gestation, increasing steadily throughout pregnancy until ≈ 32 weeks[492].

Abnormally elevated serum AFP may occur in Ca of ovary, stomach, lung, colon, pancreas, as well as in cirrhosis or hepatitis and in the majority of gravid women carrying a fetus with an open neural tube defect (see *Prenatal detection of neural tube defects*, page 113). Serum AFP > 500 ng/ml usually means primary hepatic tumor.

CSF-AFP is elevated in some pineal region germ-cell tumors (*see page 477*). 16-25% of patients with testicular tumors get cerebral mets and elevated CSF AFP levels are reported in some.

CARCINOEMBRYONIC ANTIGEN (CEA)

A glycoprotein, MW ≈ 200,000. Normally present in fetal endodermal cells. Originally described with colorectal adeno-Ca, now known to be elevated in many malignant and nonmalignant conditions (including cholecystitis, colitis, diverticulitis, hepatic involvement from any tumor, with 50-90% of terminal patients having elevation).

CSF CEA: levels > 1 ng/ml are reported with leptomeningeal spread of lung Ca (89%), breast Ca (60-67%), malignant melanoma (25-33%), and bladder Ca. May be normal even in CEA secreting cerebral mets if they don't communicate with the subarachnoid space. Only carcinomatous meningitis from lung or breast Ca consistently elevates CSF CEA in the majority of patients.

S-100 PROTEIN

Serum S-100 protein levels rise after head trauma, and possibly after other insults to the brain. Levels may also be elevated in Creutzfeldt-Jakob disease (*see page 230*).

17.11. Neurocutaneous disorders

Formerly called **phakomatoses**. Neurocutaneous disorders **(NCD)** are a group of conditions, each with unique neurologic findings and benign cutaneous lesions (both skin and the CNS derive embryologically from ectoderm), usually with dysplasia of other organ systems (often including the eyes). With the exception of ataxia-telangiectasia (not discussed here) all exhibit autosomal dominant inheritance. There is also a high rate of spontaneous mutations. These syndromes should be kept in mind in a pediatric patient with a tumor, and other stigmata of these syndromes must be sought.

NCDs that are more likely to come to the attention of a neurosurgeon:
1. neurofibromatosis: *see below*
2. tuberous sclerosis: *see page 504*
3. von Hippel-Lindau disease: *see page 459*
4. Sturge Weber syndrome: *see page 505*
5. racemose angioma (Wyburn-Mason syndrome): midbrain and retinal AVMs

17.11.1. Neurofibromatosis

Neurofibromatosis **(NFT)** is the most common of the NCDs. There are as many as 6 distinct types, the two most common of which are compared in *Table 17-64* (variant forms also occur).

There is no cure for NFT. Treatment consists of amelioration of symptoms. Ketotifen (which inhibits histamine release from mast-cells) may relieve some pruritus and local tenderness, **Rx** 2-4 mg/d for 30-40 months[493].

Table 17-64 Comparison of neurofibromatosis types 1 and 2

current designation →	Neurofibromatosis 1	Neurofibromatosis 2
alternate term	von Recklinghausen's	bilateral acoustic NFT
obsolete term	peripheral NFT	central NFT
U.S. prevalence	100,000 people	≈ 3000 people
incidence	1/2500-3300 births (Michigan)	1 in 50,000
acoustic neuromas	almost never bilateral	bilateral acoustic neuromas are the hallmark

NEUROFIBROMATOSIS 1
(NFT-1 AKA VON RECKLINGHAUSEN'S DISEASE[494])

CLINICAL FEATURES
More common than NFT-2, representing > 90% of cases of neurofibromatosis.

Diagnostic criteria[495]: two or more of the following:
1. ≥ 6 **café au lait spots**[A], each ≥ 5 mm in greatest diameter in prepubertal individuals, or ≥ 15 mm in greatest diameter in postpubertal patients
2. ≥ 2 neurofibromas of any type, or one plexiform neurofibroma (neurofibromas are usually not evident until age 10-15 yrs). May be painful
3. freckling (hyperpigmentation) in the axillary or intertriginous (inguinal) areas
4. optic glioma: *see below*
5. ≥ 2 Lisch nodules: pigmented iris hamartomas that appear as translucent yellow/brown elevations that tend to become more numerous with age
6. distinctive osseous abnormality, such as sphenoid dysplasia or thinning of long bone cortex with or without pseudarthrosis (e.g. of tibia or radius)
7. a first degree relative (parent, sibling or offspring) with NFT-1 by above criteria

Associated conditions:
- Schwann-cell tumors on any nerve (but bilateral AN are virtually nonexistent)
- spinal and/or peripheral-nerve neurofibromas

A. café au lait spots: hyperpigmented oval light brown skin macules (flat). May be present at birth, increase in number and size during 1st decade. Are present in > 99% of NFT-1 cases. Rare on face

- multiple skin neurofibromas
- aqueductal stenosis: *see page 110*
- macrocephaly
- intracranial tumors: hemispheric astrocytomas are the most common, solitary or multicentric meningiomas (usually in adults)
- unilateral defect in superior orbit → pulsatile exophthalmos
- neurologic or cognitive impairment
- kyphoscoliosis (seen in 2-10%, often progressive which then requires surgical stabilization)
- visceral manifestations from involvement of autonomic nerves or ganglia within the organ
- syringomyelia
- malignant tumors that have increased frequency in NFT: neuroblastoma, ganglioglioma, sarcoma, leukemia, Wilm's tumor
- pheochromocytoma: unusual. Never seen in children

GENETICS

Simple autosomal dominant inheritance with variable expressivity but almost 100% penetrance after age 5 years. The NFT-1 gene is on chromosome 17q11.2 which codes for neurofibromin (which may suppress tumor growth)[496]. The spontaneous mutation rate is high, with 30-50% of cases represent new somatic mutations[496].

Counselling: prenatal diagnosis is possible by linkage analysis only if there are 2 or more affected family members[496]. 70% of NFT-1 gene mutations can be detected.

MANAGEMENT
- optic gliomas
  - A. unlike optic gliomas in the absence of NFT, these are rarely chiasmal (usually involving the nerve), are often multiple, and have a better prognosis
  - B. most are non progressive, and should be followed ophthalmologically and with serial imaging (MRI or CT)
  - C. surgical intervention probably does not alter visual impairment. Therefore, surgery is reserved for special situations (large disfiguring tumors, pressure on adjacent structures...)
- other neural tumors in patients with NFT-1 should be managed in the same manner as in the general population
  - A. focal, resectable, symptomatic lesions should be surgically removed
  - B. intracranial tumors in NFT-1 may often be unresectable, and in these cases chemotherapy and/or radiation therapy may be appropriate, with surgery reserved for cases with increasing ICP
  - C. when malignant degeneration is suspected (rare, but incidence of sarcomas and leukemias is increased), biopsy with or without internal decompression may be indicated

NEUROFIBROMATOSIS 2
(NFT-2 AKA BILATERAL ACOUSTIC NFT[497])

CLINICAL

Diagnostic criteria[495]
An individual who has:
1. bilateral eighth nerve masses on imaging (MRI or CT)
2. OR a first degree relative (parent, sibling or offspring) with NFT-2 and either:
   A. unilateral eighth nerve mass
   B. OR two of the following:
      1. neurofibroma
      2. meningioma
      3. glioma: includes astrocytoma, ependymoma
      4. schwannoma: including spinal root schwannoma
      5. juvenile posterior subcapsular lenticular cataract or opacity

Other clinical features:
1. seizures or other focal deficits
2. skin nodules, dermal neurofibromas, café au lait spots (less common than in NFT-1)

3. multiple intradural spinal tumors are common (less common in NFT-1)[498]: including intramedullary (especially ependymomas) and extramedullary (schwannomas, meningiomas…)
4. antigenic nerve growth factor is increased (does not occur with NFT-1)

GENETICS
Autosomal dominant inheritance. NFT-2 is due to a mutation at chromosome 22q12.2 which results in the inactivation of schwannomin (AKA merlin, a semi-acronym for moesin-, ezrin-, and radixin-like proteins).

MANAGEMENT CONSIDERATIONS
- bilateral acoustic neuromas:
    ♦ chance of preserving hearing is best when tumor is small. Thus, one should attempt to remove smaller tumor. If hearing is serviceable in that ear after surgery, then consider removing the second tumor, otherwise follow the second tumor as long as possible and perform a subtotal removal in an attempt to prevent total deafness
    ♦ stereotactic radiosurgery therapy may be a treatment option
- prior to surgery, obtain MRI of cervical spine to R/O intraspinal tumors that may cause cord injuries during other operations
- NB: pregnancy may accelerate the growth of eighth nerve tumors

17.11.2. Tuberous sclerosis

❡ Key features
- clinical triad: seizures, mental retardation and sebaceous adenomas
- typical CNS finding: subependymal nodule ("tuber"), a hamartoma
- common neoplasm that develops: subependymal giant cell astrocytoma
- CT shows intracerebral calcifications (usually subependymal)

Tuberous sclerosis (TS), AKA Bourneville's disease, is a neurocutaneous disorder characterized by hamartomas of many organs including the skin, brain, eyes and kidneys. In the brain, the hamartomas may manifest as cortical tubers, glial nodules located subependymally or in deep white matter, or giant cell astrocytomas. Associated findings include pachygyria or microgyria

EPIDEMIOLOGY
Incidence: ≈ 1 in 178,000 person-years. Point prevalence: 10.6 per 100,000 persons (both figures from Rochester, MN[499]).
Autosomal dominant inheritance, however spontaneous mutation is common. The responsible gene may be on chromosome 9.

DIAGNOSIS
In the infant, the earliest finding is of "ash leaf" macules (hypomelanotic, leaf shaped) that are best seen with a Wood's lamp. 3 or more of these macules > 1 cm in length together with the presence of infantile myoclonus is diagnostic of TS.
In older children or adults, the myoclonus is often replaced by generalized tonic-clonic or partial complex seizures. Facial adenomas are not present at birth, but appear in > 90% by age 4 yrs (these are not really adenomas of the sebaceous glands, but are small hamartomas of cutaneous nerve elements that are yellowish-brown and glistening and tend to arise in a butterfly malar distribution usually sparing the upper lip).
Retinal hamartomas occur in ≈ 50% (central calcified hamartoma near the disc or a more subtle peripheral flat salmon-colored lesion). A distinctive depigmented iris lesion may also occur.

Plain skull x-rays
May show calcified cerebral nodules.

CT scan[500]
Intracerebral calcifications are the most common (97% of cases) and characteristic finding. Primarily located subependymally along the lateral walls of the lateral ventri-

cles or near the foramina of Monro.

Low density lesions that do not enhance are seen in 61%. Probably represent heterotopic tissue or defective myelination. Most common in occipital lobe.

Hydrocephalus **(HCP)** may occur even without obstruction. In the absence of tumor, HCP is usually mild. Moderate HCP usually occurs only in the presence of tumor.

Subependymal nodules are usually calcified, and protrude into the ventricle (**"candle guttering"** the appearance on pneumoencephalography).

Paraventricular tumors (mostly giant cell astrocytomas, *see below*) are essentially the only enhancing lesion in TS.

PATHOLOGY

Subependymal nodules ("tubers") are benign hamartomas that are almost always calcified, and protrude into the ventricles.

Giant cell astrocytoma: a transformation lesion. Almost always located at the foramen of Monro. Occurs in 7-23% of patients with TS. Histology shows fibrillary areas alternating with cells containing generous amounts of eosinophilic cytoplasm. Areas of necrosis and abundant mitotic figures may be seen, but are not associated with the typical malignant aggressiveness that these features usually denote[501].

TREATMENT

Paraventricular tumors should be followed, and removed only if they are symptomatic. The transcallosal route is recommended by some.

Infantile myoclonus may respond to steroids. Seizures are treated with AEDs.

Surgery for intractable seizures may be considered when a particular lesion is identified as a seizure focus. Better seizure control, not cure, is the goal in TS.

17.11.3. Sturge-Weber syndrome

⚑ Key features
* cardinal signs: 1) localized cerebral cortical atrophy and calcifications, 2) ipsilateral port-wine facial nevus (usually in distribution of V_1)
* contralateral seizures usually present
* plain skull films classically show "tram-tracking"

AKA encephalotrigeminal angiomatosis. A neurocutaneous disorder consisting of:
1. cardinal features:
    A. localized cerebral cortical atrophy and calcifications (especially cortical layers 2 and 3, with a predilection for the occipital lobes):
        1. calcifications appear as curvilinear double parallel lines (**"tram-tracking"**) on plain x-rays
        2. cortical atrophy usually causes contralateral hemiparesis, hemiatrophy, and homonymous hemianopia (with occipital lobe involvement)
    B. ipsilateral port-wine facial nevus (**nevus flammeus**) usually in distribution of 1st division of trigeminal nerve (rarely bilateral)
2. other findings that may be present:
    A. ipsilateral exophthalmos and/or glaucoma, coloboma of the iris
    B. oculomeningeal capillary hemangioma
    C. convulsive seizures: contralateral to the facial nevus and cortical atrophy. Present in most patients starting in infancy
    D. retinal angiomas

GENETICS

Most cases are sporadic. Other cases are suggestive of recessive inheritance, with chromosome 3 being implicated.

TREATMENT

Treatment is supportive. Anticonvulsants are used for seizures. Lobectomy or hemispherectomy may be needed for refractory seizures. XRT: complications are common and benefits are lacking. Laser surgery for the cutaneous nevus is disappointing; better results obtain from masking the nevus with a skin colored tattoo.

17.12. Spine and spinal cord tumors

15% of primary CNS tumors are intraspinal (the intracranial:spinal ratio for astro-cytomas is 10:1; for ependymomas it's 3-20:1)[502]. There is disagreement over the preva-lence, prognosis, and optimal treatment. Most primary CNS spinal tumors are benign (unlike the case with intracranial tumors). Most present by compression rather than invasion[503].

TYPES OF SPINAL TUMORS
May be classified in 3 groups. Although metastases may be found in each category, they are usually extradural. Frequencies quoted below are from a general hospital, ex-tradural lesions are less common in neurosurgical clinics because of relative exclusion of extradural lymphomas, metastatic Ca, etc.:
1. **extradural (ED)** (55%): arise outside cord in vertebral bodies or epidural tissues
2. **intradural extramedullary (ID-EM)** (40%): arise in leptomeninges or roots. Primarily meningiomas and neurofibromas (together = 55% of ID-EM tumors)
3. **intramedullary spinal cord tumors (IMSCT)** (5%): arise in SC substance. In-vade and destroy tracts and grey matter, *see page 508*

DIFFERENTIAL DIAGNOSIS OF SPINAL CORD TUMORS
See also *Myelopathy* on page 902 for nonneoplastic causes of spinal cord dysfunction (e.g. spinal meningeal cyst, epidural hematoma, transverse myelitis…).
1. extradural spinal cord tumors (55%): arise in vertebral bodies or epidural tissues
   A. metastatic: comprise the majority of ED tumors
      1. most cause bony destruction (see *Spinal epidural metastases*, page 516). Common ones include:
         a. lymphoma: most cases represent spread of systemic disease (secondary lymphoma), however some cases may be primary (*see below*)
         b. lung
         c. breast
         d. prostate
      2. metastases that may be osteoblastic:
         a. in men: prostate Ca is the most common
         b. in women: breast Ca is the most common
   B. primary spinal tumors (very rare)
      1. chordomas: *see page 464*
      2. neurofibromas: usually dilate neural foramen (dumbbell tumors)
      3. osteoid osteoma: *see page 511*
      4. osteoblastoma: *see page 511*
      5. **aneurysmal bone cyst**: peak incidence is in 2nd decade of life. Char-acteristic appearance is a cavity of highly vascular honeycomb sur-rounded by a thin cortical shell which may expand. High recurrence rate (25-50%) if not completely excised
      6. chondrosarcoma: a malignant tumor of cartilage. Lobulated tumors with calcified areas
      7. osteochondroma (chondroma): benign tumors of bone that arise from mature hyaline cartilage. Most common during adolescence. An en-chondroma is a similar tumor arising within the medullary cavity
      8. vertebral hemangioma: *see page 512*
      9. **giant cell tumors** of bone: AKA osteoclastoma (*see page 516*)
      10. osteogenic sarcoma: rare in spine
   C. miscellaneous
      1. plasmacytoma: *see page 514*
      2. multiple myeloma: *see page 514*
      3. eosinophilic granuloma (**EG**) AKA vertebra plana: osteolytic defect with progressive vertebral collapse. C-spine is the most commonly af-fected region. Isolated EG associated with systemic conditions (Let-terer-Siwe or Hand-Schüller-Christian disease) are treated with biopsy and immobilization. Collapse or neurologic deficit from com-

pression may require decompression and/or fusion. Low-dose RTX may also be effective[504, 505]

    4.   Ewing's sarcoma: aggressive malignant tumor with a peak incidence during 2nd decade of life. Spine mets are more common than primary spine lesions. Treatment is mostly palliative: radical excision followed by RTX and chemotherapy[506]

    5.   chloroma: focal infiltration of leukemic cells

    6.   angiolipoma: ≈ 60 cases reported in literature

    7.   Masson's vegetant intravascular hemangioendothelioma[507] (*see page 497*)

2. intradural extramedullary spinal cord tumors (40%)
    A. meningiomas
    B. neurofibromas
    C. many lipomas are extramedullary with intramedullary extension
    D. miscellaneous: only ≈ 4% of spinal metastases involve this compartment

3. tumors that are usually intradural, but may be partly or wholly extradural:
    A. meningiomas: 15% of spinal meningiomas are extradural
    B. neurofibromas

4. intramedullary spinal cord tumors (5%): *see below*
    A. astrocytoma 30%
    B. ependymoma 30%
    C. miscellaneous 30%, includes:
        1. malignant glioblastoma
        2. dermoid
        3. epidermoid
        4. teratoma
        5. lipoma
        6. hemangioblastoma (*see page 509*)
        7. neuroma (very rare intramedullary)
        8. syringomyelia (not neoplastic)
        9. extremely rare tumors
           a. lymphoma
           b. oligodendroglioma
           c. cholesteatoma
           d. intramedullary metastases: involves only ≈ 2% of spinal mets

SPINAL MENINGIOMAS[508]

Epidemiology

Peak age: 40-70 years. Female:male ratio = 4:1 overall, but the ratio is 1:1 in the lumbar region. 82% thoracic, 15% cervical, 2% lumbar. 90% are completely intradural, 5% are extradural, and 5% both intra- and extra-dural. 68% are lateral to the spinal cord, 18% posterior, 15% anterior. Multiple spinal meningiomas occur rarely.

Clinical

Symptoms

		At onset	At time of first surgery
1.	local or radicular pain:	42%	53%
2.	motor deficits:	33%	92%
3.	sensory symptoms:	25%	61%
4.	sphincter disturbance:		50%

Signs prior to surgery (only 1 of 174 patients was intact)[508]
    1. motor
        A. pyramidal signs only: 26%
        B. walks with aid: 41%
        C. antigravity strength:17%
        D. flexion-extension with gravity removed: 6%
        E. paralysis: 9%
    2. sensory
        A. radicular: 7%
        B. long tract: 90%
    3. sphincter deficit: 51%

Outcome

Recurrence rate with complete excision is 7% with a minimum of 6 years follow-up (relapses occurred from 4 to 17 years post-op)[508].

SPINAL LYMPHOMA
1. epidural
    A. metastatic or secondary lymphoma: the most common form of spinal lymphoma. Spinal involvement occurs in 0.1-10% of patients with non-Hodgkin's lymphoma
    B. primary spinal epidural non-Hodgkin's lymphoma: rare. Completely epidural with no bony involvement. The existence of this entity is controversial, and some investigators feel that it represents extension of undetected retroperitoneal or vertebral body lymphoma. May have a better prognosis than secondary lymphoma[509]
2. intramedullary
    A. secondary: *see page 509*
    B. primary: very rare (*see below*)

17.12.1. Intramedullary spinal cord tumors

TYPES OF INTRAMEDULLARY SPINAL CORD TUMORS
The following list excludes metastases (*see below*) and lipomas (of questionable neoplastic origin[510], and most are actually extramedullary intradural, *see below*).
1. astrocytoma (nonmalignant): 30% (the most common intramedullary spinal cord tumors **(IMSCT)** outside the filum terminale[503])
2. ependymoma: 30%
3. miscellaneous: 30%, including:
    A. malignant glioblastoma
    B. dermoid
    C. epidermoid (including iatrogenic from LP without stylet)[511, 512]
    D. teratoma
    E. hemangioblastoma (*see below*)
    F. hemangioma
    G. neuroma (very rarely intramedullary)
    H. extremely rare tumors
        1. primary lymphoma (only 6 case reports, all non-Hodgkin type[513])
        2. oligodendroglioma, only 38 cases in world literature[514]
        3. cholesteatoma
        4. paraganglioma

SPECIFIC INTRAMEDULLARY SPINAL CORD TUMORS

EPENDYMOMA
The most common glioma of lower cord, conus and filum. Slow-growing. Benign. Slight male predominance; slight peak in 3rd to 6th decade. Over 50% in filum, next most common location is cervical. Histologically: papillary, cellular, epithelial, or mixed (in filum, myxopapillary ependymoma is most common, *see below*). Cystic degeneration in 46%. May expand spinal canal in filum[515]. Usually encapsulated and minimally vascular (papillary: may be highly vascular; may cause SAH). Symptoms present > 1 yr prior to diagnosis in 82% of cases[366].

Myxopapillary ependymoma
Papillary, with microcystic vacuoles, mucosubstance; connective tissue. No anaplasia, but CSF dissemination occurs rarely. Rare reports of systemic mets[502].
Surgical removal of filum tumors consists of coagulating and dividing the filum terminale just above and below the lesion (see *Distinguishing features of the filum terminale*, page 121), and excising it in total. The filum is first cut <u>above</u> the lesion to prevent retraction upwards.

ASTROCYTOMA
Uncommon in first year. Peak: 3rd - 5th decade. Male:female = 1.5:1. The ratio of benign:malignant = 3:1 in all ages[515]. Occurs at all levels, thoracic most common, then cervical. 38% are cystic; cyst fluid usually has high protein.

DERMOID AND EPIDERMOID

Epidermoids are rare before late childhood. Slight female predominance. Cervical and upper thoracic rare; conus common. Usually ID-EM, but conus/cauda equina may have IM component (completely IM lesions rare).

LIPOMA

May occur in conjunction with spinal dysraphism (see *Lipomyeloschisis*, page 117). The following considers lipomas that occur in the absence of spinal dysraphism.

Peak occurrence: 2nd, 3rd and 5th decade. Technically hamartomas. No sex predominance. Usually ID-EM (a sub-type is truly IM and essentially replaces the cord[516]), cervicothoracic region is the most common location. NB: unlike other IMSCT's, most common symptom is ascending mono- or para-paresis (c.f. pain). Sphincter disturbance is common with low lesions. Local subcutaneous masses or dimples are frequent. Malis recommends early subtotal removal at about 1 year age in asymptomatic patient[516]. Superficial extrasacral removal is inadequate, as patients then develop dense scarring intraspinally leading to fairly rapid severe neurological damage with poor salvageability even after the definitive procedure.

HEMANGIOBLASTOMA

Cannot incise nor core because of vascularity. Requires microsurgical approach similar to AVM, possibly with intraoperative hypotension. Usually non-infiltrating, well demarcated, may have cystic caps.

METASTASES

Most spinal mets are extradural, only a few hundred case reports of IMSCT mets exist[517], accounting for 3.4% of symptomatic metastatic spinal cord lesions[518]. Primaries include: small cell lung Ca[519], breast Ca, malignant melanoma, lymphoma and colon Ca[518, 520]. Ca rarely presents first as an intramedullary spinal met.

PRESENTATION

1. pain: the most common complaint. Almost always present in filum tumors (exception: lipomas)[511]. Possible pain patterns:
   * radicular: increases with Valsalva maneuver and spine movement. Suspect SCT if dermatome is unusual for disk herniation
   * local: stiff neck or back, Valsalva maneuver increases.
     ★ Pain during recumbency ("nocturnal pain") suggests SCT
   * medullary (as in syrinx): oppressive, burning, dysesthetic, non-radicular, often bilateral, unaffected by Valsalva maneuver
2. motor disturbances
   * weakness is 2nd or 3rd most common complaint. Usually follows sensory symptoms temporally
   * children present most frequently with gait disturbances
   * syringomyelic syndrome: suggests IMSCT. Findings: UE segmental weakness, decreased DTR, dissociative anesthesia (see below)
   * long-tract involvement ▸ clumsiness and ataxia (distinct from weakness)
   * atrophy, muscle twitches, fasciculations
3. non-painful sensory disturbances
   * dissociated sensory loss: decreased pain and temperature, preserved light touch (as in Brown-Séquard syndrome, see page 716). There is disagreement whether this is common[503] or uncommon[521] in IMSCT. ± non-radicular dysesthesias (early), with upward extension[522]
   * paresthesias: either radicular or "medullary" distribution
4. sphincter disturbances
   * usually urogenital (anal less common) → difficulty evacuating, retention, incontinence, and impotence. Early in conus/cauda equina lesions, especially lipomas (pain not prominent)
   * sphincter dysfunction common in age < 1 yr due to frequency of lumbosacral lesions (dermoids, epidermoids, etc.)
5. miscellaneous symptoms:
   * scoliosis or torticollis
   * SAH
   * visible mass over spine

Onset usually insidious, but abruptness occurs (benign lesions in children occasionally progress in hours). The onset is often erroneously attributed to coincidental injury. Temporal progression[A] has been divided into 4 stages[523]:
1. pain only (neuralgic)
2. Brown-Séquard syndrome
3. incomplete transectional dysfunction
4. complete transectional dysfunction

DIAGNOSIS

It is usually difficult to distinguish IMSCT, ID-EM and ED on clinical grounds[503]. Schwannomas often start with radicular symptoms that later progress to cord involvement. Most IMSCTs are located posteriorly in cord which may cause sensory findings to predominate early[510].

DIAGNOSTIC STUDIES

Plain radiographs: vertebral body destruction, enlarged intervertebral foramina, or increases in interpedicular distances suggests ED SCT.

Lumbar puncture: Elevated protein is the most common abnormality[502] seen in ≈ 95%. The reported range with primary IMSCTs is 50-2,240 mg%. Glucose is normal except with meningeal tumor. SCT can cause complete block, indicated by:
- **Froin's syndrome**: clotting (due to fibrinogen) and xanthochromia of CSF
- **Queckenstedt's test** (failure of jugular vein compression to increase CSF pressure, which it normally does in the absence of block)
- barrier to flow of myelographic contrast media

MRI: mainstay of diagnosis. MRI may sometimes be misleading in falsely identifying cord edema (as with necrosis) as a cystic lesion. Ependymomas enhance intensely and are often associated with hemorrhage and cysts.

Myelography: classically shows fusiform cord widening (may be normal early). Distinct from ED tumors which produce hourglass deformity (with incomplete block) or paintbrush effect (with complete block), or ID-EM tumors which produce a capping effect with a sharp cutoff (meniscus sign) (see page 518).

CT: some IMSCTs enhance with IV contrast. Metrizamide CT distinguishes IMSCT from ID-EM (poor in differentiating IMSCT subtypes).

Spinal angiography: rarely indicated, except in hemangioblastoma (may be suspected on myelography by prominent vascular markings). MRI may obviate this test.

DIFFERENTIAL DIAGNOSIS

In addition to tumors discussed above (also see DDx for *Myelopathy* on page 902):
- vascular lesions (e.g. AVM): selective spinal angiography may be useful[503]
- demyelinating disease (e.g. multiple sclerosis)
- inflammatory myelitis
- paraneoplastic myelopathy
- diseases causing pain over certain body segments (e.g. cholecystitis, pyelonephritis, intestinal pathology). To differentiate from these, look for dermatomal distribution, increase with Valsalva maneuver, and accompanying sensory and/or motor changes in LEs which suggest cord/radicular lesion. Radiographic studies are frequently required to differentiate
- diseases of vertebral structures (e.g. Paget's disease, giant cell tumors of bone (see page 516), etc.)

MANAGEMENT

Surgery should be performed as soon as possible after diagnosis since surgical results correlate with the preoperative neurologic condition, and it makes no sense to follow the patient as they develop neurologic deficit[524] (some of which may be irreversible).

Astrocytomas: for low grade lesions, if a plane can be developed between the tumor and spinal cord (when it can, it usually consists of a thin gliotic layer traversed by small

---

A. 78% (of 23) ependymomas, 74% (of 42) gliomas, all 7 dermoids, and 50% (of 8) lipomas reached latter 2 stages before diagnosis (not affected by location in cross-sectional nor longitudinal dimension of SC (excludes conus lesions - more frequently diagnosed in 1st stage) (a pre-CT study)

blood vessels and adhesions[510]), an attempt at total excision is an option[525]. For high grade astrocytomas or for low-grade astrocytomas without a plane of separation, biopsy alone or biopsy plus limited excision is recommended[525].

For high-grade lesions, post-op RTX (± chemotherapy) is recommended[525]. RTX is not supported following radical resection of low grade gliomas[525].

Ependymomas: an attempt at gross total removal should be attempted. XRT is not recommended following gross total removal[525].

PROGNOSIS

No well designed studies give long term functional results with microsurgery, laser and radiotherapy. Better results occur with lesser initial deficits[510]. Recurrence depends on totality of removal, and on growth pattern of the specific tumor.

Ependymomas: total extirpation improves functional outcome, and myxopapillary ependymomas fare better than the "classic" type[366]. Best functional outcome occurs with modest initial deficits, symptoms < 2 years duration[526], and total removal. Survival is independent of extent of excision.

Astrocytomas: radical removal rarely possible (cleavage plane unusual even with microscope). Long term functional results poorer than ependymomas. There is 50% recurrence rate in 4-5 yrs.

17.12.2. Bone tumors of the spine

OSTEOID OSTEOMA AND OSTEOBLASTOMA

❢ Key features
- both are benign bone tumors
- histologically identical, differentiation depends on size (≤1 cm = osteoid osteoma, > 1 cm = osteoblastoma)
- can occur in the spine and may cause neurologic symptoms (esp. osteoblastoma)
- high cure rate with complete excision

Benign osteoblastic lesions of bone may be divided into two types: osteoid osteoma **(OO)** and benign osteoblastoma **(BOB)** (see Table 17-65).

Characteristically cause night pain and pain that is relieved by aspirin (see Clinical below). The two are indistinguishable histologically, and must be differentiated based on size and behavior.

Osteoblastoma is a rare, benign, locally recurrent tumor with a predilection for spine, that may rarely undergo sarcomatous change (to osteosarcoma)[528]. More vascular than OO[529].

Differential diagnosis:
(for lesions with similar symptoms and increased uptake on radionuclide bone scan)
1. osteoid osteoma: more pronounced sclerosis of adjacent bone than BOB
2. benign osteoblastoma
3. osteogenic sarcoma:

Table 17-65 Comparison of osteoid osteoma and benign osteoblastoma[527]

	Osteoid osteoma	Benign osteoblastoma
percent of primary bone tumors	3.2%	
percent of primary vertebral tumors	1.4%	
percent that occur in spine	10%	35%
size limitations	≤ 1 cm	> 1 cm
growth pattern	confined, self limiting	more extensive, may extend into spinal canal
location within spine (83 patients)		
% in cervical spine	27%	25%
% in thoracic spin		35%
% in lumbar region	59%	35%
location within vertebra (81 patients)		
lamina only	33%	16%
pedicle only	15%	32%
articular facet only	19%	0
vertebral body **(VB)** only	7%	5%
transverse process only	6%	8%
spinous process	5%	5%
> 1 element of neural arch	6%	19%
combined posterior elements & VB	0	11%

rare in spine
4. aneurysmal bone cyst: usually shows trabeculae in central, lucent region
5. unilateral pedicle/laminar ne-
crosis

CLINICAL

See *Table 17-66* for signs and symptoms. Tenderness confined to vicinity of the lesion occurs in ≈ 60%. 28% of patients with BOB presented with myelopathy. OO presented with neurologic deficit in only 22%.

Table 17-66 Signs and symptoms in 82 patients[527]

	Osteoid osteoma	Benign os-teoblastoma
pain on presentation	100%	100%
pain increased by motion	49%	74%
pain increased by Valsalva	17%	36%
nocturnal pain	46%	36%
pain relieved by aspirin	40%	25%
radicular pain	50%	44%
scoliosis	66%	36%
neurologic abnormalities	22%	54%
myelopathy	0	28%
weakness	12%	51%
atrophy	9%	15%

EVALUATION

Bone scans are a very sensitive means for detecting these lesions. Once localized, CT or MRI may better define the lesion in that region.

Osteoid osteoma

Radiolucent area with or without surrounding density, often isolated to pedicle or facet. May not show up on tomograms.

Osteoblastoma

Most are expansile, destructive lesions, with 17% having moderate sclerosis. 31% have areas of ↑ density, 20% surrounded by calcified shell. Often a contralateral spondylolysis[528].

TREATMENT

In order to obtain a cure, these lesions must be <u>completely</u> excised. The role of radiation therapy is poorly defined in these lesions, but is probably ineffective[528].

Osteoid osteoma

Cortical bone may be hardened and thickened, with granulomatous mass in underlying cavity.

Osteoblastoma

Hemorrhagic, friable, red to purple mass well circumscribed from adjacent bone. Complete excision → complete pain relief in 93%. Curettage only → pain relief, with more likely recurrence. Recurrence rate with total excision is ≈ 10%.

VERTEBRAL HEMANGIOMA

AKA spinal hemangioma, cavernous hemangioma, or hemangiomatous angioma. Vertebral hemangiomas **(VH)** are benign lesions of the spine with an estimated incidence of 9-12%[530, 531]. One third of cases have up to 5 levels involved, often noncontiguous. The lumbar and lower thoracic spine are the most common locations, cervical lesions are rare. Lesions involve only the vertebral bodies in ≈ 25%, posterior spinal arch in ≈ 25%, and both areas in ≈ 50%. Occasional cases of purely extradural lesions have been described[532]. Intramedullary lesions are even less common[533].

Malignant degeneration has <u>never</u> been reported. Blood vessels replace normal marrow, producing hypertrophic sclerotic bony trabeculations oriented in a rostral-caudal direction in one of two forms: cavernous or capillary (difference in subtype carries no prognostic significance).

PRESENTATION

1. incidental: most VH are asymptomatic, these require no follow-up (*see below*)
2. symptomatic: there may be a hormonal influence (unproven) that may cause symptoms to increase with pregnancy (could also be due to increased blood volume and/or venous pressure)[534] or to vary with the menstrual cycle
   A. pain: occasionally VH may present with pain localized to the level of in-

volvement with no radiculopathy. Pain is more often due to other pathology
(herniated disc, spinal stenosis…) rather than the VH

B. progressive neurologic deficit: this occurs rarely, and usually takes the form
of thoracic myelopathy. Deficit may be caused by the following mechanisms
1. subperiosteal (epidural) growth of tumor into the spinal canal
2. expansion of the bone (cortical "blistering") with widening of the pedicles and lamina producing a "bony" spinal stenosis
3. compression by vessels feeding or draining the lesion
4. compression fracture of the involved vertebra (very rare)[535]
5. spontaneous hemorrhage producing spinal epidural hematoma[536] (also very rare)
6. spinal cord ischemia due to "steal"

EVALUATION

Plain x-rays: classically show coarse vertically oriented striations or a "honeycomb"
appearance. At least ~ one third of the VB must be involved to produce these findings.

Bone scan: hemangiomas usually do not light up unless a compression fracture has
occurred (may help distinguish VH from metastatic disease).

CT: diagnostic procedure of choice. "Polka-dot" pattern represents cross-sectional
cuts through thickened trabeculae.

MRI: may help distinguish lesions that tend not to evolve (mottled increased signal
on T1WI and T2WI, possibly due to adipose tissue) from those that tend to be symptomatic (isointense on T1WI, hyperintense on T2WI).

Spinal angiography: also may help distinguish nonevolutive (normal or slight increased vascularity compared to adjacent bone) from symptomatic (moderate to marked
hypervascularity) lesions. Therapeutic: if the feeding artery does not also supply the anterior spinal artery, it may be embolized preoperatively or sacrificed at surgery.

TREATMENT[530]

1. asymptomatic VH require no routine follow up or evaluation unless pain or neurologic deficit develop, which are rare occurrences in incidentally discovered VH
2. biopsy: may be indicated in cases where diagnosis is uncertain (e.g. when metastases are a strong consideration). In spite of highly vascular nature, there have
been no reported bleeding complications with CT guided biopsy
3. those presenting with pain or neurologic deficit
A. radiation therapy: may be used alone for painful lesions, preoperatively as
a surgical adjunct, or post-op following incomplete removal. VH are radiosensitive and undergo sclerotic obliteration. Total dosage should be ≤ 40
Gy to reduce risk of radiation myelopathy. Improvement in pain may take
months to years, and no radiographic evidence of response may occur
B. embolization: provides more rapid relief of pain than RTX, can also be used
pre-op as surgical adjunct. Risks spinal cord infarction if major radicular artery (e.g. artery of Adamkiewicz, see page 76) is embolized
C. vertebroplasty: see page 750
D. surgery: for painful lesions that fail to respond to above measures, or for lesions with progressive neurologic deficit (see below)

Surgical treatment

Table 17-67 Recommendations for surgical management of VH*[530]

VH involvement	Approach	Post-op RTX?
posterior elements only	radical excision via posterior approach	not for total excision
VB involvement with anterior canal compression (with or without ST in canal)	anterior corpectomy with strut graft	
VB involved but no expansion, ST in lateral canal	laminectomy with removal of soft-tissue	follow serial CT, give RTX if VB expansion or ST expansion
extensive involvement of anterior and posterior vertebral elements with circumferential bone expansion, no ST compression	laminectomy	either RTX, or close follow-up with CT and RTX for ST recurrence or progressive VB expansion
extensive anterior and posterior involvement with ST in anterior canal	anterior corpectomy with strut graft	

* abbreviations: VB = vertebral body, ST = soft-tissue component of VH, RTX = radiation treatment

Indications are given above. Recommended management is shown in *Table 17-67*.

Major risks of surgery: blood loss, destabilization of the spine, neurologic deficit (during surgery, or postoperatively usually from epidural hematoma). Recurrence rate is 20-30% after subtotal resection, usually within 2 yrs. Patients with subtotal resection should have RTX which lowers recurrence rate to ≈ 7%.

MULTIPLE MYELOMA

Multiple myeloma **(MM)** (sometimes simply referred to as *myeloma*) is a neoplasm of a single clone of plasma cells characterized by proliferation of plasma cells in bone marrow, infiltration of adjacent tissues with mature and immature plasma cells, and the production of an immunoglobulin, usually monoclonal IgG or IgA (referred to collectively as M-protein[537]). Circulating pre-myeloma cells lodge in appropriate microenvironments (e.g. in bone marrow) where they differentiate and expand. Although MM is often referred to in the context of "metastatic lesions" to bone, it is also sometimes considered a primary bone tumor.

If only a single lesion is identified, then it is referred to as a **plasmacytoma** (there must be no other lesions on complete skeletal survey, bone marrow aspirate must show no evidence of myeloma, and serum and urine electrophoresis should show no M-protein). Patients with a solitary plasmacytoma will almost always show involvement with MM within ≈ 10 yrs.

MM presents as a result of the following (underscored items are characteristic for MM):
1. proliferation of plasma cells: interferes with normal immune system function → increased susceptibility to infection
2. bone involvement
   A. bone marrow involvement → destruction of hematopoietic capacity → normocytic normochromic anemia, leukopenia, thrombocytopenia
   B. bone resorption
      1. → weakening of the bone → pathologic fractures (*see below*)
      2. → hypercalcemia (present initially in 25% of MM patients, *see below*)
   C. swelling or local tenderness of bone
   D. bone pain: characteristically induced by movement, and absent at rest
   E. spinal involvement
      1. invasion of spinal canal in ≈ 10% of cases → spinal cord compression → myelopathy (*see page 516*)
      2. nerve root compression (radiculopathy)
3. the overproduction of certain proteins by plasma cells. May lead to:
   A. hyperviscosity syndrome
   B. cryoglobulinemia
   C. amyloidosis
   D. renal failure: multifactorial, but monoclonal light chains play a role

EPIDEMIOLOGY

In the U.S., incidence is ≈ 1-2 per 100,000 in caucasians, and is ≈ twice that in blacks. MM accounts for 1% of malignancies, and 10% of hematologic cancers. The peak age of occurrence is 60-70 yrs of age, with < 2% of patients being < 40 yrs old. Slightly more common in males. Monoclonal gammopathy without MM occurs in ≈ 0.15% of the population, and in long-term follow-up 16% of these develop MM with an annual rate of 0.18%[538].

SKELETAL DISEASE

MM involvement is by definition multiple, and is usually restricted to sites of red marrow: ribs, sternum, spine, clavicles, skull, or proximal extremities. Lesions of the spine and/or skull are the usual reasons for presentation to the neurosurgeon.

Bone resorption in MM is not due simply to mechanical erosion by plasma cells. Increased osteoclastic activity has been observed.

Plasma cell tumors of the skull involving the cranial vault usually do not produce neurologic symptoms. Cranial nerve palsies can arise from skull base involvement. Orbital involvement may produce proptosis (exophthalmos).

NEUROLOGIC INVOLVEMENT

Neurologic manifestations can occur as a result of:

---

1. spinal or skull involvement with tumor (*see above*) with compression of brain, cranial nerves, or spinal cord or roots
2. deposition of amyloid within the flexor retinaculum of the wrist → carpal tunnel syndrome (the median nerve itself does not contain amyloid, and therefore responds well to surgical division of the transverse carpal ligament, *see page 568*)
3. diffuse progressive sensorimotor polyneuropathy: occurs in 3-5% of patients with MM
    A. about half are due to amyloidosis (*see page 560*)
    B. polyneuropathy can also occur without amyloidosis, especially in the rare osteosclerotic variant of MM
4. multifocal leukoencephalopathy has been described in MM[539]
5. hypercalcemia: may produce a dramatic encephalopathy with confusion, delerium or coma. Neurologic symptoms of hypercalcemia associated with MM are more common than in hypercalcemia of other etiologies
6. very rare: intraparenchymal metastases[540]

EVALUATION

The diagnostic criteria for MM is shown in *Table 17-68*. Tests that may be used in evaluating patients with MM or suspected MM include:

1. 24 hour urine for kappa Bence-Jones protein[A] present in 75%
2. bloodwork: serum protein electrophoresis (**SPEP**) and immune electrophoresis (**IEP**) (looking for IgG kappa band)[A]
3. skeletal radiologic survey. Characteristic x-ray finding: multiple, round, "punched-out" (sharply demarcated) lytic lesions in the bones typically involved (*see above*). Osteosclerotic lesions are seen in < 3% of patients with MM. Diffuse osteoporosis may also be seen
4. CBC: anemia eventually develops in most patients with MM. It is usually of moderate severity (Hgb ≈ 7-10 gm%) with a low reticulocyte count
5. technetium-99m nuclear bone scan is usually <u>negative</u> in untreated MM (due to rarity of spontaneous new bone formation) and is less sensitive than conventional radiographs. Therefore it is not usually helpful except perhaps to implicate etiologies *other* than MM to explain the observed findings. After treatment, bone scan may become positive as osteoblastic activity ensues ("flare" response)
6. serum creatinine: for prognostication
7. bone marrow biopsy: virtually all MM patients have "myeloma cells" (although sensitive, this is not specific and other diagnostic criteria should be sought)

Table 17-68 Criteria for diagnosis of MM*

1. cytologic criteria
A. marrow morphology: plasma cells and/or myeloma cells ≥ 10% of 1000 or more cells
B. biopsy proven plasmacytoma
2. clinical and laboratory criteria
A. myeloma protein (M-component) in serum (usually > 3 gm/dl) or urine IEP
B. osteolytic lesions on x-ray (generalized osteoporosis qualifies if marrow contains > 30% plasma or myeloma cells)
O. myeloma cells in ≥ 2 peripheral blood smears

* diagnosis requires[541]: A 1 & 2, or A1 or A2 and B1, B2, or B3

TREATMENT

Many aspects of treatment fall into the purvey of the oncologist (*see review*[538]). Some aspects pertinent to neurosurgical care include:

1. mobilization: immobilization due to pain and fear of pathologic compression fractures leads to further detrimental increases in serum calcium and weakness
2. pain control: mild pain often responds well to salicylates (contraindicated in thrombocytopenia). Local XRT is also effective (*see below*)
3. local XRT for pain due to readily identifiable bone lesions. XRT may allow pathologic fractures to heal and is effective in spinal cord compression (*see page 489*)
4. percutaneous vertebroplasty (*see page 750*) may be used for some spine lesions
5. therapy for hypercalcemia usually improves symptoms related to that
6. biphosphonates inhibit bone resorption and rapidly reduces hypercalcemia (*see page 342*). Pamidronate is currently preferred over older agents
7. bortezomib (Velcade®): the first proteasome inhibitor, indicated for treatment of refractory MM

A. monoclonal proteins cannot be detected in the urine or serum of ≈ 1% of MM patients. Two or more monoclonal bands are produced in ≈0.5-2.5% of patients with MM[542]

Untreated MM has a 6 month median survival. Solitary plasmacytoma has a 50% 10-year survival. If there is an solitary site of involvement but M-protein is present (i.e. essentially a plasmacytoma except for the M-protein), elimination of the M-protein following XRT indicates a 50-60% chance of remaining free of MM, if the M-protein doesn't resolve, there is a high chance of developing MM.

GIANT CELL TUMORS OF BONE

AKA osteoclastoma (cells arise from osteoclasts). In the same general category as aneurysmal bone cysts. Typically arise in adolescence. Most common in knees and wrists. Those that come to the attention of the neurosurgeon generally arise in the skull (especially the skull base, and in particular the sphenoid bone), or in the vertebral column (≈ 4% occur in sacrum).

Pathology
Lytic with bony collapse. Almost always benign with pseudomalignant behavior (recurrence is common, and pulmonary mets can occur).

Evaluation
Work-up includes chest CT because of possibility of pulmonary mets.

Treatment
Intratumoral curettage, possibly aided by pre-op embolization. Recurrence rate with this treatment (even if resection is subtotal) is only ≈ 20%. Role of RTX is controversial[504] because of the possibility of malignant degeneration (therefore use RTX only for non-resectable recurrence). Use of osteoclast inhibiting drugs (biphosphonates e.g. pamidronate, *see page 342*) has met with some success following subtotal resection For gross residual disease after resection, re-resection is a consideration.

Cryosurgery with liquid nitrogen has been employed in long bones. Its use is limited in neurosurgical cases because of risk of injury to adjacent neural structures (brain, spinal cord) and cryotherapy induced fractures, although it has been described for use in the sacrum[543].

Close follow-up is require due to propensity for recurrence. MRI or CT q 3 months is suggested.

17.12.3.   Spinal epidural metastases

ℓ Key features
  • suspected in a cancer patient with back pain that persists in recumbency
  • occurs in ≈ 10% of all cancer patients
  • 80% of primary sites: lung, breast, GI, prostate, melanoma and lymphoma
  • no treatment prolongs survival, but may reduce pain and neurologic deficit

Spinal epidural metastases **(SEM)** occur in up to 10% of cancer patients at some time[544], and are the most common spinal tumor. 5-10% of malignancies present initially with cord compression. *Table 17-69* shows primary tumor types that give rise to SEM. For other etiologies of spinal cord compression, see items marked with a dagger (†) under *Myelopathy* on page 902.

Routes of metastasis: arterial, venous (via spinal epidural veins (**Batson's plexus**[546])) and perinervous (direct spread). Usual route of spread is hematogenous dissemination to vertebral body with erosion back through pedicles and subsequent extension into the epidural space. May also initially metastasize to lateral or posterior aspect of canal. Most mets are epidural, only 2-4% are intradural, and only 1-2% are intramedullary. Distribution between cervical, thoracic and lumbar spine is ≈ proportional to the length of the segment, thus thoracic spine is the most common site (50-60%).

Presentation
Pain is the first symptom in 95% of patients with SEM. It may be focal, radicular (commonly bilateral in thoracic region) or referred. Pain may be exacerbated by movement, recumbency (especially at night, a characteristic finding), neck-flexion, straight-leg-raising, coughing, sneezing, or straining. Patients may also present with pathologic fracture. Bone metastases can sometimes produce hypercalcemia (a medical emergency).

As cord involvement develops: leg stiffness/weakness, paresthesias, autonomic disturbances (urinary urgency or hesitancy, constipation, impotence).

The greater the neurologic deficit when treatment is initiated, the worse the chances for recovery of lost function. 76% of patients have weakness by the time of diagnosis[544]. 15% are paraplegic on initial presentation, and < 5% of these can ambulate after treatment. Median time from onset of symptoms to diagnosis is 2 mos.

Metastases to the upper cervical spine

For differential diagnosis, see *Foramen magnum lesions*, page 924 and *Axis (C2) vertebra lesions* on page 924.

Metastases to the C1-2 region comprise only ≈ 0.5% of spinal mets[547]. They typically present initially with suboccipital and posterior cervical pain, and as the lesion progresses patients develop a characteristic pain that makes it difficult to sit up (some will hold their heads in their hands to stabilize it). Possibly as a result of the capacious spinal canal at this level, only ≈11-15% of patients present with neurologic symptoms. 15% develop spinal cord compression[548], and quadriplegia from atlantoaxial subluxation occurred in ≈ 6%[548].

Table 17-69 Sources of spinal epidural metastases causing cord compression

Site of primary	Series A	Series B*	Series C†
lung	17%	14%	31%
breast	16%	21%	24%
prostate	11%	19%	8%
kidney	9%		1%
unknown site	9%	5%	2%
sarcoma	8%		2%
lymphoma	6%	12%	6%
GI tract	6%		9%
thyroid	6%		
melanoma	2%		4%
others (including multiple myeloma)	13%	29%‡	13%

* series B: retrospective study of 58 patients undergoing MRI evaluation for SEM[544]

† series C: 75 patients with SEM out of 140 patients evaluated prospectively for back pain[545]

‡ in series B, "other" includes GI, GU, skin, ENT, CNS

Anterior approaches for stabilization at this location are difficult. Pathologic fractures due to osteoblastic types of tumors (e.g. prostate, some breast) may heal with radiation treatment and immobilization. For others, good pain relief and stabilization may be achieved with radiation followed by posterior fusion[548].

EVALUATING SPINAL METASTASES

Table 17-70 Features distinguishing conus lesions from cauda equina lesions[549]

	Conus medullaris lesions	Cauda equina lesions
spontaneous pain	rare; when present, is usually bilateral & symmetric in perineum or thighs	may be most prominent symptom; severe; radicular type; in perineum, thighs & legs, back or bladder
sensory deficit	saddle; bilateral; usually symmetric; sensory dissociation	saddle; no sensory dissociation; may be unilateral & asymmetric
motor loss	symmetric; not marked; fasciculations may be present	asymmetric; more marked; atrophy may occur; fasciculations rare
autonomic symptoms (including bladder dysfunction, impotency…)	prominent early	late
reflexes	only ankle jerk absent (preserved knee jerk)	ankle jerk & knee jerk may be absent
onset	sudden and bilateral	gradual and unilateral

There is no difference in outcome between lesions above or below the conus; thus spinal cord, conus medullaris, or cauda equina mets are considered together here as epidural spinal cord compression (**ESCC**).

GRADING FUNCTION

There is prognostic significance in the presenting neurologic condition. Grading scales such as that of Brice and McKissock (*see Table 17-71*) have been proposed.

MANAGEMENT

Patients are categorized into one of the three following groups below based on the rapidity and seriousness of the neurologic findings[549]. Follow the recommendations for that group listed below.

A metastatic workup is initiated as time permits (see *Metastatic workup*, page 520) (a cursory workup, e.g. a CXR and physical exam may be all that can be ini-

Table 17-71   Grading spinal cord function with spinal metastases (Brice & McKissock)[550]

Group	Grade	Description
1	mild	patient able to walk
2	moderate	able to move legs, but not antigravity
3	severe	slight residual motor and sensory function
4	complete	no motor, sensory, or sphincter function below level of lesion

tially obtained for patients in Group I, whereas more complete workup can be done in others).

GROUP I

> Signs/symptoms **(S/S)** of new or progressive (hours to days) cord compression (e.g. urinary urgency, ascending numbness). These patients have a high risk of rapid deterioration and require immediate evaluation.

Management
1. dexamethasone **(DMZ)** (Decadron®): 100 mg IV STAT (reduces pain in 85%, may produce transient neurologic improvement)
2. radiographic evaluation
   A. plain x-rays of entire spine: 67-85% will be abnormal. Possible findings: pedicle erosion (defect in "owl's eyes" on LS spine AP view) or widening, pathological compression fracture, vertebral body **(VB)** scalloping, VB sclerosis, osteoblastic changes (may occur with prostate Ca, Hodgkin's disease, occasionally with breast Ca, and rarely with multiple myeloma)
   B. if available and patient can tolerate, emergency MRI (see *MRI in evaluating SEM*, page 520)
   C. **emergency myelogram**: this is done if MRI is not immediately available (include the possibility of a C1-2 puncture when obtaining the consent). Start with a so-called "**blockogram**" to R/O complete block: instill small volume of contrast (e.g. iohexol, *see page 127*) via LP and run the dye all the way up the spinal column (CSF is usually xanthochromic with complete block, see *Froin's syndrome*, page 510)
      1. if there is not a complete block: withdraw 10 cc of CSF and send for cytology, protein & glucose. One may then inject more contrast to complete the study
      2. if complete block: do not remove CSF (pressure shifts via LP caused neurologic deterioration in ≈ 14% of patients with complete block[551], whereas there was no deterioration after C1-2 puncture)
         a. in some cases, contrast can be "squeezed" past a "complete" block by injecting 5-10 ml of room air through a millipore filter[552] OR
         b. perform a lateral C1-2 puncture (*see page 618*) and instill contrast to delineate the superior extent of the lesion
      3. with myelography, epidural lesions classically produce **hourglass deformity** with smooth edges if block is incomplete, or **paintbrush effect** (feathered edges) if block is complete, unlike the sharp margins (**capping** or **meniscus sign**) of intradural extramedullary lesion, or fusiform cord widening of intramedullary tumors
   D. bone scan will be abnormal in ≈ 66% of patients with spine mets
3. treatment based on results of radiographic evaluation
   A. if no epidural mass: treat primary tumor (e.g. systemic chemotherapy). Local radiation therapy **(XRT)** to bony lesion if present. Analgesics for pain
   B. if epidural lesion, either surgery or start XRT (usually 30-40 Gy in 10 treatments over 7-10 d with ports extending 2 levels above and below lesion). XRT is usually as effective as laminectomy with fewer complications (for further discussion see *Treatment for SEM*, page 520). Thus, surgery instead of XRT is considered only for the indications shown in *Table 17-72*
   C. urgency of treatment (surgery or XRT) based on degree of block and rapidity of deterioration:
      1. if > 80% block or rapid progression of deficit: emergency treatment

ASAP (if treating with XRT instead of surgery, continue DMZ next day at 24 mg IV q 6 hrs x 2 days, then taper during XRT over 2 wks)
2. if < 80% block: treatment on "routine" basis (for XRT, continue DMZ 4 mg IV q 6 hrs, taper during treatment as tolerated)

Table 17-72 Indications and contraindications for surgery for spinal metastases

Indications	Relative contraindications
1. unknown primary and no tissue diagnosis (consider needle biopsy first if lesion is accessible) NB: lesions such as spinal epidural abscess can occur in patients with a history of Ca and can be mistaken for metastases[553] 2. unstable spine 3. deficit due to spinal deformity or compression by bone rather than by tumor (e.g. due to compression fracture with collapse and retropulsed bone) 4. failure of XRT (usual trial at least 48 hrs, unless significant or rapid deterioration). Usually occurs with radio-resistant tumors such as renal-cell carcinoma or melanoma 5. recurrence after maximal XRT	1. very radiosensitive tumors (multiple myeloma, lymphoma...) not previously radiated 2. total paralysis (Brice and McKissock group 4), present greater than 24 hrs duration (after this, there is essentially no chance of recovery and surgery is not indicated) 3. expected survival ≤ 4 months 4. multiple lesions at multiple levels 5. patient unable to tolerate surgery

GROUP II

Mild and stable signs/symptoms of cord compression (e.g. isolated Babinski), or either plexopathy or radiculopathy without evidence of cord compression. Admit and evaluate within 24 hrs.

Management
1. for suspected ESCC, manage as in Group I except on less emergent basis. Use low dose dexamethasone (**DMZ**) unless radiographic evaluation shows > 80% block
2. for radiculopathy alone (radicular pain, weakness or reflex changes in one myotome or sensory changes in one dermatome): if plain x-rays show bony lesion then 70-88% will have ESCC on myelography. If the plain film is normal, only 9-25% will have ESCC. Obtain MRI or myelogram and manage as for suspected ESCC
3. for plexopathy (brachial or lumbosacral): pain is the most common early symptom, distribution not limited to single dermatome, commonly referred to elbow or ankle. May mask coexistent radiculopathy, distinguish by EMG (denervation of paraspinal muscles occurs in radiculopathy) or presence of proximal signs and symptoms (Horner's syndrome in cervical region, ureteral obstruction in lumbar region). Management:
   A. MRI is initial diagnostic procedure (CT if MRI unavailable): C4 through T4 for brachial plexopathy, L1 through pelvis for lumbosacral
   B. if CT shows bony lesion or paraspinal mass (with negative CT, plain films and bone scan are rarely helpful; however, if done, and plain x-ray shows malignant appearing bony lesion, or if bone scan shows vertebral abnormality, perform MRI or myelogram within 24 hrs)
   (give dexamethasone if ESCC suspected or MRI/myelogram delayed). Management as in Group I based on degree of block, XRT ports extended laterally to include any mass shown on CT
   C. if no bony nor paraspinal lesion on MRI/CT, primary treatment of plexus tumor; analgesics for pain

GROUP III

Back pain without neuro signs/symptoms. Can be evaluated as outpatient over several days (modify based on ability of patient to travel, reliability, etc.).

Management
1. plain spine x-ray (AP, lat, oblique)
   A. if focal bony pathology demonstrated: obtain MRI or myelogram (66% of patients with isolated LBP and X-ray abnormalities had SEM; in 81% with vertebral collapse > 50%, in 31% with pedicle erosion only, and in 7% with vertebral body lesion without collapse). Proceed as in Group I based on results of MRI/myelogram
   B. if plain films normal: bone scan (bone scan positive in up to 20% of patients with normal plain films with ESCC). Consider MRI or myelogram if bone

scan abnormal in absence of benign x-ray lesion
2. CT: if bony lesion or paraspinal mass, proceed to MRI or myelogram, otherwise primary tumor treatment and analgesics

METASTATIC WORKUP

The appropriateness of the following tests depends on the amount of time available as well as clinical information that may rule some primaries in or out.
1. CXR: to rule out lung primary or other mets to lung
2. CT of chest (if CXR is negative) and abdomen
3. serum prostate specific antigen (**PSA**) in males
4. mammogram in females
5. for multiple myeloma: *see page 515*
6. careful physical exam of lymph nodes

MRI IN EVALUATING SEM

Advantages of MRI over myelography[544]:
1. non-invasive. Doesn't require second procedure (C1-2 puncture) if complete block
2. no risk of neurologic deterioration from LP in patient with complete block
3. detects lesions that do not cause bony destruction or distortion of the spinal sub-arachnoid space
4. up to 20% of patients with SEM have at least two sites of cord compression, MRI can evaluate region between two complete blocks, myelography cannot
5. demonstrates paraspinal lesions

Disadvantages of MRI versus myelography:
1. does not obtain CSF for cytological study

MRI findings in spinal epidural metastases:
1. vertebral mets are slightly hypointense compared to normal bone marrow on T1WI, and are slightly hyperintense on T2WI
2. axial cuts typically show lesion involving the posterior vertebral body with invasion into one or both pedicles
3. when myelopathy or radiculopathy are present, there is usually tumor extension into the spinal canal (may not occur in lesions presenting only with local pain)

TREATMENT FOR SEM

No treatment for SEM has been shown to prolong life. Goal of treatment is pain control, preservation of spinal stability, and maintenance of sphincter control and ability to ambulate. As yet, no chemotherapy found useful for SEM (may help with primary). Main decision is between surgery, surgery + post-op XRT, or XRT alone.

The most important factor affecting prognosis, regardless of treatment modality, is ability to walk at the time of initiation of therapy. Loss of sphincter control is a poor prognosticator and is usually irreversible.

Surgery alone appears least effective for pain control (36%, compared to 67% for surgery + XRT, and 76% for XRT alone)[554]. Deterioration in one of the 3 major criteria (pain, continence, ambulation) occurred in 26% of patients treated with laminectomy alone, 20% of laminectomy + XRT, and 17% of XRT alone (roughly comparable). However, surgery had the attendant complications of anesthetic risk, post-op pain, wound problems in 11% (further complicated by radiation), and 9% incidence of spinal instability[554]. Therefore, laminectomy appears best reserved for those situations outlined in *Table 17-72*, page 519. This data is based mostly on *laminectomy* as the surgical treatment. Anterior or posterolateral approaches for anteriorly situated tumors may offer more than laminectomy, and are indicated as primary therapy especially for radioresistant tumors[555], but these operations may not be tolerated by a significant number of patients and a randomized prospective study has yet to be done[556].

RADIATION THERAPY

Usual dose: 30 Gy delivered in 3 Gy fractions over 10 days (2 working weeks) to ports extending at least 1 vertebral level above and below the extent of the lesion.

There is a theoretical risk of radiation induced edema causing or accelerating neurologic deterioration. This has not been born out by experimental studies with the usual small daily fractions utilized. Deterioration is more likely to be due to tumor progression[557].

SURGICAL TREATMENT

See *Table 17-72*, page 519 for indications for surgery.

TECHNIQUE

The traditional technique which has been used for comparison has been laminectomy, which is <u>poor</u> for many spinal metastases since the pathology is usually <u>anterior</u> to the cord. Furthermore, laminectomy may have a significant destabilizing effect when there is metastatic involvement of the vertebral body[555, 558].

If the posterior elements are intact, a transthoracic approach with corpectomy and stabilization (e.g. with methylmethacrylate and Steinmann pins[559], or with spinal instrumentation) followed by XRT improves neurologic function in ≈ 75% and pain in ≈ 85%. A posterolateral approach (e.g. costotransversectomy) may be used for anterolateral tumor[560], but this may destabilize the spine and instrumentation may be necessary[561].

17.13.   References

1. Kleihues P, Burger P C, Scheithauer B W: The new WHO classification of brain tumors. **Brain Pathol** 3: 255-68, 1993.
2. Escourolle R, Poirier J: **Manual of basic neuropathology**. 2nd ed. W. B. Saunders, Philadelphia, 1971.
3. Mahaley M S, Mettlin C, Natarajan N, *et al.*: National survey of patterns of care for brain-tumor patients. **J Neurosurg** 71: 826-36, 1989.
4. Whittle I R, Pringle A-M, Taylor R: Effects of resective surgery for left-sided intracranial tumors on language function: A prospective study. **Lancet** 351: 1014-8, 1998.
5. Forsyth P A, Posner J B: Headaches in patients with brain tumors. A study of 111 patients. **Neurology** 43: 1678-83, 1993.
6. Paraf F, Jothy S, Van Meir E G: Brain tumor-polyposis syndrome: Two genetic diseases. **J Clin Oncol** 15: 2744-58, 1997.
7. Galicich J H, French L A: Use of dexamethasone in the treatment of cerebral edema resulting from brain tumors and brain surgery. **Am Pract Dig Treat** 12: 169-74, 1961.
8. French L A, Galicich J H: The use of steroids for control of cerebral edema. **Clin Neurosurg** 10: 212-23, 1964.
9. Glantz M J, Cole B F, Forsyth P A, *et al.*: Practice parameter: Anticonvulsant prophylaxis in patients with newly diagnosed brain tumors. Report of the quality standards subcommittee of the American academy of neurology. **Neurology** 54: 1886-93, 2000.
10. Chicoine M R, Silbergeld D L: Pharmacology for neurosurgeons. Part I: Anticonvulsants, chemotherapy, antibiotics. **Contemp Neurosurg** 18 (9): 1-6, 1996.
11. Prados M D, Berger M S, Wilson C B: Primary central nervous system tumors: Advances in knowledge and treatment. **CA Cancer J Clin** 48: 331-60, 1998.
12. Stewart D J: A critique of the role of the blood-brain barrier in the chemotherapy of human brain tumors. **J Neurooncol** (20): 121-39, 1994.
13. Salcman M, Broadwell R D: *The blood brain barrier*. In **Neurobiology of brain tumors**, Salcman M, (ed.). Williams and Wilkins, Baltimore, 1991, Vol. 4: pp 229-50.

14. Madajewicz S, Chowhan N, Tfayli A, *et al.*: Therapy for patients with high graqde astrocytoma using intraarterial chemotherapy and radiation therapy. **Cancer** 88: 2350-6, 2000.
15. Barker F G, Prados M D, Chang S M, *et al.*: Radiation response and survival time in patients with glioblastoma multiforme. **J Neurosurg** 84: 442-8, 1996.
16. Laohaprasit V, Silbergeld D L, Ojemann G A, *et al.*: Postoperative CT contrast enhancement following lobectomy for epilepsy. **J Neurosurg** 73: 392-5, 1990.
17. Jeffries B F, Kishore P R, Singh K S, *et al.*: Contrast enhancement in the posoperative brain. **Radiology** 139: 409-13, 1981.
18. Gerber A M, Savolaine E R: Modification of tumor enhancement and brain edema in computerized tomography by corticosteroids: Case report. **Neurosurgery** 6: 282-4, 1980.
19. Hatam A, Bergström M, Yu Z Y, *et al.*: Effect of dexamethasone treatment in volume and contrast enhancement of intracranial neoplasms. **J Comput Assist Tomogr** 7: 295-300, 1983.
20. Albright L, Reigel D H: Management of hydrocephalus secondary to posterior fossa tumors. Preliminary report. **J Neurosurg** 46: 52-5, 1977.
21. Berger M S, Baumeister B, Geyer J R, *et al.*: The risks of metastases from shunting in children with primary central nervous system tumors. **J Neurosurg** 74: 872-7, 1991.
22. McLaurin R L, Venes J L, (eds.): **Pediatric neurosurgery**. 2nd ed., W. B. Saunders, Philadelphia, 1989.
23. Daumas-Duport C, Scheithauer B W, Kelly P J: A histologic and cytologic method for the spatial definition of gliomas. **Mayo Clin Proc** 62: 435-49, 1987.
24. Gunel M, Piepmeier J M: Management of low-grade gliomas. **Contemp Neurosurg** 19 (9): 1-6, 1997.
25. Packer R J, Lange B, Ater J, *et al.*: Carboplatin and vincristine for recurrent and newly diagnosed low-grade gliomas of childhood. **J Clin Oncol** 11: 850-6, 1993.
26. Daumas-Duport C, Scheithauer B W, Chodkiewicz J-P, *et al.*: Dysembryoplastic neuroepithelial tumor: A surgically curable tumor of young patients with intractable seizures. **Neurosurgery** 23: 545-56,

1988.

27. Daumas-Duport C, Varlet P, Bacha S, *et al*.: Dysembryoplastic neuroepithelial tumors: Nonspecific histological forms -- a study of 40 cases. **J Neurooncol** 41 (3): 267-80, 1999.

28. Adada B, Sayed K: Dysembryoplastic neuroepithelial tumors. **Contemp Neurosurg** 26 (23): 1-5, 2004.

29. Kepes J J, Rubinstein L J, Eng L F: Pleomorphic xanthoastrocytoma: A distinctive meningeal glioma of young subjects with relatively favorable prognosis. A study of 12 cases. **Cancer** 44: 1839-52, 1979.

30. Weldon-Linne C M, Victor T A, Groothuis D R, *et al*.: Pleomorphic xanthoastrocytoma: Ultrastructural and immunohistochemical study of a case with a rapidly fatal outcome following surgery. **Cancer** 52: 2055-63, 1983.

31. Russell D S, Rubenstein L J: In **Pathology of tumours of the nervous system**. Williams and Wilkins, Baltimore, 5th ed., 1989: pp 83-161.

32. Kernohan J W, Mabon R F, Svien H J, *et al*.: A simplified classification of the gliomas. **Proc Staff Meet Mayo Clin** 24: 71-5, 1949.

33. Burger P C, Vogel F S, Green S B, *et al*.: Glioblastoma multiforme and anaplastic astrocytoma: Pathologic criteria and prognostic implications. **Cancer** 56: 1106-11, 1985.

34. Daumas-Duport C, Scheithauer B, O'Fallon J, *et al*.: Grading of astrocytomas: A simple and reproducible method. **Cancer** 62: 2152-65, 1988.

35. Kim T S, Halliday A L, Hedley-Whyte T, *et al*.: Correlates of survival and the Daumas-Duport grading system for astrocytomas. **J Neurosurg** 74: 27-37, 1991.

36. Shafqat S, Hedley-Whyte E T, Henson J W: Age-dependent rate of anaplastic transformation in low-grade astrocytoma. **Neurology** 52: 867-9, 1999.

37. Berger M S: *Role of surgery in diagnosis and management*. In **Benign cerebral glioma**, Apuzzo M L J, (ed.). Neurosurgical topics. American Association of Neurological Surgeons, Park Ridge, Illinois, 1995, Vol. 2: pp 293-307.

38. Laws E R, Taylor W F, Clifton M B, *et al*.: Neurosurgical management of low-grade astrocytoma of the cerebral hemispheres. **J Neurosurg** 61: 665-73, 1984.

39. Kopelson G, Linggood R: Infratentorial glioblastoma: The role of neuraxis irradiation. **Int J Radiation Oncology Biol Phys** 8: 999-1003, 1982.

40. Narayan P, Olson J J: Management of anaplastic astrocytoma. **Contemp Neurosurg** 23 (24): 1-6, 2001.

41. Kondziolka D, Lunsford L D, Martinez A J: Unreliability of contemporary neurodiagnostic imaging in evaluating suspected adult supratentorial (low-grade) astrocytoma. **J Neurosurg** 79: 533-6, 1993.

42. Zee C S, Conti P, Destian S, *et al*.: *Imaging features of benign gliomas*. In **Benign cerebral glioma**, Apuzzo M L J, (ed.). Neurosurgical topics. American Association of Neurological Surgeons, Park Ridge, Illinois, 1995, Vol. 2: pp 247-74.

43. Chamberlain M C, Murovic J, Levin V A: Absence of contrast enhancement on CT brain scans of patients with supratentorial malignant gliomas. **Neurology** 38: 1371-3, 1988.

44. Greene G M, Hitchon P W, Schelper R L, *et al*.: Diagnostic yield in CT-guided stereotactic biopsy of gliomas. **J Neurosurg** 71: 494-7, 1989.

45. Scherer H J: The forms of growth in gliomas and their practical significance. **Brain** 63: 1-35, 1940.

46. Choucair A K, Levin V A, Gutin P H, *et al*.: Development of multiple lesions during radiation therapy and chemotherapy. **J Neurosurg** 65: 654-8, 1986.

47. Erlich S S, Davis R L: Spinal subarachnoid metastasis from primary intracranial glioblastoma multiforme. **Cancer** 42: 2854-64, 1978.

48. Artigas J, Cervos-Navarro J, Iglesias J R, *et al*.: Gliomatosis cerebri: Clinical and histological findings. **Clin Neuropathol** 4: 135-48, 1985.

49. Wilson N W, Symon L, Lantos P L: Gliomatosis cerebri: Report of a case presenting as a focal cerebral mass. **J Neurol** 234: 445-7, 1987.

50. Barnard R O, Geddes J F: The incidence of multifocal cerebral gliomas: A histological study of large hemisphere sections. **Cancer** 60: 1519-31, 1987.

51. van Tassel P, Lee Y-Y, Bruner J M: Synchronous and metachronous malignant gliomas: CT findings. **AJNR** 9: 725-32, 1988.

52. Harsh G R, Wilson C B: *Nuroepithelial tumors of the adult brain*. In **Neurological surgery**, Youmans J R, (ed.). W. B. Saunders, Philadelphia, 3rd ed., 1990, Vol. 3: pp 3040-136.

53. Cairncross J G, Laperriere N J: Low-grade glioma: To treat or not to treat? **Arch Neurol** 46: 1238-9, 1989.

54. Shaw E G: Low-grade gliomas: To treat or not to treat? A radiation oncologist's viewpoint. **Arch Neurol** 47: 1138-9, 1990.

55. Karim A B M F, Maat B, Hatlevoll R, *et al*.: A randomized trial on dose-response in radiation therapy of low-grade cerebral glioma: European organization for research and treatment of cancer (EORTC) study 22844. **Int J Radiation Oncology Biol Phys** 36: 549-56, 1996.

56. Shibamoto Y, Kitakabu Y, Takahashi M, *et al*.: Supratentorial low-grade astrocytoma. Correlation of computed tomography findings with effect of radiation therapy and prognostic variables. **Cancer** 72: 190-5, 1993.

57. Kelly P J: *Role of stereotaxis in the management of low-grade intracranial gliomas*. In **Benign cerebral glioma**, Apuzzo M L J, (ed.). Neurosurgical topics. American Association of Neurological Surgeons, Park Ridge, Illinois, 1995, Vol. 2: pp 275-92.

58. Philippon J H, Clemenceau S H, Fauchon F H, *et al*.: Supratentorial low-grade astrocytomas in adults. **Neurosurgery** 32: 554-9, 1993.

59. Shaw E G, Daumas-Duport C, Scheithauer B W, *et al*.: Radiation therapy in the management of low-grade supratentorial astrocytomas. **J Neurosurg** 70: 853-61, 1989.

60. Morantz R A: Radiation therapy in the treatment of cerebral astrocytoma. **Neurosurgery** 20: 975-82, 1987.

61. Quinn J A, Reardon D A, Friedman A H, *et al*.: Phase II trial of temozolomide in patients with progressive low-grade glioma. **J Clin Oncol** 21 (4): 646-51, 2003.

62. Leibel S A, Sheline G E: Radiation therapy for neoplasms of the brain. **J Neurosurg** 66: 1-22, 1987.

63. Keles G E, Anderson B, Berger M S: The effect of extent of resection on time to tumor progression and survival in patients with glioblastoma multiforme of the cerebral hemisrphere. **Surg Neurol** 52: 371-9, 1999.

64. Apuzzo M L J: Comment on Coffey R J, et al.: Survival after stereotactic biopsy of malignant gliomas. **Neurosurgery** 22: 472-3, 1988.

65. Quigley M R, Maroon J C: The relationship between survival and the extent of resection in patients with supratentorial malignant gliomas. **Neurosurgery** 29: 385-9, 1991.

66. Kelly P J, Hunt C H: The limited value of cytoreductive surgery in elderly patients with malignant gliomas. **Neurosurgery** 33: 62-7, 1994.

67. Shapiro W R, Green S B, Burger P C, *et al*.: Randomized trial of three chemotherapy regimens and two radiotherapy regimens in postoperative treatment of malignant glioma: Brain tumor cooperative group trial 8001. **J Neurosurg** 71: 1-9, 1989.

68. Sneed P K, McDermott M W, Gutin P H: Interstitial brachytherapy procedures for brain tumors. **Semin Surg Oncol** 13: 157-66, 1997.

69. Kornblith P L: The role of cytotoxic chemotherapy

in the treatment of malignant brain tumors. **Surg Neurol** 44: 551-2, 1995.

70. Fine H A, Dear K B, Loeffler J S, *et al.*: Meta-analysis of radiation therapy with and without adjuvant chemotherapy for malignant gliomas in adults. **Cancer** 71: 2585-97, 1993.

71. Kornblith P L: Chemotherapy for malignant brain tumors. **J Neurosurg** 68: 1-17, 1988.

72. Esteller M, Garcia-Foncillas J, Andion E, *et al.*: Inactivation of the DNA-repair gene *MGMT* and the clinical response of gliomas to alkylating agents. **N Engl J Med** 343: 1350-4, 2000.

73. Bleehen N M, Stenning S P: A medical research Council trial of two radiotherapy doses in the treatment of grades 3 and 4 astrocytoma. The medical research Council brain tumour working party. **Br J Cancer** 64 (4): 769-74, 1991.

74. Stewart L A: Chemotherapy in adult high-grade glioma: A systematic review and meta-analysis of individual patient data from 12 randomised trials. **Lancet** 359 (9311): 1011-8, 2002.

75. Hochberg F H, Pruitt A A, Beck D O, *et al.*: The rationale and methodology for intra-arterial chemotherapy with BCNU as treatment for glioblastoma. **J Neurosurg** 63: 876-80, 1985.

76. Bashir R, Hochberg F H, Linggood R M, *et al.*: Pre-irradiation internal carotid artery BCNU in treatment of glioblastoma multiforme. **J Neurosurg** 68: 917-9, 1988.

77. Grossman S A, Reinhard C S, Colvin O M, *et al.*: The intracerebral distribution of BCNU delivery by surgically implanted biodegradable polymers. **J Neurosurg** 76: 640-7, 1992.

78. Brem H, Piantadosi S, Burger P C, *et al.*: Placebo-controlled trial of safety and efficacy of intraoperative controlled delivery by biodegradable polymers of chemotherapy for recurrent gliomas. **Lancet** 345: 1008-12, 1995.

79. Valtonen S, Timonen U, Toivanen P, *et al.*: Interstitial chemotherapy with carmustine-loaded polymers for high-grade gliomas: A randomized double-blind study. **Neurosurgery** 41: 44-9, 1997.

80. Gliadel wafers for treatment of brain tumors. **Med Letter** 40 (1035): 92, 1998.

81. Friedman H S, McLendon R E, Kerby T, *et al.*: DNA mismatch repair and O^6-alkylguanine-DNA alkyltransferase analysis and response to temodal in newly diagnosed malignant glioma. **J Clin Oncol** 16: 3851-7, 1998.

82. Harsh G R, Levin V A, Gutin P H, *et al.*: Reoperation for recurrent glioblastoma and anaplastic astrocytoma. **Neurosurgery** 21: 615-21, 1987.

83. Ammirati M, Galicich J H, Arbit E, *et al.*: Reoperation in the treatment of recurrent intracranial malignant gliomas. **Neurosurgery** 21: 607-14, 1987.

84. Wen P Y, Fine H A, Black P M, *et al.*: High-grade astrocytomas. **Neurol Clin** 13: 875 96, 1995.

85. Coffey R J, Lunsford L D, Taylor F H: Survival after stereotactic biopsy of malignant gliomas. **Neurosurgery** 22: 465-73, 1988.

86. Thomson A-M, Taylor R, Fraser D, *et al.*: Stereotactic biopsy of nonpolar tumors in the dominant hemisphere: A prospective study of effects on language functions. **J Neurosurg** 89: 923-6, 1997.

87. Burger P C, Scheithauer B W: **Atlas of tumor pathology. Tumors of the central nervous system**. Armed Forces Institute of Pathology, Washington, D.C., 1994.

88. Pollack I F, Hoffman H J, Humphreys R P, *et al.*: The long-term outcome after surgical treatment of dorsally exophytic brain-stem gliomas. **J Neurosurg** 78: 859-63, 1993.

89. Coakley K J, Huston J, Scheithauer B W, *et al.*: Pilocytic astrocytomas: Well-demarcated magnetic resonance appearance despite frequent infiltration histologically. **Mayo Clin Proc** 70: 747-51, 1995.

90. Hayostek C J, Shaw E G, Scheithauer B, *et al.*: Astrocytomas of the cerebellum: A comparative clinicopathologic study of pilocytic and diffuse astrocytomas. **Cancer** 72: 856-69, 1993.

91. Bernell W R, Kepes J J, Seitz E P: Late malignant recurrence of childhood cerebellar astrocytoma. **J Neurosurg** 37: 470-4, 1972.

92. Schwartz A M, Ghatak N R: Malignant transformation of benign cerebellar astrocytoma. **Cancer** 65: 333-6, 1990.

93. Zimmerman R A, Bilaniuk C T, Bruno L A, *et al.*: CT of cerebellar astrocytoma. **Am J Roentgenol** 130: 929-33, 1978.

94. Section of Pediatric Neurosurgery of the American Association of Neurological Surgeons, (ed.) **Pediatric neurosurgery**. 1st ed., Grune and Stratton, New York, 1982.

95. Youmans J R, (ed.) **Neurological surgery**. 3rd ed., W. B. Saunders, Philadelphia, 1990.

96. Ringertz N, Nordenstam H: Cerebellar astrocytoma. **J Neuropathol Exp Neurol** 10: 343-67, 1951.

97. Gol A: Cerebellar astrocytomas in children. **Am J Dis Child** 106: 21-4, 1963.

98. Winston K, Gilles F H, Leviton A, *et al.*: Cerebellar gliomas in children. **J Natl Cancer Inst** 58: 833-8, 1977.

99. Austin E J, Alvord E C: Recurrences of cerebellar astrocytomas: A violation of Collins' law. **J Neurosurg** 68: 41-7, 1988.

100. Bucy P C, Thieman P W: Astrocytomas of the cerebellum. A study of patients operated upon over 28 years ago. **Arch Neurol** 18: 14-9, 1968.

101. Stein B M, Tenner M S, Fraser R A R: Hydrocephalus following removal of cerebellar astrocytomas in children. **J Neurosurg** 36: 763-8, 1972.

102. Packer R J, Nicholson H S, Vezina L G, *et al.*: Brainstem gliomas. **Neurosurg Clin N Am** 3 (4): 863-79, 1992.

103. Laurent J P, Cheek W R: Brain tumors in children. **J Pediatr Neurosci** 1: 15-32, 1985.

104. Reigel D H, Scarff T B, Woodford J E: Biopsy of pediatric brain stem tumors. **Childs Brain** 5: 329-40, 1979.

105. Epstein F J, Farmaer J-P: Brain-stem glioma growth patterns. **J Neurosurg** 78: 408-12, 1993.

106. Epstein F, McCleary E L: Intrinsic brain-stem tumors of childhood: Surgical indications. **J Neurosurg** 64: 11-5, 1986.

107. Garcia C A, McGarry P A, Collada M: Ganglioglioma of the brain stem. Case report. **J Neurosurg** 60: 431-4, 1984.

108. Albright A L, Packer R J, Zimmerman R, *et al.*: Magnetic resonance scans should replace biopsies for the diagnosis of diffuse brain stem gliomas: A report from the children's cancer group. **Neurosurgery** 33: 1026-30, 1993.

109. Hoffman H J, Becker L, Craven M A: A clinically and pathologically distinct group of benign brain-stem gliomas. **Neurosurgery** 7: 243-8, 1980.

110. Kyoshima K, Kobayashi S, Gibo H, *et al.*: A study of safe entry zones via the floor of the fourth ventricle for brain-stem lesions. **J Neurosurg** 78: 987-93, 1993.

111. Stark A M, Fritsch M J, Claviez A, *et al.*: Management of tectal glioma in childhood. **Pediatr Neurol**, 2005.

112. Bognar L, Turjman F, Villanyi E, *et al.*: Tectal plate gliomas. Part II: CT scans and MR imaging of tectal gliomas. **Acta Neurochir (Wien)** 127 (1-2): 48-54, 1994.

113. Pollack I F, Pang D, Albright A L: The long-term outcome in children with late-onset aqueductal stenosis resulting from benign intrinsic tectal tumors. **J Neurosurg** 80 (4): 681-8, 1994.

114. Grant G A, Avellino A M, Loeser J D, *et al.*: Management of intrinsic gliomas of the tectal plate in children. A ten-year review. **Pediatr Neurosurg** 31 (4): 170-6, 1999.

115. Oka K, Kin Y, Go Y, et al.: Neuroendoscopic approach to tectal tumors: A consecutive series. J Neurosurg 91 (6): 964-70, 1999.

116. Kihlstrom L, Lindquist C, Lindquist M, et al.: Stereotactic radiosurgery for tectal low-grade gliomas. Acta Neurochir Suppl 62: 55-7, 1994.

117. Mork S J, Lindegaard K F, Halvorsen T B, et al.: Oligodendroglioma: Incidence and biological behavior in a defined population. J Neurosurg 63: 881-9, 1985.

118. Daumas-Duport C, Tucker M-L, Kolles H, et al.: Oligodendrogliomas: Part II - A new grading system based on morphological and imaging criteria. J Neurooncol 34: 61-78, 1997.

119. Coons S W, Johnson P C, Scheithauer B W, et al.: Improving diagnostic accuracy and interobserver concordance in the classification and grading of primary gliomas. Cancer 79: 1381-93, 1997.

120. Daumas-Duport C, Varlet P, Tucker M-L, et al.: Oligodendrogliomas: Part I - patterns of growth, histological diagnosis, clinical and imaging correlations: A study of 153 cases. J Neurooncol 34: 37-59, 1997.

121. Chin H W, Hazel J J, Kim T H, et al.: Oligodendrogliomas. I. A clinical study of cerebral oligodendrogliomas. Cancer 45: 1458-66, 1980.

122. Roberts M, German W: A long term study of patients with oligodendrogliomas. J Neurosurg 24: 697-700, 1966.

123. Coons S W, Johnson P C, Pearl D K, et al.: The prognostic significance of Ki-67 labeling indices for oligodendrogliomas. Neurosurgery 41: 878-85, 1997.

124. Fortin D, Cairncross G J, Hammond R R: Oligodendroglioma: An appraisal of recent data pertaining to diagnosis and treatment. Neurosurgery 45: 1279-91, 1999.

125. Hart M N, Petito C K, Earle K M: Mixed gliomas. Cancer 33: 134-40, 1974.

126. Rutka J T, Murakami M, Dirks P B, et al.: Role of glial filaments in cells and tumors of glial origin: A review. J Neurosurg 87: 420-30, 1997.

127. Kros J M, Schouten W C D, Janssen P J A, et al.: Proliferation of gemistocytic cells and glial fibrillary acidic protein (GFAP)-positive oligodendroglial cells in gliomas: A MIB-1/GFAP double labeling study. Acta Neuropathol (Berl) 91: 99-103, 1996.

128. Smith M T, Ludwig C L, Godfrey A D, et al.: Grading of oligodendrogliomas. Cancer 52: 2107-14, 1983.

129. Cairncross J G, Macdonald D, Ludwin S, et al.: Chemotherapy for anaplastic oligodendroglioma. J Clin Oncol 12: 2013-21, 1994.

130. Cairncross J G, Ueki K, Zlatescu M C, et al.: Specific genetic predictors of chemotherapeutic response and survival in patients with anaplastic oligodendrogliomas. J Natl Cancer Inst 90: 1473-9, 1998.

131. Levin V A, Edwards M S, Wright D C, et al.: Modified procarbazine, CCNU and vincristine (PCV-3) combination chemotherapy in the treatment of malignant brain tumors. Cancer Treat Rep 64: 237-44, 1980.

132. Glass J, Hochberg F H, Gruber M L, et al.: The treatment of oligodendrogliomas and mixed oligodendroglioma-astrocytomas with PCV chemotherapy. J Neurosurg 76: 741-5, 1992.

133. Yung W K, Prados M D, Yaya-Tur R, et al.: Multicenter phase II trial of temozolomide in patients with anaplastic astrocytoma or anaplastic oligoastrocytoma at first relapse. Temodal brain tumor group. J Clin Oncol 17: 2761-71, 1999.

134. Berger M S, Rostomily R C: Low grade gliomas: Functional mapping resection strategies, extent of resection, and outcome. J Neurooncol 34: 85-101, 1997.

135. Gonzales M, Sheline G E: Treatment of oligoden-

drogliomas with or without postoperative radiation. J Neurosurg 68: 684-8, 1988.

136. Reedy D P, Bay J W, Hahn J F: Role of radiation therapy in the treatment of cerebral oligodendroglioma. Neurosurgery 13: 499-503, 1983.

137. Taphoorn M J, Heimans J J, Snoek F J, et al.: Assessment of quality of life in patients treated for low-grade glioma: A preliminary report. J Neurol Neurosurg Psychiatry 55: 372-6, 1992.

138. Sgouros S, Carey M, Aluwihare N, et al.: Central neurocytoma: A correlative clinicopathologic and radiologic analysis. Surg Neurol 49 (2): 197-204, 1998.

139. Tong C Y, Ng H K, Pang J C, et al.: Central neurocytomas are genetically distinct from oligodendrogliomas and neuroblastomas. Histopathology 37 (2): 160-5, 2000.

140. Brat D J, Scheithauer B W, Eberhart C G, et al.: Extraventricular neurocytomas: Pathologic features and clinical outcome. Am J Surg Pathol 25 (10): 1252-60, 2001.

141. Jackson T R, Regine W F, Wilson D, et al.: Cerebellar liponeurocytoma. Case report and review of the literature. J Neurosurg 95 (4): 700-3, 2001.

142. George D H, Scheithauer B W: Central liponeurocytoma. Am J Surg Pathol 25 (12): 1551-5, 2001.

143. Bertalanffy A, Roessler K, Dietrich W, et al.: Gamma knife radiosurgery of recurrent central neurocytomas: A preliminary report. J Neurol Neurosurg Psychiatry 70 (4): 489-93, 2001.

144. Tyler-Kabara E, Kondziolka D, Flickinger J C, et al.: Stereotactic radiosurgery for residual neurocytoma. Report of four cases. J Neurosurg 95 (5): 879-82, 2001.

145. Brandes A A, Amist inverted question marka P, Gardiman M, et al.: Chemotherapy in patients with recurrent and progressive central neurocytoma. Cancer 88 (1): 169-74, 2000.

146. Kulali A, Ilcayto R, Rahmanli O: Primary calvarial ectopic meningiomas. Neurochirurgia (Stuttg) 34 (6): 174-7, 1991.

147. Mahmood A, Caccamo D V, Tomecek F J, et al.: Atypical and malignant meningiomas: A clinicopathological review. Neurosurgery 33: 955-63, 1993.

148. Sheehy J P, Crockard H A: Multiple meningiomas: A long-term review. J Neurosurg 59: 1-5, 1983.

149. Nakasu S, Hirano A, Shimura T, et al.: Incidental meningiomas in autopsy studies. Surg Neurol 27: 319-22, 1987.

150. Wara W M, Sheline G E, Newman H, et al.: Radiation therapy of meningiomas. AJR 123: 453-8, 1975.

151. Yamashita J, Handa H, Iwaki K, et al.: Recurrence of intracranial meningiomas, with special reference to radiotherapy. Surg Neurol 14: 33-40, 1980.

152. Cushing H, Eisenhardt L: Meningiomas of the sphenoidal ridge. A. Those of the deep or clinoidal third. In Meningiomas: Their classification, regional behaviour, life history, and surgical end results. Charles C Thomas, Springfield, Illinois, 1938: pp 298-319.

153. Eskandary H, Hamzel A, Yasamy M T: Foot drop following brain lesion. Surg Neurol 43: 89-90, 1995.

154. Al-Mefty O: Tuberculum sella and olfactory groove meningiomas. In Surgery of cranial base tumors, Sekhar L N and Janecka I P, (eds.). Raven Press, New York, 1993, Chapter 36: pp 507-19.

155. George B, Lot G, Velut S: Tumors of the foramen magnum. Neurochirurgie 39: 1-89, 1993.

156. George B, Lot G, Boissonnet H: Meningioma of the foramen magnum: A series of 40 cases. Surg Neurol 47: 371-9, 1997.

157. Kuratsu J-I, Kochi M, Ushio Y: Incidence and clinical features of asymptomatic meningiomas. J Neurosurg 92: 766-70, 2000.

158. Zulch K J: **Histologic typing or tumors of the central nervous system. International histological classification of tumors, no. 21**. World Health Organization, Geneva, 1979: pp 17-57.

159. Russell D S, Rubenstein L J: **Pathology of tumours of the nervous system**. 5th ed. Williams and Wilkins, Baltimore, 1989.

160. Michaud J, Gagné F: Microcystic meningoma. Clinicopathologic report of eight cases. **Arch Pathol Lab Med** 107: 75-80, 1983.

161. Thomas H G, Dolman C L, Berry K: Malignant meningioma: Clinical and pathological features. **J Neurosurg** 55: 929-34, 1981.

162. Zimmerman R D, Fleming C A, Saint-Louis L A, et al.: Magnetic resonance of meningiomas. **AJNR** 6: 149-57, 1985.

163. Taylor S I., Barakos J A, Harsh G R, et al.: Magnetic resonance imaging of tuberculum sellae meningiomas: Preventing preoperative misdiagnosis as pituitary macroadenoma. **Neurosurgery** 31: 621-7, 1992.

164. Mirimanoff R O, Dosoretz D E, Lingood R M, et al.: Meningioma: Analysis of recurrence and progression following neurosurgical resection. **J Neurosurg** 62. 18-24, 1985.

165. Adegbite A V, Khan M I, Paine K W E, et al.: The recurrence of intracranial meningiomas after surgical treatment. **J Neurosurg** 58: 51-6, 1983.

166. Jaaskelainen J: Seemingly complete removal of histologically benign intracranial meningioma: Late recurrence R. **Surg Neurol** 26: 461-9, 1986.

167. Simpson D: The recurrence of intracranial meningiomas after surgical treatment. **J Neurol Neurosurg Psychiatry** 20: 22-39, 1957.

168. Barbaro N M, Gutin P H, Wilson C B, et al.: Radiation therapy in the treatment of partially resected meningiomas. **Neurosurgery** 20: 525-8, 1987.

169. Zuccarello M, Sawaya R, deCourten-Myers: Glioblastoma occurring after radiation therapy for meningioma. Case report and review of literature. **Neurosurgery** 19: 114-9, 1986.

170. National Institutes of Health Consensus Development Conference: *Acoustic neuroma: Consensus statement*. **NIH Consens Dev Conf Consens Statement**. Bethesda, MD: Public Health Service, U.S. Department of Health and Human Services. Vol. 9, 1991.

171. Eldridge R, Parry D: Summary: Vestibular schwannoma (acoustic neuroma) consensus development conference. **Neurosurgery** 30: 962-4, 1992.

172. Harner S G, Laws E R: Clinical findings in patients with acoustic neuromas. **Mayo Clin Proc** 58: 721-8, 1983.

173. Flickinger J C, Lunsford L D, Coffey R J, et al.: Radiosurgery of acoustic neurinomas. **Cancer** 67. 345-53, 1991.

174. Jaffe B. Clinical studies in sudden deafness. **Adv Otorhinolaryngol** 20: 221-8, 1973.

175. Byl F: Seventy-six cases of presumed sudden hearing loss occurring in 1973: Prognosis and incidence. **Laryngoscope** 87: 817-24, 1977.

176. Berenholz L P, Eriksen C, Hirsh F A: Recovery from repeated sudden hearing loss with corticosteroid use in the presence of an acoustic neuroma. **Ann Otol Rhinol Laryngol** 101: 827-31, 1992.

177. Moskowitz D, Lee K J, Smith H W: Steroid use in idiopathic suden sensorineuroal hearing loss. **Laryngoscope** 94: 664-6, 1984.

178. Tarlov E C: Microsurgical vestibular nerve section for intractable Meniere's disease. **Clin Neurosurg** 33: 667-84, 1985.

179. House W F, Brackmann D E: Facial nerve grading system. **Otolaryngol Head Neck Surg** 93: 184-93, 1985.

180. Bederson J B, von Ammon K, Wichmann W W, et al.: Conservative treatment of patients with acoustic tumors. **Neurosurgery** 28: 646-51, 1991.

181. Pollock B E, Lunsford L D, Flickinger J C, et al.: Vestibular schwannoma management. Part I. Failed microsurgery and the role of delayed stereotactic radiosurgery. **J Neurosurg** 89: 944-8, 1998.

182. Yamamoto M, Hagiwara S, Ide M, et al.: Conservative management of acoustic neurinomas: Prospective study of long-term changes in tumor volumes and auditory function. **Minim Invasive Neurosurg** 41: 86-92, 1998.

183. Gardner G, Robertson J H: Hearing preservation in unilateral acoustic neuroma surgery. **Ann Otol Rhinol Laryngol** 97: 55-66, 1988.

184. Silverstein H, McDaniel A, Norrell H, et al.: Hearing preservation after acoustic neuroma surgery with intraoperative direct eighth cranial nerve monitoring: Part II. A classification of results. **Otolaryngol Head Neck Surg** 95, 1986.

185. Committee on Hearing and Equilibrium of the American Academy of Otolaryngology-Head and Neck Surgery Foundation: Guidelines for the evaluation of hearing preservation in acoustic neuroma (vestibular schwannoma). **Otolaryngol Head Neck Surg** 113 (3): 179-80, 1995.

186. Hardy D G, Macfarlane R, Baguley D, et al.: Surgery for acoustic neurinoma: An analysis of 100 translabyrinthine operations. **J Neurosurg** 71: 799-804, 1989.

187. Chiappa K H: **Evoked potentials in clinical medicine**. Raven Press, New York, 1983.

188. Niranjan A, Lunsford L D, Flickinger J C, et al.: Dose reduction improves hearing preservation rates after intracanalicular acoustic tumor radiosurgery. **Neurosurgery** 45: 753-65, 1999.

189. Samii M, Tatagiba M, C M: Acoustic neurinoma in the elderly: Factors predictive of postoperative outcome. **Neurosurgery** 31: 615-20, 1992.

190. Ojemann R G: Microsurgical suboccipital approach to cerebellopontine angle tumors. **Clin Neurosurg** 25: 461-79, 1978.

191. Rhoton A L, Jr.: The cerebellopontine angle and posterior fossa cranial nerves by the retrosigmoid approach. **Neurosurgery** 47 (3 Suppl): S93-129, 2000.

192. Sheptak P E, Jannetta P J: The two-stage excision of huge acoustic neuromas. **J Neurosurg** 51: 37-41, 1979.

193. Lownie S P, Drake C G: Radical intracapsular removal of acoustic neurinomas. Long-term follow-up review of 11 cases. **J Neurosurg** 74: 422-5, 1991.

194. Wazen J, Silverstein H, Norrell H, et al.: Preoperative and postoperative growth rates in acoustic neuromas documented with CT scanning. **Otolaryngol Head Neck Surg** 93: 151-5, 1985.

195. Yasargil M G, Fox J L: The microsurgical approach to acoustic neuromas. **Surg Neurol** 2: 393-8, 1974.

196. Rhoton A L: Microsurgical anatomy of the brainstem surface facing an acoustic neuroma. **Surg Neurol** 25: 326-39, 1986.

197. House W F: Surgical exposure of the internal auditory canal and its contents through the middle, cranial fossa. **Laryngoscope** 71: 1363-85, 1961.

198. Nutik S L, Korol H W: Cerebrospinal fluid leak after acoustic neuroma surgery. **Surg Neurol** 43: 553-7, 1995.

199. Symon L, Pell M F: Cerebrospinal fluid rhinorrhea following acoustic neurinoma surgery: Technical note. **J Neurosurg** 74: 152-3, 1991.

200. Ojemann R G: Management of acoustic neuromas (vestibular schwannomas). **Clin Neurosurg** 40: 498-539, 1993.

201. Ebersold M J, Harner S G, Beatty C W, et al.: Current results of the retrosigmoid approach to acoustic neurinoma. **J Neurosurg** 76: 901-9, 1992.

202. Sekhar L N, Gormely W B, Wright D C: The best treatment for vestibular schwannoma (acoustic neuroma): Microsurgery or radiosurgery? **Am J Otol** 17: 676-89, 1996.

203. Wiegand D A, Fickel V: Acoustic neuromas. The patient's perspective. Subjective assessment of symptoms, diagnosis, therapy, and outsome in 541 patients. **Laryngoscope** 99: 179-87, 1989.

204. Gormley W B, Sekhar L N, Wright D C, *et al.*: Acoustic neuroma: Results of current surgical management. **Neurosurgery** 41: 50-60, 1997.

205. Samii M, Matthies C: Management of 1000 vestibular schwannomas (acoustic neuromas): Surgical management with an emphasis on complications and how to avoid them. **Neurosurgery** 40: 11-23, 1997.

206. Wilkins R H, Rengachary S S, (eds.): **Neurosurgery**. McGraw-Hill, New York, 1985.

207. Flickinger J C, Lunsford L D, Pollock B E, *et al.*: Evolution in technique for vestibular schwannoma radiosurgery and effect on outcome. **Int J Radiation Oncology Biol Phys** 36: 275-80, 1996.

208. Harner S G, Daube J R, Ebersold M J, *et al.*: Improved preservation of facial nerve function with use of electrical monitoring during removal of acoustic neuromas. **Mayo Clin Proc** 62: 92-102, 1987.

209. Moller A R, Jannetta P J: Preservation of facial function during removal of acoustic neuromas: Use of monopolar constant-voltage stimulation and EMG. **J Neurosurg** 61: 757-60, 1984.

210. Hirsch A, Norén G: Audiological findings after stereotactic radiosurgery in acoustic neuromas. **Acta Otolaryngol (Stockh)** 106: 244-51, 1988.

211. Pollock B E, Lunsford L D, Kondziolka D, *et al.*: Outcome analysis of acoustic neuroma management: A comparison of microsurgery and stereotactic radiosurgery. **Neurosurgery** 36: 215-29, 1995.

212. Ojemann R G: Comment on Pollock B E, et al.: Outcome analysis of acoustic neuroma management: A comparison of microsurgery and stereotactic radiosurgery. **Neurosurgery** 36: 225-6, 1995.

213. Glasscock M E, Hays J W, Minor L B, *et al.*: Preservation of hearing in surgery for acoustic neuromas. **J Neurosurg** 78: 864-70, 1993.

214. Ojemann R G, Levine R A, Montgomery W M, *et al.*: Use of intraoperative auditory evoked potentials to preserve hearing in unilateral acoustic neuroma removal. **J Neurosurg** 61: 938-48, 1984.

215. Brackmann D E, House J R I, Hitselberger W E: *Technical modifications to the middle cranial fossa approach in removal of acoustic neuromas.* **Spring Scientific Meeting of the American Neurotolgy Society.** Los Angeles, CA: 1993.

216. Shelton C, House W F: Hearing improvement after acoustic tumor removal. **Otolaryngol Head Neck Surg** 103: 963-5, 1990.

217. Wallner K E, Sheline G E, Pitts L H, *et al.*: Efficacy of irradiation for incompletely excised acoustic neurilemomas. **J Neurosurg** 67: 858-63, 1987.

218. Pitts L H, Jackler R K: Treatment of acoustic neuromas. **N Engl J Med** 339: 1471-3, 1998 (editorial).

219. Noren G, Hirsch A, Mosskin M: Long-term efficacy of gamma knife radiosurgery in vestibular schwannomas. **Acta Neurochir** 122: 164, 1993 (abstract).

220. Linskey M E, Lunsford L D, Flickinger J C: Neuroimaging of acoustic nerve sheath tumors after stereotactic radiosurgery. **AJNR** 12: 1165-75, 1991.

221. Pollock B E, Lunsford L D, Kondziolka D, *et al.*: Vestibular schwannoma management. Part II. Failed radiosurgery and the role of delayed microsurgery. **J Neurosurg** 89: 949-55, 1998.

222. Slattery W H, Brackmann D E: Results of surgery following stereotactic irradiation for acoustic neuromas. **Am J Otol** 16: 315-21, 1995.

223. Wiet R J, Micco A G, Bauer G P: Complications of the gamma knife. **Arch Otolaryngol Head Neck Surg** 122: 414-6, 1996.

224. Yakulis R, Manack L, Murphy A I: Postradiation malignant triton tumor: A case report and review of the literature. **Arch Pathol Lab Med** 120: 541-8,

1996.

225. Comey C H, McLaughlin M R, Jho H D, *et al.*: Death from a malignant cerebellopontine angle triton tumor despite stereotactic radiosurgery. **J Neurosurg** 89: 653-8, 1998.

226. Lustig L R, Jackler R K, Lanser M J: Radiation-induced tumors of the temporal bone. **Am J Otol** 18: 230-5, 1997.

227. Beatty C W, Ebersold M J, Harner S G: Residual and recurrent acoustic neuromas. **Laryngoscope** 97: 1168-71, 1987.

228. Nutkiewicz A, DeFeo D R, Kohout R I, *et al.*: Cerebrospinal fluid rhinorrhea as a presentation of pituitary adenoma. **Neurosurgery** 6: 195-7, 1980.

229. Ebersold M J, Quast L M, Laws E R, *et al.*: Longterm results in transsphenoidal removal of nonfunctioning pituitary adenomas. **J Neurosurg** 64: 713-9, 1986.

230. Reid R L, Quigley M E, Yen S C: Pituitary apoplexy: A review. **Arch Neurol** 42: 712-9, 1985.

231. Cardoso E R, Peterson E W: Pituitary apoplexy: A review. **Neurosurgery** 14: 363-73, 1984.

232. Onesti S T, Wisniewski T, Post K D: Pituitary hemorrhage into a Rathke's cleft cyst. **Neurosurgery** 27: 644-6, 1990.

233. Liu J K, Couldwell W: Pituitary apoplexy: Diagnosis and management. **Contemp Neurosurg** 25 (12): 1-5, 2003.

234. Wakai S, Fukushima T, Teramoto A, *et al.*: Pituitary apoplexy: Its incidence and clinical significance. **J Neurosurg** 55: 187-93, 1981.

235. Rovit R L, Fein J M: Pituitary apoplexy, A review and reappraisal. **J Neurosurg** 37: 280-8, 1972.

236. Bills D C, Meyer F B, Laws E R, Jr., *et al.*: A retrospective analysis of pituitary apoplexy. **Neurosurgery** 33 (4): 602-8; discussion 608-9, 1993.

237. Melmed S: Acromegaly. **N Engl J Med** 322: 966-77, 1990.

238. Acromegaly Therapy Consensus Development Panel: Consensus statement: Benefits versus risks of medical therapy for acromegaly. **Am J Med** 97: 468-73, 1994.

239. Wilson C B: *Neurosurgical management of large and invasive pituitary tumors.* In **Clinical management of pituitary disorders**, Tindall G T and Collins W F, (eds.). Raven Press, New York, 1979: pp 335-42.

240. Hardy J: *Transsphenoidal surgery of hypersecreting pituitary tumors.* In **Diagnosis and treatment of pituitary tumors**, Kohler P O and Ross G T, (eds.). Excerpta Medica/American Elsevier, New York, 1973: pp 179-94.

241. Hardy J: *Transsphenoidal surgery of intracranial neoplasm.* In **Adv neurol**, Thompson R A and Green R, (eds.). Raven Press, New York, 1976, Vol. 15: Neoplasia in the Central Nervous System: pp 261-74.

242. Krisht A F: Giant invasive pituitary adenomas. **Contemp Neurosurg** 21 (1): 1-6, 1999.

243. Laws E R: Comment on Knosp E, et al.: Pituitary adenomas with invasion of the cavernous sinus space: A magnetic resonance imaging classification compared with surgical findings. **Neurosurgery** 33: 617, 1993.

244. Scotti G, Yu C Y, Dillon W P, *et al.*: MR imaging of cavernous sinus involvement by pituitary adenomas. **AJR** 151: 799-806, 1988.

245. Barlas O, Bayindir C, Hepgul K, *et al.*: Bromocriptine-induced cerebrospinal fluid fistula in patients with macroprolactinomas: Report of three cases and a review of the literature. **Surg Neurol** 41 (6): 486-9, 1994.

246. Wilson C B: Endocrine-inactive pituitary adenomas. **Clin Neurosurg** 38: 10-31, 1992.

247. Walsh F B, Hoyt W F, (eds.): **Clinical neuro-ophthalmology**. 3rd ed., Williams and Wilkins, Baltimore, 1969.

248. Tindall G T, Barrow D L: Current management of pituitary tumors: Part I. **Contemp Neurosurg** 10: 1-6, 1988.

249. Watts N B: Cushing's syndrome: An update. **Contemp Neurosurg** 17 (18): 1-7, 1995.

250. Watts N B, Tindall G T: Rapid assessment of corticotropin reserve after pituitary surgery. **JAMA** 259: 708-11, 1988.

251. Bilaniuk L T, Moshang T, Cara J, *et al.*: Pituitary enlargement mimicking pituitary tumor. **J Neurosurg** 63: 39-42, 1985.

252. Atchison J A, Lee P A, Albright L: Reversible suprasellar pituitary mass secondary to hypothyroidism. **JAMA** 262: 3175-7, 1989.

253. Watanakunakorn C, Hodges R E, Evans T C: Myxedema. A study of 400 cases. **Arch Intern Med** 116: 183-90, 1965.

254. Kallenberg G A, Pesce C M, Norman B, *et al.*: Ectopic hyperprolactinemia resulting from an ovarian teratoma. **JAMA** 263: 2472-4, 1990.

255. Randall R V, Scheithauer B W, Laws E R, *et al.*: Pituitary adenomas associated with hyperprolactinemia. **Mayo Clin Proc** 60: 753-62, 1985.

256. Tyrell J B, Aron D C, Forsham P H: *Glucocorticoids and adrenal androgens*. In **Basic and clinical endocrinology**, Greenspan F S, (ed.). Appleton and Lange, Norwalk, 3rd ed., 1991: pp 323-62.

257. Yanovski J A, Cutler G B, Chrousos G P, *et al.*: Corticotropin-releasing sormone stimulation following low-dose dexamethasone administration: A new test to distinguish Cushing's syndrome from pseudo-Cushing's states. **JAMA** 269: 2232-8, 1993.

258. Liddle G W: Tests of pituitary-adrenal suppressibility in the diagnosis of Cushing's syndrome. **J Clin Endocrinol Metab** 20: 1539-60, 1960.

259. McCutcheon J E, Oldfield E H: *Cortisol: Regulation, disorders, and clinical evaluation*. In **Neuroendocrinology**, Barrow D L and Selman W, (eds.). Concepts in neurosurgery. Williams and Wilkins, Baltimore, 1992, Vol. 5: pp 117-73.

260. Chrousos G P, Schulte H M, Oldfield E H, *et al.*: The corticotropin-releasing factor stimulation test: An aid in the evaluation of patients with Cushing's syndrome. **N Engl J Med** 310: 622-6, 1984.

261. Abboud C F: Laboratory diagnosis of hypopituitarism. **Mayo Clin Proc** 61: 35-48, 1986.

262. Clemmons D R, Van Wyk J J, Ridgway E C, *et al.*: Evaluation of acromegaly by radioimmunoassay of somatomedin-C. **N Engl J Med** 301: 1138, 1979.

263. Peyster R G, Hoover E D, Viscarello R R, *et al.*: CT appearance of the adolescent and preadolescent pituitary gland. **AJNR** 4: 411-4, 1983.

264. Watson J C, Shawker T H, Nieman L K, *et al.*: Localization of pituitary adenomas by using intraoperative ultrasound in patients with Cushing's disease and no demonstrable pituitary tumor on magnetic resonance imaging. **J Neurosurg** 89: 927-32, 1998.

265. Barrow D L, Mizuno J, Tindall G T: Management of prolactinomas associated with very high serum prolactin levels. **J Neurosurg** 68: 554-8, 1988.

266. Blevins L S: Medical management of pituitary adenomas. **Contemp Neurosurg** 19 (11): 1-6, 1997.

267. Landolt A M, Osterwalder V: Perivascular fibrosis in prolactinomas: Is it increased by bromocriptine? **J Clin Endocrinol Metab** 58: 1179-83, 1984.

268. Cabergoline for hyperprolactinemia. **Med Letter** 39: 58-9, 1997.

269. Webster J, Piscitelli G, Polli A, *et al.*: A comparison of cabergoline and bromocriptine in the treatment of hyperprolactinemic amenorrhea. **N Engl J Med** 331: 904-9, 1994.

270. van der Lely A J, Hutson R K, Trainer P J, *et al.*: Long-term treatment of acromegaly with pegvisomant, a growth hormone receptor antagonist. **Lancet** 358 (9295): 1754-9, 2001.

271. Pegvisomant (Somavert) for acromegaly. **Med Letter** 45: 55-6, 2003.

272. Sheehan J M, Vance M L, Sheehan J P, *et al.*: Radiosurgery for Cushing's disease after failed transsphenoidal surgery. **J Neurosurg** 93 (5): 738-42, 2000.

273. Ciric I, Mikhael M, Stafford T, *et al.*: Transsphenoidal microsurgery of pituitary macroadenomas with long-term follow-up results. **J Neurosurg** 59: 395-401, 1983.

274. Breen P, Flickinger J C, Kondziolka D, *et al.*: Radiotherapy for nonfunctional pituitary adenoma: Analysis of long-term tumor control. **J Neurosurg** 89: 933-8, 1998.

275. Schmidek H H, Sweet W H, (eds.): **Operative neurosurgical techniques**. 1st ed., Grune and Stratton, New York, 1982.

276. Powell M, Lightman S L, (eds.): **Management of pituitary tumours: A handbook**. Churchill Livingstone, New York, 1996.

277. Decker R E, Chalif D J: Progressive coma after the transsphenoidal decompression of a pituitary adenoma with marked suprasellar extension: Report of two cases. **Neurosurgery** 28: 154-8, 1991.

278. Domingue J N, Wilson C B: Pituitary abscesses. **J Neurosurg** 46: 601-8, 1977.

279. Robinson B: Intrasellar abscess after transsphenoidal pituitary adenectomy. **Neurosurgery** 12: 684-6, 1983.

280. Verbalis J G, Robinson A G, Moses A M: Postoperative and post-traumatic diabetes insipidus. **Front Horm Res** 13: 247-65, 1985.

281. Teng M M H, Huang C I, Chang T: The pituitary mass after transsphenoidal hypophysectomy. **AJNR** 9: 23-6, 1988.

282. Cohen A R, Cooper P R, Kupersmith M J, *et al.*: Visual recovery after transsphenoidal removal of pituitary adenoma. **Neurosurgery** 17: 446-52, 1985.

283. Davis D H, Laws E R, Ilstrup D M, *et al.*: Results of surgical treatment for growth hormone-secreting pituitary adenomas. **J Neurosurg** 79: 70-5, 1993.

284. Klein H J, Rath S A: Removal of tumors of the III ventricle using lamina terminalis approach: Three cases of isolated growth of craniopharyngiomas in the III ventricle. **Childs Nerv Syst** 5: 144-7, 1989.

285. Manaka S, Teramoto A, Takakura K: The efficacy of radiotherapy for craniopharyngioma. **J Neurosurg** 62: 648-56, 1985.

286. Maggio W W, Cail W S, Brookeman J R, *et al.*: Rathke's cleft cyst: Computed tomographic and magnetic resonance imaging appearances. **Neurosurgery** 21: 60-2, 1987.

287. Nishio S, Mizuno J, Barrow D L, *et al.*: Pituitary tumors composed of adenohypophysial adenoma and Rathke's cleft cyst elements: A clinicopathological study. **Neurosurgery** 21: 371-7, 1987.

288. Voelker J L, Campbell R L, Muller J: Clinical, radiographic, and pathological features of symptomatic Rathke's cleft cysts. **J Neurosurg** 74: 535-44, 1991.

289. Little J R, MacCarty C S: Colloid cysts of the third ventricle. **J Neurosurg** 39: 230-5, 1974.

290. Ciric I, Zivin I: Neuroepithelial (colloid) cysts of the septum pellucidum. **J Neurosurg** 43: 69-73, 1975.

291. Guner M, Shaw M D M, Turner J W, *et al.*: Computed tomography in the diagnosis of colloid cyst. **Surg Neurol** 6: 345-8, 1976.

292. Ryder J W, Kleinschmidt B K, Keller T S: Sudden deterioration and death in patients with benign tumors of the third ventricle area. **J Neurosurg** 64: 216-23, 1986.

293. Mamourian A C, Cromwell L D, Harbaugh R E: Colloid cyst of the third ventricle: Sometimes more conspicuous on CT than MR. **AJNR** 19: 875-8, 1998.

294. Torkildsen A: Should extirpation be attempted in cases of neoplasm in or near the third ventricle of the brain? Experiences with a palliative method. **J Neurosurg** 5: 249-75, 1948.

295. Bosch D A, Rahn T, Backlund E O: Treatment of

colloid cyst of the third ventricle by stereotactic aspiration. **Surg Neurol** 9: 15-8, 1978.

296. Rivas J J, Lobato R D: CT-assisted stereotaxic aspiration of colloid cysts of the third ventricle. **J Neurosurg** 62: 238-42, 1985.

297. Mathiesen T, Grane P, Lindquist C, *et al.*: High recurrence rate following aspiration of colloid cysts in the third ventricle. **J Neurosurg** 78: 748-52, 1993.

298. Musolino A, Fosse S, Munari C, *et al.*: Diagnosis and treatment of colloid cysts of the third ventricle by stereotactic drainage. Report on eleven cases. **Surg Neurol** 32: 294-9, 1989.

299. Apuzzo M L J, Chandrasoma P T, Zelman V, *et al.*: Computed tomographic guidance stereotaxis in the management of lesions of the third ventricular region. **Neurosurgery** 15: 502-8, 1984.

300. Apuzzo M L J: Comment on Garrido E, et al.: Cerebral venous and sagittal sinus thrombosis after transcallosal removal of a colloid cyst of the third ventricle: Case report. **Neurosurgery** 26: 542, 1990.

301. Kondziolka D, Lunsford L D: Stereotactic management of colloid cysts: Factors predicting success. **J Neurosurg** 75: 45-51, 1991.

302. Hall W A, Lunsford L D: Changing concepts in the treatment of colloid cysts. An 11-year experience in the CT era. **J Neurosurg** 66: 186-91, 1987.

303. Go R C P, Lamiell J M, Hsia Y E, *et al.*: Segregation and linkage analysis of von Hippel-Lindau disease among 220 descendents from one kindred. **Am J Human Genet** 36: 131-42, 1984.

304. Glenn G M, Linehan W M, Hosoe S, *et al.*: Screening for von Hippel-Lindau disease by DNA polymorphism analysis. **JAMA** 267: 1226-31, 1992.

305. Ho V B, Smirniotopoulos J G, Murphy F M, *et al.*: Radiologic-pathologic correlation: Hemangioblastoma. **AJNR** 13: 1343-52, 1992.

306. Wakai S, Inoh S, Ueda Y, *et al.*: Hemangioblastoma presenting with intraparenchymatous hemorrhage. **J Neurosurg** 61: 956-60, 1984.

307. Silver M L, Hennigar G: Cerebellar hemangioma (hemangioblastoma). A clinicopathological review of 40 cases. **J Neurosurg** 9: 484-94, 1952.

308. O'Neill B P, Illig J J: Primary central nervous system lymphoma. **Mayo Clin Proc** 64: 1005-20, 1989.

309. Kawakami Y, Tabuchi K, Ohnishi R, *et al.*: Primary central nervous system lymphoma. **J Neurosurg** 62: 522-7, 1985.

310. Jellinger K, Radaszkiewicz T: Involvement of the central nervous system in malignant lymphomas. **Virchows Arch (Pathol Anat)** 370: 345-62, 1976.

311. Helle T L, Britt R H, Colby T V: Primary lymphoma of the central nervous system. **J Neurosurg** 60: 94-103, 1984.

312. Alic L, Haid M: Primary lymphoma of the brain: A case report and review of the literature. **J Surg Oncol** 26: 115-21, 1984.

313. Eby N L, Grufferman S, Flannelly C M, *et al.*: Increasing incidence of primary brain lymphoma in the U.S. **Cancer** 62: 2461-5, 1988.

314. Murray K, Kun L, Cox J: Primary malignant lymphoma of the central nervous system: Results of treatment of 11 cases and review of the literature. **J Neurosurg** 65: 600-7, 1986.

315. Penn I: Development of cancer as a complication of clinical transplantation. **Transplant Proc** 9: 1121-7, 1977.

316. Levy R M, Bredesen D E, Rosenblum M L: Neurological manifestations of the acquired immunodeficiency syndrome (AIDS): Experience at UCSF and review of the literature. **J Neurosurg** 62: 475-95, 1985.

317. Jean W C, Hall W A: Management of cranial and spinal infections. **Contemp Neurosurg** 20 (9): 1-10, 1998.

318. Hochberg F H, Miller G, Schooley R T, *et al.*: Central-nervous-system lymphoma related to Epstein-Barr virus. **N Engl J Med** 309: 745-8, 1983.

319. MacMahon E M E, Glass J D, Hayward S D, *et al.*: Epstein-Barr virus in AIDS-related primary central nervous system lymphoma. **Lancet** 338: 969-73, 1991.

320. Burger P C, Scheithauer B W, Vogel F S: **Surgical pathology of the nervous system and its coverings**. 4th ed. Churchill Livingstone, New York, 2002.

321. Calamia K T, Miller A, Shuster E A, *et al.*: Intravascular lymphomatosis: A report of ten patients with central nervous system involvement and a review of the disease process. **Adv Exp Med Biol** 455: 249-65, 1999.

322. Glass J, Hochberg F H, Miller D C: Intravascular lymphomatosis. A systemic disease with neurologic manifestations. **Cancer** 71 (10): 3156-64, 1993.

323. So Y T, Beckstead J H, Davis R L: Primary central nervous system lymphoma in acquired immune deficiency syndrome: A clinical and pathological study. **Ann Neurol** 20: 566-72, 1986.

324. Poon T, Matoso I, Tchertkoff V, *et al.*: CT features of primary cerebral lymphoma in AIDS and non-AIDS patients. **J Comput Assist Tomogr** 13: 6-9, 1989.

325. DeAngelis L M: Cerebral lymphoma presenting as a nonenhancing lesion of computed tomographic/magnetic resonance scan. **Ann Neurol** 33: 308-11, 1993.

326. Enzmann D R, Krikorian J, Norman D, *et al.*: Computed tomography in primary reticulum cell sarcoma of the brain. **Radiology** 130: 165-70, 1979.

327. Vaquero J, Martinez R, Rossi E, *et al.*: Primary cerebral lymphoma: The 'ghost tumor'. **J Neurosurg** 60: 174-6, 1984.

328. Gray R s, Abrahams J J, Hufnagel T J, *et al.*: Ghost-cell tumor of the optic chiasm; primary CNS lymphoma. **J Clin Neuroophthalmol** 9: 98-104, 1989.

329. O'Neill B P, Kelly P J, Earle J D, *et al.*: Computer-assisted stereotactic biopsy for the diagnosis of primary central nervous system lymphoma. **Neurology** 37: 1160-4, 1987.

330. DeAngelis L M, Yahalom J, Heinemann M-H, *et al.*: Primary central nervous system lymphomas: Combined treatment with chemotherapy and radiotherapy. **Neurology** 40: 80-6, 1990.

331. DeAngelis L M, Yahalom J, Thaler H T, *et al.*: Combined modality therapy for primary CNS lymphomas. **J Clin Oncol** 10: 635-43, 1992.

332. O'Marcaigh A S, Johnson C M, Smithson W A, *et al.*: Successful treatment of intrathecal methotrexate overdose by using ventriculolumbar perfusion and intrathecal instillation of carboxypeptidase G_2. **Mayo Clin Proc** 71: 161-5, 1996.

333. Hochberg F H, Miller D C: Primary central nervous system lymphoma. **J Neurosurg** 68: 835-53, 1988.

334. Baumgartner J E, Rachlin J R, Beckstead J H, *et al.*: Primary central nervous system lymphomas: Natural history and response to radiation therapy in 55 patients with acquied immunodeficiency syndrome. **J Neurosurg** 73: 206-11, 1990.

335. Formenti S C, Gill P S, Lean E, *et al.*: Primary central nervous system lymphoma in AIDS: Results of radiation therapy. **Cancer** 63: 1101-7, 1989.

336. O'Neill P, Bell B A, Miller J D, *et al.*: Fifty years of experience with chordomas in southeast Scotland. **Neurosurgery** 16: 166-70, 1985.

337. Heffelfinger M J, Dahlin D C, MacCarty C S, *et al.*: Chordomas and cartilaginous tumors at the skull base. **Cancer** 32: 410-20, 1973.

338. Boriani S, Chevalley F, Weinstein J N, *et al.*: Chordoma of the spine above the sacrum. Treatment and outcome in 21 cases. **Spine** 21: 1569-77, 1996.

339. Hug E B, Loredo L N, Slater J D, *et al.*: Proton radiation therapy for chordomas and chondrosarcomas of the skull base. **J Neurosurg** 91: 432-9, 1999.

340. Meyer J E, Lepke R A, Lindfors K K, *et al.*: Chor-

domas: Their CT appearance in the cervical, thoracic and lumbar spine. **Radiology** 153: 693-6, 1984.

341. Schwarz S S, Fisher W S, Pulliam M W, *et al*.: Thoracic chordoma in a patient with paraparesis and ivory vertebral body. **Neurosurgery** 16: 100-2, 1985.

342. Wold L E, Laws E R: Cranial chordomas in children and young adults. **J Neurosurg** 59: 1043-7, 1983.

343. Azzarelli A, Quagliuolo V, Cerasoli S, *et al*.: Chordoma: Natural history and treatment results in 33 cases. **J Surg Oncol** 37: 185-91, 1988.

344. Mindell E R: Current concepts review. Chordoma. **J Bone Joint Surg** 63A: 501-5, 1981.

345. Cheng E Y, Özerdemoglu R A, Transfeldt E E, *et al*.: Lumbosacral chordoma. Prognostic factors and treatment. **Spine** 24: 1639-45, 1999.

346. Samson I R, Springfield D S, Suit H D, *et al*.: Operative treatment of sacrococcygeal chordoma. A review of twenty-one cases. **J Bone Joint Surg** 75: 1476-84, 1993.

347. Klekamp J, Samii M: Spinal chordomas - results of treatment over a 17-year period. **Acta Neurochir (Wien)** 138: 514-9, 1996.

348. Suit H D, Goitein M, Munzenrider J, *et al*.: Definitive radiation therapy for chordoma and chondrosarcoma of base of skull and cervical spine. **J Neurosurg** 56: 377-85, 1982.

349. Rich T A, Schiller A, Mankin H J: Clinical and pathologic review of 48 cases of chordoma. **Cancer** 56: 182-7, 1985.

350. Rubinstein L J: **Tumors of the central nervous system. Atlas of tumor pathology, second series, fascicle 6**. Armed Forces Institute of Pathology, Washington, DC, 1972: pp 158-60.

351. Demierre B, Stichnoth F A, Hori A, *et al*.: Intracerebral ganglioglioma. **J Neurosurg** 65: 177-82, 1986.

352. Kalyan-Raman U P, Olivero W C: Ganglioglioma: A correlative clinicopathological and radiological study of ten surgically treated cases with follow-up. **Neurosurgery** 20: 428-33, 1987.

353. Sutton L N, Packer R J, Rorke L B, *et al*.: Cerebral gangliogliomas during childhood. **Neurosurgery** 13: 124-8, 1983.

354. Miller D C, Lang F F, Epstein F J: Central nervous system gangliogliomas. Part 1: Pathology. **J Neurosurg** 79: 859-66, 1993.

355. Lang F F, Epstein F J, Ransohoff J, *et al*.: Central nervous system gangliogliomas. Part 2: Clinical outcome. **J Neurosurg** 79: 867-73, 1993.

356. Russell D S, Rubenstein L J: Ganglioglioma: A case with a long history and malignant evolution. **J Neuropathol Exp Neurol** 21: 185-93, 1962.

357. Chretien P B, Engelman K, Hoye R C, *et al*: Surgical management of intravascular glomus jugulare tumor. **Am J Surg** 122: 740-3, 1971.

358. Jackson C G, Harris P F, Glasscock M E I, *et al*.: Diagnosis and management of paragangliomas of the skull base. **Am J Surg** 159: 389-93, 1990.

359. Farrior J B, Hyams V J, Benke R, *et al*.: Carcinoid apudoma arising in a glomus jugulare tumor: Review of endocrine activity in glomus jugulare tumors. **Laryngoscope** 90: 110-9, 1980.

360. Jensen N F: Glomus tumors of the head and neck: Anesthetic considerations. **Anesth Analg** 78: 112-9, 1994.

361. Jackson C G, Glasscock M E, Nissen A J, *et al*.: Glomus tumor surgery: The approach, results, and problems. **Otolaryngol Clin North Am** 15: 897-916, 1982.

362. Kim J-A, Elkon D, Lim M-L, *et al*.: Optimum dose of radiotherapy for chemodectomas of the middle ear. **Int J Radiation Oncology Biol Phys** 6: 815-9, 1980.

363. Cummings B J, Beale F A, Garrett P G, *et al*.: The treatment of glomus tumors in the temporal bone by megavoltage radiation. **Cancer** 53: 2635-40, 1984.

364. Spector G J, Fierstein J, Ogura J H: A comparison of therapeutic modalities of glomus tumors in the temporal bone. **Laryngoscope** 86: 690-6, 1976.

365. Hatfield P M, James A E, Schulz M D: Chemodectomas of the glomus jugulare. **Cancer** 30: 1164-8, 1972.

366. Mork S J, Loken A C: Ependymoma: A follow-up study of 101 cases. **Cancer** 40: 907-15, 1977.

367. Duffner P K, Cohen M E, Freeman A I: Pediatric brain tumors: An overview. **Ca** 35: 287-301, 1985.

368. Youmans J R, (ed.) **Neurological surgery**. 2nd ed., W. B. Saunders, Philadelphia, 1982.

369. Shaw E G, Evans R G, Scheithauer B W, *et al*.: Postoperative radiotherapy of intracranial ependymoma in pediatric and adult patients. **Int J Radiation Oncology Biol Phys** 13: 1457-62, 1987.

370. Vanuytsel L, Brada M: The role of prophylactic spinal irradiation in localized intracranial ependymoma. **Int J Radiation Oncology Biol Phys** 21: 825-30, 1991.

371. Sutton L N, Goldwein J, Perilongo G, *et al*.: Prognostic factors in childhood ependymomas. **Pediatr Neurosurg** 16: 57-65, 1990.

372. Ross G W, Rubinstein L J: Lack of histopathological correlation of malignant ependymomas with postoperative survival. **J Neurosurg** 70: 31-6, 1989.

373. Tomita T, McLone D G: Spontaneous seeding of medulloblastoma: Results of cerebrospinal fluid cytology and arachnoid biopsy from the cisterna magna. **Neurosurgery** 12: 265-7, 1983.

374. Allen J C: Childhood brain tumors: Current status of clinical trials in newly diagnosed and recurrent disease. **Ped Clin N Am** 32: 633-51, 1985.

375. Kessler L A, Dugan P, Concannon J P: Systemic metastases of medulloblastoma promoted by shunting. **Surg Neurol** 3: 147-52, 1975.

376. Tomita T, McLone D G: Medulloblastoma in childhood: Results of radical resection and low-dose radiation therapy. **J Neurosurg** 64: 238-42, 1986.

377. Evans A E, Jenkins R D, Sposto R, *et al*.: The treatment of medulloblastoma: Results of a prospective randomized trial of radiation therapy with and without CCNU, vincristine, and prednisone. **J Neurosurg** 72: 572-82, 1990.

378. Mork S J, Rubinstein L J: Ependymoblastoma. A reappraisal of a rare embryonal tumor. **Cancer** 55: 1536-42, 1985.

379. Guidetti B, Gagliardi F M: Epidermoids and dermoid cysts. **J Neurosurg** 47: 12-8, 1977.

380. Berger M S, Wilson C B: Epidermoid cysts of the posterior fossa. **J Neurosurg** 62: 214-9, 1985.

381. Fleming J F R, Botterell E H: Cranial dermoid and epidermoid tumors. **Surg Gynecol Obstet** 109: 57-79, 1959.

382. Alvord E C: Growth rates of epidermoid tumors. **Ann Neurol** 2: 367-70, 1977.

383. Sabin H I, Bardi L T, Symon L: Epidermoid cysts and cholesterol granulomas centered on the posterior fossa: Twenty years of diagnosis and management. **Neurosurgery** 21: 798-803, 1987.

384. Altschuler E M, Jungreis C A, Sekhar L N, *et al*.: Operative treatment of intracranial epidermoid cysts and cholesterol granulomas: Report of 21 cases. **Neurosurgery** 26: 606-14, 1990.

385. Friedman I: Epidermoid cholesteatoma and cholesterol granuloma: Experimental and human. **Ann Otol Rhinol Laryngol** 68: 57-79, 1959.

386. de Chadarevian J, Becker W J: Mollaret's recurrent aseptic meningitis: Relationship and ultrastructural studies of the cerebrospinal fluid. **J Neuropathol Exp Neurol** 39: 661-9, 1980.

387. Abramson R C, Morawetz R B, Schlitt M: Multiple complications from an intracranial epidermoid cyst: Case report and literature review. **Neurosurgery** 24: 574-8, 1989.

388. Szabo M, Majtenyi C, Gusea A: Contribution to the background of Mollaret's meningitis. **Acta Neuropathol** 59: 115-8, 1983.

---

389. Chambers A A, Lukin R R, Tomsick T A: Cranial epidermoid tumors: Diagnosis by computed tomography. **Neurosurgery** 1: 276-80, 1977.
390. Keville F J, Wise B L: Intracranial epidermoid and dermoid tumors. **J Neurosurg** 16: 564-9, 1959.
391. Ringertz N, Nordenstam H, Flyger G: Tumors of the pineal region. **J Neuropathol Exp Neurol** 13: 540-61, 1954.
392. Regis J, Bouillot P, Rouby-Volot F, et al.: Pineal region tumors and the role of stereotactic biopsy: Review of the mortality, morbidity, and diagnostic rates in 370 cases. **Neurosurgery** 39: 907-14, 1996.
393. Di Costanzo A, Tedeschi G, Di Salle F, et al.: Pineal cysts: An incidental MRI finding? **J Neurol Neurosurg Psychiatry** 56: 207-8, 1993.
394. Hasegawa A, Ohtsubo K, Mori W: Pineal gland in old age: Quantitative and qualitative morphological study of 168 human autopsy cases. **Brain Res** 409: 343-9, 1987.
395. Torres A, Krisht A F, Akouri S: Current management of pineal cysts. **Contemp Neurosurg** 27 (7): 1-5, 2005.
396. Maurer P K, Ecklund J, Parisi J E, et al.: Symptomatic pineal cysts: Case report. **Neurosurgery** 27: 451-4, 1990.
397. Wisoff J H, Epstein F: Surgical management of symptomatic pineal cysts. **J Neurosurg** 77: 896-900, 1992.
398. Klein P, Rubinstein L J: Benign symptomatic glial cysts of the pineal gland: A report of seven cases and review of the literature. **J Neurol Neurosurg Psychiatry** 52: 991-5, 1989.
399. Mamourian A C, Towfighi J: Pineal cysts: MR imaging. **AJNR** 7: 1081-6, 1986.
400. Di Chirico A, Di Rocco F, Velardi F: Spontaneous regression of a symptomatic pineal cyst after endoscopic third-ventriculostomy. **Childs Nerv Syst** 17 (1-2): 42-6, 2001.
401. Hoffman H J, Ostubo H, Hendrick E B, et al.: Intracranial germ-cell tumors in children. **J Neurosurg** 74: 545-51, 1991.
402. Edwards M S B, Hudgins R J, Wilson C B, et al.: Pineal region tumors in children. **J Neurosurg** 68: 689-97, 1988.
403. Todo T, Kondo T, Shinoura N, et al.: Large cysts of the pineal gland: Report of two cases. **Neurosurgery** 29: 101-6, 1991.
404. Stern J D, Ross D A: Stereotactic management of benign pineal region cysts: Report of two cases. **Neurosurgery** 32: 310-4, 1993.
405. Musolino A, Cambria S, Rizzo G, et al.: Symptomatic cysts of the pineal gland: Stereotactic diagnosis and treatment of two cases and review of the literature. **Neurosurgery** 32: 315-21, 1993.
406. Kelly P J: Comment on Musolino A, et al.: Symptomatic cysts of the pineal gland: Stereotactic diagnosis and treatment of two cases and review of the literature. **Neurosurgery** 32: 320-1, 1993.
407. Dempsey P K, Kondziolka D, Lunsford L D: Stereotactic diagnosis and treatment of pineal region tumors and vascular malformations. **Acta Neurochir** 116: 14-22, 1992.
408. Kelly P J: Comment on Regis J, et al.: Pineal region tumors and the role of stereotactic biopsy: Review of the mortality, morbidity, and diagnostic rates in 370 cases. **Neurosurgery** 39: 912-3, 1996.
409. Boyd M C, Steinbok P: Choroid plexus tumors: Problems in diagnosis and management. **J Neurosurg** 66: 800-5, 1987.
410. Ellenbogen R G, Winston K R, Kupsky W J: Tumors of the choroid plexus in children. **Neurosurgery** 25: 327-35, 1989.
411. Savitz M H, Anderson P J: Primary melanoma of the leptomeninges: A review. **Mt Sinai J Med** 41: 774-91, 1974.
412. Gibson J B, Burrows D, Weir W P: Primary melanoma of the meninges. **J Pathol Bacteriol** 74: 419-38,

1957.
413. Jooma R, Hayward R D, Grant D N: Intracranial neoplasms during the first year of life: Analysis of one hundred consecutive cases. **Neurosurgery** 14: 31-41, 1984.
414. Wakai S, Arai T, Nagai M: Congenital brain tumors. **Surg Neurol** 21: 597-609, 1984.
415. Thomas J E, Baker H L: Assessment of roentgenographic lucencies of the skull: A systematic approach. **Neurology** 25: 99-106, 1975.
416. Rawlings C E, Wilkins R H: Solitary eosinophilic granuloma of the skull. **Neurosurgery** 15: 155-61, 1984.
417. Mitnick J S, Pinto R S: CT in the diagnosis of eosinophilic granuloma. **J Comput Assist Tomogr** 4: 791-3, 1980.
418. Hasegawa T, Ito H, Yamamoto S, et al.: Unilateral hyperostosis frontalis interna: Case report. **J Neurosurg** 59: 710-3, 1983.
419. Willison C D, Schochet S S, Voelker J L: Cranial epidural fibrous tumor associated with hyperostosis: A case report. **Surg Neurol** 40: 508-11, 1993.
420. Fulton J D, Shand J, Ritchie D, et al.: Hyperostosis frontalis interna, acromegaly and hyperprolactinemia. **Postgrad Med J** 66: 16-9, 1990.
421. Bavazzano A, Del Bianco P L, Del Bene E, et al.: A statistical evaluation of the relationships between headache and internal frontal hyperostosis. **Res Clin Stud Headache** 3: 191-7, 1970.
422. Floyd J L, Jackson D E, Carretta R: Appearance of hyperostosis frontalis interna on indium-111 leukocyte scans: Potential diagnostic pitfall. **J Nucl Med** 27: 495-7, 1986.
423. Oates E: Spectrum of appearance of hyperostosis frontalis interna on in-111 leukocyte scans. **Clin Nucl Med** 13: 922-3, 1988.
424. Mintz A P, Cairncross J G: Treatment of a single brain metastasis. The role of radiation following surgical excision. **JAMA** 280: 1527-9, 1998 (editorial).
425. Voorhies R M, Sundaresan N, Thaler H T: The single supratentorial lesion: An evaluation of preoperative diagnosis. **J Neurosurg** 53: 364-8, 1980.
426. Patchell R A, Posner J B: Neurologic complications of systemic cancer. **Neurol Clin** 3: 729-50, 1985.
427. Zimm S, Galen L, Wampler G L, et al.: Intracerebral metastases in solid-tumor patients: Natural history and results of treatment. **Cancer** 48: 384-94, 1981.
428. DeAngelis L M: Management of brain metastases. **Cancer Invest** 12: 156-65, 1994.
429. Davis P C, Hudgins P A, Peterman S B, et al.: Diagnosis of cerebral metastases: Double-dose delayed CT versus contrast-enhanced MR imaging. **AJNR** 12: 293-300, 1991.
430. Weiss H D, Richardson E P: Solitary brainstem metastasis. **Neurology** 28: 562-6, 1978.
431. Nugent J L, Bunn P A, Matthews M J, et al.: CNS metastses in small-cell bronchogenic carcinoma: Increasing frequency and changing pattern with lengthening survival. **Cancer** 44: 1885-93, 1979.
432. Vieth R G, Odom G L: Intracranial metastases and their neurosurgical treatment. **J Neurosurg** 23: 375-83, 1965.
433. Kindt G W: The pattern of location of cerebral metastatic tumors. **J Neurosurg** 21: 54-7, 1964.
434. Figlin R A, Piantadosi S, Feld R, et al.: Intracranial recurrence of carcinoma after complete resection of stage I, II, and III non-small-cell lung cancer. **N Engl J Med** 318: 1300-5, 1988.
435. Sampson J H, Carter J H, Friedman A H, et al.: Demographics, prognosis, and therapy in 702 patients with brain metastases from malignant melanoma. **J Neurosurg** 88: 11-20, 1998.
436. Solis O J, Davis K R, Adair L B, et al.: Intracerebral metastatic melanoma: CT evaluation. **Comput Tomogr** 1: 135-43, 1977.
437. Kondziolka D, Bernstein M, Resch L, et al.: Significance of hemorrhage into brain tumors: Clinico-

pathological study. **J Neurosurg** 67: 852-7, 1987.

438. Patchell R A, Tibbs P A, Walsh J W, *et al.*: A randomized trial of surgery in the treatment of single metastases to the brain. **N Engl J Med** 322: 494-500, 1990.

439. Pollock B E: Management of patients with multiple brain metastases. **Contemp Neurosurg** 21 (18): 1-6, 1999.

440. Horton J: *Treatment of metastases to the brain.* **Current Concept Oncology.** 1984, pp 18-22.

441. Jackson D V, Richards F, Cooper M R, *et al.*: Prophylactic cranial irradiation in small cell carcinoma of the lung: A randomized study. **JAMA** 237: 2730-3, 1977.

442. Patchell R A, Tibbs P A, Regine W F, *et al.*: Postoperative radiotherapy in the treatment of single metastases to the brain; A randomized trial. **JAMA** 280: 1485-9, 1998.

443. Kramer S, Hendrickson F, Zelen M, *et al.*: Therapeutic trials in the management of metastatic brain tumors by different time/dose fraction schemes. **Natl Cancer Inst Monogr** 46: 213-21, 1977.

444. DeAngelis L M, Mandell L R, Thaler H T, *et al.*: The role of postoperative radiotherapy after resection of single brain metastases. **Neurosurgery** 24: 798-804, 1989.

445. Smalley S R, Schray M F, Laws E R, *et al.*: Adjuvant radiation therapy after surgical resection of solitary brain metastasis: Association with pattern of failure and survival. **Int J Radiation Oncology Biol Phys** 13: 1611-6, 1987.

446. Shaw E: Comment on DeAngelis L M, et al.: The role of postoperative radiotherapy after resection of single brain metastases. **Neurosurgery** 24: 804-5, 1989.

447. Smalley S R, Laws E R, O'Fallon J R, *et al.*: Resection for solitary brain metastasis: Role of adjuvant radiation and prognostic variables in 229 patients. **J Neurosurg** 77: 531-40, 1992.

448. Bindal R K, Sawaya R, Leavens M E, *et al.*: Surgical treatment of multiple brain metastases. **J Neurosurg** 79: 210-6, 1993.

449. Tobler W D, Sawaya R, Tew J M: Successful laser-assisted excision of a metastatic midbrain tumor. **Neurosurgery** 18: 795-7, 1986.

450. Markesbery W R, Brooks W H, Gupta G D, *et al.*: Treatment for patients with cerebral metastases. **Arch Neurol** 35: 754-6, 1978.

451. Ruderman N B, Hall T C: Use of glucocorticoids in the palliative treatment of metastatic brain tumors. **Cancer** 18: 298-306, 1965.

452. Posner J B: Surgery for metastases to the brain. **N Engl J Med** 322. 544-5, 1990 (editorial).

453. Galicich J H, Sundaresan N, Thaler H T: Surgical treatment of single brain metastasis. Evaluation of results by CT scanning. **J Neurosurg** 53: 63-7, 1980.

454. Alexander E, Moriarty T M, Davis R B, *et al.*: Stereotactic radiosurgery for the definitive noninvasive treatment of brain metastases. **J Natl Cancer Inst** 87: 34-40, 1995.

455. Bindal A K, Bindal R K, Hess K R, *et al.*: Surgery versus radiosurgery in the treatment of brain metastasis. **J Neurosurg** 84: 748-54, 1996.

456. Fuller B G, Kaplan I D, Adler J, *et al.*: Stereotactic radiosurgery for brain metastases: The importance of adjuvant whole brain irradiation. **Int J Radiation Oncology Biol Phys** 23: 413-8, 1992.

457. Sze G, Soletsky S, Bronen R, *et al.*: MR imaging of the cranial meninges with emphasis on contrast enhancement and meningeal carcinomatosis. **AJNR** 10: 965-75, 1989.

458. Radhakrishnan K, Ahlskog J E, Garrity J A, *et al.*: Idiopathic intracranial hypertension. **Mayo Clin Proc** 69: 169-80, 1994.

459. Digre K B, Corbett J J: Pseudotumor cerebri in men. **Arch Neurol** 45: 866-72, 1988.

460. Durcan F J, Corbett J J, Wall M: The incidence of pseudotumor cerebri: Population studies in Iowa and Louisiana. **Arch Neurol** 45: 875-7, 1988.

461. Radhakrishnan K, Ahlskog J E, Cross S A, *et al.*: Idiopathic intracranial hypertension (pseudotumor cerebri): Descriptive epidemiology in Rochester, Minn, 1976 to 1990. **Arch Neurol** 50: 78-80, 1993.

462. Rush J A: Pseudotumor cerebri: Clinical profile and visual outcome in 63 patients. **Mayo Clin Proc** 55: 541-6, 1980.

463. King J O, Mitchell P J, Thomson K R, *et al.*: Manometry combined with cervical puncture in idiopathic intracranial hypertension. **Neurology** 58 (1): 26-30, 2002.

464. Ahlskog J E, O'Neill B P: Pseudotumor cerebri. **Ann Int Med** 97: 249-56, 1982.

465. Corbett J J, Mehta M P: Cerebrospinal fluid pressure in normal obese subjects and patients with pseudotumor cerebri. **Neurology** 33: 1386-8, 1983.

466. Jacobson D M, Karanjia P N, Olson K A, *et al.*: Computed tomography ventricular size has no predictive value in diagnosing pseudotumor cerebri. **Neurology** 40: 1454-5, 1990.

467. Bejjani G K, Cockerham K P, Pless M, *et al.*: Idiopathic intracranial hypertension. **Contemp Neurosurg** 24 (9): 1-8, 2002.

468. Giuseffi V, Wall M, Siegel P Z, *et al.*: Symptoms and disease associations in idiopathic intracranial hypertension (pseudotumor cerebri): A case-control study. **Neurology** 41 (2 (Pt 1)): 239-44, 1991.

469. Round R, Keane J R: The minor symptoms of increased intracranial hypertension: 101 patients with benign intracranial hypertension. **Neurology** 38 (9): 1461-4, 1988.

470. Wang S J, Silberstein S D, Patterson S, *et al.*: Idiopathic intracranial hypertension without papilledema: A case control study in a headache center. **Neurology** 51: 245-9, 1998.

471. Sher N A, Wirtschafter J, Shapiro S K, *et al.*: Unilateral papilledema in 'benign' intracranial hypertension (pseudotumor cerebri). **JAMA** 250: 2346-7, 1983.

472. Wall M, George D: Idiopathic intracranial hypertension: A prospective study of 50 patients. **Brain** 114: 155-80, 1991.

473. Digre K B: *Epidemioligy of idiopathic intracranial hypertension.* **Annual meeting of the North American Neuro-Ophthalmoligical Society (NANOS).** 1992

474. Farb R I, Vanek I, Scott J N, *et al.*: Idiopathic intracranial hypertension: The prevalence and morphology of sinovenous stenosis. **Neurology** 60: 1418-24, 2003.

475. Johnston I, Hawke S, Halmagyi M, *et al.*: The pseudotumor syndrome: Disorders of cerebrospinal fluid circulation causing intracranial hypertension without ventriculomegaly. **Arch Neurol** 48: 740-7, 1991.

476. Powers J M, Schnur J A, Baldree M E: Pseudotumor cerebri due to partial obstruction of the sigmoid sinus by a cholesteatoma. **Arch Neurol** 43: 519-21, 1986.

477. Wen D Y, Hardten D R, Wirtschafter J D, *et al.*: Elevated intracranial pressure from cerebral venous obstruction by Masson's vegetant intravascular hemangioendothelioma. **J Neurosurg** 75: 787-90, 1991.

478. Johnson L N, Krohel G B, Madsen R W, *et al.*: The role of weight loss and acetazolamide in the treatment of idiopathic intracranial hypertension (pseudotumor cerebri). **Ophthalmology** 105 (12): 2313-7, 1998.

479. Newberg B: Pseudotumor cerebri treated by rice/reduction diet. **Arch Intern Med** 133: 802-7, 1974.

480. Weisberg L A: Benign intracranial hypertension. **Medicine (Baltimore)** 54: 197-207, 1975.

481. Hahn F J, McWilliams F E: The small ventricle in

pseudotumor cerebri: Demonstration of the small ventricle in benign intracranial hypertension. **CT** 2: 249-53, 1978.

482. Higgins J N, Owler B K, Cousins C, *et al.*: Venous sinus stenting for refractory benign intracranial hypertension. **Lancet** 359 (9302): 228-30, 2002.

483. Brourman N D, Spoor T C, Ramocki J M: Optic nerve sheath decompression for pseudotumor cerebri. **Arch Ophthalmol** 106: 1384-90, 1988.

484. Sergott R C, Savino P J, Bosley T M: Modified optic nerve sheath decompression provides long-term visual improvement for pseudotumor cerebri. **Arch Ophthalmol** 106: 1384-90, 1988.

485. Corbett J J, Nerad J A, Tse D, *et al.*: Optic nerve sheath fenestration for pseudotumor cerebri: The lateral orbitotomy approach. **Arch Ophthalmol** 106: 1391-7, 1988.

486. Kelman S E, Heaps R, Wolf A, *et al.*: Optic nerve decompression surgery improves visual function in patients with pseudotumor cerebri. **Neurosurgery** 30: 391-5, 1992.

487. Kelman S E, Sergott R C, Cioffi G A, *et al.*: Modified optic nerve decompression in patients with functioning lumboperitoneal shunts and progressive visual loss. **Ophthalmology** 98: 1449-53, 1991.

488. Spoor T C, Ramocki J M, Madion M P, *et al.*: Treatment of pseudotumor cerebri by primary and secondary optic nerve sheath decompression. **Am J Ophthalmol** 112: 177-85, 1991.

489. Kaufman B: The "empty" sella turcica - A manifestation of the intrasellar subarachnoid space. **Radiology** 90: 931-41, 1968.

490. Lee W M, Adams J E: The empty sella syndrome. **J Neurosurg** 28: 351-6, 1968.

491. McKeever P E: *Immunohistochemistry of the nervous system*. In **Diagnostic immunohistochemistry**, Dabbs D J, (ed.). Churchill Livingstone, New York, 2002, Chapter 18: pp 559-624.

492. Burton B K: Alpha-fetoprotein screening. **Adv Pediatr** 33: 181-96, 1986.

493. Riccardi V M: Mast-cell stabilization to decrease neurofibroma growth: Preliminary experience with ketotifen. **Arch Dermatol** 123: 1011-6, 1987.

494. Riccardi V M: Von Recklinghausen neurofibromatosis. **N Engl J Med** 305: 1617-27, 1981.

495. National Institutes of Health Consensus Development Conference: Neurofibromatosis: Conference statement. **Arch Neurol** 45: 575-8, 1988.

496. Karnes P S: Neurofibromatosis: A common neurocutaneous disorder. **Mayo Clin Proc** 73: 1071-6, 1998.

497. Martuza R L, Eldridge R: Neurofibromatosis 2: (bilateral acoustic neurofibromatosis). **N Engl J Med** 318: 684-8, 1988.

498. Egelhoff J C, Bates D J, Ross J S, *et al.*: Spinal MR findings in neurofibromatosis types 1 and 2. **AJNR** 13: 1071-7, 1992.

499. Wiederholt W C, Gomez M R, Kurland L T: Incidence and prevalence of tuberous sclerosis in Rochester, Minnesota, 1950 through 1982. **Neurology** 35: 600-3, 1985.

500. McLaurin R L, Towbin R B: Tuberous sclerosis: Diagnostic and surgical considerations. **Pediat Neurosci** 12: 43-8, 1985.

501. Chow C W, Klug G L, Lewis E A: Subependymal giant-cell astrocytoma in children: An unusual discrepancy between histological and clinical features. **J Neurosurg** 68: 880-3, 1988.

502. Kopelson G, Linggood R M, Kleinman G M, *et al.*: Management of intramedullary spinal cord tumors. **Radiology** 135: 473-9, 1980.

503. Adams R D, Victor M: *Intraspinal tumors*. In **Principles of neurology**. McGraw-Hill, New York, 2nd ed., 1981: pp 638-41.

504. Dunn E J, Davidson R I, Desai S: *Diagnosis and management of tumors of the cervical spine*. In **The cervical spine**, The Cervical Spine Research Soci-

ety Editorial Committee, (ed.). JB Lippincott, Philadelphia, 2nd ed., 1989: pp 693-722.

505. Menezes A H, Sato Y: Primary tumors of the spine in children - natural history and management. **Concepts Pediatr Neurosurg** 10: 30-53, 1990.

506. Grubb M R, Currier B L, Pritchard D J, *et al.*: Primary Ewing's sarcoma of the spine. **Spine** 19: 309-13, 1994.

507. Porter D G, Martin A J, Mallucci C L, *et al.*: Spinal cord compression due to Masson's vegetant intravascular hemangioendothelioma: Case report. **J Neurosurg** 82: 125-7, 1995.

508. Solero C L, Fornari M, Giombini S, *et al.*: Spinal meningiomas: Review of 174 operated cases. **Neurosurgery** 25 (2): 153-60, 1989.

509. Lyons M K, O'Neill B P, Kurtin P J, *et al.*: Diagnosis and management of primary spinal epidural non-Hodgkin's lymphoma. **Mayo Clin Proc** 71: 453-7, 1996.

510. Stein B: Intramedullary spinal cord tumors. **Clin Neurosurg** 30: 717-41, 1983.

511. Stern W E: Localization and diagnosis of spinal cord tumors. **Clin Neurosurg** 25: 480-94, 1977.

512. DeSousa A L, Kalsbeck J E, Mealey J, *et al.*: Intraspinal tumors in children. A review of 81 cases. **J Neurosurg** 51: 437-43, 1979.

513. Hautzer N W, Aiyesimoju A, Robitaille Y: Primary spinal intramedullary lymphomas: A review. **Ann Neurol** 14: 62-6, 1983.

514. Alvisi C, Cerisoli M, Giuloni M: Intramedullary spinal gliomas: Long term results of surgical treatment. **Acta Neurochir** 70: 169-79, 1984.

515. Dorwart R H, LaMasters D G, Watanabe T J: *Tumors*. In **Computed tomography of the spine and spinal cord**, Newton T H and Potts D G, (eds.). Clavadal Press, San Anselmo, 1983: pp 115-31.

516. Malis L I: Intramedullary spinal cord tumors. **Clin Neurosurg** 25: 512-39, 1978.

517. Smaltino F, Bernini F P, Santoro S: Computerized tomography in the diagnosis of intramedullary metastases. **Acta Neurochir** 52: 299-303, 1980.

518. Edelson R N, Deck M D F, Posner J B: Intramedullary spinal cord metastases. **Neurology** 22: 1222-31, 1972.

519. Murphy K C, Feld R, Evans W K, *et al.*: Intramedullary spinal cord metastases from small cell carcinoma of the lung. **J Clin Onc** 1: 99-106, 1983.

520. Jellinger K, Kothbauer P, Sunder-Plassmann, *et al.*: Intramedullary spinal cord metastases. **J Neurol** 220: 31-41, 1979.

521. Stein B: Surgery of intramedullary spinal cord tumors. **Clin Neurosurg** 26: 473-9, 1979.

522. Sebastian P R, Fisher M, Smith T W, *et al.*: Intramedullary spinal cord metastasis. **Surg Neurol** 16: 336-9, 1981.

523. Nittner K: In **Handbuch der neurochirurgie**, Olivecrona H and Tonnis W, (eds.). Springer-Verlag, New York, 1972, Vol. VII 2: pp 1-606.

524. Post K D, Stein B M: *Surgical management of spinal cord tumors and arteriovenous malformations*. In **Operative neurosurgical techniques**, Schmidek H H and Sweet W H, (eds.). W.B. Saunders, Philadelphia, 3rd ed., 1995, Vol. 2, Chapter 163: pp 2027-48.

525. Nadkarni T D, Rekate H L: Pediatric intramedullary spinal cord tumors: Critical review of the literature. **Childs Nerv Syst** 15: 17-28, 1999.

526. Guidetti B, Mercuri S, Vagnozzi R: Long-term results of the surgical treatment of 129 intramedullary spinal gliomas. **J Neurosurg** 54: 323-30, 1981.

527. Janin Y, Epstein J A, Carras R, *et al.*: Osteoid osteomas and osteoblastomas of the spine. **Neurosurgery** 8: 31-8, 1981.

528. Amacher A L, Eltomey A: Spinal osteoblastoma in children and adolescents. **Childs Nerv Syst** 1: 29-32, 1985.

529. Lichtenstein L, Sawyer W R: Benign osteoblastoma.

J Bone Joint Surg 46A: 755-65, 1964.

530. Fox M W, Onofrio B M: The natural history and management of symptomatic and asymptomatic vertebral hemangiomas. J Neurosurg 78: 36-45, 1993.

531. Healy M, Herz D A, Pearl L: Spinal hemangiomas. Neurosurgery 13: 689-91, 1983.

532. Richardson R R, Cerullo L J: Spinal epidural cavernous hemangioma. Surg Neurol 12: 266-8, 1979.

533. Cosgrove G R, Bertrand G, Fontaine S, et al.: Cavernous angiomas of the spinal cord. J Neurosurg 68: 31-6, 1988.

534. Tekkök I H, Açikgöz B, Saglam A, et al.: Vertebral hemangioma symptomatic during pregnancy - report of a case and review of the literature. Neurosurgery 32: 302-6, 1993.

535. Graham J J, Yang W C: Vertebral hemangioma with compression fracture and paraparesis treated with preoperative embolization and vertebral resection. Spine 9: 97-101, 1984.

536. Kosary I A, Braham J, Shacked I, et al.: Spinal epidural hematoma due to hemangioma of vertebra. Surg Neurol 7: 61-2, 1977.

537. Keren D F, Alexanian R, Goeken J A, et al.: Guidelines for clinical and laboratory evaluation of patients with monoclonal gammopathies. Arch Pathol Lab Med 123: 106-7, 1999.

538. Bataille R, Harousseau J-L: Multiple myeloma. N Engl J Med 336: 1657-64, 1997.

539. McCarthy J, Proctor S J: Cerebral involvement in multiple myeloma. Case report. J Clin Pathol 31: 259-64, 1978.

540. Norum J, Wist E, Dahil I M: Cerebral metastases from multiple myeloma. Acta Oncol 30: 868-9, 1991 (letter).

541. Costa G, Engle R L, Schilling A, et al.: Melphalan and prednisone: An effective combination for the treatment of multiple myeloma. Am J Med 54: 589-99, 1973.

542. Foerster J. Multiple myeloma. In Wintrobe's clinical hematology, Lee G R, Bithell T C, Foerster J, et al., (eds.). Lea and Febiger, Philadelphia, 9th ed., 1993, Vol. 2: pp 2219-49.

543. Marcove R C, Sheth D S, Brien E W, et al.: Conservative surgery for giant cell tumors of the sacrum. The role of cryosurgery as a supplement to curettage and partial excision. Cancer 74 (4): 1253-60, 1994.

544. Godersky J C, Smoker W R K, Knutzon R: Use of MRI in the evaluation of metastatic spinal disease. Neurosurgery 21: 676-80, 1987.

545. Rodichok L D, Ruckdeschel J C, Harper G R, et al.: Early detection and treatment of spinal epidural metastases: The role of myelography. Ann Neurol 20: 696-702, 1986.

546. Batson O V: The function of the vertebral veins and their role in the spread of metastases. Ann Surg 112: 138, 1940.

547. Sherk H H: Lesions of the atlas and axis. Clin Orthop 109: 33-41, 1975.

548. Nakamura M, Toyama Y, Suzuki N, et al.: Metastases to the upper cervical spine. J Spinal Disord 9: 195-201, 1996.

549. Portenoy R K, Lipton R B, Foley K M: Back pain in the cancer patient: An algorithm for evaluation and management. Neurology 37: 134-8, 1987.

550. Brice J, McKissock W: Surgical treatment of malignant extradural spinal tumors. Br Med J 1: 1341-4, 1965.

551. Hollis P H, Malis L I, Zappulla R A: Neurological deterioration after lumbar puncture below complete spinal subarachnoid block. J Neurosurg 64: 253-6, 1986.

552. Lee Y-Y, Glass J P, Wallace S: Myelography in cancer patients: Modified technique. AJR 145: 791-5, 1985.

553. Danner R L, Hartman B J: Update of spinal epidural abscess: 35 cases and review of the literature. Rev Infect Dis 9: 265-74, 1987.

554. Findlay G F G: Adverse effects of the management of malignant spinal cord compression. J Neurol Neurosurg Psychiatry 47: 761-8, 1984.

555. Cooper P R, Errico T J, Martin R, et al.: A systematic approach to spinal reconstruction after anterior decompression for neoplastic disease of the thoracic and lumbar spine. Neurosurgery 32: 1-8, 1993.

556. Sonntag V K H, Marcotte P J: Comment on Cooper P R et al.: A systematic approach to spinal reconstruction after anterior decompression for neoplastic disease of the thoracic and lumbar spine. Neurosurgery 32: 8, 1993.

557. Rubin P: Extradural spinal cord compression by tumor: Part I. Experimental production and treatment trials. Radiology 93: 1243-8, 1969.

558. Onimus M, Schraub S, Bertin D, et al.: Surgical treatment of vertebral metastasis. Spine 11: 883-91, 1986.

559. Sundaresan N, Galicich J H, Lane J M, et al.: Treatment of neoplastic epidural cord compression by vertebral body resection and stabilization. J Neurosurg 63: 676-84, 1985.

560. Overby M C, Rothman A S: Anterolateral decompression for metastatic epidural spinal cord tumors: Results of a modified costrotransversectomy approach. J Neurosurg 62: 344-8, 1985.

561. Shaw B, Mansfield F L, Borges L: One-stage posterolateral decompression and stabilization for primary and metastatic vertebral tumors in the thoracic and lumber spine. J Neurosurg 70: 405-10, 1989.

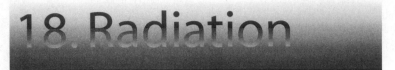
18. Radiation

Ionizing radiation[2] includes x-rays and gamma rays (both of which transmit their energy via photons) and particulate radiation. The goal of XRT in treating tumors is to cause cell death or to stop cell replication. Photons impart critical energy to achieve this result by the photoelectric effect (at lower energies, < 0.05 MeV), by Compton scattering (at higher energies of 0.1-10 MeV, e.g. in linear accelerators and Gamma knives), or by pair-production (at the highest energies)[1]. In the Compton effect, the initial collision of the photon with an atom creates a free electron which then ionizes other atoms and breaks chemical bonds. The absorption of radiation by indirect ionization in the presence of water produces free radicals (containing an unpaired electron) which causes cellular injury (usually by damaging DNA) within the tumor.

Radiation absorption

Radiation doses can be quantitated by the amount of energy absorbed per unit mass, where 1 Gray (Gy) equals 1 joule/kg. *Table 18-1* shows the conversion factor between Grays and rads. The biological effect of radiation can be described by the roentgen-equivalent man (**REM**) or Sievert (Sv) where 1 Sv = 100 REM. 1 REM is estimated to cause ≈ 300 additional cases of cancer per million persons (one third of which are fatal). The average annual exposure to radiation is 360 mREM (about 30 mREM are due to background cosmic radiation). A CXR produces about 10-40 mREM of exposure, a CAT scan of the head ≈ 18-40 REM (1.25 REM/slice), a cerebral arteriogram ≈ 10-20 REM (including fluoroscopy), and a transcontinental airline flight ≈ 5 mREM[1].

Table 18-1 Conversion factors between Grays and rads

1 Gy (Gray) = 100 cGy = 100 rads
1 cGy (centigray) = 1 rad

18.1. Conventional external beam radiation

Fractionation

The practice in which the total radiation dose is delivered in a series of smaller brief applications. This is one means of increasing the therapeutic ratio (the ratio of the effectiveness of XRT on tumor cells to that of normal cells). Radiation injury is a function of the dose, the exposure time, and the area exposed. Radiation oncologists refer to the four "R's" of radiobiology[2]:

1. **R**epair of sublethal damage
2. **R**eoxygenation of tumor cells that were hypoxic before XRT: oxygenated cells are more sensitive than hypoxic cells because oxygen combines with unpaired electrons to form peroxides which are more stable and lethal than free radicals
3. **R**epopulation of tumor cells following treatment
4. **R**edistribution (or reassortment) of cells within the cell cycle: cells in the mitotic phase are the most sensitive

Dosing

The biologically effective dose of fractionated radiation is often modeled by the linear-quadratic equation (LQ-model) shown in *Eq 18-1*, where D = the total dose of radiation, d = dose per fraction, and the factors α & β are used to describe the cell response to radiation. An α/β ratio of 10 is designated as early-responding tissue such as tumor cells, and a ratio of 3 is used for late-responding tissue, such as normal brain and also AVMs.

$$\text{biologically effective dose (Gy)} = D \times \left[1 + \frac{d}{\alpha/\beta}\right] \qquad \textbf{Eq 18-1}$$

18.1.1. Cranial radiation

Following surgery for tumor (craniotomy or spinal surgery), most surgeons wait ≈ 7-10 days before instituting XRT to the surgical site (allows initiation of healing).

Two CNS tumors that "melt away" with XRT but tend to recur later:
1. lymphoma
2. germ cell tumors

RADIATION INJURY AND NECROSIS

Radiation necrosis (RN) may mimic recurrent (or denovo) tumor both clinically and radiographically. Differences in prognosis and treatment make it important to distinguish between tumor and RN.

PATHOPHYSIOLOGY

As radiation is selectively toxic to more rapidly dividing cells, the two normal cell types within the CNS most vulnerable to RN are vascular endothelium (which have a turnover time of ≈ 6-10 mos) and oligodendroglial cells. Vascular injury may be the primary limiting factor to the tolerance of cranial XRT[3]. Injury from XRT occurs at lower doses when given concurrently with chemotherapy (especially methotrexate).

Radiation effects are divided into 3 phases[4]:
1. acute: occur during treatment. Rare. Usually an exacerbation of symptoms already present. Probably secondary to edema. Treat with ↑ steroids
2. early delayed: few weeks to 2-3 mos following completion of XRT. In spinal cord → Lhermitte's sign. In brain → post-irradiation lethargy & memory difficulties
3. late delayed: 3 mos-12 yrs (most within 3 years). Due to small artery injury → thrombotic occlusion → white matter atrophy or frank coagulative necrosis

Manifestations of radiation effects:
1. decreased cognition
   A. dementia may develop following XRT[5]
   B. children: may attain lower IQ by ≈ 25 points, especially with > 40 Gy whole brain XRT. Measurable IQ differences occur in children radiated before age 7, but more subtle deficits occur even in older children[6]
2. injury to anterior optic pathways
3. injury to hypothalamic-pituitary axis → hypopituitarism → growth retardation in children
4. primary hypothyroidism (especially in children)
5. may induce formation of new tumor: tumors most commonly identified as having increased incidence following radiation treatment are gliomas (including glioblastoma multiforme[8]), meningiomas[8], and nerve sheath tumors[9]. Skull base tumors have been reported following EBRT[10]
6. malignant transformation: e.g. after SRS for acoustic neuromas (see page 437)
7. leukoencephalopathy: profound demyelinating/necrotizing reaction 4-12 mos after combined RXT and methotrexate, especially in children with acute lymphoblastic leukemia (ALL) and adults with primary CNS tumors

EVALUATION

CT & MRI

Cannot reliably differentiate some cases of radiation necrosis from tumor (especially astrocytoma; RN occasionally resembles glioblastoma multiforme) even with contrast. Often see periventricular lucency and ventricular dilatation (difficult to distinguish from hydrocephalus). Dynamic FLASH-MRI shows some promise.

MR spectroscopy (see page 137) was reliable in distinguishing tumor from RN when either pure tumor or pure RN was present, but was less definitive with mixed tumor/necrosis[11].

Nuclear brain scan

Some reports of success with thallium-201 and technetium-99m brain scans.

Computerized radionuclide studies

PET (positron emission tomography) scan: because positron emitting isotopes have short half lives, PET scanning requires a nearby cyclotron to generate the radiopharma-ceuticals at great expense. Utilizing [18F]-fluorodeoxyglucose (FDG), regional glucose metabolism is imaged and is generally increased with recurrent tumor, and is decreased with RN. Specificity for distinguishing RN from tumor recurrence is > 90%, but sensitiv-ity may be too low to make it reliable[12]. Amino acid tracers such as [11C]methionine and [18F]tyrosine are taken up by most brain tumors[13], especially gliomas, and may also be used to help differentiate tumor from necrosis. Accuracy may be increased by fusing PET scan with MRI[14].

SPECT (single positron emission computed tomography): "poor man's PET scan". Uses radio-labeled amphetamine. Uptake depends on presence of intact neurons and the condition of cerebral blood vessels (including blood brain barrier). Decreased radionu-clide uptake indicates necrosis, whereas tumor recurrence has no decreased uptake.

TREATMENT

Symptoms from any form of radiation toxicity often respond initially to steroids.

Reoperation and excision is appropriate if there is deterioration from mass effect, regardless of whether the mass effect is from recurrent tumor or RN (the decision to re-operate should be based on the patient's Karnofsky rating, *see page 899*). Although some benefit has been shown, most reoperation studies are biased because they often select the patients who are doing better.

Other forms of therapy include: hyperbaric oxygen and anticoagulation.

Patients with documented tumor recurrence (as opposed to RN) may also be consid-ered for additional radiation (external beam, interstitial brachytherapy, or stereotactic radiosurgery (SRS)) or chemotherapy.

PREVENTION

Injury is dependent on total radiation dose, number of treatments or fractions (less damage occurs with more frequent small treatments), and volume treated.

Various studies to determine the tolerance of normal brain to XRT have estimated that 65-75 Gy given over 6.5-8 wks in 5 fractions/week is usually tolerated (radiation ne-crosis will occur in ≈ 5% after 60 Gy fractionated in 30 treatments over 6 weeks). Other studies have shown tolerance to 45 Gy for 10 fractions, 60 Gy for 35 fractions, and 70 Gy for 60 fractions[4].

18.1.2. Spinal radiation

SIDE EFFECTS

1. radiation myelopathy: *see below*
2. those due to overlap with GI tract: N/V, diarrhea
3. bone marrow suppression
4. growth retardation in children[15]
5. risk of developing cavernous malformations of the spinal cord (*see page 841*)

RADIATION MYELOPATHY

Radiation myelopathy (RM) typically occurs in patients with spinal cord included in radiation therapy (XRT) ports used to treat cancer outside the spinal cord, includes breast, lung, thyroid, and epidural mets. Radiation neuropathy may occur with irradia-tion in the region of the axilla for carcinoma of the breast (*see page 555*). In the lower ex-tremities, XRT for pelvic or bone tumors (e.g. of the femur) may produce lumbar plexopathy. In addition to permanent changes, radiation therapy may also produce spi-nal cord edema which may resolve after completion of radiation therapy.

EPIDEMIOLOGY

Incidence difficult to estimate due to the fact that the onset is typically delayed to-gether with the poor survival of patients with malignant disease requiring XRT.

Most cases reported involve the cervical cord in spite of the higher frequency with which the thoracic cord is exposed to XRT (perhaps due to higher XRT doses to the head and neck and longer survival than with lung Ca)[16]. Delay between completion of XRT and onset of symptoms is usually ≈ 1 yr (reported range: 1 mos-5 yrs).

Important factors relating to the occurrence of RM include[16]:
1. rate of application (probably the most important factor)
2. total radiation dose
3. extent of cord shielding
4. individual susceptibility and variability
5. amount of tissue radiated
6. vascular supply to the region radiated
7. source of radiation

PATHOPHYSIOLOGY
Effects of XRT on the spinal cord that lead to RM are:
1. direct injury to cells (including neurons)
2. vascular changes, including endothelial cell proliferation → thrombosis
3. hyalinization of collagen fibers

CLINICAL
Clinical types of radiation myelopathy
Four clinical types have been described and are shown in *Table 18-2*.

Table 18-2   Types of radiation myelopathy

Type	Description
1	benign form; commonly several mos following XRT (reported as late as 1 yr). Usually resolves completely within several mos. Mild sensory symptoms (frequently limited to a Lhermitte's sign) without objective neurological findings
2	injury to anterior horn cells → lower motor neuron signs in arms or legs
3	described only in experimental animals after doses larger than normal XRT. Complete cord lesion within hours due to injury to blood vessels
4	the type commonly reported. Chronic, progressive myelopathy (*see text*)

Onset is usually insidious, but abruptness has also been described; the presentation often mimics epidural mets. First symptoms: usually paresthesias and hypesthesia of LEs, and Lhermitte's sign. Then spastic weakness of LEs with hyperreflexia develops. A Brown-Séquard syndrome is not uncommon.

Approximately 50% of patients developing RM also have dysphagia from esophageal strictures requiring dilatations (the dysphagia often predates the myelopathy).

EVALUATION
Essentially a diagnosis of exclusion. Radiographic imaging (CT, myelography) will be normal. MRI may show spinal cord infarction. The history of previous radiation is key. The differential diagnosis is included in *Acute paraplegia or quadriplegia* on page 913.

PROGNOSIS
Prognosis for Type 4 RM is poor. Usually progresses to complete (or near complete) cord lesion. Paraplegia and/or sphincter involvement are poor signs.

PREVENTION
Maximum recommended cord radiation dose depends on size of port, and varies with investigator. With large field techniques (> 10 cm of cord), the risk of RM is negligible with ≤ 3.3 Gy in 42 days (0.55 Gy/wk), and with small field techniques ≤ 4.3 Gy in 42 days (0.717 Gy/wk). Larger doses may possibly be given safely if fractionated over longer periods. Recommended upper limit: 0.2 Gy/fraction.

18.2.   Stereotactic radiosurgery

❢ Key features
- uses stereotactic localization to precisely focus a large dose of radiation onto a lesion, usually in a single treatment
- best accepted indication: AVM ≤ 3 cm diameter with compact nidus for which surgical removal is not appropriate (deep location, proximity to eloquent brain)

- advantage: low immediate procedural morbidity
- disadvantages: delayed complications of radiation. With AVM: long latency (1-3 years) to obliteration creates period with risk of hemorrhage

Conventional fractionated XRT capitalizes on the differential response of normal tissue from tumor cells to radiation (see *Fractionation*, page 534). Additionally, in cases where there is a localized lesion, XRT also takes advantage of averaging multiple treatment beams delivered through independent radiation ports in order to allow a larger dose of radiation to be applied to the lesion while exposing surrounding (normal) tissues to a lesser dose. The term "stereotactic radiosurgery" (**SRS**) describes the use of stereotactic localization to administer large radiation doses with a very steep gradient to a precise intracranial locus while exposing normal structures to safely tolerated doses. Unlike conventional external beam radiation therapy (**EBRT**), the dose is usually administered in a single treatment session (for exceptions to this, see *Fractionated SRS*, page 539).

INDICATIONS

In general, SRS is useful for well circumscribed lesions less than approximately **2.5-3** cm diameter (the "classic" lesion for which SRS is used is for appropriate AVMs, *see below*). For larger lesions, the radiation dose must be reduced because of anatomic and radiobiological constraints, and the precision of the stereotactic technique is offset due to overlap.

Published uses of stereotactic radiosurgery include:
1. AVMs: *see below*
2. tumors: *see below*
   A. acoustic neuromas: *see below*
   B. pituitary adenomas: conventional EBRT (fractionated over ≈ 5 wks) is generally preferred to SRS as the initial form of XRT
   C. craniopharyngiomas
   D. pineal tumors
   E. metastases
   F. high grade gliomas: *see below*
   G. meningiomas of the cavernous sinus[17]
3. functional neurosurgery
   A. for control of chronic pain[18] including trigeminal neuralgia[19, 20] (*see page 382*)
   B. pallidotomies for Parkinson's disease: usually <u>not</u> a technique of choice because of inability to perform physiologic stimulation prior to lesioning to verify target location which may vary by several millimeters. May be a consideration for the rare patient who cannot undergo placement of a stimulating/lesioning needle (e.g. refractory coagulopathy)
4. for treating patients refusing open surgery for various conditions

AVMs

SRS is best accepted for the treatment of small (< 3 cm) AVMs that are deep or border on eloquent brain and have a "compact" (i.e. sharply demarcated) nidus[21-23]. This includes those incompletely excised with previous surgery. The radiation induces endothelial cell proliferation which produces thickening of the vascular wall and ultimately obliteration of the lumen over a period of ≈ 1-2 years. SRS is of no benefit for venous angiomas (*see page 839*). SRS probably reduces the rebleeding risk for cavernous malformations[24]. For a comparison of treatment options for AVMs *see page 838*.

Larger AVMs (up to 5 cm) have also been treated with SRS with some success. Tentorial dural AVMs (*see page 843*) have also shown promising response to SRS[25].

TUMORS

The use of SRS for tumors is controversial. It is not advisable for use on benign tumors in young patients because of possible delayed side-effects following radiation (see *Delayed morbidity*, page 542) (possible exception: bilateral acoustic neuromas, *see below*).

Infiltrating tumors

Generally not indicated for infiltrating tumors, e.g gliomas (poorly defined tumor margins defeats the advantage of precisely localized radiation) although it has been used for recurrent lesions following traditional treatment (surgical excision and fractionated external beam radiation). One of the arguments for SRS in these tumors is the fact that 90% of recurrences are within the original radiographic solid tumor volume[26]. RTOG trial

9305 showed no benefit with upfront use of SRS added to EBRT and BCNU chemotherapy in treating glioblastoma multiforme (http://www.rtog.org/closedsummaries/9305.html).

Acoustic neuromas

For most cases, the optimal treatment for an acoustic neuroma (AN) is surgery[A]. Possible indications for SRS for AN: poor operative candidates (due to poor medical condition and/or advanced age, some use > 65 or 70 yrs as a cutoff), patient refusing surgery, bilateral ANs, post-operative treatment of incompletely removed ANs that continue to grow on serial imaging, or recurrences following surgical removal (also see *Acoustic neuromas* under *Results* below).

CONTRAINDICATIONS

Compressive tumors of the spinal cord or medulla: even with the sharp isodose fall-off curves of SRS, there is still significant radiation delivered within a few millimeters of the margins of the lesion. This, together with the slight swelling of lesions that commonly follows SRS creates significant risk of neurologic injury, especially over the long term (which is even more likely with benign lesions in young individuals).

COMPARISON OF SRS TECHNOLOGIES

Various methods are available, differing mostly on the source of the radiation and the technique for increasing the dose delivered to the lesion. A photon beam that is produced by electron acceleration is called an x-ray, whereas if it is produced by natural radioactive decay it is called a gamma ray. Although photons are identical regardless of how they are produced, gamma rays have a narrower distribution of energy than x-rays. The spatial accuracy of the gamma knife may be slightly better than linac systems, but the small difference does not seem critical because the error inherent in selecting the target margins exceeds the typical linac imprecision of ≈ 1 mm[28]. The linac has greater flexibility in dealing with non-spherical lesions and is much more economical than the gamma knife. For small lesions (< 3 cm diameter) both photon and charged particle beam sources have similar results.

Gamma knife

Different sized collimators and exposure times, using more than one isocenter, and plugging collimators that would pass radiation thorough sensitive structures are used to modify the treatment plan.

Linac

Standard linacs usually require modifications to provide the required precision (e.g. precision bearings, external collimators...).

Different sized collimators, different beam energies (arc weighting), and alterations of the arc paths and the number of arcs are used to modify treatments.

FRACTIONATED SRS

Most SRS to date has been done with single fraction treatment. AVMs share some characteristics of what radiation oncologists call "late responding" lesions based on the linear quadratic model (LQ-model), and there is little rationale for fractionated protocols (although the LQ-model may not apply to SRS). Some slow growing tumors may also be similar to late responding tissue, but there may regions of hypoxic cells where XRT will be less effective, and where the reoxygenation phenomenon would improve response (see the *Four "R's" of radiobiology, page 534*). Also, if there is some uncertainty regarding the tumor margins on CT or MRI and there is the possibility that some normal brain may be included in the treatment plan (or fear that constricting the treatment margins would exclude some tumor) this is again a situation where fractionation will help.

Accelerated fractionation (2-3 fractions/d x 1 week) are being investigated but are not appropriate in the vicinity of radiosensitive structures and may be inconvenient and expensive. **Hypofractionation** (1 fraction/d x 1 week) may be a better compromise.

For malignancies, fractionated schemes will almost always improve effectiveness of XRT. Research into fractionated SRS employs various methods to reposition the stereotactic frame, including masks, dental molds, etc. Displacement errors can be as high as

---

A. e.g. see the many comments following the article by Pollock, et al.[27], also *see page 433*

2-8 mm with mask systems, whereas recommended tolerances are 0.3 mm and 3°.

Although the optimal protocol has not yet been determined, fractionated SRS may have significant advantages for pituitary adenomas, peri-chiasmal lesions, in children (where it is even more desirable to minimize radiation of the normal brain), and in acoustic neuromas considered for SRS where there is useful hearing.

TREATMENT PLANNING

For a selected isocentric radiation dose to be delivered to a given volume, computer simulation programs help radiosurgeons select the number of arcs or beams, collimator width, etc., to keep exposure of nearby normal brain to acceptable limits, and limit radiation to particularly sensitive structures. *Table 18-3* shows maximum recommended doses of various organs for a single fraction. In the brain, critical radiation sensitive structures include: optic vitreous, nerve, and chiasm, brain stem, and pituitary gland.

Cranial nerves: special sensory nerves (optic, vestibulocochlear) are the most radiosensitive. Somatic afferents (trigeminal), visceral efferents (facial), and somatic efferents (oculomotor, hypoglossal) are the next most radiosensitive[30].

SRS treatment may also have a deleterious effect in structures sensitive to swelling, such as brain stem. Most radiosurgeons decline to use SRS for lesions in the region of the optic chiasm. However, in general it is <u>not</u> the radiosensitive structures located at a distance from the lesion that are at greatest risk. Rather, it is that tissue included in the higher dose isocenters immediately adjacent to the lesion.

For the linac, optimal dose drop-off usually occurs when ≥ **500° total degree-arc** is used (e.g. 5 arcs of 100° each). Using more than 5 arcs rarely produces a significant difference out to the 20% isodose curve.

Table 18-3 Maximum recommended radiation dose of critical organs
(delivered in a single fraction)

Structure	Maximum dose (cGy)	% of maximum (at a prescribed dose of 50 Gy)
eye lens (cataract induction begins at 500 cGy)	100	2%
optic nerve[29]	100	2%
skin in beam	50	1%
thyroid	10	0.2%
gonads	1	0.02%
breast	3	0.06%

Doses

Doses specify the amount of radiation delivered to the isocenter (or to a specified isodose curve, e.g. 18 Gy to the 50% isodose curve) and relating the isodose curve to a specific region of the lesion (e.g. at the edge of the AVM nidus). **Dose-volume relation**: the dose of radiation that can be tolerated is highly dependent on the volume being treated (larger treatment volumes require lower doses to avoid complications).

Dose selection is made based on known information or is estimated from dose-volume-relationship. If uncertain, err on the side of a lower dose. Previous XRT must also be taken into account by the radiation physicist. Adjacent structures within ≈ 2.5 mm of the target will receive injurious radiation and the total dose should reduced.

Target localization

CT: the optimal imaging modality for SRS. Accuracy is never better than ≈ 0.6 mm which is the pixel size.

Stereotactic angiography: rarely required, and may even introduce errors in treatment planning. Stereotactic angiography should not be used alone because of problems including: the true geometry of the lesion cannot be fully appreciated, vessels may be obscured by other vessels or bone, etc.[31-34]. *Digital* subtraction angiography is even more problematic because it warps the image and requires an "unwarping" algorithm to be used for SRS.

MRI: has a 1-2 mm shift due to spatial distortion artifact from the magnet. If MRI is required to visualize the lesion, it is probably better to use image fusion techniques with a stereotactic-CT and a *non-stereotactic* MRI.

Conformational planning

The shape of the treatment volume can be influenced to some degree by covering some sources (with gamma-knife units) or by choosing arcs with certain orientations (with linac based systems).

With linac systems, the <u>height</u> of the treatment volume is controlled by the horizontal arc collimator size, and the width is controlled by the vertical arc collimator size.

Lesions that are not round or ellipsoid in shape require multiple isocenters. Lower total doses for each isocenter must then be used.

AVMs

If embolization is used before SRS, wait ≈ 30 days between the two procedures. DO NOT use radio-opaque material in embolization mixture (*see page 839*). Some experts find that target selection after embolization is extraordinarily difficult because of multiple small residual "nidi".

A bolus-enhanced stereotactic CT is usually employed (except for those AVMs that are difficult to see on CT or when metal clips from previous surgery or radio-opaque substance from embolization creates too much artifact). Caution with stereotactic angiography (*see above*).

A general consensus is that **15 Gy to the periphery** of the AVM is optimal (range: 10-25). At McGill with linac SRS, they use 25-50 Gy delivered to 90% isodose curve at the edge of the nidus. With Bragg-peak, complications occurred less frequently with doses ≤ 19.2 Gy compared to doses above that (this may reduce the obliteration rate or increase the latency period)[35].

Due to the fact that AVMs are benign lesions that are often treated in young patients, conformal planning is critical to avoid injury to nearby normal brain.

Cavernous malformations (CM)

Iron is a relatively potent radiation sensitizer, therefore the hemosiderin ring around the CM should be **excluded** from the treatment plan. Dosimetry depends on volume and location of the lesion, an average of ≈ 15-16 Gy to the 50% isodose curve is used.

Tumors

Acoustic neuromas (and meningiomas):

For 1 isocenter: 10-15 Gy with the tumor at the 80% isodose line (current recommended maximum dose[36, 37]:**14 Gy**) is associated with a lower incidence of cranial nerve palsies than higher doses[38]. For 2 isocenters: treat 10-15 Gy at the 70% isodose line.

Metastases:

Median dose of 15 Gy (range: 9-25 Gy) at the center with the tumor contained in the 80% isodose curve has been recommended. One literature review found a reported range of 13-18 Gy at the center with good local control[39].

RESULTS

AVMs

At 1 year, 46-61% of AVMs were completely obliterated on angiography, and at 2 years 86% were obliterated. There was no reduction in size in < 2% of cases. Smaller lesions have higher obliteration rates (with Bragg-peak in AVMs < 2 cm diameter, 94% thrombosed at 2 yrs, and 100% at 3 yrs[35]). AVMs > 25 mm diameter have only ≈ 50% chance of obliteration with 1 SRS treatment.

Although the immediate "procedural" mortality is 0%, Bragg-peak proton beam treatment of AVMs affords no protection against hemorrhage in the first 12-14 months following treatment[23] (the so-called "**incubation period**"); this is similar to the 12-24 month latency for photon radiation[21]. Hemorrhages have occurred during the incubation period even in AVMs that had never bled before[35], and the question has been raised whether a partially thrombosed AVM is more likely to bleed because of increased outflow resistance.

Factors associated with treatment failures include[40]: incomplete angiographic definition of the nidus (the most frequent factor, responsible for 57% of cases), recanalization of the nidus (7%), masking of nidus by hematoma, and a theorized "radiobiological resistance". In some, no discernible reason for failure could be identified. In this series the complete obliteration rate was ≤ 64%, possibly because arteriography was heavily relied upon for treatment planning instead of emphasizing stereotactic CT.

If AVM persists 2-3 yrs after SRS, retreatment with SRS is an option[40] (usually the residual is smaller).

Acoustic neuromas

In 111 tumors ≤ 3 cm in size[41], 44% decreased in size, 42% did not change, and 14% increased. Although retardation of growth is observed in the majority of cases, long-term results are not available to fully assess therapeutic efficacy and complication rate at this time[42]. Use in **recurrent** ANs following microsurgery is endorsed by some (*see page 438*). Also see *Outcome & follow-up*, page 436 for a comparison of outcomes with SRS versus microsurgery.

Gliomas
Median survival for large GBMs is so poor that SRS did not appear to have any benefit. Following SRS for gliomas, there is rarely reduction of enhancing volume (it is more common to have *enlargement*, sometimes with increased neurologic deficit).

Metastases
There has not been a randomized study to compare surgery to SRS. *See page 490* for comparison of outcomes with cerebral mets with various treatments including SRS. Radiographic local control rate of ≈ 88% (reported range: 82-100%) has been cited[39].

The advantage of SRS is that there is no risk from the treatment of hemorrhage, infection, or mechanical spread of tumor cells. Disadvantages include not obtaining tissue for diagnosis (11% of the time the lesions may not be mets, *see page 488*).

No significant difference has been found with SRS between tumors considered "radiosensitive" and those that are "radioresistant" as defined by standards developed for EBRT (see *Table 17-58*, page 489) (however, histology may affect the *rate* of response). The lack of significance of "radioresistance" may be due in part to the fact that the sharp dose drop-off with SRS allows higher doses to be delivered to tumors than would be used with EBRT.

Supratentorial control is better than infratentorial. Also, there is no significant difference in local control between single and dual mets. The RTOG has identified 3 or fewer mets as a more favorable prognosticator.

TREATMENT MORBIDITY AND MORTALITY

Immediate morbidity
Immediate mortality from the actual treatments themselves is probably zero. Morbidity: all but ≈ 2.5% of patients were discharged home within 24 hrs. Many centers do not admit patients overnight. Some immediate adverse reactions include[43]:
1. 16% of patients require analgesics for post-procedural headaches and antiemetics for nausea/vomiting
2. at least 10% of patients with subcortical AVMs had focal or generalized seizures within 24 hrs of treatment (only one was on subtherapeutic AEDs. All were controllable with additional AEDs)

Premedication: The Pittsburgh Gamma Knife group gives methylprednisolone 40 mg IV and phenobarbital 90 mg IV immediately after the radiation dose to patients with tumors or AVMs to reduce these adverse effects[43].

Delayed morbidity
Long-term morbidity directly related to the radiation may occur, and just as with conventional XRT, is more frequent with larger doses and treatment volumes. Another risk particular to AVMs is that of hemorrhage during the latency period, which is 3-4% during the first year and is <u>not</u> higher following SRS. Radiation complications [44]:
1. white matter changes: occurred 4-26 mos (mean 15.3) post-SRS. Seen on imaging (high intensity on MRI T2WI, or low density on CT) in ≈ 50% of patients, symptomatic in only 20% of patients[35]. Associated with radiation necrosis in ≈ 3% of cases
2. vasculopathy: diagnosed by narrowing seen on angiography or by ischemic changes on imaging in ≈ 5% of cases
3. cranial nerve deficits: occur in ≈ 1% of all cases. Incidence is higher with tumors of CPA or skull base
4. induced tumors: only 6 reported malignant tumors in over 80,000 radiosurgical procedures for benign disease[45]. Estimated incidence: < 1 in 1000
5. normal perfusion pressure breakthrough[46]: classically occurs following conventional microsurgery for AVMs (*see page 839*), it has also been described following SRS[47]

18.3.   Interstitial brachytherapy

Technique whereby radioactive implants are used to deliver locally high doses of radiation directly to tumors while exposing nearby normal brain to less toxic doses. At present, the numbers are too small and the follow-up too short to determine the efficacy of interstitial brachytherapy[48]. Controlled prospective studies have not yet been completed.

Interstitial brachytherapy **(IB)** may reduce the rate of tumor growth, but it rarely produces clinical improvement. Patients are generally not considered for IB unless their Karnofsky score is ≥ 70.

Techniques include:
1. insertion of high activity iodine-125 pellets which remain in place (either by conventional open surgery or by stereotactic technique)
2. insertion of catheters (so-called afterloading catheters) containing radioactive source (such as gold or I^{125}) by stereotactic technique, which are then removed at a predetermined time (usually 1-7 days)
3. instillation of radioactive liquids (e.g. phosphorous isotope) into a cyst cavity

I^{125} has several characteristics that favor its use: it emits low-energy gamma rays which are absorbed by surrounding tissues minimizing radiation exposure of the normal brain, medical personnel and visitors. It is available as low-activity (< 5 mCi) or high-activity (5-40 mCi) seeds.

Treatment planning is devised to deliver 60 Gy to the edge of a volume that extends 1 cm beyond the contrast-enhancing tumor, with variations included to spare radiosensitive structures (e.g. optic chiasm). Usual delivery rates are 40-50 cGy/hr to the tumor margin (30 cGy/hr is the critical dose for cessation of human tumor growth) requiring that the seeds stay in the afterloading catheter ≈ 6 days.

RADIATION NECROSIS

Symptomatic radiation necrosis **(RN)** occurs in ≈ 40% of cases, and may occur as early as several months after IB. It may be impossible to differentiate from recurrent tumor in many cases. Symptomatic treatment is often achieved with increased corticosteroid dosages. Continued neurologic deterioration may require craniotomy.

OUTCOME

IB is often used as a "last ditch" effort in a patient with a recurrent malignant tumor who has received maximal external beam irradiation and who is not a candidate for reoperation (as expected, the results in patients with such poor prognoses are not good). However, patients eligible for IB are usually better than those who are not candidates, and this may bias the results towards a better outcome[49]. Some studies with early (primary treatment) use have shown possible benefit[50].

18.4. References

1. Thompson T P, Maitz A H, Kondziolka D, et al.: Radiation, radiobiology, and neurosurgery. **Contemp Neurosurg** 21 (13): 1-5, 1999.
2. Hall E J, Cox J D: Physical and biologic basis of radiation therapy. In **Moss' radiation oncology**, Cox J D, (ed.). Mosby-Year Book, Inc.; St. Louis, Missouri, 7th ed., 1994: pp 3-66.
3. O'Connor M M, Mayberg M R: Effects of radiation on cerebral vasculature: A review. **Neurosurgery** 46: 138-51, 2000.
4. Leibel S A, Sheline G E: Radiation therapy for neoplasms of the brain. **J Neurosurg** 66: 1-22, 1987.
5. Duffner P K, Cohen M E, Thomas P: Late effects of treatment on the intelligence of children with posterior fossa tumors. **Cancer** 51: 233-7, 1983.
6. Radcliffe J, Packer R J, Atkins T E, et al.: Three- and four-year cognitive outcome in children with non-cortical brain tumors treated with whole-brain radiotherapy. **Ann Neurol** 32: 551-4, 1992.
7. Zuccarello M, Sawaya R, deCourten-Myers: Glioblastoma occurring after radiation therapy for meningioma: Case report and review of literature. **Neurosurgery** 19: 114-9, 1986.
8. Mack E E, Wilson C B: Meningiomas induced by high-dose cranial irradiation. **J Neurosurg** 79: 28-31, 1993.
9. Ron E, Modan B, Boice J D, et al.: Tumors of the brain and nervous system after radiotherapy in childhood. **N Engl J Med** 319: 1033-9, 1988.
10. Lustig L R, Jackler R K, Lanser M J: Radiation-induced tumors of the temporal bone. **Am J Otol** 18: 230-5, 1997.
11. Rock J P, Hearshen D, Scarpace L, et al.: Correlations between magnetic resonance spectroscopy and image-guided histopathology, with special attention to radiation necrosis. **Neurosurgery** 51 (4): 912-9; discussion 919-20, 2002.
12. Thompson T P, Lunsford L D, Kondziolka D: Distinguishing recurrent tumor and radiation necrosis with positron emission tomography versus stereotactic biopsy. **Stereotact Funct Neurosurg** 73 (1-4): 9-14, 1999.
13. Ericson K, Lilja A, Bergstrom M, et al.: Positron emission tomography with ([^{11}C]methyl)-L-methionine, [^{11}C]D-glucose, and [^{68}Ga]EDTA in supratentorial tumors. **J Comput Assist Tomogr** 9: 683-9, 1985.
14. Thiel A, Pietrzyk U, Sturm V, et al.: Enhanced accuracy in differential diagnosis of radiation necrosis by positron emission tomography-magnetic resonance imaging coregistration: Technical case report. **Neurosurgery** 46: 232-4, 2000.

15. Tomita T, McLone D G: Medulloblastoma in childhood: Results of radical resection and low-dose radiation therapy. **J Neurosurg** 64: 238-42, 1986.
16. Eyster E F, Wilson C B: Radiation myelopathy. **J Neurosurg** 32: 414-20, 1970.
17. Duma C M, Lunsford L D, Końdziolka D, *et al.*: Stereotactic radiosurgery of cavernous sinus meningiomas as an addition or alternative to microsurgery. **Neurosurgery** 32: 699-705, 1993.
18. Steiner L, Forster D, Leksell L, *et al.*: Gammathalamotomy in intractable pain. **Acta Neurochir** 52: 173-84, 1980.
19. Leksell L: Stereotactic radiosurgery in trigeminal neuralgia. **Acta Chir Scand** 137: 311-4, 1971.
20. Lunsford L D: Comment on Taha J M and Tew J M: Comparison of surgical treatments for trigeminal neuralgia: Reevaluation of radiofrequency rhizotomy. **Neurosurgery** 38: 871, 1996.
21. Saunders W M, Winston K R, Siddon R L, *et al.*: Radiosurgery for arteriovenous malformations of the brain using a standard linear accelerator: Rationale and technique. **Int J Radiation Oncology Biol Phys** 13: 441-7, 1988.
22. Poulsen M G: Arteriovenous malformations: A summary of 6 cases treated with radiation therapy. **Int J Radiation Oncology Biol Phys** 13: 1553-7, 1987.
23. Kjellberg R N, Hanamura T, Davis K R, *et al.*: Bragg-peak proton-beam therapy for arteriovenous malformations of the brain. **N Engl J Med** 309: 269-74, 1983.
24. Pollock B E, Garces Y I, Stafford S L, *et al.*: Stereotactic radiosurgery for cavernous malformations. **J Neurosurg** 93 (6): 987-91, 2000.
25. Lewis A I, Tomsick T A, Tew J M: Management of tentorial dural arteriovenous malformations: Transarterial embolization combined with stereotactic radiation or surgery. **J Neurosurg** 81: 851-9, 1994.
26. Choucair A K, Levin V A, Gutin P H, *et al.*: Development of multiple lesions during radiation therapy and chemotherapy. **J Neurosurg** 65: 654-8, 1986.
27. Pollock B E, Lunsford L D, Kondziolka D, *et al.*: Outcome analysis of acoustic neuroma management: A comparison of microsurgery and stereotactic radiosurgery. **Neurosurgery** 36: 215-29, 1995.
28. Luxton G, Petrovich Z, Jozsef G, *et al.*: Stereotactic radiosurgery: Principles and comparison of treatment methods. **Neurosurgery** 32: 241-59, 1993.
29. Leber K A, Berglöff J, Pendi G: Dose-response tolerance of the visual pathways and cranial nerves of the cavernous sinus to stereotactic radiosurgery. **J Neurosurg** 88: 43-50, 1998.
30. Tishler R B, Loeffler J S, Lunsford L D, *et al.*: Tolerance of cranial nerves of the cavernous sinus to radiosurgery. **Int J Radiation Oncology Biol Phys** 27: 215-21, 1993.
31. Blatt D L, Friedman W A, Bova F J: Modifications based on computed tomographic imaging in planning the radiosurgical treatment of arteriovenous malformations. **Neurosurgery** 33: 588-96, 1993.
32. Bova F J, Friedman W A: Stereotactic angiography: Pitfalls and problems. **Int J Radiation Oncology Biol Phys** 20: 891-5, 1991.
33. Spiegelmann R, Friedman W A, Bova F J: Limitations of angiographic target localization in radiosurgical treatment planning. **Neurosurgery** 30: 619-

24, 1992.
34. Friedman W A: Comment on Pollock B E, et al.: Repeat stereotactic radiosurgery of arteriovenous malformations: Factors associated with incomplete outcomes. **Neurosurgery** 38: 323, 1996.
35. Steinberg G K, Fabrikant J I, Marks M P, *et al.*: Stereotactic heavy-charged-particle Bragg-peak radiation for intracranial arteriovenous malformations. **N Engl J Med** 323: 96-101, 1990.
36. Kondziolka D, Lunsford L D, McLaughlin M R, *et al.*: Long-term outcomes after radiosurgery for acoustic neuromas. **N Engl J Med** 339: 1426-33, 1998.
37. Niranjan A, Lunsford L D, Flickinger J C, *et al.*: Dose reduction improves hearing preservation rates after intracanalicular acoustic tumor radiosurgery. **Neurosurgery** 45: 753-65, 1999.
38. Linskey M E, Lunsford L D, Flickinger J C: Radiosurgery for acoustic neuromas: Early experience. **Neurosurgery** 26: 736-45, 1990.
39. Fuller B G, Kaplan I D, Adler J, *et al.*: Stereotactic radiosurgery for brain metastases: The importance of adjuvant whole brain irradiation. **Int J Radiation Oncology Biol Phys** 23: 413-8, 1992.
40. Pollock B E, Kondziolka D, Lunsford L D, *et al.*: Repeat stereotactic radiosurgery of arteriovenous malformations: Factors associated with incomplete outcomes. **Neurosurgery** 38: 318-24, 1996.
41. Hirsch A, Norén G: Audiological findings after stereotactic radiosurgery in acoustic neuromas. **Acta Otolaryngol (Stockh)** 106: 244-51, 1988.
42. National Institutes of Health Consensus Development Conference: *Acoustic neuroma: Consensus statement*. **NIH Consens Dev Conf Consens Statement.** Bethesda, MD: Public Health Service, U.S. Department of Health and Human Services. Vol. 9, 1991.
43. Lunsford L D, Flickinger J, Coffey R J: Stereotactic gamma knife radiosurgery. Initial North American experience in 207 patients. **Arch Neurol** 47: 169-75, 1990.
44. Marks M P, Delapaz R L, Fabrikant J I, *et al.*: Intracranial vascular malformations: Imaging of charged-particle radiosurgery. Part II. Complications. **Radiology** 168: 457-62, 1988.
45. Loeffler J S, Niemierko A, Chapman P H: Second tumors after radiosurgery: Tip of the iceberg or a bump in the road? **Neurosurgery** 52 (6): 1436-40; discussion 1440-2, 2003.
46. Spetzler R F, Wilson C B, Weinstein P, *et al.*: Normal perfusion pressure breakthrough theory. **Clin Neurosurg** 25: 651-72, 1978.
47. Pollock B E: Occlusive hyperemia: A radiosurgical phenomenon? **Neurosurgery** 47: 1178-84, 2000.
48. Bernstein M, Laperriere N, Leung P, *et al.*: Interstitial brachytherapy for malignant brain tumors: Preliminary results. **Neurosurgery** 26: 371-80, 1990.
49. Florell R C, Macdonald D R, Irish W D, *et al.*: Selection bias, survival, and brachytherapy for glioma. **J Neurosurg** 76: 179-83, 1992.
50. Gutin P H, Prados M D, Phillips T L, *et al.*: External irradiation followed by an interstitial high activity iodine-125 implant "boost" in the initial treatment of malignant gliomas: NCOG study 6G-82-2. **Int J Radiation Oncology Biol Phys** 21: 601-6, 1991.

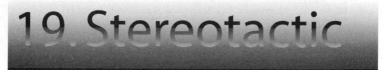

19. Stereotactic

Stereotactic (Greek: *stereo* = 3-dimensional, *tactic* = to touch) surgery was used for surgery performed in humans, usually for thalamic lesioning to treat Parkinsonism (see *Surgical treatment of Parkinson's disease*, page 365), where the target site to be lesioned was located relative to landmarks with intraoperative pneumoencephalography or contrast ventriculography. Use of this procedure fell off dramatically in the late 1960's with the introduction of L-dopa for Parkinsonism[1].

Current techniques would be more appropriately termed image-guided stereotactic surgery. Usually performed under local anesthesia (except in certain patients, e.g. some pediatrics). In the first part of the procedure, a CT scan or MRI (or occasionally, angiogram) is performed with a localizing device affixed to the patient's head, allowing the target to be precisely localized in space. Frameless systems used bony landmarks and sometimes fiducial markers to register the patient's skull relative to radiographic images (CT or MRI scans).

The second part of the procedure utilizes a set of guides oriented to the same coordinate system to direct biopsy needles, etc., to the target location. At this point, different stereotactic systems will require that the second part of the procedure be completed in the CT scan suite, or may permit it to be performed in the O.R.

Advantages of completing the procedure in the CT scan suite include:
1. verification of instrument placement at the desired target
2. immediate identification of problems such as hemorrhage
3. selection of entirely new coordinates if the first set yields undesirable results (some systems, such as the Leksell, permit coordinates to be read directly off the printed CT scan images)

Disadvantages of completing the procedure in the CT scan suite include:
1. longer time commitment of the CT scanner
2. possibly less sterile conditions
3. the need to get other equipment from the O.R. that is forgotten or needed for a unique reason (adds time to the procedure)
4. need to move the patient to the O.R. if a complication develops needing emergent craniotomy
5. difficult to use for procedures much more extensive than twist drill or bull hole

INDICATIONS FOR STEREOTACTIC SURGERY
1. biopsy (also, *see below*)
   A. deeply located cerebral lesions: especially near eloquent brain
   B. brain stem lesions: may be approached through the cerebral hemisphere[2]
   C. multiple small lesions (e.g. in some AIDS patients, *see page 234*)
   D. patient medically unable to tolerate general anesthesia for open biopsy
2. catheter placement
   A. drainage of deep lesions: colloid cyst, abscess
   B. indwelling catheter placement for intratumoral chemotherapy
   C. radioactive implants for interstitial radiation brachytherapy[3]
   D. shunt placement: for hydrocephalus (rarely used) or to drain cyst
3. electrode placement
   A. depth electrodes for epilepsy
   B. "deep brain stimulation" for chronic pain (requires electrophysiologic stimulation)
4. lesion generation
   A. movement disorders: Parkinsonism (*see page 366*), dystonia, hemiballismus
   B. treatment of chronic pain
   C. treatment of epilepsy (rarely used)
5. evacuation of intracerebral hemorrhage
   A. using an Archimedes' screw device[4,5]
   B. with adjunctive urokinase[6,7] or recombinant tissue-plasminogen activator[8]

(see page 860)

6. stereotactic "radiosurgery" (see *Stereotactic radiosurgery*, page 537)
7. to localize a lesion for open craniotomy (e.g. AVM[9], deep tumor)
    A. using a ventricular-type catheter
    B. using a blunt biopsy needle or introducer[10]
    C. systems using visible light laser beam for guidance
8. transoral biopsy of C2 (axis) vertebral body lesions[11]
9. "experimental" or unconventional applications
    A. stereotactic clipping of aneurysms[12]
    B. stereotactic laser surgery
    C. CNS transplantation[13]: e.g. for Parkinsonism (*see page 365*)
    D. foreign body removal[14]

STEREOTACTIC BIOPSY

This section presents information regarding stereotactic brain biopsy **(SBB)** in general. For SBB in specific conditions, see the index entry for that condition. May be performed under local or general anesthesia. For indications, *see above*.

Contraindications

1. coagulation disorders
    A. coagulopathies: bleeding diatheses, iatrogenic (heparin or coumadin)
    B. low platelet count **(PC)**: PC < 50,000/ml is an absolute contraindication, it is desirable to get the PC ≥ 100,000
2. inability to tolerate general anesthesia and to cooperate for local anesthesia

Yield

The yield rate (i.e. the ability to make a diagnosis from a SBB) reported in large series in the literature ranges from 82-99% in nonimmunocompromised **(NIC)** patients, and is slightly lower in AIDS patients at 56-96%. Higher yield rates in AIDS may result from improved surgical technique and histologic evaluation[15].

The yield rate is higher for lesions that enhance with contrast on CT or MRI (99% in NIC patients) than with lesions that do not enhance (74%)[16].

Complications

The most frequent complication is hemorrhage, although most are too small to have clinical impact. The risk of a *major* complication (mostly due to hemorrhage) in NIC patients ranges from 0-3% (with most < 1%), and 0-12% in AIDS[16]. Higher complication rates seen in AIDS patients in some series may be due to reduced platelet count or function, and to vessel fragility in primary CNS lymphoma. In NIC patients, multifocal high grade gliomas had the highest complication rate.

19.1. References

1. Gildenberg P L: Whatever happened to stereotactic surgery? **Neurosurgery** 20: 983-7, 1987.
2. Hood T W, Gebarski S S, McKeever P E, *et al*.: Stereotactic biopsy of intrinsic lesions of the brain stem. **J Neurosurg** 65: 172-6, 1986.
3. Coffey R J, Friedman W A: Interstitial brachytherapy of malignant brain tumors using computed tomography-guided stereotaxis and available imaging software: Technical report. **Neurosurgery** 20: 4-7, 1987.
4. Backlund E-O, von Holst H: Controlled subtotal evacuation of intracerebral hematomas by stereotactic technique. **Surg Neurol** 9: 99-101, 1978.
5. Tanikawa T, Amano K, Kawamura H, *et al*.: CT-guided stereotactic surgery for evacuation of hypertensive intracerebral hematoma. **Appl Neurophysiol** 48: 431-9, 1985.
6. Niizuma H, Otsuki T, Johkura H, *et al*.: CT-guided stereotactic aspiration of intracerebral hematoma - result of a hematoma-lysis method using urokinase. **Appl Neurophysiol** 48: 427-30, 1985.
7. Niizuma H, Shimizu Y, Yonemitsu T, *et al*.: Results of stereotactic aspiration in 175 cases of putaminal hemorrhage. **Neurosurgery** 24: 814-9, 1989.
8. Schaller C, Rohde V, Meyer B, *et al*.: Stereotactic puncture and lysis of spontaneous intracerebral hemorrhage using recombinant tissue-plasminogen activator. **Neurosurgery** 36: 328-35, 1995.
9. Sisti M B, Solomon R A, Stein B M: Stereotactic craniotomy in the resection of small arteriovenous malformations. **J Neurosurg** 75: 40-4, 1991.
10. Moore M R, Black P M, Ellenbogen R, *et al*.: Stereotactic craniotomy: Methods and results using the Brown-Roberts-Wells stereotactic frame. **Neurosurgery** 25: 572-8, 1989.
11. Patil A A: Transoral stereotactic biopsy of the second cervical vertebral body: Case report with technical note. **Neurosurgery** 25: 999-1002, 1989.
12. Kandel E I, Peresedov V V: Stereotaxic clipping of arterial aneurysms and arteriovenous malformations. **J Neurosurg** 46: 12-23, 1977.
13. Backlund E-O, Granberg P-O, Hamberger B, *et al*.: Transplantation of adrenal medullary tissue to striatum in parkinsonism: First clinical trials. **J Neuro-**

surg 62: 169-73, 1985.

14. Blacklock J B, Maxwell R E: Stereotactic removal of a migrating ventricular catheter. **Neurosurgery** 16: 230-1, 1985.

15. Levy R M, Russell E, Yungbluth M, *et al.*: The efficacy of image-guided stereotactis brain biopsy in neurologically symptomatic acquired immunodefi-

ciency syndrome patients. **Neurosurgery** 30: 186-90, 1992.

16. Nicolato A, Gerosa M, Piovan E, *et al.*: Computerized tomography and magnetic resonance guided stereotactic brain biopsy in non-immunocompromised and AIDS patients. **Surg Neurol** 48: 267-77, 1997.

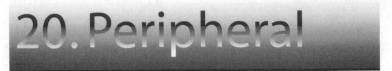
20. Peripheral

The peripheral nervous system (**PNS**) consists of those structures (including cranial nerves III-XII, spinal nerves, nerves of the extremities, and the cervical, brachial and lumbosacral plexi) containing nerve fibers or axons that connect the central nervous system (**CNS**) with motor and sensory, somatic and visceral, end organs[1].

Table 20-1   Muscle strength grading scale*

Grade	Strength	
0	no contraction (total paralysis)	
1	flicker or trace contraction (palpable or visible)	
2	active movement with gravity eliminated	
3	active movement against gravity	4- slight resistance
4	active movement against resistance; subdivisions →	4 moderate resistance
5	normal strength (against full resistance)	4+ strong resistance
NT	not testable	

*   Royal Medical Research Council of Great Britain, modified

Table 20-2   Upper vs. lower motor neuron paralysis

	Upper motor neuron paralysis	Lower motor neuron paralysis
possible etiologies	stroke (motor strip, internal capsule…), spinal cord injury	herniated intervertebral disk, nerve entrapment syndrome, polio
muscle tone	initially flaccid; later spastic with clasp-knife resistance	flaccid
tendon reflexes	hyperactive; clonus may be present	absent
pathologic reflexes (e.g. Babinski, Hoffman)	present (after days to weeks)	absent
muscle manifestations	spontaneous spasms may occur; some atrophy of disuse may occur	fibrillations (need EMG to detect), fasciculations; atrophy after days to weeks as a result of trophic influence

MUSCLE INNERVATION

Table 20-3   Muscle innervation - shoulder & upper extremity *

	Muscle	Action to test	Roots†	Trunk‡	Cord§	Nerve
	deep neck	flex, ext, rotation of neck	C1-4	–	–	cervical
	trapezius	elevates shoulder	XI, C3, 4			(spinal acc + roots)
	diaphragm	inspiration	C3-5			phrenic
•	serratus anterior	forward shoulder thrust	C5-7	–	–	long thoracic
	levator scapulae	elevate scapula	C3, 4, **5**			dorsal scapular
	rhomboids	adduct & elevate scapula	C4, 5			" " "
	supraspinatus	abduct arm (0-90°)	C4, **5**, 6	S		suprascapular
•	infraspinatus	rotate arm out	**C5**, 6	S	–	" " "
	latissimus dorsi	adduct arm	C5, 6, **7**, 8			thoracodorsal
	teres major, subscapularis	" " "	C5-7			subscapular
•	deltoid	abduct arm (> 90°)	**C5**, 6	S	P	axillary
	teres minor	lat arm rotation	C4,5			" "

Table 20-3 Muscle innervation - shoulder & upper extremity (continued)*

Muscle	Action to test	Roots†	Trunk‡	Cord§	Nerve
• biceps brachii	flex & supinate forearm	**C5**, **C6**	S	L	musculocutaneous
coracobrachialis	adduct arm/flex forearm	C5-7			" " "
brachialis	flex forearm	C5, 6			" " "
• flexor carpi ulnaris	ulnar flexion of hand	C7, **8**, T1	M, I	M	ulnar
• flexor digitorum profundus III & IV (ulnar part)	flex distal phalanx of fingers 4-5	C7, **8**, T1	M, I	M	" "
adductor pollicis	thumb adduction	C8, **T1**		M	" "
abductor digiti minimi	abduction little finger	C8, T1		M	" "
opponens digiti minimi	opposition little finger	C7, 8, T1			" "
flexor digiti minimi brevis	flexion little finger	C7, **8**, **T1**		M	" "
• interossei	flex proximal phalanx, extend 2 distal phalanges, abduct or adduct fingers	C8, **T1**	I	M	" "
lumbricals 3 & 4	flex proximal phalanges & extend 2 distal phalanges of fingers 4-5	C7, **8**			" "
• pronator teres	forearm pronation	C6,7	S,M	L	median
• flexor carpi radialis	radial flexion of hand	" "	S,M	L	" "
palmaris longus	hand flexion	C7, 8, T1			" "
• flexor digitorum superficialis	flexion middle phalanx fingers 2-5, flex hand	C7, **8**, T1	M, I	M	" "
• abductor pollicis brevis	abduct thumb metacarpal	C8, **T1**	I	M	" "
flexor pollicis brevis	flex prox phalanx thumb	C8, **T1**			" "
• opponens pollicis	opposes thumb metacarp	C8, **T1**	I	M	" "
lumbricals 1 & 2	flex proximal phalanx & extend 2 distal phalanges fingers 2-3	C8, **T1**			" "
• flexor digitorum profundus I & II (radial part)	flex distal phalanx of fingers 2-3; flex hand	C7, **8**, T1	M, I	M	anterior interosseous
• flexor pollicis longus	flex distal phalanx thumb	C7, **8**, T1			" " "
• triceps brachii	forearm extension	C6, **7**, 8	all	P	radial
• brachioradialis	forearm flexion (with thumb pointed up)	C5, **6**	S	P	" "
• extensor carpi radialis	radial hand extension	C5, **6**	S,M	P	" "
• supinator	forearm supination	C6, 7	S	P	" "
• extensor digitorum	extension of hand & phalanges of fingers 2-5	**C7**, C8	M, I	P	posterior interosseous (PIN)
extensor carpi ulnaris	ulnar hand extension	**C7**, C8			" " "
• abductor pollicis longus	abduction thumb metacarpal & radial hand extens.	**C7**, C8	M, I	P	" " "
extensor pollicis brevis & longus	thumb extension & radial hand extension	**C7**, C8			" " "
extensor indicis proprius	index finger extension & hand extension	**C7**, C8			" " "
pectoralis major: clavicular head	push arm forward against resistance	**C5**, 6			lateral pectoral
pectoralis major: sternocostal head	adduct arm	C6, **7**, 8			lateral & medial pectoral

* NB: items marked with a bullet (•) are clinically important muscle/nerves.
  NB: U.S. finger numbering convention: 1=thumb, 2=index, 3=middle, 4=ring, 5=little.

† Major innervation is indicated in **boldface**. Differing opinions exist, most shown are based on reference².

‡ **Trunk** (trunks of brachial plexus): S = superior, M = middle, I = inferior, all = all three.

§ **Cord** (cords of brachial plexus): P = posterior, L = lateral, M = medial.

THUMB

Flexion/extension occurs in the plane of the palm. Abduction/adduction occur in a plane at right angles to palm.

Opponens (bringing the thumb across the hand) may occasionally be anomalously innervated by the ulnar nerve.

Table 20-4 The 3 innervations of the thumb

Action	Nerve
abduction/flex/opposition	median
adduction	ulnar
extension	radial*

* via the posterior interosseous nerve

Table 20-5 Muscle innervation - hip & lower extremity *

	Muscle	Action	Roots†	Plexus‡	Nerves
•	iliopsoas§	hip flexion	**L1, 2,** 3	L	femoral & L1, 2, 3
	sartorius	hip flex & thigh evert	L2, 3		femoral
•	quadriceps femoris	leg (knee) extension	**L2, 3, 4**	L	" "
	pectineus	thigh adduction	L2, 3		obturator
•	adductor longus	" " "	**L2, 3,** 4	L	"
	adductor brevis	" " "	L2-4		" "
	adductor magnus	" " "	L3, 4		" "
	gracilis	" " "	L2-4		" "
	obturator externus	thigh adduction & lateral rotation	L3, 4		" "
•	gluteus medius/minimus	thigh abduction & medial rotation	**L4, 5,** S1	S	superior gluteal
	tensor fasciae lata	thigh flexion	L4, 5		" " "
	piriformis	lateral thigh rotation	L5, S1		" " "
•	gluteus maximus	thigh abduction (patient prone)	**L5, S1,** 2	S	inferior gluteal
•	obturator internus	lateral thigh rotation	L5, S1	S	muscular branches
	gemelli	" " " "	L4, 5, S1	S	" " "
	quadratus femoris	" " " "	L4, 5, S1	S	" " "
•	biceps femorisΔ	leg flex (& assist thigh extension)	L5, **S1,** 2		sciatic (trunk)
•	semitendinosusΔ	" " " "	L5, **S1,** 2		" " "
•	semimembranosusΔ	" " " "	L5, **S1,** 2		" " "
•	tibialis anterior	foot dorsiflex & supination	L4, 5¶	S	deep peroneal
•	extensor digitorum longus	extension toes 2-5 & foot dorsiflexion	**L5,** S1		" " "
•	extensor hallucis longus (EHL)**	great toe extension & foot dorsiflexion	L5¶, S1	S	" " "
•	extensor digitorum brevis	extension great toe & toes 2-5	**L5,** S1	S	" " "
•	peroneus longus & brevis	P-flex pronated foot & eversion	L5, S1	L/S	superficial peroneal
•	posterior tibialis	P-flex supinated foot & inversion	L4, 5	S	tibial
	flexor digitorum longus	P-flex sup foot, flex terminal phalanx toes 2-5	L5, **S1, 2**		" "
	flexor hallucis longus	P-flex sup foot, flex terminal phalanx great toe	L5, **S1, 2**		" "
	flexor digitorum brevis	flex mid phalanx toes 2-5	S2, 3		" "
	flexor hallucis brevis	flex proximal phalanx great toe	L5, S1, 2		" "
•	gastrocnemius	knee flexion, ankle P-flex	**S1,** 2	S	" "
	plantaris	" " " " "	**S1,** 2		" "
•	soleus	ankle P-flex	**S1,** 2	S	" "
•	abductor hallucis††	(cannot test††)	**S1,** 2	S	
	perineal & sphincters	voluntary contract pelvic floor	S2-4		pudendal

* Abbreviations: P-flex = plantarflexion, D-flex = dorsiflexion, phlnx = phalanx.

† Major innervation is indicated in **boldface** type. E.g. when roots are shown as L4, **5**, this indicates L5 is the main innervation, but both L4 & L5 contribute.

‡ **Plexus**: L = lumbar, S = sacral

§ iliopsoas is the term for the combined iliacus and psoas major muscles

Δ **"hamstrings"**: familiar term for the grouped: semitendinosus and semimembranosus (together, the medial hamstrings) and the biceps femoris (lateral hamstrings)

¶ although many references, including some venerable ones, cite AT as being primarily L4, many clinicians agree that L5 innervation is probably more significant

** EHL is the <u>best</u> L5 muscle to test clinically (although S1 radiculopathy can also weaken this muscle)

†† abductor hallicus <u>cannot</u> be tested clinically, but is important for EMG

20.1. Brachial plexus

Formed by <u>ventral</u> rami (the dorsal rami innervate the paraspinal muscles), most commonly of nerve roots C5-T1. Schematically depicted in *Figure 20-1*.

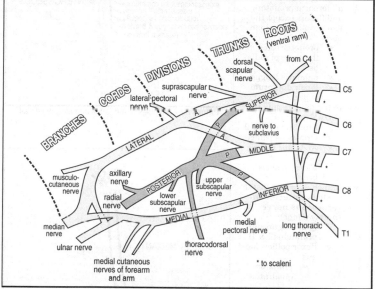

Figure 20-1 Schematic diagram of the brachial plexus
(By Permission: Churchill Livingstone, Edinburgh, 1973,
R. Warwick & P. Williams: Gray's Anatomy 35th Edition © Longman Group UK Limited)

BRACHIAL PLEXUS BRANCHES

Table 20-3 shows action, etc. of specific muscles. Also see *Figure 20-1*. "∕" indicates that the nerve supplies the muscles listed; "➥" denotes a branch of the preceding nerve.

Radial nerve (C5-C8) (see *Figure 20-2*)
Radial nerve (and its branches) innervate of arm and forearm extensors:
- ∕ triceps (all 3 heads)
- ∕ brachioradialis
- ∕ extensor carpi radialis longus & brevis (latter originates ≈ at terminal branch)
- ∕ supinator (originates near the terminal branch)
- ➥ continues into forearm as **posterior interosseous nerve** (C7, C8)

- ✗ extensor carpi ulnaris
- ✗ extensor digitorum
- ✗ extensor digiti minimi
- ✗ extensor pollicis brevis & longus
- ✗ abductor pollicis longus
- ✗ extensor indicus

Axillary nerve (C5, C6)
See *Figure 20-2*.
- ✗ teres minor
- ✗ deltoid

Median nerve (C5-T1)
See *Figure 20-3*.
1. nothing in arm
2. all forearm pronators and flexors except the two supplied by ulnar nerve
   - ✗ pronator teres
   - ✗ flexor carpi radialis
   - ✗ palmaris longus
   - ✗ flexor digitorum superficialis
3. in the hand ⇒ only the "**LOAF** muscles"
   - ✗ **L**umbricals 1 & 2
   - ✗ **O**pponens pollicis
   - ✗ **A**bductor pollicis brevis
   - ✗ **F**lexor pollicis brevis
- ➥ branch at or just distal to elbow **anterior interosseous nerve** (purely <u>motor</u>)
   - ✗ flexor digitorum profundus I & II
   - ✗ flexor pollicis longus
      - ✗ pronator quadratus

Ulnar nerve (C8, T1)
See *Figure 20-3*.
1. nothing in arm
2. only 2 muscles in forearm:
   - ✗ flexor carpi ulnaris
   - ✗ flexor digitorum profundus III & IV
3. all hand muscles excluding "LOAF" muscles (*see above*)
   - ✗ adductor pollicis
   - ✗ flexor pollicis brevis
   - ✗ all dorsal & palmar interossei

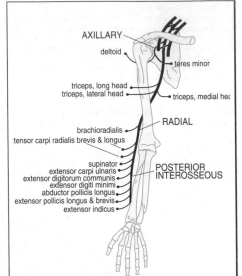

AXILLARY

deltoid

teres minor

triceps, long head
triceps, lateral head

triceps, medial head

brachioradialis

RADIAL

extensor carpi radialis brevis & longus

supinator
extensor carpi ulnaris
extensor digitorum communis
extensor digiti minimi
abductor pollicis longus
extensor pollicis longus & brevis
extensor indicus

POSTERIOR
INTEROSSEOUS

Figure 20-2 Muscles of the radial and axillary nerves

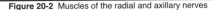

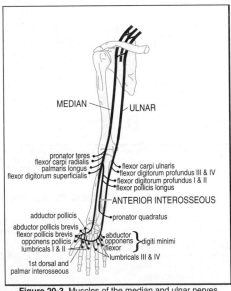

MEDIAN

ULNAR

pronator teres
flexor carpi radialis
palmaris longus
flexor digitorum superficialis

flexor carpi ulnaris
flexor digitorum profundus III & IV
flexor digitorum profundus I & II
flexor pollicis longus

ANTERIOR INTEROSSEOUS

adductor pollicis

pronator quadratus

abductor pollicis brevis
flexor pollicis brevis
opponens pollicis
lumbricals I & II

abductor
opponens
flexor

} digiti minimi

lumbricals III & IV

1st dorsal and
palmar interosseous

Figure 20-3 Muscles of the median and ulnar nerves

    ✗ lumbricals 3 & 4
    ✗ hypothenar muscles (abductor, opponens & flexor digiti minimi)

Musculocutaneous nerve (C5, C6)
Supplies arm flexors
    ✗ coracobrachialis
    ✗ biceps
    ✗ brachialis
    ➥ **lateral cutaneous nerve of the forearm** (terminal branch) supplies cutaneous
        sensation to radial aspect of forearm

Dorsal scapular nerve (C4, C5)
    ✗ rhomboids (major & minor)
    ✗ levator scapulae

Suprascapular nerve (C5, C6)
    ✗ supraspinatus
    ✗ infraspinatus

Subscapular nerve (C5-7)
    ✗ teres major
    ✗ subscapularis

Thoracodorsal nerve (C6, C7, C8)
    ✗ latissimus dorsi

Long thoracic nerve (C5-7)
Originates off of proximal nerve roots
    ✗ serratus anterior (holds scapula to chest wall): lesion → **winging of the scapula**
        (to test: patient leans forward against wall with arms outstretched, scapula sep-
        arates from posterior chest wall if the serratus anterior is not contracting)

20.2.   Peripheral neuropathies

DEFINITIONS

peripheral neuropathy	sometimes the term polyneuropathy is also used; diffuse lesions of peripheral nerves producing weakness, sensory disturbance, and/or reflex changes
mononeuropathy	a disorder of a single nerve, often due to trauma or entrapment
mononeuropathy multiplex	involvement of 2 or more nerves, usually due to a systemic abnormality (e.g. vasculitis, DM...)

A mnemonic for etiologies of peripheral neuropathies is "DANG THE RAPIST" (*see Table 20-6*). Diabetes, alcoholism, and Guillain-Barré (underscored) account for 90% of cases. Other etiologies include: arteritis/vasculitis, monoclonal gammopathy of uncertain significance (MGUS), hepatitis C virus-associated cryoglobulinemia, acute idiopathic polyneuritis, Sjögren's syndrome (disease).

Table 20-6 Mnemonic for etiologies of peripheral neuropathy

Diabetes (*see below*) or **D**rugs (*see page 557*)	**R**enal (uremic neuropathy - *see page 560*) or **R**adiation
Alcoholism (*see below*)	**A**myloid (*see page 560*) or **A**IDS (*see page 558*)
Nutritional (B$_{12}$ deficiency...)	**P**orphyria or **P**sychiatric or **P**araneoplastic (*see below*) or **P**seudoneuropathy (*see below*) or **P**MR (*see page 59*)
Guillain-Barré (*see page 53*)	
Traumatic	**I**nfectious/post-infectious (e.g. Hansen's disease)
Hereditary	**S**arcoidosis (neurosarcoidosis, *see page 56*) or "**S**ystemic"
Endocrine or **E**ntrapment	**T**oxins (including heavy metals, e.g lead toxicity (plumbism), *see page 753*)

Evaluation
Initial (generic) workup for peripheral neuropathies of unknown etiology:
    1. bloodwork: Hgb-A1C, TSH, ESR and vitamin B$_{12}$
    2. EMG

Classification
1. inherited neuropathies
   A. **Charcot-Marie-Tooth (CMT)** (AKA peroneal muscular atrophy, AKA Hereditary Motor and Sensory Neuropathy (**HMSN**)): the most common inherited disorder of peripheral nerves. Several forms, (the most common form is autosomal dominant, but there are also X-linked recessive forms). The most common forms involve demyelination. Progressive loss of motor and sensory function with atrophy in UEs & LEs. Earliest findings: pes cavus with hammer toes, foot drop and frequent ankle sprains. Patients are more susceptible to entrapment neuropathies due to underlying compromise of peripheral nerves
   B. hereditary neuropathy with liability to pressure palsies (**HNPP**): similar to CMT but due to focal areas of irregular thickening of myelin sheaths ("tomaculous" changes), mild trauma or pressure can produce nerve palsies that may last for months
2. acquired neuropathies: see sections below for details
   A. acquired pure <u>sensory</u> neuropathies (in the absence of autonomic dysfunction) are rare. May be seen with pyridoxine therapy or paraneoplastic syndromes (*see below*)
   B. entrapment neuropathies: *see page 563*
3. pseudoneuropathy
   A. **definition**: psychogenic somatoform disorders or malingering, reproducing the pains, paresthesias, hyperalgesia, weakness, and even objective findings such as changes in color and temperature which may mimic neuropathic symptoms[3]

PARANEOPLASTIC SYNDROMES AFFECTING THE NERVOUS SYSTEM

Occurs in < 1% of cancer patients. Peripheral <u>sensory</u> neuropathy of unknown etiology has been associated with cancer since its earliest description[4]. Therefore, in patients with **sensory neuropathy** of unknown etiology, occult neoplasms should be ruled out. If the workup is negative, the patient should be followed since up to 35% of patients will be found to have cancer after a mean interval of 28 months [5].

ALCOHOL NEUROPATHY
Characteristically produces a diffuse sensory neuropathy, with absent achilles reflexes.

BRACHIAL PLEXUS NEUROPATHY[6 (P 918)]
Differential diagnosis of etiologies of brachial plexopathy:
1. tumor: e.g. Pancoast's syndrome (almost always lower plexus lesion)
2. (idiopathic) brachial plexitis: most commonly upper plexus or diffuse (*see below*)
3. viral
4. following radiation treatment: often diffuse (*see below*)
5. diabetes
6. vasculitis
7. inherited: dominant genetics
8. trauma (*see page 561*)

Evaluation: when the etiology is unclear, check CXR (with apical lordotic view), glucose, ESR and ANA. Idiopathic brachial plexitis will usually start to show some improvement by about 4 weeks. Obtain MRI through the plexus if no improvement by ≈ this time.

IDIOPATHIC BRACHIAL PLEXUS NEUROPATHY
AKA (paralytic) **brachial neuritis**, AKA brachial plexitis, AKA neuralgic amyotrophy, AKA Parsonage-Turner syndrome, among others. Idiopathic. Not clearly infectious or inflammatory; allergic mechanism possible. Prognosis is generally good.

In a classic review of 99 cases[7]: male:female = 2.4:1. Antecedent or concurrent upper respiratory tract infection occurred in 25%. May follow vaccination. 34% had bilateral involvement.

Predominant symptom is acute onset of intense pain, with weakness developing simultaneously or after a variable period (70% occur within 2 weeks of pain) usually as the pain lessened. Weakness never preceded pain, onset of weakness was sudden in 80%. Pain was usually constant, and described as "sharp", "stabbing", "throbbing" or "aching". Arm movement exacerbated pain, and muscle soreness was noted in 15%. Pain lasted hours to several weeks. Paresthesias occurred in 35%. Pain usually lacked radicular features. When bilateral, weakness is usually asymmetric.

EMG/NCV may help localize the portion of the plexus involved, and may detect subclinical involvement of the contralateral extremity. Must wait ≥ 3 weeks from onset.

Exam

Weakness or paralysis in 96%, confined to shoulder girdle in 50%. In descending order of involvement: deltoid, spinati, serratus anterior, biceps brachii, and triceps. Winging of the scapula occurred in 20%. Sensory loss occurred in 60% of plexus lesions, of mixed variety (superficial cutaneous and proprioceptive). Sensory loss most common in outer surface of upper arm (circumflex nerve distribution) and radial aspect of forearm. Reflexes were variable.

Overall distribution judged to predominantly involve <u>upper</u> plexus in 56%, diffuse plexus in 38%, and lower in 6%.

Outcome

Functional recovery is better in patients with primarily upper plexus involvement. After 1 year, 60% of upper plexus lesions were functioning normally, whereas none with lower involvement were (latter took 1.5-3 years). Rate of recovery estimated to be 36% within 1 year, 75% within 2, and 89% by 3 years. Recurrence was seen in only 5%. No evidence that steroids altered the course of the disease.

RADIATION NEUROPATHY

Often follows external beam irradiation in the region of the axilla for breast carcinoma. Produces sensory loss with or without weakness. CT or MRI may be needed to rule-out tumor invasion of the brachial plexus.

LUMBOSACRAL PLEXUS NEUROPATHY[8]

Analogous to idiopathic brachial plexitis (*see above*). It is controversial whether this actually exists in isolation without diabetes. Often starts with LE pain of abrupt onset, followed in days or a few weeks by weakness with or without muscle atrophy. Sensory symptoms are less prominent, and usually involve paresthesias. Objective sensory loss is only occasionally seen. There may be tenderness over the femoral nerve.

Differential diagnosis

May be confused with femoral neuropathy or L4 radiculopathy when quadriceps weakness and wasting occurs. Similarly, L5 radiculopathy or peroneal neuropathy may be erroneously suspected when foot drop is seen. Straight leg raising may occasionally be positive. Conspicuously absent are: back pain, exacerbation of pain by Valsalva maneuver or back motion, and significant sensory involvement. For differential diagnosis of foot drop, *see page 909*. For other causes of sciatica, *see page 905*.

Etiologies

Other etiologies are similar to that for brachial plexus neuropathy (*see above*) except that under tumor, a pelvic mass should be considered (check prostate on rectal exam).

Evaluation

Evaluation is as for brachial plexus neuropathy (*see above*), except that instead of a brachial plexus MRI, a lumbar MRI and pelvic CT should be done to rule out masses.

EMG is key to diagnosis: evidence of patchy denervation (fibrillation potentials, and motor unit potentials that are either decreased in number or increased in amplitude or duration and polyphasic) involving at least 2 segmental levels with <u>sparing</u> of the paraspinal muscles is highly diagnostic (once diabetes, etc. have been ruled-out).

Recovery from pain precedes return of strength. Improvement is generally monophasic, slow (years), and incomplete.

DIABETIC NEUROPATHY

≈ 50% of patients with DM develop neuropathic symptoms or show slowing of nerve conduction velocities on electrodiagnostic testing. Diabetic neuropathy is reduced by tight control of blood glucose[9]. Disagreement exists over the number of distinct clinical syndromes; there is probably a continuum[10] and they likely occur in various combina-

tions. Some of the more readily identified syndromes include:
1. **primary sensory polyneuropathy**: symmetric, affecting feet and legs more than hands. Chronic, slowly-progressive. Often with accelerated loss of distal vibratory sense (normal loss with aging is ≈ 1% per year after age 40). Presents as pain, paresthesias, and dysesthesias. Soles of feet may be tender to pressure
2. autonomic neuropathy: involving bladder, bowel, and circulatory reflexes (resulting in orthostatic hypotension). May produce impotence, impaired micturition, diarrhea, constipation, impaired pupillary light response
3. **diabetic plexus neuropathy**[11] or proximal neuropathy: possibly secondary to vascular injury to nerves (similar to a diabetic mononeuritis):
   A. one that occurs in patients > 50 years old with mild diabetes type II that is often confused with femoral neuropathy. Causes severe pain in the hip, anterior thigh, knee, and sometimes medial calf. Weakness of the quadriceps, iliopsoas, and occasionally thigh adductors. Loss of knee jerk. Possible sensory loss over medial thigh and lower leg. Pain usually improves in weeks, the weakness in months

   ★ B. **diabetic amyotrophy**: occurs in similar patient population often with recently diagnosed DM. Alternative names include[12]: **Bruns-Garland syndrome**, ischemic mononeuropathy multiplex…[13]. Abrupt onset of asymmetric pain (usually deep aching/burning with superimposed lancinating paroxysms, most severe at night) in back, hip, buttocks, thigh, or leg. Progressive weakness in proximal or proximal and distal muscles, often preceded by weight loss. Patellar reflexes are absent or reduced. Sensory loss is minimal. Proximal muscles (especially thigh) may atrophy. EMG findings consistent with demyelination invariably accompanied by axonal degeneration, with involvement of paraspinals and no evidence of myopathy. Symptoms may progress steadily or stepwise for weeks or even up to 18 months, and then gradually resolve. Opposite extremity may become involved during the course or may occur months or years later. Sural nerve biopsy may suggest demyelination
   C. diabetic proximal neuropathy (**DPN**): fairly similar findings to diabetic amyotrophy except for subacute onset of symmetric LE involvement that usually start with weakness may be a variant[14]. *Table 20-7* (adapted[14]) compares DPN to diabetic amyotrophy and chronic inflammatory demyelinating polyradiculoneuropathy (**CIDP**)

Table 20-7 Comparison of diabetic amyotrophy, diabetic proximal neuropathy (DPN), and CIDP

Description	Diabetic amyotrophy	DPN	CIDP
Onset	acute	subacute	gradual
Initial symptoms	asymmetric pain→ weakness	symmetric weakness	symmetric weakness
UE weakness	no	uncommon	yes
Sensory loss	minimal	minimal	moderate
Areflexia	LE	LE	generalized
CSF protein	variable	increased	increased
Axonal pathologic changes	common	typical	uncommon
Conduction slowing	patchy	patchy	diffuse
Prognosis	good	good	poor without treatment
Response to immunotherapy	unknown	possible	yes
Course	monophasic	monophasic	progressive

TREATMENT

Treatment of the Bruns-Garland syndrome is primarily expectant, although immunotherapy (steroids, immune globulin, or plasma exchange) may be considered in severe or progressive cases (efficacy is unproven)[14].

For sensory polyneuropathy, good control of blood sugar contributes to reduction of symptoms. Adjunctive agents that have been used include:
1. **mexiletine** (Mexitil®): start at 150 mg q 8 hrs, and titrate to symptoms to a maximum of 10 mg/kg/d
2. **amitriptyline** (Elavil®) and fluphenazine (Prolixin®): start with 25 mg amitriptyline PO q hs and 1 mg fluphenazine PO TID; and work up to 75 mg amitriptyline PO q hs[15] (≈ 100 mg qd amitriptyline alone may also be effective[16]).
   Usefulness has been challenged[17], but many studies do show benefit[16, 18]. SIDE EF-

FECTS: that may limit use include sedation, confusion, fatigue, malaise, hypomania, rash, urinary retention, and orthostatic hypotension

3. **desipramine** (Norpramin®): more selective blocker of norepinephrine reuptake (which seems more effective for this condition than serotonin reuptake blockers). Effectiveness at mean doses of 110 mg/day ≈ same as amitriptyline and therefore may be useful for patients unable to tolerate amitriptyline[16]. SIDE EFFECTS: include insomnia (may be minimized by AM dosing), orthostatic hypotension, rash, bundle branch block, tremor, pyrexia. Available in 10, 25, 50, 75, 100 & 150 mg tablets

4. **capsaicin** (Zostrix®): effective in some (see *Capsaicin*, on page 389)

5. **paroxetine** (Paxil®): a selective serotonin reuptake inhibitor **(SSRI)** antidepressant. *Rx*: 20 mg PO q AM. If necessary, increase by 10 mg/d q week up to a maximum of 50 mg/day (except in elderly, debilitated, or renal or hepatic failure where maximum is 40 mg/day). Available in 20 mg (scored) & 30 mg tablets

6. **gabapentin** (Neurontin®) doses of 1800-3600 mg/d produces at least moderate pain relief from painful diabetic neuropathy in 60% of patients[19] and was ≈ as efficacious as amitriptyline[20]

DRUG INDUCED NEUROPATHY

Many drugs have been implicated as possible causes of peripheral neuropathy. Those that are better established or more notorious include:

1. thalidomide: neuropathy may occur with chronic use, and may be irreversible[21]
2. metronidazole (Flagyl®)
3. phenytoin (Dilantin®)
4. amitriptyline (Elavil®)
5. dapsone: a rare complication reported with use in nonleprosy patients is a reversible peripheral neuropathy that may be due to axonal degeneration, producing a Guillain-Barré-like syndrome (*see page 53* for Guillain-Barré syndrome)
6. nitrofurantoin (Macrodantin®): may additionally cause optic neuritis
7. cholesterol lowering drugs: e.g. lovastatin (Mevacor®), indapamide (Lozol®), gemfibrozil (Lopid®)
8. thallium: may produce tremors, leg pains, paresthesias in the hands and feet, polyneuritis in the LE, psychosis, delerium, seizures, encephalopathy
9. arsenic: may produce numbness, burning and tingling of the extremities
10. chemotherapy: cisplatin, vincristine…

FEMORAL NEUROPATHY

Manifests as:
1. motor deficits:
   A. wasting and weakness of the quadriceps femoris (knee extension)
   B. weakness of iliopsoas (hip flexion): if present, indicates very proximal pathology (lumbar root or plexus lesion) as the branches to the iliopsoas arise just distal to the neural foramina
2. diminution of the patellar (knee jerk) reflex
3. sensory findings:
   A. sensory loss over the anterior thigh and medial calf
   B. pain in same distribution may occur
4. mechanical signs: positive femoral stretch test (*see page 303*)

Differential diagnosis:
1. L4 radiculopathy: L4 radiculopathy should not cause iliopsoas weakness (see *L4 involvement*, page 907)
2. diabetic plexus neuropathy (see *Diabetic neuropathy* above)
3. (idiopathic) lumbosacral plexus neuropathy (*see above*)

Etiologies:
1. diabetes: the most frequent cause
2. femoral nerve entrapment: rare
   A. may occur secondary to inguinal hernia or may be injured by deep sutures placed during herniorrhaphy
   B. secondary to prolonged pelvic surgery from retractor compression (usually bilateral)
3. intraabdominal tumor

4. femoral arterial catheterization: see *Neuropathy after cardiac catheterization* below
5. retroperitoneal hematoma (e.g. in hemophiliac or on anticoagulants)
6. during surgery (*see page 559*)

AIDS NEUROPATHY

3.3% of patients with AIDS will develop peripheral nerve disorders[22] (whereas none who were just HIV positive developed neuropathy). The most common disorder is distal symmetric polyneuropathy (**DSP**), usually consisting of vague numbness and tingling, and sometimes painful feet (although it may also be painless). There may be subtle reduction of light tough and vibratory sense. Other neuropathies include mononeuropathies (usually meralgia paresthetica, *see page 573*), mononeuropathy multiplex, or lumbar polyradiculopathy. Drugs used to treat HIV can also cause neuropathies (*see below*).

The DSP in AIDS patients is often associated with CMV infection, *Mycobacterium avium intracellulare* infection, or may be due to lymphomatous invasion of the nerve or lymphomatous meningitis. May demonstrate a mixed axonal demyelinating type of neuropathy on electrodiagnostic testing.

Neuropathies associated with drugs used to treat HIV:
1. nucleoside reverse transcriptase inhibitors
   A. zidovudine (Retrovir®) (formerly AZT)
   B. didanosine (ddI; Videx®): can cause a painful dose-related neuropathy[23]
   C. stavudine (d4T; Zerit®): can cause sensory neuropathy which usually improves when d4T is discontinued, and may not recur if restarted at lower dose[23]
   D. zalcitabine (ddC; Hivid®): dose-related neuropathy can be severe and persistent. More common in patients with DM or didanosine treatment[23]
2. protease inhibitors
   A. ritonavir (Norvir®): can cause peripheral paresthesias
   B. amprenavir (Agenerase®): can cause perioral paresthesias

PERIOPERATIVE NEUROPATHIES

Also, see *Neuropathy after cardiac catheterization* below. Most often involves ulnar nerve or brachial plexus. In many cases, a nerve that is abnormal but asymptomatic may become symptomatic as a result of any of the following factors: stretch or compression of the nerve, generalized ischemia or metabolic derangement. The injury may be permanent or temporary. Occurs almost exclusively in adults[24].

1. **ulnar neuropathy**: controversial. Often blamed on external nerve compression or stretch as a result of malpositioning. Although this may be true in some cases, in one series this was a factor in only ≈ 17%[25]. Patient-related characteristics are shown in *Table 20-8*[26]. Many of these patients have abnormal contralateral nerve conduction, suggesting a possible predisposing condition[27]. Many patients do not complain of symptoms until > 48 hours post-op[26-28]. Risk may be reduced by padding the arm at, and especially distal to, the elbow, and avoiding flexion of the elbow (avoid > 110° flexion which tightens the cubital tunnel retinaculum) and by reducing the amount of time convalescing in the recumbent position[28]

   Table 20-8 Patient-related characteristics in anesthesia-related ulnar neuropathy

male gender
obesity (body mass index ≥ 38)
prolonged post-op bed rest

2. **brachial plexus neuropathy**: may be mistaken for ulnar neuropathy. Does not appear to be related to arm position or padding. May be associated with:
   A. median sternotomy (most common with internal mammary dissection). Posterior sternal retraction displaces the upper ribs and may stretch or compress the C6 through T1 roots (major contributors to the ulnar nerve)
   B. head-down positions where the patient is stabilized with a shoulder brace. The brace should be placed over the acromioclavicular joint(s), and non-slip mattresses and flexion of the knees may be used as adjuncts[24]
   C. prone position (rare): especially with shoulder abduction and elbow flexion with contralateral head rotation[24]

3. **median neuropathy**: perioperative median nerve injury may result from stretch of the nerve. Seems to occur primarily in middle-aged muscular males. Padding should be placed under the forearms and hands to maintain mild elbow flexion[24]

4. lower extremity neuropathies: most occur in patients undergoing procedures in the lithotomy position[24]. Frequency of involvement in a large series of patients undergoing procedures in the lithotomy position[29]: common peroneal 81%, sciatic 15%, and femoral 4%. Risk factors other than position: prolonged duration of procedure, extremely thin body habitus, and cigarette smoking in the preoperative period

    A. common peroneal neuropathy: susceptible to injury in the posterior popliteal fossa where it wraps around the fibular head. May be compressed by leg holders, which should be padded in this area

    B. femoral neuropathy: compression of the nerve by self-retaining abdominal wall retractor or rendering the nerve ischemic by occlusion of the external iliac artery[24]. Hemorrhage into the iliopsoas muscle may also compress the nerve. Cutaneous branches of the femoral nerve may be injured during labor and/or delivery[30] (most are transient)

    C. sciatic neuropathy: stretch injuries may occur with hyperflexion of the hip and extension of the knee as may occur in the lithotomy position

    D. meralgia paresthetica[81]: tends to occur bilaterally in young, slender males positioned prone, with operations lasting 6-10+ hours. Onset: 1-8 days postop. Spontaneous recovery typically occurs over an average of 5.8 months

Management

Once a neuropathy is detected, determine if it is sensory, motor, or both. Pure sensory neuropathies are more often temporary than motor[26], and expectant management for ≈ 5 days is suggested (have the patient avoid postures or activities that may further injure the nerve). Neurologic consultation should be requested (usually to include EMG evaluation) for all motor neuropathies and for sensory neuropathies persisting > 5 days[24].

OTHER NEUROPATHIES

Neuropathy after cardiac catheterization

In a series of ≈ 10,000 patients followed after femoral artery catheterization[31] (e.g. for coronary angiography or angioplasty), neuropathy occurred in 0.2% (with an estimated range in the literature up to ≈ 3%). Risk factors identified include: patients developing retroperitoneal hematomas or pseudoaneurysms after the procedure, procedures requiring larger introducer sheaths (e.g. angioplasty & stent placement > diagnostic catheterization), excessive anticoagulation (PTT > 90 for at least 12 hours).

Two groups of patients were identified and are shown in *Table 20-9*.

Excruciating pain after the catheterization procedure often preceded the development or recognition of neuropathy.

Treatment:

After considering available information, the recommendation is to repair pseudoaneurysms surgically, but to treat the neuropathy conservatively. A case could <u>not</u> be made that surgical drainage of hematoma reduced the risk of neuropathy. Weakness from femoral or obturator neuropathy was treated with inpatient rehabilitation.

Table 20-9 Neuropathy after cardiac catheterization (N = 9585)[31]

Catheterization complication	Neurologic complication
Group I (4 patients)	
groin hematoma or pseudoaneurysm	sensory neuropathy in all 4 cases • in distribution of medial & intermediate femoral cutaneous nerves → isolated sensory neuropathy (dysesthesia & sensory loss) of the anterior and medial thigh • no motor deficit
Group II (16 patients)	
large retroperitoneal hematoma	femoral neuropathy • sensory in all 16 cases: dysesthesia of the anterior/medial thigh & medial calf • motor in 13 cases: iliopsoas & quadriceps weakness
	obturator neuropathy in 4 cases • sensory: upper medial thigh • motor: obturator weakness
	lateral femoral cutaneous nerve → meralgia paresthetica

Outcome:
    Group I patients all had resolution in < 5 mos. In group II, 50% had complete resolution in 2 mos. 6 patients had persistent symptoms, 5 had mild femoral <u>sensory</u> neuropathy (1 of whom felt it was at least somewhat disabling), 1 had mild persistent quadriceps weakness and occasionally walks with a cane.

Amyloid neuropathy
    Amyloid is an insoluble extracellular protein aggregate that can be deposited in peripheral nerves. Amyloidosis occurs in a number of conditions, e.g. in ≈ 15% of patients with <u>multiple myeloma</u> (also, *see page 514*). The neuropathy predominantly produces a progressive autonomic neuropathy and symmetric dissociated sensory loss (reduced pain and temperature, preserved vibratory sense). There is usually less prominent motor involvement. May predispose to pressure injury of nerves (especially carpal tunnel syndrome, *see page 567* for laboratory tests).

Uremic neuropathy
    Occurs in chronic renal failure. Early symptoms include calf cramps ("Charlie horses"), dysesthetic pain in feet (similar to painful diabetic neuropathy) and "restless legs". Achilles reflexes are lost. A stocking sensory loss is followed later by LE weakness that starts distally and ascends. The offending toxin is not known. Dialysis or renal transplantation relieves the symptoms.

PERIPHERAL NERVE INJURIES

ANATOMY OF PERIPHERAL NERVES *(see Figure 20-4)*
    Endoneurium surrounds myelinated and unmyelinated axons. These bundles are gathered into **fascicles** surrounded by **perineurium**. The **epineurium** encases the nerve trunk, containing fascicles separated by interfascicular epineurium or **mesoneurium**.

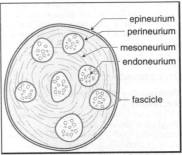

Figure 20-4 Anatomy of a peripheral nerve

NERVE REGENERATION
    Peripheral nerves regenerate ≈ 1 mm/day (about 1 inch/month). Divide this figure into distance that the nerve has to traverse (from knowledge of anatomy) for guide as to how long to wait before considering failure of therapy (either operative or non-operative). However, this rule may not be applicable to long distances (> ≈ 12 inches) and there may be fibrosis of the muscle beyond salvage.

PERIPHERAL NERVE INJURY CLASSIFICATION *(see Table 20-10)*

Table 20-10   Classification of peripheral nerve injury*

Seddon system	Sunderland system
Neuropraxia	**First-degree**
Features common to both systems Physiologic transection (nerve in continuity). Basement membrane intact. Compression or ischemia → local conduction block (impaired axonal transport). ★ <u>No</u> wallerian degeneration†. Motor involvement is typically > sensory. Autonomic function is preserved	
Recovers in hours to months; average is 6-8 weeks	Focal demyelination may occur. Recovery is usually complete in 2-3 weeks (not the "1 mm/day rule")
Axonotmesis	**Second-degree**
Features common to both systems Complete interruption of axons and myelin sheaths. Supporting structures (including endoneurium) intact. ★ Wallerian degeneration† occurs	
	Recovers at 1 mm/day as axon follows "tubule". Sometimes may only be diagnosed retrospectively. Recovery is poor in lesions requiring > 18 months to reach target muscle

Table 20-10   Classification of peripheral nerve injury* (continued)

Seddon system	Sunderland system
	Third-degree
	Endoneurium disrupted, epineurium & perineurium intact. Nerve may not appear seriously damaged on gross inspection. Recovery may range from poor to complete and depends on degree of intrafascicular fibrosis
	Fourth-degree
	Interruption of all neural & supporting elements. Epineurium intact. Grossly: nerve is usually indurated & enlarged
Neurotmesis	**Fifth-degree**
Nerve completely severed or disorganized by scar tissue. Spontaneous regeneration impossible	Complete transection with loss of continuity
	Sixth-degree‡
	Mixed lesion. Combination of elements of first through fourth degree. There may be some preserved sensory fascicles (may produce a positive Tinel's sign)

* there are numerous classification systems. This table shows and compares approximate equivalence of the Seddon classification (an older 3-tiered system) and the Sunderland systems (which has 5 tiers, essentially dividing neurotmesis into 3 subgroups, others have added a 6th category as shown)

† **wallerian degeneration** AKA orthograde degeneration, AKA secondary degeneration: degeneration of the axon <u>distal</u> to a focal lesion

‡ not part of original Sunderland system

BRACHIAL PLEXUS INJURIES
Etiologies include:
1. penetrating trauma
2. traction (stretch injuries): more likely to affect the posterior and lateral cords than the medial cord and median nerve
3. first rib fractures
4. compression by hematoma

Initial exam seeks to differentiate preganglionic injuries (proximal to dorsal root ganglion) which cannot be repaired surgically, from postganglionic injuries. Clues to a **preganglionic injury** include:
1. Horner's syndrome: pre-ganglionic injury interrupts white rami communicantes
2. paralysis of serratus anterior (long thoracic nerve): produces winging of scapula
3. paralysis of rhomboids (dorsal scapular nerve)
4. early neuropathic pain suggests nerve root avulsion
5. EMG: requires ≥ 3 weeks from injury for some findings. Look for:
   A. denervation potentials in paraspinal muscles due to loss of neural input. The posterior ramus of the spinal nerve originates just distal to the dorsal root ganglion. Due to overlap, cannot localize to a specific segment
   B. normal sensory nerve action potential (**SNAP**): preganglionic injuries leave the dorsal ganglion sensory cell body and the distal axon intact, so that normal SNAP can be recorded proximally even in an anesthetic region
6. meningocele on myelography or MRI (suggests, but does not prove, that lesions at adjacent levels are also probably very proximal)

(Duchene)-Erb's palsy
Upper brachial plexus injury (C5 & 6, some authors include C7) e.g. from forceful separation of humeral head from shoulder, commonly due to difficult parturition (*see below*) or motorcycle accident. Paralysis of deltoid, biceps, rhomboids, brachioradialis, supra- & infra-spinatus, and occasionally supinator.

Motor: arm hangs at side internally rotated & extended at elbow ("**Bellhop's tip position**"). Hand motion is unaffected.

Klumpke's palsy
Injury to lower brachial plexus (C8 & T1, some authors include C7), from traction of abducted arm e.g. in catching oneself during a fall from a height, or by Pancoast's syndrome (lung apex tumor - check CXR with apical lordotic view). Characteristic claw deformity (also seen with ulnar nerve injury) with weakness and wasting of small hand

muscles. Possible Horner's syndrome if T1 involved.

Perinatal brachial plexus palsy (PBPP)

Incidence is 0.3-2.0 per 1000 live births (0.1% in infants with birthweight < 4000 gm[32]). Rarely, a congenital case may be mistaken for so-called "obstetrical" palsy[33].

Classification of PBPP injuries: Upper plexus injuries are most common, with about half having C5 & C6 injuries, and 25% involving C7 also[34]. Combined upper and lower lesions occur in ≈ 20%. Pure lower lesions (C7-T1) are rare, constituting only ≈ 2%. Lesions are bilateral in ≈ 4%. A 4-level scale of intensity is shown in *Table 20-11*[35].

Risk factors:
1. high birth weight
2. primiparous mother
3. shoulder dystocia
4. forceps[36] or vacuum assisted delivery
5. breech presentation[37]
6. prolonged labor
7. previous birth complicated by PBPP

One mechanism is lowering of the shoulder with opposite inclination of the cervical spine[33].

Table 20-11   Perinatal brachial plexs injury

Group	Lesion	Manifestation	Spontaneous recovery rate
1	C6 or C6 roots or superior trunk	paralyisis of shoulder abduction, elbow flexsion & forearm supination. Finger flexion is norma	90%
2	above + involvement of C7 or medial trunk	above + paralysis of of finger extensors (but not flexors)	65%
3	above + finger flexors	essentially no hand movement. No Horner's syndrome	≈ < 50%
4	complete brachial plexus	flail arm + Horner's syndrome	0%
	"dominant C7" paralysis variant	selective loss of shoulder abduction & elbow extension	

Management of PBPP: Unless a Group 4 injury is clearly present at birth, conservative treatment is suggested. If there is no spontaneous recovery by 3 months, the electrophysiological evaluation should be performed, and if nerve root avulsion is confirmed, surgical treatment should be considered[38].

Surgery is not favored in the presence of signs of preganglionic injury (*see above*). When EMG shows signs of reinnervation, some also recommend continued expectant management.

MANAGEMENT OF BRACHIAL PLEXUS INJURIES

1. most injuries show maximal deficit at onset. Progressive deficit is usually due to vascular injuries (pseudoaneurysm, A-V fistula, or expansile clot), these should be explored immediately
2. clean, sharp, relatively fresh lacerating injuries (usually iatrogenic, scalpel induced) should be explored acutely and repaired with tension-free end-to-end anastamoses within 72 hrs
3. penetrating injuries with severe or complete deficit should be explored as soon as the primary wound heals
4. gunshot wounds (GSW) to the brachial plexus rarely divide nerves. Deficit is usually due to axonotmesis or neurotmesis (*see below*). Nerves showing partial function usually recover spontaneously; those with complete dysfunction rarely do so. Surgery is of little benefit for discrete injuries to the lower trunk, medial cord, or C8/T1 roots. Most are managed conservatively for 2-5 months. Indications for surgery are shown in *Table 20-12*

Table 20-12   Indications for neurosurgical intervention in GSW to the brachial plexus[39]

1. complete loss in the distribution of at least one element
   A. no improvement clinically or on EMG in 2-5 months
   B. deficit in distribution that is responsive to surgery (e.g. C5, C6, C7, upper or middle trunk, lateral or posterior cords or their outflows)
   C. injuries with loss only in lower elements are not operated
2. incomplete loss with failure to control pain medically
3. pseudoaneurysm, clot or fistula involving plexus
4. true causalgia requiring sympathectomy

5. traction injuries: incomplete postganglionic injuries tend to improve spontaneously. Injuries in adults without satisfactory recovery at 3-4 months are explored
6. neuromas in continuity: those that conduct a SNAP are managed by neurolysis. Those that do not conduct a SNAP have complete internal disruption and require resection and grafting

20.2.1. Missile injuries of peripheral nerves

Most injuries from a single bullet are due to shock and cavitation from the missile causing axonotmesis or neurotmesis, and are not from direct nerve transection. Approximately 70% will recover with expectant management.

However, if there is a lack of improvement on serial examinations including electrodiagnostic studies, intervention should be undertaken by about 5-6 months to avoid further difficulties due to nerve fibrosis and muscle atrophy.

See *Table 20-12* for indications for surgery for missile injuries of the brachial plexus.

20.2.2. Entrapment neuropathies

Entrapment neuropathy is a peripheral nerve injury resulting from compression either by external forces or from nearby anatomic structures. Mechanism can vary from one or two significant compressive insults to many localized, repetitive mild compressions of a nerve. Certain nerves are particularly vulnerable at specific locations by virtue of being superficial, fixed in position, traversing a confined space, or in proximity to a joint. The most common symptom is pain (frequently at rest, more severe at night, often with retrograde radiation causing more proximal lesion to be suspected) with tenderness at the point of entrapment. May be associated with:
1. diabetes mellitus
2. hypothyroidism: due to glycogen deposition in Schwann cells
3. acromegaly
4. amyloidosis: primary or secondary (as in multiple myeloma)
5. carcinomatosis
6. polymyalgia rheumatica: *see page 61*
7. rheumatoid arthritis: 45% incidence of 1 or more entrapment neuropathies
8. gout

Mechanism of injury

Brief compression primarily affects myelinated fibers, and classically spares unmyelinated fibers (except in cases of *severe* acute compression). Acute compression compromises axoplasmic flow which can reduce membrane excitability. Chronic compression affects both myelinated and unmyelinated fibers and can produce segmental demyelination in the former, and if the insult persists, axolysis and wallerian degeneration will occur in both types. The issue of ischemia is more controversial[40]. Some contend that simultaneous venous stasis at the site of compression can produce ischemia which can lead to edema outside the axonal sheath which may further exacerbate the ischemia. Eventually, fibrosis, neuroma formation, and progressive neuropathy can occur.

OCCIPITAL NERVE ENTRAPMENT

Greater occipital nerve (nerve of Harnold) is a sensory branch of C2 (see *Figure 16-1*, page 378 for cutaneous distribution). Entrapment presents as **occipital neuralgia**: pain in occiput usually with a trigger point near the superior nuchal line. Pressure here reproduces pain radiating up along back of head towards vertex.

More common in women.

Differential diagnosis:
1. headache
   A. may be mimicked by migraine headache
   B. may be part of muscle contraction (tension) headache
2. myofascial pain[41]: the pain may be separated from the trigger point
3. vertebrobasilar disease including aneurysm and SAH
4. cervical spondylosis
5. pain from Chiari I malformation (*see page 104*)

Possible causes of entrapment:
1. trauma
   A. direct trauma (including iatrogenic placement of suture through the nerve during surgical procedures, e.g. in closing a posterior fossa craniectomy)
   B. following traumatic cervical extension[42] which may crush the C2 root and ganglion between the C1 arch and C2 lamina
   C. fractures of the upper cervical spine (*see page 725* and *page 725*)
2. atlanto-axial subluxation (**AAS**) (e.g. in rheumatoid arthritis) or arthrosis
3. entrapment by hypertrophic C1-2 (epistrophic) ligament[43]
4. neuromas
5. arthritis of the C2-3 zygapophyseal joint

TREATMENT

> Σ Available evidence is from small, retrospective, case series studies and is insufficient to conclude that either local injection or surgery are effective. Nerve blocks with steroids and local anesthetics provide only temporary relief. Surgical procedures such as nerve root decompression or neurectomy may provide effective pain relief for some patients; however, patient-selection criteria for these procedures have not been defined, and recurrence is common.

When there is no neurologic deficit, the condition is usually self limited.

Non surgical treatment
1. greater occipital nerve block with local anesthetic and steroids
   A. may provide relief typically lasting ≈ 1 month[44] (*see below*)
   B. is no longer considered diagnostic because it is not sufficiently specific
2. physical therapy: massage and daily stretching exercises
3. TENS unit: provided ≥ 50% relief in 13 patients for up to 5 yrs[45]
4. oral antiinflammatory agents
5. centrally acting pain medications: Neurontin, Paxil, Elavil...
6. botulinum toxin injection[46]: although this study had quite a few placebo responders

If these measures do not provide permanent relief in <u>disabling</u> cases, surgical treatment may be considered, although caution is advised by many due to poor results[41, 47]. Alcohol neurolysis may be tried. A collar is <u>not</u> indicated as it may irritate the condition.

Surgical treatment options:
1. peripheral occipital nerve procedures: these may not be effective for proximal compression of the C2 root or ganglion:
   A. occipital neurectomy
      1. peripheral avulsion of the nerve
      2. avulsion of the greater occipital nerve as it exits between the transverse process of C2 and the inferior oblique muscle
   B. alcohol injection of greater occipital nerve
2. release of the nerve within the trapezius muscle. Immediate results: relief in 46%, improvement in 36%. Only 56% reported improvement at 14.5 mos[48]
3. decompression of C2 nerve root if compressed between C1 and C2[43]
4. intradural division of the C2 dorsal route via a posterior intradural approach
5. in cases of AAS, atlanto-axial fusion (*see page 623*) may relieve the pain
6. ganglionectomy

Occipital nerve block
Inject trigger point(s) if one or more can be identified (there is usually a trigger point near the superior nuchal line). The nerve may also be blocked at the point where it emerges from the dorsal neck muscles.

If the pathology is more proximal (e.g. at C2 spinal ganglion), then block of the ganglion may be required. Technique[49] (done under fluoroscopy): shave hair below the mastoid process; prep with iodine; infiltrate with local; insert a 20 gauge spinal needle midway between C1 and C2, halfway between the midline and the lateral margin of the dorsal neck muscles. Aim rostrally, the final target is the midpoint of the C1-2 joint on AP fluoro, and almost but not touching the inferior articular process of C1. Infiltrate 1-3 ml of anesthetic and check for analgesia in the C2 distribution.

Occipital neurectomy
The occipital nerve usually pierces the cervical muscles ≈ 2.5 cm lateral to the midline, just below the inion. Palpation or doppler localization of the pulse of the accompa-

nying greater occipital artery sometimes helps to locate the nerve. However, relief only occurs in ≈ 50%, and recurrence, usually within a year, is common.

MEDIAN NERVE ENTRAPMENT

Two most common sites of entrapment of the median nerve:
- at the wrist by transverse carpal ligament: carpal tunnel syndrome (*see below*)
- in upper forearm by pronator teres: pronator teres syndrome (*see page 566*)

ANATOMY

The median nerve has contributions from C5 through T1. In the upper forearm it passes between the two heads of the pronator teres and supplies this muscle. Just beyond this point, it branches to form the purely motor anterior interosseous nerve which supplies all but 2 muscles of finger and wrist flexion. It descends adherent to deep surface of flexor digitorum superficialis (**FDS**), lying on the flexor digitorum profundus. Near the wrist, it emerges from the lateral edge of FDS becoming more superficial, lying medial to the tendon of flexor carpi radialis, just lateral to and partially under the cover of the palmaris longus tendon. It passes under the transverse carpal ligament (**TCL**) through the **carpal tunnel** which also contains the tendons of the flexor digitorum profundus and superficialis deep to the nerve. The motor branch arises deep to the TCL, but may anomalously pierce the TCL. It supplies the "LOAF muscles" (**L**umbricals 1 & 2, **O**pponens pollicis, and **A**bductor and **F**lexor pollicis brevis).

The TCL attaches medially to pisiform and hook of hamate, laterally to trapezium and tubercles of scaphoid. TCL is continuous proximally with fascia over FDS and antebrachial fascia, distally with the flexor retinaculum. The TCL extends distally into the palm to ≈ 3 cm beyond the distal wrist crease. The palmaris longus tendon, which is absent in 10% of population, partially attaches to the TCL.

Palmar cutaneous branch (PCB) of median nerve, arises from radial aspect of median nerve approximately 5.5 cm proximal to styloid process of radius, underneath the cover of FDS of the middle finger. It crosses wrist above the TCL to provide sensory innervation to the base of the thenar eminence.

The sensory distribution of the average median nerve is shown in *Figure 20-5*.

CARPAL TUNNEL SYNDROME

Carpal tunnel syndrome (**CTS**) is the most common entrapment neuropathy in the upper extremity. The median nerve is compressed within its course through the carpal tunnel just distal to the wrist crease.

Usually occurs in middle aged patients. Ratio of female:male = 4:1. It is bilateral in over 50% of cases, but is usually worse in the dominant hand.

COMMON ETIOLOGIES[50]

In most cases, no specific etiology can be identified. CTS is very common in the geriatric population. The following etiologies tend to be more common in younger patients:
A. "classic" CTS: chronic time course, usually over a period of months to years
   1. trauma: often job-related (may also be associated with avocations)
      A. repetitive movements of hand or wrist
      B. repeated forceful grasping or pinching of tools or other objects
      C. awkward positions of hand and/or wrist, including wrist extension, ulnar deviation, or especially forced wrist flexion

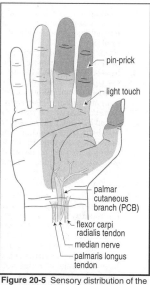

Figure 20-5 Sensory distribution of the median nerve

D. direct pressure over carpal tunnel

E. use of vibrating hand tools

2. systemic conditions: in addition to systemic causes listed for entrapment neuropathies on page 563 (especially rheumatoid arthritis, diabetes), also consider:

A. obesity

B. local trauma

C. may transiently appear during pregnancy

D. mucopolysaccharidosis V

E. tuberculous tenosynovitis

3. patients with A-V dialysis shunts in the forearm have an increased incidence of CTS, possibly on an ischemic basis or possibly from the underlying renal disorder

B. "acute" CTS: an uncommon condition where the symptoms of CTS appear suddenly and severely, usually following some type of exertion or trauma. Etiologies:

1. median artery thrombosis: a persistent median artery is present in < 10% of the population

2. hemorrhage or hematoma in the transverse carpal ligament

SIGNS AND SYMPTOMS

The physical exam for CTS is fairly insensitive.

Signs and symptoms may include:

1. dysesthesias:

A. characteristically patients are awakened at night by a painful numbness in the hand that often subjectively feels like a loss of circulation of blood. They often seek relief by: shaking or dangling or swinging the hand, opening and closing or rubbing the fingers, running hot or cold water over the hand, or pacing the floor. It may radiate up the arm, occasionally as far as shoulder

B. daytime activities that characteristically may bring on symptoms: holding a book or newspaper to read, driving a car, holding a telephone receiver

C. distribution of symptoms:

1. on palmar side in radial 3.5 fingers (palmar side of thumb, index finger, middle finger, and radial half of ring finger)

2. dorsal side of these same fingers distal to the PIP joint

3. radial half of palm

4. subjective involvement of little finger occurs not infrequently

2. weakness of hand, especially grip. May be associated with thenar atrophy (late change, severe atrophy is seldom seen with current awareness of CTS by most physicians). An occasional patient may present with severe atrophy and no history of pain

3. clumsiness of the hand or difficulty with fine motor skills: due mostly to numbness more than a motor deficit. Often presents as difficulties buttoning buttons...

4. hypesthesia in median nerve sensory distribution: usually best appreciated in finger tips, loss of 2-point discrimination may be more sensitive test

5. **Phalen's test**: 30-60 secs of complete wrist flexion exaggerates or reproduces pain or tingling. Positive in 80% of cases[51]

6. **Tinel's sign** at the wrist: paresthesias or pain in median nerve distribution produced by gently percussing over the carpal tunnel. Positive in 60% of cases. May also be present in other conditions. Reverse Tinel's sign: produces symptoms radiating up the forearm for variable distance

7. ischemic testing: place blood pressure cuff proximal to wrist, inflation **x** 30-60 seconds may reproduce CTS pain

DIFFERENTIAL DIAGNOSIS

Differential diagnosis includes (modified[52]):

1. cervical radiculopathy: coexists in 70% of patients with either median or ulnar neuropathy (C6 radiculopathy may mimic CTS). Usually relieved by rest, and exacerbated by neck movement. Sensory impairment has dermatomal distribution. It has been postulated that cervical nerve root compression may interrupt axoplasmic flow and predispose the nerve to compressive injury distally (the term **double-crush syndrome** was coined to describe this[53]), and although this has been challenged[54] it has not been disproven

2. thoracic outlet syndrome: loss of bulk in hand muscles other than thenar. Sensory impairment in ulnar side of hand and forearm (see page 576)

3. pronator teres syndrome: more prominent palmar pain than with CTS (median palmar cutaneous branch does not pass through carpal tunnel, see page 569)

---

4. **de Quervain's syndrome**: tenosynovitis of the abductor pollicus longus and extensor pollicus brevis tendons often caused by repetitive hand movements. Results in pain and tenderness in the wrist near the thumb. Onset in 25% of cases is during pregnancy, and many in 1st postpartum year. Usually responds to wrist splints and/or steroid injections. NCVs should be normal. Finkelstein's test: thumb passively abducted while thumb abductors are palpated, positive if this aggravates the pain[55]
5. **reflex sympathetic dystrophy**: may respond to sympathetic block (*see page 627*)
6. **tenosynovitis of any of the flexor ligaments**: may occasionally be due to TB or fungus. Usually a long, indolent course. Fluid accumulation may be present

DIAGNOSTIC TESTS

Electrodiagnostics

Electromyogram (**EMG**) and nerve conduction velocities (**NCV**): may help distinguish CTS from cervical root abnormalities and from tendonitis.

NCV: reportedly, can be normal in 15-25% of cases of CTS[A]. Sensory latencies are more sensitive than motor (*see Table 20-13 for values*). In uncertain cases, compare median nerve sensory conduction velocity to that of the ulnar nerve: normal median nerve should be at least 4 m/sec faster than the

Table 20-13 Distal conduction latencies through carpal tunnel (assumes normal proximal NCV)

Degree of involvement	Sensory latency* (mSec)	Motor latency† (mSec)
normal	< 3.7	< 4.5
mild involvement	3.7-4.0	4.4-6.9
moderate	4.1-5.0	7.0-9.9
severe	> 5 or unobtainable	> 10

*   to index finger
†   to abductor pollicis brevis

ulnar, reversal of this pattern suggests median nerve injury. Alternatively, the sensory latencies for the *palmar* median and ulnar nerves can be compared, the median nerve latency should not be ≥ 0.3 mS longer than the ulnar.

EMG: normal in up to 31% of cases of CTS. In relatively advanced CTS, it may show increased polyphasicity, positive waves, fibrillation potentials, and decreased motor unit numbers on maximal thenar muscle contraction. Helps detect cervical radiculopathy if present.

Laboratory tests

Recommended in cases where etiology is unclear (e.g. young individual with no history of repetitive hand movement).
1. thyroid hormone levels (T_4 (total or free) & TSH): to R/O myxedema
2. CBC: anemia is common in multiple myeloma, also to R/O amyloidosis
3. electrolytes:
   A. to R/O chronic renal failure that could cause uremic neuropathy
   B. blood glucose: R/O diabetes
4. in cases suspicious for multiple myeloma: (*see page 515* for full details)
   A. 24 hour urine for kappa Bence-Jones protein
   B. bloodwork: serum protein electrophoresis (**SPEP**) and immune electrophoresis (**IEP**) (looking for IgG kappa band)
   C. skeletal radiologic survey
   D. anemia is common on the CBC

NON-SURGICAL MANAGEMENT

Recommended for cases of recent onset, mild involvement, or where exacerbating phenomena are expected to be corrected (e.g. correction of hypothyroidism)[56 (p 1776)]
1. rest
2. non-steroidal anti-inflammatory drugs
3. neutral position splints: 50% of cases improve when involvement is only mild to moderate. Relapse is common. A trial of at least 2-4 weeks is recommended
4. steroid injection: 33% relapse within 15 mos. Repeat injections are possible
   A. use 10-25 mg hydrocortisone. Avoid local anesthetics (may mask symptoms of intra-neural injection)
   B. inject into carpal tunnel (deep to transverse carpal ligament) to ulnar side of palmaris longus to avoid median nerve (in patients without palmaris lon-

---

A. NB: great reservation should be used in considering operating on CTS with normal NCVs

gus, inject in line with fourth digit)
C. median nerve injuries have been reported with this technique[57], primarily due to intra-neural injection (all steroids are neurotoxic upon intrafascicular injection, and so are some of the carrier agents)

SURGICAL TREATMENT
The operation is termed neurolysis of the median nerve at the wrist. It is reserved for cases refractory to non-surgical therapy, or where severe sensory loss or thenar atrophy is present. Surgical treatment of cases due multiple myeloma is also effective.

With bilateral CTS, in general one operates on the more painful hand first. However if the condition is severe in both hands (on EMG) and if it has progressed beyond the painful stage and is only causing weakness and/or numbness, it may be best to operate on the "better" hand first in order to try and maximize recovery of the median nerve at least on that side. Simultaneous bilateral procedures may also be done[58].

Surgical techniques
A number of techniques are popular, including: incision through palm of hand, transverse incision through wrist crease (with or without a retinaculatome[59]), and endoscopic techniques (using single or dual incisions).

Complications of carpal tunnel surgery[60]
1. pain due to neuroma formation following transection of palmar cutaneous branch (PCB) of median nerve
   - branches of PCB may cross interthenar crease
   - avoid by: using magnification, avoiding transverse wrist incision, and making incision slightly to ulnar side of interthenar crease
   - treated by ligating this branch where it originates from median nerve in forearm (results in small area of numbness at base of thenar eminence)
2. neuroma of dorsal sensory branch of radial nerve
   - caused by extending incision proximally and radially
   - may be treated by neurolysis of neuroma
3. injury to recurrent thenar (motor) branch of median nerve
   - anomaly may cause nerve to lie above or to pierce TCL
   - avoided by: staying to ulnar side of midline
4. direct injury to median nerve
5. volar displacement and entrapment of median nerve in healing edges of TCL
6. hypertrophic scar causing compression of median nerve
   - usually caused by incision crossing wrist perpendicular to flexion crease
   - avoid by not crossing flexion crease, or in cases where necessary cross wrist obliquely at 45° angle directed toward ulnar side[60]
7. failure to improve symptoms
   - incorrect diagnosis: if EMG or NCV not done pre-op, they should be done after surgical failure (to R/O e.g. cervical root involvement (look for posterior myotome involvement), or generalized peripheral neuropathy)
   - incomplete transection of TCL: the most common cause for failure if diagnosis is correct (also possibility of accessory ligament or fascial band proximal to TCL). When this is identified on re-exploration, 75% of patients will be cured or improved after division is completed
8. joint stiffness
   - caused by excessively long immobilization of wrist and fingers
9. injury to superficial palmar arch (arterial): usually results from "blind" distal division of TCL
10. bowstringing of flexor tendons
11. **reflex sympathetic dystrophy**: exact incidence is unknown, reported in 4 of 132 patients in one series (probably too high, most surgeons will see only one or two cases in their career). Treatment with IV phentolamine has been suggested, but most cases are self limited after ≈ 2 weeks
12. infection: usually causes exquisite tenderness
13. hematoma: also usually quite painful and tender

INJURIES TO THE MAIN TRUNK OF THE MEDIAN NERVE
The median nerve descends the upper arm adjacent to the lateral side of the brachial artery. It crosses to the medial side of the artery at the level of the coracobrachialis. In the cubital fossa, the median nerve passes behind the lacertus fibrosus (bicipital apo-

neurosis) and enters the forearm between the two heads of the pronator teres. It then descends underneath the fibrous bridge of the flexor digitorum superficialis (sublimis).

Above the elbow, the median nerve may rarely be compressed by Struther's ligament. At the elbow and forearm, the median nerve may rarely be trapped at any of three sites: 1) lacertus fibrosus (bicipital aponeurosis)[61], 2) pronator teres, 3) sublimis bridge. Neuropathy may also result from direct or indirect trauma or external pressure ("**honeymoon paralysis**")[61]. Longstanding compression of the main trunk of the median nerve produces a "**benediction hand**" when trying to make a fist (index finger extended, middle finger partially flexed; due to weakness of flexor digitorum profundus I & II).

STRUTHER'S LIGAMENT

The supracondylar process **(SCP)** is an anatomical variant located 5-7 cm above medial epicondyle, present in 0.7-2.7% of population. Struther's ligament bridges the SCP to the medial epicondyle. The median nerve and brachial artery pass underneath, the ulnar nerve may also. Usually asymptomatic, but occasionally may cause typical median nerve syndrome.

PRONATOR (TERES) SYNDROME

From direct trauma or repeated pronation with tight hand-grip. Trapped where nerve dives between 2 heads of pronator teres. Causes vague aching and easy fatiguing of forearm muscles with weak grip and poorly localized paresthesias in index finger and thumb. Nocturnal exacerbation is absent. Pain in palm distinguishes this from CTS since median palmar cutaneous branch **(PCB)** exits before TCL and is spared in CTS.

Treat with resting forearm. Surgical decompression indicated for cases that progress while on rest or when continued trauma is unavoidable.

ANTERIOR INTEROSSEOUS NEUROPATHY

| Key features
| • loss of flexion of the distal phalanges of the thumb and index finger
| • no sensory loss

The anterior interosseous nerve is a primarily motor branch of the median nerve that arises in the upper forearm where it supplies the flexor digitorum profundus **(FDP)** I & II and flexor pollicus longus. In the distal forearm it supplies the pronator quadratus.

Neuropathy results in weakness of flexion of distal phalanges of thumb (weak flexor pollicus longus), index and middle finger (weak FDP I & II). In trying to pinch the tips of the index finger and thumb, the terminal phalanges extend and instead of the tips, the pulps touch ("**pinch sign**")[62]. There is no sensory loss.

In the absence of an identifiable cause of nerve injury, expectant management is recommended for 8-12 weeks, following which exploration is indicated which may reveal a constricting band near the origin.

ULNAR NERVE ENTRAPMENT

Ulnar nerve has components of C7, C8 and T1 nerve roots. Even though this is the second most prevalent entrapment neuropathy after CTS, it is still relatively uncommon.

Motor findings include:
1. wasting of the interossei may occur, and is most evident in the first dorsal interosseous (in the thumb web space)
2. Wartenberg's sign: one of the earliest findings of ulnar nerve entrapment (abducted little finger due to weakness of the third palmar interosseous muscle)
3. **Froment's prehensile thumb sign**: grasping a sheet of paper between thumb and index finger results in extension of the proximal phalanx of the thumb and flexion of the distal phalanx as a result of substituting flexor pollicus longus (innervated by anterior interosseous nerve) for the weak adductor pollicis[63 (p 18)]
4. **claw deformity** of the hand (**main en griffe**): in severe ulnar nerve injuries on attempted finger extension (some have called this "benediction hand", which differs from that with the same name in median nerve injury where this sign occurs on trying to make a fist). Fingers 4 and 5 and to a lesser extent 3 are hyperextended at the MCP joints (extensor digitorum is unopposed by interossei and "ulnar" lumbricals III & IV) and flexed at the interphalyngeal joints (due to pull of long

flexor muscles)

May occur with injury to the medial cord of the brachial plexus.

In the upper arm, the ulnar nerve descends anterior to the medial head of triceps; in 70% of people it passes under **arcade of Struthers** (distinct from Struther's ligament) a flat, thin, aponeurotic band. This is not normally a point of entrapment, but may cause kinking after ulnar nerve transposition if not adequately divided[56 (p 1781)].

ENTRAPMENT AT ELBOW

AKA **tardy ulnar palsy** because initial case reports occurred 12 or more years following injury at the elbow, and the majority commence over 10 years following the original injury. The elbow is the most vulnerable point of ulnar nerve: here the nerve is superficial, fixed, and crosses a joint. Most cases are idiopathic, although there may be a history of elbow fracture (especially lateral condyle of the humerus, with associated cubitus valgus

Table 20-14 McGowan classification of ulnar nerve injury

Grade	Description
1	purely subjective symptoms & mild hypesthesia
2	sensory loss & weakness of intrinsic hand muscles ± slight wasting
3	severe sensorimotor deficit

deformity), dislocation, arthritis, or repeated minor trauma. May also be injured during anesthesia[64] (*see page 558*). May be graded by the McGowan classification[65] as shown in *Table 20-14*.

Causes discomfort (pain, numbness and/or tingling) in little finger and ulnar half of ring finger, elbow pain, and hand weakness. Early symptoms may be purely motor (see *Froment's sign* and *claw deformity* above), may be exacerbated by the cold, and are often somewhat vague and may be described as a loss of finger coordination or clumsiness. Cramping and easy fatiguing of the ulnar innervated muscles of the hand may occur. Pain may not be a significant feature, but if present tends to be aching in nature along the ulnar aspect of the elbow or forearm. Atrophy of interossei is common.

The ulnar nerve is usually tender and palpably enlarged in the ulnar groove.

NCV: abnormal results include a velocity < 48 m/sec across the elbow, or a velocity across the elbow > 10 m/sec slower than the velocity above or below the elbow. Amplitude attenuation may occur even with normal velocities.

NON-SURGICAL TREATMENT

Avoid elbow trauma (patient education, an elbow pad may help). Results are often better when definite traumatic etiology can be identified and eliminated.

SURGICAL TREATMENT

Surgical options primarily consist of:
1. simple nerve decompression without transposition[66] (*see below*)
2. nerve decompression and transposition (extent of surgery differs because degree of entrapment varies; all forms of transposition require fashioning a sling to retain the nerve in its new location). Transposition may be to:
    A. subcutaneous tissue: this leaves the nerve fairly superficial and vulnerable
    B. within the flexor carpi ulnaris muscle (intramuscular transposition): some contend this actually worsens the condition due to intramuscular fibrosis
    C. a submuscular position: see below
3. medial epicondylectomy. Usually combined with decompression. May be best reserved for patients with a bony deformity

Submuscular transposition

Placement under pronator teres, within a groove fashioned in the flexor carpi ulnaris **(FCU)**.

Transposition vs. decompression

Has not been subjected to prospective randomized studies. Advantages of simple decompression vs. transposition include[67]: shorter operation that can be done more easily under local anesthesia, avoidance of nerve kinking and muscular fibrosis around the transposed nerve, and preservation of cutaneous branches, ulnar branches, and nourish-

---

ing blood vessels that sometimes may be sacrificed with transposition, rendering portions of the nerve ischemic. Generally recommended except in the case of bony deformity or subluxation of the nerve[67, 68].

Results with surgery

Not as good as with CTS, possibly due in part to the fact that patients tend to present much later. Overall, a good to excellent result is obtained in 60%, fair result in 25%, and a poor result (no improvement or worsening) in 15%[69 (p 2530)]. These results may be worse in patients with symptoms present > 1 year, with only 30% of these symptomatically improved in one series[66]. Lower success rate is also seen in older patients and those with certain medical conditions (diabetes, alcoholism…). Pain and sensory changes respond better than muscle weakness and atrophy.

ENTRAPMENT IN THE FOREARM

Just distal to the elbow, the ulnar nerve passes from the groove between the medial epicondyle and the olecranon process to enter between the two heads of the flexor carpi ulnaris (**FCU**) under the fascial band connecting the two heads (the cubital tunnel) but superficial to the flexor superficialis. Entrapment in the cubital tunnel at or just distal to the elbow produces the **cubital tunnel syndrome**, which is very rare. Findings are similar to tardy ulnar nerve palsy (*see above*).

Surgical treatment consists of steps outlined for nerve *distal* to the elbow in ulnar nerve decompression. A technique for locating the course of the ulnar nerve distal to the elbow is to place the proximal phalanx of the surgeon's little finger (using the hand contralateral to the patient's being decompressed) in the ulnar groove aiming it toward the ulnar side of the wrist[39 (p 262)].

ENTRAPMENT IN THE WRIST OR HAND

At the wrist, the terminal ulnar nerve enters **Guyon's canal**, the roof of which is the palmar fascia and palmaris brevis, the floor is the flexor retinaculum of the palm (key: the canal is above the transverse carpal ligament that produces carpal tunnel syndrome) and the pisohamate ligament. The canal has no tendons, only the ulnar nerve and artery. At the middle of the canal the nerve divides into deep and superficial branch. The superficial branch is mostly sensory (except for the branch to palmaris brevis), and supplies hypothenar eminence and ulnar half of ring finger. The deep (muscular) branch innervates hypothenar muscles, lumbricals 3 & 4, and all interossei. Occasionally the abductor digiti minimi branch arises from the main trunk or superficial branch.

Shea and McClain[70] divided lesions of the ulnar nerve in Guyon's canal into 3 types shown in *Table 20-15*. Injury to the distal motor branch can also occur in the palm and produces findings similar to a Type II injury.

Table 20-15   Types of ulnar nerve lesions in Guyon's canal

Type	Location of compression	Weakness	Sensory deficit
Type I	just proximal to or within Guyon's canal	all intrinsic hand muscles innervated by ulnar n.	palmar ulnar distribution*
Type II	along deep branch	muscles innervated by deep branch†	none
Type III	distal end of Guyon's canal	none	palmar ulnar distribution*

*   palmar ulnar distribution: the hypothenar eminence and ulnar half of ring finger, both on the palmar surface only (the dorsum is innervated by the dorsal cutaneous nerve)

†   depending on the location, may spare hypothenar muscles

Injury is most often due to a ganglion of the wrist[71], but also may be due to trauma (pneumatic drill, pliers, repetitively slamming a stapler, leaning on palm while riding bicycle). Symptoms are similar to those of ulnar nerve involvement at the elbow, except there will never be sensory loss in the <u>dorsum</u> of the hand in the ulnar nerve territory because the dorsal cutaneous branch leaves the nerve in the forearm 5-8 cm proximal to the wrist (sparing of flexor carpi ulnaris and flexor digitorum profundus III & IV is not helpful in localizing because these are so rarely involved even in proximal lesions). Electrodiagnostics are usually helpful in localizing the site of the lesion. Pain, when present, may be exacerbated by tapping over pisiform (Tinel's sign). It may also radiate up the forearm.

Surgical decompression may be indicated in refractory cases.

Arises from the posterior divisions of the 3 trunks of the brachial plexus. Receives contributions from C5 to C8. The nerve winds laterally along the spiral groove of the radius. Distinguish from brachial plexus posterior cord injury by sparing of deltoid (axillary nerve) and latissimus dorsi (thoracodorsal nerve).

AXILLARY COMPRESSION

Less common than compression in mid-upper arm.

Etiologies: crutch misuse; poor arm position during drunken sleep.

Clinical: weakness of triceps and more distal muscles innervated by radial nerve.

MID-UPPER ARM COMPRESSION

Sites of compression: in spiral groove, at intermuscular septum, or just distal to this.

Etiologies:
1. improper positioning of arm in sleep (especially when drunk), AKA "**Saturday night palsy**"
2. from positioning under general anesthesia
3. from callus due to old humeral fracture

Clinical: weakness of wrist extensors (**wrist drop**) and finger extensors, key: <u>triceps is normal</u>; involvement of distal nerve is variable, may include thumb extensor palsy and paresthesias in radial nerve distribution. Differential diagnosis: isolated wrist and finger extensor weakness can also occur in lead poisoning.

FOREARM COMPRESSION

The radial nerve enters the anterior compartment of the arm just above the elbow. It gives off branches to brachialis, brachioradialis, and extensor carpi radialis (**ECR**) longus before dividing into the posterior interosseous nerve and the superficial radial nerve. The posterior interosseous nerve dives into the supinator muscle through a fibrous band known as the **arcade of Frohse** (*see page 551* for muscles supplied).

POSTERIOR INTEROSSEOUS NEUROPATHY

Posterior interosseous neuropathy ("**PIN**") may result from: lipomas, ganglia, fibromas, arthritis, entrapment at the arcade of Frohse (rare), and strenuous use of arm.

Clinical: marked extensor weakness of thumb and fingers (**finger drop**). Distinguished from radial nerve palsy by less wrist extensor weakness (<u>no wrist drop</u>) due to sparing of ECR brevis and longus (there will be radial deviation due to palsy of extensor carpi ulnaris). <u>No sensory loss</u>.

Treatment: cases that do not respond to 4-8 weeks of expectant management should be explored, and any constrictions lysed (including arcade of Frohse).

RADIAL TUNNEL SYNDROME

AKA **supinator tunnel syndrome**. The "radial tunnel" extends from just above the elbow to just distal to it, and is composed of different structures (muscles, fibrous bands...) depending on the level[72]. It contains the radial nerve and its two main branches (posterior interosseous and superficial radial). Repeated forceful supination or pronation or inflammation of supinator muscle attachments (as in tennis elbow) may traumatize the nerve (sometimes by ECR brevis). Characteristic finding: pain in the region of the common extensor origin at the lateral epicondyle on resisted extension of the middle finger which tightens the ECR brevis. May be mistakenly diagnosed as resistant "tennis elbow". There may also be peristhesias in the distribution of the superficial radial nerve and local tenderness along the radial nerve anterior to the radial head. Even though the site of entrapment is similar to PIN, unlike PIN, there is usually no muscle weakness. This syndrome responds to nerve decompression[72].

INJURY IN THE HAND

The distal cutaneous branches of the superficial radial nerve cross the extensor pollicus longus tendon, and can often be palpated at this point with the thumb in extension. Injury to the medial branch of this nerve occurs commonly e.g. with handcuff injuries, and causes a small area of sensory loss in the dorsal web-space of the thumb.

AXILLARY NERVE INJURIES

Isolated neuropathy of the axillary nerve may occur in the following situations[73]:
1. sleeping in the prone position with the arms abducted above the head
2. compression from a thoracic harness
3. injection injury in the high posterior aspect of the shoulder
4. entrapment of the nerve in the quadrilateral space (bounded by the teres major and minor muscles, long head of triceps, and neck of humerus) which contains the axillary nerve and the posterior humeral circumflex artery. Arteriogram may show loss of filling of the artery with the arm abducted and externally rotated
5. shoulder dislocation: the nerve is tethered to the joint capsule[74]

SUPRASCAPULAR NERVE

The suprascapular nerve is a mixed peripheral nerve arising from the superior trunk of the brachial plexus, with contributions from C5 & C6. Suprascapular palsy is usually due to entrapment of the nerve within the suprascapular notch beneath the **transverse scapular** (suprascapular) **ligament (TSL)**[75]. There is often a history of frozen shoulder or shoulder trauma. Entrapment results in weakness & atrophy of infra- and supra-spinatus (**IS & SS**) and deep, poorly localized (referred) shoulder pain (the sensory part of the nerve innervates the posterior joint capsule but has no cutaneous representation).

Differential diagnosis includes[75]:
1. rotator cuff injuries (distinction may be very difficult)
2. adhesive capsulitis
3. bicipital tenosynovitis
4. arthritis
5. cases of Parsonage-Turner syndrome limited to the suprascapular nerve (see *Idiopathic brachial plexus neuropathy*, page 554)
6. cervical radiculopathy (≈ C5)   NB: these two will also produce rhomboid
7. upper brachial plexus lesion } and deltoid weakness and, usually, cutaneous sensory loss

Diagnosis requires temporary relief with nerve block, and EMG abnormalities of SS & IS (in rotator cuff tears, fibrillation potentials will be absent). Transient pain relief with a suprascapular nerve block helps verify the diagnosis[76].

Surgical treatment is indicated for documented cases that fail to improve with expectant management.

MERALGIA PARESTHETICA

Originally known as the **Bernhardt-Roth syndrome**, and sometimes called "swashbuckler's disease", meralgia paresthetica (**MP**) (Greek: *meros* - thigh, *algos* - pain) is a condition caused by entrapment of the **lateral femoral cutaneous nerve (LFCN)** of the thigh, (a purely sensory branch with contributions from L2 and L3 nerve roots, see *Figure 3-7*, page 75 for distribution) where it enters the thigh though the opening between the inguinal ligament and its attachment to the anterior superior iliac spine (**ASIS**). Anatomic variation is common, and the nerve may actually pass through the ligament, and as many as four branches may be found.

Signs and symptoms
Burning dysesthesias in the lateral aspect of the upper thigh, occasionally just above the knee, usually with increased sensitivity to clothing (hyperpathia). There may be decreased sensation in this distribution. Spontaneous rubbing or massaging the area in order to obtain relief is very characteristic[77]. MP may be bilateral in up to 20% of cases. Sitting or lying prone usually ameliorates the symptoms.

There may be point tenderness at the site of entrapment (where pressure may reproduce the pain), which is often located where the nerve exits the pelvis medial to the

ASIS. Hip extension may also cause pain.

Occurrence

Usually seen in obese patients, may be exacerbated by wearing tight belts or girdles, and by prolonged standing or walking. Recently found in long distance runners. Higher incidence in diabetics. May also occur post-op in slender patients positioned prone, tends to be <u>bilateral</u> (*see page 559*).

Possible etiologies are too numerous to list, more common ones include: tight clothing or belts, surgical scars post-abdominal surgery, cardiac catheterization (*see page 559*), pregnancy, iliac crest bone graft harvesting, ascites, obesity, metabolic neuropathies, and abdominal or pelvic mass.

DIFFERENTIAL DIAGNOSIS

1. femoral neuropathy: sensory changes tend to be more anteromedial than MP
2. L2 or L3 radiculopathy: look for motor weakness (thigh flexion or knee extension)
3. nerve compression by abdominal or pelvic tumor (suspected if concomitant GI or GU symptoms)

The condition can usually be diagnosed on clinical grounds. When it is felt to be necessary, confirmatory tests may help, including: EMG (may be difficult, the electromyographer cannot always find the nerve), MRI or CT/myelography when disc disease is suspected, pelvic imaging (MRI or CT), somatosensory evoked potentials, or the response to local anesthetic injections.

TREATMENT

Tends to regress spontaneously, but recurrence is common. Nonsurgical measures achieve relief in ≈ 91% of cases and should be tried prior to considering surgery[78]:

1. remove offending articles (constricting belts, braces, casts, tight garments...)
2. in obese patients: weight loss and exercises to strengthen the abdominal muscles is usually effective, but is rarely achieved by the patient
3. elimination of activities involving hip extension
4. application of ice to the area of presumed constriction **x** 30 minutes TID
5. NSAID of choice **x** 7-10 days
6. capsaicin ointment applied TID (*see page 389*)
7. if the above measures fail, injection of 5-10 ml of local anesthetic (with or without steroids) at the point of tenderness, or medial to the ASIS may provide temporary or sometimes long lasting relief, and confirms the diagnosis

Surgical treatment

Options include:

1. surgical decompression (neurolysis) of the nerve: higher failure and recurrence rate than neurectomy
2. decompression and transposition
3. division of the nerve (neurectomy) is more effective, but may cause denervation pain, and leaves an anesthetic area (usually a minor nuisance)

Technique[78]:

OBTURATOR NERVE ENTRAPMENT

Composed of L2-4 roots. Courses along pelvic wall to provide sensation to the inner thigh, and motor to the thigh adductors (gracilis and adductors longus, brevis, and magnus). It may be compressed by pelvic tumors, also from the pressure of the fetal head or forceps during parturition.

The result is numbness of the medial thigh and weak thigh adduction.

FEMORAL NERVE ENTRAPMENT

Composed of roots L2-4. Entrapment is a rare cause of femoral neuropathy. See *Femoral neuropathy* on page 557.

COMMON PERONEAL NERVE PALSY

The peroneal nerve is the most common nerve to develop *acute* compression palsy. The **sciatic nerve** (L4-S3) contains 2 separate nerves within a common sheath, the **common peroneal nerve (CPN)** (AKA lateral popliteal nerve) and the **posterior tibial nerve** (AKA medial popliteal nerve). At a variable location in the thigh, the two branches separate (see *Table 32-4*, page 910), the CPN passes behind the fibular head where it is superficial and fixed, making it vulnerable to pressure or trauma (e.g. from crossing the legs at the knee). Just distal to this, it divides into:

- **deep peroneal nerve** (AKA anterior tibial nerve): primarily motor
  - A. motor: foot and toe extensors (EHL, tibialis anterior, extensor digitorum longus)
  - B. sensory: very small area between great toe and second toe
- **superficial peroneal nerve** (AKA musculocutaneous nerve)
  - A. motor: foot evertors (peroneus longus and brevis)
  - B. sensory: lateral distal leg and dorsum of foot

Findings in peroneal nerve palsy
- sensory changes (uncommon): involves lateral aspect of lower half of leg
- muscle involvement: *see Table 20-16*

Common peroneal nerve palsy (most common) produces weak ankle dorsiflexion (foot drop) due to anterior tibialis palsy, weak foot eversion, and sensory impairment in areas innervated by deep and superficial peroneal nerve (lateral calf and dorsum of foot). There may be a Tinel's sign with percussion of the nerve near the fibular neck. Occasionally, only the deep peroneal nerve is involved, resulting in foot drop with minimal sensory loss. Must differentiate from other causes of foot drop (see *Foot drop*, page 909).

Table 20-16 Muscle involvement in peroneal nerve palsy

Muscle	Involvement
EHL	most commonly involved
tibialis anterior	↓
toe extensors	↓
peroneal muscle (foot eversion)	least commonly involved (often spared)

Causes of common peroneal nerve injury
1. entrapment as it crosses the fibular neck or as it penetrates the peroneus longus
2. diabetes mellitus and other metabolic peripheral neuropathies
3. inflammatory neuropathy: including Hansen's disease (leprosy)
4. traumatic: e.g. clipping injury in football players, stretch injury due to dislocating force applied to the knee, fibular fracture
5. masses in the area of the fibular head/proximal lower leg: popliteal fossa cysts, anterior tibial artery aneurysm[79] (rare)
6. pressure at fibular head: e.g. from crossing the legs at the knee, casts, obstetrical stirrups (*see page 559*)...
7. traction injuries: severe inversion sprains of the ankle
8. intraneural tumors: neurofibroma, schwannoma, ganglion cysts
9. vascular: venous thrombosis
10. weight loss

Evaluation

EMG: It takes 2-4 weeks from the onset of symptoms for the EMG to become positive. Stimulate above and below fibular head for prognostic information: if absent in both sites, bad prognosis (indicates retrograde degeneration has occurred). Wallerian degeneration takes ≈ 5 days to cause deterioration. The short head of the biceps femoris is spared in cases of compression of the peroneal nerve at the fibular head due to the fact that the nerve takeoff is proximal to the popliteal fossa. EMG can also differentiate L5 radiculopathy.

MRI: May demonstrate causes such as a ganglion cyst arising from the superior tibiofibular articulation.

Treatment
When a reversible cause can be eliminated, the outcome is usually good. Surgical exploration and decompression may be considered when there is no reversible cause or when improvement does not occur.

Entrapment of **(posterior) tibial nerve** may occur in the tarsal tunnel, posterior and inferior to medial malleolus. The tunnel is covered by the flexor retinaculum (lancinate ligament) which extends downward from the medial malleolus to the tubercle of the calcaneus. There is often (but not necessarily) a history of old ankle dislocation or fracture. The nerve may be trapped at the retinacular ligament. This results in pain and paresthesias in the toes and sole of foot (often sparing the heel because the sensory branches often originate proximal to the tunnel), typically worse at night. May cause clawing of toes secondary to weakness of intrinsic foot muscles.

Percussion of nerve at medial malleolus produces paresthesias that radiate distally (Tinel's sign).

Diagnosis

EMG and NCV studies may help.

Treatment

External ankle support to improve foot mechanics.
Surgical decompression is indicated for confirmed cases that fail to improve.

20.3. Thoracic outlet syndrome

The thoracic outlet is a confined area at the apex of the lung bordered by the 1st rib below and the clavicle above through which passes the subclavian artery, vein, and brachial plexus.

Thoracic outlet syndrome **(TOS)** is a term implying compression of one or more of the enclosed structures producing a heterogeneous group of disorders. TOS tends to be diagnosed more often by general and vascular surgeons than by neurologists and neurosurgeons. Four unrelated conditions with different structures involved:

1. arterial vascular: producing arm, hand and finger pallor and ischemia
2. venous vascular: producing arm swelling and edema
3. true neurologic: compressing the lower trunk or median cord of the brachial plexus (*see below*)

"noncontroversial", with characteristic symptom complex, reproducible clinical findings, confirmatory laboratory tests. Low incidence[80]

4. disputed neurologic: (*see below*)

Differential diagnosis

1. herniated cervical disc
2. cervical arthrosis
3. lung cancer (pancoast tumor)
4. tardy ulnar nerve palsy
5. carpal tunnel syndrome
6. orthopedic shoulder problems
7. complex regional pain syndrome (reflex sympathetic dystrophy)

TRUE NEUROLOGIC TOS

A rare condition primarily affecting adult women, usually unilateral.

Neurologic structures involved
1. most common: compression of the C8/T1 roots
2. or proximal lower trunk of the brachial plexus **(BP)**
3. less common: compression of the median cord of the BP

Etiologies
1. constricting band extending from the first rib to a rudimentary "cervical rib" or to an elongated C7 transverse process
2. scalenus (anticus) syndrome: controversial (see *Disputed neurologic TOS* below)
3. compression beneath the pectoralis minor tendon under the coracoid process: may result from repetitive movements of the arms above the head (shoulder elevation and hyperabduction)

Signs & symptoms include:
1. ★ sensory changes in distribution of median cord (mainly along medial forearm), sparing median nerve sensory fibers (pass through upper and middle trunks)
2. hand clumsiness or weakness and wasting, especially abductor pollicis brevis and ulnar hand intrinsics
3. there may be tenderness over Erb's point (2 to 3 cm above the clavicle in front of the C6 transverse process)
4. may be painless
5. usually unilateral

Confirmatory tests:
1. EMG: unreliable (may be negative)
2. MRI does not show bony abnormalities well, but may occasionally demonstrate a kink in the lower BP. Can also rule-out conditions that may mimic TOS such as herniated cervical disc
3. cervical spine x-rays with obliques and apical lordotic CXR may demonstrate bony abnormalities. However, not every cervical rib produces symptoms.

Treatment

Controversial. Conservative treatment (usually including stretching and physical therapy) is about as effective as surgery and avoids attendant risks.

Decompression can be achieved by removing the muscles that surround the nerves (scalenectomy), by transaxillary first rib resection, or both.

DISPUTED NEUROLOGIC TOS

Controversial. May be similar to the scalenus anticus syndrome (or just scalenus syndrome) more popularly diagnosed in the 1940's and 50's. There seems to be a lack of consensus regarding the pathophysiology (including structures involved), clinical presentation, helpful tests, and optimal treatment. Removal of first thoracic rib is often advocated for treatment, frequently via a transaxillary approach. Unfortunately, injuries especially to the lower trunk of the brachial plexus, may result from the surgery for 1st rib resections.

Other variations include an "upper plexus" type for which total anterior scalenectomy is advocated.

20.4. Miscellaneous peripheral nerve

Nerve block

For example, to block greater occipital nerve in occipital neuralgia.

Rx: add 40 mg methylprednisolone aqueous suspension (Depo-Medrol®) to 10 ml of 0.75% bipuvicaine (Marcaine®) and inject into region of irritated or inflamed nerve.

20.5. References

1. Fernandez E, Pallini R, La Marca F, *et al*.: Neurosurgery of the peripheral nervous system - part I: Basic anatomic concepts. **Surg Neurol** 46: 47-8, 1996.
2. Medical Research Council: **Aids to the examination of the peripheral nervous system**. Her Majesty's Stationery Office, London, 1976.
3. Ochoa J L, Verdugo R J: Reflex sympathetic dystrophy: A common clinical avenue for somatoform expression. **Neurol Clin** 13: 351-63, 1995.
4. Denny-Brown D: Primary sensory neuropathy with muscular changes associated with carcinoma. **J Neurol Neurosurg Psychiatry** 11: 73-87, 1948.
5. Camerlingo M, Nemni R, Ferraro B, *et al*: Malignancy and sensory neuropathy of unexplained cause: A prospective study of 51 patients. **Arch Neurol** 55: 981-4, 1998.
6. Adams R D, Victor M: **Principles of neurology**.

2nd ed. McGraw-Hill, New York, 1981.
7. Tsairis P, Dyck P J, Mulder D W: Natural history of brachial plexus neuropathy: Report on 99 patients. **Arch Neurol** 27: 109-17, 1972.
8. Evans B A, Stevens J C, Dyck P J: Lumbosacral plexus neuropathy. **Neurology** 31: 1327-30, 1981.
9. The Diabetes Control and Complications Trial Research Group: The effect of intensive treatment of diabetes on the development and progression of long-term complications in insulin-dependent diabetes mellitus. **N Engl J Med** 329: 977-86, 1993.
10. Asbury A K: Proximal diabetic neuropathy. **Ann Neurol** 2: 179-80, 1977.
11. Dyck P J, Thomas P K: **Peripheral neuropathy**. 2nd ed. W. B. Saunders, Philadelphia, 1984.
12. Garland H: Diabetic amyotrophy. **BMJ** 2: 1287-90, 1955.

13. Barohn R J, Sahenk Z, Warmolts J R, *et al.*: The Bruns-Garland syndrome (diabetic amyotrophy): Revisited 100 years later. **Arch Neurol** 48: 1130-5, 1991.

14. Pascoe M K, Low P A, Windebank A J: Subacute diabetic proximal neuropathy. **Mayo Clin Proc** 72: 1123-32, 1997.

15. Davis J L, Lewis S B, Gerich J E, *et al.*: Peripheral diabetic neuropathy treated with amitriptyline and fluphenazine. **JAMA** 21: 2291-2, 1977.

16. Max M B, Lynch S A, Muir J, *et al.*: Effects of desipramine, amitriptyline, and fluoxetine on pain in diabetic neuropathy. **N Engl J Med** 326: 1250-6, 1992.

17. Mendel C M, Klein R F, Chappell D A, *et al.*: A trial of amitriptyline and fluphenazine in the treatment of painful diabetic neuropathy. **JAMA** 255: 637-9, 1986.

18. Mendel C M, Grunfeld C: Amitriptyline and fluphenazine for painful diabetic neuropathy. **JAMA** 256: 712-4, 1986.

19. Backonja M, Beydoun A, Edwards K R, *et al.*: Gabapentin for the symptomatic treatment of painful neuropathy in patients with diabetes mellitus: A randomized controlled trial. **JAMA** 280 (21): 1831-6, 1998.

20. Morello C M, Leckband S G, Stoner C P, *et al.*: Randomized double-blind study comparing the efficacy of gabapentin with amitriptyline on diabetic peripheral neuropathy pain. **Arch Intern Med** 159 (16): 1931-7, 1999.

21. New uses of thalidomide. **Med Letter** 38: 15-6, 1996.

22. Fuller G N, Jacobs J M, Guiloff R J: Nature and incidence of peripheral nerve syndromes in HIV infection. **J Neurol Neurosurg Psychiatry** 56: 372-81, 1993.

23. Drugs for HIV infection. **Med Letter** 42 (1069): 1-6, 2000.

24. Warner M A: Perioperative neuropathies. **Mayo Clin Proc** 73: 567-74, 1998.

25. Wadsworth T G, Williams J R: Cubital tunnel external compression syndrome. **Br Med J** 1: 662-6, 1973.

26. Warner M A, Marner M E, Martin J T: Ulnar neuropathy: Incidence, outcome, and risk factors in sedated or anesthesthetized patients. **Anesthesiology** 81: 1332-40, 1994.

27. Alvine F G, Schurrer M E: Postoperative ulnar-nerve palsy: Are there predisposing factors? **J Bone Joint Surg** 69A: 255-9, 1987.

28. Stewart J D, Shantz S H: Perioperative ulnar neuropathies: A medicolegal review. **Can J Neurol Sci** 30: 15-9, 2003.

29. Warner M A, Martin J T, Schroeder D R, *et al.*: Lower-extremity motor neuropathy associated with surgery performed on patients in a lithotomy position. **Anesthesiology** 81: 6-12, 1994.

30. O'Donnell D, Rottman R, Kotelko D, *et al.*: Incidence of maternal postpartum neurologic dysfunction. **Anesthesiology** 81 (Suppl): A1127, 1994 (abstract).

31. Kent C K, Moscucci M, Gallagher S G, *et al.*: Neuropathies after cardiac catheterization: Incidence, clinical patterns, and long-term outcome. **J Vasc Surg** 19: 1008-14, 1994.

32. Rouse D J, Owen J, Goldenberg R L, *et al.*: The effectiveness and costs of elective cesarean delivery for fetal macrosomia diagnosed by ultrasound. **JAMA** 276 (18): 1480-6, 1996.

33. Gilbert A, Brockman R, Carlioz H: Surgical treatment of brachial plexus birth palsy. **Clin Orthop** 264: 39-47, 1991.

34. Boome R S, Kaye J C: Obstetric traction injuries of the brachial plexus: Natural history, indications for surgical repair and results. **J Bone Joint Surg** 70B: 571-6, 1988.

35. van Ouwerkerk W J, van der Sluijs J A, Nollet F, *et al.*: Management of obstetric brachial plexus lesions: State of the art and future developments. **Childs Nerv Syst** 16 (10-11): 638-44, 2000.

36. Piatt J H, Hudson A R, Hoffman H J: Preliminary experiences with brachial plexus explorations in children: Birth injury and vehicular trauma. **Neurosurgery** 22: 715-23, 1988.

37. Hunt D: Surgical management of brachial plexus birth injuries. **Dev Med Child Neurol** 30: 821-8, 1988.

38. Anand P, Birch R: Restoration of sensory function and lack of long-term chronic pain syndromes after brachial plexus injury in human neonates. **Brain** 125 (Pt 1): 113-22, 2002.

39. Kline D G, Hudson A R: **Nerve injuries: Operative results for major nerve injuries, entrapments, and tumors**. W. B. Saunders, Philadelphia, 1995.

40. Neary D, Ochoa J L, Gilliatt R W: Subclinical entrapment neuropathy in man. **J Neurol Sci** 24: 283-98, 1975.

41. Graff-Radford S B, Jaeger B, Reeves J L: Myofascial pain may present clinically as occipital neuralgia. **Neurosurgery** 19: 610-3, 1986.

42. Hunter C R, Mayfield F H: Role of the upper cervical roots in the production of pain in the head. **Am J Surg** 48: 743-51, 1949.

43. Poletti C E, Sweet W H: Entrapment of the C2 root and ganglion by the atlanto-epistrophic ligament: Clinical syndrome and surgical anatomy. **Neurosurgery** 27: 288-91, 1990.

44. Anthony M: Headache and the greater occipital nerve. **Clin Neurol Neurosurg** 94 (4): 297-301, 1992.

45. Weiner R L, Reed K L: Peripheral neurostimulation for control of intractable occipital neuralgia. **Neuromodulation** 2 (3): 217-21, 1999.

46. Freund B J, Schwartz M: Treatment of chronic cervical-associated headache with botulinum toxin A: A pilot study. **Headache** 40 (3): 231-6, 2000.

47. Weinberger L M: Cervico-occipital pain and its surgical treatment. **Am J Surg** 135: 243-7, 1978.

48. Bovim G, Fredriksen T A, Stolt-Nielsen A, *et al.*: Neurolysis of the greater occipital nerve in cervicogenic headache. A follow up study. **Headache** 32 (4): 175-9, 1992.

49. Bogduk N: Local anesthetic blocks of the second cervical ganglion. A technique with application in occipital headache. **Cephalalgia** 1: 41-50, 1981.

50. Feldman R G, Goldman R, Keyserling W M: Classical syndromes in occupational medicine: Peripheral nerve entrapment syndromes and ergonomic factors. **Am J Ind Med** 4: 661-81, 1983.

51. Phalen G S: The carpal tunnel syndrome. Clinical evaluation of 598 hands. **Clin Ortho Rel Res** 83: 31, 1972.

52. Sandzen S C: Carpal tunnel syndrome. **Am Fam Physician** 24: 190-204, 1981.

53. Upton R M, McComas A J: The double crush in nerve entrapment syndromes. **Lancet** 11: 359-62, 1973.

54. Wilbourn A J, Gilliatt R W: Double-crush syndrome: A critical analysis. **Neurology** 49: 21-9, 1997.

55. Rempel D M, Harrison R J, Barnhart S: Work-related cumulative trauma disorders of the upper extremity. **JAMA** 267: 838-42, 1992.

56. Wilkins R H, Rengachary S S, (eds.): **Neurosurgery**. McGraw-Hill, New York, 1985.

57. Linskey M E, Segal R: Median nerve injury from local steroid injection in carpal tunnel syndrome. **Neurosurgery** 26: 512-5, 1990.

58. Pagnanelli D M, Barrer S J: Bilateral carpal tunel release at one operation: Report of 228 patients. **Neurosurgery** 31: 1030-4, 1992.

59. Pagnanelli D M, Barrer S J: Carpal tunnel syndrome: Surgical treatment using the Paine retinaculatome. **J**

Neurosurg 75: 77-81, 1991.

60. Louis D S, Greene T L, Noellert R C: Complications of carpal tunnel surgery. **J Neurosurg** 62: 352-6, 1985.

61. Laha R K, Lunsford L D, Dujovny M: Lacertus fibrosus compression of the median nerve. **J Neurosurg** 48: 838-41, 1978.

62. Nakano K K, Lundergan C, Okihiro M: Anterior interosseous nerve syndromes: Diagnostic methods and alternative treatments. **Arch Neurol** 34: 477-80, 1977.

63. Brazis P W, Masdeu J C, Biller J: **Localization in clinical neurology**. 2nd ed. Little Brown and Company, Boston, 1990.

64. Bonney G: Iatrogenic injuries of nerves. **J Bone Joint Surg** 68B: 9-13, 1986.

65. McGowan A J: The results of transposition of the ulnar nerve for traumatic ulnar neuritis. **J Bone Joint Surg** 32B: 293-301, 1950.

66. Le Roux P D, Ensign T D, Burchiel K J: Surgical decompression without transposition for ulnar neuropathy: Factors determining outcome. **Neurosurgery** 27: 709-14, 1990.

67. Tindall S C: Comment on LeRoux P D, et al.: Surgical decompression without transposition for ulnar neuropathy: Factors determining outcome. **Neurosurgery** 27: 714, 1990.

68. Bartels R H M A, Mcnovsky T, Van Overbccke J J, et al.: Surgical management of ulnar nerve compression at the elbow: An analysis of the literature. **J Neurosurg** 89: 722-7, 1988.

69. Youmans J R, (ed.) **Neurological surgery**. 3rd ed., W. B. Saunders, Philadelphia, 1990.

70. Shea J D, McClain E J: Ulnar-nerve compression syndromes at and below the wrist. **J Bone Joint Surg** 51A: 1095-103, 1969.

71. Cavallo M, Poppi M, Martinelli P, et al.: Distal ulnar neuropathy from carpal ganglia: A clinical and electrophysiological study. **Neurosurgery** 22: 902-5, 1988.

72. Roles N C, Maudsley R H: Radial tunnel syndrome: Resistant tennis elbow as a nerve entrapment. **J Bone Joint Surg** 54B: 499-508, 1972.

73. McKowen H C, Voorhies R M: Axillary nerve entrapment in the quadrilateral space: Case report. **J Neurosurg** 66: 932-4, 1987.

74. de Laat E A T, Visser C P J, Coene L N J E M, et al.: Nerve lesions in primary shoulder dislocations and humeral neck fractures. **J Bone Joint Surg** 76B: 381-3, 1994.

75. Hadley M N, Sonntag V K H, Pittman H W: Suprascapular nerve entrapment: A summary of seven cases. **J Neurosurg** 64: 843-8, 1986.

76. Callahan J D, Scully T B, Shapiro S A, et al.: Suprascapular nerve entrapment: A series of 27 cases. **J Neurosurg** 74: 893-6, 1991.

77. Stevens H I: Meralgia paresthetica. **Arch Neurol Psychiatry** 77: 557-74, 1957.

78. Williams P H, Trzil K P: Management of meralgia paresthetica. **J Neurosurg** 74: 76-80, 1991.

79. Kars H Z, Topaktas S, Dogan K: Aneurysmal peroneal nerve compression. **Neurosurgery** 30: 930-1, 1992.

80. Wilbourn A J: The thoracic outlet syndrome is overdiagnosed. **Arch Neurol** 47: 328-30, 1990.

81. Sanabria E A M, Nagashima T, Yamashita H, et al.: Postoperative bilateral meralgia paresthetica after spine surgery: An overlooked entity? **Spinal Surgery** 17 (3): 195-202, 2003.

21. Neurophthalmology

21.1. Nystagmus

Involuntary rhythmic oscillation of the eyes, usually conjugate. Most common form is jerk nystagmus, in which the direction of the nystagmus is defined for the direction of the fast (cortical) component (which is not the abnormal component). Horizontal or upward gaze-provoked nystagmus may be due to sedatives or AEDs; otherwise **vertical nystagmus** is indicative of posterior fossa pathology.

LOCALIZING LESION FOR VARIOUS FORMS OF NYSTAGMUS
1. **seesaw nystagmus**: intorting eye moves up, extorting eye moves down, pattern then reverses. Lesion in diencephalon. Also reported with chiasmal compression (occasionally accompanied with bitemporal hemianopia in parasellar masses)
2. **convergence nystagmus**: slow abduction of eyes followed by adducting (converging) jerks, usually associated with features of Parinaud's syndrome. May be associated with nystagmus retractorius (*see below*) with similar location of lesion
3. **nystagmus retractorius**: resulting from co-contraction of all EOM's. May accompany convergence nystagmus. Lesion in upper midbrain tegmentum (usually vascular disease or tumor, especially pinealoma)
4. **downbeat nystagmus**: nystagmus with the fast phase downward while in primary position. Most patients have a structural lesion in the posterior fossa, especially at the cervicomedullary junction (foramen magnum **(FM)**)[1], including Chiari I malformation, basilar impression, p-fossa tumors, syringobulbia[2]. Uncommonly occurs in multiple sclerosis, spinocerebellar degeneration, and in some metabolic conditions (hypomagnesemia, thiamine deficiency, alcohol intoxication or withdrawal, or treatment with phenytoin, carbamazepine or lithium[3])
5. **upbeat nystagmus**: lesion in medulla
6. **abducting** nystagmus occurs in INO. Lesion in pons (MLF)
7. **Brun's** nystagmus: lesion in pontomedullary junction **(PMJ)**
8. **vestibular** nystagmus: lesion in PMJ
9. **ocular myoclonus**: lesion in myoclonic triangle
10. **periodic alternating** nystagmus **(PAN)**: lesion in FM and cerebellum
11. **square wave jerks**, macro square wave jerks, macro saccadic oscillations. Lesion in cerebellar pathways
12. "nystagmoid" eye movements (not true nystagmus)
    A. **ocular bobbing**: lesion in pontine tegmentum (*see page 588*)
    B. **ocular dysmetria**: overshoot of eye on attempted fixation followed by diminishing oscillations until eye "hones in" on target. Lesion in cerebellum or pathways (may be seen in Friedreich's ataxia)
    C. ping-pong gaze: *see page 158*
    D. "windshield wiper eyes": *see page 158*

21.2. Papilledema

AKA choked (optic) disk. Thought to be caused by axoplasmic stasis. One theory: elevated ICP is transmitted through the subarachnoid space of the optic nerve sheath to the region of the optic disc. Elevated ICP will usually obliterate retinal venous pulsation if the pressure is transmitted to the point where the central retinal vein passes through the subarachnoid space (≈ 1 cm posterior to the globe). Papilledema may also be dependent on the ratio of retinal arterial to retinal venous pressure, with ratios < 1.5:1 more commonly associated with papilledema than higher ratios.

Elevated ICP generally causes bilateral papilledema (*see below* for *unilateral* papilledema). Papilledema may appear similar to optic neuritis on funduscopy, but the latter is usually associated with more severe visual loss and tenderness to pressure over the eye.

Papilledema typically takes 24-48 hours to develop following a sustained rise in ICP. It is rarely seen as early as ≈ 6 hours after onset, but not earlier. Papilledema does not cause visual blurring or reduction of visual fields unless very severe and prolonged.

Differential diagnosis of <u>unilateral</u> papilledema:
1. compressive lesions
   A. orbital tumors
   B. tumors of optic nerve sheath (meningiomas)
   C. optic nerve tumors (optic gliomas)
2. local inflammatory disorder
3. Foster-Kennedy syndrome: *see page 85*
4. demyelinating disease (e.g. multiple sclerosis)
5. elevated ICP (as in pseudotumor cerebri) with some form of blockage on the normal appearing side which prevents transmission of elevated CSF pressure to that optic disc[4]
6. eye prosthesis (artificial eye)

21.3.   Pupillary diameter

PUPILODILATOR (SYMPATHETIC)
Pupilodilator muscle fibers are arranged radially in the iris.

First-order sympathetic nerve fibers arise in the posterolateral hypothalamus, and descend uncrossed in the lateral tegmentum of the midbrain, pons, medulla and cervical spinal cord to the intermediolateral cell column of the spinal cord from C8 T2 (ciliospinal center of Budge). Here they synapse with lateral horn cells (neurotransmitter: ACh) and give off 2nd order neurons (preganglionics).

Second-order neurons enter the sympathetic chain and ascend but do not synapse until they reach the superior cervical ganglion, where they give rise to 3rd order neurons.

Third-order neurons (postganglionics) course upward with the common carotid artery, those that mediate sweat in the face split off with the ECA. The rest travel with the ICA passing over the carotid sinus. Some fibers accompany V1 (ophthalmic division of trigeminal nerve), passing through (without synapsing) the ciliary ganglion, reaching the pupilodilator muscle of the eye as 2 long ciliary nerves (neurotransmitter: NE). Other fibers from the ICA travel with the ophthalmic artery to innervate the lacrimal gland and Müller's muscle (AKA the orbital muscle).

PUPILLOCONSTRICTOR (PARASYMPATHETIC)
Pupilloconstrictor muscle fibers are arranged as a sphincter in the iris.

Parasympathetic preganglionic fibers arise in the **Edinger-Westphal nucleus** (in high midbrain, superior colliculus level). They synapse in the ciliary ganglion and give off postganglionics which travel within the substance of the third cranial nerve (located peripherally) to innervate the sphincter pupillae and ciliary muscle (parasympathetic stimulation of the latter relaxes the lens which "thickens" and accommodates).

PUPILLARY LIGHT REFLEX
Mediated by rods and cones of the retina which are stimulated by light, and transmit via their axons in the optic nerve. As with the visual path, temporal retinal fibers remain ipsilateral, whereas nasal retinal fibers decussate in the optic chiasm. Fibers subserving the light reflex bypass the lateral geniculate body **(LGB)** (unlike fibers for vision which enter the LGB) to synapse in the **pretectal nuclear complex** at the level of the superior colliculus. Intercalating neurons connect to both Edinger-Westphal parasympathetic motor nuclei. The preganglionic fibers travel within the third nerve to the ciliary ganglion as described above under *Pupilloconstrictor (parasympathetic)*.

Monocular light normally stimulates bilaterally symmetric (i.e. equal) pupillary constriction (ipsilateral response is called *direct*, contralateral response is *consensual*).

A complete bedside pupillary exam consists of:
1. measuring pupil size in a lighted room
2. measuring pupil size in a darkened room
3. noting the reaction to bright light (direct and consensual)
4. near response: it is necessary to check this only if the light reaction is not good: the pupil normally constricts on convergence, and this response should be greater than the light reflex (accommodation is not necessary, and a visually handicapped patient can be instructed to follow their own finger as it is brought in)
    A. **light-near dissociation**: pupillary constriction on convergence and absent light response, classically described in syphilis (**Argyll Robertson pupil**)
5. **swinging flashlight test**: alternate the flashlight from one eye to the other with as little delay as possible in moving to the other side; wait at least 5 seconds for the pupil to redilate (dilation after initial constriction is called **pupillary escape** and is a normal phenomenon due to retinal adaptation). Normally the direct and consensual light reflexes are equal; if the consensual reflex is stronger than the direct (enlargement of the pupil on direct illumination compared to its size with consensual response), this is an **afferent pupillary defect** (*see below*)

21.3.1. Alterations in pupillary diameter

MARCUS GUNN PUPIL

AKA **afferent pupillary defect (APD)**, AKA amaurotic pupil. Finding: consensual reflex is stronger than the direct (opposite of normal). Contrary to some textbooks, the amaurotic pupil is <u>not</u> larger than the other[5]. The presence of the consensual reflex is evidence of a preserved third nerve (with parasympathetics) on the side of the impaired direct reflex. Best detected with the swinging flashlight test (*see above*).

Etiologies

Lesion ipsilateral to the side of the impaired direct reflex, <u>anterior to the chiasm</u>:
1. either in the retina (e.g. retinal detachment, retinal infarct e.g. from embolus)
2. or optic nerve, as may occur in:
    A. optic or retrobulbar neuritis: commonly seen in MS, but may also occur after vaccinations or viral infections, and usually improves gradually
    B. trauma to the optic nerve: indirect (*see page 645*) or direct

ANISOCORIA

Key point: an afferent pupillary defect (**APD**) together with anisocoria indicates two separate lesions (i.e. an APD alone does <u>not</u> produce anisocoria) (*see below*).

Differential diagnosis:
1. physiologic anisocoria: < 1 mm difference in pupil size that is the same in a light and dark room. Seen in ≈ 20% of population (more common in people with a light iris)
2. Horner's syndrome: interruption of sympathetics to pupilodilator (*see page 583*). Here the abnormal pupil is the <u>smaller</u> pupil (miosis)
3. Adie's pupil (AKA tonic pupil): *see below*
4. third nerve palsy (*see page 585*)
    A. oculomotor neuropathy (a "peripheral" neuropathy of the third nerve): usually spares pupil. Etiologies: DM (usually resolves in ≈ 8 weeks), EtOH…
    B. compression: including by the following (tends <u>not</u> to spare pupil)
        1. aneurysm:
            a. p-comm: the most common aneurysm to cause this
            b. basilar bifurcation: occasionally compresses posterior III nerve
        2. uncal herniation: see *Oculomotor nerve compression* below
5. local trauma to the eye: so-called traumatic iridoplegia can occur in isolation (may result in traumatic mydriasis or miosis)
6. pharmacologic pupil: *see below*
7. light-near dissociation: *see above*
    A. Argyll Robertson pupil: classically described in syphilis (*see page 582*)
    B. Parinaud's syndrome: dorsal midbrain lesion (*see page 86*)
    C. oculomotor neuropathy (usually causes a tonic pupil as in oculomotor compression, *see below*): DM, EtOH
    D. Adie's pupil: *see below*

8. eye prosthesis (artificial eye)

ADIE'S PUPIL (TONIC PUPIL)

An iris palsy resulting in a dilated pupil, due to impaired postganglionic parasympathetics. Thought to be due to a viral infection of the ciliary ganglion. When associated with loss of all muscle tendon reflexes it is called Holmes-Adie's (is not limited to knee jerks, as some texts indicate). Typically seen in a woman in her twenties.

Slit-lamp exam shows some parts of iris contract and others don't.

These patients exhibit light-near dissociation (see above): in checking near response it is necessary to wait a few seconds. Dilute pilocarpine (0.1-0.125%), a parasympathomimetic, causes miosis (constriction) in Adie's pupil possibly because of denervation supersensitivity (normal pupils will react only to ≈ 1% pilocarpine).

PHARMACOLOGIC PUPIL

Occurs following administration of a mydriatic agent. This sometimes may be "occult" when other care providers have not been alerted that a mydriatic agent has been used, or when health care personnel unwittingly inoculate agents, such as scopolamine, into a patient's eye or into their own eye. May present with accompanying H/A, and if it is unknown that a mydriatic is involved, this may be misinterpreted e.g. as a warning of an expanding p-comm aneurysm.

A pharmacologically dilated pupil is very large (7-8 mm), which is even larger than mydriasis due to third nerve compression (5-6 mm).

Management: Can admit and observe overnight, pupil should normalize. May also differentiate this from a third nerve lesion by instilling 1% pilocarpine (a parasympathomimetic) in both eyes (for comparison): a pharmacologic pupil does not constrict, whereas the normal side and a dilated pupil from a third nerve palsy will.

Using mydriatic agents to produce pupillary dilatation

Indications: to improve the ability to examine the retina. NB: ability to follow bedside examination of pupils will be lost for duration of drug effect. This could mask pupillary dilatation from third nerve compression due to herniation (see page 161 and page 162). Always alert other caregivers and place a note in the chart that the pupil has been pharmacologically dilated (see above), including the agent(s) used and the time administered.

Rx: 2 gtt of 0.5% or 1% tropicamide (Mydriacyl®) blocks the parasympathetic supply to pupil, and produces a mydriasis that lasts a couple hrs to half a day. This can be augmented with 1 gtt 2.5% phenylephrine ophthalmic (Mydfrin®, Neofrin®, Phenoptic® and others) which stimulates the sympathetics.

OCULOMOTOR NERVE COMPRESSION

Third nerve compression may manifest initially with a mildly dilated pupil (5-6 mm). Possible etiologies include uncal herniation or expansion of a p-comm or basilar bifurcation aneurysm. However, within 24 hours, most of these cases will also develop an oculomotor palsy (with down and out deviation of the eye and ptosis). These pupils respond to mydriatics and to miotic agents (the latter helps differentiate this from a pharmacologic pupil, see above).

Although it is possible for a unilaterally dilated pupil alone to be the initial presentation in uncal herniation, in actuality almost all of these patients will have some other finding, e.g. alteration in mental status (confusion, agitation, etc.) before midbrain compression occurs (i.e. it would be rare for a person undergoing early uncal herniation to be awake, talking, appropriate and neurologically intact).

NEUROMUSCULAR BLOCKING AGENTS (NMBAS)

Due to the absence of nicotinic receptors on the iris, non-depolarizing muscle blocking agents, such as pancuronium (Pavulon®) do not alter pupillary reaction to light[6] except in large doses where some of the first and second order neurons may be blocked.

HORNER'S SYNDROME

Horner's syndrome (HS) is caused by interruption of sympathetics to the eye and face anywhere along their path (see *Pupilodilator (sympathetic)*, page 581). Unilateral findings on the involved side in a fully developed Horner's syndrome are shown in *Table 21-1*.

Miosis (pupillary constriction) in HS

The miosis in Horner's syndrome is only ≈ 2-3 mm. This will be brought out by darkening the room, which causes the normal pupil to dilate.

Table 21-1 Findings in Horner's syndrome
• miosis (constricted pupil)
• ptosis
• enophthalmos
• hyperemia of eye
• anhidrosis of half of face

Ptosis and enophthalmos

Ptosis is due primarily to paralysis of the superior and inferior tarsal muscles (weakness of the inferior tarsal muscle is actually considered "inverse ptosis"). Enophthalmos is due to **Müller's muscle** paralysis, which also contributes a maximum of ≈ 2 mm to the ptosis. Ptosis in HS is partial, if complete ptosis is present, it is due to weakness of levator palpebra superioris which is not involved in Horner's syndrome.

ANATOMY

1st order neuron (central neuron): Interruption between hypothalamus and intermediolateral cell column of C8-T2 spinal cord. Often accompanied by other brainstem abnormalities. Etiologies: infarction from vascular occlusion (usually PICA), syringobulbia, intraparenchymal neoplasm.

2nd order neuron (preganglionic): Interruption between spinal cord and superior cervical ganglion. Etiologies: lateral sympathectomies, significant chest trauma, apical pulmonary neoplasms[7] (Pancoast's tumor).

3rd order neuron (postganglionic): Interruption after superior cervical ganglion (sympathetics travel on carotid artery); most common type. Etiologies: neck trauma, carotid vascular disease/studies (e.g. carotid dissections, *see page 885*), cervical bony abnormalities, migraine, skull base neoplasms. With involvement only of fibers on ICA, anhidrosis does not occur (i.e. sweating is preserved) on ipsilateral face since fibers to facial sweat glands travel with ECA.

PHARMACOLOGIC TESTING IN HORNER'S SYNDROME

Establishing the diagnosis

Cocaine is used if the diagnosis of a Horner's syndrome is in doubt (not necessary when a pupil lag upon darkening the room can be demonstrated in the affected eye). Has no localizing value. *Rx*: 1 gtt 4% cocaine OU (not the 10% solution that is commonly used in ENT procedures which will also anesthetize the sphincter pupillae, thus preventing miosis), repeat in 10 min. Observe pupils over 30 min. Cocaine blocks the NE re-uptake of postganglionics at the neuroeffector junction. In HS, no NE is released and cocaine will not dilate eye. If pupil dilates normally, no HS. Delayed dilatation occurs in partial HS.

Localizing the site of the lesion

First order HS usually is accompanied by other hypothalamic, brainstem, or medullary findings.

To differentiate a second from third-order: 1% hydroxyamphetamine (Paradrine®) releases NE from nerve endings at neuroeffector junction causing dilation of pupil except in 3rd order neuron lesions (injured postganglionics do not release NE).

21.4. Extraocular motor system

Cr. N. III innervates the ipsilateral medial rectus **(MR)**, inferior rectus **(IR)**, inferior oblique **(IO)**, and contralateral superior rectus **(SR)**. Cr. N IV (the only cranial nerve that decussates; may decussate internally) innervates the contralateral superior oblique **(SO)** (depresses the adducted eye). Cr. N. VI innervates the ipsilateral lateral rectus **(LR)**.

The **frontal eye field** is the cortical area that initiates voluntary (supranuclear) lateral saccadic eye movements ("pre-programmed", rapid, ballistic) to the opposite side, and is located in Brodmann's area 8 (in the frontal lobe, anterior to the primary motor cortex, see *Figure 3-1*, page 68). These corticobulbar fibers pass through the genu of the internal capsule to the paramedian pontine reticular formation **(PPRF)**, which sends fibers to the ipsilateral abducens/para-abducens (VI) nuclear complex, and via the medial longitudinal fasciculus **(MLF)** to the contralateral III nucleus to innervate the contralateral MR. Inhibitory fibers go to the ipsilateral third nerve to inhibit the antagonist MR muscle. Thus, the right PPRF controls lateral eye movements to right.

INTERNUCLEAR OPHTHALMOPLEGIA

Internuclear ophthalmoplegia (INO) is due to a lesion of the MLF (*see above*) rostral to the abducens nucleus, and produces the following:
1. the eye ipsilateral to the lesion fails to ADDuct completely on attempting to look to the opposite side
2. adduction nystagmus in the contralateral eye (monocular nystagmus) often with some weakness of ABDuction (together with #1 produces a lateral gaze palsy)
3. convergence is not impaired in isolated MLF lesions (INO is not an EOM palsy)

The most common causes of INO:
1. MS: the most common cause of bilateral INO in young adults
2. brainstem stroke: the most common cause of unilateral INO in the elderly

OCULOMOTOR (CR. N. III) NERVE PALSY (OMP)

May include peripherally located fibers mediating pupillary constriction (parasympathetics), and motor fibers to the following EOMs: SR, MR, IR, IO.

Oculomotor nerve motor palsy causes ptosis with eye deviated "down & out". Nuclear involvement of 3rd nerve is rare. NB: 3rd nerve palsy alone can cause up to 3 mm exophthalmos (proptosis) from relaxation of the rectus muscles.

Also see *Painful ophthalmoplegia* and *Painless ophthalmoplegia* below. For brainstem syndromes, see *Benedikt's syndrome*, page 86 and *Weber's syndrome* on page 85. Also, see *Anisocoria*, page 582.

The rule of the pupil in third nerve palsy

Elucidated in 1958 by Rucker. In effect, states "Extrinsic compression of the third nerve impairs pupillary constriction." However it is often overlooked that in 3% the pupil was spared and there was slight impairment of the extraocular muscles[8].

Pupil sparing oculomotor palsy (pupils react to light): Usually from intrinsic vascular lesions occluding vaso-nervorum causing central ischemic infarction. Spares parasympathetic fibers located peripherally in 3rd nerve in 62-83% of cases[8]. Etiologies include:
1. diabetic neuropathy
2. atherosclerosis (as seen in chronic HTN)
3. vasculopathies: including giant cell arteritis (temporal arteritis) - *see page 58*
4. chronic progressive ophthalmoplegia: usually bilateral
5. myasthenia gravis

Rarely, pupil-sparing OMP has been described following an intra-axial lesion, as in a midbrain infarction[9].

Non pupil-sparing oculomotor palsy: Usually from extrinsic compression.
1. tumor: the most common tumors affecting 3rd nerve:
   A. chordomas
   B. clival meningiomas
2. vascular: the most common vascular lesions:
   A. aneurysms of p-comm artery (pupil sparing with aneurysmal oculomotor palsy occurs in < 1%). ★ Development of a new 3rd nerve palsy ipsilateral to a p-comm aneurysm may be a sign of expansion with the possibility of imminent rupture, and is traditionally considered an indication for urgent treatment (*see page 805*)
   B. aneurysms of the distal basilar artery or bifurcation (basilar tip)
3. uncal herniation
4. cavernous sinus lesions: usually cause additional cranial nerve findings (V_1, V_2, IV, VI; see *Cavernous sinus syndrome*, page 918). Classically the third nerve palsy e.g. from enlarging cavernous aneurysm will not produce a dilated pupil because the sympathetics which dilate the pupil are also paralyzed[1 (p 1492)]

Other causes of oculomotor palsy

Trauma, uncal herniation, laterally expanding pituitary adenomas, Lyme disease, cavernous sinus lesions: usually cause additional cranial nerve findings (see *Multiple cranial nerve palsies (cranial neuropathies)*, page 917).

Lesions within the orbit tend to affect 3rd nerve branches unequally. Superior division lesion → ptosis and impaired elevation; inferior division lesion → impairment of depression, adduction and pupillary reaction.

ABDUCENS (VI) PALSY

Produces a lateral rectus palsy. Clinically produces diplopia that is exaggerated with lateral gaze to the side of the palsy. Etiologies of isolated 6th nerve palsy include[10]:
1. vasculopathy: including diabetes and giant cell arteritis. Most cases resolve within 3 months (alternative cause should be sought in cases lasting longer)
2. **increased intracranial pressure**: palsy may occur with increased ICP even in the absence of direct compression of the nerve (a "false localizing" sign in this setting). Postulated to occur due to the fact that the VI nerve has a long intracranial course which may render it more sensitive to increased pressure. May be bilateral. Etiologies include:
   A. traumatically increased ICP: *see page 637*
   B. increased ICP due to hydrocephalus (e.g. from p-fossa tumor): *see page 404*
   C. idiopathic intracranial hypertension (pseudotumor cerebri): *see page 493*
3. cavernous sinus lesions: cavernous carotid aneurysm (*see page 818*), neoplasm (meningioma...), carotid cavernous fistula (*see page 845*)
4. inflammatory:
   A. Gradenigo's syndrome (involvement at Dorello's canal): *see page 588*
   B. sphenoid sinusitis: (involvement at Dorello's canal)
5. intracranial neoplasm: e.g. clivus chordoma, chondrosarcoma
6. pseudoabducens palsy: may be due to
   A. thyroid eye disease: the most common cause of chronic VI palsy. Will have positive forced duction test (eye cannot be moved by examiner)
   B. myasthenia gravis: responds to edrophonium (Tensilon®) test
   C. long-standing strabismus
   D. Duane's syndrome
   E. fracture of the medial wall of the orbit with medial rectus entrapment
7. following lumbar puncture: almost invariably unilateral (*see page 616*)
8. fracture through clivus: *see page 665*
9. idiopathic

MULTIPLE EXTRAOCULAR MOTOR NERVE INVOLVEMENT

Lesions in cavernous sinus (*see below*) involve cranial nerves III, IV, VI and V_1 & V_2 (ophthalmic and maxillary divisions of trigeminal nerve), and spare II and V_3.
Superior orbital fissure syndrome: dysfunction of nerves III, IV, VI and V_1.
Orbital apex syndrome: involves II, III, IV, VI and partial V_1.
4th nerve palsy may result from a contrecoup injury in frontal head trauma.

PAINFUL OPHTHALMOPLEGIA

Definition: pain and dysfunction of ocular motility (may be due to involvement of one or more of cranial nerves III, IV, V & VI).

ETIOLOGIES
1. intraorbital
   A. inflammatory pseudotumor (idiopathic orbital inflammation): *see below*
   B. contiguous sinusitis
   C. invasive fungal sinus infection producing orbital apex syndrome. Rhinocerebral <u>mucormycosis</u> (AKA zygomycosis): sinusitis with painless black palatal or nasal septal ulcer or eschar with hyphal invasion of blood vessels by fungi of the order *Mucorales*, especially *rhizopus*[11]. Usually seen in diabetic or immunocompromised patients, occasionally in otherwise healthy patients[12]. Often involves dural sinuses and may cause cavernous sinus thrombosis
   D. mets
   E. lymphoma
2. superior orbital fissure/anterior cavernous sinus
   A. Tolosa-Hunt syndrome: *see below*
   B. mets

C. nasopharyngeal Ca
D. lymphoma
E. herpes zoster
F. carotid-cavernous fistula
G. cavernous sinus thrombosis
H. intracavernous aneurysm
3. parasellar region
A. pituitary adenoma
B. mets
C. nasopharyngeal Ca
D. sphenoid sinus mucocele
E. meningioma/chordoma
F. apical petrositis (Gradenigo's syndrome): *see below*
4. posterior fossa
A. p-comm aneurysm
B. basilar artery aneurysm (rare)
5. miscellaneous
A. diabetic ophthalmoplegia
B. migrainous ophthalmoplegia
C. cranial arteritis
D. tuberculous meningitis: may cause ophthalmoplegia, usually incomplete, most often primarily oculomotor nerve

PAINLESS OPHTHALMOPLEGIA
Differential diagnosis:
1. chronic progressive ophthalmoplegia: pupil sparing, usually bilateral, slowly progressive
2. myasthenia gravis: pupil sparing, responds to edrophonium (Tensilon®) test
0. myositis: usually also produces symptoms in other organ systems (heart, gonads...)

PSEUDOTUMOR (OF THE ORBIT)
AKA **"chronic granuloma"** (a misnomer, since true epithelioid granulomas are rarely found). An idiopathic inflammatory disease confined to the orbit that may mimic a true neoplasm. Usually unilateral.

Typically presents with rapid onset of proptosis, pain, and EOM dysfunction (painful ophthalmoplegia with diplopia). Most commonly involves the superior orbital tissues.

Differential diagnosis:
See *Orbital lesions* on page 929 for list.
Key points for Grave's disease **(GD)**: the histologic appearance of GD (hyperthyroidism) may be indistinguishable from pseudotumor. Involvement with GD is usually bilateral.

TREATMENT
Surgery tends to cause a flare up, and is thus usually best avoided.
Steroids are the treatment of choice. **Rx**: 50-80 mg prednisone q d. Severe cases may necessitate treatment with 30-40 mg/d for several months.
Radiation treatment with 1000-2000 rads may be needed for cases of reactive lymphocytic hyperplasia.

TOLOSA-HUNT SYNDROME
Nonspecific inflammation in the region of the superior orbital fissure, often with extension into the cavernous sinus, sometimes with granulomatous features. A diagnosis of exclusion. May be a topographical variant of orbital pseudotumor (*see above*). Clinical diagnostic criteria:
1. painful ophthalmoplegia
2. involvement of any nerve traversing the cavernous sinus. The pupil is usually spared (frequently not the case with aneurysms, specific inflammation, etc.)
3. symptoms last days to weeks
4. spontaneous remission, sometimes with residual deficit

5. recurrent attacks with remissions of months or years
6. no systemic involvement (occasional N/V, due to pain?)
7. dramatic improvement with systemic steroids: 60-80 mg prednisone PO q day (slow taper), relief within about 1 day
8. occasional inflammation of rectus muscle from contiguous inflammation

RAEDER'S PARATRIGEMINAL NEURALGIA

Two essential components[13]:
1. unilateral oculosympathetic paresis (AKA partial Horner's syndrome (HS), this usually lacks anhidrosis, and in this syndrome, possibly ptosis also)
2. homolateral trigeminal nerve involvement (usually tic-like pain, but may be analgesia or masseter weakness; pain, if present, must be tic-like and does not include e.g. unilateral head, face or vascular pain)

Localizing value: region adjacent to trigeminal nerve in middle fossa. The cause is often not determined, but may rarely be due to aneurysm[14] compressing V_1 with sympathetics.

GRADENIGO'S SYNDROME

AKA apical petrositis. Mastoiditis with involvement of petrous apex (if pneumatized). Usually seen by ENT physicians. Classic triad:
1. abducens palsy: from inflammation of 6th nerve at Dorello's canal, which is where it enters the cavernous sinus just medial to the petrous apex
2. retro-orbital pain: due to inflammation of V_1
3. draining ear

21.5. Miscellaneous neurophthalmologic signs

Corneal mandibular reflex: eliciting the corneal reflex produces a jaw jerk or contralateral jaw movement (ipsilateral pterygoid contraction). A primitive pontine reflex, may be seen in a variety of insults to the brain (trauma, intracerebral hemorrhage...).

Hippus: spasmodic, rhythmic pupillary movement. A "normal" variant. May confuse examination when checking pupillary responses; record the initial response.

Marcus Gunn phenomenon: not to be confused with Marcus Gunn *pupil* (*see page 582*). Opening the mouth causes opening of a ptotic eye (abnormal reflex between proprioception of pterygoid muscles and third nerve). Reverse Marcus Gunn phenomenon: normal eye that closes with opening the mouth. Seen only in patients with peripheral facial nerve injuries, and probably results from aberrant regeneration.

Ocular bobbing[15]: abrupt, spontaneous, conjugate downward eye deviation with slow return to midposition, 2 to 12 times per min; associated with bilateral paralysis of horizontal gaze, including to doll's-eyes and calorics. Most commonly seen with destructive lesions of the pontine tegmentum (usually hemorrhage, but also infarction, glioma, trauma), but has also been described with compressive lesions[16]. Atypical bobbing is similar except that horizontal gaze is preserved, and can be seen with cerebellar hemorrhage, hydrocephalus, trauma, metabolic encephalopathy...

Opsoclonus[17]: (rare) rapid, conjugate, irregular, non-rhythmic (differentiates this from nystagmus) eye movements vertically or horizontally, persist (attenuated) during sleep (opsochoria if dysconjugate). Usually associated with diffuse myoclonus (fingers, chin, lips, eyelid, forehead, trunk and LEs); also, malaise, fatigability, vomiting and some cerebellar findings. Often resolves spontaneously within 4 mos.

Oscillopsia: visual sensation that stationary objects are swaying side-to-side or vibrating[18]. Rarely the sole manifestation of Chiari I malformation[19] (often associated with downbeat nystagmus). Other causes include MS, or injury to both vestibular nerves (e.g. aminoglycoside ototoxicity[20], bilateral vestibular neurectomies (see *Dandy's syndrome*, page 591)).

Chronic, progressive optic atrophy is due to a compressive lesion (aneurysm, meningioma, osteopetrosis...) until proven otherwise.

21.6. References

1. Wilkins R H, Rengachary S S, (eds.): **Neurosurgery**. McGraw-Hill, New York, 1985.
2. Pinel J F, Larmande P, Guegan Y, *et al.*: Down-beat nystagmus: Case report with magnetic resonance imaging and surgical treatment. **Neurosurgery** 21: 736-9, 1987.
3. Williams D P, Troost B T, Rogers J: Lithium-induced downbeat nystagmus. **Arch Neurol** 45: 1022-3, 1988.
4. Sher N A, Wirtschafter J, Shapiro S K, *et al.*: Unilateral papilledema in 'benign' intracranial hypertension (pseudotumor cerebri). **JAMA** 250: 2346-7, 1983.
5. Walsh F B, Hoyt W F, (eds.): **Clinical neuro-ophthalmology**. 3rd ed., Williams and Wilkins, Baltimore, 1969.
6. Widjicks E F: Determining brain death in adults. **Neurology** 45: 1003-11, 1995.
7. Lepore F E: Diagnostic pharmacology of the pupil. **Clin Neuropharmacol** 8: 27-37, 1985.
8. Trobe J D: Third nerve palsy and the pupil. Footnotes to the rule. **Arch Ophthalmol** 106 (5): 601-2, 1988.
9. Breen L A, Hopf H C, Farris B K, *et al.*: Pupil-sparing oculomotor nerve palsy due to midbrain infarction. **Arch Neurol** 48: 105-6, 1991.
10. Galetta S L, Smith J L: Chronic isolated sixth nerve palsies. **Arch Neurol** 46: 79-82, 1989.
11. DeShazo R D, Chapin K, Swain R E: Fungal sinusitis. **N Engl J Med** 337: 254-9, 1997.
12. Radner A B, Witt M D, Edwards J E: Acute invasive rhinocerebral zygomycosis in an otherwise healthy patient: Case report and review. **Clin Infect Dis** 20: 163-6, 1995.
13. Mokri B: Raeder's paratrigeminal syndrome. **Arch Neurol** 39: 395-9, 1982.
14. Kashihara K, Ito H, Yamamoto S, *et al.*: Raeder's syndrome associated with intracranial internal carotid artery aneurysm. **Neurosurgery** 20: 49-51, 1987.
15. Fisher C M: Ocular bobbing. **Arch Neurol** 11: 543-6, 1964.
16. Sherman D G, Salmon J H: Ocular bobbing with superior cerebellar artery aneurysm: Case report. **J Neurosurg** 47: 596-8, 1977.
17. Smith J L, Walsh F B: Opsoclonus - ataxic conjugate movements of the eyes. **Arch Ophthalm** 64: 244-50, 1960.
18. Brickner R: Oscillopsia: A new symptom commonly occurring in multiple sclerosis. **Arch Neurol Psychiatry** 36: 586-9, 1936.
19. Gingold S I, Winfield J A: Oscillopsia and primary cerebellar ectopie: Case report and review of the literature. **Neurosurgery** 29: 932-6, 1991.
20. Mann T R, Reynolds N C, Stoddard J J: Subjective oscillopsia ("jiggling vision") presumably due to aminoglycoside ototoxicity: A report of two cases. **J Clin Neuro Ophthalmol** 8: 35-8, 1988.

22. Neurotology

22.1.   Dizziness and vertigo

Differential diagnosis of dizziness:
1. near syncope: some overlap with syncope (see *Syncope and apoplexy*, page 914)
   A. orthostatic hypotension
   B. cardiogenic hypotension
       1. arrhythmia
       2. valvular disease
   C. vasovagal episode
   D. hypersensitive carotid sinus: (see *Syncope and apoplexy*, page 914)
2. dysequilibrium
   A. multiple sensory deficits: e.g. peripheral neuropathy, visual impairment
   B. cerebellar degeneration
3. vertigo: sensation of movement (usually spinning)
   A. inner ear dysfunction
       1. labyrinthitis
       2. Meniere's disease (*see below*)
       3. trauma: endolymphatic leak
       4. drugs: especially aminoglycosides
       5. **benign (paroxysmal) positional vertigo**[1]: AKA cupulolithiasis.
           Attacks of severe vertigo when the head is turned to certain positions
           (usually in bed). Due to calcium concretions in the semicircular ca-
           nals. Self limited (most cases do not last > 1 year). No hearing loss
       6. syphilis
       7. vertebrobasilar insufficiency: *see page 881*
   B. vestibular nerve dysfunction
       1. vestibular neuronitis: sudden onset of vertigo, gradual improvement
       2. compression:
           a. meningioma
           b. acoustic neuroma: usually slowly progressive ataxia instead of
               severe vertigo. BSAER latencies usually abnormal. CT or MRI
               usually abnormal
   C. **disabling positional vertigo**: as described by Jannetta et al.[2], constant
       disabling positional vertigo or dysequilibrium, causing ≈ constant nausea,
       no vestibular dysfunction nor hearing loss (tinnitus may be present). One
       possible cause is vascular compression of the vestibular nerve which may
       respond to microvascular decompression
   D. brainstem dysfunction
       1. vascular disease (see *Vertebrobasilar insufficiency*, page 881): less dis-
           tinct vestibular symptoms, prominent nonvestibular symptoms
       2. migraine: especially basilar artery migraine
       3. demyelinating disease: e.g. multiple sclerosis
       4. drugs: anticonvulsants, alcohol, sedatives/hypnotics, salicylates
   E. dysfunction of cervical proprioceptors: as in cervical osteoarthritis
4. poorly defined lightheadedness: mostly psychiatric. May also include:
   A. hyperventilation
   B. hypoglycemia
   C. anxiety neurosis
   D. hysterical

VESTIBULAR NEURECTOMY
Complete loss of vestibular function from one side is thought to produce transient

vertigo due to the mismatch of vestibular input from the two ears. Theoretically, a central compensatory mechanism (the "**cerebellar clamp**") results in the amelioration of symptoms. In cases of unilateral fluctuating vestibular dysfunction, this compensatory mechanism may be impaired. Unilateral selective vestibular neurectomy **(SVN)** may convert the fluctuating or partial loss to a complete cessation of input and facilitate compensation. Bilateral SVN is often complicated by oscillopsia (*see page 588*, AKA **Dandy's syndrome**, with difficulty in maintaining balance in the dark due to loss of the vestibulo-ocular reflex) and is to be avoided.

Indications

The two conditions for which SVN is most commonly employed are Meniere's disease (*see below*) and partial vestibular injury (viral or traumatic). SVN may be indicated in disabling cases refractory to medical or non-destructive surgical treatment when vestibular studies demonstrate continued or progressive uncompensated vestibular dysfunction[3].

SVN preserves hearing and in Meniere's disease is > 90% effective in eliminating episodic vertiginous spells (≈ 80% success rate in non-Meniere's cases), but is unlikely to improve stability with rapid head movement.

Surgical approaches for SVN

1. **retrolabyrinthine**, AKA postauricular approach: anterior to sigmoid sinus. Primary choice in patients with Meniere's disease who have not had previous endolymphatic sac **(ELS)** procedures since it permits simultaneous SVN and decompression of the endolymphatic sac. Requires mastoidectomy with skeletonization of the semicircular canals and ELS. The dural opening is bounded anteriorly by the posterior semicircular canal, posteriorly by the sigmoid sinus. Watertight dural closure is difficult
2. **retrosigmoid**, AKA posterior fossa, AKA suboccipital approach: posterior to sigmoid sinus. The original approach plied by Dandy in pre-microsurgical era, usually sacrificed hearing, and occasionally facial nerve function. Better results today with microscopic techniques. Indicated for cases other than Meniere's disease where there is no need for identification of the ELS. Also the best approach for positive identification of eighth nerve
3. **middle fossa** (extradural) approach: the fibers of the vestibular division may be more segregated from the cochlear fibers in the IAC than in the CPA, thus permitting more complete section of the vestibular nerve. May be appropriate for failed response to SVN by the above approaches. Disadvantages: requires temporal lobe retraction, does not allow exposure of ELS, and higher morbidity and risk of damage to facial nerve[4] than retrolabyrinthine approach

Surgical considerations for selective vestibular neurectomy

(Also see *Figure 3-5*, page 72)

- the vestibular nerve is in the superior half of the eighth nerve complex, and is slightly more gray in color than the cochlear division (due to less myelin[5]). They may be separated by a small vessel or by an indentation in the bundle
- facial (VII) nerve:
  - whiter than the VIII nerve complex
  - lies anterior and superiorly to the VIII nerve
  - EMG monitoring of the facial nerve is recommended
  - direct stimulation confirms the identification
- any vessels present on eighth nerve bundle must be preserved to save hearing (primarily, the artery of the auditory canal must be preserved)
- if no plane of cleavage can be defined between vestibular & cochlear divisions, the superior half of the nerve bundle is divided
- the endolymphatic sac lies ≈ midway between the posterior edge of the internal auditory meatus and the sigmoid sinus

---

22.2. Meniere's disease

Probably due to a derangement of endolymphatic fluid regulation (a consistent finding is **endolymphatic hydrops**: increased endolymphatic volume and pressure with dilatation of endolymph spaces), with resultant fistulization into the perilymphatic spaces.

Clinical triad
- attacks of violent vertigo (due to vestibular nerve dysfunction): usually the earliest and the most disabling symptom. Nausea, vomiting, and diaphoresis are frequent concomitants. Severe attacks may cause prostration. Vertigo may persist even after complete deafness. Balance is normal between attacks
- tinnitus: often described as resembling the sound of escaping steam, not a true "ringing"
- fluctuating low frequency hearing loss: may fluctuate for a periods of weeks to years, and may progress to permanent deafness if untreated (a sensation of fullness in the ear is commonly described[6], however, this is nonspecific and may occur with hearing loss for any reason)

Drop attacks ("otolithic crises of Tumarkin") occasionally occur.

Attack duration: $\approx$ 5-30 minutes (some say 2-6 hours), with a "post-ictal" period of fatigue lasting several hrs.

Frequency: varies from one or two attacks a year to several times per week.

Two subtypes differ from classical form: vestibular Meniere's (episodic vertigo with normal hearing) and cochlear Meniere's (few vestibular symptoms).

Natural course of syndrome is characterized by periods of remission. Eventually the vertiginous attacks either progress in severity, or "burn out" (being replaced by constant unsteadiness[6]).

Incidence $\approx$ 1 per 100,000 population[7]. Most cases have onset between 30-60 years of age, rarely in youth or in the elderly. May become bilateral in 20%.

(Also see *Differential diagnosis: Dizziness and vertigo* on page 590 for more details)
1. benign (paroxysmal) positional vertigo: AKA cupulolithiasis. Self limited (most cases last < 1 year). No hearing loss
2. disabling positional vertigo: constant disabling positional vertigo or dysequilibrium, $\approx$ constant nausea, no vestibular dysfunction nor hearing loss (tinnitus may be present)
3. acoustic neuroma: usually slowly progressive ataxia instead of episodic severe vertigo. BSAER latencies usually abnormal. CT or MRI usually positive
4. vestibular neuronitis: sudden onset of vertigo with gradual improvement
5. vertebrobasilar insufficiency (VBI): less distinct vestibular symptoms, and prominence of nonvestibular symptoms (*see page 881*)

1. electronystagmography (ENG) with bithermal caloric stimulation usually abnormal, may show blunted thermal responses
2. audiogram: low frequency hearing loss, fairly good preservation of discrimination and loudness recruitment, negative tone decay on impedance testing
3. BSAER usually shows normal latencies
4. radiographic imaging (CT, MRI, etc.): no findings in Meniere's disease
5. in bilateral cases, a VDRL should be checked to R/O luetic disease

TREATMENT

1. reduced intake of salt (strict salt restriction is as effective as any medication) and caffeine
2. diuretics: taken daily until ear fullness abates, then PRN ear pressure (usually once or twice weekly suffices)
    A. acetazolamide: *Rx* Diamox® sequels 500 mg p.o. q d x 1 week, increase to BID if symptoms persist. D/C if paresthesias develop. Do not use during 1st rimester of pregnancy
3. vestibular suppressants
    A. diazepam (Valium®): probably the most effective
    B. meclizine HCl (Antivert®): *Rx* Adult dose for vertigo associated with the

vestibular system (during attacks): 25-100 mg/day PO divided. Dose for motion sickness: 25-50 mg PO one hr prior to stimulus. Supplied: 12.5, 25 & 50 mg tabs. SIDE EFFECTS: drowsiness

4. vasodilators: postulated to be mediated by increased cochlear blood flow: inhalation of 5-10% CO_2 works well, but relief is short lived

SURGICAL TREATMENT

Reserved for <u>incapacitating</u> cases <u>refractory</u> to medical management. When functional hearing exists, procedures that spare hearing are preferred because of high incidence of bilateral involvement. Procedures include:

1. endolymphatic shunting procedures: to mastoid cavity (Arenberg shunt) or to subarachnoid space. Reserved for cases with serviceable hearing. ≈ 65% success rate (*see below*). If symptoms are relieved ≥ 1 year, then a recurrence would be treated by shunt revision, if < 1 year then vestibular neurectomy
2. direct application of corticosteroids to the inner ear
3. nonselective vestibular ablation (in cases with nonserviceable hearing on the side of involvement)
   A. surgical labyrinthectomy
   B. middle ear perfusion with gentamicin
   C. translabyrinthine section of the 8th nerve
4. selective vestibular neurectomy (in cases with serviceable hearing): *see page 590*

OUTCOME

ENDOLYMPH SHUNTING PROCEDURES

Outcomes from 112 endolymphatic shunting procedures are shown in *Table 22-1*.

NEURECTOMY PROCEDURES

Vestibulocochlear nerve section (based on early posterior fossa surgery by Dandy; entire eighth nerve bundle was sectioned in 587 patients; all were deaf post-op): 90% relieved of vertigo, 5% unchanged and 5% worse; 9% incidence of facial paralysis (3% incidence of permanent paralysis).

Table 22-1 Outcome*[6]

	Vertigo	Tinnitus	Hearing†	Ear pressure
improved	79 (70%)‡	53 (47%)	19 (17%)	57 (51%)
stable	33 (29%)	49 (43%)	50 (45%)	24 (21%)
worse	(none)	10 (10%)	39 (35%)	31 (28%)

*   in 112 endolymphatic-subarachnoid shunts

†   improved hearing considered serviceable (50 dB pure tone, 70% speech discrimination); additional 4 patients had improved but non-serviceable hearing

‡   5 patients had recurrence of vertigo after 1-3 years

Selective vestibular nerve section (sparing cochlear portion, 95 patients from Dandy): 10% had improved hearing, 28% unchanged, 48% worse, 14% deaf.

Retrolabyrinthine approach: in 32 patients with Meniere's syndrome (25 failed endolymph shunt) responding to survey, 85% had complete relief of vertigo, 6% improved, 9% no relief (one of whom responded to middle fossa neurectomy)[5].

Complications and untoward effects

Patients with little vestibular nerve function pre-op (determined by ENG) usually have little difficulty immediately following vestibular neurectomy; patients with more function may have a transient worsening post-op until they accommodate.

Among 42 patients undergoing retrolabyrinthine approach: none lost hearing as a result of surgery, no facial weakness, one CSF rhinorrhea requiring re-operation, and one meningitis with good outcome[5].

In post-op failures, check ENG. If any vestibular nerve function is demonstrated on operated side, then the nerve section was incomplete; consider re-operating.

22.3.   Facial nerve palsy

Severity of facial palsy is graded with the House and Brackmann scale (see *Table*

17-24, page 431).

LOCALIZING SITE OF LESION

Central facial palsy (AKA supranuclear facial palsy)

The cortical representation for facial movement occurs in the motor strip along the lateral aspect (just above the most inferior opercular portion of the precentral gyrus). The keys to differentiating central paralysis (due to <u>supranuclear</u> lesions) from peripheral facial palsy are that <u>central</u> palsies:

1. are confined primarily to the lower face due to some bilateral cortical representation of upper facial movement
2. may spare emotional facial expression[8] (e.g. smiling at a joke)

Nuclear facial palsy

The motor nucleus of the seventh nerve is located at the pontomedullary junction. Motor fibers ascend within the pons and form a sharp bend ("internal genu") around the sixth nerve nucleus, forming a visible bump in the floor of the 4th ventricle (facial colliculus). Nuclear VII palsy results in paralysis of all VII nerve motor function. In nuclear facial palsies, other neurologic findings also often occur from involvement of adjacent neural structures by the underlying process (stroke, tumor...), e.g. in Millard-Gubler syndrome, there is ipsilateral abducens palsy + contralateral limb weakness (*see page 86*). Tumors invading the floor of the 4th ventricle (e.g. medulloblastoma) may also cause nuclear facial palsy (from involvement of facial colliculus in the floor of 4th ventricle).

Facial nerve lesion

The seventh nerve exits from the brain stem at the ponto-medullary junction where it may be involved in CPA tumors. It enters the supero-anterior portion of the internal auditory canal (see *Figure 3-5*, page 72). The geniculate ganglion ("external genu") is located within the temporal bone. The first branch from the ganglion is the greater superficial petrosal nerve **(GSPN)** which passes to the pterygopalatine ganglion and innervates the nasal and palatine mucosa and the lacrimal gland of the eye; lesions proximal to this point produce a dry eye. The next branch is the branch to the stapedius muscle; lesions proximal to this point produce hyperacusis. Next, the chorda tympani joins the facial nerve bringing taste sensation from the anterior two thirds of the tongue. Basal skull fractures may injure the nerve just proximal to this point. Travelling with the chorda tympani are fibers to the submandibular and sublingual glands. The facial nerve exits the skull at the stylomastoid foramen. It then enters the parotid gland, where it splits into the following branches to the facial muscles (cranial to caudal): temporal, zygomatic, buccal, mandibular, and cervical. Lesions within the parotid gland (e.g. parotid tumors) may involve some branches but spare others.

ETIOLOGIES

These etiologies produce primarily facial nerve palsy, also see *Multiple cranial nerve palsies (cranial neuropathies)*, page 917.

1. Bell's palsy: *see below*
2. herpes zoster oticus (auris): *see page 596*
3. trauma: basal skull fracture

   } 90-95% of all cases of facial palsy[9]

4. birth:
   A. congenital
      1. bilateral facial palsy (facial diplegia) of Möbius syndrome*: unique in that it affects upper face more than lower face (*see page 917*)
      2. congenital facial diplegia may be part of facioscapulohumeral or myotonic muscular dystrophy*
   B. traumatic
5. otitis media: with acute otitis media, facial palsy usually improves with antibiotics; with chronic suppurative otitis surgical intervention is required
6. central facial paralysis and nuclear facial paralysis: see *Localizing site of lesion* above
7. neoplasm: usually causes hearing loss, and (unlike Bell's palsy) <u>slowly progressive</u> facial paralysis
   A. most are either benign schwannomas of the facial or auditory nerve, or malignancies metastatic to the temporal bone. Facial neuromas account for ≈ 5% of peripheral facial nerve palsies[10]; the paralysis tends to be slowly progressive (*see page 922*)
   B. parotid tumors may involve some branches but spare others
   C. Masson's vegetant intravascular hemangioendothelioma (*see page 497*)

8. neurosarcoidosis*: VII is the most commonly affected cranial nerve (*see page 56*)
9. diabetes: 17% of patients > 40 yrs old with peripheral facial palsy (**PFP**) have abnormal glucose tolerance tests. Diabetics have 4.5 times the relative risk of developing PFP than nondiabetics[11]
10. Lyme disease*: a spirochetal disease[12], facial diplegia is a hallmark
11. Guillain-Barré syndrome*: facial diplegia occurs in ≈ 50% of fatal cases
12. occasionally seen in Klippel-Feil syndrome

* items with an asterisk are often associated with facial diplegia (i.e. bilateral facial palsy)

BELL'S PALSY

Bell's palsy (**BP**), AKA idiopathic peripheral facial palsy (**PFP**), is the most common cause of facial paralysis (50-80% of PFPs). Incidence: 150-200/1-million/yr.

Etiology: by definition, PFP is called Bell's palsy when it is not due to known causes of PFP (e.g. infection, tumor or trauma) and there are no other neurological (e.g. involvement of other cranial nerves) or systemic manifestations (e.g. fever, diabetes, possibly hypertension[13])[14]. Thus, true BP is idiopathic, and is a diagnosis of exclusion. Most cases probably represent a viral inflammatory demyelinating polyneuritis[15] usually due to the herpes simplex virus[16]. Facial palsy due to Lyme disease can usually be recognized on clinical grounds[17]. Severity may be graded on the House & Brackmann grading scale (see *Table 17-24*, page 431).

PRESENTATION

A viral prodrome is frequent: URI, myalgia, hypesthesia or dysesthesia of the trigeminal nerve, N/V, diarrhea... Paralysis may be incomplete and remain so (Type I); it is complete at onset in 50% (Type II), the remainder progress to completion in 1 week. Usually exhibits distal to proximal progression: motor branches, then chorda tympani (loss of taste and decreased salivation), then stapedial branch (hyperacusis), then geniculate ganglion (decreased tearing). Associated symptoms are shown in *Table 22-2*, and are usually, but not always, ipsilateral.

Table 22-2 Associated symptoms with Bell's palsy

Symptom	%
facial & retroauricular pain	60%
dysgeusia	57%
hyperacusis	30%
reduced tearing	17%

Herpes zoster vesicles develop in 4% of patients 2-4 days after onset of paralysis; and in 30% of patients 4-8 days after onset. During the recovery phase excessive lacrimation may occur (aberrant nerve regeneration).

PROGNOSIS

All cases show some recovery (if none by 6 mos, other etiologies should be sought). Extent of recovery: 75-80% of cases recover completely, 10% partial, remainder poor. If recovery begins by 10-21 d, tends to be complete; if not until 3-8 wks → fair, if not until 2-4 mos → poor recovery. If paralysis is complete at onset, 50% will have incomplete recovery. Cases of incomplete paralysis at onset that do not progress to complete paralysis → complete recovery; incomplete paralysis at onset that progresses to complete → incomplete recovery in 75%. A worse prognosis is associated with: more proximal involvement, hyperacusis, decreased tearing, age > 60 yrs, diabetes, HTN, psychoneuroses, and aural, facial or radicular pain.

MANAGEMENT

Patients with PFP should be examined at an early stage to optimize outcome.

Electrodiagnostics: EMG may detect re-innervation potentials, aids prognostication. Nerve conduction study: electrical stimulation of the facial nerve near the stylomastoid foramen while recording EMG in facial muscles (a facial nerve may continue to conduct for up to ≈ 1 week even after complete transection).

Eye protection: protection of the eye is critical. Artificial tears during the day, eye ointment at night, avoid bright light (using dark glasses during the day).

Steroids: dramatically reduces the pain of BP. Prednisone is frequently used[9], and reduces the number of patients with complete denervation[18] (dose: prednisone 1 mg/kg per day divided BID; after 5-6 days if paralysis is incomplete taper over 5 days, if paralysis is complete after the first 5-6 days then continue another 10 days and then taper over 5 days; never D/C abruptly to avoid rebound inflammation).

Surgical decompression: controversial. The definitive study has not been done. Rarely utilized. Indications may include:

1. complete facial nerve degeneration without response to nerve stimulation (although this absence is also used as an argument against surgery[9])
2. progressively deteriorating response to nerve stimulation
3. no clinical nor objective (nerve testing) improvement after 8 wks (however, in cases where the diagnosis of Bell's palsy is felt to be certain, the active disease will have abated by ≈ 14 days after onset[9])

HERPES ZOSTER OTICUS FACIAL PARALYSIS

Symptoms are more severe than Bell's palsy, herpetic vesicles are usually present, and antibody titers to varicella-zoster virus rise. These patients have a higher risk of facial nerve degeneration.

SURGICAL TREATMENT OF FACIAL PALSY

For cases with focal injury to the facial nerve (e.g. trauma, injury during surgery for CPA tumor…), dynamic reconstruction by nerve anastamoses are usually considered superior to static methods[19]. For nonfocal causes, e.g. Bell's palsy, only "static" methods may be applicable. A functional neural repair is not possible if the facial muscles have atrophied or fibrosed.

Surgical treatment options include:
1. for intracranial injury to facial nerve (e.g. during CPA tumor surgery): intracranial reapproximation (with or without graft) offers the best hope for the most normal facial reanimation
    A. timing
        1. at time of tumor removal (for a divided facial nerve during removal of acoustic neuroma[20-22]): the best result that can be achieved with this is House-Brackmann Grade III. The operation fails to produce good results in ≈ 33% of cases[22]
        2. in delayed fashion, especially if the nerve was left in anatomic continuity
    B. techniques
        1. direct reanastamosis: difficult due to the frail nature of the VII nerve (especially when it has been stretched by a tumor)
        2. cable graft: e.g. using greater auricular nerve[23] or sural nerve
2. extracranial facial nerve anastamosis
    A. hypoglossal nerve (Cr. N. XII)-facial nerve anastamosis: (*see below*)
    B. spinal accessory nerve (Cr. N. XI)-facial nerve anastamosis: (*see below*)
    C. phrenic nerve-facial nerve anastamosis
    D. glossopharyngeal (Cr. N. IX)-facial nerve anastamosis
    E. crossface grafting (VII-VII): results have not been very good
3. "mechanical" or "static" means
    A. facial suspension: e.g. with polypropylene (Marlex®) mesh[24]
    B. eye closure techniques (protects the eye from exposure and reduced tearing)
        1. tarsorrhaphy: partial or complete
        2. gold weights in eyelid
        3. stainless-steel spring in eyelid

Timing of surgery

If the facial nerve is known to be interrupted (e.g. transected during removal of acoustic neuroma) then early surgical treatment is indicated. When the status of the nerve is unknown or if in continuity but not functioning, then several months of observation and electrical testing should be allowed for spontaneous recovery. Very late attempts at anastamosis have less chance for recovery due to facial muscle atrophy.

HYPOGLOSSAL NERVE-FACIAL NERVE (XII-VII) ANASTAMOSIS

Cannot be used bilateral in patients with facial diplegia or in those with other lower cranial nerve deficits (or potential for same). In spite of some suggestions to the contrary, sacrificing the XII nerve does create some morbidity (tongue atrophy with difficulty speaking, mastication and swallowing in ≈ 25% of cases, exacerbated when the facial muscles do not function on that side; aspiration may occur if vagus (Cr. N. X) dysfunction coexists with loss of XII).

Not as effective as it would theoretically seem possible. The resultant facial reanimation is often less than ideal (may permit mass movement). To avoid severe disappointment, the patient should thoroughly understand the likely side effects and that the facial movement will probably be much less than normal, often with poor voluntary control.

Usually performed in conjunction with anastamosis of the descendens hypoglossi to the distal hypoglossal nerve to try and reduce hemiatrophy of the tongue. Atrophy may also be reduced by using a "jump graft" without completely interrupting XII[25].

Technique

Variations:
1. interposition jump grafts: spares function in the XII nerve (to minimize glottic denervation, the incision of XII should be distal to the descendens hypoglossi[25])
    A. using cutaneous nerve jump graft[25]
    B. using muscle interposition jump graft[26]
2. mobilizing the intratemporal portion of VII out of the fallopian canal (as previously described[27]) and then anastamosing it using a bevelled cuts to a partially incised XII[28]

Outcome

Results are better if performed early, although good results can occur up to 18 mos after injury. In 22 cases, 64% had good results, 14% fair, 18% poor, and 1 patient had no evidence of reinnervation. In 59% of cases, evidence of reinnervation was seen by 3-6 mos, in the remaining patients with reinnervation improvement was noted by 8 mos[29]. Recovery of forehead movement occurs in only ≈ 30%. Return of tone precedes movement by ≈ 3 months.

SPINAL ACCESSORY NERVE-FACIAL NERVE (XI-VII) ANASTAMOSIS

First described in 1895 by Sir Charles Ballance[30]. Sacrifices some shoulder movement rather than use of tongue. Initial concerns about significant shoulder disability and pain resulted in the technique of using only the SCM branch of XI[31], however these problems have not occurred in the majority of patients even with use of the major division[32].

22.4. Hearing loss

Two anatomic types: conductive and sensorineural.
1. conductive hearing loss
    A. patients tend to speak with normal or low volume
    B. findings:
        1. <u>Rinne test</u> with 256 Hz tuning fork will be negative (i.e. abnormal, air conduction < bone conduction)
        2. <u>Weber test</u> will lateralize to side of hearing loss
        3. abnormal middle ear impedance measurements
    C. etiologies: anything that interferes with ossicular movement, including: otitis media with middle ear effusion, otoslcerosis
2. sensorineural hearing loss
    A. patients tend to speak with loud voice
    B. clinical findings:
        1. <u>Rinne test</u> will be positive (i.e. normal, air conduction > bone conduction)
        2. <u>Weber test</u> will lateralize to side of better hearing
    C. further divided into sensory or neural. Distinguished by otoacoustic emissions (only produced by a cochlea with functioning hair cells) or BSAERs
        1. sensory: loss of outer hair cells in the cochlea. Etiologies: cochlear damage (usually causes high-frequency hearing loss) from noise exposure, ototoxic drugs (e.g. aminoglycosides), senile cochlear degeneration, viral labyrinthitis. Speech discrimination may be relatively preserved
        2. neural: due to compression of the 8th cranial nerve. Etiologies: CP angle tumor (e.g. acoustic neuroma). Typically loss of word discrimination out of proportion to pure tone audiogram abnormalities

    • Sensory and neural hearing loss may be distinguished by otoacoustic emissions (only produced by a cochlea with functioning hair cells) or BSAERs. An elevated stapedial reflex threshold out of proportion to PTA abnormalities is also highly diagnostic of a retrocochlear (neural) lesion

22.5. References

1. Brandt T, Daroff R B: The multisensory physiological and pathological vertigo syndromes. **Ann Neurol** 7: 195-203, 1980.
2. Jannetta P J, Moller M B, Moller A R: Disabling positional vertigo. **N Engl J Med** 310: 1700-5, 1984.
3. Arriaga M A, Chen D A: Vestibular nerve section in the treatment of vertigo. **Contemp Neurosurg** 19 (14): 1-6, 1997.
4. McElveen J T, House J W, Hitselberger W E, *et al.*: Retrolabyrinthine vestibular nerve section: A viable alternative to the middle fossa approach. **Otolaryngol Head Neck Surg** 92: 136-40, 1984.
5. House J W, Hitelsberger W E, McElveen J, *et al.*: Retrolabyrinthine section of the vestibular nerve. **Otolaryngol Head Neck Surg** 92: 212-5, 1984.
6. Glassock M E, Miller G W, Drake F D, *et al.*: Surgical management of Meniere's disease with the endolymphatic subarachnoid shunt. **Laryngoscope** 87: 1668-75, 1977.
7. Tarlov E C: Microsurgical vestibular nerve section for intractable Meniere's disease. **Clin Neurosurg** 33: 667-84, 1985.
8. Shambaugh G E: *Facial nerve decompression and repair.* In **Surgery of the ear.** W. B. Saunders, Philadelphia, 1959: pp 543-71.
9. Adour K K: Diagnosis and management of facial paralysis. **N Engl J Med** 307: 348-51, 1982.
10. Shambaugh G E, Clemis J D: *Facial nerve paralysis.* In **Otolaryngology,** Paparella M M and Schumrick D A, (eds.). W. B. Saunders, Philadelphia, 1973, Vol. 2: pp 275.
11. Adour K K, Wingerd J, Doty H E: Prevalence of concurrent diabetes mellitus and idiopathic facial paralysis (Bell's palsy). **Diabetes** 24: 449-51, 1975.
12. Treatment of Lyme disease. **Med Letter** 30: 65-6, 1988.
13. Abraham-Inpijn L, Devriese P P, Hart A A M: Predisposing factors in Bell's palsy: A clinical study with reference to diabetes mellitus, hypertension, clotting mechanism and lipid disturbance. **Clin Otolaryngol** 7: 99-105, 1982.
14. Devriese P P, Schumacher T, Scheide A, *et al.*: Incidence, prognosis and recovery of Bell's palsy: A survey of about 1000 patients (1974-1983). **Clin Otolaryngol** 15: 15-27, 1990.
15. Adour K K, Byl F M, Hilsinger R L, *et al.*: The true nature of Bell's palsy: Analysis of 1000 consecutive patients. **Laryngoscope** 88: 787-801, 1978.
16. Adour K K, Bell D N, Hilsinger R L: Herpes simplex virus in idiopathic facial paralysis (Bell palsy). **JAMA** 233: 527-30, 1975.
17. Kuiper H, Devriese P P, de Jongh B M, *et al.*: Absence of Lyme borreliosis among patients with presumed Bell's palsy. **Arch Neurol** 49: 940-3, 1992.
18. Adour K K, Wingerd J: Idiopathic facial paralysis (Bell's palsy): Factors affecting severity and outcome in 446 patients. **Neurology** 24: 1112-6, 1974.
19. Conley J, Baker D C: Hypoglossal-facial nerve anastamosis for reinnervation of the paralyzed face. **Plast Reconstr Surg** 63: 63-72, 1979.
20. Pluchino F, Fornari M, Luccarelli G: Intracranial repair of interrupted facial nerve in course of operation for acoustic neuroma by microsurgical technique. **Acta Neurochir** 79: 87-93, 1986.
21. Stephanian E, Sekhar L N, Janecka I P, *et al.*: Facial nerve repair by interposition nerve graft: Results in 22 patients. **Neurosurgery** 31: 73-7, 1992.
22. King T T, Sparrow O C, Arias J M, *et al.*: Repair of facial nerve after removal of cerebellopontine angle tumors: A comparative study. **J Neurosurg** 78: 720-5, 1993.
23. Alberti P W R M: The greater auricular nerve. Donor for facial nerve grafts: A note on its topographical anatomy. **Arch Otolaryngol** 76: 422-4, 1962.
24. Strelzow V V, Friedman W H, Katsantonis G P: Reconstruction of the paralyzed face with the polypropylene mesh template. **Arch Otolaryngol** 109: 140-4, 1983.
25. May M, Sobol S M, Mester S J: Hypoglossal-facial nerve interpositional-jump graft for facial reanimation without tongue atrophy. **Otolaryngol Head Neck Surg** 104: 818-25, 1991.
26. Drew S J, Fullarton A C, Glasby M A, *et al.*: Reinnervation of facial nerve territory using a composite hypoglossal nerve-muscle autograft-facial nerve bridge. An experimental model in sheep. **Clin Otolaryngol** 20: 109-17, 1995.
27. Hitselberger W E: *Hypoglossal-facial anastamosis.* In **Acoustic tumors: Management,** House W F and Luetje C M, (eds.). University Park Press, Baltimore, 1979, Vol. II: pp 97-103.
28. Atlas M D, Lowinger D S G: A new technique for hypoglossal-facial nerve repair. **Laryngoscope** 107: 984-91, 1997.
29. Pitty L F, Tator C H: Hypoglossal-facial nerve anastamosis for facial nerve palsy following surgery for cerebellopontine angle tumors. **J Neurosurg** 77: 724-31, 1992.
30. Duel A B: Advanced methods in the surgical treatment of facial paralysis. **Ann Otol Rhinol Laryngol** 43: 76-88, 1934.
31. Poe D S, Scher N, Panje W R: Facial reanimation by XI-VII anastamosis without shoulder paralysis. **Laryngoscope** 99: 1040-7, 1989.
32. Ebersold M J, Quast L M: Long-term results of spinal accessory nerve-facial nerve anastamosis. **J Neurosurg** 77: 51-4, 1992.

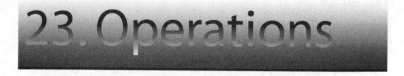
23. Operations

This section provides information useful in the O.R. that apply to a number of different topics. Some items that are pertinent to only one topic will be found in that section instead (e.g. *transsphenoidal tumor removal* is found in the section on *pituitary tumors*).

REMEMBER: before performing any invasive procedure, know the patient's coagulation status (history, and if indicated: PT, PTT, bleeding time, platelets, FDP...).

23.1.   Intraoperative dyes

This section covers visible dyes that may be useful in the operating room. For radio-opaque dyes, see *Contrast agents in neuroradiology*, page 126. There is little information available in the literature regarding the intrathecal (**IT**) use of the following agents.

Indigo carmine: is a blue dye which has been used intrathecally to locate CSF leaks. There are few published reports, and no accounts of adverse effects. In 1933 a report[1] of IT injection of 5 ml of 0.6% indigo carmine solution produced blue-green discoloration of the CSF draining through a fistula into the nose within 15 minutes, lasting for 5 hours, with no indication of toxicity. It is excreted in the urine (and not in mucous membranes). The consensus is that it should be relatively safe for IT use, but the manufacturer did not recommend this application.

✱ **Methylene blue**: although it had been used for years, methylene blue is probably <u>cytotoxic</u> and appears to become fixed to neural tissue. It should therefore <u>not</u> be used as a stain in neurosurgical operations or diagnostic tests. CNS damage (some permanent) occurred in 14 patients given an IT injection of a 1% solution. Symptoms included: para-paresis, quadriplegia, multiple cranial nerve involvement (including anosmia and optic atrophy), dementia and hydrocephalus[2].

Fluorescein: although intrathecal injection (e.g. to look for CSF leak) has been used by ENT surgeons with apparently acceptable results, there is a risk of seizures. 2.5% fluorescein is diluted 1:10 with CSF or saline and ~ 6 ml is injected into the spinal subarachnoid space (or 0.5 ml of 5% fluorescein mixed with 5-10 ml of CSF[3]).

Fluorescein has also been used <u>IV</u> (adult dose: 1 amp IV) to help mark areas where there is breakdown of the blood brain barrier (e.g. in tumors, *see page 84*), however, this substance is eventually excreted in mucus, urine, etc., and just about everything turns orange. It has also been used to perform intraoperative "visible angiograms" during the removal of AVMs.

23.2.   Operating room equipment

OPERATING MICROSCOPE

For spine cases, the ideal location of the observer eyepiece is usually directly opposite the surgeon. For intracranial work, the observer's (assistant's) eyepiece is placed to right of operator's except in the following:
1.   transsphenoidal surgery (when the surgeon stands to the patient's right)
2.   <u>right</u> posterior fossa craniotomy in the lateral oblique (suboccipital) position

For all intracranial vascular operations, most posterior cervical operations (laminectomies, wiring/fusions…) and many tumor operations, firm head fixation is required.

23.3.   Surgical hemostasis

Methods include:
1. thermocoagulation
   A. electrical coagulation: Bovie cautery (monopolar), bipolar cautery
   B. thermal units: e.g. AccuTemp® disposable eye cautery units (particularly useful to coagulate dura when inserting a ventriculostomy in the ICU)
   C. laser: especially neodymium:yttrium-aluminum-garnet (Nd:YAG) laser
2. mechanical
   A. bone wax: originated by Sir Victor Horsely. Also <u>inhibits bone formation</u>
   B. ligature: less commonly used in neurosurgery than other specialties
   C. "silver clips" (e.g. HemoClips®)
3. chemical hemostasis: *see below*

CHEMICAL HEMOSTASIS
See review[4] for more information. Some key points:
1. gelatin sponge (Gelfoam®): no intrinsic coagulating effect. Absorbs 45 times its weight in blood which causes it to expand and tamponade bleeding. Absorbable
2. oxidized cellulose (Oxycel®) and oxidized regenerated cellulose (Surgicel®): absorbable. Acidic material that reacts with blood to form a reddish brown "pseudoclot". Bactericidal to over 20 different organisms. May retard bone growth. Oxycel® interferes with epithelialization more than Surgicel®
3. microfibrillar collagen (Avitene®): promotes adhesion and aggregation of platelets. Loses effectiveness in severe thrombocytopenia (< 10,000/ml). May be used on bone bleeding. Remove excess material to reduce risk of infection
4. thrombin (Thrombostat®): does not depend on any intermediate physiological agent. Caution: thrombin may cause significant edema when placed on brain where the pia has been disrupted

23.4.   Anterior approaches to the spine

In the following presentation, it may be necessary to take into account the possibility of overlap (e.g. a tumor of C7 which requires access down to at least T1 to permit stabilization).

Approaches
1. cervical spine
   A. anterior odontoid screw: *see page 625*
   B. C1-3: transoral approach
   C. C3-C7: typical anterior cervical discectomy approach
2. thoracic spine
   A. T1-3: sternal splitting anterior approach
   B. T4-11:
      1. right thoracotomy
         a. the patient needs to be able to tolerate deflation of the right lung
         b. approach often by cardiovascular or chest surgeon
         c. T3-4: often involves mobilizing some of the shoulder muscles which adds to complexity of exposure
         d. practical points:
            i. determining level in spine: counting down from the top in surgery is very difficult. Since pre-op MRI usually counts from the top down, and in surgery it is often necessary to count from the bottom up, check on plain pre-op x-rays that patient has 5 lumbar and 12 thoracic vertebrae
      2. endoscopic approaches

3. lumbar spine
  A. L1-5
    1. indications: tumor, fracture
    2. practical points
      a. aortic bifurcation located at the mid body of L3: a true anterior approach is therefore not practical. Therefore a **retroperitoneal approach** is used
      b. iliac crests may prevent a pure lateral approach to L4 and especially L5, which limits the placement of screws for the compression plate
      c. if a 360° fusion with pedicle screws is to be employed: potential problem with screws from compression plate hitting pedicle screws. There is some leeway in angulation of the pedicle screws to compensate for this
      d. complications to avoid:
        i. injury to great vessels, especially the left iliac vein
        ii. unnecessary sacrifice of intercoastal nerve which can cause atrophy of the abdominal muscles and eventration of the abdominal wall (not a true incisional hernia)
        iii. do not enter the peritoneum
        iv. injury to the kidney and ureter
        v. ✖ anterior instrumentation must be avoided to prevent delayed vascular injury from repeated pulsations
    3. position
      a. **left sided approach** is preferred (i.e. right lateral decubitus position). Exceptions where a left sided approach is used:
        i. primarily right-sided pathology
        ii. CT or MRI shows there is not enough room because of the location of the aorta
      b. level of pathology is positioned over the break in table (to get the iliac crest out of the way during initial approach - remember to unbreak table before final instrumentation!). Key: shoulders and pelvis true vertical for x-ray localization
      c. axillary roll
      d. flex the upper thigh (to relax psoas muscle) & knee
      e. stabilized with bean bag (keep patient exposed from midline anterior to posterior) and wide adhesive tape over pads at shoulder and thigh (keep iliac crest exposed for donor bone)
      f. use a fluoro compatible table, or place patient on table reversed to permit access by C-arm
    4. incision[5]
      a. to access L2 and below: oblique incision starting anteroinferiorly at the edge of the rectus muscle extending cephalad and posteriorly through the bed of the 12th rib, ending posteriorly at the vertebral musculature
      b. exposure of L1: e.g. for instrumentation, requires extending the incision cephalad through the bed of the 10th rib, and may require radical takedown of the diaphragm for full exposure
    5. approach[5]
      a. the 12th rib can be divided or disarticulated posteriorly, and may be used as a source of bone for fusion
      b. the kidney and ureter are retracted anteriorly, the psoas muscle is retracted laterally
      c. segmental vessels are ligated or coagulated at the midportion of the VB
      d. Bookwalter retractor is useful
    6. surgical aspects
      a. to get the lateral compression plate true lateral, place it as "posterior" as possible (also keeps it away from the great vessels)
    7. post op
      a. TLSO for 3 months
      b. increase activity slowly in brace
      c. some bulging of the flank muscles is normally associated with this approach

---

23.5. Craniotomies

CRANIOTOMY PRE- & POST-OP MANAGEMENT

RISKS

Many risks cannot be generalized for all craniotomies and are specific to various tumors, aneurysms, etc. General information:

1. post-operative hemorrhage
   A. overall risk of post-operative hemorrhage[6, 7]: 0.8-1.1%. 43-60% of the hematomas were intraparenchymal, 28-33% epidural, 5-7% subdural, 5% intrasellar, 8% mixed, 11% confined to superficial wound. Overall mortality was 32%
   B. hematoma may occur at the surgical site or in remote locations, e.g. intracerebellar hemorrhage after pterional[8] and temporal[9] craniotomies (*see page 852*)
2. in craniotomy for brain tumor[10]:
   A. risk of anesthetic complications: 0.2%
   B. increased neurologic deficit in 1st 24 hours post-op: ≈ 10%
   C. wound infection: 2%
3. postoperative headache (*see page 604*)

PRE-OP ORDERS

1. for tumor: if patient on steroids, give ≈ 50% higher dose 6 hrs before and on-call to O.R. (stress doses); if not on steroids give dexamethasone 10 mg PO 6 hrs before and on call to O.R. (in A.M., give with sip water)
2. if already on antiepileptic drugs (**AEDs**) continue same doses. If not on AEDs, and cortical incision anticipated, load with oral PHT (may give 300 mg PO q 4 hrs **x 3** doses (total 900 mg) to load orally)
3. prophylactic antibiotics on call to O.R. (*optional*)
4. recommended: pneumatic compression boots or knee-high TED® hose

POST-OP ORDERS

Guidelines (individualize as appropriate)

1. admit PACU, transfer to ICU (neuro unit if available) when stable
2. VS: q 15 min x 4 hrs, then q 1 hr. Temperature q 4 hrs x 3 d, then q 8 hrs. Neuro check q 1 hr
3. activity: bed rest (BR) with HOB elevated 20-30°
4. remove elastic leg wraps (if present) and replace with knee high TED hose or use pneumatic compression boots
5. I & O q 1 hr (if no Foley: straight cath q 4 hrs PRN bladder distension)
6. incentive spirometry q 2 hrs while awake (do not use following transsphenoidal surgery)
7. diet: NPO except minimal ice chips and meds as ordered
8. IVF: NS + 20 mEq KCl/L @ 90 ml/hr
9. O$_2$: 2 L per NC
10. meds:
    A. dexamethasone (Decadron®): if not on chronic steroids, give 4 mg IV q 6 hrs. Otherwise give stress doses based on patients current dose and length of treatment (*see page 10*)
    B. H$_2$ antagonist, e.g. ranitidine 50 mg IVPB q 8 hrs
    C. phenytoin (Dilantin®) 100 mg slow IVP q 8 hrs. Maintain therapeutic levels of AEDs for 2-3 months post-op for most supratentorial craniotomies, with the exception of aneurysm, AVM, head injury or meningioma where 6-12 months may be more reasonable[11]
    D. nitroprusside (**NTP**) (Nipride®): titrate to keep SBP < 160 mm Hg and/or DBP < 100 mm Hg (use cuff pressures, may use A-line pressures if they cor-

relate with cuff pressures)

    E. codeine 30-60 mg IM q 3-4 hrs PRN H/A

    F. acetaminophen (Tylenol®) 650 mg PO/PR q 4 hrs PRN temperature > 100.5° F (38 C)

    G. *continue prophylactic antibiotics if used:* (e.g. cefazolin (Kefzol®) 500-1000 mg IVPB q 6 hrs x 24 hrs, then D/C)

11. labs:
    A. CBC once stabilized in ICU and q d thereafter
    B. renal profile once stabilized in ICU and q 12 hrs thereafter
    C. ABG once stabilized in ICU and q 12 hrs x 2 days, then D/C (also check ABG after any ventilator change if patient on ventilator)

12. call M.D. if any deterioration in crani checks, for T > 101° (38.5 C), sudden increase in SBP, SBP < 120, U.O. < 60 ml/2-hrs

POST-OP COMPLICATIONS

POSTOPERATIVE DETERIORATION

When the postoperative neurologic status is worse than pre-op, especially in a patient who deteriorates after initially doing well, emergency evaluation and treatment is indicated.

Possible etiologies:
1. hematoma (see *Risks*, page 602)
    A. intracerebral hemorrhage **(ICH)**
    B. epidural hematoma: at or remote from surgical site
    C. subdural hematoma
2. cerebral infarction
    A. arterial
    B. venous infarction: especially with surgery on or around the venous sinuses (e.g. see page 811)
3. postoperative seizure: may be due to inadequate anticonvulsant levels, and may be exacerbated by any of the above (*see below for management*)
4. acute hydrocephalus
5. pneumocephalus (also see *Pneumocephalus*, page 667):
    A. tension pneumocephalus: see *Tension pneumocephalus*, page 668
    B. simple pneumocephalus: the simple presence of air in the cranium can cause neurologic symptoms even if not under tension. Symptoms include: lethargy, confusion, severe headache, nausea & vomiting, seizures. Air may be located over the cerebral convexities, in the p-fossa, and/or in the ventricles and usually resorbs with symptomatic improvement in 1-3 days
6. edema: may improve with steroids
    A. worsening of cerebral edema: moderate post-op worsening of cortical function of immediately adjacent brain is not unexpected in many operations, and is usually transient. However, reversible etiologies (such as subdural hematoma) must be ruled out
    B. traction or manipulation of cranial nerves may cause dysfunction that may be temporary. Division of cranial nerves can cause permanent dysfunction
7. persistent anesthetic effect (including paralytics): unlikely in a patient who deteriorates after initially doing well post-op. Consider reversing medication given during surgery (caution re hypertension and agitation), e.g. naloxone, flumazenil (*see page 156*), or reversal of pharmacologic muscle block (*see page 3*)
8. vasospasm: following SAH or may be due to manipulation of blood vessels

POSTOPERATIVE SEIZURES

Management:
1. intubate if patient does not rapidly regain consciousness, is not protecting airway, or has labored respirations
2. CT scan: rule out hematoma (intracerebral or extra-axial) or hydrocephalus
3. anticonvulsants:
    A. draw blood for appropriate anticonvulsant level
    B. bolus with additional anticonvulsants: do not wait for levels

Persistent headache **(H/A)** is well described following posterior fossa craniectomy (incidence range: 0-83%[12]). The time course in one series[13] was: 23% at 3 mos, 16% at 1 yr, and 9% at 2 yrs.

Persistent H/A may also be observed following supratentorial craniotomy[14] (prevalence 1 year after anterior temporal lobectomy for seizures: 12%[14]). The **"syndrome of the trephined"**: headache and sometimes pulsatile pain (usually localized to the area of the skull defect), amnesia, inability to concentrate, insomnia… similar in some ways to postconcussive syndrome (*see page 682*).

These H/A have been attributed to: traction on the dura when the bone is not replaced, tension on the dura due to tight dural closure, temporalis or nuchal muscle dissection, nerve entrapment in the closing sutures or in the healing scar, intradural blood and/or bone dust, CSF leak[14].

Prevention

No single method or group of methods has been successful in completely eliminating the complaint of post-op H/A[15, 16]. Until further research can further advance the understanding of the cause and prevention of these H/A, it seems reasonable to employ the following measures as much as possible in an attempt to minimize these debilitating symptoms: restoring function of the temporalis or suboccipital musculature, rigid fixation of bone flaps, cranioplasty for large craniectomies, meticulous tension-free dural closure (using duraplasty when necessary), and keeping intradural blood clot and bone dust to the minimum possible[17].

Treatment

Initially, symptomatic treatment is indicated. Referral to a H/A specialist may be appropriate when it becomes apparent that the H/A are not resolving spontaneously after ≈ 3 months[17].

23.5.1.   Posterior fossa (suboccipital) craniectomy

INDICATIONS

To gain access to the cerebellum, cerebellopontine angle **(CPA)**, to one vertebral artery, or using extreme lateral posterior fossa approach to the antero-lateral brain stem. See paramedian (*page 605*) and midline (*page 606*) suboccipital craniectomies for details.

TECHNIQUE

POSITION

Position options include:
1. sitting position: *see below*
2. lateral oblique, AKA **"park bench"** position: patient three-quarters oblique (almost prone)
3. semi-sitting
4. supine with shoulder roll, head almost horizontal
5. prone
6. Concorde position: prone, thorax elevated, neck flexed and tilted away from the side on which the surgeon will be standing

SITTING POSITION

Used less frequently than in the past because of associated complications and acceptable alternative positions (except for some specific circumstances). However, some experts feel that the risks of the sitting position have been greatly overstated[18].

Advantages
1. improved drainage of blood and CSF out of surgical site
2. enhanced venous drainage which helps reduce venous bleeding and also ICP
3. easy ventilation due to unencumbered chest
4. patient's head may be kept exactly midline, aiding operator orientation, and reducing risk of kinking of vertebral arteries

Disadvantages/risks
1. possible air embolism (*see below*)
2. fatigue of operators hands
3. increased surgical risks from placement of CVP catheter (required to treat possible AE): e.g. pneumothorax with subclavian vein catheterization, thrombosis
4. risk of post-op hematoma at the operative site may be increased since potential venous bleeders may remain occult while the patient is sitting, but may become manifest when patient returns to a horizontal position post-op. However, one study found no such increased incidence[6]
5. risk of post-op subdural hematoma: 1.3% of p-fossa cases[19]
6. possible brachial plexus injury: prevent this by not allowing patient's arms to hang at the side. Instead, fold them across abdomen
7. midcervical quadriplegia[20, 21]: presumably due to flexion myelopathy[22-24]. The combination of the sitting position with hypotension[25] or neck flexion with possible compression of the anterior spinal artery, ± cervical bar, and elevation of the head thus reducing the arterial pressure may all contribute
8. sciatic nerve injury (**piriformis syndrome**)[26]: prevent this by flexing patient's knees (reduces tension on sciatic nerve)
9. extent of post-op pneumocephalus is more pronounced, and may increase the risk of tension pneumocephalus[27] (see *Pneumocephalus*, page 667)
10. venous pooling of blood in the LEs under anesthesia may cause relative hypovolemia and should be counteracted by binding the LEs prior to positioning
11. decreased cerebral blood flow due to lower hemodynamic arterial pressure[28]

Air embolism (AE): A potentially fatal complication of any operation when an opening to air occurs in a non-collapsible vein (e.g. diploic vein or a dural sinus) when there is a negative pressure in the vein (e.g. when the head is elevated above the heart)[29]. Air is entrained in the vein and can become trapped in the right atrium which may impair venous return causing hypotension. May also produce cardiac arrhythmias. **Paradoxical air embolism** can occur in the presence of a patent foramen ovale[30] or pulmonary AV fistula, and may produce ischemic cerebral infarction.

Greater negative pressures occur in the sitting position due to the extreme elevation of the head, but AE can occur in any operation with the head elevated higher than the heart. Incidence: a wide range has been quoted in the literature, and depends on the monitoring method used: ≈ 7-25% incidence with the sitting position using Doppler monitoring is an estimate[19].

Operations with significant risk of AE (i.e. sitting position) require the use of precordial Doppler monitoring and placement of a right atrial CVP line.

Diagnosis and treatment:

The earliest clue to the occurrence of AE may be a <u>fall</u> in the end tidal pCO_2. Machinery sounds in the precordial Doppler also suggest AE. Hypotension may develop. Measures shown in *Table 23-1* should be immediately instituted.

Table 23-1   Treatment for air embolism

1. find and occlude site of air entry, or else rapidly pack wound with sopping wet sponges/laps and wax bone edges
2. lower patient's head if at all possible (30° or less from horizontal)
3. jugular venous compression (bilateral best; second choice: right only)
4. rotate patient <u>LEFT</u> side down (attempt to trap air in right atrium)
5. aspirate air from right atrium via CVP catheter
6. ventilate patient with 100% O_2
7. discontinue nitrous oxide if used (may expand AE)[31]
8. use pressors and volume expanders to maintain BP
9. PEEP is <u>ineffective</u> in preventing or treating AE; may increase the risk of paradoxical AE[29]

PARAMEDIAN SUBOCCIPITAL CRANIECTOMY
Indications:
1. access to the cerebellopontine angle (**CPA**)
   A. CPA tumors, including:
      1. acoustic neuroma
      2. CPA meningioma
      3. epidermoids
   B. microvascular decompression

1. trigeminal neuralgia
2. hemifacial spasm
3. miscellaneous: geniculate neuralgia, glossopharyngeal neuralgia
2. lesions of one cerebellar hemisphere:
    A. tumors: metastases, hemangioblastomas…
    B. hemorrhage within cerebellar hemisphere
3. access to vertebral artery
    A. aneurysms: PICA, vertebrobasilar junction
    B. vertebral endarterectomy
4. access to antero-lateral brainstem tumors (extreme lateral p-fossa approach)
    A. foramen magnum tumors, including: chordomas, meningiomas

MIDLINE SUBOCCIPITAL CRANIECTOMY
Indications: access to the midline or both sides of the posterior fossa
1. midline posterior fossa lesions
    A. cerebellar vermian and paravermian lesions, including: vermian AVM, cerebellar astrocytoma near the midline
    B. tumors of the fourth ventricle: ependymoma, medulloblastoma
    C. pineal region tumors
    D. brainstem lesions: brainstem vascular lesions (e.g. cavernous angioma)
2. decompressive craniectomies
    A. for Chiari malformation
3. cerebellar tumors: metastases, hemangioblastoma, cystic astrocytoma…

EXTREME LATERAL POSTERIOR FOSSA APPROACH
Allows access to antero-lateral region of brain stem. Differs from above in that the skin incision is designed to get the bulk of the skin and muscle flap out of the way.

Key: remove the lip of the foramen magnum as far laterally as possible, best done with a diamond drill.

POST-OP CONSIDERATIONS FOR P-FOSSA CRANI'S

POST-OP CHECK
In addition to routine, the following should be checked:
❑ 1. respirations: rate, pattern (see *Intubation* below)
❑ 2. follow closely for hypertension (*see below*)
❑ 3. evidence of CSF leak through wound

POST-OP MANAGEMENT

Intubation
Post-op intubation for 24-48 hours is sometimes maintained on a precautionary basis: many complications often have respiratory arrest as the initial manifestation (*see below*), and the patient may deteriorate precipitously from this point. There is a trade-off as the stimulus of the endotracheal tube may exacerbate hypertension and patient agitation, and so sedation is often required, which may obscure the neuro exam and depress respirations. If the patient wakes up extremely well from an uncomplicated p-fossa crani and it is not late at night, most surgeons will extubate.

Hypertension
Hypertension should be avoided at all costs to prevent bleeding from tenuous vessels (e.g. nitroprusside should be prepared prior to termination of the operation, and should be hanging and ready to titrate to keep SBP ≤ 160 mm Hg during the reversal of anesthesia and post-op).
Physician should be called for any sudden changes in BP post-op (may indicate elevated pressure in posterior fossa, *see below*).

Posterior fossa edema and/or hematoma

In the posterior fossa, a small amount of mass effect can be rapidly fatal due to the paucity of room and the immediate transmission of pressure directly to the brain stem. It can also occlude CSF circulation through the aqueduct and cause acute hydrocephalus with the attendant risk of tonsillar herniation. Increased pressure in the p-fossa is usually heralded by sudden increases in BP or changes in respiratory pattern (pupillary reflexes, level of consciousness and ICP are not affected until late). See *Table 23-2* for emergency treatment measures.

Table 23-2 Emergency treatment for p-fossa swelling

★ Rapid intubation, ventricular tap (through previously placed burr hole, if possible, *see below*), and reoperation is indicated. The wound should be opened immediately wherever patient is (recovery room, ICU, floor…). CT scanning may cost valuable minutes; it is rarely appropriate to delay treatment for this (must be judged on an individual basis).

To expedite ventricular taps, a prophylactic occipital burr hole (**Frazier burr hole**) is often placed during posterior fossa surgery to permit drainage of CSF from the lateral ventricles in the event of acute hydrocephalus from blockage of the 4th ventricle or aqueduct. If acute hydrocephalus develops (e.g. from a hematoma), an emergent percutaneous ventricular tap with ventricular needle (or, if not available, spinal needle) is performed, passing the needle through the burr hole aiming for the middle of the forehead. In the presence of acute hydrocephalus, CSF should be encountered at a depth of 3-5 cm. NB: this maneuver may provide a few more minutes while preparing for the definitive treatment of re-opening the wound; however, hydrocephalus may not initially be present since it takes some time to develop.

CSF fistula

Occurs in 5-17% of cases. A potential source of meningitis, thus CSF leak must be treated immediately. A CSF leak may indicate abnormal CSF hydrodynamics (i.e. hydrocephalus), and maneuvers to stem the leak will likely fail until the CSF is shunted or hydrodynamics normalizes.

A CSF leak may occur through:
1. the skin incision
2. via the eustachian tube (*see page 435* for possible routes of egress following suboccipital acoustic neuroma removal):
   A. through the nose (CSF rhinorrhea)
   B. down the back of the throat
3. the ear (CSF otorrhea) in cases with perforated TM

Treatment:
Initial treatment measures to temporize in the hope that CSF hydrodynamics will normalize and/or that the leak site will scar closed within a few days:
1. elevate the HOB
2. lumbar subarachnoid drainage
3. if the leak occurs through the skin incision:
   A. reinforce the incision with sutures, e.g. running locked 3-0 nylon after preparation of the skin with antimicrobial and local anesthetic
   B. alternatively, the incision may be painted with several coats of collodion

If persistent, a CSF fistula requires surgical correction, see *CSF fistula*, page 174 for general information, *see page 436* for CSF fistula following suboccipital removal of acoustic neuroma.

Fifth or seventh nerve injuries

Causes diminished corneal reflex with potential corneal ulceration; initially managed with isotonic eye drops (e.g. Natural Tears® q 2-4 hrs & PRN, or with a moisturizing insert (e.g. Lacricert®) q day, and at night with an eye patch or taping eyelid shut.

Miscellaneous

Supratentorial intracerebral hemorrhage has been described, and may result from transient hypertension[32].

23.5.2. Pterional craniotomy

INDICATIONS
1. aneurysms
   A. all aneurysms of anterior circulation
   B. basilar tip aneurysms
2. direct surgical approach to cavernous sinus
3. suprasellar tumors
   A. pituitary adenoma (when there is a large suprasellar component)
   B. craniopharyngioma

23.5.3. Temporal craniotomy

INDICATIONS
1. temporal lobe biopsy: herpes simplex encephalitis
2. temporal lobectomy: for resection of seizure focus, decompression post-trauma...
3. hematoma (epidural or subdural) overlying temporal lobe
4. tumors of the temporal lobe
5. small, laterally located acoustic neuromas[33]
6. access to the floor of the middle cranial fossa (including foramen ovale/Meckel's cave, the labyrinthine and upper tympanic portion of the facial nerve)
7. access to **medial temporal lobe** e.g. for amygdalo-hippocampectomy (*see page 285*) or for mesial temporal sclerosis (*see page 257*)

TECHNIQUE
Two basic methods for temporal craniotomy:
1. small craniotomy or craniectomy through a linear skin incision: good for cortical biopsy or draining chronic subdural hematoma. Also permits access to floor of middle fossa. Simple quick closure
2. question-mark skin incision with standard craniotomy flap: useful for temporal lobe exposure for tumor or acute hematoma

TEMPORAL LOBECTOMY
✱ Danger points:
1. dominant hemisphere: Wernicke's speech area. Although variable (see *Temporal lobectomy*, page 284), one can usually safely resect up to 4-5 cm from temporal tip
2. non-dominant hemisphere: one can resect up to 6-7 cm before running the risk of injuring the optic radiation
3. sylvian fissure (middle cerebral artery): it is best to amputate the temporal lobe backward from the tip for the extent of the desired resection, and then work deep
4. medially, the incisura should be identified to avoid injury to the brain stem which lies just medial to this

23.5.4. Frontal craniotomy

INDICATIONS
1. access to frontal lobe: e.g. for tumor, frontal lobectomy (*see below*)
2. approach to third ventricle or to sellar region tumors in some situations, includ-

ing craniopharyngiomas, planum sphenoidale meningiomas
3. repair of ethmoidal CSF fistula

FRONTAL LOBECTOMY

✱ Danger points:
1. anterior cerebral arteries in the midline (deep)
2. superior sagittal sinus (SSS) in the midline (note: the SSS may be sacrificed in its anterior third without engendering venous infarction in most cases, whereas venous infarction will almost always occur with division of the SSS posterior to that)
3. avoid inadvertently crossing the midline into the contralateral hemisphere through the corpus callosum
4. dominant hemisphere: Broca's (motor speech) area is located in the inferior frontal gyrus

23.5.5. Skull base surgery

The term "skull base surgery" has been used to describe a resurgence of interest and a concomitant development of numerous surgical techniques to provide access to difficult areas at the base of the skull. While beyond the scope of this book, some information and literature citations are presented here (refer to standard references[34]).

DOLENC APPROACH

A pterional craniotomy with extradural removal of anterior clinoid[A], which facilitates:
1. intradural exposure of the proximal carotid artery (removal of the anterior clinoid exposes an additional ≈ 6 mm of carotid[35])
2. the extradural 7 mm of carotid artery (between the cavernous sinus and the point where it enters the dura) is also accessible
3. access to petrous carotid (by drilling off the bone over Glasscock's triangle)
4. access to the cavernous sinus
5. lateral access to the sella

INDICATIONS
1. carotid-ophthalmic aneurysms
2. cavernous sinus lesions
   A. vascular lesions[36] (e.g. carotid cavernous fistula)
   B. cavernous sinus tumors
3. skull base tumors

23.5.6. Petrosal craniotomy

INDICATIONS
1. lesions of the petrous apex (e.g. petroclival meningiomas)
2. lesions of the clivus (e.g. chordomas) with both posterior fossa and supratentorial components

---

A. NB: this may be more difficult, and in the case of aneurysm, more dangerous than the classic intradural removal of the clinoid

Advantages
Spares sinus and otologic apparatuses. Minimizes cerebellar and temporal lobe retraction.

TECHNIQUE
See reference[37]

23.5.7. Approaches to the lateral ventricle

Classic review[38 (p 561-74)] summarized:
1. atrium (AKA trigone); numerous approaches include:
   A. middle temporal gyrus: through the dilated temporal horn
   B. lateral temporal parietal
   C. superior parietal occipital
   D. transcallosal (*see below*)
   E. transtemporal horn: access to temporal horn is via lobectomy of the temporal tip
   F. occipital lobe incision or occipital lobectomy: recommended only if patient has homonymous hemianopsia pre-op
2. frontal horn
   A. middle frontal gyrus
3. midventricular body
   A. transcallosal
   B. middle frontal gyrus: usually prevents access to vascular supply until most of the tumor is removed (especially for tumors supplied primarily by posterior choroidal artery)
4. temporal horn
   A. middle temporal gyrus
   B. transtemporal horn

23.5.8. Approaches to the third ventricle

Classic references review the microsurgical anatomy[39] and surgical approaches[40], and are briefly summarized below.

Alternative approaches for lesions of the anterior third ventricle[41]:
1. transcortical: approach is through the lateral ventricle and is feasible only in the presence of hydrocephalus; especially useful if the tumor extends from the third ventricle into one of the lateral ventricles. Risk of seizures is 5% (higher then with transcallosal). *See page 611*
2. transcallosal: may be preferable in the absence of hydrocephalus (*see below*)
   A. anterior transcallosal: good visualization of both walls of third ventricle; risk of bilateral fornicial damage
   B. posterior transcallosal: allows approach to quadrigeminal plate or pineal region; risk of damage to deep veins
3. subfrontal: allows four different approaches
   A. subchiasmatic: between optic nerve and optic chiasm
   B. optico-carotid: through the triangular space bordered by optic nerve medially, carotid artery laterally, and ACA posteriorly
   C. lamina terminalis: above the optic chiasm[42]
   D. transsphenoidal: requires removal of tuberculum sellae, planum sphenoidale, and anterior wall of the sella turcica
4. transsphenoidal
5. subtemporal
6. stereotactic: may be useful for aspiration of colloid cysts (see *Stereotactic drainage of colloid cysts*, page 459)

Summarized[40]. During the approach, deep veins should be preserved at all costs, even if it means stretching them to the point that they may rupture.

It is helpful to place a suture through the tumor capsule to act as a tether.

The tumor should first be removed from within the capsule; techniques include aspiration, and then opening the capsule and debulking from within. The capsule may then be collapsed and dissected from adherent structures. If the capsule adhesions seem unyielding, the most likely cause is incomplete intracapsular evacuation.

Vessels on the surface of the tumor should be presumed to be supplying normal brain, and should be dissected off the capsule once it is completely emptied.

TRANSCALLOSAL APPROACH TO LATERAL OR THIRD VENTRICLE

Performed through an interhemispheric approach to the corpus callosum (**CC**) via a parietal craniotomy, usually right sided in a left-hemisphere dominant patient.

INDICATIONS

Primarily for tumors or lesions of the lateral or third ventricle, including:
1. colloid cysts
2. craniopharyngiomas
3. cysticercosis cysts
4. thalamic glioma
5. AVM

TECHNIQUE[39, 40, 43]

Disconnection syndrome: more common with posterior callosotomy (near the splenium) where more visual information crosses. The risk is reduced by creating a callosotomy < **2.5 cm** in length extending posteriorly from a point 1-2 cm behind the tip of the genu[44]. For an interfornicial approach, the callosotomy must be perfectly midline.

COMPLICATIONS

1. venous infarction, may be due to:
   A. sacrifice of critical cortical draining veins: plan the flap to avoid this with preoperative angiography, or with sagittal T2WI MRI images[45]
   B. superior sagittal sinus (**SSS**) thrombosis[46]. Factors that may contribute to sinus injury include[47]:
      1. injury from retractor: avoid placing retractor on sinus (deformation of midline should not exceed 5 mm)
      2. over-retraction of the dural sinus flap or on SSS itself (lateral deformation should be < 2 cm)
      3. injury during the opening of the bone in the region of the sinus
      4. over-use of bipolar coagulation in the region of the SSS
      5. hypercoagulable state of the patient, including dehydration
2. transient mutism as a result of bilateral cingulate gyrus retraction or thalamic injury in conjunction with section of the midportion of the callosum[45]

TRANSCORTICAL APPROACH TO LATERAL OR THIRD VENTRICLE

INDICATIONS

In the absence of hydrocephalus, it is difficult to navigate through the ventricular

system. Thus, with normal sized ventricles, the third ventricle and region of the foramen of Monro are better approached transcallosally (*see page 611*).
1. tumors of the atrium of the lateral ventricle
2. tumors of the roof of the third ventricle
3. third ventricular tumors with significant extension into one lateral ventricle

APPROACHES
1. posterior parietal
2. middle temporal gyrus: useful when temporal horn of lateral ventricle is dilated due to hydrocephalus caused by the tumor; access is through the temporal horn
3. **middle frontal gyrus approach**: a 4 cm incision is made parallel to the axis of the middle frontal gyrus, above and anterior to the expressive speech center (Broca's area) and anterior to the motor strip[40] (about the same point as used for frontal ventriculostomy, see *Kocher's point*,page 620)

23.5.9.   Interhemispheric approach

INDICATIONS
For lesions abutting on midline, deep to surface, but superficial to corpus callosum (lesions that can "fall away" from midline). Similar to transcallosal approach above, except that the pathology can be placed on the down side, which allows gravity to retract the hemisphere and thus minimizes pressure necrosis injury from mechanical retractors.

23.5.10.   Occipital craniotomy

INDICATIONS
Occipital lobe tumors including posterior falx meningiomas or tentorial meningiomas with only supratentorial component. Occipital lobe intracerebral hemorrhages.

23.6.   Cranioplasty

Indications
1. cosmetic restoration of external skull symmetry
2. relief of symptoms due to craniotomy defect (*see page 604*)
3. protection from trauma (blunt or penetrating) in area of skull defect from craniotomy or posttraumatic

Timing
In certain cases, no consensus is possible. To avoid the risk of infection, authors recommend delaying cranioplasty with a "foreign body" at least 6 months after an open (i.e. contaminated) wound or one that traverses the nasal sinuses. Others perform primary closure at the time of repair of the skull fracture. In "clean" cases (e.g. repair of defect after removing hemangioma of the skull) there is little argument against immediate cranioplasty.

Material
Options for material include methylmethacrylate, and tantalum mesh. Split thickness calvaria may also be used. Any foreign material that is used should be perforated

(methacrylate may be multiply drilled) to prevent the accumulation of fluid (either underneath the flap, or between the flap and the skull).

23.7. Anterior approaches to the spine

23.7.1. Transoral approach to anterior craniocervical junction

Primarily useful for <u>extradural</u> lesions (approach to intradural lesions has been described[48], but the use has been extremely limited because of difficulties obtaining watertight closure and increased risk of meningitis). Refinements in techniques and equipment (e.g. flexible reinforced oral endotracheal tube, McGarver or Crockard retractor, operating microscope, and suturing transnasal red-rubber catheters to the uvula to aid in retraction) allows access from as high as the cervicomedullary junction to as low as C4 vertebral body without need for tracheostomy or splitting of the tongue[49].

Transoral odontoidectomy: 75% of patients undergoing transoral removal of the odontoid process required posterior fusion[50] afterwards, due to ligamentous instability[51, 52].

23.7.2. Anterior access to the cervico-thoracic junction/upper thoracic spine

Access with a lateral approach is poor due to small amount of room in pulmonary apices. Utilizing a sternal splitting procedure, one can access down to T3 (occasionally as far as T5) from an anterior midline approach.

23.7.3. Anterior access to mid & lower thoracic spine

Position the patient on the O.R. on a bean-bag table with the break in the table under the level of pathology (remember to unbreak the table prior to instrumenting). Stabilize the patient using adhesive tape over surgical towels. An axillary roll is placed. A double-lumen endotracheal tube is used to permit dropping the lung on the side of the thoracotomy.

To increase the exposure, a rib may be resected. Generally, the level opened and the rib removed are one or two levels above the level of pathology (e.g. for T7 VB tumor, the T6 or T5 rib are removed).

ANTERIOR ACCESS TO MID THORACIC SPINE
Unless pathology is predominantly left-sided, a right-sided thoracotomy is preferred because the heart does not impede access.

ANTERIOR ACCESS TO LOWER THORACIC SPINE
Unless pathology is predominantly right-sided, a left-sided thoracotomy is preferred (easier to mobilize aorta than vena cava).

23.7.4. Anterior access to thoracolumbar junction

Unless pathology is predominantly left-sided, a right-sided retroperitoneal approach is preferred (eliminates liver from impeding access).

23.7.5. Anterior access to the lumbar spine

Trans-abdominal approach through a Pfannenstiel's incision.

The location of the bifurcation of the inferior vena cava generally ranges from just above to just below the L4-5 disc space. When the bifurcation is at or below the disc space, procedures such as L4-5 ALIF van be very difficult if the veins cannot be mobilized off the vertebrae.

At L5-S1, the anterior sacral artery runs down the middle and has to be sacrificed to do an ALIF.

23.8. Percutaneous access to the CNS

23.8.1. Percutaneous ventricular puncture

INDICATIONS

In pediatrics, may be used to remove hemorrhagic ventricular fluid following intraventricular hemorrhage, or to obtain CSF specimen in cases of suspected ventriculitis. May be used emergently in pediatrics or adult as a temporizing measure in patient herniating from hydrocephalus.

PEDS

Shave hair. 5 minute Betadine® prep.

The right side is preferred. Enter through coronal suture just lateral to anterior fontanelle **(AF)** using a 20-22 Ga. spinal needle. If a CT scan has been done, it may be used to help judge angulation (usually varies between contra- and ipsi-lateral medial canthus and intersection with EAM).

ADULT[53]

Only used emergently. Takes advantage of thin orbital roof in adult.

Prep conjunctiva and skin with antiseptic. Elevate the eyelid and depress the globe. Using a 16-18 Ga. spinal needle, penetrate the anterior third of orbital roof (1-2 cm behind orbital rim) with firm pressure (may need gentle tapping). Aim at coronal suture in the midline. The frontal horn should be about 3-4 cm deep.

23.8.2. Subdural tap

Indications

Utilized in pediatrics. Used to be done for diagnostic purposes, but this has been supplanted by CT, ultrasound… Currently, this procedure may be used emergently for decompression, and to drain subdural collections and to obtain fluid for diagnostic tests, such as culture (repeat taps may be used, but surgery should be considered after ≈ 5-6).

Technique

Shave hair. Prep 5 minutes with povidone iodine (Betadine®). Using a short 20-21 Ga. spinal needle, penetrate the lateral margin of the anterior fontanelle **(AF)** or coronal suture at least 2 cm off midline. With bilateral fluid collections, bilateral taps should be done.

23.8.3.　Lumbar puncture

1. known or suspected intracranial mass ⎫
2. non-communicating hydrocephalus　⎬ risk of tonsillar herniation (*see below*)
3. infection in region desired for puncture: choose another site if possible
4. coagulopathy
    A. platelet count should be > 50,000/mm³ (*see page 19*)
    B. patient should not be on anticoagulants because of risk of epidural hematoma (*see page 353*) or subarachnoid hemorrhage[54] with secondary cord compression
5. caution in suspected aneurysmal SAH: excessive lowering of the CSF pressure increases the transmural pressure (pressure across the aneurysm wall) and may precipitate rerupture
6. caution in patients with complete spinal block: 14% will deteriorate after LP[55]

* elevated ICP and/or papilledema by themselves are <u>NOT</u> contraindications (e.g. LP is actually used diagnostically and as a treatment in idiopathic intracranial hypertension, *see below*)

TECHNIQUE

Background and anatomy

　The spinal cord and column are the same length in a 3-month fetus, after that the spinal column grows faster than the cord. As a result, the conus medullaris is located rostral to the termination of the thecal sac in the adult. The conus is located between the middle thirds of the vertebral bodies of L1 and L2 in 51-68% of adults (the most common location), T12-L1 in ≈ 30%, and L2-3 in ≈ 10% (with 94% of cords terminating within the territory of L1 and L2 vertebral bodies)[56]. The thecal sac ends ≈ S2. The intercristal line (connecting the superior border of the iliac crests) crosses the spine at the L4 spinous process or between the L4 and L5 spinous processes in most adults.

Procedure

　For adult LP: use the L4-5 interspace in most cases (located at or just below the intercristal line) or 1 level higher (L3-4). Peds: L4-5 is preferred over L3-4.

　The needle is always advanced with the <u>stylet in place</u> at least through the skin and some subcutaneous tissue to avoid introducing epidermal cells which may cause iatrogenic <u>epidermoid tumors</u> (see*Complications following LP* below). The needle is aimed slightly cranially (to parallel the spinous processes) and usually a little down towards the bed (aiming towards the umbilicus). If a Quincke LP (standard) needle is used, the bevel is turned parallel to the length of the spinal column to reduce the risk of post-LP H/A (see *needle type*, page 617). In general, if bone is encountered it is more often due to deviation from a true midline trajectory rather than a failure to aim correctly in the rostral-caudal direction. The needle should be withdrawn to just below the skin surface before attempting a new trajectory.

　If during insertion of the needle the patient experiences pain radiating down one LE, this usually indicates that a nerve root has been encountered. The needle should be withdrawn immediately and reinserted aiming more towards the side contralateral to the extremity that experienced the pain.

　At the end of the procedure, the stylet should be replaced before the needle is withdrawn (to reduce post-LP H/A, *see below*).

OPENING PRESSURE

　The opening pressure **(OP)** should be measured and recorded for every LP. To be meaningful, the patient should be lying down and as relaxed as possible (should not be in forced fetal position), with the bed flat. The variation of pressure with respirations is usually a good indication of a communicating fluid column (the fluctuation is in-phase with the respiratory pressures in the inferior vena cava, rising with inspiration and falling with expiration[57]). See *Table 10-1*, page 171 for normal values.

　Queckenstedt's test: if a subarachnoid block is suspected (e.g. from spinal tumor), compress the jugular vein **(JV)** first on one side then on both (do not compress carotid arteries). If there is no block, the pressure will rise to 10-20 cm of fluid, and will drop to the original level within 10 seconds of release of the JV[58 (p 11)]. Do <u>not</u> do JV compression if intracranial disease is suspected.

Routinely, three tubes are sent for analysis as shown in *Table 23-3*. See *Table 10-4*, page 172 for interpreting the results of the laboratory analysis.

If the tap is possibly *traumatic* (i.e. bloody), or if having an accurate cell count is essential (e.g. to R/O SAH) then 4 tubes are collected, and the first and last are sent for cell counts and are compared (see *Traumatic tap*, page 173).

If special cultures are required (e.g. acid fast, fungal, viral) they are also specified on the tube for culture & sensitivity (C & S).

Table 23-3   Routine tests for CSF

Test	If there is no concern about possible traumatic tap	If there is special concern about traumatic tap
cell count		Tube 1
gram stain + C & S	Tube 1	Tube 2
protein and glucose	Tube 2	Tube 3
cell count	Tube 3	Tube 4

If CSF for *cytology* is desired (e.g. to R/O carcinomatous meningitis or CNS lymphoma), then at least 10 ml of CSF must be sent in one tube to pathology.

COMPLICATIONS FOLLOWING LP

The overall risk of disabling or persistent symptoms (defined as severe H/A lasting > 7 days, cranial nerve palsies, major exacerbation of pre-existing neurological disease, prolonged back pain, aseptic meningitis, and nerve root or peripheral nerve injuries) has been estimated at 0.1-0.5%[59]. Severe side effects, which include brainstem herniation, infection, subdural hematoma or effusion, and SAH, are rare[60 (p 171-2)].

Possible complications include:
1. tonsillar herniation
   A. acute herniation in the presence of mass lesion (*see below*)
   B. chronic tonsillar herniation (acquired Chiari 1 malformation): reported after multiple traumatic LPs with presumed post-LP CSF leak[61]
2. infection (spinal meningitis)
3. "spinal headache": usually positional (diminishes with recumbency) (*see below*)
4. spinal epidural hematoma: usually seen only with coagulopathy (*see page 353*)
5. spinal epidural CSF collection: may be fairly common in patients with post-LP H/A. Usually resolves spontaneously
6. epidermoid tumor: risk may be increased by advancing LP needle without stylet (transplanting a core of epidermal tissue)[62-64]
7. impinging nerve root with needle: usually causes transient radicular pain, may cause permanent radiculopathy in some
8. intracranial subdural hygroma or hematoma[65, 66] (rare)
9. vestibulocochlear dysfunction[67]:
   A. subclinical (demonstrated on audiogram) or moderate reduction in hearing may occur, and seems to correlate with post-procedure CSF leakage
   B. sudden hearing loss may occur. Perform audiogram to quantify loss. Treat with bed rest for several days, prednisone 60 mg/d tapered over 2-3 weeks
   C. pathogenesis: reduced CSF pressure may reduce perilymph pressure through the cochlear aqueduct[68], producing endolymphatic hydrops
10. ocular abnormalities
    A. abducens palsy: almost invariably unilateral. Often delayed 5-14 days post-LP, usually recovers after 4-6 wks[69]
11. dural sinus thrombosis[70] (usually with underlying thrombophilia)

RISK OF ACUTE TONSILLAR HERNIATION FOLLOWING LUMBAR PUNCTURE

The question of when to tap first (to save time) and when to obtain CT scan first to R/O intracranial mass (for safety) before performing an LP is controversial.

Issues

The time delay to initiating antibiotics is the most important variable in the outcome of meningitis. Time may be more crucial in community acquired meningitis, than in post-op neurosurgical meningitis.

The theoretical risk in performing an LP with an intracranial mass is that the resultant shift in pressure may precipitate tonsillar herniation.

Starting antibiotics without first having a CSF specimen risks the difficulties in managing partially treated meningitis, or a suboptimal choice of antibiotic medication.

Clinical evaluation for possible contraindication to LP is unreliable. Papilledema takes a minimum of 6 hrs to develop after the onset of increased ICP, and in most cases it requires up to 24 hrs. Therefore, its absence does not insure normal intracranial pressure. Furthermore, papilledema may be seen in conditions where there is not a contraindication to LP (e.g. idiopathic intracranial hypertension, where LP is one of the accepted treatments, *see page 493*).

The availability of CT scans, often within the emergency department itself, may involve a delay of only a few minutes, if qualified personnel to interpret the study are also immediately available.

Historical information

Herniation following LP was more common prior to ≈ 1950, long before CT scans were available, where the procedure was performed even when some patients had clear evidence of ↑ ICP, large bore spinal needles (12-16 gauge) were more commonly employed, and large quantities of CSF were removed for therapeutic purposes. In a report in 1969 of 30 patients who deteriorated after LP[71], 73% had localizing signs (hemiparesis, anisocoria…) and 30% had papilledema. None of 5 patients with cerebral abscess deteriorated after the first of multiple LPs.

In a series of 129 patients with ↑ ICP[72], the complication rate reported was 6%; however, some of these complications were probably unrelated to LP, and many of these patients were in extremis. In 7 series totalling 418 patients, a complication rate of 1.2% was calculated[72].

Σ Herniation as a result of LP is consistently reported only in patients with severe non-infectious processes, often with accompanying signs of mass effect (localizing signs, papilledema). Thus, in cases of suspected meningitis in the absence of focal findings and papilledema, if a CT scan cannot be performed and interpreted within a few minutes, the benefits of performing an LP with a needle ≤ 20 gauge and removing only a few ml of CSF probably outweigh the small risk of herniation. In the unlikely event that there is acute deterioration associated with the withdrawal of a few ml of CSF, the (anecdotal) recommendation is to immediately replace the fluid through the LP needle.

HEADACHE FOLLOWING LUMBAR PUNCTURE

For characteristics of the H/A and treatment *see page 46*. Risk of post-LP H/A (**PLPHA**) is related to a number of factors including:

Factors outside the control of the physician:
1. age: ↑ in younger patients
2. sex: ↑ in females
3. prior headache history (including previous PLPHA)
4. body size: ↑ with small body mass index = weight/height[273]
5. pregnancy

Variables that have been shown to influence the incidence of PLPHA:
1. needle size: larger needles carry increased risk[74]
2. bevel orientation: orienting the bevel parallel to the longitudinally running fibers of the dura reduces the risk of PLPHA[75]
3. replacing the stylet prior to needle removal lowers the incidence[73]
4. the number of dural punctures (may not be totally under the physician's control)

Variables that may or may not influence the incidence of PLPHA:
1. needle type
   A. Quincke needle: bevelled edge with cutting tip (the standard LP needle). Incidence of PLPHA with 20 and 22 gauge Quincke needles: 36%[76])
   B. atraumatic needles: a number of types are available. Most are "pencil pointed" and may produce a hole with a lower incidence of transdural leak[77]. Unproven[73]

Factors found <u>not</u> to affect the incidence of PLPHA:
1. the position of the patient after LP (does not seem to prevent PLPHA, but may delay the onset of symptoms[78, 79])
2. volume of fluid removed at the time of LP
3. hydration following LP[73]

23.8.4.   C1-2 puncture and cisternal tap

Indications

Situations where CSF specimen is required but access via LP is difficult or contraindicated (lumbar arachnoiditis, marked obesity...), or to instill contrast to demonstrate the rostral extent of a block documented by dye injected via LP. Spinal headache is less common with these procedures than with LP. C1-2 puncture is safer than cisternal tap.

✖ Contraindicated: in patient with Chiari malformation (often present in myelomeningocele) due to low lying cerebellar tonsils and medullary kink.

Normal CSF values for glucose and protein differ only slightly from CSF obtained by lumbar puncture. Opening pressures averaged 18 cm of fluid with lateral puncture.

C1-2 PUNCTURE

AKA lateral cervical puncture. Equipment: LP tray (useful for the specimen tubes, extension tube for contrast injection under fluoroscopy, lidocaine, and spinal needle) with a standard 20 Ga spinal needle, contrast if needed (e.g. Iohexol®). It is preferred to perform the procedure under fluoro, however it has also been described without fluoroscopic guidance with a completely cooperative patient[80].

Patient position: supine in bed without a pillow, with the head straight up. Avoid any head rotation which may bring the vertebral artery

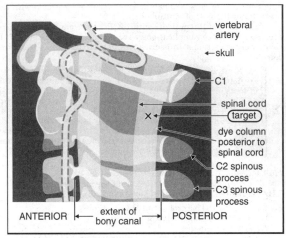

Figure 23-1 C1-2 puncture target*

*   composite diagram of a myelogram and vertebral arteriogram illustrating the relative location of the spinal cord, CSF space, and VA. Only bony landmarks will be visible with fluoroscopy

(**VA**) into the needle path[81]. Place head within lateral fluoroscopy unit (since this is rarely available, a C-arm fluoro positioned horizontally may be used).

If iodinated dye is being injected for myelography, the head should be elevated to prevent contrast from running into posterior fossa; in cases with cervical spine injury, one can put the entire bed in reverse Trendelenburg.

Entry point: 1 cm caudal and 1 cm posterior (dorsal) to the tip of the mastoid process. **Needle insertion**: use a 25 Ga. needle to anesthetize the skin at the entry point. Under fluoro, advance a larger needle (e.g. 21 Ga.) towards the C1-2 interspace while injecting local anesthetic: aim for a target in the middle of the posterior third of the bony spinal canal (or, alternatively, 2-3 mm anterior to the posterior margin of the bony canal) ("**X**" in *Figure 23-1*). Leave this needle in as a marker. Insert the 20 Ga. spinal needle parallel to the marker needle. Verify the course with fluoro. If fluoro is not used, insert the spinal needle at the entry point, and advance it parallel to the plane of the bed, perpendicular to the neck[80]. If the needle penetrates deeply without encountering bone or CSF, it is most likely that the tip is too par posterior. If bone is encountered, redirect the needle in the rostrocaudal plane.

Several "pops" may be felt, and the stylet should be removed after each to check for CSF return. The subarachnoid space is ≈ 5-6 cm deep to the skin surface in most adults[82].

The needle must be supported more than with a lumbar puncture.

To inject iodinated contrast, use e.g. ≈ 5 ml of 180 mg% Iohexol® for cervical myelogram, watch dye on fluoro (should be able to see it in subarachnoid space).

Risks

Case report of a death from subdural hematoma due to puncture of an anomalous vertebral artery[83] (found in ≈ 0.4% of population). If the VA is penetrated, the needle is withdrawn and local pressure is applied. Penetration of the upper spinal cord/lower medulla (risk of serious neurologic sequelae, even from this, is small). Herniation (as with LP) when there is increased ICP.

CISTERNAL TAP

Suboccipital access to the cisterna magna. Usually done with patient sitting, with neck slightly flexed[84]. Overlying hair should be shaved. Local anesthetic is infiltrated. A 22 gauge spinal needle is inserted exactly in the midline between the inion and the C2 spinous process, directed superiorly towards the glabella until the needle strikes the occiput or enters the cisterna magna. If the occiput is encountered, the needle is withdrawn slightly and reinserted directed slightly inferiorly, the process is repeated ("walking down the occiput") until the cisterna magna is entered (a "pop" will be felt).

The distance from the skin surface to the cisterna magna is 4-6 cm, and from the dura to the medulla is ≈ 2.5 cm. However, due to tenting of the dura, the needle may be very close to the medulla before entering the subarachnoid space.

Risks

1. hemorrhage in the cisterna magna: may be due to perforation of a large vessel[80]
2. piercing the medulla oblongata: may cause vomiting, respiratory arrest...
3. positioning may compromise blood flow in the vertebral artery in elderly patients

23.9.   CSF diversionary procedures

23.9.1.   Ventricular catheterization

Most common sites[85 (p 151-3)]:

★   1.   **occipital-parietal** region: commonly used for CSF shunt
   A.   entry site: a number of means have been described, including:
       1.   **Frazier burr hole**: placed prophylactically before p-fossa crani for emergency ventriculostomy in event of post-op swelling. Location: 3-4 cm from midline, 6-7 cm above inion[38 (p 520)] (caution: an error in locating the inion could put the catheter in an undesirable location if this method alone is used)
       2.   **parietal boss**: flat portion of parietal bone
       3.   follow point from mid-pupillary line parallel to sagittal suture until it intersects line extending posteriorly from the top of the pinna
       4.   ≈ 3 cm above and ≈ 3 cm posterior to top of pinna
   B.   trajectory: insert the catheter parallel to skull base:
       1.   initially aim for middle of forehead
       2.   if this fails, aim for ipsilateral medial canthus
   C.   insertion length: ideally, the tip should be just anterior to the foramen of Monro in the frontal horn[86]. Ventriculoscopic guidance (if available) increases the accuracy to a significant degree. In the absence of this:
       1.   intracranial length should be ≈ two thirds of the length of the skull (this is short enough to prevent penetration of frontal brain parenchyma, but long enough to take tip beyond the foramen of Monro to prevent catheter from ending up in the temporal horn where choroid plexus increases the chance of obstruction)
       2.   in adults without macrocrania the inserted length is usually ≈ 12 cm when the burr hole is in line with the axis of the lateral ventricle[87] (lengths > 12 cm are rarely required). In hydrocephalic infants usually ≈ 7-8 cm is required

3. use the stylet for the initial ≈ 6 cm of insertion, then remove it and insert the remaining length (keeps the catheter straight during penetration of occipital parenchyma and prevents the tip from dropping into the temporal horn where there is choroid plexus, also the temporal horn may collapse and occlude the catheter when the HCP is resolved)

2. **Keen's point** (posterior parietal): (placement in trigone) 2.5-3 cm posterior and 2.5-3 cm superior to pinna (was the usual site of occurrence of cerebral abscesses arising from otitis media, and was often used to tap these)

3. **Dandy's point**: 2 cm from midline, 3 cm above inion (may be more prone to damage visual pathways than above)

★ 4. **Kocher's point** (coronal): places catheter in frontal horn. The right side is usually used. Commonly employed for ICP monitors

A. entry site: 2-3 cm from midline which is approximately the mid-pupillary line with forward gaze, 1 cm anterior to coronal suture (to avoid motor strip)

B. trajectory: direct catheter perpendicular to surface of brain, which can be approximated by aiming in coronal plane towards medial canthus of ipsilateral eye and in AP plane towards EAM

C. insertion length: advance catheter with stylet until CSF is obtained (should be < 5-7 cm depth; this may be 3-4 cm with markedly dilated ventricles). Advance catheter without stylet 1 cm deeper. ✖ CAUTION: if CSF is not obtained until very long insertion length (e.g. ≥8 cm) the tip is probably in a cistern (e.g. prepontine cistern) which is undesirable

23.9.2. Ventriculostomy/ICP monitor

AKA intraventricular catheter **(IVC)** or external ventricular drainage **(EVD)**.

INSERTION TECHNIQUE

Unless contraindicated (e.g. right ventricular bleed), the right (non-dominant) side is preferred. Shave entire ipsilateral hemicranium and contralateral frontal portion. Five minute Betadine prep.

Site: approximately Kocher's point (*see above*). To avoid motor strip, enter 1-2 cm anterior to coronal suture (estimated position of coronal suture: follow line up midway between lateral canthus and EAM), and to avoid the sagittal sinus, 2-3 cm lateral to midline (2 fingerbreadths or ≈ 3 cm is commonly employed as an approximation). Incision oriented in sagittal plane (in case it needs to be incorporated in flap); elevate periosteum; place self-retaining retractor; make twist drill hole. Bone-wax edges to stop bone bleeding; cauterize dura with bipolar coagulator; incise dura in cruciate fashion with #11 scalpel blade; cauterize incised dural edges and then pia/arachnoid with bipolar.

For ventriculostomy: insert catheter perpendicular to brain surface[88] to a depth of 5-7 cm (most catheters are marked at 5 and 10 cm). With any ventricular enlargement, CSF should flow at least by 3-4 cm depth (with normal ventricles, this may be 4-5 cm). If no CSF is encountered here and the catheter is passed further until CSF is obtained, it is unlikely to be due to catheterization of frontal horn of lateral ventricle (in this case, at ≈ 9-11 cm the tip will often be in the pre-pontine cistern, a subarachnoid space, which is undesirable). If unsuccessful after a maximum of three attempted passes, then place a subarachnoid bolt or intraparenchymal monitor.

For (Richmond) subarachnoid bolt: screw in until tip is flush with inner table.

"SUMP DRAINAGE"

The tip of a 25 gauge butterfly may be bent at a 90° angle, and inserted into a subcutaneous reservoir for prolonged ventricular drainage[89]. In one series OF 34 patients, this was used for prolonged periods (up to 44 days) with acceptably low infection rate[90]. The use of a one-way valve, continuous antibiotics (ampicillin and cloxacillin) and meticulous technique was credited for the lack of infection.

23.9.3. Ventricular shunts

Ventricular catheter

Occipital burr hole is used in most cases for insertion site of ventricular catheter (see *Ventricular catheterization page 619* for technique). Some prefer a frontal burr hole

(Kocher's point) citing a lower incidence of failure from choroid plexus occlusion (this is controversial). The use of flanged catheters (designed to keep choroid plexus away from catheter holes) is discouraged because these actually have a higher incidence of choroid plexus occlusion and these catheters can become so entangled that removal is impossible without significant risk of hemorrhage.

VENTRICULOPERITONEAL SHUNT

Peritoneal catheter

For small children, use at least 30 cm length of intraperitoneal tubing to allow for continued growth (120 cm total length of peritoneal tubing was associated with a lower revision rate for growth without significant increase in other complications[91]). A silver clip is placed at the point where the catheter enters the peritoneum so that the amount of residual intraperitoneal catheter can be determined on later films (more important in growing children).

Distal slits on the peritoneal catheter may increase the risk of distal obstruction[92], and should probably be trimmed off. Wire reinforced catheters should not be used because of excessively high rate of viscus perforation, and this tubing was designed to prevent kinking which is not a problem with modern shunts.

VP SHUNT, POST-OP ORDERS (ADULT)

1. flat in bed (to avoid overshunting and possible subdural hematoma)
2. if peritoneal end is new or revised, do not feed until bowel sounds resume (usually at least 24 hrs, due to ileus from manipulation of peritoneum)
3. shunt series (AP & lateral skull, and chest/abdominal x-ray) as baseline for future comparison (some surgeons obtain these films immediately post-op in case some immediate revision is indicated, e.g. ventricular catheter tip in temporal horn)

VENTRICULO-ATRIAL SHUNT INSERTION

A growing patient is followed with annual CXRs. When the catheter tip is above ≈ T4, the catheter must be lengthened or converted to a VP shunt.

VENTRICULOPLEURAL SHUNT INSERTION

See reference[93].

23.9.4.   Ventricular access device

An indwelling ventricular catheter connected to a reservoir that is situated under the scalp for the purpose of chronic access to the intrathecal space (or some other compartment). Sometimes referred to as an Ommaya® reservoir.

INDICATIONS

Indications for insertion:
1. administration of intrathecal **(IT)** antineoplastic chemotherapy:
    A. for CNS neoplasms, including: carcinomatous meningitis, CNS lymphoma or leukemia (*see page 464*)
    B. IT chemotherapy is often used for the following even in the *absence* of CNS involvement because of the high relapse rate in the CNS: acute lymphoblastic leukemia, lymphoblastic lymphoma, Burkitt's lymphoma
2. administration of intrathecal antibiotic for chronic meningitis
3. chronic removal of CSF from infants with intraventricular hemorrhage
4. for fluid aspiration from a chronic tumor cyst that is resistant to therapy (radiation or surgery)

TECHNIQUE OF INSERTION

See reference[94]

RESERVOIR PUNCTURE
The scalp is prepped with antimicrobial scrub, and using sterile technique, a 25 gauge or smaller butterfly needle is introduced at an oblique angle, preferably with a non-coring needle. The original (Ommaya®) reservoir has firm plastic bottom surface which can be penetrated if too much force is applied.

23.9.5. Third ventriculostomy

See page 187 for indications and complications.
Older techniques include a subfrontal approach, opening the chiasmatic and lamina terminalis cisterns, and making a 5-10 mm opening in the lamina terminalis. Stereotactic third ventriculostomy (using contrast ventriculography[95] or CT guided) has also been described. Current technique consists of fenestrating the floor of the third ventricle using the ventriculoscope.

23.9.6. LP shunt

TECHNIQUE OF INSERTION
See reference[96].

LP SHUNT EVALUATION
Evaluation of function is more difficult than with VP shunt since an access device is not always inserted.
1. it is sometimes possible to tap the tubing with a 27 gauge butterfly needle
2. "shunt-o-gram"
   A. with injection of water-soluble contrast[97]: perform LP just above or below level of lumbar catheter. The pressure may be 0 or negative, and it may be necessary to aspirate CSF to confirm placement. Inject 10 ml of iohexol or 250 mg metrizamide and monitor the flow of contrast fluoroscopically as the patient is brought vertical. Coughing or valsalva maneuver will accelerate the flow of contrast
   B. one can inject radio-isotope via LP and look for subsequent tracer activity in peritoneal cavity
3. one can also get indirect evidence of shunt function just by measuring the pressure via LP, it should be low (only helpful in cases where shunt was placed for elevated CSF pressure, e.g. pseudotumor cerebri; not helpful in NPH)

23.10. Sural nerve biopsy

Although a number of peripheral nerves may be biopsied, the sural nerve fulfills the criteria of being well studied, expendable with minimal deficit, easily accessible, and often involved in the pathologic process in question.

INDICATIONS
Nerve biopsy plays a small role in diagnosing peripheral neuropathies, but may be very accurate for vasculitis, amyloidosis, Hansen's disease, metachromatic and globoid leukodystrophy, neoplastic infiltration of peripheral nerve, and relapsing polyneuritis[98] (p 316). May help distinguish the two types of Charcot-Marie-Tooth syndrome. May show demyelination in diabetic amyotrophy (*see page 556*).

RISKS OF PROCEDURE
1. sensory loss in the sural nerve distribution is *expected*, but often does not persist

for more than several weeks (unless the underlying disease process prevents this)
2. problems with wound healing: the ankle is a notorious region for poor circulation and the loss of sensation (from the disease or biopsy) may render the area subject to repeated trauma without the patient being aware. Furthermore, many patients with an undiagnosed systemic disease requiring a sural nerve biopsy will have poor wound healing (a significant number are also diabetic)
3. failure to make a diagnosis: although biopsy may be able to exclude some contingencies, it often does not make a specific diagnosis

23.11. Surgical fusion of the cervical spine

Techniques include:
1. C1 and C2
    A. atlantoaxial fusion (*see below*), sometimes with incorporation of the occiput
        1. wiring/fusion techniques
            a. Brooks fusion: *see page 624*
            b. Gallie fusion: *see page 624*
            c. fusion technique of Dickman and Sonntag: *see page 624*
        2. plates/clamps
            a. Halifax clamps
            b. hook plates
        3. atlanto-axial transarticular facet screw fixation: *see page 626*
    B. odontoid screw fixation: best suited for odontoid Type II fractures < 6 months old with intact transverse ligament: *see page 625*
2. subaxial spine
    A. posterior lateral mass screw-plate fixation
    B. anterior vertebral body screw-plate fixation

23.11.1. Upper cervical spine

ATLANTOAXIAL FUSION (C1-2 ARTHRODESIS)

INDICATIONS
1. instability of the C1-2 joints, including:
    A. atlantoaxial dislocation due to disruption of the transverse ligament: e.g. due to rheumatoid arthritis, local infection, or trauma
    B. incompetence of the odontoid process
        1. odontoid fractures meeting surgical criteria (*see page 728*), including
            a. Type II fractures with > 6 mm displacement
            b. instability at the fracture site in halo-vest traction
            c. chronic nonunion of odontoid fractures
            d. disruption of the transverse ligament
        2. following transoral odontoidectomy
        3. tumors destroying the odontoid process
2. vertebrobasilar insufficiency with head turning (bow hunter's sign): *see page 882*

TECHNICAL CONSIDERATIONS
Surgical options include:
1. posterior cervical wiring and fusion:
    A. C1-C2 or C1-C3 posterior wiring and fusion: if C1 is intact, or has only lateral mass fractures or a unilateral ring fracture, then this is usually the procedure of choice. C1-2 arthrodesis results in ≈ 50% reduction of head rotation (≈ 35° of lateral mobility in each direction of head turning is lost) regardless of which of the following techniques is used:
        1. Brooks fusion technique and its modifications: lateral wires sublaminar to both C1 and C2, with wedge bone grafts (*see below*)
        2. Gallie fusion technique and its modifications: midline wire under the

arch of C1 with an "H" bone graft (*see below*)
3.   interspinous fusion technique of Dickman and Sonntag: *see page 624*
B.   occipitocervical fusion: *see below*
2.   C1-C2 lateral mass fusion: useful in cases of incompetent C1 where only the posterior arch is compromised
3.   Halifax clamps with fusion[99]: these clamps are effective in minimizing movement in flexion, but are less stable in extension or with rotation
4.   C1-2 posterior transarticular facet screws (**TAS**)[100-102]: an adjunct to C1-2 wiring/fusion (*see page 626*)
5.   anterior fusion techniques: may preserve more mobility:
A.   combined anterolateral and posterior bone grafting[103]
B.   odontoid compression screw fixation for odontoid fractures (may be done anterolaterally[103] or transorally) (*see page 625*)
6.   combining anterior (transoral) decompression with posterior fusion: indicated when a significant anterior mass is present causing neural compression and/or making passage of sublaminar wires at C1 unsafe

OCCIPITOCERVICAL FUSION

Incorporation of the occiput is usually unnecessary.

Indication for occipitocervical fusion (versus C1-2 fusion)[104]:
1.   widespread bone destruction
2.   absence of a complete arch of C1
A.   congenital
B.   post-decompression[A]
C.   posttraumatic: "bursting" C1 fracture (bilateral or multiple C1 ring fractures)[A]. NB: some feel that this may be satisfactorily treated with halo immobilization until the atlas fracture heals (as they almost all do) followed by C1 to C2 wiring/fusion[105]
3.   congenital anomalies of the occipitocervical joints
4.   upward migration of the odontoid into the foramen magnum
5.   marked irreducible shifts of C1 or C2

Disadvantages of occipitocervical fusion (versus C1-2 fusion):
1.   loss of movement at the occipitoatlantal junction reduces the range of motion of the neck as follows[106]:
A.   flexion/extension: reduced by ≈ 30% (13° occurs at occiput-C1 junction)
B.   lateral rotation: 10° are lost
C.   lateral bending: 8° are lost
2.   non-union rate is higher[107]

TECHNIQUES OF POSTERIOR ATLANTOAXIAL FUSION

BROOKS FUSION

Method of Brooks[108] (originally described as the **Smith-Robinson** technique) as modified by Griswold[109] consists of C1 to C2 sublaminar wiring with 2 wedge bone grafts:
1.   more immediate stability and more rotational stability than Gallie fusion
2.   associated risks:
A.   spinal cord and/or brain stem infarction
B.   injury to spinal cord while passing C2 sublaminar wires[110]
C.   nonunion (≈ 10% failure rate; 20% if occiput is included)

GALLIE FUSION

An "H" graft is obtained from the iliac crest and is placed between C2 and either C1 or occiput. A wire is passed sublaminar to C1 only.

INTERSPINOUS FUSION TECHNIQUE OF DICKMAN AND SONNTAG

Somewhat of a blend of the Brook's and Gallie method. A single bicortical graft is used, and the wire is passed sublaminar to C1 only. The bone graft is wedged between C1 and C2 (trapping it between the loops of wire)[111, 112]. This technique may have less ten-

---

A.   alternatively, C1-2 lateral mass fusion (with or without lateral mass screws, *see page 626*) may be used in these cases if only the posterior arch of C1 is compromised

dency to pull C1 posteriorly than Gallie, and yet avoids the inherent danger of C2 sub-laminar wires as in Brooks fusion.

Postoperative immobilization

Halo brace provides optimal immobilization (reduces 90–95% of motion in C-spine) and is mandatory with rheumatoid arthritis **(RA)** (*see page 337*) or osteopenia. Also recommended for non-rigid immobilization (e.g. cables and grafts).

If for some reason the patient cannot tolerate a Halo, in non-RA cases a good SOMI brace represents a slightly less effective alternative. Must be maintained for 3-4 months. Sonntag recommends a halo for 12 weeks, then check flexion-extension films with the halo ring still on the head but disconnected from the vest, if stable then remove the ring and use a Philadelphia collar for 4-6 weeks.

A hard collar may be used for rigid internal immobilization (screws) as long as there is no osteopenia or RA.

OUTCOME

The frequency of osseous fusion with the Brooks or Gallie fusion has been quoted from 70-85% (wider range of 60-100% in small series). A 97% union rate was reported with the Dickman and Sonntag technique in 36 patients immobilized post-op as above[112]. When posterior techniques are used for late nonunion, there is still a significant failure rate reported from 20-80% (some of these results predate Brooks type fusion which lowered nonunion rates). In odontoid nonunion, even with successful C1-2 arthrodesis, the dens may never fuse.

Nonunion

Nonunion rates are higher in the presence of rheumatoid arthritis[113]. Other factors felt to be associated with nonunion include: inadequate post-op immobilization, lack of use of autologous bone, malnutrition, cigarette smoking, osteoporosis, and drugs that inhibit bone fusion (steroids, NSAIDs, cytotoxic or immunosuppressive drugs, nicotine...)[113].

Pseudarthrosis occurs mostly at the interface between the graft and C1, or at both the C1 and the C2 graft interface (rarely at the C2-graft interface alone). There may also be complete resorption of bone graft[113].

Treatment strategies for nonunion include modifying correctable risk factors such as: stopping suppressive drugs 1 week before and for 2 weeks after surgery, cessation of smoking without nicotine patches or supplements (nicotine interferes with vascularization of healing bone grafts), improving nutrition…. Surgical component of treatment includes revision of arthroses using autologous bone grafts with meticulous preparation of the graft site, occipitocervical fusion, transarticular screws, and post-op halo immobilization[113]. Complications associated with revisions include dural tears (with or without CSF leak post-op), wound infection, and cellulitis at a halo-pin site.

ANTERIOR ODONTOID SCREW FIXATION

Introduction

50% of axial rotation of the head occurs at the C1-C2 complex. Treatment of odontoid fractures by fusing C1 to C2 significantly reduces this mobility (although subaxial articulations will compensate somewhat over time). Odontoid screw fixation **(OSF)** attempts to treat odontoid fractures by restoring the structural integrity of the odontoid process without sacrificing the normal mobility.

Stability of the C1-2 joint depends on the integrity of the odontoid process and the atlantal transverse ligament (which is the most important structure holding the odontoid process in position against the anterior arch of C1 - *see page 719*).

Evaluation

A full set of C-spine x-rays is needed, including an open-mouth odontoid view. MRI is recommended to rule-out disruption of atlantal transverse ligament. Reformatted coronal and sagittal CT reconstructions are also recommended to demonstrate the orientation of the fracture path and to verify the integrity of the posterior elements. Complex motion tomography may be used if the CT findings are unclear.

Indications

Reducible odontoid Type II fracture (and Type III fractures where the fracture line is in the cephalad portion of the body of C2 in an elderly patient who may not fuse as well with immobilization as a younger patient[114]) with an intact transverse ligament. A con-

---

troversial requirement is age of fracture < 6 months old.

Contraindications

1. fractures of the C2 vertebral body (except cephalad Type III fracture)
2. disruption of atlantal transverse ligament: as demonstrated on MRI. Also may be suggested if the sum of the overhang of the lateral masses of C1 on C2 exceeds 7 mm (rule of Spence, *see page 723*)
3. large odontoid fracture gap
4. irreducible fracture
5. some authors consider a nonunion ≥ 3 wks old as a contraindication due to the lower success rate
6. patients with short, thick necks and/or barrel chest: makes it difficult to achieve the proper angle. May be circumvented by the instrumentation distributed by Richard-Nephew which utilize a cannulated flexible drill, tap and screwdriver
7. pathologic odontoid fracture
8. fracture line in oblique orientation to frontal plane (shearing forces can cause malalignment during screw tightening)

Post-op

Postoperative immobilization: the immediate post-op strength of the odontoid + screw is only ≈ 50% of the normal odontoid. Therefore, a cervical brace is recommended for 6 weeks[114] (although some authors some don't use one[115]). If the patient has significant osteoporosis, a halo brace is recommended.

Results

Healing takes ≈ 3 months (or longer with chronic nonunion). With fractures < 6 months old, the union rate was 95%. Chronic nonunions > 6 months old have a significant risk of hardware failure (screw breakage or pull-out), with a bony union rate of 31%, and 38% rate of presumed fibrous union[115]. Thus, in cases of chronic nonunion > 6 months old, C1-2 arthrodesis is probably a better choice unless the need to maintain motion is worth the risk of needing a second operation if this one fails.

The average technical complication rate is ≈ 6% (2% screw malposition, 1.5% screw breakout).

C1-2 TRANSARTICULAR FACET SCREWS (TAS)

May be used as an adjunct to posterior C1-2 wiring and bone graft (e.g. technique of Dickman and Sonntag, *see page 624*) to achieve immediate stabilization without the need for postoperative external orthosis, or in cases where the posterior arch of C1 is fractured or absent. ✖ A major risk of the procedure is vertebral artery (VA) injury.

Selection of candidates

May be appropriate in elderly patients or those with rheumatoid arthritis, in whom there may be slow fusion, or for those who have failed a previous attempt at C1-2 wiring/fusion. Also in young individuals who have ligamentous laxity.

All patients must have thin cut CT scans from the occipital condyles through C3 with sagittal reconstruction through the C1-2 facet on both sides to look for the presence of a vertebral artery in the intended path of the screw. Also, risk of VA injury can be reduced using CT scans reconstructed along the planned trajectory of the screw (aiming from a point 4 mm above the inferior C2 facet to a point in the anterior C1 button on CT[116]).

Results

A fusion rate of up to 99% has been reported[100] with no complications. Injury to the vertebral artery is the main potential complication.

23.12.   Bone graft

Used mostly for spine fusions. Most common sources for allograft: bone removed during decompression, iliac crest, rib[117]. Autologous or autogenous fibula may also be used.

Successful fusion involves:
1. osteogenesis: native capacity to form bone by osteoblasts (found in living marrow)
2. osteoinduction: factors (including bone morphogenetic protein (**BMP**)) that influence osteoblasts to form bone
3. osteoconduction: the structure of the graft that acts as a scaffold upon which new bone forms

Allograft can provide only osteoconduction. Autograft has all 3 features.

Allografts are an acceptable source of bone for structural grafts such as in anterior spinal interbody fusion. However, for onlay grafts such as those used in posterior intertransverse fusion, autografts are essential.

Potential complications associated with procuring autograft:
1. persistent post-op donor site pain: occurs in as many as 34% of patients (the severity of which was graded as "unacceptable" in 3%)[118]. Reconstruction with absorbable mesh may help[119]
2. wound infection
3. fracture
4. cosmetic deformity
5. increased time to procure
6. neurovascular complications: numbness, blood loss, hematoma…

23.13. Nerve blocks

Also see *Occipital nerve block*, page 564.

23.13.1 Stellate ganglion block

Do not perform this bilaterally (can get bilateral laryngeal paralysis → respiratory compromise). Stellate ganglion is actually closer to C7 than C6, but risks at C7 are much higher (closer to pleura → pneumothorax, vertebral artery → arterial injection → seizures and/or hematoma, recurrent laryngeal nerve → unilateral vocal cord paralysis → hoarseness (common), brachial plexus → UE weakness). Other complications: intradural injection → spinal anesthesia, phrenic nerve block.

Technique
Patient supine; interscapular roll; head tilted backward, mouth slightly open to relax strap muscles. Displace SCM and carotid sheath laterally, insert 1.5 inch 22 Ga. needle to contact **Chassaignac's tubercle** (anterior tubercle of transverse process of C6) AKA **carotid tubercle** (the most prominent in the C-spine) usually at the level of the cricoid cartilage, approximately 1.5-2 inches above clavicle.

Withdraw needle 1-2 mm and aspirate (do not inject intravascularly). Inject small test dose, then full 10 ml of 0.5% bipuvicaine (Marcaine®) or 20 ml of 1% lidocaine. Remove needle and elevate patient's head on pillow to facilitate spread.

Verify block by Horner's syndrome, and anhidrosis and increased warmth of ipsilateral hand.

23.13.2. Lumbar sympathetic block

Technique
Patient prone on fluoro table. Use local anesthetic to allow insertion of 20-22 gauge spinal needles (10 to 12.5 cm long) at L2, L3 and L4 levels. Needle inserted 4.5-5 cm lateral to spinous process until transverse process contacted, then redirected caudally and inserted to a depth 3.5-4 cm deeper than transverse process. Final needle tip position should be just anterolateral to vertebral bodies. At each level, instill ≈ 8 ml of 1% lidocaine local after verifying that nothing can be aspirated.

Keep patient on bed rest for several hours, then ambulate with assist; watch for orthostatic hypotension due to vascular pooling in blocked lower extremity.

23.13.3. Intercostal nerve block

INDICATIONS
1. postthoracotomy pain
2. intercostal neuralgia
3. postherpetic neuralgia
4. pain from rib fractures

PROCEDURE
In order to obtain good anesthesia, the following should be noted:
1. a good site for injection is in the <u>posterior axillary line</u> (**PAL**) because
    A. this is proximal to the origin of the lateral cutaneous nerve (which originates ≈ in the anterior axillary line)
    B. this avoids the scapula for nerves above ≈ T7
    C. this reduces the risk of pneumothorax from injecting closer to the spine (the latter requires a longer needle path and there is increased difficulty palpating landmarks)
2. due to overlap, at least 3 intercostal nerves usually need to be blocked to achieve at least some area of anesthesia; it is usually necessary to block 1-2 intercostal nerves both above and below the affected dermatome
3. the intercostal nerves lie on the undersurface of the corresponding rib in close proximity to the pleura; the order of structures from top down is: rib, vein, artery, nerve

Technique
1. after raising a skin wheal at the desired level in the PAL, insert a 22 Ga. or smaller needle directly against the rib
2. walk the needle down the rib millimeter by millimeter until the needle just slips under the rib; to avoid pleural puncture, do not advance the needle more than one-eighth inch deep to the anterior surface of the rib
3. aspirate to be certain that there is no air (from lung penetration) or blood (from entering the intercostal artery or vein)
4. if no air or blood returns, inject 3-5 ml of local anesthetic
5. if there is any question about lung penetration, obtain a portable CXR to R/O pneumothorax

23.14. References

1. Fox N: Cure in a case of cerebrospinal rhinorrhea. **Arch Otolaryngol** 17: 85-7, 1933.
2. Evans J P, Keegan H R: Danger in the use of intrathecal methylene blue. **JAMA** 174: 856-9, 1960.
3. Calcaterra T C: Extracranial repair of cerebrospinal rhinorrhea. **Ann Otol Rhinol Laryngol** 89: 108-16, 1980.
4. Arand A G, Sawaya R: Intraoperative chemical hemostasis. **Neurosurgery** 23: 223-33, 1986.
5. Rechtine G R, McAllister E W: *Flank retroperitoneal approach to the lumbar spine*. In **Anterior approaches to the spine**, Zdeblick T A, (ed.). Quality Medical Publishing, Inc., St. Louis, Missouri, 1999: pp 193-201.
6. Kalfas I H, Little J R: Postoperative hemorrhage: A survey of 4992 intracranial procedures. **Neurosurgery** 23: 343-7, 1988.
7. Palmer J D, Sparrow O C, Iannotti F I: Postoperative hematoma: A 5-year survey and identification of avoidable risk factors. **Neurosurgery** 35: 1061-5, 1994.
8. Papanastassiou V, Kerr R, Adams C: Contralateral cerebellar hemorrhagic infarction after pterional craniotomy: Report of five cases and review of the literature. **Neurosurgery** 39: 841-52, 1996.
9. Toczek M T, Morrell M J, Silverberg G A, *et al.*: Cerebellar hemorrhage complicating temporal lobectomy: Report of four cases. **J Neurosurg** 85: 718-22, 1996.
10. Mahaley M S, Mettlin C, Natarajan N, *et al.*: National survey of patterns of care for brain-tumor patients. **J Neurosurg** 71: 826-36, 1989.
11. North J B, Penhall R K, Hanieh A, *et al.*: Phenytoin and postoperative epilepsy: A double-blind study. **J Neurosurg** 58: 672-7, 1983.
12. Driscoll C L, Beatty C W: Pain after acoustic neuroma surgery. **Otolaryngol Clin North Am** 30: 893-903, 1997.
13. Harner S G, Beatty C W, Ebershold M J: Headache after acoustic neuroma excision. **Am J Otolaryngol** 14: 552-5, 1993.
14. Kaur A, Selwa L, Fromes G, *et al.*: Persistent headache after supratentorial craniotomy. **Neurosurgery** 47: 633-6, 2000.
15. Catalano P J, Jacobowitz O, Post K D: Prevention of headache after retrosigmoid removal of acoustic tumors. **Am J Otol** 17: 904-8, 1996.
16. Lovely T J, Lowry D W, Jannetta P J: Functional outcome and the effect of cranioplasty after retromastoid craniectomy for microvascular decompression. **Surg Neurol** 51: 191-7, 1999.
17. Long D M: Comment on Kaur A et al.: Persistent

headache after supratentorial craniotomy. **Neurosurgery** 47: 636, 2000.

18. Fager C A: Comment on Zeidman S M and Ducker T B: Posterior cervical laminoforaminotomy for radiculopathy: Review of 172 cases. **Neurosurgery** 33: 362, 1993.

19. Standefer M S, Bay J W, Trusso R: The sitting position in neurosurgery. **Neurosurgery** 14: 649-58, 1984.

20. Kurze T: Microsurgery of the posterior fossa. **Clin Neurosurg** 26: 463-78, 1979.

21. Hitselberger W E, House W F: A warning regarding the sitting position for acoustic tumor surgery. **Arch Otolaryngol** 106: 69, 1980.

22. Wilder B L: Hypothesis: The etiology of midcervical quadriplegia after operation with the patient in the sitting position. **Neurosurgery** 11: 530-1, 1982.

23. Iwasaki Y, Tashiro K, Kikuchi S, et al.: Cervical flexion myelopathy: A "tight dural canal mechanism". **J Neurosurg** 66: 935-7, 1987.

24. Haisa T, Kondo T: Midcervical flexion myelopathy after posterior fossa surgery in the sitting position: Case report. **Neurosurgery** 38: 819-22, 1996.

25. Epstein N E, Danto J, Nardi D: Evaluation of intraoperative somatosensory-evoked potential monitoring during 100 cervical operations. **Spine** 18: 737-47, 1993.

26. Brown J A, Braun M A, Namey T C: Pyriformis syndrome in a 10-year-old boy as a complication of operation with the patient in the sitting position. **Neurosurgery** 23: 117-9, 1988.

27. Lunsford L D, Maroon J C, Sheptak P E, et al.: Subdural tension pneumocephalus: Report of two cases. **J Neurosurg** 50: 525-7, 1979.

28. Tindall G T, Craddock A, Greenfield J C: Effects of the sitting position on blood flow in the internal carotid artery of man during general anesthesia. **J Neurosurg** 26: 383-9, 1967.

29. Grady M S, Bedford R F, Park T S: Changes in superior sagittal sinus pressure in children with head elevation, jugular venous compression, and PEEP. **J Neurosurg** 65: 199-202, 1986.

30. Black S, Cucchiara R F, Nishimura R A, et al.: Parameters affecting occurrence of paradoxical air embolism. **Anesthesiology** 71: 235-41, 1989.

31. Munson E S, Merrick H C: Effect of nitrous oxide on venous air embolism. **Anesthesiology** 27: 783-7, 1966.

32. Haines S J, Maroon J C, Jannetta P J: Supratentorial intracerebral hemorrhage following posterior fossa surgery. **J Neurosurg** 49: 881-6, 1978.

33. Brackmann D E: *The middle fossa approach*. In **Surgery of cranial base tumors**, Sekhar L N and Janecka I P, (eds.). Raven Press, New York, 1993, Chapter 24: pp 367-77.

34. Sekhar L N, Janecka I P, (eds.): **Surgery of cranial base tumors**. Raven Press, New York, 1993.

35. Nutik S L: Removal of the anterior clinoid process for exposure of the proximal intracranial carotid artery. **J Neurosurg** 49: 529-34, 1988.

36. Dolenc V: Direct microsurgical repair of intracavernous vascular lesions. **J Neurosurg** 58: 824-31, 1983.

37. Al-Mefty O, Fox J L, Smith R R: Petrosal approach to petroclival meningiomas. **Neurosurgery** 22: 510-7, 1988.

38. Schmidek H H, Sweet W H, (eds.): **Operative neurosurgical techniques**. 1st ed., Grune and Stratton, New York, 1982.

39. Yamamoto I, Rhoton A L, Peace D A: Microsurgery of the third ventricle: Part 1. **Neurosurgery** 8: 334-56, 1981.

40. Rhoton A L, Yamamoto I, Peace D A: Microsurgery of the third ventricle: Part 2. Operative approaches. **Neurosurgery** 8: 357-73, 1981.

41. Carmel P W: Tumors of the third ventricle. **Acta Neurochir** 75: 136-46, 1985.

42. Klein H J, Rath S A: Removal of tumors of the III ventricle using lamina terminalis approach: Three cases of isolated growth of craniopharyngiomas in the III ventricle. **Childs Nerv Syst** 5: 144-7, 1989.

43. Shucart W A, Stein B M: Transcallosal approach to the anterior ventricular system. **Neurosurgery** 3: 339-43, 1978.

44. Apuzzo M L J, Chikovani O K, Gott P S, et al.: Transcallosal, interforniceal approaches for lesions affecting the third ventricle: Surgical considerations and consequences. **Neurosurgery** 10: 547-54, 1982.

45. Apuzzo M L J: Surgery of masses affecting the third ventricular chamber: Techniques and strategies. **Clin Neurosurg** 34: 499-522, 1988.

46. Garrido E, Fahs G R: Cerebral venous and sagittal sinus thrombosis after transcallosal removal of a colloid cyst of the third ventricle: Case report. **Neurosurgery** 26: 540-2, 1990.

47. Apuzzo M L J: Comment on Garrido E, et al.: Cerebral venous and sagittal sinus thrombosis after transcallosal removal of a colloid cyst of the third ventricle: Case report. **Neurosurgery** 26: 542, 1990.

48. Crockard H A, Sen C N: The transoral approach for the management of intradural lesions at the craniovertebral junction: Review of 7 cases. **Neurosurgery** 28: 88-98, 1991.

49. Hadley M N, Spetzler R F, Sonntag V K H: The transoral approach to the superior cervical spine. A review of 53 cases of extradural cervicomedullary compression. **J Neurosurg** 71: 16-23, 1989.

50. Menezes A H, VanGilder J C: Transoral-transpharyngeal approach to the anterior craniocervical junction. **J Neurosurg** 69: 895-903, 1988.

51. Dickman C A, Locantro J, Fessler R G: The influence of transoral odontoid resection on stability of the craniocervical junction. **J Neurosurg** 77: 525-30, 1992.

52. Dickman C A, Crawford N R, Brantley A G U, et al.: Biomechanical effects of transoral odontoidectomy. **Neurosurgery** 36: 1146-53, 1995.

53. Navarro I M, Renteria J A G, Peralta V H R, et al.: Transorbital ventricular puncture for emergency ventricular decompression. **J Neurosurg** 54: 273-4, 1981.

54. Brem S S, Hafler D A, Van Uitert R L, et al.: Spinal subarachnoid hematoma: A hazard of lumbar puncture resulting in reversible paraplegia. **N Engl J Med** 303: 1020-1, 1981.

55. Hollis P H, Malis L I, Zappulla R A: Neurological deterioration after lumbar puncture below complete spinal subarachnoid block. **J Neurosurg** 64: 253-6, 1986.

56. Reimann A E, Anson B J: Vertebral level of termination of the spinal cord with a report of a case of sacral cord. **Anat Rec** 88: 127, 1944.

57. Antoni N: Pressure curves from the cerebrospinal fluid. **Acta Med Scand Suppl** 170: 439-62, 1946.

58. Adams R D, Victor M: **Principles of neurology**. 2nd ed. McGraw-Hill, New York, 1981.

59. Wiesel J, Rose D N, Silver A L, et al.: Lumbar puncture in asymptomatic late syphilis. An analysis of the benefits and risks. **Arch Intern Med** 145: 465-8, 1985.

60. Fishman R A: **Cerebrospinal fluid in diseases of the nervous system**. W. B. Saunders, Philadelphia, 1992.

61. Sathi S, Stieg P E: "Acquired" Chiari I malformation after multiple lumbar punctures: Case report. **Neurosurgery** 32: 306-9, 1993.

62. Stern W E: Localization and diagnosis of spinal cord tumors. **Clin Neurosurg** 25: 480-94, 1977.

63. DeSousa A L, Kalsbeck J E, Mealey J, et al.: Intraspinal tumors in children. A review of 81 cases. **J Neurosurg** 51: 437-45, 1979.

64. McDonald J V, Klump T E: Intraspinal epidermoid tumors caused by lumbar puncture. **Arch Neurol**

43: 936-9, 1986.

65. Pavlin J, McDonald J S, Child B, *et al.*: Acute subdural hematoma: An unusual sequela to lumbar puncture. **Anesthesiology** 52: 338-40, 1979.

66. Rudehill A, Gordon E, Rahu T: Subdural hematoma: A rare but life threatening complication after spinal anesthesia. **Acta Anaesthesiol Scand** 17: 376-7, 1983.

67. Sundberg A, Wang L P, Fog J: Influence on hearing of 22 G Whitacre and 22 G Quincke needles. **Anaesthesia** 47: 981-3, 1992.

68. Michel O, Brusis T: Hearing loss as a sequel of lumbar puncture. **Ann Otol Rhinol Laryngol** 101: 390-4, 1992.

69. Kestenbaum A: **Clinical methods of neuroophthalmologic examination**. 2nd ed. Grune and Stratton, New York, 1961.

70. Wilder-Smith E, Kothbauer-Margreiter I, Lämmle B, *et al.*: Dural puncture and activated protein C resistance: Risk factors for cerebral venous sinus thrombosis. **J Neurol Neurosurg Psychiatry** 63: 351-6, 1997.

71. Duffy G P: Lumbar puncture in the presence of raised intracranial pressure. **Brit Med J** 1: 407-9, 1969.

72. Korein J, Cravioto H, Leicach M: Reevaluation of lumbar puncture: A study of 129 patients with papilledema or intracranial hypertension. **Neurology** 9: 290-7, 1959.

73. Evans R W, Armon M D, Frohman M H S, *et al.*: Assessment: Prevention of post-lumbar puncture headaches: Report of the therapeutics and technology assessment subcommittee of the American academy of neurology. **Neurology** 55: 909-14, 2000.

74. Tourtellotte W W, Henderson W G, Tucker R P, *et al.*: A randomized, double blind clinical trial comparing the 22 versus 26 gauge needle in the production of the post-lumbar puncture syndrome in normal individuals. **Headache** 12: 73-8, 1972.

75. Mihic D N: Postspinal headache and relationship of needle bevel to longitudinal dural fibres. **Reg Anesth** 10: 76-81, 1985.

76. Kuntz K M, Kokmen E, Stevens J C, *et al.*: Post-lumbar puncture headaches: Experience in 501 consecutive procedures. **Neurology** 42: 1884-07, 1992.

77. Carson D, Serpell M: Choosing the best needle for diagnostic lumbar puncture. **Neurology** 47: 33-7, 1996.

78. Hilton-Jones D, Harrad R A, Gill M W, *et al.*: Failure of postural maneuvers to prevent lumbar puncture headache. **J Neurol Neurosurg Psychiatry** 45: 743-6, 1982.

79. Carbaat P A T, van Crevel H: Lumbar puncture headache: Controlled study on the preventive effect of 24 hours bed rest. **Lancet** 1: 1133-5, 1981.

80. Zivin J A: Lateral cervical puncture: An alternative to lumbar puncture. **Neurology** 28: 616-8, 1978.

81. Penning L: Normal movements of the cervical spine. **AJR** 130: 317-26, 1978.

82. Section of Pediatric Neurosurgery of the American Association of Neurological Surgeons, (ed.) **Pediatric neurosurgery**. 1st ed., Grune and Stratton, New York, 1982.

83. Rogers L A: Acute subdural hematoma and death following lateral cervical spinal puncture. **J Neurosurg** 58: 284-6, 1983.

84. Ward E, Orrison W W, Watridge C B: Anatomic evaluation of cisternal puncture. **Neurosurgery** 25: 412-5, 1989.

85. Wilkins R H, Rengachary S S, (eds.): **Neurosurgery**. McGraw-Hill, New York, 1985.

86. Becker D P, Nulsen F E: Control of hydrocephalus by valve-regulated venous shunt: Avoidance of complications in prolonged shunt maintenance. **J Neurosurg** 28: 215-26, 1968.

87. Keskil S I, Ceviker N, Baykaner K, *et al.*: Index for optimum ventricular catheter length: Technical

note. **J Neurosurg** 75: 152-3, 1991.

88. Ghajar J B G: A guide for ventricular catheter placement: Technical note. **J Neurosurg** 63: 985-6, 1985.

89. Mann K S, Yue C P, Ong G B: Percutaneous sump drainage: A palliation for oft-recurring intracranial cystic lesions. **Surg Neurol** 19: 86-90, 1983.

90. Chan K H, Mann K S: Prolonged therapeutic external ventricular drainage: A prospective study. **Neurosurgery** 23: 436-8, 1988.

91. Couldwell W T, LeMay D R, McComb J G: Experience with use of extended length peritoneal shunt catheters. **J Neurosurg** 85: 425-7, 1996.

92. Cozzens J W, Chandler J P: Increased risk of distal ventriculoperitoneal shunt obstruction associated with slit valves or distal slits in the peritoneal catheter. **J Neurosurg** 87: 682-6, 1997.

93. McComb J G: *Techniques for CSF diversion*. In **Hydrocephalus**, Scott R M, (ed.). Williams and Wilkins, Baltimore, 1990: pp 47-65.

94. Leavens M E, Aldama-Luebert A: Ommaya reservoir placement: Technical note. **Neurosurgery** 5: 264-6, 1979.

95. Hoffman H J: Technical problems in shunts. **Monogr Neural Sci** 8: 158-69, 1982.

96. Spetzler R, Wilson C B, Schulte R: Simplified percutaneous lumboperitoneal shunting. **Surg Neurol** 7: 25-9, 1977.

97. Ishiwata Y, Yamashita T, Ide K, *et al.*: A new technique for percutanous study of lumboperitoneal shunt patency. **J Neurosurg** 68: 152-4, 1988.

98. Youmans J R, (ed.) **Neurological surgery**. 3rd ed., W. B. Saunders, Philadelphia, 1990.

99. Aldrich E F, Crow W N, Weber P B, *et al.*: Use of MR imaging-compatible Halifax interlaminar clamps for posterior cervical fusion. **J Neurosurg** 74: 185-9, 1991.

100. Grob D, Jeanneret B, Aeb M, *et al.*: Atlanto-axial fusion with transarticular screw fixation. **J Bone Joint Surg** 73B: 972-6, 1991.

101. Stillerman C B, Wilson J A: Atlanto-axial stabilization with posterior transarticular screw fixation: Technical description and report of 22 cases. **Neurosurgery** 32: 948-55, 1993.

102. Marcotte P, Dickman C A, Sonntag V K H, *et al.*: Posterior atlantoaxial facet screw fixation. **J Neurosurg** 79: 234-7, 1993.

103. Bohler J: Anterior stabilization for acute fractures and non-unions of the dens. **J Bone Joint Surg** 64: 18-28, 1982.

104. Fielding J W: The status of arthrodesis of the cervical spine. **J Bone Joint Surg** 70A: 1571-4, 1988.

105. Lipson S J: Fractures of the atlas associated with fractures of the odontoid process and transverse ligament ruptures. **J Bone Joint Surg** 59A: 940-3, 1977.

106. White A, Panjabi M: *Kinematics of the spine*. In **Clinical biomechanics of the spine**, White A A, (ed.). J.B. Lippincott, Philadelphia, 2nd ed., 1990: pp 85-126.

107. Roberts A, Wickstrom J: Prognosis of odontoid fractures. **J Bone Joint Surg** 54A: 1353, 1972.

108. Brooks A L, Jenkins E B: Atlanto-axial arthrodesis by the wedge compression method. **J Bone Joint Surg** 60A: 279-84, 1978.

109. Griswold D M, Albright J A, Schiffman E, *et al.*: Atlanto-axial fusion for instability. **J Bone Joint Surg** 60A: 285-92, 1978.

110. Geremia G K, Kim K S, Cerullo L, *et al.*: Complications of sublaminar wiring. **Surg Neurol** 23: 629-34, 1985.

111. Papadopoulos S M, Dickman C A, Sonntag V K H: Atlantoaxial stabilization in rheumatoid arthritis. **J Neurosurg** 74: 1-7, 1991.

112. Dickman C A, Sonntag V K H, Papadopoulos S M, *et al.*: The interspinous method of posterior atlanto-axial arthrodesis. **J Neurosurg** 74: 190-8, 1991.

113. Dickman C A, Sonntag V K H: Surgical manage-

ment of atlantoaxial nonunions. **J Neurosurg** 83: 248-53, 1995.

114. Morone M A, Rodts G R, Erwood S, *et al.*: Anterior odontoid screw fixation: Indications, complication avoidance, and operative technique. **Contemp Neurosurg** 18 (18): 1-6, 1996.

115. Apfelbaum R I: Screw fixation of the upper cervical spine: Indications and techniques. **Contemp Neurosurg** 16 (7): 1-8, 1994.

116. Paramore C G, Dickman C A, Sonntag V K H: The anatomical suitability of the C1-2 complex for transarticular screw fixation. **J Neurosurg** 85: 221-4, 1996.

117. Galler R M, Sonntag V K H: Bone graft harvest. **BNI Quarterly** 19 (4): 13-9, 2003.

118. Heary R F, Schlenk R P, Sacchieri T A, *et al.*: Persistent iliac crest donor site pain: Independent outcome assessment. **Neurosurgery** 50 (3): 510-6; discussion 516-7, 2002.

119. Wang M Y, Levi A D O, Shah S, *et al.*: Polylactic acid mesh reconstruction of the anterior iliac crest after bone harvesting reduces early postoperative pain after anterior cervical fusion surgery. **Neurosurgery** 51: 413-6, 2002.

DEFINITIONS

concussion	alteration of consciousness as a result of closed head injury (*see text* for details)
contusion (cerebral)	On CT: high density (AKA "hemorrhagic contusions") or low density (representing associated edema). High density areas on CT usually show less mass effect than their apparent size. Most common in areas where sudden deceleration of the head causes the brain to impact on bony prominences (e.g. temporal, frontal and occipital poles). Surgical decompression may sometimes be considered if herniation threatens. *See page 669*
contrecoup injury	(French: "counter blow") in addition to the potential injury to the brain directly under the point of impact, the force imparted to the head may cause the brain to be thrust against the skull directly opposite the blow. May result in contusions typically in locations described above
diffuse axonal injury (**DAI**) (AKA diffuse axonal shearing)	a *primary* lesion of rotational acceleration/deceleration head injury[1]. In its severe form, hemorrhagic foci occur in the corpus callosum and dorsolateral rostral brain stem with microscopic evidence of diffuse injury to axons (axonal retraction balls, microglial stars, and degeneration of white matter fiber tracts). Often cited as the cause of loss of consciousness in patients rendered immediately comatose following head injury in the absence of a space occupying lesion on CT[2] (although DAI may also be present with subdural[3] or epidural hematomas[4])

CONCUSSION

AKA mild traumatic brain injury (**MTBI**).

Definition: An alteration of consciousness as a result of nonpenetrating traumatic injury to the brain.

Some specify a time element to the alteration stating it should be brief, however, there is no consensus on the length of time considered to be "brief". In general, there are no gross or microscopic parenchymal abnormalities. CT is normal or significant only for mild swelling which is thought to represent hyperemia[6]. MRI will demonstrate abnormalities in up to 25% of cases where CT is normal[7]. The term contusion should be used when there are areas of low attenuation on CT (edema associated with contusion) or high attenuation areas (hemorrhagic contusions, which may progress to frank parenchymal hemorrhages). Authorities generally concur that *loss* of consciousness is **not** necessary[5, 8-10] (*see Table 24-2* for grading scales). Alterations in consciousness may include confusion, amnesia (the hallmarks of concussion), or loss of consciousness (**LOC**). Neurobehavioral features frequently observed in concussion are shown in *Table 24-1*.

Table 24-1 Findings commonly observed in concussion[5]

- vacant stare or befuddled expression
- delayed verbal & motor responses: slow to answer questions or follow instructions
- easy distractability, difficulty focusing attention, inability to perform normal activities
- disorientation: walking in the wrong direction, unaware of date, time or place
- speech alterations: slurred or incoherent, disjointed or incomprehensible statements
- incoordination: stumbling, inability to tandem walk
- exaggerated emotionality: inappropriate crying, distraught appearance
- memory deficits: repeatedly asking same question that has been answered, cannot name 3 out of 3 objects after 5 minutes
- any period of LOC: paralytic coma, unresponsiveness to stimuli

Confusion may be evident immediately following the blow, or may take several minutes to develop[11]. When there is LOC, the fact that it is often virtually instantaneous (there may be a latency of a few seconds), and the usually rapid return of function with no evidence of microscopic changes suggests that the LOC is due to a transient disturbance in neuronal function. Levels of glutamate (an excitatory neurotransmitter) rise after concussion and the brain enters a hyperglycolytic and hypermetabolic state which can sometimes be demonstrated up to 7-10 days after the injury. It is also during this period that the brain may be more susceptible than normal to a second insult (so-called second impact syndrome, *see below*) which, due in part to impairment of cerebral autoregulation, may produce much more severe sequelae (including possible malignant cerebral edema, *see page 636*) than it would have acting alone.

Also, *see below* for sports-related concussion.

Concussion may be followed by post-concussive syndrome (*see page 682*).

SPORTS RELATED CONCUSSION

≈ 10% of head and spinal injuries are a result of a sports-related event[12]. Concussion, AKA mild traumatic brain injury (**MTBI**), is very different from the severe types of head injuries commonly seen by neurosurgeons in the E/R and office. The widest experience in studying this entity derives from athletics, and generalization to other types of trauma must be done circumspectly.

Concussion grading

The Glasgow coma scale is too insensitive for minor brain injuries. Other grading systems have been proposed, the two most widely used are those of Cantu[13, 14], and that of the American Academy of Neurology (**AAN**)[10] (based on the guidelines of the Colorado Medical Society[15]) both of which are shown in *Table 24-2*. Some data suggest that LOC by itself may not be a significant discriminant (e.g. prolonged confusion > 30 minutes may be worse than a LOC for a few seconds). Most systems consider a concussion to be mild if there is a change in sensorium without loss of consciousness, however they differ mostly in the definition of "change in sensorium".

At present, there is no scientific basis to recommend one system over any other. It is therefore suggested that one system be selected and used consistently (the AAN system may become more widely recognized). However, undue emphasis should not be placed on grading.

Table 24-2 Concussion grading

Grade	Cantu system*	★ AAN system*
1 (mild)	1. PTA < 30 mins 2. no LOC	1. transient confusion 2. no LOC 3. symptoms resolve in < 15 mins
2 (moderate)	1. LOC < 5 mins, or 2. PTA > 30 mins	as above, but symptoms last > 15 mins (still no LOC) (PTA is common)
3 (severe)	1. LOC ≥ 5 mins, or 2. PTA ≥ 24 hrs	any LOC, whether brief (seconds) or prolonged

* abbreviations: LOC = loss of consciousness; PTA = posttraumatic amnesia

Second impact syndrome (SIS)

A rare condition that has been described primarily in athletes who sustain a second head injury apparently while still symptomatic from an earlier injury, and in whom subsequent malignant cerebral edema develops which is refractory to essentially all treatment efforts and carries a 50-100% mortality. Classically, the athlete walks off the field under his or her own power after the second injury, only to deteriorate to coma within 1-5 minutes and then, due to vascular engorgement, progresses to herniation.

The existence of a syndrome compatible with SIS was first described by Schneider[16] in 1973, and was later called the "second impact syndrome of catastrophic head injury" in 1984[17]. Even though it has been contended that SIS is rare (if it exists at all) and may be overdiagnosed[18], its predilection for teenagers and children still warrants extra precaution following concussion.

Return to play guidelines

No system of return to play (**RTP**) guidelines has been rigorously tested and proven to be scientifically sound (a number of trials are in progress). Regardless of the system used, one universal recommendation of experts is:

★ a symptomatic player should not return to competition.

Cerebral contraindications for RTP are shown in *Table 24-3*[19].

Table 24-3 Cerebral contraindications for return to contact sports

1. persistent postconcussion symptoms
2. permanent CNS sequelae from head injury (e.g. organic dementia, hemiplegia, homonymous hemianopsia)
3. hydrocephalus
4. spontaneous SAH from any cause
5. symptomatic (neurologic or pain producing) abnormalities about the foramen magnum (e.g. Chiari malformation)

When none of these contraindications are present, suggestions for RTP are shown in *Table 24-4* based on the AAN guidelines. Also *see page 743* for spine-related RTP guidelines.

Options[10]: recommendations are considered practice options and are summarized in *Table 24-4*

The rationale for the waiting periods following grade 2 or 3 concussions is due to the potentially increased vulnerability of the brain to injury following a concussion (see *Second impact syndrome*, page 633). Almost all players with mild concussions should be able to return to the contest. Some also allow players with moderate concussions to return if they become symptom-free at rest and with exertion using provocative tests. **Exertion**: to evaluate under exertion, commonly utilized provocative tests include the 40-yard run, sit-ups, push-ups, and/or deep knee-bends[12]. In the E/R, exertion may be administered by having the patient lie on the exam table and tip the head backward slightly off the edge. The development of any symptoms during exertion is considered abnormal and precludes return to the present contest.

Table 24-4 Management options for a single sports-related concussion

AAN grade	Management options[10]
1 mild	1. remove from contest 2. examine q 5 mins for amnesia or postconcussive symptoms* 3. may return to contest if symptoms clear within 15 mins
2 moderate	1. remove from contest 2. disallow return that day 3. examine on-site frequently for signs of evolving intracranial pathology 4. reexamination the next day by a trained individual 5. CT or MRI if H/A or other symptoms worsen or last > 1 week† 6. return to practice after 1 full week without symptoms*
3 severe	1. ambulance transport from field to E/R if still unconscious or for concerning signs (C-spine precautions if indicated) 2. emergent neuro exam. Neuroimaging as appropriate 3. may go home with head-injury instructions (see *Table 24-9*, page 638) if normal findings at time of initial neuro exam 4. admit to hospital for any signs of pathology or for continued abnormal mental status 5. assess neuro status daily until all symptoms have stabilized or resolved 6. prolonged unconsciousness, persistent mental status alterations, worsening post-concussion symptoms, or abnormalities on neurologic exam → urgent neurosurgical evaluation or transfer to a trauma center 7. after brief (< 1 minute) grade 3 concussion, do not return to practice until asymptomatic for 1 full week* 8. after prolonged (> 1 minute) grade 3 concussion, return to practice only after 2 full weeks without symptoms*‡ 9. CT or MRI if H/A or other symptoms worsen or last > 1 week†

*   evaluation at rest and with exertion (*see text*)
†   season is terminated for that player if CT/MRI shows edema, contusion, or other acute intracranial pathology. Return to play in any contact sports in the future should be seriously discouraged
‡   some experts also require a normal CT scan

Multiple concussions:

Multiple concussions in a short period of time are potentially dangerous (*see above*). Recommendations[12] for multiple concussions in the same season are shown in *Table 24-5*. Also, see *Chronic traumatic encephalopathy*, page 683 for long-term effects of multiple concussions.

Neuroimaging

The need for neuroimaging (e.g. CT scan) in the athlete with resolved or improving symptoms is controversial, and is felt to be best left to the judgement of the treating physician. Suggested indications:
1. a severe concussion
2. symptoms persisting > 1

Table 24-5 Recommendations for multiple sports-related concussions in the same season

Concussion		Guidelines to be met before return to competition
No.	Severity	
2	mild	1 week*
	moderate or severe	1 month* + normal CT or MRI†
3	mild	most consider this a season ending injury and recommend CT or MRI†
	moderate	season ending injury, consideration for ending all participation in contact sports
2	severe	

*   without symptoms at rest and with exertion (*see text*)
†   if any acute abnormalities on CT/MRI: terminate season. Consider ending all participation in contact sports

week, even if mild
3. before returning to competition after a 2nd or 3rd concussion in the same season

GRADING HEAD INJURIES

Despite many (valid) criticisms, the initial post-resuscitation Glasgow Coma Scale (**GCS**) score (see *Table 8-1*, page 154) remains the most widely used and perhaps best replicated scale employed in the assessment of head trauma.

Stratification: There are a number schemes to stratify the *severity* of head injury. Any such categorization is arbitrary. A simple system based only on GCS score is as follows: GCS 14 -15 = mild, GCS 9-13 = moderate, and GCS ≤ 8 = severe.

A more involved system[20] incorporates other factors in addition to the GCS score as shown in *Table 24-6*.

A classification system based on CT scan[21] is shown in *Table 24-7*.

Table 24-6 Categorization of head injury severity

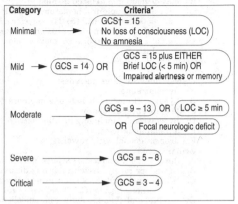

Category	Criteria*
Minimal →	GCS† = 15 / No loss of consciousness (LOC) / No amnesia
Mild →	GCS = 14 OR / GCS = 15 plus EITHER / Brief LOC (< 5 min) OR / Impaired alertness or memory
Moderate →	GCS = 9 – 13 OR / LOC ≥ 5 min / OR / Focal neurologic deficit
Severe →	GCS = 5 – 8
Critical →	GCS = 3 – 4

* all criteria in any oval must be met to qualify in that category
† GCS = Glasgow coma scale (see *Table 8-1*, page 154)

GENERAL

56-60% of patients with GCS score ≤ 8 have 1 or more other organ system injured[22]. 25% have "surgical" lesions. There is a 4-5% incidence of associated spine fractures with significant head injury (mostly C1 to C3).

When a detailed history is unavailable,

Table 24-7 CT classification of head injury

Category	Definition	Mortality
Diffuse Injury I	no visible intracranial abnormality	10%
Diffuse Injury II	cisterns present., 0-5 mm midle shift and/or lesion densities present	14%
Diffuse Injury III	cisterns compressed or absent, 0-5 mm midline shift, no high or mixed density lesion > 25 cc	34%
Diffuse Injury IV	midline shift > 5 mm, no high or mixed density lesion > 25 cc	56%

remember: the loss of consciousness may have preceded (and possibly have caused) the trauma. Therefore, maintain an index of suspicion for e.g. aneurysmal SAH, hypoglycemia, etc. in the differential diagnosis of the causes of trauma and associated coma.

Brain injury from trauma results from two distinct processes:
1. **impact damage** (primary injury): includes cortical contusions, lacerations, bone fragmentation, diffuse axonal injury, and brainstem contusion
2. **secondary injury**: develops subsequent to the impact damage. Includes injuries from intracranial hematomas, edema, hypoxemia, ischemia (primarily due to elevated intracranial pressure (**ICP**) and/or shock)

Hypotension: Hypotension[A] (shock) is rarely attributable to head injury except:
1. in terminal stages (i.e. with dysfunction of medulla and cardiovascular collapse)
2. in infancy, where enough blood can be lost intracranially or into the subgaleal space to cause shock
3. where enough blood has been lost from scalp wounds to cause hypovolemia

---

A. SBP < 90 mm Hg may impair CBF and exacerbate brain injury and should be avoided *see page 657*

DELAYED DETERIORATION

~ 15% of patients who do not initially exhibit signs of significant brain injury may deteriorate in a delayed fashion, sometimes referred to as patients who "talk and deteriorate" or when more lethal, patient who "**talk and die**"[23]. Etiologies:
1. ~ 75% will exhibit an intracranial hematoma
   A. may be present on initial evaluation
   B. may develop in a delayed fashion
      1. delayed epidural hematoma (**EDH**): *see page 671*
      2. delayed subdural (**SDH**): *see page 673*
      3. delayed traumatic contusions: *see page 669*
2. posttraumatic diffuse cerebral edema: *see below*
3. hydrocephalus
4. tension pneumocephalus
5. seizures
6. metabolic abnormalities, includes:
   A. hyponatremia
   B. hypoxia: etiologies include pneumothorax, MI, CHF...
   C. hepatic encephalopathy
   D. hypoglycemia: including insulin reaction
   E. adrenal insufficiency
   F. drug or alcohol withdrawal
7. vascular events
   A. dural sinus thrombosis: *see page 888*
   B. carotid (or rarely, vertebral) artery dissection: *see page 885*
   C. SAH: due to rupture of aneurysm (spontaneous or posttraumatic) or carotid-cavernous fistula (**CCF**) (*see page 845*)
   D. cerebral embolism: including fat embolism syndrome
8. meningitis
9. hypotension (shock)

POSTTRAUMATIC BRAIN SWELLING

This term encompasses two distinct processes:
1. increased cerebral blood volume: may result from loss of cerebral vascular autoregulation (*see page 648*). This hyperemia may sometimes occur with extreme rapidity, in which case it is loosely referred to as diffuse or "**malignant cerebral edema**"[24] which carries close to 100% mortality and may be more common in children. Management consists of aggressive management to maintain ICP < 20 mm Hg and CPP > 60 mm Hg[25]A
2. true cerebral edema: classically at autopsy these brains "weep fluid"[26]. Both vasogenic and cytotoxic cerebral edema (*see page 85*) can occur within hours of head injury[26, 27]

Table 24-8 Factors to assess in head injured patients

Clinical concern	Items to check	Steps to remedy
hypoxia or hypoventilation	ABG, respiratory rate	intubate any patient who has hypercarbia, hypoxemia, or is not localizing
hypotension or hypertension	BP, Hgb/Hct	transfuse patients with significant loss of blood volume
anemia	Hgb/Hct	transfuse patients with significant anemia
seizures	electrolytes, AED levels	correct hyponatremia or hypoglycemia; administer AEDs when appropriate*
infection or hyperthermia	WBC, temperature	LP if meningitis is possible and no contraindications (*see page 615*)
spinal stability	spine x-rays	spine immobilization (spine board, cervical collar & sandbags...); patients with locked facets should be reduced if possible before transfer

* see *Seizures*, page 256, as well as *Posttraumatic seizures* on page 260

A. CPP ≥ 70 mm Hg is generally recommended (see *ICP treatment threshold*, page 655)

24.1.   Transfer of trauma patients

It is sometimes necessary for a neurosurgeon to accept a trauma patient in transfer from another institution that is not equipped to handle major neurologic injuries, or to transfer patients to other facilities for a variety of reasons. *Table 24-8* lists factors that should be assessed and stabilized (if possible) prior to transfer. These items should also be evaluated in trauma patients on whom a neurosurgeon is consulted in his or her own E/R as well as in patients with other CNS abnormalities besides trauma.

24.2.   Management in E/R

24.2.1.   Neurosurgical exam in trauma

The following describes some features that should be assessed under certain circumstances with the understanding that this <u>must be individualized</u>. This addresses only craniospinal injuries.

General physical condition (oriented towards neuro assessment)
1. visual inspection of cranium:
    A. evidence of basal skull fracture (see *Basal skull fractures*, page 665):
        1. raccoon's eyes: periorbital ecchymoses
        2. Battle's sign: postauricular ecchymoses (around mastoid air sinuses)
        3. CSF rhinorrhea/otorrhea. see page 171
        4. hemotympanum or laceration of external auditory canal
    B. check for facial fractures
        1. LeFort fractures (*see page 667*): palpate for instability of facial bones, including zygomatic arch
        2. orbital rim fracture: palpable step-off
    C. periorbital edema, proptosis
2. cranio-cervical auscultation
    A. auscultate over carotid arteries: bruit may be associated with carotid dissection
    B. auscultate over globe of eye: bruit may indicate traumatic carotid-cavernous fistula (see *Carotid-cavernous fistula*, page 845)
3. physical signs of trauma to spine
4. evidence of seizure: single, multiple, or continuing (status epilepticus)

Neurologic exam
1. cranial nerve exam
    A. optic nerve function
        1. if conscious: serial quantitation of vision in each eye is important[28] (*see page 645*). A Rosenbaum near vision card is ideal (*see inside back cover*), otherwise use any printed material. If patient cannot see this, check if they can count fingers. Failing this, check for hand motion vision and lastly light perception. Children may develop transient cortical blindness lasting 1-2 days, usually after a blow to the back of the head
        2. if unconscious: check for afferent pupillary defect (*see page 582*), best demonstrated with swinging flashlight test (*see page 582*). Indicates possible optic nerve injury
    B. pupil: size in ambient light; reaction to light
    C. VII: check for peripheral VII palsy (facial asymmetry of unilateral upper <u>and</u> lower facial muscles): see *Posttraumatic facial palsy*, page 666
    D. abducens (VI nerve) palsy: may occur as a result of ↑ ICP (*see page 586*) or with clival fractures (*see page 665*)
    E. funduscopic exam: check for papilledema, pre-retinal hemorrhages, retinal detachment, abnormalities of the retina suggestive of anterior optic nerve injury. If a detailed exam is required, pharmacologic dilatation with mydri-

atics may be employed, however, this will preclude following the pupils for a variable period of time, and should be undertaken advisedly (*see page 583*)
2. level of consciousness/mental status
   A. Glasgow coma scale for quantitating level of consciousness in poorly responsive patient (see *Table 8-1*, page 154)
   B. check orientation in patient able to communicate
3. motor exam (assesses motor tracts from motor cortex through spinal cord)
   A. if patient is cooperative: check motor strength in all 4 extremities
   B. if uncooperative: check for movement of all 4 extremities to noxious stimulus (differentiate voluntary movement from posturing or stereotypical spinal cord reflex). This also assesses sensation in an unresponsive patient
   C. if any doubt about integrity of spinal cord: check "resting" tone of anal sphincter on rectal exam, evaluate voluntary sphincter contraction if patient can cooperate, check anal wink, and assess bulbocavernosus reflex (see *Neurological assessment*, page 710 for details)
4. sensory exam
   A. cooperative patient:
      1. check pinprick on trunk and in all 4 extremities, touch on major dermatomes (C4, C6, C7, C8, T4, T6, T10, L2, L4, L5, S1, sacrococcygeal)
      2. check posterior column function: joint position sense of LEs
   B. uncooperative patient: check for central response to noxious stimulus (e.g. grimace, vocalization…, as opposed to flexion-withdrawal which could be a spinal cord mediated reflex)
5. reflexes
   A. muscle stretch ("deep tendon") reflexes if patient is not thrashing: e.g. preserved reflex indicates that a flaccid limb is due to CNS injury and not nerve root injury (and vice versa)
   B. check plantar reflex for upgoing toes (Babinski sign)
   C. in suspected spinal cord injury: the anal wink and bulbocavernosus reflex are checked on the rectal exam (*see above*)

CLINICAL CATEGORIZATION OF RISK FOR INTRACRANIAL INJURY

A multidisciplinary panel[29] prospectively followed 7,035 patients with head trauma to determine the probability of an intracranial injury (**ICI**) (and to evaluate the utility of skull x-rays (**SXR**) in head trauma, discussed only briefly here, *see page 641* for more). The panel stratified patients into one of three groups based on the likelihood of intracranial injury as outlined in the following sections. The breakdown is fairly similar to a 4 tier system based on an analysis of 10,000 patients in Italy[30].

1. LOW RISK FOR INTRACRANIAL INJURY

In this group, there is an extremely low likelihood of intracranial injury (**ICI**), even if a skull fracture is present on SXR (incidence of ICI: ≤ 8.5 in 10,000 cases with 95% confidence level[29]). NB: this category **excludes** patients with a history of loss of consciousness. Possible findings are shown in *Table 24-10*.

Table 24-10   Findings with low risk of ICI

• asymptomatic
• H/A
• dizziness
• scalp hematoma, laceration, contusion, or abrasion
• no moderate nor high risk criteria (*see Table 24-11* and *Table 24-13*) (no loss of consciousness, etc.)

Recommendations
Observation at home with written head-injury discharge instructions, e.g as illustrated in *Table 24-9*.

Table 24-9   Sample discharge instructions for head injuries

Seek medical attention for any of the following:
• a change in level of consciousness (including difficulty in awakening)
• abnormal behavior
• increased headache
• slurred speech
• weakness or loss of feeling in an arm or leg
• persistent vomiting
• enlargement of one or both pupils (the black round part in the middle of the eye) that does not get smaller when a bright light is shined on it
• seizures (convulsions or fits)
• significant increase in swelling at injury site
Do not take sedatives or pain medication stronger than Tylenol for 24 hours. Do not take aspirin or other anti-inflammatory medications.

CT scan is not usually indicated. Plain SXRs are not recommended: 99.6% of SXRs in this group are normal. Linear non-displaced skull fractures in this group require no treatment, although in-hospital observation (at least overnight) may be considered.

2. *MODERATE RISK FOR INTRACRANIAL INJURY*

Possible findings are shown in *Table 24-11*.

Table 24-11 Findings with moderate risk of ICI

- history of change or loss of consciousness on or after injury
- progressive H/A
- EtOH or drug intoxication
- posttraumatic seizure
- unreliable or inadequate history
- age < 2 yr (unless trivial injury)
- vomiting
- posttraumatic amnesia
- signs of basilar skull fracture
- multiple trauma
- serious facial injury
- possible skull penetration or depressed fracture
- suspected child abuse.
- significant subgaleal swelling[30]

Table 24-12 Criteria for observation at home

1. normal cranial CT[31]
2. initial GCS ≥ 14
3. no high risk criteria (*see Table 24-13*)
4. no moderate risk criteria (*see Table 24-11*) except loss of consciousness
5. patient is now neurologically intact (amnesia for the event is acceptable)
6. there is a responsible, sober adult that can observe the patient
7. patient has reasonable access to return to the hospital E/R if needed
8. no "complicating" circumstances (e.g. no suspicion of domestic violence, including child abuse)

Recommendations
1. brain CT scan (unenhanced): clinical grounds alone may miss important lesions in this group[31], & 46% of patients with minor head injury **(MHI)** have an intracranial lesion (the most frequent finding was hemorrhagic contusion)[32]
2. SXR: not recommended (*see page 641*) unless CT scan not available. Useless if normal. A SXR is helpful only if positive (a clinically unsuspected depressed skull fracture might be important)
3. observation
   A. at home, if the patient meets the criteria outlined in *Table 24-12*. Provide caregiver with written head-injury discharge instructions (sometimes called "subdural precautions"), as shown in *Table 24-9*
   B. in-hospital observation to rule-out neurologic deterioration if patient does not meet criteria in *Table 24-12* (including cases where CT scan is not done).

Managing patients with in-hospital observation and CT scan only in cases of deterioration (GCS score ≤ 13) is as sensitive as CT in detecting intracranial hematomas[32-36], but is less cost effective than routinely performing an early CT scan and discharging patients who have a normal CT and no other indication for hospitalization[32]

3. *HIGH RISK FOR INTRACRANIAL INJURY*

Possible findings are shown in *Table 24-13*.

Recommendations
CT scan. Admit. If there are focal findings, notify operating room to be on standby. For rapid deterioration, consider emergency burr holes (see *Exploratory burr holes*, page 645). Determine if intracranial monitor is indicated (*see page 649*).

SXR: a fracture is rarely surprising, and a SXR is inadequate for assessing for intracranial injury. A SXR is possibly useful for localizing a radio-opaque penetrating foreign body (knife blade, bullet...) for the O.R. (omit if significant delay required).

Table 24-13 Findings with high risk of ICI

- depressed level of consciousness not clearly due to EtOH, drugs, metabolic abnormalities, postictal, etc.
- focal neurological findings
- decreasing level of consciousness
- penetrating skull injury or depressed fracture

OTHER RISK FACTORS

Occipital vs. frontal fractures
Patients with occipital fractures may be at higher risk of significant intracranial in-

jury **(ICI)**. May be related to the fact that in forward trauma, one may protect oneself with the outstretched arms. Furthermore, the facial bones and air sinuses exert an impact absorbing effect.

24.2.2. Radiographic evaluation

CT SCANS IN TRAUMA
Almost without exception, an unenhanced (i.e. non-contrast) CT scan of the brain suffices for patients seen in the emergency department presenting after trauma or with a new neurologic deficit. Enhanced CT or MRI may be appropriate after the unenhanced CT, but are not usually required emergently (exceptions include: significant brain edema due to suspected neoplasm that is not demonstrated without contrast, spinal MRI in patients with spinal cord injuries or compression e.g. from neoplasm).

The main emergent conditions to rule out (and brief descriptions):
1. blood (hemorrhages or hematomas):
    A. extra-axial blood: surgical lesions are usually ≥ 1 cm maximal thickness
       1. epidural hematoma **(EDH)** (*see page 669*): usually biconvex and are due to arterial bleeding
       2. subdural hematoma **(SDH)** (*see page 672*): usually crescentic, and due to venous bleeding. May cover larger surface area than EDH. Chronology of SDH: acute = high density, subacute ≈ isodense, chronic ≈ low density
    B. subarachnoid blood (SAH): high density spread thinly over convexity and filling sulci or basal cisterns. Trauma is the most common cause of SAH. However, when the history of trauma is not clear, an arteriogram may be indicated to R/O a ruptured aneurysm (possibly precipitating the trauma)
    C. intracerebral hemorrhage **(ICH)**: increased density in brain parenchyma
    D. hemorrhagic contusion (*see page 669*): often "fluffy" inhomogeneous high-density areas within brain parenchyma adjacent to bony prominences (frontal and occipital poles, sphenoid wing). Less well defined than ICH
    E. intraventricular hemorrhage: present in ≈ 10% of severe head injuries[37]. Associated with poor outcome, however, may be a marker for severe injury rather than the *cause* of the poor outcome. Use of intraventricular rt-PA has been reported for treatment[38] (*see page 860*)
2. hydrocephalus
3. cerebral swelling: obliteration of basal cisterns (*see page 681*), compression of ventricles and sulci...
4. evidence of cerebral anoxia: loss of gray-white interface, signs of swelling
5. skull fractures:
    A. basal skull fractures (including temporal bone fracture)
    B. orbital blow-out fracture
    C. calvarial fracture (CT may miss some linear nondisplaced skull fractures)
       1. linear vs. stellate
       2. open vs. closed
       3. diastatic (separation of sutures)
       4. depressed vs. nondepressed: CT helps assess need for surgery
6. ischemic infarction: findings are minimal or subtle if < 24 hrs since CVA
7. pneumocephalus: may indicate skull fracture (basal or open convexity)
8. shift of midline structures (due to extra- or intra-axial hematomas or asymmetric cerebral edema): shift can cause altered levels of consciousness (*see page 155*)

Indications for initial CT
1. presence of any moderate[39] or high risk criteria (*see Table 24-11* and *Table 24-13*) which include: GCS ≤ 14, unresponsiveness, focal deficit, amnesia for injury, altered mental status (including those that are significantly inebriated), deteriorating neuro status, signs of basal or calvarial skull fracture
2. assessment prior to general anesthesia for other procedures (during which neurologic exam cannot be followed in order to detect delayed deterioration)

Follow-up CT
Routine follow-up CT (when there is no indication for *urgent* follow-up CT, *see below*):
1. for patients with <u>severe</u> head injuries:
    A. for <u>stable</u> patients, follow-up CTs are usually obtained between day 3 to 5,

(some recommend at 24 hrs also) and again between day 10 to 14
   B. some recommend routine follow-up CT several hours after the "time zero"
      CT (i.e. initial CT done within hours of the trauma) to rule-out delayed EDH
      (*see page 671*), SDH (*see page 673*), or traumatic contusions[40] (*see page 669*)
2. for patients with mild to moderate head injuries:
   A. with an abnormal initial CT, the CT scan is repeated prior to discharge
   B. stable patients with mild head injury and normal initial CT do not require
      follow-up CT

Urgent follow-up CT: performed for neurological deterioration (loss of 2 or more points
on the GCS, development of hemiparesis or new pupillary asymmetry), persistent vomiting, worsening H/A, seizures or unexplained rise in intracranial pressure (**ICP**).

SPINE FILMS

1. cervical spine: must be cleared radiographically from the cranio-cervical junction
down through and including the C7-T1 junction. Spinal injury precautions (cervical collar...) are continued until the C-spine is cleared. The steps in obtaining adequate films are outlined in *Spine injuries, Radiographic evaluation and initial
C-spine immobilization* on page 705
2. thoracic and lumbosacral spine films should be obtained based on physical findings and on mechanism of injury (see *Spine injuries, Radiographic evaluation
and initial C-spine immobilization* on page 705)

SKULL X-RAYS

    A skull fracture increases the probability of an surgical intracranial injury (**ICI**) (in
a comatose patient it is a 20-fold increase, in a conscious patient it is a 400-fold increase
[41, 42]). However, significant ICI can occur with a normal SXR (SXR was normal in 75% of
minor head injury patients found to have intracranial lesions on CT, attesting to the insensitivity of SXRs[02]). SXRs affect management of only 0.4-2% of patients in most
reports[29].

A SXR may be helpful in the following:
1. in patients with moderate risk for intracranial injury (see *Table 24-11*, page 639)
by detecting an unsuspected depressed skull fracture (however, most of these patients will get a CT scan, which obviates the need for SXR)
2. if a CT scan cannot be obtained, a SXR may identify significant findings such as
pineal shift, pneumocephalus, air-fluid levels in the air sinuses, skull fracture
(depressed or linear)... (however, sensitivity for detecting ICI is very low)
3. in patients with penetrating missile injuries

MRI SCANS IN TRAUMA

    Usually not appropriate for acute head injures. While MRI is more sensitive than
CT, there were no <u>surgical</u> lesions demonstrated on MRI that were not evident on CT [43].
    MRI may be helpful later after the patient is stabilized, e.g. to evaluate brainstem
injuries, small white matter changes[44] (e.g. punctate hemorrhages in the corpus callosum
seen in diffuse axonal injury, *see page 632*)...

ARTERIOGRAM IN TRAUMA

    Cerebral arteriogram: useful with non missile penetrating trauma (*see page 687*).
Also may be useful in experienced hands if CT is unavailable for diagnosing EDH...

24.2.3.   E/R management specifics

PRACTICE PARAMETER 24-2 INITIAL RESUSCITATION AND BP MANAGEMENT
Guidelines[45]: hypotension (SBP < 90 mm Hg) or hypoxia (apnea, cyanosis, or O_2 saturation < 90% in the field, or PaO_2 < 60 mm Hg) must be monitored and avoided/corrected as soon as possible

ADMITTING ORDERS FOR MINOR OR MODERATE HEAD INJURY

Admitting orders for <u>minor</u> head injury (GCS ≥ 14[A])[B]

1. activity: BR with HOB elevated 30-45°
2. neuro checks q 2 hrs (q 1 hr if more concerned; consider ICU for these patients). Contact physician for neurologic deterioration
3. NPO until alert; then clear liquids, advance as tolerated
4. isotonic IVF (e.g. NS + 20 mEq KCl/L) run at maintenance: ≈ 100 cc/hr for average size adult (peds: 2000 cc/m^2/d)[C]
5. mild analgesics: acetaminophen (PO, or PR if NPO), codeine if necessary
6. anti-emetic: give infrequently to avoid excessive sedation, avoid phenothiazine anti-emetics (which lower the seizure threshold); e.g. use trimethobenzamide (Tigan®) 200 mg IM q 8 hrs PRN for adults

Admitting orders for <u>moderate</u> head injury (GCS 9-13)[B]

1. orders as for minor head injury (*see above*) except patient is kept NPO in case surgical intervention is needed (including ICP monitor)
2. for GCS = 9-12 admit to ICU. For GCS = 13, admit to ICU if CT shows any significant abnormality (hemorrhagic contusions unless very small, rim subdural...)
3. patients with normal or near-normal CTs should improve within hours. Any patient who fails to reach a GCS of 14-15 within 12 hrs should have a repeat CT at that time[39]

EARLY USE OF PARALYTICS AND SEDATION (PRIOR TO ICP MONITORING)

PRACTICE PARAMETER 24-3 EARLY SEDATION AND PARALYSIS

Options[46]: sedation and neuromuscular blockade (NMB) can be helpful for transporting the head-injured patient, but they interfere with the neuro exam

Options[46]: NMB should be used when sedation alone is inadequate

The routine use of sedatives and paralytics in neurotrauma patients may lead to a higher incidence of pneumonia, longer ICU stays, and possibly sepsis[47]. These agents also impair neurologic assessment[46, 48]. Use should therefore be reserved for cases with clinical evidence of intracranial hypertension (*see Table 24-14*), or where use is necessary for transport or to permit evaluation of the patient[49].

Table 24-14   Clinical signs of IC-HTN*

1.	unilateral or bilateral pupillary dilatation
2.	asymmetric pupillary reaction to light
3.	decerebrate or decorticate posturing (usually contralateral to blown† pupil)
4.	progressive deterioration of the neurologic exam not attributable to extracranial factors

*   Items A-C represent clinical signs of herniation. The most convincing clinical evidence of IC-HTN is the witnessed evolution of 1 or more of these signs. IC-HTN may produce a bulging fontanelle in an infant.

†   "blown pupil" : fixed & dilated pupil

INTUBATION AND HYPERVENTILATION

PRACTICE PARAMETER 24-4 INTUBATION

Options[45]: secure the airway (usually by endotracheal intubation) in patients with GCS ≤ 8 who are unable to maintain their airway or who remain hypoxic despite supplemental O$_2$

Indications for <u>intubation</u> in trauma:

A. traditionally, mild head injury has been defined as GCS ≥ 13. However, the increased frequency of both surgical lesions and CT scan abnormalities in patients with GCS = 13 suggests that they would be better classified with the *moderate* rather than mild head injuries[31]
B. see *Clinical categorization of risk for intracranial injury* on page 638 for admitting criteria
C. the concept of "running the patient dry" is considered obsolete (*see page 657*)

1. depressed level of consciousness (patient cannot protect airway): usually GCS ≤ 7
2. need for hyperventilation (**HPV**): *see below*
3. severe maxillofacial trauma: patency of airway tenuous
4. need for pharmacologic paralysis for evaluation or management

Cautions regarding intubation:
1. if basal skull fracture is possible, avoid nasotracheal intubation (to avoid intracranial entry of tube through cribriform plate). Use orotracheal intubation
2. prevents assessment of patient's ability to verbalize[48] e.g. for determining Glasgow Coma Scale score

Hyperventilation (HPV)

PRACTICE PARAMETER 24-5 EARLY HYPERVENTILATION

Options[46]: hyperventilation before ICP monitoring is established should be reserved for patients with signs of transtentorial herniation (*see Table 24-14*) or progressive neurologic deterioration not attributable to extracranial causes

1. due to possible exacerbation of cerebral ischemia, HPV should not be used prophylactically (*see page 659*)
2. prior to ICP monitoring, HPV should only be used briefly when CT or clinical signs of IC-HTN are present[49] (*see Table 24-14* for clinical signs)
   A. when appropriate indications are met: HPV to $pCO_2 = 30\text{-}35$ mm Hg
   B. HPV should not be used to the point that $pCO_2 < 30$ mm Hg (this further reduces CBF but does not necessarily reduce ICP)
3. acute alkalosis increases protein binding of calcium (decreases ionized Ca^{++}). Patients being hyperventilated may develop ionized hypocalcemia with tetany (despite normal total [Ca])

MANNITOL IN E/R

PRACTICE PARAMETER 24-6 EARLY USE OF MANNITOL

Options[46]: the use of mannitol before ICP monitoring is established should be reserved for patients who are adequately volume-resuscitated with signs of transtentorial herniation (*see Table 24-14*) or progressive neurologic deterioration not attributable to extracranial causes

Indications in E/R (also *see page 660* for more details):
1. evidence of intracranial hypertension (*see Table 24-14*)
2. evidence of mass effect (focal deficit, e.g. hemiparesis)
3. sudden deterioration prior to CT (including pupillary dilatation)
4. after CT, if a lesion that is associated with increased ICP is identified
5. after CT, if going to O.R.
6. to assess "salvageability": in patient with no evidence of brainstem function, look for return of brainstem reflexes

Contraindications:
1. prophylactic administration is not recommended due to its volume-depleting effect. Use only for appropriate indications (*see above*)
2. hypotension or hypovolemia: hypotension can negatively influence outcome[49]. Therefore, when intracranial hypertension (**IC-HTN**) is present, first utilize sedation and/or paralysis, and CSF drainage. If further measures are needed, fluid resuscitate the patient before administering mannitol. Use hyperventilation in hypovolemic patients until mannitol can be given
3. relative contraindication: mannitol may slightly impede normal coagulation
4. CHF: before causing diuresis, mannitol transiently increases intravascular volume. Use with caution in CHF, may need to pre-treat with furosemide (Lasix®)

Rx: bolus with 0.25-1 gm/kg over < 20 min (for average adult: ≈ 350 ml of 20% solution). Peak effect occurs in ≈ 20 minutes (*see page 660* for follow-up dosing).

PROPHYLACTIC ANTIEPILEPTIC DRUGS (AEDs)

PRACTICE PARAMETER 24-7 PROPHYLACTIC ANTICONVULSANTS AFTER TBI

Standards[50, 51]: prophylactic phenytoin, carbamazepine, phenobarbital or valproate[52] is not recommended for preventing *late* PTS

Options[50, 51]: AEDs may be used as a treatment option to prevent *early* PTS in patients at high risk of seizures after TBI (*see Table 24-15*), however, there is no evidence that this improves outcome. Phenytoin and carbamazepine are effective in preventing early PTS[52]

The routine use of prophylactic anticonvulsants in traumatic brain injury (**TBI**) does not prevent the late development of posttraumatic seizures (**PTS**) i.e. epilepsy, and has been shown not to be useful except in certain circumstances[50, 51].

See page 261 for details on using and discontinuing prophylactic AEDs following TBI. (*Table 24-15* reiterates the markers for patients at increased risk of early PTSs).

Table 24-15 Conditions with increased risk of posttraumatic seizures

1. acute subdural, epidural, or intracerebral hematoma
2. open-depressed skull fracture with parenchymal injury
3. seizure within the first 24 hrs after injury
4. Glasgow Coma Scale score < 10
5. penetrating brain injury
6. history of significant alcohol abuse
7. ± cortical (hemorrhagic) contusion on CT

POSTTRAUMATIC SUBARACHNOID HEMORRHAGE

Trauma is the most common cause of SAH. There is some evidence that nimodipine (Nimotop®) may improve outcome in head-injured patients with subarachnoid blood detected on CT[53]. ***Rx:*** 60 mg PO or per NG q 4 hrs, hold for hypotension (*see page 799*).

PATIENTS WITH ASSOCIATED SEVERE SYSTEMIC INJURIES

Hypotension (defined as a single SBP < 90 mm Hg) doubles mortality, hypoxia (apnea or cyanosis, or PaO_2 < 60 mm Hg on ABG) also increases mortality[54], and the combination of both triples mortality and increases the risk bad outcome.

In centers where diagnostic peritoneal lavage (**DPL**) is used to assess for intra-abdominal hemorrhage, if the initial fluid is not grossly bloody and the patient is hemodynamically stable, the patient should be taken for cranial CT while the remainder of the lavage fluid is collecting for quantitative analysis.

Patients with grossly positive DPL and/or hemodynamic instability may need to be rushed to the O.R. for emergent laparotomy by trauma surgeons without benefit of cerebral CT. These guidelines are offered:

✖ CAUTION: many patients with severe trauma may be in DIC (either due to systemic injuries, or directly related to severe head injury possibly because the brain is rich in thromboplastin[55]). Operating on patients in DIC is usually disastrous. At the least, check the PT/PTT

1. if neuro-exam is relatively good (i.e. GCS > 8, which implies at least localizing)
    A. operative neurosurgical intervention is probably not required
    B. utilize good neuroanesthesia techniques (elevate head of bed, judicious administration of IV fluids, avoiding prophylactic hyperventilation...)
    C. obtain a head CT scan immediately post-op
2. if patient has focal neurologic deficit, an exploratory burr-hole should be placed in the O.R. simultaneously with the treatment of other injuries. Placement is guided by the pre-op deficit (see *Exploratory burr holes*, page 645)
3. if there is severe head injury (GCS ≤ 8) without localizing signs, or if initial burr hole is negative, or if there is no pre-op neuro exam, then
    A. measure the ICP: insert a ventriculostomy catheter (if the lateral ventricle cannot be entered after 3 passes, an intraparenchymal fiber-optic monitor or subarachnoid bolt should be used)
        1. normal ICP: unlikely that a surgical lesion exists. Manage ICP medically and, if a IVC was inserted, with CSF drainage
        2. elevated ICP (≥ 20 mm Hg): inject 3-4 cc of air into ventricles through IVC, then obtain portable intraoperative AP skull x-ray (intra-operative pneumoencephalogram) to determine if there is any midline shift

a. mass effect with ≥ 5 mm of midline shift is explored[56] with burr-hole(s) on the side opposite the direction of shift
b. if no mass effect, intracranial hypertension is managed medically and with CSF drainage
B. routine use of exploratory burr holes for children with GCS = 3 has been found not to be justified[57]

INDIRECT OPTIC NERVE INJURY

≈ 5% of head trauma patients manifest an associated injury to some portion of the visual system. Approximately 0.5-1.5% of head trauma patients will sustain *indirect* injury (as opposed to penetrating trauma) to the optic nerve, most often from an ipsilateral blow to the head (usually frontal, occasionally temporal, rarely occipital)[28]. The optic nerve may be divided into 4 segments: intraocular (1 mm in length), intraorbital (25-30 mm), intracanalicular (10 mm), and intracranial (10 mm). The intracanalicular segment is the most common one damaged with closed head injuries. Funduscopic abnormalities visible on initial exam indicates anterior injuries (injury to the intraocular segment (optic disc) or the 10-15 mm of the intraorbital segment immediately behind the globe where the central retinal artery is contained within the optic nerve), whereas posterior injuries (occurring posterior to this but anterior to the chiasm) takes 4-8 weeks to show signs of disc pallor and loss of the retinal nerve fiber layer.

Treatment[28]: No prospective study has been carried out. Optic nerve decompression has been advocated for indirect optic nerve injury, however, the results are not clearly better than expectant management with the exception that documented <u>delayed</u> visual loss appears to be a strong indication for surgery. Transethmoidal is the accepted route, and is usually done within 1-3 weeks from the trauma[58]. The use of "megadose steroids" may be appropriate as an adjunct to diagnosis and treatment.

POST-TRAUMATIC HYPOPITUITARISM

Trauma is a rare cause of hypopituitarism. It may follow closed head injury (with or without basilar skull fracture) or penetrating trauma[59]. In 20 cases in the literature[60] all had deficient growth hormone and gonadotropin, 95% had corticotropin deficiency, 85% had reduced TSH, 63% had elevated PRL. Only 40% had transient or permanent DI.

24.2.4. Exploratory burr holes

In a trauma patient, the clinical triad of altered mental status, unilateral pupillary dilatation with loss of light reflex, and contralateral hemiparesis is most often due to upper brainstem compression by uncal transtentorial herniation which, in the majority of trauma cases, is due to an extraaxial intracranial hematoma. Furthermore, the prognosis of patients with traumatic herniation is poor. Outcome may possibly be improved slightly by increasing the rapidity with which decompression is undertaken, however, an upper limit of salvageability is probably still only ≈ 20% satisfactory outcome.

Burr holes are primarily a <u>diagnostic tool</u>, as bleeding cannot be controlled and most acute hematomas are too congealed to be removed through a burr hole. However, if the burr hole is positive, it is possible that modest decompression may be performed, and then the definitive craniotomy can be undertaken incorporating the burr hole(s).

With widespread availability of quickly accessible CT scanning, exploratory burr holes are infrequently indicated.

INDICATIONS
1. clinical criteria: based on deteriorating neurologic exam. Indications in E/R (rare): patient dying of rapid transtentorial herniation (*see below*) or brainstem compression that does not improve or stabilize with mannitol and hyperventilation[61].
   • indicators of transtentorial herniation/brainstem compression:
      1. sudden drop in Glasgow Coma Scale (**GCS**) score
      2. one pupil fixes and dilates
      3. paralysis or decerebration (usually contralateral to blown pupil)
   • recommended situations where criteria should be applied:
      1. neurologically stable patient undergoes <u>witnessed</u> deterioration as described above
      2. awake patient undergoes same process in transport, and changes are

well documented by competent medical or paramedical personnel
2. other criteria
    A. some patients needing emergent surgery for systemic injuries (e.g. positive peritoneal lavage + hemodynamic instability) where there is not time for a brain CT (see *Patients with associated severe systemic injuries*, page 644)

MANAGEMENT

Controversial. The following should serve only as guidelines:
1. if patient fits the above criteria (emergent operation for systemic injuries or deterioration with failure to improve with mannitol and hyperventilation), and CT scan cannot be performed and interpreted immediately, then treatment should not wait for CT scan
    A. in general, if the O.R. can be immediately available, burr holes are preferably done there (equipped to handle craniotomy, better lighting and sterility, dedicated scrub nurse...) especially in older patients (> 30 yrs) not involved in MVAs (see *Literature* below). This may more rapidly diagnose and treat extraaxial hematomas in herniating patients, although no difference in outcome has been proven
    B. if delay in getting to the O.R. is foreseen, emergency burr holes in the E/R should be performed
2. placement of burr-hole(s) as outlined under *Technique* below)

TECHNIQUE

Position

Shoulder roll, head turned with side to be explored up. Three pin skull-fixation used if concern about possible aneurysm or AVM (to allow for retractors and increased stability) or if additional stability is desired (e.g. with unstable cervical fractures), otherwise a horse-shoe head-holder suffices and saves time and permits rapid access to the other side.

Choice of side for initial burr hole

Start with a temporal burr hole (*see below*) on the side:
1. ipsilateral to a blown pupil. This will be on the correct side in > 85% of epidurals[62] and other extra-axial mass lesions[63]
2. if both pupils are dilated, use the side of the first dilating pupil (if known)
3. if pupils are equal, or it is not known which side dilated first, place on side of obvious external trauma
4. if no localizing clues, place hole on left side (to evaluate and decompress the dominant hemisphere)

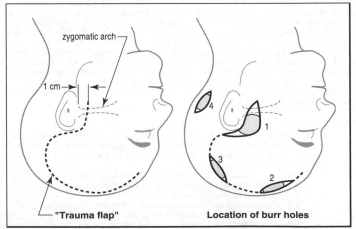

Figure 24-1 Technique to convert burr-hole(s) into trauma flap (adapted[63, 64])

Approach
   Burr holes are placed along a path that can be connected to form a "trauma flap" if a craniotomy becomes necessary (*see Figure 24-1*). The "trauma flap" is so-called because it provides wide access to most of the cerebral convexity permitting complete evacuation of acute blood clot and control of most bleeding.

First outline the trauma flap with a skin marker:
1. start at the zygomatic arch < 1 cm anterior to the tragus (spares the branch of the facial nerve to the frontalis muscle and the anterior branch of the superficial temporal artery)
2. proceed superiorly and then curve posteriorly at the level of top of the pinna
3. 4-6 cm behind the pinna it is taken superiorly
4. 1-2 cm ipsilateral to the midline (sagittal sinus) curve anteriorly to end behind the hairline

Burr hole locations
1. first (temporal) burr-hole: over middle cranial fossa (#1 in *Figure 24-1*) just superior to the zygomatic arch. Provides access to middle fossa (the most common site of epidural hematoma) and usually allows access to most convexity subdural hematomas, as well as proximity to middle meningeal artery in region of pterion
2. if no epidural hematoma, the dura is opened if it has bluish discoloration (suggests subdural hematoma) or if there is a strong suspicion of a mass lesion on that side
3. if completely negative, usually perform temporal burr hole on contralateral side
4. if negative, further burr holes should be undertaken if a CT cannot now be done
5. proceed to ipsilateral frontal burr hole (#2 in *Figure 24-1*)
6. subsequent burr holes may be placed at parietal region (#3 in *Figure 24-1*) and lastly in posterior fossa (#4 in *Figure 24-1*)

LITERATURE
   In 100 trauma patients undergoing transtentorial herniation or brainstem compression[63], exploratory burr holes (bilateral temporal, frontal and parietal, done in the O.R.) were positive in 56%. Lower rates in younger patients (< 30 yrs) and those in MVAs (as opposed to falls or assaults). SDH was the most common extraaxial mass lesion (alone and unilateral in 70%, bilateral in 11%, and in combination with EDH or ICH in > 9%).
   When burr holes were positive, the first burr hole was on the correct side 86% of the time when placed as above. Six patients had significant extraaxial hematomas missed with exploratory burr holes (mostly due to incomplete burr hole exploration). Only 3 patients had the above neurologic findings as a result of intraparenchymal hematomas.

Outcome
   Mean follow-up: 11 mos (range: 1-37). 70 of the 100 patients died. No morbidity or mortality was directly attributable to the burr holes. Four patients with good outcome and 4 with moderate disability had positive burr holes.

24.3.   Intracranial pressure

24.3.1.   General information about ICP

CEREBRAL PERFUSION PRESSURE (CPP) AND CEREBRAL AUTOREGULATION
   Secondary brain injury (i.e. following the initial trauma) is attributable in part to cerebral ischemia (see *Secondary injury*, page 635). The critical parameter for brain function and survival is not actually ICP, rather it is adequate cerebral blood flow **(CBF)** to meet $CMRO_2$ demands (for a discussion of CBF & $CMRO_2$, *see page 763*). CBF is difficult to quantitate, and can only be measured continuously at the bedside with specialized equipment and difficulty[65]. However, CBF depends on cerebral perfusion pressure **(CPP)**, which is related to ICP (which is more easily measured) as shown in *Eq 24-1*.

$$\frac{\text{cerebral perfusion}}{\text{pressure}} = \frac{\text{mean arterial}}{\text{pressure}*} - \frac{\text{intracranial}}{\text{pressure}}$$

OR

$$\text{CPP} = \text{MAP}* - \text{ICP}$$

Eq 24-1

* note: the actual pressure of interest is the **mean carotid pressure (MCP)** which may be approximated as the MAP with the transducer zeroed ≈ at the level of the foramen of Monro[66]

Normal adult CPP is > 50 mm Hg. **Cerebral autoregulation** is a mechanism whereby over a wide range, large changes in systemic BP produce only small changes in CBF. Due to autoregulation, CPP would have to drop below 40 in a normal brain before CBF would be impaired.

In the head injured patient, recent evidence suggests that elevated ICP (≥ 20 mm Hg) may be more detrimental than changes in CPP (as long as CPP is > 60 mm Hg[67])[25] (higher levels of CPP were not protective against significant ICP elevations[25]).

INTRACRANIAL PRESSURE

The following are approximations to help simplify understanding ICP (these are only models, and as such are not entirely accurate):
1. the modified **Monro-Kellie** hypothesis states that the sum of the intracranial volumes of blood (CBV), brain, CSF, and other components (e.g. tumor, hematoma) is constant, and that an increase in any one of these must be offset by an equal decrease in another, or else pressure will rise
2. these volumes are contained in an inelastic, completely closed skull
3. pressure is distributed evenly throughout the intracranial cavity

NORMAL ICP

The normal range of ICP varies with age. Values for pediatrics are not well established. Guidelines are shown in *Table 24-16*.

Table 24-16 Normal ICP

Age group	Normal range (mm Hg)
adults and older children*	< 10-15
young children	3-7
term infants†	1.5-6

* the age of transition from "young" to "older" child is not precisely defined

† may be subatmospheric in newborns[68]

INTRACRANIAL HYPERTENSION (IC-HTN)

Traumatic IC-HTN may be due any of the following (alone or in various combinations):
1. cerebral edema
2. hyperemia: the normal response to head injury[69]. Possibly due to vasomotor paralysis (loss of cerebral autoregulation). May be more significant than edema in raising ICP[24] (*see page 655*)
3. traumatically induced masses
   A. epidural hematoma
   B. subdural hematoma
   C. intraparenchymal hemorrhage (hemorrhagic contusion)
   D. foreign body (e.g. bullet)
   E. depressed skull fracture
4. hydrocephalus due to obstruction of CSF absorption or circulation
5. hypoventilation (causing hypercarbia → vasodilatation)
6. systemic hypertension (HTN)
7. venous sinus thrombosis
8. increased muscle tone and valsalva maneuver as a result of agitation or posturing
9. sustained posttraumatic seizures (status epilepticus)

A secondary increase in ICP is sometimes observed 3-10 days following the trauma, and may be associated with a worse prognosis[70]. Possible causes include:
1. delayed hematoma formation
   A. delayed epidural hematoma: *see page 671*
   B. delayed acute subdural hematoma: *see page 673*
   C. delayed traumatic intracerebral hemorrhage[40] (or hemorrhagic contusions) with perilesional edema: usually in older patients, may cause sudden deterioration. May be severe enough to require evacuation (*see page 669*)
2. cerebral vasospasm[71]
3. severe adult respiratory distress syndrome (**ARDS**) with hypoventilation
4. delayed edema formation: more common in pediatric patients

5. hyponatremia

Indications to treat IC-HTN

Various cutoff values are used at different centers above which treatment measures for intracranial hypertension **(IC-HTN)** are initiated. Although 15, 20 and 25 have been quoted, most centers use **ICP ≥ 20-25 mm Hg** as the upper limit[49]. There is high mortality and worse outcome[25] among patients with ICP persistently > 20 compared to 20% in those where ICP could be kept < 20[72]. Better control may be possible by treating early rather than waiting and trying to control higher ICPs or when plateau waves occur[22].

"Deadly" ICP (in adult), i.e. likely to be fatal if uncontrolled: > 25-30 mm Hg.

Cushing's triad

Cushing's triad is shown in *Table 24-17*, and may be seen with IC-HTN regardless of cause. However, the full triad is only seen in ≈ 33% of cases of IC-HTN.

Table 24-17   Cushing's triad

A.	hypertension
B.	bradycardia
C.	respiratory irregularity

CT scan and elevated ICP

Whereas CT findings may be correlated with a *risk* of IC-HTN, no combination of CT findings has been shown to allow accurate estimates of actual ICP. 60% of patients with closed head injury and an abnormal CT[A] will have IC-HTN[73].

Only 13% of patients with a normal CT scan will have IC-HTN[73]. However, patients with a normal CT *AND* 2 or more risk factors identified in *Table 24-18* will have ≈ 60% risk of IC-HTN. If only 1 or none are present, ICP will be increased in only 4%.

Table 24-18   Risk factors for IC-HTN with a normal CT

- age > 40 yrs
- SBP < 90 mm Hg
- decerebrate or decorticate posturing on motor exam (unilateral or bilateral)

24.3.2.   ICP monitoring

INDICATIONS FOR ICP MONITORING

> **PRACTICE PARAMETER 24-8 INDICATIONS FOR ICP MONITORING**
>
> **Guidelines**[74, 75]: patients with a GCS ≤ 8 and either an abnormal admitting brain CT[A] or ≥ 2 of the risk factors in *Table 24-18*

★ 1.   neurologic criteria[75]: severe head injury (GCS ≤ 8 after cardiopulmonary resuscitation) and either:
      A.   an abnormal admitting head CT[A]
      OR
      B.   a normal CT, but with ≥ 2 of the risk factors in *Table 24-18*

- some centers monitor patients who don't follow commands. Rationale: patients who follow commands (GCS ≥ 9) are at low risk for IC-HTN, and one can follow sequential neurologic exams in these patients and institute further evaluation or treatment based on neurologic deterioration
- some monitor patients who don't localize, and follow neuro exam on others
2.   multiple systems injured with altered level of consciousness (especially where therapies for other injuries may have deleterious effects on ICP, e.g. high levels of PEEP or the need for large volumes of IV fluids or the need for heavy sedation)
3.   with traumatic intracranial mass
      A.   a physician may choose to monitor ICP in some of these patients[74, 75]
      B.   post-op, subsequent to removal

CONTRAINDICATIONS (RELATIVE)

1.   "awake" patient: monitor usually not necessary, can follow neuro exam
2.   coagulopathy (including DIC): frequently seen in severe head injury. If an ICP monitor is essential, take steps to correct coagulopathy (FFP, platelets...) and

---

A. "abnormal" CT: demonstrates hematomas (EDH, SDH or ICH), contusions[73], compression of basal cisterns (*see page 681*) or edema[74]

consider <u>subarachnoid bolt</u> or <u>epidural monitor</u> (an IVC or intraparenchymal monitor is contraindicated) (for recommended range of PT or INR, *see page 22*)

DURATION OF MONITORING

D/C monitor when ICP normal x 48-72 hrs after withdrawal of ICP therapy. Caution: IC-HTN may have delayed onset (often starts on day 2-3, and day 9-11 is a common second peak especially in peds). Also see *Delayed deterioration*, page 636. Avoid a false sense of security imparted by a normal early ICP.

COMPLICATIONS OF ICP MONITORS

See *Table 24-19* for a summary of complication rates for various types of monitors[49].

1. infection: *see below*
2. hemorrhage[49]: overall incidence is 1.4% for all devices (*see Table 24-19* for breakdown). Risk of significant hematoma requiring surgical evacuation is ≈ 0.5%[73, 77]
3. malfunction or obstruction: with fluid coupled devices, higher rates of obstruction occur at ICPs > 50 mm Hg
4. malposition: 3% of IVCs require operative repositioning

Table 24-19   Complications rates with various types of ICP monitors

Monitor type	Bacterial colonization*	Hemorrhage	Malfunction or obstruction
IVC	ave: 10-17% range[Smith, 1976 #781; 76: 0-40%	1.1%	6.3%
subarachnoid bolt	ave: 5% range: 0-10%	0	16%
subdural	ave: 4% range: 1-10%	0	10.5%
parenchymal	ave: 14% (two reports, 12% & 17%)	2.8%	9-40%

*   some studies report this as infection, but do not distinguish between clinically significant infection and colonization of ICP monitor

INFECTION WITH ICP MONITORS

There is no consensus regarding use of prophylactic antibiotics (**PAB**) with ICP monitors, and adequate controlled prospective randomized trials have not been done[78] (72% of respondents to a survey used PABs). Colonization of the device is much more common than clinically significant infection (ventriculitis or meningitis). See *Table 24-19* for colonization rates. Fever, leukocytosis and CSF pleocytosis have low predictive value (CSF cultures are more helpful).

Duration: One study[79] found periprocedural antibiotics (cefuroxime 1.5 gm IV q 8 hrs for ≤ 3 doses) were as effective as continuing antibiotics for the entire duration of EVD, and were less expensive.

Risk factors identified[76, 80]:
1. intracerebral hemorrhage with intraventricular extension
2. ICP > 20 mm Hg
3. duration of monitoring: one study found an increased risk with monitor duration > 5 days (infection risk reaches 42% by day #11)[77, 80] and the recommendation was made to prophylactically change catheters at 5 day intervals. A recent analysis[76] found a non-linear increase of risk during the first 10-12 days after which the rate diminished rapidly, with no significant reduction in infection rate in patients undergoing prophylactic change of monitors at ≤ 5 days
4. neurosurgical operation: including operations for depressed skull fracture
5. irrigation of system
6. other infections: septicemia, pneumonia

Factors not associated with increased incidence of infection:
1. insertion of IVC in neuro intensive care unit (instead of O.R.)
2. previous IVC
3. drainage of CSF
4. use of steroids

Treatment of infection:
Removal of device if at all possible (if continued ICP monitoring is required consideration may be given to inserting a monitor at another site) and appropriate antibiotics.

TYPES OF MONITORS

1. **intraventricular catheter (IVC)**: AKA external ventricular drainage (**EVD**), connected to an external pressure transducer via fluid-filled tubing. The standard by which others are judged (also see *Intraventricular catheter (IVC)* below)[A]
   A. advantages:
      1. relatively lower cost
      2. in addition to measuring pressure, allows therapeutic CSF drainage
      3. may be recalibrated to minimize measurement drift
   B. disadvantages
      1. may be difficult to insert into compressed or displaced ventricles
      2. obstruction of the fluid column (e.g. by blood clot) may cause inaccuracy
      3. some effort is required to check and maintain function (e.g. see *IVC problems*, page 654 and *IVC trouble shooting* on page 654)
      4. transducer must be consistently maintained at a fixed reference point relative to patient's head (must be moved as HOB is raised/lowered)
2. **intraparenchymal monitor** (e.g. Camino labs or Honeywell/Phillips[81, 82]): similar to IVC but more expensive. Some are subject to measurement drift[83, 84], others may not be[85]
3. less accurate monitors
   A. **subarachnoid screw** (bolt): risk of infection 1%, rises after 3 days. At high ICPs (often when needed most) surface of brain may occlude lumen → false readings (usually lower than actual, may still show ≈ normal waveform)
   B. **subdural**: may utilize a fluid coupled catheter (e.g. Cordis Cup catheter), fiberoptic tipped catheter, or strain gauge tipped catheter
   C. **epidural**: may utilize a fluid coupled catheter, or fiberoptic tipped catheter (Ladd fiberoptic). Accuracy is questionable
   D. in infants, one can utilizing an open anterior fontanelle (**AF**):
      1. **fontanometry**[86]: probably not very accurate
      2. **aplanation principle**: may be used in suitable circumstances (viz.: if the fontanelle is concave with the infant upright, and convex when flat or head down) to estimate the ICP within 1 cm H_2O[68]. The infant is placed supine, and the AF is visualized and palpated while the head is raised and lowered. When the AF is flat, the ICP equals atmospheric pressure, and ICP can be estimated in cm H_2O as the distance from the AF to the point where the venous pressure is 0 (for a recumbent infant, the midpoint of the clavicle usually suffices). If the AF is not concave with the infant erect, then this method cannot be used because either the ICP exceeds the distance from the AF to the venous zero point, or the scalp may be too thick

Conversion factors between mm Hg and cm H_2O are shown in *Eq 24-2* and *Eq 24-3*.

$$1 \text{ mm Hg (torr)} = 1.36 \text{ cm } H_2O \qquad \text{Eq 24-2}$$

$$1 \text{ cm } H_2O = 0.735 \text{ mm Hg (torr)} \qquad \text{Eq 24-3}$$

INTRAVENTRICULAR CATHETER (IVC)
See *Types of monitors* above for some basic information.

Insertion technique
For technique to place catheter in frontal horn, see *Kocher's point* on *page 620*. The right side is usually used unless specific reasons to use the left are present (e.g. blood clot in right lateral ventricle which might occlude IVC).

Set-up
Figure 24-2 shows a typical external ventricular drainage (**EVD**) system/ ventriculostomy ICP monitor. Not every system will have the same components. Note that the effect of having an opening on the top of the drip chamber (through an air-filter) is the same as having the drip nozzle open to air, and therefore as long as this filter is not wet or plugged the pressure in the IVC is regulated by the height of the nozzle (as read on the pressure scale; note that the "0" is level with the nozzle).

The external auditory canal (**EAC**) is often used as a convenient external landmark

---

A. other options for IVCs utilize transducers tipped with fiberoptic or strain gauge devices which are located within the intraventricular catheter; in this discussion, "IVC" does not refer to this type

for "0" (approximates the level of the foramen of Monro). In *Figure 24-2* the drip chamber is illustrated at 8 cm above the EAC.

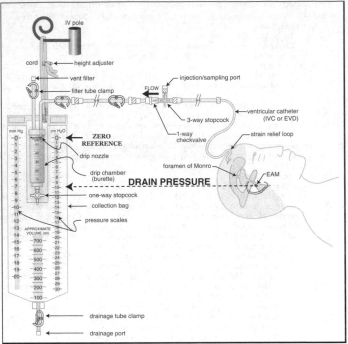

Figure 24-2 Medtronic® ventricular drainage system/ICP monitor

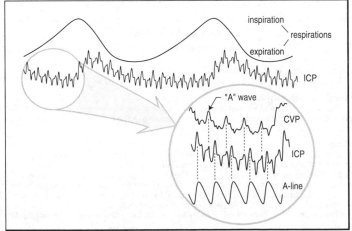

Figure 24-3 Normal ICP waveform

Types of ICP waveforms
Normal waveforms
The normal ICP waveform (as occurs with normal blood pressure and in the absence of IC-HTN) as illustrated in *Figure 24-3* is rarely seen since ICP is usually monitored only when it is elevated. The origin of the variations seen in the normal tracing is somewhat in dispute. One explanation describes these two types of waveforms[87]:
1. small pulsations transmitted from the systemic blood pressure to the intracranial cavity
    A. large (1-2 mm Hg) peak corresponding to the arterial systolic pressure wave, with a small dicrotic notch
    B. this peak is followed by smaller and less distinct peaks
    C. followed by a peak corresponding to the central venous "A" wave from the right atrium
2. blood pressure pulsations are superimposed on slower respiratory variations. During expiration, the pressure in the superior vena cava increases which reduces venous outflow from the cranium causing an elevation in ICP. This may be reversed in a mechanically ventilated patients, and is opposite to that in the lumbar subarachnoid space which follows the pressure in the inferior vena cava

Pathological waveforms
As ICP rises and cerebral compliance decreases, the venous components disappear and the arterial pulses become more pronounced. In right atrial cardiac insufficiency, the CVP rises and the ICP waveform takes on a more "venous" or rounded appearance and the venous "A" wave begins to predominate.

A number of "pressure waves" that are more or less pathologic have been described. Currently, this classification is not considered to be of great clinical utility, with more emphasis being placed on recognizing and successfully treating elevations of ICP. Plateau waves will rarely be seen because they are usually aborted at the onset by instituting treatments outlined herein (*see page 655*). A brief description of some of these waveforms is included here for general information[88].

1. **Lundberg A waves** AKA **plateau waves** (of Lundberg): (*see Figure 24-4*) ICP elevations ≥ 50 mm Hg for 5-20 minutes. Usually accompanied by a simultaneous increase in MAP (it is debated whether the latter is cause or effect)
2. **Lundberg B waves** AKA pressure pulses: amplitude of 10-20 mm Hg is lower than A waves. Variation with types of periodic breathing. Last 30 secs - 2 mins
3. **Lundberg C waves**: frequency of 4-8/min. Low amplitude C waves (AKA Traube-Hering waves) may sometimes be seen in the normal ICP waveform. High amplitude C-waves may be pre-terminal, and may sometimes be seen on top of plateau waves

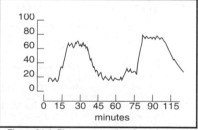

Figure 24-4 Plateau waves (Lundberg A waves)

Normal functioning of the IVC system
The system should be checked for proper functioning at least every 2-4 hours, and any time there is a change in: ICP (increase or decrease), neuro exam, or CSF output (for systems open to drainage).
1. check for presence of good waveform with respiratory variations and transmitted pulse pressures
2. IVCs: to check for patency, open the system to drain and lower the drip chamber below level of head and observe for 2-3 drops of CSF (normally do not allow more than this to drain)
3. for systems open to drainage:
    A. volume of CSF in drip chamber should be indicated every hour with a mark on a piece of tape on the drip chamber, and the volume should increase with time unless ICP is less than the height of the drip chamber (under these circumstances the system would usually not be left open to drainage).
    NB: the maximum expected output from a ventriculostomy would be ≈ 450-

700 ml per day in a situation where none of the produced CSF is absorbed by the patient. This is not commonly encountered. A typical amount of drainage would be ≈ 75 ml every 8 hrs

B. drip chamber should be emptied into drainage bag regularly (e.g. q 4 or 8 hours) and any time the chamber begins to get full (record volume)

4. in cases where there is a question whether the monitor is actually reflecting ICP, lowering the HOB towards 0° should increase ICP. Gentle pressure on both jugular veins simultaneously should also cause a gradual rise in ICP over 5-15 seconds that should drop back down to baseline when the pressure is released

IVC problems

The following represents some of the error or pitfalls that commonly occur with external ventricular drainage. Some also apply to ICP monitoring in general.

1. air filter on drip chamber gets wet
   A. fluid cannot drain freely into drip chamber (the pressure is no longer regulated by the height of the drip nozzle)
      1. if the outflow from the drip chamber is clamped, then no flow at all is possible
      2. if the clamp on the drip chamber outlet is open, then the pressure is actually regulated by the height of the nozzle in the <u>collection bag</u> and not the drip chamber
   B. solution: if a fresh filter is available, then replace the wet one. Otherwise one must improvise (with the risk of exposing the system to contamination): e.g. replace the wet filter with a filter from an IV set, or with a sterile gauze taped over the opening
2. air filter on collection bag gets wet: this will make it difficult to empty the drip chamber into the bag
   A. this is not usually an urgent problem unless the drip chamber is full and the collection bag is distended tensely with air
   B. the filter will dry out with time and will usually start to work again
   C. if it is necessary to empty the drip chamber before the filter is dry, then using sterile technique insert a needle into the bag drainage port and decompress the bag of fluid and air
3. improper connections: a pressurized irrigation bag with or without heparinized solution should <u>never</u> be connected to an ICP monitor
4. changing position of head of bed: must move drip chamber to keep it level the same relative to external landmarks:
   A. when open to drainage, this will assure the correct pressure will be maintained
   B. when opened to pressure transducer, will maintain correct zero
5. when open to drain, pressure reading from transducer is not meaningful: the pressure cannot exceed the height of the drip chamber in this situation
6. drip chamber falls to floor:
   A. overdrainage, possible seizures and/or subdural hematoma formation
   B. solution: securely tape chamber to pole, bed-rail..., check position regularly

IVC trouble shooting

See also *IVC problems* above.

1. IVC no longer works
   A. manifestation of problem:
      1. dampening or loss of normal waveform
      2. no fluid drains into drip chamber (applies only when catheter has been opened to drain)
   B. possible causes:
      1. occlusion of catheter proximal to transducer
         a. slide clamp closed or stopcock closed
         b. catheter occluded by brain particles, blood cells, protein
      2. IVC pulled out of ventricle
   C. test: temporarily lower drip nozzle and watch for 2-3 drops CSF
   D. solution:
      1. verify all clamps are open
      2. flush no more than 1.5 ml of non-bacteriostatic saline (AKA preservative-free saline) with very gentle pressure into ventricular catheter (NB: in elevated ICP the compliance of the brain is abnormally low and small volumes can cause large pressure changes)
         a. if no return then brain or clot is probably plugging catheter. If it

is known that the ventricles are ≈ completely collapsed then the IVC may be OK and CSF should still drain over time. Otherwise this is a non-functioning catheter, and if a monitor/drain is still indicated then a new catheter may need to be inserted (CT may be considered first if the status of the ventricles is not known). If catheter is clotted by intraventricular hemorrhage, rt-PA may sometimes be used[38] (*see page 860*)

2. ICP waveform dampened
   A. possible causes:
      1. occlusion of catheter proximal to transducer: *see above*
      2. IVC pulled out of ventricle: no fluid will drain
      3. air in system:
         a. solution: allow CSF to drain and expel air
         b. caution: do not allow excessive amount of CSF to drain (may allow obstruction of catheter, subdural formation...). Do not inject fluid to flush air into brain
      4. following decompressive craniectomy: due to the fact that the monitor is no longer in a closed space, this is a normal finding in this setting

ADJUNCTS TO ICP MONITORING

There are a number of experimental monitoring techniques, some of which are not widely available. Measurements of CBF have utilized xenon enhanced CT (for regional CBF), PET scanning... Other techniques are listed below.

JUGULAR VENOUS MONITORING

Jugular venous oxygen saturation (**SJO$_2$**) sampled from the jugular bulb has been utilized as an adjunct to ICP monitoring to gain additional data of cerebral perfusion. Monitoring by intermittent sampling is required since currently available continuous monitoring systems are plagued with significant artifacts and single measurements are of little value due to fluctuations[89]. Although normal values (SJO$_2$ > 50%) may sometimes be associated with poor outcomes, multiple venous desaturations (< 50%), or sustained or profound desaturation episodes are usually associated with poor outcome[90, 91]. Sustained desaturations should prompt an evaluation for correctable etiologies: kinking of jugular vein, poor catheter position, CPP < 60, vasospasm, surgical lesion, PaCO$_2$ < 28 mm Hg.

Also sometimes utilized is the **arterial-jugular venous oxygen content difference (AVdO$_2$)**[92]. AVdO$_2$ > 9 ml/dl (vol%) probably indicates global cerebral ischemia[93, 94], while values < 4 ml/dl indicate cerebral **hyperemia**[89] ("luxury perfusion" in excess of the brain's metabolic requirement[94]).

24.3.3. ICP treatment measures

PRACTICE PARAMETER 24-9 ICP TREATMENT THRESHOLD
Guidelines[95]: ICP treatment should be initiated for ICP > 20-25 mm Hg
Options[95]: interpretation & treatment of ICP based on any threshold should be corroborated by frequent clinical examination & CPP data
Options[96]: CPP should be maintained ≥ 70 mm Hg

This section presents a general protocol for treating documented (or sometimes clinically suspected) intracranial hypertension (**IC-HTN**). *The Guidelines for the Management of Severe Head Injury*[49] are generally adhered to (published in the *Journal of Neurotrauma*[97]). *Table 24-20* summarizes a protocol (see *Measures to lower ICP* below for details).

Table 24-20 Summary of measures to control IC-HTN*
Goals: keep **ICP** < 20 mm Hg, and **CPP** ≥ 70 mm Hg

Step	Rationale
GENERAL MEASURES (should be utilized routinely)	
elevate HOB to 30-45°	reduces ICP by enhancing venous outflow, but also reduces mean carotid pressure → no net change in CBF
keep neck straight, avoid tight trach tape	constriction of jugular venous outflow increases ICP
avoid hypotension (SBP < 90 mm Hg)	• normalize intravascular volume • use pressors if needed
control hypertension if present	• nitroprusside if not tachycardic • beta-blocker if tachycardic (labetalol, esmolol…) • avoid overtreatment → hypotension
avoid hypoxia (pO₂ < 60 mm Hg) (maintain airway and adequate oxygenation)	hypoxia may cause further ischemic brain injury
ventilate to normocarbia (pCO₂ = 35-40 mm Hg)	avoid prophylactic hyperventilation (*see page 659*)
light sedation: codeine 30-60 mg IM q 4 hrs PRN	(same as *heavy sedation, see below*)
unenhanced head CT scan for ICP problems†	rule out surgical condition
SPECIFIC MEASURES FOR IC-HTN	
(proceed to successive steps if documented IC-HTN persists - each step is <u>ADDED</u> to the previous measure)	
heavy sedation (e.g. fentanyl 1-2 ml or MSO₄ 2-4 mg IV q 1 hr) and/or paralysis (e.g. vecuronium 8-10mg IV)	reduces elevated sympathetic tone and HTN induced by movement, tensing abdominal musculature…
drain 3-5 ml CSF if IVC present	reduces intracranial volume
mannitol 0.25-1 gm/kg, then 0.25 mg/kg q 6 hrs, increase dose if IC-HTN persists & serum osmol ≤ 320 (NB: skip this step if hypovolemia or hypotension)	expands plasma volume, increases serum tonicity which draws fluid out of brain, may improve rheologic properties of blood
if there is "osmotic room" (i.e. serum osmol < 320) bolus with 10-20 ml of 23.4% hypertonic saline (HS)	some patients refractory to mannitol will respond to HS
hyperventilate to pCO₂ = 30-35 mm Hg	"blow off" (reduce) pCO₂ → ↓ CBF → ↓ ICP
If IC-HTN persists, consider unenhanced head CT† & EEG‡. Proceed to "second tier" therapy (*see page 658*).	

* see text for details (beginning on *page 657*). As IC-HTN subsides, carefully withdraw treatment

† if IC-HTN persists, and especially for a sudden unexplained rise in ICP or loss of previously controlled ICP, give strong consideration to repeating cranial CT to rule out a surgical condition, i.e. "clot" (SDH, EDH, or ICH) or hydrocephalus

‡ EEG to rule-out subclinical status epilepticus which is a rare cause of sustained IC-HTN

Dosages are given for an average adult, unless specified as mg/kg. Treatment may be initiated prior to insertion of a monitor if there is acute neurologic deterioration or clinical signs of IC-HTN, but continued treatment requires documentation of persistent IC-HTN.

For persistent IC-HTN consider "second tier" therapies shown on *page 658*.

Additional measures which may be used to treat an acute ICP *crisis* are shown in *Table 24-21*.

ICP MANAGEMENT PROTOCOL

Goals of therapy:
1. keep ICP < 20 mm Hg (prevents "plateau waves" from compromising cerebral blood-flow (**CBF**) and causing cerebral ischemia and/or brain death[98])
2. keep CPP > 70 mm Hg[49] (i.e. avoid hypotension). The primary goal is to control ICP, simultaneously, CPP should supported by maintaining adequate MAP[99].

SURGICAL TREATMENT
1. any subdural or epidural hematoma larger than ≈ 1 cm maximal thickness should be removed surgically to eliminate the contribution of this to IC-HTN
2. patients with hemorrhagic contusions ("pulped brain") showing progressive deterioration may need to have the contused brain tissue surgically removed (*see page 659*)

---

3. decompressive craniectomy may be considered for IC-HTN that cannot be controlled medically

Table 24-21 Measures to treat an acute ICP crisis*

Step	Rationale
check airway, position…(see general measures in *Table 24-20*). For resistant or sudden IC-HTN, consider unenhanced head CT	
be sure patient is sedated and paralyzed (*see Table 24-20*)	(*see Table 24-20*)
drain 3-5 ml CSF if IVC present	↓ intracranial volume
mannitol† 1 gm/kg IV bolus or 10-20 ml of 23.4% saline	↑ plasma volume → ↑ CBF → ↓ ICP, ↑ serum osmolality → ↓ brain water
hyperventilate with Ambu® bag (keep pCO₂ > 25 mm Hg)	"blow off" (reduce) pCO₂ → ↓ CBF → ↓ ICP. CAUTION: due to reduced CBF, uco for no more than several minutes (*see page 659*)
pentobarbital‡ 100 mg slow IV or thiopental 2.5 mg/kg IV over 10 minutes	sedates, ↓ ICP (NB: also myocardial depressant → ↓ MAP), treats seizures, may be neuroprotective

* for measures to treat ICP that is trending up over a longer period, *see Table 24-20* or information starting on *page 657*

† skip this step and go to hyperventilation if hypotensive, volume depleted, or if serum osmolality > 320 mOsm/L

‡ the availability of pentobarbital in the U.S. has been reduced, and other sedatives may need to be substituted, *see page 662*

GENERAL CARE

Major goals:
1. avoid hypoxia (pO₂ < 60 mm Hg)
2. avoid hypotension (SBP ≤ 90 mm Hg): 67% positive-predictive value (PPV) for poor outcome (79% PPV when combined with hypoxia)[100]

Specific treatment measures
1. prophylaxis against steroid ulcers (if steroids are used) and Cushing's (stress) ulcers (seen in severe head injury and in increased ICP, accompanied by hypergastrinemia)[101-105] for all patients (see *Prophylaxis for stress ulcers*, page 40)
    A. elevating gastric pH. titrated antacid and/or H₂ antagonist (e.g. ranitidine 50 mg IV q 8 hrs). Avoid cimetidine if phenytoin is also being given
    B. sucralfate
2. aggressive control of fever (fever is a potent stimulus to increase CBF, and may also increase plateau waves)[98]
3. arterial line for BP monitoring and frequent ABGs
4. CVP or PA line if high doses of mannitol are needed (to help keep patient euvolemic)
5. IV fluids
    A. choice of fluids:
        1. isolated head injury: IVF of choice is isotonic (e.g. NS + 20 mEq KCl/L)
        2. avoid hypotonic solutions (e.g. lactated ringers) which may impair cerebral compliance[106]
    B. fluid volume:
        1. provide adequate fluid resuscitation to avoid hypotension
        2. normalization of intravascular fluid volume is not detrimental to ICP
        3. although fluid restriction reduces the amount of mannitol needed to control ICP[107], the concept of "running patients dry" is obsolete[108]
        4. if mannitol is required, patient should be maintained at euvolemia
        5. also exercise caution in restricting fluids following SAH (see *Cerebral salt wasting*, page 14)
        6. if injuries to other systems are present (e.g. perforated viscus), they may dictate fluid management
    C. pressors (e.g. dopamine) are preferable to IV fluid boluses in head injury

MEASURES TO LOWER ICP

General measures that should be routine
1. positioning:
    A. elevate HOB 30-45° (*see below*)
    B. keep head midline (to prevent kinking jugular veins)
2. light sedation: codeine 30-60 mg IM q 4 hrs PRN, or lorazepam (Ativan®) 1-2 mg IV q 4-6 hrs PRN
3. avoid hypotension (SBP < 90 mm Hg): normalize intravascular volume, support with pressors if needed

4. control HTN (in ICH, aim for patient's baseline, see *Initial management of ICH*, page 856)
5. prevent hyperglycemia: (aggravates cerebral edema) usually present in head injury[109, 110], may be exacerbated by steroids
6. intubate patients with GCS ≤ 8 or with respiratory distress (give IV lidocaine first, see *Adjunctive measures* below)
7. avoid hyperventilation: keep pCO$_2$ at the low end of eucapnia (35 mm Hg)

Measures to use for documented IC-HTN

First, check *General measures that should be routine* above. Proceed to each step if IC-HTN persists.
1. heavy sedation and/or paralysis when necessary (also assists treatment of HTN) e.g. when patient is agitated, or to blunt the elevation of ICP that occurs with certain maneuvers such as moving the patient to CT table. Caution: with heavy sedation or paralysis, the ability to follow the neurologic exam is lost (follow ICPs)
    A. for heavy sedation (intubation recommended to avoid respiratory depression → elevation of pCO$_2$ → ↑ ICP): e.g. one of the following:
        1. fentanyl 1-2 ml IV q 1 hr
        2. MSO$_4$ 2-4 mg IV q 1 hr
        3. propofol drip (*see page 37*)
        4. "low dose" pentobarbital (adult: 100 mg IV q 4 hrs; peds: 2-5 mg/kg IV q 4 hrs)
    B. for paralysis (intubation mandatory): e.g. vecuronium 8-10 mg IV q 2-3 hrs
2. CSF drainage (when IVC is being utilized to measure ICP): 3-5 ml of CSF should be drained with the drip chamber at ≤ 10 cm above EAC. Works immediately by removal of CSF (reducing intracranial volume) and possibly by allowing edema fluid to drain into ventricles[111] (latter point is controversial)
3. "osmotic therapy" when there is evidence of IC-HTN:
    A. mannitol (also *see below*) 0.25-1 gm/kg bolus (over < 20 mins) followed by 0.25 gm/kg IVP (over 20 min) q 6 hrs PRN ICP > 20. May "alternate" with: furosemide (Lasix®) (also *see below*): adult 10-20 mg IV q 6 hrs PRN ICP > 20. Peds: 1 mg/kg, 6 mg max IV q 6 hrs PRN ICP > 20
    B. keep patient euvolemic to slightly hypervolemic
    C. if IC-HTN persists and serum osmolarity is < 320 mOsm/L, increase mannitol up to 1 gm/kg, and shorten the dosing interval
    D. if ICP remains refractory to mannitol, consider hypertonic saline, either continuous 3% saline infusion or as bolus of 10-20 ml of 23.4% saline (D/C after ≈ 72 hours to avoid rebound edema)
    E. hold osmotic therapy if serum osmolarity is ≥ **320 mOsm/L** (higher tonicity may have no advantage and risks renal dysfunction (*see below*)) or SBP < 100
4. hyperventilation **(HPV)** to **pCO$_2$ = 30-35 mm Hg** (for details, *see below*)
    A. ✖ do not use prophylactically
    B. ✖ avoid aggressive HPV (pCO$_2$ ≤ 25 mm Hg) at all times
    C. use only for
        1. short periods for acute neurologic deterioration
        2. or chronically for documented IC-HTN unresponsive to sedation, paralytics, CSF drainage and osmotic therapy
    D. avoid HPV during the first 24 hrs after injury if possible
5. ✖ steroids: the routine use of glucocorticoids is not recommended for treatment of patients with head injuries (*see below*)

"Second tier" therapy for persistent IC-HTN

If IC-HTN remains refractory to the above measures, and especially if there is loss of previously controlled ICP, strong consideration should be given to repeating a head CT to rule out a surgical condition before proceeding with "second tier" therapies which are either effective but with significant risks (e.g. high-dose barbiturates), or are unproven in terms of benefit on outcome. Also consider an EEG to rule-out status epilepticus that is not clinically evident (*see page 266* for treatment measures for status epilepticus; some medications are effective for both seizures and IC-HTN, e.g. pentobarbital, propofol...).
1. high dose barbiturate therapy: initiate if ICP remains > 20-25 mm Hg (see *High-dose barbiturate therapy*, page 662)
2. hyperventilate to pCO$_2$ = 25-30 mm Hg. Monitoring SjO$_2$, AVdO$_2$, and/or CBF is recommended (*see below*)
3. hypothermia[112, 113]: patients must be monitored for a drop in cardiac index, throm-

bocytopenia, elevated creatinine clearance, and pancreatitis. Avoid shivering which raises ICP[113]

4. decompressive craniectomy:
   A. removal of portion of calvaria[114] and/or large areas of contused hemorrhagic brain (makes room immediately; removes region of disrupted BBB). Controversial (may enhance cerebral edema formation[115]). Flap must be at least 12 cm in diameter, and duroplasty is mandatory
   B. if contused, consider temporal tip lobectomy (no more than 4-5 cm on dominant side, 6-7 cm on non-dominant) (total temporal lobectomy[116] is probably too aggressive) or frontal lobectomy. Has not shown great therapeutic promise. Also, see *Hemicraniectomy for malignant MCA territory infarction*, page 772
5. lumbar drainage: showing some promise. Watch for "cerebral sag"
6. hypertensive therapy

ADJUNCTIVE MEASURES
1. <u>lidocaine</u>: 1.5 mg/kg IVP (watch for hypotension, reduce dose if necessary) at least one minute before endotracheal intubation or suctioning. Blunts the rise in ICP as well as tachycardia and systemic HTN (based on patients with brain tumors undergoing intubation under light barbiturate-nitrous oxide anesthesia; extrapolation to trauma patients is unproven)[117]
2. high frequency (jet) ventilation: consider if high levels of PEEP are required[118] (NB: patients with reduced lung compliance, e.g. pulmonary edema, transmit more of PEEP through lungs to thoracic vessels and may raise ICP). Levels of PEEP up to 10 cm H_2O do not cause clinically significant increases in ICP[119]. Higher levels of PEEP > 15-20 cm $H2O$ are not recommended. Also, rapid elimination of PEEP may cause a sudden increase in circulating blood volume which may exacerbate cerebral edema and also elevate ICP

DETAILS OF SOME MEASURES OUTLINED ABOVE

ELEVATING HEAD OF BED (HOB)
   Early data indicated that keeping the HOB at 30-45° optimized the trade-off between the following two factors as the HOB is elevated: reducing ICP (by enhancing venous outflow and by promoting displacement of CSF from the intracranial compartment to the spinal compartment) and reducing MAP (and thus CPP) at the level of the carotid arteries.
   Recent data[120] indicate that although mean carotid pressure (**MCP**) is reduced, the ICP is also reduced and the CBF is unaffected by elevating the HOB to 30°. The onset of action of raising the HOB is immediate.

HYPERVENTILATION
   Hyperventilation (**HPV**) lowers ICP by reducing pCO_2 which causes cerebral vasoconstriction, thus reducing the cerebral blood volume (**CBV**)[121]. Of concern, vasoconstriction also lowers CBF which could produce focal ischemia in areas with preserved cerebral autoregulation as a result of shunting[122, 123]. However, ischemia does not necessarily follow as the O_2 extraction fraction (**OEF**) may also increase, up to a point[124].

PRACTICE PARAMETER 24-10 HYPERVENTILATION FOR **ICP** MANAGEMENT
Standards[125]: in the absence of IC-HTN, chronic prolonged hyperventilation (**HPV**) (PaCO2 ≤ 25 mm Hg) should be avoided
Guidelines[125]: the use of *prophylactic** HPV (PaCO2 ≤ 35 mm Hg) during the 1st 24 hrs after severe TBI should be avoided because it can compromise cerebral perfusion
Options[125]: HPV may be necessary for brief periods when there is acute neurologic deterioration, or for longer periods if there is IC-HTN refractory to sedation, paralysis, CSF drainage and osmotic diuretics

*   italics added

✱ Hyperventilation (**HPV**), once considered among first-line defense measures against IC-HTN, must now be regarded as a method to be used in moderation only in specific situations[49] (*see below*). *Prophylactic*[A] HPV may actually be associated with a <u>worse</u> outcome[126]. When indicated, use HPV only to pCO_2 = 30-35 mm Hg (see *Caveats for hyperventilation* below). CBF in severe head trauma patients is already about half of normal during the first 24 hrs after injury[127-130]. In one study, the use of HPV to pCO_2 = 30 mm Hg within 8-14 hrs of severe head injury did not impair *global* cerebral metabolism[124], but *focal* changes

Table 24-22   Summary of recommendations for pCO_2 following head trauma (*see text* for details)

pCO_2 (mm Hg)	Description
35-40	**normocarbia**. Use routinely
30-35	**hyperventilation**. Do not use prophylactically. Use only as follows: briefly for clinical evidence of IC-HTN (neurologic deterioration) or chronically for documented IC-HTN unresponsive to other measures
25-30	**augmented hyperventilation**. A second tier treatment. Use only when other methods fail to control IC-HTN. Additional monitoring recommended to R/O cerebral ischemia
< 25	**aggressive hyperventilation**. No documented benefit. Significant potential for ischemia

were not studied. Hyperventilation to $PaCO_2$ < 30 mm Hg further reduces CBF, but does not consistently reduce ICP and may cause loss of cerebral autoregulation[94]. If carefully monitored, there may be occasion to use this. A summary of the ranges of pCO_2 and the recommendations is shown in *Table 24-22*.

Reducing pCO_2 from 35 to 29 mm Hg lowers ICP 25-30% in most patients. Onset of action: ≤ 30 seconds. Peak effect at ≈ 8 mins. Duration of effect is occasionally as short as 15-20 mins. Effect may be blunted by 1 hour (based on patients with intracranial tumors), after which it is difficult to return to normocarbia without rebound elevation of ICP[131, 132]. Thus, HPV must be weaned slowly[98].

Indications for hyperventilation (HPV)
1. for brief periods (minutes) at the following times
   A. prior to insertion of ICP monitor: if there are clinical signs of IC-HTN (see *Table 24-14*, page 642)
   B. after insertion of a monitor: if there is a sudden increase in ICP and/or acute neurologic deterioration, HPV may be used while evaluating patient for a treatable condition (e.g. delayed intracranial hematoma)
2. for longer periods when there is documented IC-HTN unresponsive to sedation, paralytics, CSF drainage (when available) and osmotic diuretics
3. HPV may be appropriate for IC-HTN resulting primarily from hyperemia (*see page 655*)

Caveats for hyperventilation
1. avoid during the first 5 days after head injury if possible (especially first 24 hrs)
2. do not use prophylactically (i.e. without appropriate indications, *see above*)
3. if documented IC-HTN is unresponsive to other measures, hyperventilate only to pCO_2 = 30-35 mm Hg
4. if prolonged HPV to pCO_2 of 25-30 mm Hg is deemed necessary, consider monitoring SJO_2, $AVdO_2$, or CBF to rule-out cerebral ischemia (*see page 655*)
5. <u>never</u> reduce pCO_2 < 25 mm Hg

MANNITOL
The mechanism(s) by which mannitol provides its beneficial effects is still controversial, but probably includes some combination of the following
1. lowering ICP
   A. immediate plasma expansion[134-136]: reduces the hematocrit and blood viscosity (improved rheology) which increases CBF and O_2 delivery. This reduces ICP within a few minutes, and is most marked in patients with CPP < 70 mm Hg
   B. osmotic effect: increased serum tonicity draws edema fluid from cerebral parenchyma. Takes 15-30 minutes until gradients are established[134]. Effect lasts 1.5-6 hrs, depending on the clinical condition[49, 137, 138]

A. *prophylactic* HPV implies cases where there are no clinical signs of IC-HTN and where IC-HTN unresponsive to other measures has not been documented by ICP monitoring

2. supports the microcirculation by improving blood rheology (*see above*)
3. possible free radical scavenging[139]

With bolus administration, onset of ICP lowering effect occurs in 1-5 minutes; peaks at 20-60 minutes. When urgent reduction of ICP is needed, an initial dose of 1 gm/kg should be given over 30 minutes. When long-term reduction of ICP is intended, the infusion time should be lengthened to 60 minutes[140] and the dose reduced (e.g. 0.25-0.5 gm/kg q 6 hrs).

Cautions with mannitol
1. mannitol opens the BBB, and mannitol that has crossed the BBB may draw fluid into the CNS (this may be minimized by repeated bolus administration vs. continuous infusion[135, 141]) which can aggravate vasogenic cerebral edema[142]. Thus, when it is time to D/C mannitol, it should be tapered to prevent ICP rebound[140]
2. caution: corticosteroids + phenytoin + mannitol may cause hyperosmolar nonketotic state with high mortality[98]
3. excessively vigorous bolus administration may → HTN and if autoregulation is defective → increased CBF which may promote herniation rather than prevent it[143]
4. high doses of mannitol carries the risk of acute renal failure (acute tubular necrosis), especially in the following[69, 144]: serum osmolarity > 320 mOsm/L, use of other potentially nephrotoxic drugs, sepsis, pre-existing renal disease
5. large doses prevents diagnosing DI by use of urinary osmols or SG (*see page 17*)
6. because it may further increase CBF[145], the use of mannitol may be deleterious when IC-HTN is due to hyperemia (*see page 655*)

FUROSEMIDE

The use of furosemide (Lasix®) has been advocated, but little data exists to support this[49]. Loop acting diuretics may reduce ICP[146] by reducing cerebral edema[147] (possibly by increasing serum tonicity), and may also slow the production of CSF[148]. They also act synergistically with mannitol[149] (see *Mannitol* above).

Rx: 10-20 mg IV q 6 hrs, may be alternated with mannitol such that the patient receives one or the other q 3 hrs. Hold if serum osmolarity > 320 mOsm/L.

HYPERTONIC SALINE

May reduce ICP in patients refractory to mannitol[320, 321], although no improvement in outcome over mannitol has been demonstrated[321, 322]. Potentially deleterious effect on stroke penumbra in animal studies.

Rx: Continuous infusion: 3% saline. Bolus: 10-20 ml of 7.5-23.4% saline. Must be given through a central line. HS should be discontinued after ≈ 72 hours to avoid rebound edema[321]. Hold if serum osmolarity > 320 mOsm/L.

STEROIDS

Although glucocorticoids reduce **vasogenic cerebral edema** (e.g. surrounding brain tumors) and may be effective in lowering ICP in pseudotumor cerebri, they have little effect on **cytotoxic cerebral edema** which is more prevalent following trauma (see *Cerebral edema*, page 85).

Significant side effects may occur[152] including coagulopathies, hyperglycemia[153] with its undesirable effect on cerebral edema (see *Possible deleterious side effects of steroids*, page 10), and increased incidence of infection.

The use of non-glucocorticoid steroids (e.g. 21-aminosteroids, AKA lazaroids) are currently being investigated.

24.3.4.   High-dose barbiturate therapy

> **PRACTICE PARAMETER 24-13** BARBITURATES IN SEVERE HEAD INJURY
>
> **Guidelines**[154]: high-dose barbiturates may be considered in hemodynamically stable salvageable severe TBI with IC-HTN refractory to maximal medical and surgical ICP lowering therapy

Theoretical benefits of barbiturates in head injury derive from vasoconstriction in normal areas (shunting blood to ischemic brain tissue), decreased metabolic demand for O_2 ($CMRO_2$) with accompanying reduction of CBF, free radical scavenging, reduced intracellular calcium, and lysosomal stabilization[155]. There is little question that barbiturates lower ICP, even when other treatments have failed[156], but regarding outcome, studies have shown both benefits[157, 158] and lack of same[159, 160]. Patients that do respond have a lower mortality (33%) than those in whom ICP control could not be accomplished (75%)[158].

The limiting factor for therapy is usually <u>hypotension</u> due to barbiturate induced reduction of sympathetic tone[161 (p 354)] (causing peripheral vasodilatation) and direct mild myocardial depression. Hypotension occurs in ≈ 50% of patients in spite of adequate blood volume and use of dopamine[159].

NB: the ability to follow the neurologic exam is lost, and one must follow ICP.

"Barbiturate coma" vs. high-dose therapy: If barbiturates are given until there is burst suppression on EEG, this is considered true "barbiturate coma". This results in near maximal reductions in $CMRO_2$ and CBF[49]. However, most regimens should technically be called "high dose intravenous therapy" since they simply try to establish target serum barbiturate levels (e.g. 3-4 mg% for pentobarbital), even though there is poor correlation between serum level, therapeutic benefit, and systemic complications[49].

Adjunctive measures to administration of high-dose barbiturates:
1. consider a Swan-Ganz (PA) catheter placed during the first hour of loading dose
2. high-dose barbiturates cause paralytic ileus: therefore NG tube to suction & IV hyperalimentation are usually needed

INDICATIONS

The use of barbiturates should be reserved for situations where the ICP cannot be controlled by the previously outlined measures[158], as there is evidence that <u>prophylactic</u> barbiturates do not favorably alter outcome, and are associated with significant side effects, mostly hypotension[159], that can cause neurologic deterioration.

CHOICE OF AGENTS

A number of agents have been studied, however, there is inadequate data to recommend one drug over another. The most information is available on pentobarbital (*see below*). Alternative agents which have not been as well studied: thiopental (*see below*), phenobarbital (*see page 275*), propofol (*see page 663*), or the non-barbiturate agent etomidate (*see page 808*).

pentobarbital (Nembutal®)   DRUG INFO

Pentobarbital has a fast onset (full effects within ≈ 15 minutes), short duration of action (3-4 hrs), and a half life of 15-48 hrs.

Protocols for pentobarbital therapy in adults

There are many protocols. A simple one from a randomized clinical trial[162]:
* loading dose:
  A. pentobarbital 10 mg/kg IV over 30 minutes
  B. then 5 mg/kg q hr **x** 3 doses
* maintenance: 1 mg/kg/hr

A more elaborate protocol:
1. loading dose: pentobarbital 10 mg/kg/hr IV over 4 hrs as follows:
   A. FIRST HOUR: 2.5 mg/kg slow IVP q 15 min **x** 4 doses (total: 10 mg/kg in first hr), follow BP closely
   B. next 3 hours: 10 mg/kg/hr continuous infusion (put 2500 mg in 250 ml of appropriate IVF, run at **K** ml/hr **x** 3 hrs (**K** = patient's weight in kg))
2. maintenance: 1.5 mg/kg/hr infusion (put 250 mg in 250 ml IVF and run at 1.5 **x K** ml/hr)
3. check serum pentobarbital level 1 hr after loading dose completed; usually 3.5-5.0 mg%
4. check serum pentobarbital level q day thereafter
5. if level ever > 5 mg% and ICP acceptable, reduce dose
6. baseline brain stem auditory evoked response (**BSAER**) early in treatment. May be omitted on clinical grounds. Repeat BSAER if pentobarbital level ever > 6 mg%. Reduce dose if BSAER deteriorates (caution: hemotympanum may interfere with BSAER)
7. goal: ICP < 24 mm Hg and pentobarbital level 3-5 mg%. Consider discontinuing pentobarbital due to ineffectiveness if ICP still > 24 with adequate drug levels **x** 24 hrs
8. if ICP < 20 mm Hg, continue treatment **x** 48 hrs, then taper dose. Backtrack if ICP rises

Table 24-23 CNS effects of various pentobarbital levels*

Degree of CNS depression	mg%	µg/ml
level for valid brain death exam	≤ 1	≤ 10
sedated, relaxed, easily aroused	0.05-0.3	0.5-3
heavy sedation, difficult to arouse, respiratory depression	2	20
"coma" level (burst suppression occurs in most patients)	5	50

* levels reported are for intolerant patients; there is significant variability between patients and tolerant patients may not be sedated even at levels as high as 100 µg/ml

Neuro function takes ≈ 2 days off pentobarbital to return (*see Table 24-23*). Level should be ≈ ≤ 10 µg/ml before brain death exam is valid.

---

thiopental (Pentothal®)   DRUG INFO

May be useful when a rapidly acting barbiturate is needed (e.g. intra-op) or when large doses of pentobarbital are not available. One of many protocols follows (note: thiopental has not been as well studied for this indication, but is theoretically similar to pentobarbital[163, 164]):
1. loading dose: thiopental 5 mg/kg (range: 3-5) IV over 10 minutes
2. follow with continuous infusion of 5 mg/kg/hr (range: 3-5) for 24 hours
3. may need to rebolus with 2.5 mg/kg as needed for ICP control
4. after 24 hours, fat stores become saturated, reduce infusion to 2.5 mg/kg/hr
5. titrate to control ICP or use EEG to monitor for electrocerebral silence
6. "therapeutic" serum level: 6-8.5 mg/dl

---

propofol (Diprivan®)   DRUG INFO

Not well studied for ICP management. Suggest utilizing protocol for sedation (reproduced here): start at 5-10 µg/kg/min. Increase by 5-10 µg/kg/min q 5-10 minutes PRN ICP control. Has been used for neuroprotection during aneurysm surgery up to doses of 170 µg/kg/min (*see page 808*). May also cause hypotension.

24.4.   Skull fractures

Table 24-24 shows some differentiating features to distinguish linear skull fractures. See also *Clinical categorization of risk for intracranial injury* on page 638.

90% of pediatric skull fractures are linear and involve the calvaria.

Diastatic fractures extend into and separate sutures. More common in young children[165].

Table 24-24   Differentiating linear skull fractures from normal <u>plain</u> film findings

Feature	Linear skull fracture	Vessel groove	Suture line
density	dark black	grey	grey
course	straight	curving	follows course of known suture lines
branching	usually none	often branching	joins other suture lines
width	very thin	thicker than fracture	jagged, wide

24.4.1.   Depressed skull fractures

Classified as either closed (**simple fracture**) or open (**compound fracture**).

ADULT
Criteria to elevate a depressed skull fracture in an adult:
1. > 8-10 mm depression (or > thickness of skull)^A
2. deficit related to underlying brain
3. CSF leak (i.e. dural laceration)
4. ± open (compound) depressed fracture
5. ✖ more conservative treatment is recommended for fractures overlying a major dural venous sinus

There is no evidence that elevating a depressed skull fracture will reduce the subsequent development of posttraumatic seizures[166], which are probably more related to the initial brain injury.

PEDIATRIC[167]
Most common in frontal and parietal bones. One third are closed, and these tend to occur in younger children as a result of the thinner, more deformable skull. Open fractures tended to occur with MVAs, closed fractures tended to follow accidents at home. Dural lacerations are more common in compound fractures.

Simple depressed skull fractures
No difference in outcome (seizures, neurologic dysfunction or cosmetic appearance) in surgical vs. nonsurgical treatment. In the younger child, remodelling of the skull as a result of brain growth tends to smooth out the deformity.
Indications for surgery for pediatric simple depressed skull fracture:
1. definite evidence of dural penetration
2. persistent cosmetic defect in the older child after the swelling has subsided
3. ± focal neurologic deficit related to the fracture (this group has a higher incidence of dural laceration, although it is usually trivial)

"Ping-pong ball" fractures[168]
A green-stick type of fracture → caving in of a focal area of the skull as in a crushed area of a ping-pong ball. Usually seen only in the newborn due to the plasticity of the skull.

Indications for surgery
No treatment is necessary when these occur in the temporoparietal region in the ab-

---

A. exception: depressed fractures overlying and depressing one of the dural sinuses may be dangerous to elevate, and if the patient is neurologically intact, and no indication for operation (e.g. CSF leak mandates surgery) may be best managed conservatively

sence of underlying brain injury as the deformity will usually correct as the skull grows.
1. radiographic evidence of intraparenchymal bone fragments
2. associated neurologic deficit (rare)
3. signs of increased intracranial pressure
4. signs of CSF leak deep to the galea
5. difficulty with long-term follow-up

Technique
Frontally located lesions may be corrected for cosmesis by a small linear incision behind the hairline, opening the cranium adjacent to the depression, and pushing it back out e.g. with a Penfield #3 dissector.

24.4.2. Basal skull fractures

Most basal (AKA basilar) skull fractures **(BSF)** are extensions of fractures through the cranial vault.

DIAGNOSIS

Radiographic diagnosis

CT scan is often poor for directly demonstrating BSF. Plain skull x-rays and clinical criteria (*see below*) are usually more sensitive. Sensitivity of CT diagnosis can be increased by the use of bone windows together with thin cuts ($\leq$ 5 mm) and coronal images. BSF appear as linear lucencies through the skull base.

Indirect radiographic findings (on CT or plain films) that suggest BSF include: pneumocephalus (diagnostic of BSF in the absence of an open fracture of the cranial vault), air/fluid level within or opacification of air sinus with fluid (suggestive). Other related findings include: fractures of the cribriform plate or orbital roof.

Clinical diagnosis
Some of these signs may take several hours to develop. Signs include:
1. CSF otorrhea or rhinorrhea
2. hemotympanum or laceration of external auditory canal
3. postauricular ecchymoses (Battle's sign)
4. periorbital ecchymoses (raccoon's eyes) in the absence of direct orbital trauma, especially if bilateral
5. cranial nerve injury:
   A. VII and/or VIII: usually associated with temporal bone fracture
   B. olfactory nerve (Cr. N. I) injury: often occurs with anterior fossa BSF and results in anosmia, this fracture may extend to the optic canal and cause injury to the optic nerve (Cr. N. II)
   C. VI injury: can occur with fractures through the clivus (*see below*)

Severe basilar skull fractures may produce shearing injuries to the pituitary gland.

TREATMENT

NG tubes: ✖ Caution: cases have been reported where an NG tube has been passed intracranially[169-171] and is associated with fatal outcome in 64% of cases. Possible mechanisms include: a cribriform plate that is thin (congenitally or due to chronic sinusitis) or fractured (due to a frontal basal skull fracture or a comminuted fracture through the skull base).

Suggested contraindications to blind placement of an NG tube include: trauma with possible basal skull fracture, ongoing or history of previous CSF rhinorrhea, meningitis with chronic sinusitis.

Prophylactic antibiotics: The routine use of prophylactic antibiotics is controversial. This remains true even in the presence of a CSF fistula (see *CSF fistula*, page 174). However, most ENT physicians recommend treating fractures through the nasal sinuses as open contaminated fractures, and they use broad spectrum antibiotics (e.g. ciprofloxacin) for 7-10 days.

Treatment of the BSF: Most do not require treatment by themselves. However, conditions that may be associated with BSF which may require specific management include:

1. "traumatic aneurysms"[172] (see *Traumatic aneurysms*, page 820)
2. posttraumatic carotid-cavernous fistula (see *Carotid-cavernous fistula*, page 845)
3. CSF fistula: operative treatment may be required for persistent CSF rhinorrhea (see *CSF fistula*, page 174)
4. meningitis or cerebral abscess: may occur with BSF into air sinuses (frontal or mastoid) even in the absence of an identifiable CSF leak. May even occur many years after the BSF was sustained (see *Post craniospinal trauma meningitis (post-traumatic meningitis)*, page 212)
5. cosmetic deformities
6. posttraumatic facial palsy (see *Temporal bone fractures* below)

TEMPORAL BONE FRACTURES

Although often mixed, there are two basic types of temporal bone fractures:
1. longitudinal fracture: more common (70-90%). Usually through petro-squamosal suture, parallel to and through EAC. Can often be diagnosed on otoscopic inspection of the EAC. Usually passes between cochlea and semicircular canals (**SCC**) sparing the VII and VIII nerves, but may disrupt ossicular chain
2. transverse fracture: perpendicular to EAC. Often passes through cochlea and may place stretch on geniculate ganglion, resulting in VIII and VII nerve deficits respectively

POSTTRAUMATIC FACIAL PALSY

Posttraumatic unilateral peripheral facial nerve palsy may be associated with petrous bone fractures as noted above.

Management

Management is often complicated by multiplicity of injuries (including head injury requiring endotracheal intubation) making it difficult to determine the time of onset of facial palsy. Guidelines:
1. regardless of time of onset:
   A. steroids (glucocorticoids) are often utilized (efficacy unproven)
   B. consultation with ENT physician is usually indicated
2. immediate onset of unilateral peripheral facial palsy: facial EMG (AKA electroneuronography[173] or **ENOG**) takes at least 72 hrs to become abnormal. These cases are often followed and are possible candidates for surgical VII nerve decompression if no improvement occurs with steroids (timing of surgery is controversial, but is usually not done emergently)
3. delayed onset of unilateral peripheral facial palsy: follow serial ENOGs, if continued nerve deterioration occurs while on steroids, and activity on ENOG drops to less than 10% of the contralateral side, surgical decompression may be considered (controversial, thought to improve recovery from ≈ 40% to ≈ 75% of cases)

CLIVAL FRACTURES[174]

3 categories (75% are longitudinal or transverse):
1. longitudinal: may be associated with injuries of vertebrobasilar vessels including:
   A. dissection or occlusion: may cause brain stem infarction
   B. traumatic aneurysms
2. transverse: may be associated with injuries to the anterior circulation
3. oblique

Clival fractures are highly lethal. May be associated with:
1. cranial nerve deficits: especially III through VI; bitemporal hemianopsia
2. CSF leak
3. diabetes insipidus

24.4.3.   Craniofacial fractures

FRONTAL SINUS FRACTURES

Frontal sinus fractures account for 5-15% of facial fractures.

In the presence of a frontal sinus fracture, intracranial air (pneumocephalus) on CT even without a clinically evident CSF leak, must be presumed to be due to dural laceration (although it could also be due to a basal skull fracture, see *Pneumocephalus* below).

Anesthesia of the forehead may occur due to supratrochlear and/or supraorbital nerve involvement.

The risks of posterior wall fractures are not immediate, but may be delayed (some even by months or years) and include:
1. brain abscess
2. CSF leak with risk of meningitis
3. cyst or mucocele formation: injured frontal sinus mucosa has a higher predilection for mucocele formation than other sinuses[175]. Mucoceles may also develop as a result of frontonasal duct obstruction due to fracture or chronic inflammation. Mucoceles are prone to infection (mucopyocele) which can erode bone and expose dura with risk of infection

SURGICAL CONSIDERATIONS

Indications

Linear fractures of the anterior wall of the frontal sinus are treated expectantly.

Indications for exploration of posterior wall fractures is <u>controversial</u>[176]. Some argue that a few mm of displacement, or that CSF fistula that resolves may not require exploration. Others vehemently disagree.

Technique

LEFORT FRACTURES

*   **LeFort I**: <u>transverse</u>. Fracture line crosses pterygoid plate and maxilla just above the apices of the upper teeth
*   **LeFort II**: <u>pyramidal</u>. The transverse fracture extends upward across inferior orbital rim and orbital floor to medial orbital wall, and then across nasofrontal suture
*   **LeFort III**: <u>craniofacial dislocation</u>. Fracture involves zygomatic arches, zygomaticofrontal suture, nasofrontal suture, pterygoid plates, and orbital floors (separating maxilla from cranium)

PNEUMOCEPHALUS

AKA (intra)cranial aerocele, AKA pneumatacele, is defined as the presence of intracranial gas. It is critical to distinguished this from **tension pneumocephalus** which is gas under pressure (*see below*). The gas may be located in any of the following compartments: epidural, subdural, subarachnoid, intraparenchymal, intraventricular.

Presentation: H/A in 38%, N/V, seizures, dizziness, and obtundation[177]. An intracranial succussion splash is a rare (occurring in ≈ 7%) but pathognomonic finding. Tension pneumocephalus may additionally cause signs and symptoms just as any mass (may cause focal deficit or increased ICP).

Causes of pneumocephalus:
1. skull defects
    A. post neurosurgical procedure
        1. craniotomy: risk is higher when patient is operated in the sitting position[178]
        2. shunt insertion[179, 180]
        3. burr-hole drainage of chronic subdural hematoma[181, 182]: incidence is probably < 2.5%[182] although higher rates have been reported
    B. posttraumatic
        1. fracture through air sinus: including basal skull fracture

2. open fracture over convexity (usually with dural laceration)
   C. congenital skull defects: including defect in tegmen tympani[183]
   D. neoplasm (osteoma[184], epidermoid[185], pituitary tumor): usually caused by tumor erosion through skull
2. infection with gas-producing organisms
3. post invasive procedure:
   A. lumbar puncture
   B. ventriculostomy
   C. spinal anesthesia[186]
4. barotrauma[187]: e.g. with scuba diving (possibly through a defect in the tegmen tympani)
5. may be potentiated by a CSF drainage device in the presence of a CSF leak[188]

Tension pneumocephalus
Intracranial gas can develop elevated pressure in the following settings:
1. when nitrous oxide anesthesia is not discontinued prior to closure of the dura[189] (see *nitrous oxide (N₂O)*, page 1)
2. "ball-valve" effect due to an opening to the intracranial compartment with soft tissue (e.g. brain) that may permit air to enter but prevent exit of air or CSF
3. when trapped room temperature air expands with warming to body temperature: a modest increase of only ≈ 4% results from this effect[190]
4. in the presence of continued production by gas-producing organisms

Diagnosis
Pneumocephalus is most easily diagnosed on CT[191] which can detect quantities of air as low as 0.5 ml. Air appears dark black (darker than CSF) and has a Hounsfield coefficient of –1000. One characteristic finding is the **Mt. Fuji sign** in which the two frontal poles are surrounded by and separated by air[182]. Intracranial gas may also be evident on plain skull x-rays.

As pneumocephalus usually does not require treatment, it is critical to differentiate it from tension pneumocephalus, which may need to be evacuated if symptomatic. It may be difficult to distinguish the two; brain that has been compressed e.g. by a chronic subdural may not expand and the "gas gap" may mimic the appearance of gas under pressure.

Treatment
When due to gas-producing organisms, treatment of the primary infection is initiated and the pneumocephalus is followed.

Treatment of non-infectious simple pneumocephalus depends on the whether or not the presence of a CSF leak is suspected. If there is no leak the gas will be resorbed with time, and if the mass effect is not severe it may simply be followed. If a CSF leak is suspected, management is as with any CSF fistula (see *CSF fistula*, page 174).

Tension pneumocephalus must be evacuated; the urgency is similar to that of an intracranial hematoma. Dramatic and rapid improvement may occur with the release of gas under pressure. Options include placement of new twist drill or burr holes, or insertion of a spinal needle through a pre-existing burr hole (e.g. following a craniotomy).

24.4.4. Skull fractures in pediatric patients

This section deals with some special concerns of skull fractures in pediatrics. Also see *Child abuse*, page 689.

POSTTRAUMATIC LEPTOMENINGEAL CYSTS
AKA **growing skull fractures**. Posttraumatic leptomeningeal cysts **(PTLMC)** are distinct from arachnoid cysts (AKA leptomeningeal cysts, which are not posttraumatic). PTLMC consists of a fracture line that widens with time. Although usually asymptomatic, the cyst may cause mass effect with neurologic deficit. Traumatic aneurysm is another rare complication[192].

PTLMCs are very rare, occurring in 0.05-0.6% of skull fractures[193, 194]. Usually requires both a widely separated fracture AND a dural tear. Mean age at injury: < 1 year, over 90% occur before age 3 years[195] (formation may require the presence of a rapidly growing brain[196]) although rare adult cases have been described[197-199] (a total of 5 cases in the literature as of 1998[199]). Most often presents as scalp mass, although there are two reports of presentation with head pain alone[197]. PTLMC rarely occur > 6 mos out from the injury. Some children may develop a skull fracture that seems to grow during the initial few weeks, that is <u>not</u> accompanied by a subgaleal mass, and that heal spontaneously within several months; the term "pseudogrowing fracture" has been suggested for these[200].

X-ray appearance: widening of fracture and scalloping (or saucering) of edges.

TREATMENT

Treatment of true PTLMC is surgical, with dural closure mandatory. Since the dural defect is usually larger than the bony defect, it may be advantageous to perform a craniotomy around the fracture site, repair the dural defect, and replace the bone[198]. Pseudogrowing fractures should be followed with x-rays and operated only if expansion persists beyond several months or if a subgaleal mass is present.

SCREENING FOR DEVELOPMENT OF PTLMC

If early growth of a fracture line with no subgaleal mass is noted, repeat skull films in 1-2 months before operating (to rule-out pseudogrowing fracture). In young patients with separated skull fractures (the width of the initial fracture is rarely mentioned), consider obtaining follow-up skull film 6-12 mos post-trauma. However, since most PTLMCs are brought to medical attention when the palpable mass is noticed, routine follow-up x-rays may not be cost-effective.

24.5.   Hemorrhagic contusion

AKA traumatic intracerebral hemorrhage (**TICH**). Often considered as high density areas on CT (some exclude areas < 1 cm diameter[201]). TICH usually produce much less mass effect than their apparent size. Most commonly occur in areas where sudden deceleration of the head causes the brain to impact on bony prominences (e.g. temporal, frontal and occipital poles) in coup or contrecoup fashion.

TICH often enlarge and/or coalesce with time as seen on serial CTs. They also may appear in a delayed fashion (see *Delayed traumatic intracerebral hemorrhage* below). CT scans months later often show surprisingly minimal or no encephalomalacia.

Treatment

Surgical decompression may sometimes be considered if herniation threatens.

DELAYED TRAUMATIC INTRACEREBRAL HEMORRHAGE

Abbreviated (**DTICH**). In patients with GCS ≤ 8, incidence is ≈ 10%[202, 203] (reported incidence varies with resolution of CT scanner[40], timing of scan, and definition). Most DTICH occur within 72 hrs of the trauma[203]. Some patients seem to be doing well and then present with an apoplectic event (although DTICH accounted only for 12% of patients who "talk and deteriorate"[204]).

Factors that contribute to formation of DTICH include local or systemic coagulopathy, hemorrhage into an area of necrotic brain softening, coalescence of extravassated microhematomas[205].

Treatment is the same as for TICH (*see above*).

Outcome for patients with DTICH described in the literature is generally poor, with a mortality ranging from 50-75%[205].

24.6.   Epidural hematoma

Incidence of epidural hematoma (**EDH**): 1% of head trauma admissions (which is ≈ 50% the incidence of acute subdurals). Ratio of male:female = 4:1. It usually occurs in young adults, and is rare before age 2 yrs or after age 60 (perhaps because the dura is more adherent to the inner table in these groups).

Dogma was that a temporoparietal skull fracture disrupts the middle meningeal artery as it exits its bony groove at the pterion, causing arterial bleeding that dissects the dura from the inner table. Another possibility is that dissection of the dura from the inner table may occur first, then bleeding occurs into the space thus created.

Source of bleeding: 85% = arterial bleeding (the middle meningeal artery is the most common source of middle fossa EDHs). Many of the remainder of cases are due to bleeding from middle meningeal vein or dural sinus.

70% occur laterally over the hemispheres with their epicenter at the pterion, the rest occur in the frontal, occipital, and posterior fossa (5-10% each).

PRESENTATION WITH EDH

"Textbook" presentation (< 10%-27% have this classical presentation[62]):
* brief posttraumatic loss of consciousness (**LOC**)
* followed by a "**lucid interval**" for several hours
* then, obtundation, contralateral hemiparesis, ipsilateral pupillary dilatation

If untreated can go on to produce decerebrate rigidity, HTN, respiratory distress, and death.

Deterioration usually occurs over few hours, but may take days and rarely, weeks (longer intervals may be associated with venous bleeding).

Other presenting findings: H/A, vomiting, seizure (may be unilateral), hemi-hyperreflexia + unilateral Babinski sign, and elevated CSF pressure (LP is seldom used any longer). Bradycardia is usually a late finding. In peds, EDH should be suspected if there is a 10% drop in hematocrit after admission.

Contralateral hemiparesis is not uniformly seen, especially with EDH in locations other than laterally over the hemisphere. Shift of the brain stem away from the mass may produce compression of the opposite cerebral peduncle on tentorial notch which can produce *ipsilateral* hemiparesis (so called **Kernohan's phenomenon** or Kernohan's notch phenomenon)[206], a false localizing sign.

60% of patients with EDH have a dilated pupil, 85% of which are ipsilateral.

No initial loss of consciousness occurs in 60%. No lucid interval in 20%. Beware: lucid interval may also be seen in other conditions (including subdural hematoma).

Differential diagnosis: Includes a posttraumatic disorder described by Denny-Brown consisting of a "lucid interval" followed by bradycardia, brief periods of restlessness and vomiting, without intracranial hypertension or mass. Children especially may have H/A, and may become drowsy and confused. Theory: a form of vagal syncope, but must be distinguished from EDH.

EVALUATION

Plain skull x-rays

No fracture is identified in 40% of EDH. In these cases the patient's age was almost always < 30 yrs.

CT scan in EDH

"Classic" CT appearance occurs in 84% of cases: high density biconvex (lenticular) shape adjacent to the skull. In 11% the side against the skull is convex and that along the brain is straight, and in 5% it is crescent shaped (resembling subdural hematoma)[207]. EDH usually has uniformly density, sharply defined edges on multiple cuts, high attenuation (undiluted blood), contiguous with inner table, usually confined to small segment of calvaria. Mass effect is frequent. Occasionally, an epidural may be isodense with brain and may not show up unless IV contrast is given[207].

MORTALITY WITH EDH

Overall: 20-55% (higher rates in older series). Optimal diagnosis and treatment within few hours results in 5-10% estimated mortality (12% in a recent CT era series[208]). Mortality without lucid interval double that with. Bilateral Babinski's or decerebration pre-op → worse prognosis. Death is usually due to respiratory arrest from uncal herniation causing injury to the midbrain.

20% of patients with EDH on CT also have ASDH at autopsy or operation. Mortality with both lesions concurrently is higher, reported range: 25-90%.

TREATMENT OF EDH

MEDICAL

CT may detect small EDHs and can be used to follow them. However, in most cases, EDH is a surgical condition (see *Indications for surgery* below).

Nonsurgical management may be attempted in the following:

Small (≤ 1 cm maximal thickness) subacute or chronic EDH[209], with minimal neurological signs/symptoms (e.g. slight lethargy, H/A) and no evidence of herniation. Although medical management of p-fossa EDHs has been reported, these are more dangerous and surgery is recommended.

In 50% of cases there will be a slight transient increase in size between days 5-16, and some patients required emergency craniotomy when signs of herniation occurred[210].

Management

Management includes: admit, observe (in monitored bed if possible). Optional: steroids for several days, then taper. Follow-up CT: in 1 wk if clinically stable. Repeat in 1-3 mos if patient becomes asymptomatic (to document resolution). Prompt surgery if signs of local mass effect, signs of herniation (increasing drowsiness, pupil changes, hemiparesis…) or cardiorespiratory abnormalities.

SURGICAL

Evacuation is performed in the O.R. unless the patient herniates in E/R.

Indications for surgery

1. any symptomatic EDH
2. an acute asymptomatic EDH > 1 cm in its thickest measurement (EDHs larger than this will be exceedingly difficult for patient to resorb)
3. EDH in pediatric patients is riskier than adults since there is less room for clot. Threshold for surgery in pediatrics should be very low

Surgical objectives

1. clot removal: lowers ICP and eliminates focal mass effect
2. hemostasis: coagulate bleeding soft tissue (dural veins & arteries). Apply bone wax to intra-diploic bleeders (e.g. middle meningeal artery)
3. prevent reaccumulation: place dural tack-up sutures

DELAYED EPIDURAL HEMATOMA (DEDH)

Definition: an EDH that is not present on the initial CT scan, but is found on subsequent CT. Comprise 9-10% of all EDHs in several series[211, 212].

Theoretical risk factors for DEDH include the following (NB: many of these risk factors may be incurred after the patient is admitted following a negative initial CT):

1. lowering ICP either medically (e.g. osmotic diuretics) and/or surgically (e.g. evacuating contralateral hematoma) which reduces tamponading effect
2. rapidly correcting shock (hemodynamic "surge" may cause DEDH)[213]
3. coagulopathies

DEDH have been reported in mild head injury (GCS > 12) infrequently[214]. Presence of a skull fracture has been identified as a common feature of DEDH[214].

Key to diagnosis: high index of suspicion. Avoid a false sense of security imparted by an initial "nonsurgical" CT. 6 of 7 patients in one series improved or remained unchanged neurologically despite enlarging EDH (most eventually deteriorate). 1 of 5 with an ICP monitor did not have a heralding increase in ICP. May develop once an intracranial lesion is surgically treated, as occurred in 5 of 7 patients within 24 hrs of evacuation of another EDH. 6 of 7 patients had known skull fractures in the region where the delayed EDH developed[212], but none of 3 had a skull fracture in another report[213].

POSTERIOR FOSSA EPIDURAL HEMATOMA[215]

Comprise ≈ 5% of EDH. More common in 1st two decades of life. Although as many as 84% have occipital skull fractures, only ≈ 3% of children with occipital skull fractures develop p-fossa EDH. The source of bleeding is usually not found, but there is a high incidence of tears of the dural sinuses. Cerebellar signs are surprisingly lacking or subtle in most. Surgical evacuation is recommended for symptomatic lesions. Overall mortality is ≈ 26% (mortality was higher in patients with an associated intracranial lesion).

24.7. Subdural hematoma

24.7.1. Acute subdural hematoma

The magnitude of <u>impact damage</u> (as opposed to secondary damage, *see page 635*) is usually much higher in acute subdural hematoma (**ASDH**) than in epidural hematomas, which generally makes this lesion much more lethal. There is often associated underlying brain injury, which may be less common with EDH. Symptoms may be due to compression of the underlying brain with midline shift, in addition to parenchymal brain injury and possibly cerebral edema[216, 217].

Two common causes of traumatic ASDH:
1. accumulation around parenchymal laceration (usually frontal or temporal lobe). There is usually severe underlying primary brain injury. Often no "lucid interval". Focal signs usually occur later and are less prominent than with EDH.
2. surface or bridging vessel torn from cerebral acceleration-deceleration during violent head motion. With this etiology, primary brain damage may be less severe, a lucid interval may occur with later rapid deterioration

ASDH may also occur in patients receiving anticoagulation therapy[218, 219], usually with but sometimes without a history of trauma (the trauma may be minor). Receiving anticoagulation therapy increases the risk of ASDH 7-fold in males and 26-fold in females[218].

CT SCAN IN ASDH

Crescentic mass of increased attenuation adjacent to inner table. Edema is often present. Usually over convexity, but may also be interhemispheric, along tentorium, or in p-fossa. Membrane formation begins by about 4 days after injury[220]. Changes with time on CT (*see Table 24-25*):isodense after ≈ 2 wks, only clues may be obliteration of sulci

Table 24-25 ASDH density changes on CT with time

Category	Time frame	Density on CT
acute	1 to 3 days	hyperdense
subacute	4 days to 2 or 3 wks	≈ isodense
chronic	usually > 3 wks and < 3-4 mos	hypodense (approaching density of CSF)
	after about 1-2 months	may become lenticular shaped (similar to epidural hematoma) with density > CSF, < fresh blood

and lateralizing shift, the latter may be absent if bilateral. Subsequently becomes hypodense to brain (see *Chronic subdural hematoma*, page 674).

Differences from EDH: more diffuse, less uniform, usually <u>concave</u> over brain surface, and often less dense (from mixing with CSF).

TREATMENT

Rapid (*see below*) surgical evacuation should be considered for symptomatic subdurals that are greater than about 1 cm at the thickest point (or > 5 mm in peds). Smaller subdurals often do not require evacuation, and surgery may increase the brain injury if there is severe hemispheric swelling with herniation through the craniotomy.

A large craniotomy flap is often required to evacuate the thick coagulum and to gain access to possible bleeding sites. The actual bleeding site is often not identified at the time of surgery. One may start with a small linear dural opening and enlarge it as needed and only if brain swelling seems controllable.

MORBIDITY AND MORTALITY WITH ASDH

Mortality

Range: 50-90% (a significant percentage of this mortality is from the underlying brain injury, and not the ASDH itself).

Traditionally thought to be higher in aged patients (60%). 90-100% in patients on anticoagulants[219].

"Four hour rule"

Based on a 1981 series of 82 patients with ASDH[221], it had been widely held that:

1. patients operated within 4 hrs of injury had 30% mortality, compared to 90% mortality if surgery was delayed > 4 hrs
2. functional survival (Glasgow Outcome Scale ≥ 4, see *Table 31-3*, page 900) rate of 65% could be achieved with surgery within 4 hrs
3. other factors related to outcome in this series include:
   A. post-op ICP: 79% of patients with functional recovery had post-op ICPs that didn't exceed 20 mm Hg, whereas only 30% of patients who died had ICP < 20 mm Hg
   B. initial neuro exam
   C. age was <u>not</u> a factor (ASDH tend to occur in older patients than EDH)

However, the magnitude of the importance of rapid surgical treatment is still controversial. A study of 101 patients with ASDH found overall mortality of 66%, and functional recovery of 19%[222]. Postoperative seizures occurred in 9%, and did not correlate with outcome. The following was determined:

1. delay to surgery: delays > 4 hours increased mortality from 59% to 69% and decreased functional survival (Glasgow Outcome Scale ≥ 4, see page 900) from 26% to 16%. These differences suggested a trend but were not statistically significant
2. the following variables were identified as strongly influencing outcome:
   A. mechanism of injury: the worst outcome was with motorcycle accidents, with 100% mortality in unhelmeted patients, 33% in helmeted
   B. age: correlated with outcome only > 65 yrs age, with 82% mortality and 5% functional survival in this group (other series had similar results[223])
   C. neurologic condition on admission: the ratio of mortality to functional survival rate related to the admission Glasgow Coma Scale (GCS) is shown in *Table 24-26*
   D. postoperative ICP: patients with peak ICPs < 20 mm Hg had 40% mortality, and no patient with ICP > 45 had a functional survival

Of all the above factors, only the time to surgery and postoperative ICP can be directly influenced by the treating neurosurgeon.

Table 24-26 Outcome as related to admission GCS

GCS	Mortality	Functional survival
3	90%	5%
4	76%	10%
5	62%	18%
6 & 7	51%	44%

INTERHEMISPHERIC SUBDURAL HEMATOMA

Subdural hematoma along the falx between the two cerebral hemispheres (interhemispheric scissure)

May occur in children[224], possibly associated with child abuse[225].

In adults, a consequence of head trauma in 79-91%, ruptured aneurysm[226] in ≈ 12%, surgery in the vicinity of the corpus callosum, and rarely spontaneously[227].

Incidence is unknown. Spontaneous cases should be investigated for possible underlying aneurysm. Occasionally may be bilateral, sometimes may be delayed (*see below*)

May be asymptomatic, or may present with the so-called "falx syndrome" - paresis or focal seizures contralateral to the hematoma. Other presentations: gait ataxia, dementia, language disturbance, oculomotor palsies.

Treatment

Controversial. Small asymptomatic cases may be managed expectantly. Surgery should be considered for progressive neurological deterioration, approached through a parasagittal craniotomy.

Outcome

Reported mortality: 25-42%. Mortality is higher in the presence of altered levels of consciousness. Mortality rate may actually be lower (24%) than with all-comers[227]. This is significantly lower than SDH in other sites (*see above*).

DELAYED ACUTE SUBDURAL HEMATOMA (DASDH)

DASDHs have received less attention than delayed epidural or intraparenchymal hematomas. Incidence is ≈ 0.5% of operatively treated ASDHs[205].

Definition: ASDH not present on an initial CT (or MRI) that shows up on a subsequent study. Indications for treatment are the same as for ASDH. Neurologically stable patients with a small DASDH and medically controllable ICP are managed expectantly.

INFANTILE ACUTE SUBDURAL HEMATOMA
Infantile acute subdural hematoma (**IASDH**) is often considered as a special case of SDH. Roughly defined as an acute SDH in an infant due to minor head trauma without initial loss of consciousness or cerebral contusion[228], possibly due to rupture of a bridging vein. The most common trauma is a fall backwards from sitting or standing. The infants will often cry immediately and then (usually within minutes to 1 hour) develop a generalized seizure. Patients are usually < 2 yrs old (most are 6-12 mos, the age when they first begin to pull themselves up or walk)[229].

These clots are rarely pure blood, and are often mixed with fluid. 75% are bilateral or have contralateral subdural fluid collections. It is speculated that IASDH may represent acute bleeding into a preexisting fluid collection[229].

Skull fractures are rare. In one series, retinal and preretinal hemorrhages were seen in all 26 patients[228].

Treatment
Treatment is guided by clinical condition and size of hematoma. Minimally symptomatic cases (vomiting, irritability, no altered level of consciousness and no motor disturbance) with liquefied hematoma may be treated with percutaneous subdural tap, which may be repeated several times as needed. Chronically persistent cases may require a subduroperitoneal shunt.

More symptomatic cases with high density clot on CT require craniotomy. A subdural membrane similar to those seen in adult chronic SDH is not unusual[229]. Caution: these patients are at risk of developing intraoperative hypovolemic shock.

Outcome
8% morbidity and mortality rate in one series[228]. Much better prognosis than ASDH of all ages probably because of the absence of cerebral contusion in IASDH.

24.7.2. Chronic subdural hematoma

Chronic subdural hematomas (**CSDH**) generally occur in the elderly, with the average age being ≈ 63 yrs (exception: subdural collections of infancy, *see page 678*). Head trauma is identified in < 50% (sometimes rather trivial trauma). Other risk factors: alcohol abuse, seizures, CSF shunts, coagulopathies (including therapeutic anticoagulation[219]), and patients at risk for falls (e.g. with hemiplegia from previous CVA). CSDHs are bilateral in ≈ 20-25% of cases[230, 231].

Hematoma thickness tends to be larger in older patients due to a decrease in brain weight and increase in subdural space with age[232].

Classically CSDHs contains dark "motor oil" fluid which does not clot[233]. When the subdural fluid is clear (CSF), the collection is termed a subdural hygroma (*see page 677*).

Pathophysiology
Many CSDH probably start out as acute subdurals. Blood within the subdural space evokes an inflammatory response. Within days, fibroblasts invade the clot, and form neomembranes on the inner (cortical) and outer (dural) surface. This is followed by ingrowth of neocapillaries, enzymatic fibrinolysis, and liquefaction of blood clot. Fibrin degradation products are reincoporated into new clots and inhibit hemostasis. The course of CSDH is determined by the balance of plasma effusion and/or rebleeding from the neomembranes on the one hand and reabsorption of fluid on the other[234, 235].

Presentation
Patients may present with minor symptoms of headache, confusion, language difficulties (e.g. word-finding difficulties or speech arrest, usually with dominant hemisphere lesions), or TIA-like symptoms (*see page 916*). Or, they may develop varying degrees of coma, hemiplegia, or seizures (focal, or less often generalized). Often, the diagnosis may be unexpected prior to imaging. Specialized clinical grading systems have been published, but are not widely used.

TREATMENT

1. seizure prophylaxis: used by some. Fully load with phenytoin (17 mg/kg slow IV, see *phenytoin (PHT) (Dilantin®)*, page 271) and follow with 100 mg slow IV q 8 hrs. It may be safe to discontinue after a week or so if there are no seizure. If late seizure occurs with or without prior use of AEDs, longer-term therapy is required. Some feel that the incidence of side effects from AEDs approximates the incidence of seizures and therefore they do not recommend prophylactic AEDs
2. coagulopathies (and iatrogenic anticoagulation) should be reversed
3. surgical evacuation of hematoma indicated for:
   A. symptomatic lesions: including focal deficit, mental status changes…
   B. or subdurals with maximum thickness greater than ≈ 1 cm

SURGICAL CONSIDERATIONS

Surgical options

There is not uniform agreement on the best method to treat CSDHs. For details of techniques (burr holes, whether or not to use subdural drain…) *see below*.

1. placing two burr holes, and irrigating through and through with tepid saline until the fluid runs clear
2. single "large" burr hole with irrigation and aspiration: *see below*
3. single burr hole drainage with placement of a subdural drain, maintained for 24-48 hrs (removed when output becomes negligible)
4. twist drill craniostomy: *see below* (note that small "twist drill" drainage without subdural drain has higher recurrence rate than e.g. burr holes)
5. formal craniotomy with excision of subdural membrane (may be necessary in cases which persistently recur after above procedures, possibly due to seepage from the subdural membrane). Still a safe and valid technique[236]. No attempt should be made to remove the deep membrane adherent to the surface of brain

Techniques that promote continued drainage after the immediate procedure and that may thus reduce residual fluid and prevent reaccumulation:

1. use of a subdural drain: (*see below*)
2. using a generous burr hole under the temporalis muscle: (*see below*)
3. keeping the patient on bed-rest with the head of the bed flat (1 pillow is permitted) with mild overhydration for 24-48 hours post-op (or if a drain is used, until 24-48 hours after it is removed). May promote expansion of the brain and expulsion of residual subdural fluid
4. some advocate continuous lumbar subarachnoid infusion when the brain fails to expand, however there are possible complications[181]

TWIST DRILL CRANIOSTOMY FOR CHRONIC SUBDURALS

This method is thought to decompress the brain more slowly and avoids the presumed rapid pressure shifts that occurs following other methods, which may be associated with complications such as intraparenchymal (intracerebral) hemorrhage. May even be performed at the bedside under local anesthesia.

A ventricular catheter is inserted into the subdural space, and is drained to a standard ventriculostomy drainage bag maintained 20 cm below the level of the craniostomy site[237-239] (see *Subdural drain* below). The patient is kept flat in bed (*see above*). Serial CTs assess the adequacy of drainage. The catheter is removed when at least ≈ 20% of the collection is drained and when the patient shows signs of improvement, which occurs within a range of 1-7 days (mean of 2.1 days).

BURR HOLES FOR CHRONIC SUBDURAL HEMATOMAS

To prevent recurrence, the use of small burr holes (without a subdural drain) is not recommended. A generous (> 2.5 cm diameter - it is recommended that one actually measure this) subtemporal craniectomy should be performed, and bipolar coagulation is used to shrink the edges of the dura and subdural membrane back to the full width of the bony opening (do not try to separate these two layers as this may promote bleeding). This allows continued drainage of fluid into the temporalis muscle. A piece of Gelfoam® may be placed over the opening to help prevent fresh blood from oozing into the opening.

SUBDURAL DRAIN

Use of a subdural drain is associated with a decrease in need for repeat surgery from 19% to 10%[240]. If a subdural drain is used, a closed drainage system is recommended. Difficulties may occur with ventriculostomy catheters because the holes are small and are restricted to the tip region (so-designed to keep choroid plexus from plugging the catheter when inserted into the ventricles when used as intended as a CSF shunt), especially with thick "oily" fluid (on the positive side, slow drainage may be desirable). The drainage bag is maintained ≈ 50-80 cm below the level of the head[239, 241].

Post-op, the patient is kept flat (see above). Prophylactic antibiotics may be given until ≈ 24-48 hrs following removal of the drain, at which time the HOB is gradually elevated. CT scan prior to removal of the drain (or shortly after removal) may be helpful to establish a baseline for later comparison in the event of deterioration.

There is a case report of administration of urokinase through a subdural drain to treat reaccumulation of clot following evacuation[242].

OUTCOME

There is clinical improvement when the subdural pressure is reduced to close to zero, which usually occurs after ≈ 20% of the collection is removed[239].

Patients who have high subdural fluid pressure tend to have more rapid brain expansion and clinical improvement than patients with low pressures[241].

Residual subdural fluid collections after treatment are common, but clinical improvement does not require complete resolution of the fluid collection on CT. CTs showed persistent fluid in 78% of cases on post-op day 10, and in 15% after 40 days[241], and may take up to 6 months for complete resolution. Recommendation: do not treat persistent fluid collections evident on CT (especially before ≈ 20 days post-op) unless it increases in size on CT or if the patient shows no recovery or deteriorates.

76% of 114 patients were successfully treated with a single drainage procedure using a twist drill craniostomy with subdural ventricular catheter, and 90% with one or two procedures[237]. These statistics are slightly better than twist drill craniostomy with aspiration alone (i.e. no drain).

Complications of surgical treatment

Although these collections often appear innocuous, severe complications may occur, and include:
1. seizures (including intractable status epilepticus)
2. intracerebral hemorrhage (ICH): occurs in 0.7-5%[243]. Very devastating in this setting: one third of these patients die and one third are severely disabled
3. failure of the brain to re-expand and/or reaccumulation of the subdural fluid
4. tension pneumocephalus
5. subdural empyema: may also occur with untreated subdurals[244]

In 60% of patients ≥ age 75 yrs (and in no patients < 75 yrs), rapid decompression is associated with hyperemia in the cortex immediately beneath the hematoma, which may be related to the complications of ICH or seizures[243]. All complications are more common in elderly or debilitated patients.

Overall mortality with surgical treatment for CSDH is 0-8%[243]. In a series of 104 patients treated mostly with craniostomy[245], mortality was ≈ 4%, all of which occurred in patients > 60 yrs old and were due to accompanying disease. Another large personal series reported 0.5% mortality[246]. Worsening of neurologic status following drainage occurs in ≈ 4%[245].

24.7.3. Spontaneous subdural hematoma

Occasionally patients with no identifiable trauma will present with severe H/A with or without associated findings (nausea, seizures, lethargy, focal findings including possible ipsilateral hemiparesis[247]...) and CT or MRI discloses a subdural hematoma that may be acute, subacute or chronic in appearance. The onset of symptoms is often sudden[247].

Risk factors

Risk factors identified in a review of 21 cases in the literature[248] include:
- hypertension: present in 7 cases
- vascular abnormalities: arteriovenous malformation (AVM), aneurysm[249]
- neoplasm
- infection: including meningitis, tuberculosis
- alcoholism
- hypovitaminosis: especially vitamin C deficiency[250]
- coagulopathies: including iatrogenic (anticoagulation)

- seemingly innocuous insults (e.g. bending over) or injuries resulting in no direct trauma to the head (e.g. whiplash injuries)

ETIOLOGY

The bleeding site was determined in 14 of the 21 cases, and was arterial in each, typically involving a cortical branch of the MCA in the area of the sylvian fissure. One hypothesis is that previous inflammation results in arachnoid adhesions, which may lacerate vessels upon minor trauma.

TREATMENT

Surgical evacuation is the treatment of choice. For subacute to chronic subdurals, burr-hole evacuation is usually adequate (*see above*).

24.7.4.   Traumatic subdural hygroma

From the Greek *hygros* meaning wet. AKA traumatic subdural effusion, AKA hydroma. Excess fluid in the subdural space (may be clear, blood tinged, or xanthochromic and under variable pressure) is almost always associated with head trauma, especially alcohol-related falls or assaults[251]. Skull fractures were found in 39% of cases. Distinct from chronic subdural hematoma, which is usually associated with underlying cerebral contusion, and usually contains darker clots or brownish fluid ("motor oil" fluid), and may show membrane formation adjacent to inner surface of dura (hygromas lack membranes).

"Simple hygroma" refers to a hygroma without significant accompanying conditions. "Complex hygroma" refers to hygromas with associated significant subdural hematoma, epidural hematoma, or intracerebral hemorrhage.

On CT, the density of the fluid is similar to that of CSF.

PATHOGENESIS

Mechanism of formation of hygroma is probably a tear in the arachnoid membrane with resultant CSF leakage into the subdural compartment. Hygroma fluid contains prealbumin, which is also found in CSF but not in subdural hematomas. The most likely locations of arachnoid tears are in the sylvian fissure or the chiasmatic cistern. Another possible mechanism is post-meningitis effusion (especially influenza meningitis).

May be under high pressure. May increase in size (possibly due to a flap-valve mechanism) and exert mass effect, with the possibility of significant morbidity. Cerebral atrophy was present in 19% of patients with simple hygromas.

PRESENTATION

Table 24-27 shows clinical findings of subdural hygromas. Many present without focal findings. Complex hygromas usually present more acutely and require more urgent treatment.

TREATMENT

Asymptomatic hygromas do not require treatment. Recurrence following simple burr-hole drainage is common. Many surgeons maintain a subdural drain for 24-48 hrs post-op. Recurrent cases may require either a craniotomy to locate the site of CSF leak (may be very difficult), or a subdural-peritoneal shunt may be placed.

OUTCOME

Outcome may be more related to accompanying injuries than

Table 24-27   Major clinical features of traumatic subdural hygromas[251]

Type of hygroma	Simple	Complex	Total
number of patients	66	14	80
spontaneous eye opening	74%	57%	71%
disorientation or stupor	65%	57%	64%
mental status change without focal signs	52%	50%	51%
neurological plateau with deficit or delayed deterioration	42%	7%	36%
seizures (usually generalized)	36%	43%	38%
hemiparesis	32%	21%	30%
neck stiffness	26%	14%	24%
anisocoria (maintained light reflex)	15%	7%	14%
headache	14%	14%	14%
alert (no mental status change)	8%	0%	6%
hemiplegia	6%	14%	8%
comatose (responsive to pain only)	3%	43%	10%

to the hygroma itself.

5 of 9 patients with complex hygromas and subdural hematoma died. For simple hygromas, morbidity was 20% (12% for decreased mental status without focal findings, 32% if hemiparesis/plegia was present).

24.7.5.   Extraaxial fluid collections in children

Differential diagnosis
1. benign subdural collection in infants (*see below*)
2. chronic <u>symptomatic</u> extraaxial fluid collections or effusions (*see below*)
3. cerebral atrophy: should not contain xanthochromic fluid with elevated protein
4. "external hydrocephalus": ventricles often enlarged, fluid is CSF (*see page 181*)
5. normal variant of enlarged subarachnoid spaces and interhemispheric fissure
6. acute subdural hematoma: high density (fresh blood) on CT (occasionally these will appear as low density collections in children with low hematocrits). Will usually be unilateral (the others above are usually bilateral). These lesions may occur as birth injuries, and typically present with seizures, pallor, tense fontanelle, poor respirations, hypotension, and retinal hemorrhages
7. "craniocerebral disproportion" (head too large for the brain)[252]: extracerebral spaces enlarged up to 1.5 cm in thickness and filled with CSF-like fluid (possibly CSF), ventricles at upper limits of normal, deep sulci, widened interhemispheric fissure, normal intracranial pressure. Patients are developmentally normal. May be the same as benign extra-axial fluid of infancy (*see below*). Making this diagnosis with certainty is difficult in first few months of life

BENIGN SUBDURAL COLLECTIONS OF INFANCY

Benign subdural collections (or effusions) of infancy[253, 254], are perhaps better described by the alternate term **benign extra-axial fluid collections of infancy**, since it is difficult to distinguish whether they are subdural or subarachnoid[255]. They appear on CT as peripheral hypodensities over the frontal lobes in infants. Imaging may also show dilatation of the interhemispheric fissure, cortical sulci[256], and sylvian fissure. Ventricles are usually normal or slightly enlarged, with no evidence of transependymal absorption. Brain size is normal. Transillumination is increased over both frontal regions. The fluid is usually clear yellow (xanthochromic) with high protein content. The etiology of these is unclear, some cases may be due to perinatal trauma. They are more common in term infants than preemies. Must be differentiated from external hydrocephalus (*see page 181*).

Presentation: Mean age of presentation is ≈ 4 months[255].

May show: signs of elevated intracranial pressure (tense or large fontanelle, accelerated head growth crossing percentile curves), developmental delay usually as a result of poor head control due to the large size (developmental delay without macrocrania runs counter to the concept of "benign"[255]), frontal bossing, jitteriness. Other symptoms, such as seizures (possibly focal) are indicative of symptomatic collections (*see below*). Large collections in the *absence* of macrocrania are more suggestive of cerebral atrophy.

Treatment: Most cases gradually resolve spontaneously, often within 8-9 months. A single tap for diagnostic purposes (to differentiate from cortical atrophy and to rule out infection) may be done, and may accelerate the rate of disappearance. Repeat physical exams with OFC measurements should be done at ≈ 3-6 month intervals. Head growth usually parallels or approaches normal curves by ≈ 1-2 yrs age, and by 30-36 months orbital-frontal head circumference (**OFC**) approaches normal percentiles for height and weight. They usually catch up developmentally as OFCs normalize.

SYMPTOMATIC CHRONIC EXTRAAXIAL FLUID COLLECTIONS IN CHILDREN

These have been variously classified as hematomas (chronic subdural hematoma), effusions, or hygromas, with differing definitions associated with each. Since the appearance on imaging and the treatment is similar, Litofsky et al. proposes that they all be classified together as extraaxial fluid collections[257]. The difference between these lesions and "benign" subdural effusions may simply be the degree of clinical manifestation.

Etiologies

The following etiologies were listed in a series of 103 cases[257]:
1. 36% were thought to be the result of trauma (22 were victims of child abuse)
2. 22% followed bacterial meningitis (post-infectious)
3. 19 occurred after placement or revision of a shunt (*see page 198*)
4. no cause could be identified in 17 patients

Other causes include[252]:
1. tumors: extracerebral or intracerebral
2. post-asphyxia with hypoxic brain damage and cerebral atrophy
3. defects of hemostasis: vitamin K deficiency...

Signs and symptoms

Symptoms include: seizure (26%), large head (22%), vomiting (20%), irritability (18%), lethargy (13%), headache (older children), poor feeding, respiratory arrest...

Signs include: full fontanelle (30%), macrocrania (25%), fever (17%), lethargy (13%), hemiparesis (12%), retinal hemorrhages, coma, papilledema, developmental delay...

Evaluation

CT usually shows ventricular compression and obliteration of the cerebral sulci, unlike with benign subdural collections. The "cortical vein sign" helps to distinguish this from external hydrocephalus (*see page 181*).

Treatment

Options include:
1. observation: follow-up with serial OFC measurements, ultrasound and CT
2. serial percutaneous subdural taps: some patients require as many as 16 taps[258]. Some series show good results and others show low success rate[259, 260]
3. burr hole drainage: may include long-term external drainage. Simple burr hole drainage may not be effective with severe craniocephalic disproportion as the brain will not expand to obliterate the extra-axial space
4. subdural-peritoneal shunt: unilateral shunt is usually adequate even for bilateral effusions[257, 260, 261] (no study is required to demonstrate communication between the 2 sides[257, 262]). An extremely low pressure system should be utilized. The general practice is to remove the shunt after 2-3 months of drainage (once the collections are obliterated) to reduce the risk of associated mineralization of the dura and arachnoid and possible risk of seizures (these shunts are easily removed at this time, but may be more difficult to remove at a later date)[263]

Other recommendations:

At least one percutaneous tap should be performed to rule-out infection.

Many authors recommend observation for the patient with no symptoms or with only enlarging head and developmental delay.

24.8.   Nutrition in the head-injured patient

SUMMARY OF RECOMMENDATIONS (*SEE TEXT* FOR DETAILS)

Σ
1. by the 7th day after head injury, replace the following (enterally or parenterally):
   A. non-paralyzed patients: 140% of predicted basal energy expenditure (**BEE**)
   B. paralyzed patients: 100% of predicted BEE
2. provide ≥ 15% of calories as protein
3. nutritional replacement should begin within 72 hrs of head injury in order to achieve goal #1 by day 7
4. the enteral route is preferred (IV hyperalimentation is preferred if higher nitrogen intake is desired or if there is decreased gastric emptying)

RATIONALE

CALORIC REQUIREMENTS

Rested comatose patients with isolated head injury have a metabolic expenditure that is 140% of normal for that patient (range: 120-250%)[49, 264-266]. Paralysis with muscle blocker or barbiturate coma reduced this excess expenditure in most patients to ≈ 100-120% of normal, but some remained elevated by 20-30%[267]. Energy requirements rise during the first 2 weeks after injury, but it is not known for how long this elevation persists. Mortality is reduced in patients who receive full caloric replacement by day 7 after trauma[268].Since it generally takes 2-3 days to get nutritional replacement up to speed whether the enteral or parenteral route is utilized[49], it is recommended that nutritional supplementation begin within 72 hrs of head injury.

Enteral vs IV hyperalimentation: Caloric replacement that can be achieved is similar between enteral or parenteral routes[269]. The enteral route is preferred because of reduced risk of hyperglycemia, infection and cost[270]. IV hyperalimentation may be utilized if higher nitrogen intake is desired or if there is decreased gastric emptying. No significant difference in serum albumin, weight loss, nitrogen balance, or final outcome was found between enteral and parenteral nutrition[269].

Estimates of basal energy expenditure **(BEE)** can be obtained from the **Harris-Benedict equation**[271], shown in *Eq 24-4* through *Eq 24-6*, where W is weight in kg, H is height in cm, and A is age in years.

$$\text{Males: BEE} = 66.47 + 13.75 \times W + 5.0 \times H - 6.76 \times A \qquad \textbf{Eq 24-4}$$

$$\text{Females: BEE} = 65.51 + 9.56 \times W + 1.85 \times H - 4.68 \times A \qquad \textbf{Eq 24-5}$$

$$\text{Infants: BEE} = 22.1 + 31.05 \times W + 1.16 \times H \qquad \textbf{Eq 24-6}$$

Enteral nutrition

Isotonic solutions (such as Isocal® or Osmolyte®) should be used at full strength starting at 30 ml/hr. Check gastric residuals q 4 hrs and hold feedings if residuals exceed ≈ 125 ml in an adult. Increase the rate by ≈ 15-25 ml/hr every 12-24 hrs as tolerated until the desired rate is achieved[272]. Dilution is not recommended (may slow gastric emptying), but if it is desired, dilute with normal saline to reduce free water intake.

Cautions:
NG tube feeding may interfere with absorption of phenytoin (see *phenytoin (PHT) (Dilantin®)*, page 271). Reduced gastric emptying may be seen following head-injury[273] (NB: some may have temporarily *elevated* emptying) as well as in pentobarbital coma, patients may need IV hyperalimentation until the enteric route is usable. Others have described better tolerance of enteral feedings using jejunal administration[274].

NITROGEN BALANCE

As an estimate, for each gram of N excreted (mostly in the urine, however, some is also lost in the feces), 6.25 gm of protein have been catabolized. It is recommended that at least 15% of calories be supplied as protein. The percent of calories consumed **(PCC)** derived from protein can be calculated from *Eq 24-7*, where N is nitrogen in grams, and BEE is the basal energy expenditure[264] (*see Eq 24-4* through *Eq 24-6*).

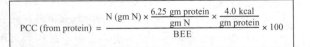

$$\text{PCC (from protein)} = \frac{N \, (\text{gm N}) \times \dfrac{6.25 \text{ gm protein}}{\text{gm N}} \times \dfrac{4.0 \text{ kcal}}{\text{gm protein}}}{\text{BEE}} \times 100 \qquad \textbf{Eq 24-7}$$

Thus, to supply PCC (protein) = 15% once the BEE is known, use *Eq 24-8*. Some enteral formulations include Magnacal® (PCC = 14%) and TraumaCal® (PCC = 22%).

$$N \, (\text{gm N}) = 0.006 \times \text{BEE} \qquad \textbf{Eq 24-8}$$

24.9. Outcome from head trauma

24.9.1. Age

In general, the degree of recovery from closed head injury is better in infants and young children than in adults. In adults, decerebrate posturing or flaccidity with loss of pupillary or oculovestibular reflex is associated with a poor outcome in most cases, these findings are not as ominous in pediatrics.

24.9.2. Outcome prognosticators

The frequency of poor outcome from closed head injury is increased with persistent ICP > 20 mm Hg after hyperventilation, increasing age, impaired or absent pupillary light response or eye movement, hypotension (SBP < 90), hypercarbia, hypoxemia, or anemia[72]. This is probably due at least in part to the fact that some of these are markers for significant injury to other body systems. One of the most important predictors for poor outcome is the presence of a mass lesion requiring surgical removal[275]. High ICP during the first 24 hrs is also a poor prognosticator.

OBLITERATION OF BASAL CISTERNS ON CT

In 218 patients with GCS ≤ 8, the condition of the basal cisterns (BC) was classified on initial CT (almost all within 48 hrs of admission) as: absent, compressed, normal, or not visualized (quality of CT too poor to tell)[276]. The relationship of outcome to the BCs is shown in *Table 24-28*.

18 patients had a shift of brain structures > 15 mm associated with

Table 24-28 Correlation of GOS* with basal cisterns

Basal cis-terns	– – – OUTCOME* – – –				
	Mortality	Vegeta-tive	Severe disability	Moderate disability	Good
	(GOS 1)	(GOS 2)	(GOS 3)	(GOS 4)	(GOS 5)
normal	22%	6%	16%	21%	35%
compressed	39%	7%	18%	17%	19%
absent	77%	2%	6%	4%	11%
not-visualized	68%	0%	11%	9%	12%

* GOS = Glasgow outcome scale, see *Table 31-3*, page 900

absent BCs, all of them died. The status of the BCs were more important within each GOS score than across scores. Also, see *Table 24-7*, page 635 for further information on CT

APOLIPOPROTEIN E (APOE) ε4 ALLELE

The presence of this genotype portends a worse prognosis following traumatic brain injury[277]. Furthermore, the incidence of severe brain injury in individuals with the apoE-4 allele greatly exceeds the rate of the allele in the general population[278]. This allele is also a risk factor for Alzheimer's disease (*see below*) as well as for chronic traumatic encephalopathy (*see page 684*).

24.9.3. Late complications from head injury

Long term complications include:
1. posttraumatic seizures: (*see page 260*)
2. communicating hydrocephalus: incidence ≈ 3.9% of severe head injuries
3. posttraumatic syndrome (or postconcussive syndrome): *see below*
4. hypogonadotropic hypogonadism[279]: also *see page 645*
5. chronic traumatic encephalopathy (*see page 683*)
6. Alzheimer's disease (**AD**): head injury (especially if severe) promotes the deposition of amyloid proteins, especially in individuals possessing the apolipoprotein E

(apoE) ε4 allele[278], which may be related to the development of AD[280-282]

POSTCONCUSSIVE SYNDROME

Variously defined collection of symptoms (*see below*) that is usually considered as a possible sequelae to minor head trauma (although some of these features can be seen following more serious head trauma). Loss of consciousness is not a prerequisite.

Controversy exists over the relative contribution of actual organic dysfunction vs. psychological factors (including conversion reaction, secondary gain which may be for attention, financial reward, drug seeking...). Furthermore, the presence of some of these symptoms can undoubtedly lead to the development of others (e.g headache can cause difficulty concentrating and thus poor job performance and thence depression).

A paradox has been noted by clinicians that the complaints following minor head injury seem out of proportion when considered in the context of the frequency of complaints after serious head injury. It has also been noted that patients with early post-traumatic complaints generally improve with time, whereas the late development of symptoms is often associated with a more protracted and fulminant course.

Symptoms commonly considered part of this syndrome include the following (with headache, dizziness and memory difficulties being the most frequent):
1. somatic
   A. headache
   B. dizziness or light-headedness
   C. visual disturbances: blurring is a common complaint
   D. anosmia
   E. hearing difficulties: tinnitus, reduced auditory acuity
   F. balance difficulties
2. cognitive
   A. difficulty concentrating
   B. dementia: more common with multiple brain injuries than with a single concussion (see *Chronic traumatic encephalopathy*, page 683)
      1. loss of intellectual ability
      2. memory problems: usually impairs short-term memory
   C. impaired judgement
3. psychosocial
   A. emotional difficulties: including depression, mood swings (emotional lability), euphoria/giddiness, easy irritability, lack of motivation, abulia
   B. personality changes
   C. loss of libido
   D. disruption of sleep/wake cycles, insomnia
   E. easy fatigability
   F. intolerance to light (photophobia) and/or loud (or even moderate) noise
   G. increased rate of job loss and divorce (may be related to any of above)

Virtually any symptom can be ascribed to the condition. Other symptoms that may be described by patients which are generally not included in the definition:
1. fainting (vaso-vagal episodes): may need to rule out posttraumatic seizures, as well as other causes of syncope
2. altered sense of taste
3. dystonia[283]

Treatment

Treatment for symptoms attributed to this syndrome tends to be supportive. Often times these patients obtain treatment from primary care physicians, neurologists, physiatrists, and/or psychiatrists/psychologists. Neurosurgical involvement in the continuing care for these patients is usually at the discretion of the individual physician based on his or her practice patterns. Recovery follows a highly variable course.

Some symptoms may need to be evaluated for possible correctable late complications (seizures, hydrocephalus, CSF leak...). Alves and Jane[284] perform a head CT, MRI, BSAER and neuropsychological battery if symptoms after minor head injury persist > 3 months. An EEG may be appropriate in cases where there is a question of seizures. If all studies are negative, "the authors tell the patient (and the lawyer) that there is no objective evidence for disease and that psychiatric evaluation is warranted." Non-correctable abnormalities on these studies prompt reassurance that significant symptoms should subside by 1 year, and that no specific treatment, other than psychological counselling, is helpful.

CHRONIC TRAUMATIC ENCEPHALOPATHY

Often described in retired boxers, chronic traumatic encephalopathy **(CTE)** encompasses a spectrum of symptoms that range from mild to a severe form AKA **dementia pugilistica**[285], or punch drunk syndrome. Symptoms involve motor, cognitive and psychiatric systems. CTE is distinct from post-traumatic dementia (which may follow a single closed head injury) or from post-traumatic Alzheimer's syndrome. Although generally accepted, not all authorities agree that repeated concussions have any long-term sequelae[286].

There are some similarities with Alzheimer's disease **(AD)**, including the presence of neurofibrillary tangles having similar microscopic characteristics and the development of amyloid angiopathy with the attendant risk of intracerebral hemorrhage[207]. EEG changes occur in one-third to one-half of professional boxers (diffuse slowing or low-voltage records).

Clinical: Clinical features of CTE are shown in *Table 24-29*[285] and include:

1. cognitive: mental slowing and memory deficits (dementia)
2. personality changes: explosive behavior, morbid jealousy, pathological intoxication with alcohol, and paranoia
3. motor: cerebellar dysfunction, symptoms of Parkinson's disease, pyramidal tract dysfunction

Grading scales have been devised to rank patients as having probable, possible, and improbable CTE.

The chronic brain injury scale **(CBIS)** assesses involvement of motor, cognitive, and psychological axes as shown in *Table 24-30*.

Risk factors for dementia pugilistica in boxing[285]:

1. risk increases with length of boxing career, especially > 10 yrs
2. age at retirement: risk goes up after age 28 yrs
3. number of bouts: especially ≥ 20 (more important than the number of knock-outs)
4. boxing style: increased risk among poorer performers, those known as sluggers rather than "scientific" boxers, those known to be hard to knock out or known to take a punch and keep going
5. age at examination: long latency causes increased prevalence with age
6. and possibly, the number of head blows

Table 24-29   CTE of boxing*

Motor	Cognitive	Psychiatric
Early (≈ 57%)		
dysarthria tremors mild incoordination especially non-dominant hand	decreased complex attention	emotional lability euphoria/hypomania irritability, suspiciousness ease of aggression & talkativeness
Middle (≈ 17%)		
parkinsonism increased dysarthria, tremors, and incoordination	slowed mental speed mild deficits in memory, attention & executive ability	magnified personality decreased spontaneity paranoid, jealous inappropriate violent outbursts
Late (< 3%)		
pyramidal signs prominent parkinsonism prominent dysarthria, tremors & ataxia	prominent slowness of thought/speech amnesia attention deficits executive dysfunction	cheerful/silly decreased insight paranoid, psychotic disinhibited, violent possible Klüver-Bucy

*   In professional boxers with ≥ 20 bouts

Table 24-30   Chronic brain injury scale

Grade involvement of each of the following axes separately: • motor • cognitive • psychological	Scoring for each axis: 0 = none 1 = mild 2 = moderate 3 = severe
Sum total points	**Severity**
0	normal
1 - 2	mild
3 - 4	moderate
> 4	severe

7. risk increases in patients with the apolipoprotein E (apo E) ε4 allele (as in Alzheimer's disease) as shown in *Table 24-31*
8. professional boxers (more risk than amateurs)

Neuro-imaging: The most common finding is cerebral atrophy. A cavum septum pellucidum **(CSP)** is observed in 13% of boxers[288]. CSP in this setting probably represents an acquired condition[289] and correlates with cerebral atrophy.

Neuropathology includes:
1. cerebral and cerebellar atrophy
2. neurofibrillary degeneration of cortical and subcortical areas
3. deposition of ß-amyloid protein
   A. forming diffuse amyloid plaques
   B. in a subset of CTE patients this involves the vessel walls giving rise to cerebral amyloid angiopathy

Table 24-31 Odds ratio for developing Alzheimer's disease

Head injury	Apo E ε4 allele	Odds ratio
–	–	1
–	+	2
+	–	1
+	+	10

24.10. Gunshot wounds to the head

Gunshot wounds to the head **(GSWH)** account for the majority of penetrating brain injuries, and comprise ≈ 35% of deaths from brain injury in persons < 45 yrs old. GSWH are the most lethal type of head injury, ≈ two thirds die at the scene, and GSWH ultimately are the proximal cause of death in > 90% of victims[290].

PRIMARY INJURY
Primary injury from GSWH results from a number of factors including:
1. injury to soft tissue
   A. direct scalp and/or facial injuries
   B. soft tissue and bacteria may be dragged intracranially, the devitalized tissue may also then support growth of the bacteria
   C. pressure waves of gas combustion may cause injury if the weapon is close
2. comminuted fracture of bone: may injure subjacent vascular and/or cortical tissue (depressed skull fracture). May act as secondary missiles
3. cerebral injuries from missile
   A. direct injury to brain tissue in path of bullet (may ricochet, fragment...)
   B. injury to tissue by shock waves and coup + contrecoup injury from missile impact (may cause injuries distant from bullet path)

Extent of primary injury is related to <u>impact velocity</u>:
- impact velocity > 100 m/s: causes explosive intracranial injury that is uniformly fatal (NB: impact velocity is less than muzzle velocity)
- low <u>muzzle</u> velocity bullets (≈ < 250 m/s): as with most handguns. Tissue injury is caused primarily by laceration and maceration along a path slightly wider than missile diameter
- high <u>muzzle</u> velocity bullets (≈ 750 m/s): from military weapons and hunting rifles. Causes additional damage by shock waves and temporary cavitation (tissue pushed away from the missile causes a conical cavity of injury that may exceed bullet diameter many-fold, and causes low-pressure region which may draw surface debris into the wound)

SECONDARY INJURY
Cerebral edema occurs similar to closed head injury. ICP may rise rapidly within minutes (higher ICPs result from higher impact velocities). Cardiac output may also fall initially. Together, ↑ ICP and ↓ MAP adversely effect cerebral perfusion pressure.
Other common complicating factors include: DIC, intracranial hemorrhage from lacerated blood vessels.

LATE COMPLICATIONS
Late complications include:
1. cerebral abscess
2. traumatic aneurysm[291]

3. seizures
4. large fragments may migrate

EVALUATION

Exam should describe visible entrance and exit wounds. In through-and-through missile wounds of the skull, the entrance wound is typically smaller than the exit wound due to bullet mushrooming. Entrance wounds may be especially small with direct contact of the muzzle to the head. At surgery or autopsy, the entrance wound will typically show bevelling of the inner table, whereas exit wounds have a beveled outer table.

GRADING SYSTEMS

The Glasgow Coma Scale is still the most widely used system and allows better comparison between series than specialized scales for GSWHs. See *Outcome* below.

MANAGEMENT

INITIAL STABILIZATION

GENERAL MEASURES
1. CPR as required; endotracheal intubation if stuporous or airway compromised
2. additional injuries (e.g. chest wounds) identified and treated appropriately
3. usual precautions taken for spine injury
4. fluids as needed to replace estimated blood loss which may be variable: care to avoid excessive hydration (to minimize cerebral edema)
5. pressors to support MAP during and after fluid resuscitation

TREATMENT OF THE INJURY

Neurological assessment as rapidly as possible and as thoroughly as time permits. Decision by experienced neurosurgeon regarding the ultimate treatment of the patient will determine appropriate steps to be taken. Patients with little CNS function (in the absence of shock) are unlikely to benefit from craniotomy. Supportive measures are indicated in most cases (for possibility of organ donation, opportunity for family to adjust to situation, and requirements for observation period to determine actual brain death).

In patients considered for further treatment, rapid deterioration at any point with signs of herniation requires immediate surgical intervention. As time permits, the following should be undertaken:

- initial steps
  A. control bleeding from scalp and associated wounds (hemostats on scalp vessels)
  B. shave scalp to identify entrance/exit sites, and to save time in the O.R.
- radiographic evaluation
  A. AP and lateral skull films to localize metal and bone fragments, and to help identify entrance/exit sites (omit if time not available)
  B. non-contrast CT scan of the brain: identifies bullet track, intracranial hematomas, intraparenchymal location of bone and metal
  C. angiography is occasionally indicated (*see below*)
- medical treatment (similar to closed head injury)
  A. assume ICP is elevated:
    1. elevate HOB 30-45° with head midline (avoids kinking jugular veins)
    2. **mannitol** (1 gm/kg bolus) as blood pressure tolerates
    3. **hyperventilate** to pCO_2 = **30-35** mm Hg if indications are met (see *Indications for hyperventilation (HPV)*, page 660)
    4. steroids: (unproven efficacy) 10 mg dexamethasone IVP
  B. prophylaxis against GI ulcers: H_2 antagonist (e.g. ranitidine 50 mg IVPB q 8 hrs), NG tube to suction
  C. begin phenytoin **(PHT)** loading: effective in controlling acute seizures, incidence of late seizures are not reduced once PHT is stopped
  D. antibiotics: generally used although no controlled study demonstrates efficacy in preventing meningitis or abscess. Most organisms are sensitive to penicillinase resistant agents, e.g. nafcillin, recommended for ≈ 5 days

E.   tetanus toxoid administration

ANGIOGRAPHY IN GSWH

Rarely performed emergently. When done, usually performed on ≈ day 2-3.

Indications[292]:
1.   unexpected delayed hemorrhage
2.   a trajectory that would likely involve named vessels in a salvageable patient
3.   large intraparenchymal hemorrhages in a salvageable patient

SURGICAL TREATMENT

Indications for surgery are controversial. Patients with minimal neurologic function, e.g. fixed pupils, decorticate or decerebrate posturing... (when not in shock and with good oxygenation) should not be operated upon, because the chance of meaningful recovery is close to zero. Patients with less severe injuries should be considered for urgent operation.

Goals of surgery
1.   debridement of devitalized tissue: less tissue is injured in civilian GSWH, but elevated ICP post-op may imply more vigorous debridement was needed, especially of non-eloquent brain (e.g. temporal tips)
2.   evacuation of hematomas: subdural, intraparenchymal...
3.   removal of accessible bone fragments[A]
4.   retrieval of bullet fragment[A] for forensic purposes (note: everyone who handles the fragments may be subpoenaed to testify as to the "chain of evidence"). Large intact fragments should be sought as they tend to migrate
5.   obtaining hemostasis
6.   watertight dural closure (usually requires graft)
7.   separation of intracranial compartment from air sinuses traversed by bullet
8.   identification of entry and exit wounds for forensic purposes (see *Evaluation* above)

Surgical technique

ICP MONITORING

ICP is often elevated after surgical debridement[293] and monitoring may be warranted.

OUTCOME

Prognostic factors
1.   level of consciousness is the most important prognostic factor: ≈ 94% of patients who are comatose with inappropriate or absent response to noxious stimulus on admission die, and half the survivors are severely disabled[294]
2.   path of the bullet. Especially poor prognosis is associated with:
     A.   bullets that cross the midline
     B.   bullets that pass through the geographic center of the brain
     C.   bullets that enter or traverse the ventricles
     D.   the more lobes traversed by the bullet
3.   hematomas seen on CT are poor prognostic findings
4.   suicide attempts are more likely to be fatal

24.11.   Non-missile penetrating trauma

This section deals with penetrating injuries to the brain (and to some extent to the spinal cord) excluding gunshot wounds to the head. Includes trauma from: knives, lawn darts, arrows...

A.   risk of infection and seizures due to retained bullet fragments is not high in civilian GSWH, therefore only accessible fragments should be sought and removed

Cases with foreign body still embedded

In penetrating trauma, it is usually not appropriate to remove any protruding part of the foreign body until the patient is in the operating room, unless it cannot be avoided. If possible, it is helpful to have another identical object for comparison in planning extrication of the embedded object[295]. To minimize extending the trauma to the CNS, the protruding object should be stabilized in some way during transportation and evaluation.

Indications for angiography
1. object passes in region of large named artery
2. object passes near dural sinuses
3. visible evidence of arterial bleeding: angiography is not appropriate if hemorrhage cannot be controlled

Surgical techniques
1. empiric antibiotic coverage is appropriate (see *Meningitis post craniospinal trauma*, page 212). Take cultures from the wound and the foreign body to guide later antibiotic therapy

---

24.12. High altitude cerebral edema

Acute high-altitude sickness (**AHAS**) is a systemic disorder that affects individuals usually within 6-48 hrs after ascent to high altitudes. **Acute mountain sickness** is the most common form of AHAS, with symptoms of nausea, headache, anorexia, dyspnea, insomnia and fatigue[296]. The incidence is ≈ 25% at 7,000 feet, and ≈ 50% at 15,000 feet. Other symptoms of AHAS include edema of feet and hands, and pulmonary edema (HAPE = high altitude pulmonary edema). Ocular findings include retinal hemorrhages[297], nerve fiber layer infarction, papilledema and vitreous hemorrhage[298]. Cerebral edema (**HACE** = high altitude cerebral edema), usually associated with pulmonary edema, may occur in severe cases of AHAS. Symptoms of HACE include: severe headache, mental dysfunction (hallucinations, inappropriate behavior, reduced mental status), and neurologic abnormalities (ataxia, paralysis, cerebellar findings).

Prevention: gradual ascent, 2-4 day acclimatization at intermediate altitudes (especially include sleeping at these levels), avoidance of alcohol or hypnotics.

Treatment of cerebral edema: immediate descent and oxygen (6-12 L/min by NC or FM) are recommended. Dexamethasone 8 mg PO or IV followed by 4 mg q 6 hrs may help temporize.

24.13. Pediatric head injury

75% of children hospitalized for trauma have a head injury. Although most pediatric head injuries are mild and involve only evaluation or brief hospital stays, CNS injuries are the most common cause of pediatric traumatic death[299]. The overall mortality for all pediatric head injuries requiring hospitalization has been reported between 10-13%[300], whereas the mortality associated with severe pediatric head injury presenting with decerebrate posturing has been reported as high as 71%[301].

Differences between adult and pediatric head injury:
1. epidemiology:
   A. children often have milder injuries than adults
   B. lower chance of a surgical lesion in a comatose child[302]
2. types of injury: injuries peculiar to pediatrics
   A. birth injuries: skull fractures, cephalhematoma (*see below*), subdural or epidural hematomas, brachial plexus injuries (*see page 562*)
   B. perambulator/walker injuries
   C. child abuse (*see below*): shaken baby syndrome...
   D. injuries from skateboarding, scooters...
   E. lawn darts
   F. cephalhematoma: *see below*
   G. leptomeningeal cysts, AKA "growing skull fractures": *see page 668*
3. response to injury

A. responses to head injury of older adolescent are very similar to adults
B. "malignant cerebral swelling": acute onset of severe cerebral swelling (probably due to hyperemia[24, 303]) following some head injuries, especially in young children (may not be as common as previously thought[304])
C. posttraumatic seizures: more likely to occur within the 1st 24 hrs in children than in adults[305] (*see page 260*)

Imaging studies

> **PRACTICE PARAMETER 24-14** IMAGING IN MINOR PEDIATRIC HEAD INJURY*
>
> **Recommendations**†[306]: CT scan for children with neurologic or cognitive dysfunction, or suspicion of a depressed or basilar skull fracture
>
> **Recommendations**† [306]: when a CT scan is not done in a child ≤ 1 year age meeting the above criteria (e.g. because of sedation concerns), a skull film may be considered

* Definitions: minor head injury: GCS ≥13; pediatrics = ages 1 month - 17 years of age. Excludes: suspicion or proof of child abuse, patients requiring hospitalization for other reasons
† based mostly prospective trials (not randomized) or large case series

≈ 22% of those with a history of loss of consciousness (**LOC**) > 5 mins have a brain injury, whereas 92% without LOC > 5 mins will have no brain injury [306].

Home observation

> **PRACTICE PARAMETER 24-15**
> HOME OBSERVATION IN MINOR PEDIATRIC HEAD INJURY*
>
> **Recommendations**†[306]: a child with GCS = 14-15 and normal CT scan‡ can be considered for home observation if neurologically stable

* Definitions: same as in *PRACTICE PARAMETER 24-14*
† mostly prospective trials (not randomized) or large case series
‡ these patients are at near zero risk of having an occult brain injury

Outcome

As a group, children fare better than adults with head injury[307]. However, very young children do not do as well as the schoolage child[308].

All aspects of neuropsychological dysfunction following head injury may not always be related to the trauma, as children who get injured may have pre-existing problems that increase their propensity to get hurt[309] (this is controversial[310]).

24.13.1. Cephalhematoma

Accumulation of blood under the scalp. Occur almost exclusively in children.

Two types:
1. **subgaleal hematoma**: may occur without bony trauma, or may be associated with linear nondisplaced skull fracture (especially in age < 1 yr). Bleeding into loose connective tissue separates galea from periosteum. May cross sutures. Usually starts as a small localized hematoma, and may become huge (with significant loss of circulating blood volume in age < 1 year, transfusion may be necessary). Inexperienced clinicians may suspect CSF collection under the scalp which does not occur. Usually presents as a soft, fluctuant mass. These do not calcify
2. **subperiosteal hematoma** (some refer to *this* as cephalhematoma): most commonly seen in the newborn (associated with parturition, may also be associated with neonatal scalp monitor[311, 312]). Bleeding elevates periosteum, extent is limited by sutures. Firmer and less ballotable than subgaleal hematoma[313 (p 312)]; scalp moves freely over the mass. 80% reabsorb, usually within 2-3 weeks. Occasionally may calcify

Infants may develop jaundice (hyperbilirubinemia) as blood is resorbed, occasionally as late as 10 days after onset.

Treatment

Treatment beyond analgesics is almost never required, and most usually resolve within 2-4 weeks. Avoid the temptation of percutaneously aspirating these as the risk of infection exceeds the risk of following them expectantly, and in the newborn removal of the blood may make them anemic. Follow serial hemoglobin and hematocrit in large lesions. If a subperiosteal hematoma persists > 6 weeks, obtain a skull film. If the lesion is calcified, surgical removal may be indicated for cosmetic reasons (although with most of these the skull will return to normal contour in 3-6 months[313 (p 315)].

24.13.2. Child abuse

At least 10% of children < 10 yrs age that are brought to E/R with alleged accidents are victims of child abuse[314]. The incidence of accidental head trauma of significant consequence below age 3 is low, whereas this is the age group in which battering is highest[315].

There are no findings that are pathognomonic for child abuse. Factors which raise the index of suspicion include:
1. retinal hemorrhage (*see below*)
2. bilateral chronic subdural hematomas in a child < 2 yrs age (*see page 678*)
3. skull fractures that are multiple or associated with intracranial injury
4. significant neurological injury with minimal signs of external trauma

SHAKEN BABY SYNDROME
Vigorous shaking of a child produces violent whiplash-like angular acceleration-decelerations of the head (the infant head is relatively large in proportion to the body, and the neck muscles are comparatively weak)[316] which may lead to significant brain injury. Some researchers believe that impact is often also involved[225].

Characteristic findings include retinal hemorrhages (*see below*), subdural hematomas (bilateral in 80%) and/or subarachnoid hemorrhage (SAH). There are usually few or no external signs of trauma (including cases with impact, although findings may be apparent at autopsy). In some cases there may be finger marks on the chest, multiple rib fractures and/or pulmonary compression ± parenchymal lung hemorrhage. Deaths in these cases are almost all due to uncontrollable intracranial hypertension. There may also be injury to the cervicomedullary junction[317].

RETINAL HEMORRHAGE (RH) IN CHILD ABUSE
"In a traumatized child with multiple injuries and an inconsistent history, the presence of RH is pathognomonic of battering"[315]. However, RH may also occur in the absence of any evidence of child abuse. 16/26 battered children < 3 yrs age had RH on funduscopy, whereas 1/32 non-battered traumatized children with head injury had RH (the single false positive: traumatic parturition, where the incidence of RH is 15-30%).

Differential diagnosis of etiologies of retinal hemorrhage:
1. child abuse (including "shaken baby syndrome", *see above*)
2. benign subdural effusion in infants (*see page 678*)
3. acute high altitude sickness (see *High altitude cerebral edema*, page 687)
4. acute increase in ICP: e.g. with a severe seizure (may be similar to Purtschers retinopathy (*see below*)
5. Purtschers retinopathy[318]: loss of vision following major trauma (chest crush injuries, airbag deployment[319]...), pancreatitis, childbirth or renal failure, among others. Posterior pole ischemia with cotton-wool exudates and hemorrhages around the optic disc due to microemboli of possibly fat, air, fibrin clots, complement-mediated aggregates or platelet clumps. No known treatment

24.14. References

1. Gennarelli T A, Thibault L E, Adams J H, *et al*.: Diffuse axonal injury and traumatic coma in the primate. **Ann Neurol** 12: 564-74, 1982.
2. Adams J H, Graham D I, Murray L S, *et al*.: Diffuse axonal injury due to nonmissile head injury in humans: An analysis of 45 cases. **Ann Neurol** 12: 557-63, 1982.
3. Sahuquillo-Barris J, Lamarca-Ciuro J, Vilalta-Castan J, *et al*.: Acute subdural hematoma and diffuse axonal injury after severe head trauma. **J Neu-**

rosurg 68: 894-900, 1988.

4. Sahuquillo-Barris, Lamarca-Ciuro J, Vilalta-Castan J, *et al.*: Epidural hematoma and diffuse axonal injury. **Neurosurgery** 17: 378-9, 1985 (letter).

5. Kelly J P, Rosenberg J H: Diagnosis and management of concussion in sports. **Neurology** 48: 575-80, 1997.

6. Alexander M P: Mild traumatic brain injury: Pathophysiology, natural history, and clinical management. **Neurology** 45: 1253-60, 1995.

7. Levin H S, Williams D H, Eisenberg H M, *et al.*: Serial MRI and neurobehavioral findings after mild to moderate closed head injury. **J Neurol Neurosurg Psychiatry** 55: 255-62, 1992.

8. Gurdjian E S, Voris H C: Report of the *ad hoc* committee to study head injury nomenclature. **Clin Neurosurg** 12: 386-94, 1966.

9. Valadka A B, Narayan R K: *Emergency room management of the head-injured patient.* In **Neurotrauma**, Narayan R K, Wilberger J E, and Povlishock J T, (eds.). McGraw-Hill, New York, 1996: pp 119-35.

10. Quality Standards Subcommittee of the American Academy of Neurology: Practice parameter: The management of concussion in sports (summary statement). **Neurology** 48: 581-5, 1997.

11. Yarnell P R, Lynch S: Retrograde memory immediately after concussion. **Lancet** 1: 863-4, 1970.

12. Flannagan P P, Bailes J E: Neurological injury in athletes. **Contemp Neurosurg** 20 (17): 1-7, 1998.

13. Cantu R C: Guidelines for return to contact sports after a cerebral concussion. **Physician Sports Med** 14: 75-83, 1986.

14. Cantu R C: Head injuries in sports. **Br J Sports Med** 30: 289-96, 1996.

15. Kelly J P, Nichols J S, Filley C M, *et al.*: Concussion in sports: Guidelines for the prevention of catastrophic outcome. **JAMA** 266: 2867-9, 1991.

16. Schneider R C: **Head and neck injuries in football.** Williams & Wilkins, Baltimore, 1973.

17. Saunders R L, Harbaugh R E: Second impact in catastrophic contact-sports head trauma. **JAMA** 252: 538-9, 1984.

18. McCrory P R, Berkovic S F: Second impact syndrome. **Neurology** 50: 677-83, 1998.

19. Cantu R C: Return to play guidelines after a head injury. **Clin Sports Med** 17: 45-60, 1998.

20. Stein S C: *Classification of head injury.* In **Neurotrauma**, Narayan R K, Wilberger J E, and Povlishock J T, (eds.). McGraw-Hill, New York, 1996: pp 31-41.

21. Marshall L F, Marshall S B, Klauber M R, *et al.*: The diagnosis of head injury requires a classification based on computed axial tomography. **J Neurotrauma** 9 Suppl 1: S287-92, 1992.

22. Saul T G, Ducker T B: Effect of intracranial pressure monitoring and and aggressive treatment on mortality in severe head injury. **J Neurosurg** 56: 498-503, 1982.

23. Reilly P L, Adams J H, Graham D I: Patients with head injury who talk and die. **Lancet** 2: 375-7, 1975.

24. Bruce D A, Alavi A, Bilaniuk L, *et al.*: Diffuse cerebral swelling following head injuries in children: The syndrome of "malignant brain edema". **J Neurosurg** 54: 170-8, 1981.

25. Juul N, Morris G F, Marshall S B, *et al.*: Intracranial hypertension and cerebral perfusion pressure: Influence on neurological deterioration and outcome in severe head injury. **J Neurosurg** 92: 1-6, 2000.

26. Kimelberg H: Current concepts of brain edema. **J Neurosurg** 83: 1051-9, 1995.

27. Bullock R, Maxwell W, Graham D: Glial swelling following cerebral contusion: An ultrastructural study. **J Neurol Neurosurg Psychiatry** 54: 427-34, 1991.

28. Kline L B, Morawetz R B, Swaid S N: Indirect injury of the optic nerve. **Neurosurgery** 14: 756-64, 1984.

29. Masters S J, McClean P M, Arcarese J S, *et al.*: Skull x-ray examination after head trauma. **N Engl J Med** 316: 84-91, 1987.

30. Arienta C, Caroli M, Balbi S: Management of head-injured patients in the emergency department: A practical protocol. **Surg Neurol** 48: 213-9, 1997.

31. Stein S C, Ross S E: The value of computed tomographic scans in patients with low-risk head injuries. **Neurosurgery** 26: 638-40, 1990.

32. Ingebrigtsen R, Romner B: Routine early CT-scan is cost saving after minor head injury. **Acta Neurol Scand** 93: 207-10, 1996.

33. Duus B R, Lind B, Christensen H, *et al.*: The role of neuroimaging in the initial management of patients with minor head injury. **Ann Emerg Med** 23: 1279-83, 1994.

34. Feuerman T, Wackym P A, Gade G F, *et al.*: Value of skull radiography, head computed tomographic scanning, and admission for observation in cases of minor head injury. **Neurosurgery** 22: 449-53, 1988.

35. Schacford S R, Wald S R, Ross S E, *et al.*: The clinical utility of computed tomographic scanning and neurologic examination in the management of patients with minor head injuries. **J Trauma** 33: 385-94, 1992.

36. Stein S C, Ross S E: Mild head injury: A plea for routine early CT scanning. **J Trauma** 33: 11-3, 1992.

37. Le Roux P D, Haglund M M, Newell D W, *et al.*: Intraventricular hemorrhage in blunt head trauma: An analysis of 43 cases. **Neurosurgery** 31: 678-85, 1992.

38. Grabb P A: Traumatic intraventricular hemorrhage treated with intraventricular recombinant-tissue plasminogen activator: Technical case report. **Neurosurgery** 43: 966-9, 1998.

39. Stein S C, Ross S E: Moderate head injury: A guide to initial management. **J Neurosurg** 77: 562-4, 1992.

40. Young H A, Gleave J R W, Schmidek H H, *et al.*: Delayed traumatic intracerebral hematoma: Report of 15 cases operatively treated. **Neurosurgery** 14: 22-5, 1984.

41. Jennett B, Teasdale G: **Management of head injuries.** Davis, Philadelphia, 1981.

42. Dacey R G, Alves W M, Rimel R W, *et al.*: Neurosurgical complications after apparently minor head injury: Assessment of risk in a series of 610 patients. **J Neurosurg** 65: 203-10, 1986.

43. Wilberger J E, Deeb Z, Rothfus W: Magnetic resonance imaging after closed head injury. **Neurosurgery** 20: 571-6, 1987.

44. Levin H S, Amparo E G, Eisenberg H M, *et al.*: Magnetic resonance imaging after closed head injury in children. **Neurosurgery** 24: 223-7, 1989.

45. The Brain Trauma Foundation. The American Association of Neurological Surgeons. The Joint Section on Neurotrauma and Critical Care: Resuscitation of blood pressure and oxygenation. **J Neurotrauma** 17 (6-7): 471-8, 2000.

46. The Brain Trauma Foundation. The American Association of Neurological Surgeons. The Joint Section on Neurotrauma and Critical Care: Initial management. **J Neurotrauma** 17 (6-7): 463-9, 2000.

47. Hsiang J K, Chesnut R M, Crisp C D, *et al.*: Early, routine paralysis for intracranial pressure control in severe head injury: Is it necessary? **Crit Care Med** 22: 1471-6, 1994.

48. Marion D W, Carlier P M: Problems with initial Glasgow coma scale assessment caused by prehospital treatment of patients with head injuries: Results of a national survey. **J Trauma** 36: 89-95, 1994.

49. Bullock R, Chesnut R M, Clifton G, *et al.*: **Guidelines for the management of severe head injury,** The Brain Trauma Foundation (New York), The American Association of Neurological Surgeons

(Park Ridge, Illinois), and The Joint Section of Neurotrauma and Critical Care, 1995.

50. Bullock R, Chesnut R M, Clifton G, *et al*.: *The role of anti-seizure prophylaxis following head injury*. In **Guidelines for the management of severe head injury**. The Brain Trauma Foundation (New York), The American Association of Neurological Surgeons (Park Ridge, Illinois), and The Joint Section of Neurotrauma and Critical Care, 1995, Chapter 15.

51. Chang B S, Lowenstein D H: Antiepileptic drug prophylaxis in severe traumatic brain injury. Report of the quality standards subcommittee of the American academy of neurology. **Neurology** 60: 10-6, 2003.

52. The Brain Trauma Foundation. The American Association of Neurological Surgeons. The Joint Section on Neurotrauma and Critical Care: Role of antiseizure prophylaxis following head injury. **J Neurotrauma** 17 (6-7): 549-53, 2000.

53. Findlay J M: Current management of cerebral vasospasm. **Contemp Neurosurg** 19 (24): 1-6, 1997.

54. Chesnut R M, Marshall L F, Klauber M R, *et al*.: The role of secondary brain injury in determining outcome from severe head injury. **J Trauma** 34: 216-22, 1993.

55. Kautman H H, Hut K-S, Mattson J C, *et al*.: Clinicopathological correlations of disseminated intravascular coagulation in patients with head injury. **Neurosurgery** 15: 34-42, 1984.

56. Becker D P, Miller J D, Ward J D, *et al*.: The outcome from severe head injury with early diagnosis and intensive management. **J Neurosurg** 47: 491-502, 1977.

57. Johnson D L, Duma C, Sivit C: The role of immediate operative intervention in severely head-injured children with a Glasgow coma scale score of 3. **Neurosurgery** 30: 320-4, 1992.

58. Niho S, Niho M, Niho K: Decompression of the optic canal by the transethmoidal route and decompression of the superior orbital fissure. **Can J Ophthalmol** 5. 22-40, 1970.

59. Vance M L: Hypopituitarism. **N Engl J Med** 330: 1651-62, 1994.

60. Edwards O M, Clark J D A: Post-traumatic hypopituitarism: Six cases and a review of the literature. **Medicine (Baltimore)** 65: 281-90, 1986.

61. Mahoney B D, Rockswold G L, Ruiz E, *et al*.: Emergency twist drill trephination. **Neurosurgery** 8: 551-4, 1981.

62. McKissock W, Taylor J C, Bloom W H, *et al*.: Extradural hematoma: Observations on 125 cases. **Lancet** 2: 167-72, 1960.

63. Andrews B T, Pitts L H, Lovely M P, *et al*.: Is CT scanning necessary in patients with tentorial herniation? **Neurosurgery** 19: 408-14, 1986.

64. Mayfield F H, McBride B H. *Differential diagnosis and treatment of surgical lesions*. In **Neurological surgery of trauma**, Coates J B and Meirowsky A M, (eds.). Office of the Surgeon General, Washington D.C., 1965: pp 55-64.

65. Sioutos P J, Orozco J A, Carter L P, *et al*.: Continuous regional cerebral cortical blood flow monitoring in head-injured patients. **Neurosurgery** 36: 943-50, 1995.

66. Rosner M J, Coley I B: Cerebral perfusion pressure, intracranial pressure, and head elevation. **J Neurosurg** 65: 636-41, 1986.

67. Unterberg A W, Kiening K L, Hartl R, *et al*.: Multimodal monitoring in patients with head injury: Evaluation of the effects of treatment on cerebral oxygenation. **J Trauma** 42 (Suppl 5): S32-7, 1997.

68. Welch K: The intracranial pressure in infants. **J Neurosurg** 52: 693-9, 1980.

69. Mendelow A D, Teasdale G M, Russell T, *et al*.: Effect of mannitol on cerebral blood flow and cerebral perfusion pressure in human head injury. **J Neurosurg** 63: 43-8, 1985.

70. Unterberg A, Kiening K, Schmiedek P, *et al*.: Long-

term observations of intracranial pressure after severe head injury. The phenomenon of secondary rise of intracranial pressure. **Neurosurgery** 32: 17-24, 1993.

71. Taneda M, Kataoka K, Akai F, *et al*.: Traumatic subarachnoid hemorrhage as a predictable indicator of delayed ischemic symptoms. **J Neurosurg** 84: 762-8, 1996.

72. Miller J D, Butterworth J F, Gudeman S K, *et al*.: Further experience in the management of severe head injury. **J Neurosurg** 54: 289-99, 1981.

73. Narayan R K, Kishore P R S, Becker D P, *et al*.: Intracranial pressure: To monitor or not to monitor? A review of our experience with severe head injury. **J Neurosurg** 56: 650-9, 1982.

74. The Brain Trauma Foundation. The American Association of Neurological Surgeons. The Joint Section on Neurotrauma and Critical Care: Indications for intracranial pressure monitoring. **J Neurotrauma** 17 (6-7): 479-91, 2000.

75. Bullock R, Chesnut R M, Clifton G, *et al*.: *Indications for intracranial pressure monitoring*. In **Guidelines for the management of severe head injury**. The Brain Trauma Foundation (New York), The American Association of Neurological Surgeons (Park Ridge, Illinois), and The Joint Section of Neurotrauma and Critical Care, 1995, Chapter 5.

76. Holloway K L, Barnes T, Choi S, *et al*.: Ventriculostomy infections: The effect of monitoring duration and catheter exchange in 584 patients. **J Neurosurg** 85: 419-24, 1996.

77. Paramore C G, Turner D A: Relative risks of ventriculostomy infection and morbidity. **Acta Neurochir** 127: 79-84, 1994.

78. Prabhu V C, Kaufman H H, Voelker J L, *et al*.: Prophylactic antibiotics with intracranial pressure monitors and external ventricular drains: A review of the evidence. **Surg Neurol** 52: 226-37, 1999.

79. Alleyne C H, Hassan M, Zabramski J M: The efficacy and cost of prophylactic end periprocedural antibiotics in patients with external ventricular drains. **Neurosurgery** 47: 1124-9, 2000.

80. Mayhall C G, Archer N H, Lamb V A, *et al*.: Ventriculostomy-related infections: A prospective epidemiologic study. **N Engl J Med** 310: 553-9, 1984.

81. Sundbarg G, Nordstrom C-H, Messetter K, *et al*.: A comparison of intraparenchymatous and intraventricular pressure recording in clinical practice. **J Neurosurg** 67: 841-5, 1987.

82. Crutchfield J S, Narayan R K, Robertson C S, *et al*.: Evaluation of a fiberoptic intracranial pressure monitor. **J Neurosurg** 72: 482-7, 1990.

83. Ostrup R C, Luersen T G, Marshall L F, *et al*.: Continuous monitoring of intracranial pressure with a miniaturized fiberoptic device. **J Neurosurg** 67: 206-9, 1987.

84. Piek J, Bock W J: Continuous monitoring of cerebral tissue pressure in neurosurgical practice - experience with 100 patients. **Intens Care Med** 16: 184-8, 1990.

85. Gopinath S P, Robertson C S, Contant C F, *et al*.: Clinical evaluation of a miniature strain-gauge transducer for monitoring intracranial pressure. **Neurosurgery** 36: 1137-41, 1995.

86. Salmon J H, Hajjar W, Bada H S: The fontogram: A noninvasive intracranial pressure monitor. **Pediatrics** 60: 721-5, 1977.

87. Hamer J, Alberti E, Hoyer S, *et al*.: Factors influencing CSF pulse waves. **J Neurosurg** 46: 36-45, 1977.

88. Lundberg N: Continuous recording and control of ventricular fluid pressure in neurosurgical practice. **Acta Psych Neurol Scand** 36S: 1-193, 1960.

89. Pickard J D, Czosnyka M: Management of raised intracranial pressure. **J Neurol Neurosurg Psychiatry** 56: 845-58, 1993.

90. Cruz J: On-line monitoring of global cerebral hypoxia in acute brain injury. Relationship to intracra-

nial hypertension. **J Neurosurg** 79: 228-33, 1993.
91. Sheinberg M, Kanter M J, Robertson C S, *et al*.: Continuous monitoring of jugular venous oxygen saturation in head-injured patients. **J Neurosurg** 76: 212-7, 1992.
92. Robertson C S, Narayan R K, Gokaslan Z L, *et al*.: Cerebral arteriovenous oxygen difference as an estimate of cerebral blood flow in comatose patients. **J Neurosurg** 70: 222-30, 1989.
93. Gotoh F, Meyer J S, Takagi Y: Cerebral effects of hyperventilation in man. **Arch Neurol** 12: 410-23, 1965.
94. Obrist W D, Langfitt T W, Jaggi J L, *et al*.: Cerebral blood flow and metabolism in comatose patients with acute head injury. Relationship to intracranial hypertension. **J Neurosurg** 61: 241-53, 1984.
95. Bullock R, Chesnut R M, Clifton G, *et al*.: *Intracranial pressure treatment threshold*. In **Guidelines for the management of severe head injury**. The Brain Trauma Foundation (New York), The American Association of Neurological Surgeons (Park Ridge, Illinois), and The Joint Section of Neurotrauma and Critical Care, 1995, Chapter 6.
96. Bullock R, Chesnut R M, Clifton G, *et al*.: *Guidelines for cerebral perfusion pressure*. In **Guidelines for the management of severe head injury**. The Brain Trauma Foundation (New York), The American Association of Neurological Surgeons (Park Ridge, Illinois), and The Joint Section of Neurotrauma and Critical Care, 1995, Chapter 8.
97. Bullock R, Chesnut R M, Clifton G, *et al*.: Guidelines for the management of severe head injury. **J Neurotrauma** 13: 639-734, 1996.
98. Ropper A H: Raised intracranial pressure in neurologic disease. **Sem Neurology** 4: 397-407, 1984.
99. Bouma G J, Muizelaar J P: Relationship between cardiac output and cerebral blood flow in patients with intact and with impaired autoregulation. **J Neurosurg** 73: 368-74, 1990.
100. The Brain Trauma Foundation. The American Association of Neurological Surgeons. The Joint Section on Neurotrauma and Critical Care: Hypotension. **J Neurotrauma** 17 (6-7): 591-5, 2000.
101. Larson D E, Farnell M B: Upper gastrointestinal hemorrhage. **Mayo Clin Proc** 58: 371-87, 1983.
102. Grosfeld J L, Shipley F, Fitzgerald J F, *et al*.: Acute peptic ulcer in infancy and childhood. **Am Surgeon** 44: 13-9, 1978.
103. Curci M R, Little K, Sieber W K, *et al*.: Peptic ulcer disease in childhood reexamined. **J Ped Surg** 11: 329-35, 1976.
104. Krasna I H, Schneider K M, Becker J M: Surgical management of stress ulcerations in childhood. **J Ped Surg** 6: 301-6, 1971.
105. Chan K-H, Lai E C S, Sun H, *et al*.: Prospective double-blind placebo-controlled randomized trial on the use of ranitidine in preventing postoperative gastroduodenal complications in high-risk neurosurgical patients. **J Neurosurg** 82: 413-7, 1995.
106. Shackford S R, Zhuang J, Schmoker J: Intravenous fluid tonicity: Effect on intracranial pressure, cerebral blood flow, and cerebral oxygen delivery in focal brain injury. **J Neurosurg** 76: 91-8, 1992.
107. Garretson H D, McGraw C P, O'Connor C, *et al*.: *Effectiveness of fluid restriction, mannitol and furosemide in reducing ICP*. In **Intracranial pressure V**, Ishii S, Nagai H, and Brock M, (eds.). Springer-Verlag, Berlin, 1983: pp 742-45.
108. Ward J D, Moulton R J, Muizelaar P J, *et al*.: *Cerebral homeostasis*. In **Neurosurgical critical care**, Wirth F P and Ratcheson R A, (eds.). Concepts in neurosurgery. Williams and Wilkins, Baltimore, 1987, Vol. I: pp 187-213.
109. De Salles A A F, Muizelaar J P, Young H F: Hyperglycemia, cerebrospinal fluid lactic acidosis, and cerebral blood flow in severely head-injured patients. **Neurosurgery** 21: 45-50, 1987.
110. Kaufman H H, Bretaudiere J-P, Rowlands B J, *et al*.: General metabolism in head injury. **Neurosurgery** 20: 254-65, 1987.
111. Cao M, Lisheng H, Shouzheng S: Resolution of brain edema in severe brain injury at controlled high and low ICPs. **J Neurosurg** 61: 707-12, 1984.
112. Metz C, Holzschuh M, Bein T, *et al*.: Moderate hypothermia in patients with severe head injury: Cerebral and extracerebral effects. **J Neurosurg** 85: 533-41, 1996.
113. Mild therapeutic hypothermia to improve the neurologic outcome after cardiac arrest. **N Engl J Med** 346 (8): 549-56, 2002.
114. Polin R S, Shaffrey M E, Bogaev C A, *et al*.: Decompressive bifrontal craniectomy in the treatment of severe refractory posttraumatic cerebral edema. **Neurosurgery** 41: 84-94, 1997.
115. Cooper P R, Hagler H, Clark W: In **Intracranial pressure IV**, Shulman K and Marmarou A, (eds.). Springer Verlag, New York, 1980: pp 277-9.
116. Nussbaum E S, Wolf A L, Sebring L, *et al*.: Complete temporal lobectomy for surgical resuscitation of patients with transtentorial herniation secondary to unilateral hemispheric swelling. **Neurosurgery** 29: 62-6, 1991.
117. Hamill J F, Bedford R F, Weaver D C, *et al*.: Lidocaine before endotracheal intubation: Intravenous or laryngotracheal? **Anesthesiology** 55: 578-81, 1981.
118. Hurst J M, Saul T G, DeHaven C B, *et al*.: Use of high frequency jet ventilation during mechanical hyperventilation to reduce ICP in patients with multiple organ system injury. **Neurosurgery** 15: 530-4, 1984.
119. Cooper K R, Boswell P A, Choi S C: Safe use of PEEP in patients with severe head injury. **J Neurosurg** 63: 552-5, 1985.
120. Feldman Z, Kanter M J, Robertson C S, *et al*.: Effect of head elevation on intracranial pressure, cerebral perfusion pressure, and cerebral blood flow in head-injured patients. **J Neurosurg** 76: 207-11, 1992.
121. Grubb R L, Raichle M E, Eichling J O, *et al*.: The effects of changes in $PaCO_2$ on cerebral blood volume, blood flow, and vascular mean transit time. **Stroke** 5: 630-9, 1974.
122. Darby J M, Yonas H, Marion D W, *et al*.: Local 'inverse steal' induced by hyperventilation in head injury. **Neurosurgery** 23: 84-8, 1988.
123. Fleischer A S, Patton J M, Tindall G T: Monitoring intraventricular pressure using an implanted reservoir in head injured patients. **Surg Neurol** 3: 309-11, 1975.
124. Diringer M N, Yundt K, Videen T O, *et al*.: No reduction in cerebral metabolism as a result of early moderate hyperventilation following severe traumatic brain injury. **J Neurosurg** 92: 7-13, 2000.
125. Bullock R, Chesnut R M, Clifton G, *et al*.: *The use of hyperventilation in the acute management of severe traumatic brain injury*. In **Guidelines for the management of severe head injury**. The Brain Trauma Foundation (New York), The American Association of Neurological Surgeons (Park Ridge, Illinois), and The Joint Section of Neurotrauma and Critical Care, 1995, Chapter 9.
126. Muizelaar J P, Marmarou A, Ward J D, *et al*.: Adverse effects of prolonged hyperventilation in patients with severe head injury: A randomized clinical trial. **J Neurosurg** 75: 731-9, 1991.
127. Bouma G J, Muizelaar J P, Choi S C, *et al*.: Cerebral circulation and metabolism after severe traumatic brain injury: The elusive role of ischemia. **J Neurosurg** 75: 685-93, 1991.
128. Bouma G J, Muizelaar J P, Stringer W A, *et al*.: Ultra early evaluation of regional cerebral blood flow in severely head injured patients using xenon enhanced computed tomography. **J Neurosurg** 77: 360-8, 1992.

129. Fieschi C, Battistini N, Beduschi A, *et al.*: Regional cerebral blood flow and intraventricular pressure in acute head injuries. **J Neurol Neurosurg Psychiatry** 37: 1378-88, 1974.

130. Schroder M L, Muizelaar J P, Kuta A J: Documented reversal of global ischemia immediately after removal of an acute subdural hematoma. **Neurosurgery** 80: 324-7, 1994.

131. James H, Langfitt T, Kumar V, *et al.*: Treatment of intracranial hypertension; analysis of 105 consecutive continuous recordings of ICP. **Acta Neurochir** 36: 189-200, 1977.

132. Lundberg N, Kjallquist A: A reduction of increased ICP by hyperventilation, a therapeutic aid in neurological surgery. **Acta Psych Neurol Scand (Suppl)** 139: 1-64, 1958.

133. Bullock R, Chesnut R M, Clifton G, *et al.*: *The use of mannitol in severe head injury*. In **Guidelines for the management of severe head injury**. The Brain Trauma Foundation (New York), The American Association of Neurological Surgeons (Park Ridge, Illinois), and The Joint Section of Neurotrauma and Critical Care, 1995, Chapter 10.

134. Barry K G, Berman A R: Mannitol infusion. Part III. The acute effect of the intravenous infusion of mannitol on blood and plasma volume. **N Engl J Med** 264: 1085-8, 1961.

135. James H E: Methodology for the control of intracranial pressure with hypertonic mannitol. **Acta Neurochir** 51: 161-72, 1980.

136. McGraw C P, Howard G: The effect of mannitol on increased intracranial pressure. **Neurosurgery** 13: 269-71, 1983.

137. Cruz J, Miner M E, Allen S J, *et al.*: Continuous monitoring of cerebral oxygenation in acute brain injury: Injection of mannitol during hyperventilation. **J Neurosurg** 73: 725-30, 1990.

138. Marshall L F, Smith R W, Rauscher L A, *et al.*: Mannitol dose requirements in brain-injured patients. **J Neurosurg** 48: 169-72, 1978.

139. Takagi H, Saito T, Kitahara T, *et al.*: *The mechanism of the ICP reducing effect of mannitol*. In **ICP V**, Ishii S, Nagai H, and Brock M, (eds.). Springer-Verlag, Berlin, 1993: pp 729-33.

140. Node Y, Yajima K, Nakazawa S: *A study of mannitol and glycerol on the reduction of raised intracranial pressure on their rebound phemonenon*. In **Intracranial pressure V**, Ishii S, Nagai H, and Brock M, (eds.). Springer-Verlag, Berlin, 1983: pp 738-41.

141. Cold G E: Cerebral blood flow in acute head injury: The regulation of cerebral blood flow and metabolism during the acute phase of head injury, and its significance for therapy. **Acta Neurochir Suppl** 49: 1-64, 1990 (review).

142. Kaufmann A M, Cardoso E R: Aggravation of vasogenic cerebral edema by multiple dose mannitol. **J Neurosurg** 77: 584-9, 1992.

143. Ravussin P, Abou-Madi M, Archer D, *et al.*: Changes in CSF pressure after mannitol in patients with and without elevated CSF pressure. **J Neurosurg** 69: 869-76, 1988.

144. Feig P U, McCurdy D K: The hypertonic state. **N Engl J Med** 297: 1444-54, 1977.

145. Muizelaar J P, Lutz H A, Becker D P: Effect of mannitol on ICP and CBF and correlation with pressure autoregulation in severely head-injured patients. **J Neurosurg** 61: 700-6, 1984.

146. Cottrell J E, Robustelli A, Post K, *et al.*: Furosemide- and mannitol-induced changes in intracranial pressure and serum osmolality and electrolytes. **Anesthesiology** 47: 28-30, 1977.

147. Tornheim P A, McLaurin R L, Sawaya R: Effect of furosemide on experimental cerebral edema. **Neurosurgery** 4: 48-52, 1979.

148. Buhrley L E, Reed D J: The effect of furosemide on sodium-22 uptake into cerebrospinal fluid and brain.

Exp Brain Res 14: 503-10, 1972.

149. Marion D W, Letarte P B: Management of intracranial hypertension. **Contemp Neurosurg** 19 (3): 1-6, 1997.

150. Bullock R, Chesnut R M, Clifton G, *et al.*: *The role of glucocorticoids in the treatment of severe head injury*. In **Guidelines for the management of severe head injury**. The Brain Trauma Foundation (New York), The American Association of Neurological Surgeons (Park Ridge, Illinois), and The Joint Section of Neurotrauma and Critical Care, 1995, Chapter 12.

151. The Brain Trauma Foundation. The American Association of Neurological Surgeons. The Joint Section on Neurotrauma and Critical Care: Role of steroids. **J Neurotrauma** 17 (6-7): 531-5, 2000.

152. Braughler J M, Hall E D: Current application of "high-dose" steroid therapy for CNS injury: A pharmacological perspective. **J Neurosurg** 62: 806-10, 1985.

153. Lam A M, Winn H R, Cullen B F, *et al.*: Hyperglycemia and neurologic outcome in patients with head injury. **J Neurosurg** 75: 545-51, 1991.

154. Bullock R, Chesnut R M, Clifton G, *et al.*: *The use of barbiturates in the control of intracranial hypertension*. In **Guidelines for the management of severe head injury**. The Brain Trauma Foundation (New York), The American Association of Neurological Surgeons (Park Ridge, Illinois), and The Joint Section of Neurotrauma and Critical Care, 1995, Chapter 11.

155. Lyons M K, Meyer F B: Cerebrospinal fluid physiology and the management of increased intracranial pressure. **Mayo Clin Proc** 65: 684-707, 1990.

156. Shapiro H M, Wyte S R, Loeser J: Barbiturate augmented hypothermia for reduction of persistent intracranial hypertension. **J Neurosurg** 40: 90-100, 1979.

157. Marshall L F, Smith R W, Shapiro H M: The outcome with aggressive treatment in severe head injuries. Part II: Acute and chronic barbiturate administration in the management of head injury. **J Neurosurg** 50: 26-30, 1979.

158. Rea G L, Rockswold G L: Barbiturate therapy in uncontrolled intracranial hypertension. **Neurosurgery** 12: 401-4, 1983.

159. Ward J D, Becker D P, Miller J D, *et al.*: Failure of prophylactic barbiturate coma in the treatment of severe head injury. **J Neurosurg** 62: 383-8, 1985.

160. Schwartz M, Tator C, Towed D, *et al.*: The university of Toronto head injury treatment study: A prospective randomized comparison of pentobarbital and mannitol. **Can J Neurol Sci** 11: 434-40, 1984.

161. Gilman A G, Goodman L S, Gilman A, (eds.): **Goodman and gilman's the pharmacological basis of therapeutics**. 6th ed., Macmillan Publishing Co., New York, 1980.

162. Eisenberg H M, Frankowski R F, Contant C F, *et al.*: High-dose barbiturate control of elevated intracranial pressure in patients with severe head injury. **J Neurosurg** 69: 15-23, 1988.

163. Boarini D J, Kassell N F, Coester H C: Comparison of sodium thiopental and methohexital for high-dose barbiturate anesthesia. **J Neurosurg** 60: 602-8, 1984.

164. Spetzler R F, Martin N, Hadley M N, *et al.*: Microsurgical endarterectomy under barbiturate protection: A prospective study. **J Neurosurg** 65: 63-73, 1986.

165. Mealey J: *Skull fractures*. In **Pediatric neurosurgery**, Section of Pediatric Neurosurgery of the American Association of Neurological Surgeons, (ed.). Grune and Stratton, New York, 1st ed., 1982: pp 289-99.

166. Jennett B: **Epilepsy after non-missile head injuries**. 2nd ed. William Heinemann, London, 1975: pp 179.

167. Steinbok P, Flodmark O, Martens D, *et al.*: Management of simple depressed skull fractures in children. **J Neurosurg** 66: 506-10, 1987.

168. Loeser J D, Kilburn H L, Jolley T: Management of depressed skull fracture in the newborn. **J Neurosurg** 44: 62-4, 1976.

169. Seebacher J, Nozik D, Mathieu A: Inadvertent intracranial introduction of a nasogastric tube. A complication of severe maxillofacial trauma. **Anesthesia** 42: 100-2, 1975.

170. Wyler A R, Reynolds A F: An intracranial complication of nasogastric intubation: Case report. **J Neurosurg** 47: 297-8, 1977.

171. Baskaya M K: Inadvertent intracranial placement of a nasogastric tube in patients with head injuries. **Surg Neurol** 52: 426-7, 1999.

172. Benoit B G, Wortzman G: Traumatic cerebral aneurysms: Clinical features and natural history. **J Neurol Neurosurg Psychiatry** 36: 127-38, 1973.

173. Esslen E: *Electrodiagnosis of facial palsy.* In **Surgery of the facial nerve,** Miehlke A, (ed.). W. B. Saunders, Philadelphia, 2nd ed., 1973: pp 45-51.

174. Feiz-Erfan I, Ferreira M A T, Rekate H L, *et al.*: Longitudinal clival fracture: A lethal injury survived. **BNI Quarterly** 17: 26, 2001 (case report).

175. Donald P J: The tenacity of the frontal sinus mucosa. **Otolaryngol Head Neck Surg** 87: 557-66, 1979.

176. Robinson J, Donald P J: *Management of associated cranial lesions.* In **Craniospinal trauma,** Pitts L H and Wagner F C, (eds.). Thieme Medical Publishers, Inc., New York, 1990, Chapter 6: pp 59-87.

177. Markham T J: The clinical features of pneumocephalus based on a survey of 284 cases with report of 11 additional cases. **Acta Neurochir** 15: 1-78, 1967.

178. Lunsford L D, Maroon J C, Sheptak P E, *et al.*: Subdural tension pneumocephalus: Report of two cases. **J Neurosurg** 50: 525-7, 1979.

179. Little J R, MacCarty C S: Tension pneumocephalus after insertion of ventriculoperitoneal shunt for aqueductal stenosis: Case report. **J Neurosurg** 44: 383-5, 1976.

180. Pitts L H, Wilson C B, Dedo H H, *et al.*: Pneumocephalus following ventriculoperitoneal shunt: Case report. **J Neurosurg** 43: 631-3, 1975.

181. Caron J-L, Worthington C, Bertrand G: Tension pneumocephalus after evacuation of chronic subdural hematoma and subsequent treatment with continuous lumbar subarachnoid infusion and craniostomy drainage. **Neurosurgery** 16: 107-10, 1985.

182. Ishiwata Y, Fujitsu K, Sekino T, *et al.*: Subdural tension pneumocephalus following surgery for chronic subdural hematoma. **J Neurosurg** 68: 58-61, 1988.

183. Dowd G C, Molony T B, Voorhies R M: Spontaneous otogenic pneumocephalus: Case report and review of the literature. **J Neurosurg** 89: 1036-9, 1998.

184. Mendelson D B, Hertzanu Y, Firedman R: Frontal osteoma with spontaneous subdural and intracerebral pneumatacele. **J Laryngol Otol** 98: 543-5, 1984.

185. Clark J B, Six E G: Epidermoid tumor presenting as tension pneumocephalus. **J Neurosurg** 60: 1312-4, 1984.

186. Roderick L, Moore D C, Artru A A: Pneumocephalus with headache during spinal anesthesia. **Anesthesiology** 62: 690-2, 1985.

187. Goldmann R W: Pneumocephalus as a consequence of barotrauma: Case report. **JAMA** 255: 3154-6, 1986.

188. Black P M, Davis J M, Kjellberg R N, *et al.*: Tension pneumocephalus of the cranial subdural space: A case report. **Neurosurgery** 5: 368-70, 1979.

189. Raggio J F, Fleischer A S, Sung Y F, *et al.*: Expanding pneumocephalus due to nitrous oxide anesthesia: Case report. **Neurosurgery** 4: 261-3, 1979.

190. Raggio J F: Comment on Black P M, et al.: Tension pneumocephalus of the cranial subdural space: A

case report. **Neurosurgery** 5: 369, 1979.

191. Osborn A G, Daines J H, Wing S D, *et al.*: Intracranial air on computerized tomography. **J Neurosurg** 48: 355-9, 1978.

192. Buckingham M J, Crone K R, Ball W S, *et al.*: Traumatic intracranial aneurysms in childhood: Two cases and a review of the literature. **Neurosurgery** 22: 398-408, 1988.

193. Ramamurthi B, Kalyanaraman S: Rationale for surgery in growing fractures of the skull. **J Neurosurg** 32: 427-30, 1970.

194. Arseni C S: Growing skull fractures of children. A particular form of post-traumatic encephalopathy. **Acta Neurochir** 15: 159-72, 1966.

195. Lende R, Erickson T: Growing skull fractures of childhood. **J Neurosurg** 18: 479-89, 1961.

196. Gadoth N, Grunebaum M, Young L W: Leptomeningeal cyst after skull fracture. **Am J Dis Child** 137: 1019-20, 1983.

197. Halliday A L, Chapman P H, Heros R C: Leptomeningeal cyst resulting from adulthood trauma: Case report. **Neurosurgery** 26: 150-3, 1990.

198. Iplikciglu A C, Kokes F, Bayar A, *et al.*: Leptomeningeal cyst. **Neurosurgery** 27: 1027-8, 1990 (letter).

199. Britz G W, Kim K, Mayberg M R: Traumatic leptomeningeal cyst in an adult: A case report and review of the literature. **Surg Neurol** 50: 465-9, 1998.

200. Sekhar L N, Scarff T B: Pseudogrowth in skull fractures of childhood. **Neurosurgery** 6: 285-9, 1980.

201. Lipper M H, Kishore P R S, Girevendulis A K, *et al.*: Delayed intracranial hematoma in patients with severe head injury. **Neuroradiology** 133: 645-9, 1979.

202. Cooper P R, Maravilla K, Moody S, *et al.*: Serial computerized tomographic scanning and the prognosis of severe head injury. **Neurosurgery** 5: 566-9, 1979.

203. Gudeman S K, Kishore P R, Miller J D, *et al.*: The genesis and significance of delayed traumatic intracerebral hematoma. **Neurosurgery** 5: 309-13, 1979.

204. Rockswold G L, Leonard P R, Nagib M: Analysis of management in thirty-three closed head injury patients who "talked and deteriorated". **Neurosurgery** 21: 51-5, 1987.

205. Cohen T I, Gudeman S K: *Delayed traumatic intracranial hematoma.* In **Neurotrauma,** Narayan R K, Wilberger J E, and Povlishock J T, (eds.). McGraw-Hill, New York, 1996: pp 689-701.

206. Kernohan J W, Woltman H W: Incisura of the crus due to contralateral brain tumor. **Arch Neurol Psychiatr** 21: 274, 1929.

207. Tsai F Y, Teal J S, Hieshima G B: **Neuroradiology of head trauma.** University Park Press, Baltimore, 1984.

208. Rivas J J, Lobato R D, Sarabia R, *et al.*: Extradural hematoma: Analysis of factors influencing the courses of 161 patients. **Neurosurgery** 23: 44-51, 1988.

209. Kaye E M, Cass P R, Dooling E, *et al.*: Chronic epidural hematomas in childhood: Increased recognition and nonsurgical management. **Pediat Neurol** 1: 255-9, 1985.

210. Pang D, Horton J A, Herron J M, *et al.*: Nonsurgical management of extradural hematomas in children. **J Neurosurg** 59: 958-71, 1983.

211. Piepmeier J M, Wagner F C: Delayed post-traumatic extracerebral hematoma. **J Trauma** 22: 455-60, 1982.

212. Borovich B, Braun J, Guilburd J N, *et al.*: Delayed onset of traumatic extradural hematoma. **J Neurosurg** 63: 30-4, 1985.

213. Bucci M N, Phillips T W, McGillicuddy J E: Delayed epidural hemorrhage in hypotensive multiple trauma patients. **Neurosurgery** 19: 65-8, 1986.

214. Riesgo P, Piquer J, Botella C, *et al.*: Delayed extradural hematoma after mild head injury: Report of

three cases. **Surg Neurol** 48: 226-31, 1997.

215. Roda J M, Giminez D, Perez-Higueras A, *et al.*: Posterior fossa epidural hematomas: A review and synthesis. **Surg Neurol** 19: 419-24, 1983.

216. Aoki N, Oikawa A, Sakai T: Symptomatic subacute subdural hematoma associated with cerebral hemispheric swelling and ischemia. **Neurol Res** 18: 145-9, 1996.

217. Nishio M, Akagi K, Abekura M, *et al.*: [A case of traumatic subacute subdural hematoma presenting symptoms arising from cerebral hemisphere edema]. **No Shinkei Geka** 26: 425-9, 1998 (Japanese).

218. Wintzen A R, Tijssen J G P: Subdural hematoma and oral anticoagulation therapy. **Ann Neurol** 39: 69-72, 1982.

219. Kawamata T, Takeshita M, Kubo O, *et al.*: Management of intracranial hemorrhage associated with anticoagulant therapy. **Surg Neurol** 44: 438-43, 1995.

220. Munro D, Merritt H H: Surgical pathology of subdural hematoma: Based on a study of one hundred and five cases. **Arch Neurol Psychiatry** 35: 64-78, 1936.

221. Seelig J M, Becker D P, Miller J D, *et al.*: Traumatic acute subdural hematoma: Major mortality reduction in comatose patients treated within four hours. **N Engl J Med** 304: 1511-8, 1981.

222. Wilberger J E, Harris M, Diamond D L: Acute subdural hematoma: Morbidity, mortality, and operative timing. **J Neurosurg** 74: 212-8, 1991.

223. Howard M A, Gross A S, Dacey R G, *et al.*: Acute subdural hematomas: An age-dependent clinical entity. **J Neurosurg** 71: 858-63, 1989.

224. Houtteville J P, Toumi K, Theoron J, *et al.*: Interhemispheric subdural hematoma: Seven cases and review of the literature. **Br J Neurosurg** 2: 357-67, 1900.

225. Duhaime A-C, Gennarelli T A, Thibault L E, *et al.*: The shaken baby syndrome: A clinical, pathological, and biomechanical study. **J Neurosurg** 66: 409-15, 1987.

226. Fein J M, Rovit R L: Interhemispheric subdural hematoma secondary to hemorrhage from a callosomarginal artery aneurysm. **Neuroradiology** 1: 183-6, 1970.

227. Rapana A, Lamaida E, Pizza V, *et al.*: Inter-hemispheric scissure, a rare location for a traumatic subdural hematoma, case report and review of the literature. **Clin Neurol Neurosurg** 99: 124-9, 1997.

228. Aoki N, Masuzawa II: Infantile acute subdural hematoma. **J Neurosurg** 61: 273-80, 1984.

229. Ikeda A, Sato O, Tsugane R, *et al.*: Infantile acute subdural hematoma. **Childs Nerv Syst** 3: 19-22, 1987.

230. Robinson R G: Chronic subdural hematoma: Surgical management in 133 patients. **J Neurosurg** 61: 263-8, 1984.

231. Wakai S, Hashimoto K, Watanabe N, *et al.*: Efficacy of closed-system drainage in treating chronic subdural hematoma: A prospective comparative study. **Neurosurgery** 26: 771-3, 1990.

232. Fogelholm R, Heiskanen O, Waltimo O: Influence of patient's age on symptoms, signs, and thickness of hematoma. **J Neurosurg** 42: 43-6, 1975.

233. Weir B K, Gordon P: Factors affecting coagulation, fibrinolysis in chronic subdural fluid collection. **J Neurosurg** 58: 242-5, 1983.

234. Labadie E L: *Fibrinolysis in the formation and growth of chronic subdural hematomas.* In **Fibrinolysis and the central nervous system**, Sawaya R, (ed.). Hanley and Belfus, Philadelphia, 1990: pp 141-8.

235. Drapkin A J: Chronic subdural hematoma: Pathophysiological basis of treatment. **Br J Neurosurg** 5: 467-73, 1991.

236. Hamilton M G, Frizzell J B, Tranmer B I: Chronic subdural hematoma: The role for craniotomy reevaluated. **Neurosurgery** 33: 67-72, 1993.

237. Camel M, Grubb R L: Treatment of chronic subdural hematoma by twist-drill craniostomy with continuous catheter drainage. **J Neurosurg** 65: 183-7, 1986.

238. Hubschmann O R: Twist drill craniostomy in the treatment of chronic and subacute hematomas in severely ill and elderly patients. **Neurosurgery** 6: 233-6, 1980.

239. Tabaddor K, Shulman K: Definitive treatment of chronic subdural hematoma by twist-drill craniostomy and closed-system drainage. **J Neurosurg** 46: 220-6, 1977.

240. Lind C R, Lind C J, Mee E W: Reduction in the number of repeated operations for the treatment of subacute and chronic subdural hematomas by placement of subdural drains. **J Neurosurg** 99: 44-6, 2003.

241. Markwalder T-M, Steinsiepe K F, Rohner M, *et al.*: The course of chronic subdural hematoma after burr-hole craniostomy and closed-system drainage. **J Neurosurg** 55: 390-3, 1981.

242. Arginteanu M S, Byun H, King W: Treatment of a recurrent subdural hematoma using urokinase. **J Neurotrauma** 16: 1235-9, 1999.

243. Ogasawara K, Koshu K, Yoshimoto T, *et al.*: Transient hyperemia immediately after rapid decompression of chronic subdural hematoma. **Neurosurgery** 45: 484-9, 1999.

244. Dill S R, Cobbs C G, McDonald C K: Subdural empyema: Analysis of 32 cases and review. **Clin Inf Dis** 20: 372-86, 1995.

245. Ernestus R-I, Beldzinski P, Lanfermann H, *et al.*: Chronic subdural hematoma: Surgical treatment and outcome in 104 patients. **Surg Neurol** 48: 220-5, 1997.

246. Sambasivan M: An overview of chronic subdural hematoma: Experience with 2300 cases. **Surg Neurol** 47: 418-22, 1997.

247. Talalla A, McKissock W: Acute 'spontaneous' subdural hemorrhage: An unusual form of cerebrovascular accident. **Neurology** 21: 19-25, 1971.

248. Hesselbrock R, Sawaya R, Means E D: Acute spontaneous subdural hematoma. **Surg Neurol** 21: 363-6, 1984.

249. Korosue K, Kondoh T, Ishikawa Y, *et al.*: Acute subdural hematoma associated with nontraumatic middle meningeal artery aneurysm: Case report. **Neurosurgery** 22: 411-3, 1988.

250. Scott M: Spontaneous nontraumatic subdural hematomas. **JAMA** 141: 596-602, 1949.

251. Stone J L, Lang R G R, Sugar O, *et al.*: Traumatic subdural hygroma. **Neurosurgery** 8: 542-50, 1981.

252. Strassburg H M: Macrocephaly is not always due to hydrocephalus. **J Child Neurol** 4 (Suppl): S32-40, 1989.

253. Briner S, Bodensteiner J: Benign subdural collections of infancy. **Pediatrics** 67: 802-4, 1980.

254. Robertson W C, Chun R W M, Orrison W W, *et al.*: Benign subdural collections of infancy. **J Pediatr** 94: 382, 1979.

255. Carolan P L, McLaurin R L, Towbin R B, *et al.*: Benign extraaxial collections of infancy. **Pediatr Neurosci** 12: 140-4, 1986.

256. Mori K, Handa H, Itoh M, *et al.*: Benign subdural effusion in infants. **J Comput Assist Tomogr** 4: 466-71, 1980.

257. Litofsky N S, Raffel C, McComb J G: Management of symptomatic chronic extra-axial fluid collections in pediatric patients. **Neurosurgery** 31: 445-50, 1992.

258. McLaurin R L, Isaacs E, Lewis H P: Results of nonoperative treatment in 15 cases of infantile subdural hematoma. **J Neurosurg** 34: 753-9, 1971.

259. Herzberger E, Rotem Y, Braham J: Remarks on thirty-three cases of subdural effusions in infancy. **Arch Dis Childhood** 31: 44-50, 1956.

260. Moyes P D: Subdural effusions in infants. **Can Med**

Assoc J 100: 231-4, 1969.

261. Aoki N, Miztani H, Masuzawa H: Unilateral subdu-ral-peritoneal shunting for bilateral chronic subdural hematomas in infancy. **J Neurosurg** 63: 134-7, 1985.

262. Aoki N: Chronic subdural hematoma in infancy. Clinical analysis of 30 cases in the CT era. **J Neuro-surg** 73: 201-5, 1990.

263. Johnson D L: Comment on Litofsky N S, et al.: Management of symptomatic chronic extra-axial fluid collections in pediatric patients. **Neuro-surgery** 31: 450, 1992.

264. Clifton G L, Robertson C S, Grossman R G, *et al.*: The metabolic response to severe head injury. **J Neurosurg** 60: 687-96, 1984.

265. Young B, Ott L, Norton J, *et al.*: Metabolic and nu-tritional sequelae in the non-steroid treated head in-jury patient. **Neurosurgery** 17: 784-91, 1985.

266. Deutschman C S, Konstantinides F N, Raup S, *et al.*: Physiological and metabolic response to isolated closed head injury. **J Neurosurg** 64: 89-98, 1986.

267. Clifton G L, Robertson C S, Choi S C: Assessment of nutritional requirements of head injured patients. **J Neurosurg** 64: 895-901, 1986.

268. Rapp R P, Young B, Twyman D, *et al.*: The favor-able effect of early parenteral feeding on survival in head injured patients. **J Neurosurg** 58: 906-12, 1983.

269. Hadley M N, Grahm T W, Harrington T, *et al.*: Nu-tritional support and neurotrauma: A critical review of early nutrition in forty-five acute head injury pa-tients. **Neurosurgery** 19: 367-73, 1986.

270. The Brain Trauma Foundation. The American Asso-ciation of Neurological Surgeons. The Joint Section on Neurotrauma and Critical Care: Nutrition. **J Neu-rotrauma** 17 (6-7): 539-47, 2000.

271. Harris J A, Benedict F G: **Biometric studies of bas-al metabolism in man**, Carnegie Institution. Publi-cation No. 279. Washington, D.C., 1919.

272. Clifton G L, Robertson C S, Contant C F, *et al.*: En-teral hyperalimantation in head injury. **J Neurosurg** 62: 186-93, 1985.

273. Ott L, Young B, Phillips R, *et al.*: Altered gastric emptying in the head-injured patient: Relationship to feeding intolerance. **J Neurosurg** 74: 738-42, 1991.

274. Grahm T W, Zadrozny D B, Harrington T: Benefits of early jejunal hyperalimantation in the head-in-jured patient. **Neurosurgery** 25: 729-35, 1989.

275. Stablein D M, Miller J D, Choi S C, *et al.*: Statistical methods for determining prognosis in severe head injury. **Neurosurgery** 6: 243-8, 1980.

276. Toutant S M, Klauber M R, Marshall L F, *et al.*: Ab-sent or compressed basal cisterns on first CT scan: Ominous predictor of outcome in severe head inju-ry. **J Neurosurg** 61: 691-4, 1984.

277. Friedman G, Froom P, Sazbon L, *et al.*: Apolipopro-tein E-ε4 genotype predicts a poor outcome in survi-vors of traumatic injury. **Neurology** 52: 244-8, 1999.

278. Nicoll J A R, Roberts G W, Graham D I: Apolipo-protein E ε4 allele is associated with deposition of amyloid ß-protein following head injury. **Nature Med** 1: 135-7, 1995.

279. Clark J D A, Raggatt P R, Edward O M: Hypotha-lamic hypogonadism following major head injury. **Clin Endocrin** 29: 153-65, 1988.

280. Mayeux R, Ottman R, Tang M X, *et al.*: Genetic sus-ceptibility and head injury as risk factors for Alzhe-imer's disease among community-dwelling elderly persons and their first degree relatives. **Ann Neurol** 33: 494-501, 1993.

281. Roberts G W, Gentleman S M, Lynch A, *et al.*: ß amyloid protein deposition in the brain after severe head injury: Implications for the pathogenesis of Alzheimer's disease. **J Neurol Neurosurg Psychia-try** 57: 419-25, 1994.

282. Mayeux R, Ottman R, Maestre G, *et al.*: Synergistic effects of traumatic head injury and apolipoprotein-ε4 in patients with Alzheimer's disease. **Neurology** 45: 555-7, 1995.

283. Lee M S, Rinne J O, Ceballos-Bauman A, *et al.*: Dystonia after head trauma. **Neurology** 44: 1374-8, 1994.

284. Alves W M, Jane J A: *Post-traumatic syndrome*. In **Neurological surgery**, Youmans J R, (ed.). W. B. Saunders, Philadelphia, 3rd ed., 1990, Vol. 3: pp 2230-42.

285. Mendez M F: The neuropsychiatric aspects of box-ing. **Int'l J Psychiatry in Medicine** 25: 249-62, 1995.

286. Parkinson D: Evaluating cerebral concussion. **Surg Neurol** 45: 459-62, 1996.

287. Jordan B D, Kanik A B, Horwich M S, *et al.*: Apoli-poprotein E ε4 and fatal cerebral amyloid angiopa-thy associated with dementia pugilistica. **Ann Neurol** 38: 698-9, 1995.

288. Jordan B D, Jahre C, Hauser W A, *et al.*: CT of 338 active professional boxers. **Radiology** 185: 509-12, 1992.

289. Jordan B D, Jahre C, Hauser W A: Serial computed tomography in professional boxers. **J Neuroimag-ing** 25: 249-62, 1992.

290. Kaufman H H: Civilian gunshot wounds to the head. **Neurosurgery** 32: 962-4, 1993.

291. Kaufman H H, Moake J L, Olson J D, *et al.*: Delayed intracerebral hematoma due to traumatic aneurysm caused by a shotgun wound: A problem in prophy-laxis. **Neurosurgery** 6: 181-4, 1980.

292. Miner M E: Comment on Benzel E C, et al.: Civilian craniocerebral gunshot wounds. **Neurosurgery** 29: 71, 1991.

293. Kaufman H H, Makela M E, Lee K F, *et al.*: Gunshot wounds to the head: A perspective. **Neurosurgery** 18: 689-95, 1986.

294. Benzel E C, Day W T, Kesterson L, *et al.*: Civilian craniocerebral gunshot wounds. **Neurosurgery** 29: 67-72, 1991.

295. Salvino C K, Origitano T C, Dries D J, *et al.*: Tran-soral crossbow injury to the cervical spine: An un-usual case of penetrating cervical spinal injury. **Neurosurgery** 28: 904-7, 1991.

296. Montgomery A B, Mills J, Luce J M: Incidence of acute mountain sickness at intermediate altitude. **JAMA** 261: 732-4, 1989.

297. Butler F K, Harris D J, Reynolds R D: Altitude ret-inopathy on mount Everest, 1989. **Ophthalmology** 99: 739-46, 1992.

298. Frayser R, Houston C S, Bryan A C, *et al.*: Retinal hemorrhage at high altitude. **N Engl J Med** 282: 1183-4, 1970.

299. Ward J D: *Pediatric head injury*. In **Neurotrauma**, Narayan R K, Wilberger J E, and Povlishock J T, (eds.). McGraw-Hill, New York, 1996: pp 859-67.

300. Zuccarello M, Facco E, Zampieri P, *et al.*: Severe head injury in children: Early prognosis and out-come. **Childs Nerv Syst** 1: 158-62, 1985.

301. Bruce D A, Raphaely R C, Goldberg A I, *et al.*: Pathophysiology, treatment and outcome following severe head injury in children. **Childs Brain** 5: 174-91, 1979.

302. Alberico A M, Ward J D, Choi S C, *et al.*: Outcome after severe head injury: Relationahip to mass le-sions, diffuse injury, and ICP course in pediatric and adult patients. **J Neurosurg** 67: 648-56, 1987.

303. Humphreys R P, Hendrick E B, Hoffman H J: The head injured child who "talks and dies". **Childs Nerv Syst** 6: 139-42, 1990.

304. Muizelaar J P, Marmarou A M, DeSalles A A, *et al.*: Cerebral blood flow in severely head-injured chil-dren: Part I. Relationship with GCS score, outcome, ICP, and PVI. **J Neurosurg** 71: 63-71, 1989.

305. Hahn Y S, Fuchs S, Flannery A M, *et al.*: Factors in-fluencing posttraumatic seizures in children. **Neuro-**

surgery 22: 864-7, 1988.
306. Health Policy & Clinical Effectiveness Program, *Evidence based clinical practice guideline for management of children with mild traumatic head injury.* 2000, Cincinnati, Ohio.
307. Luerson T G, Klauber M R, Marshall L F: Outcome from head injury related to patient's age: A longitudinal prospective study of adult and pediatric head injury. **J Neurosurg** 68: 409-16, 1988.
308. Kriel R L, Krach L E, Panser L A: Closed head injury: Comparison of children younger and older than 6 years of age. **Pediatr Neurol** 5: 296-300, 1989.
309. Bijur P E, Haslum M, Golding J: Cognitive and behavioral sequelae of mild head injury in children. **Pediatrics** 86: 337-40, 1990.
310. Pelco L, Sawyer M, Duffielf G, *et al.*: Premorbid emotional and behavioral adjustment in children with mild head injury. **Brain Inj** 6: 29-37, 1992.
311. Listinsky J L, Wood B P, Ekholm S E: Parietal osteomyelitis and epidural abscess: A delayed complication of fetal monitoring. **Pediatr Radiol** 16: 150-1, 1986.
312. Kaufman H H, Hochberg J, Anderson R P, *et al.*: Treatment of calcified cephalhematoma. **Neurosurgery** 32: 1037-40, 1993.
313. Matson D D: **Neurosurgery of infancy and childhood.** 2nd ed. Charles C Thomas, Springfield, 1969.
314. Meservy C J, Towbin R, McLaurin R L, *et al.*: Radiographic characteristics of skull fractures resulting from child abuse. **AJR** 149: 173-5, 1987.
315. Eisenbrey A B: Retinal hemorrhage in the battered child. **Childs Brain** 5: 40-4, 1979.
316. Caffey J: On the theory and practice of shaking infants. Its potential residual effects of permanent brain damage and mental retardation. **Am J Dis Child** 124: 161-9, 1972.
317. Hadley M N, Sonntag V K H, Rekate H L, *et al.*: The infant whiplash-shake injury syndrome: A clinical and pathological study. **Neurosurgery** 24: 536-40, 1989.
318. Buckley S A, James B: Purtscher's retinopathy. **Postgrad Med J** 72 (849): 409-12, 1996.
319. Shah G K, Penne R, Grand M G: Purtscher's retinopathy secondary to airbag injury. **Retina** 21 (1): 68-9, 2001.
320. Doyle J A, Davis D P, Hoyt D B: The use of hypertonic saline in the treatment of traumatic brain injury. **J Trauma** 50 (2): 367-83, 2001.
321. Ogden A T, Mayer S A, Connolly E S: Hyperosmolar agents in neurosurgical practice: The evolving role of hypertonic saline. **Neurosurgery** 57: 207-15, 2005.
322. Vialet R, Albanese J, Thomachot L, et al.: Isovolume hypertonic solutes (sodium chloride or mannitol) in the treatment of refractory posttraumatic intracranial hypertension: 2 ml/kg 7.5% saline is more effective than 2 ml/kg 20% mannitol. **Crit Care Med** 31 (6): 1683-7, 2003.

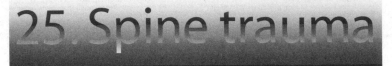
25. Spine trauma

20% of patients with a major spine injury will have a second spinal injury at another level, which may be noncontiguous. These patients often have simultaneous but unrelated injuries (e.g. chest trauma). Injuries directly associated with spinal cord injuries include arterial dissections (carotid and/or vertebral arteries).

TERMINOLOGY

SPINAL STABILITY

An adaptation of the definition of White and Panjabi of **clinical stability**: the ability of the spine under physiologic loads to limit displacement so as to prevent injury or irritation of the spinal cord and nerve roots (including cauda equina) and, to prevent incapacitating deformity or pain due to structural changes[1].

Biomechanical instability refers to the ability of the spine *ex vivo* to resist forces. For models of stability for cervical spine fractures *see page 733*, for thoracolumbar fractures *see page 744*.

LEVEL OF INJURY

There is disagreement over what should be defined as "the level" of a spinal cord injury. Some use the lowest level of completely <u>normal</u> function. However, most sources define the "level" as the most caudal segment with motor function that is at least 3 out of 5 and if pain and temperature sensation is present.

COMPLETENESS OF LESION

Incomplete lesion

Definition: any residual motor or sensory function more than 3 segments below the level of the injury[2]. Look for signs of preserved long-tract function.
Signs of incomplete lesion:
- sensation (including position sense) or voluntary movement in the LEs
- **"sacral sparing"**: sensation around the anus, voluntary rectal sphincter contraction, or voluntary toe flexion
- an injury does <u>not</u> qualify as incomplete with preserved sacral reflexes alone

Types of incomplete lesion:
- central cord syndrome: *see page 714*
- Brown-Séquard syndrome (cord hemisection): *see page 716*
- anterior cord syndrome: *see page 716*
- posterior cord syndrome: rare, *see page 716*

Complete lesion

No preservation of any motor and/or sensory function more than 3 segments below the level of the injury. About 3% of patients with complete injuries on initial exam will develop some recovery within 24 hours. The persistence of a complete spinal cord injury beyond 24 hours indicates that no distal function will recover.

SPINAL SHOCK

This term is often used in two completely different senses:
1. hypotension (shock) that follows spinal cord injury (SBP usually ≈ 80 mm Hg). See *Hypotension* page 703 for treatment. Caused by multiple factors:
    A. interruption of sympathetics
        1. loss of vascular tone (vasoconstrictors) below level of injury
        2. leaves parasympathetics relatively unopposed causing <u>bradycardia</u>
    B. loss of muscle tone due to skeletal muscle paralysis below level of injury results in venous pooling and thus a *relative* hypovolemia
    C. blood loss from associated wounds → true hypovolemia
2. transient loss of all neurologic function (including segmental and polysynaptic re-

flex activity and autonomic function) below the level of the SCI[3,4] → flaccid paralysis and areflexia lasting varying periods (usually 1-2 weeks, occasionally several months and sometimes permanently), the resolution of which yields the anticipated spasticity below the level of the lesion. A poor prognostic sign. Spinal cord reflexes immediately above the injury may also be depressed on the basis of the Schiff-Sherrington phenomenon

25.1.   Whiplash-associated disorders

"Whiplash" was initially a lay term, which is currently defined as a traumatic injury to the soft tissue structures in the region of the cervical spine (including: cervical muscles, ligaments, intervertebral discs, facet joints...) due to hyperflexion, hyperextension, or rotational injury to the neck in the absence of fractures, dislocations, or intervertebral disc herniation[5]. It is the most common non-fatal automobile injury[6]. Symptoms may start immediately, but more commonly are delayed several hours or days. In addition to symptoms related to the cervical spine, common associated complaints include headaches, cognitive impairment, and low back pain.

A proposed clinical classification system of WAD is shown in *Table 25-1*. A consensus regarding diagnosis and management of these injuries is shown in *Table 25-2* and *Table 25-3*. Keep in mind that conditions such as occipital neuralgia may occasionally follow whiplash type injuries and should be treated appropriately (*see page 563*).

Table 25-1 Clinical grading of WAD severity

Grade	Description
0	no complaints, no signs*
1	neck pain or stiffness or tenderness, no signs
2	above symptoms with reduced range of motion or point tenderness
3	above symptoms with weakness, sensory deficit, or absent deep tendon reflexes
4	above symptoms with fracture or dislocation*

*   the definition of whiplash excludes these patients[5]

Table 25-2 Evaluation of WAD

Grade 1 patients with normal mental status and physical exam do not require plain radiographs on presentation

Grade 2 & 3 patients: C spine x rays, possibly with flexion-extension views. Special imaging studies (MRI, CT, myelography...) are not indicated

Grade 3 & 4: these patients should be managed as suspected spinal cord injury (*see Initial management of spinal cord injury* below, and sections that follow)

Table 25-3   Treatment of WAD[7]*

Whiplash is usually a benign condition requiring little treatment & resolves in days to a few weeks in most cases.

Recommendation	Grade		
	1	2	3
Range of motion exercises	should be started immediately for all		
Encourage early return to regular activities	immediately	ASAP	
Cervical collars and rest†	no	not for > 72 hrs	not for > 96 hrs
Passive modality therapies: heat, ice, massage, TENS, ultrasound, relaxation techniques, acupuncture, and work alteration	no	optional if symptoms last > 3 wks	
Medications: optional use of NSAIDs and non-narcotic analgesics? (recommended for ≤ 3 wks)	no	yes	yes. Limited narcotics may also occasionally be needed
Surgery	no	no	only for progressive neurologic deficit or persisting arm pain

✖ **Not recommended:** cervical pillows and soft collars, bed rest, spray and stretch exercises, muscle relaxant medication, TENS, reflexology, magnetic necklaces, herbal remedies, homeopathy, OTC medications (except NSAIDs, *see above*), and intra-articular, intrathecal, or trigger point steroid injections

*   excluding patients with fractures, dislocations, or spinal cord injuries

†   soft foam collars are generally discouraged; if they are to be used, the narrow part should be placed in front to avoid neck extension[5]

Outcome

In a study of 117 patients < 56 years of age having WAD due to automobile accidents (excluding those with cervical fractures, dislocations, or injuries elsewhere in the body) conducted in Switzerland[8] (where all medical costs were paid by the state and there was no opportunity for litigation and no compensation for pain and suffering, although there was the possibility of permanent disability), the recovery rate was as shown in *Table 25-4*. Of the 21 patients with continued symptoms at 2 yrs, only 5 were restricted with respect to work (3 reduced to part-time work, 2 on disability). Patients with persistent symptoms were older, had more varied complaints on initial exam,

Table 25-4 Recovery of patients with WAD

Time (mos)	Percent recovered
3	56%
6	70%
12	76%
24	82%

had a more rotated or inclined head position at the time of impact, had a higher incidence of pretraumatic headaches, and had a higher incidence of certain pre-existing findings (such as radiologic evidence of cervical osteoarthritis). The amount of damage to the automobile and the speed of the cars has little relationship to the degree of injury, and outcome was not influenced by gender, vocation, or psychological factors.

25.2. Pediatric spine injuries

Spinal cord injury is fairly uncommon in children, with the ratio of head injuries to spinal cord injuries being ≈ 30:1 in pediatrics. Only ≈ 5% of spinal cord injuries occur in children. Due to ligamentous laxity together with a high head to body weight ratio, immaturity of paraspinal muscles and the underdeveloped uncinate processes, these tend to involve ligamentous rather than bony injuries (*see* SCIWORA, *page 732*). The cervical spine is the most vulnerable segment (with subaxial injuries being fairly uncommon), with 42% of injuries occurring here, 31% thoracic, and 27% lumbar. The fatality rate is higher with pediatric spine injuries than with adults (opposite to the situation with head injury), with the cause of death more often related to other severe injuries than to the spinal injury[9].

PRACTICE PARAMETER 25-1 PEDIATRIC C-SPINE INJURIES

Diagnosis

Guidelines[10]: C-spine x-rays are <u>not</u> indicated in pediatric trauma patients who are:
- alert & conversant
- neurologically intact
- without posterior midline cervical tenderness (with no distracting pain)
- and who are not intoxicated

Options[10]: for pediatric trauma patients who are: nonconversant or have altered mental status, neurologic deficit, neck pain or a painful distracting injury, are intoxicated, or have unexplained hypotension:
- patients < 9 yrs: AP & lateral C-spine x-rays
- patients ≥ 9 yrs: open-mouth odontoid view in addition to the above
- supplement these x-rays with additional thin cut CT through areas of suspicion or areas not visualized on plain x-ray
- flexion-extension C-spine x-rays or fluoroscopy may be considered to R/O ligamentous instability if there is still a suspicion of instability after the above x-rays are obtained
- consider: C-spine MRI to R/O cord or nerve root compression, evaluate ligamentous integrity, or provide information for neurologic prognosis

Treatment

Options[10]:
- children < 8 yrs age: immobilize with thoracic elevation or an occipital recess (allows more neutral alignment due to the relatively large head)
- children < 7 yrs age with injuries of the C2 dentocentral synchondrosis (*see page 142*): closed reduction and halo immobilization
- consider: primary operative treatment for isolated C-spine ligamentous injuries with associated deformity

PEDIATRIC CERVICAL SPINE INJURIES

For pediatric C-spine anatomy *see page 142*. In the age group ≤ 9 yrs, 67% of cervical spine injuries occur in the upper 3 segments of the cervical spine (occiput-C2)[11].

SYNCHONDROSES (*see page 142*)

Normal synchondroses may be mistaken for fractures (especially the dentocentral synchondrosis of the atlas (*see page 142*) which may be mistaken for an odontoid fracture). Conversely, actual fractures may occur through synchondroses[12, 13]. Recommended treatment for fractures through synchondroses: the tendency for synchondroses to fuse suggests that emergency reduction followed by external immobilization be attempted. Internal immobilization/fusion should be reserved for persistent instability[13].

PSEUDOSPREAD OF THE ATLAS[14]

Pseudospread of the atlas (defined as > 2 mm total overlap of the two C1 lateral masses on C2 on AP open-mouth view) is present in most children 3 mos to 4 yrs age. Prevalence is 91-100% during the second year of life. Youngest example at 3 mos, oldest at 5.75 yrs. The total offset is typically 2 mm during the first yr, 4 mm during the second, 6 mm during the third, and decreasing thereafter. The maximum is 8 mm. Trauma is not a contributing factor.

Neck rotation can also sometimes simulate the appearance of a Jefferson fracture.

Pseudospread is probably a result of disproportionate growth of the atlas on the axis. This could be misdiagnosed as a Jefferson fracture (*see page 723*), which rarely occurs prior to the teen-ages (owing to lower weight of children, more flexible necks, increased plasticity of skull, and shock absorbing synchondroses of C1).

When suspicion of fracture is high: CT scan through C1 can resolve the issue of whether or not there is a fracture.

PSEUDOSUBLUXATION

Either anterior displacement of C2 (axis) on C3 and/or significant angulation at this level. Seen in children (up to age 10 yrs) on lateral C-spine x-ray after trauma. Up to age 10 yrs, flexion and extension are centered at C2-3; this moves down to C4-5 or C5-6 after age 10. C2 normally moves forward on C3 up to 2-3 mm in peds[15]. When the head is flexed, displacement is expected; may be exacerbated by spasm[16]. Does not represent pathological instability. Fractures and dislocations are unusual in children, and when they do occur, they resemble those in adults.

10 cases reported between ages 4-6 yrs[17]: pain was not uncommon. In each case, either the head or neck was flexed (sometimes minimally); the pseudosubluxation corrected when x-ray was repeated with head in true neutral position.

Recommendation: treat patient for soft-tissue injury and not for subluxation.

25.3.   Initial management of spinal cord injury

The major causes of death in spinal cord injury (**SCI**) are aspiration and shock[4]. Initial survey under ATLS protocol: assessment of airway takes precedence, then breathing, then circulation & control of hemorrhage ("ABC's"). This is followed by a brief neurologic exam.

NB: other injuries (e.g. abdominal injuries) may be masked below the level of SCI.

Any of the following patients should be treated as having a SCI until proven otherwise:
1. all victims of significant trauma
2. trauma patients with loss of consciousness
3. minor trauma victims with complaints referable to the spine (neck or back pain or tenderness) or spinal cord (numbness or tingling in an extremity, weakness)
4. associated findings suggestive of SCI include
   A. abdominal breathing
   B. priapism (autonomic dysfunction)

The orientation of the management differs based on the patient's situation as follows:
1. no history of significant trauma, completely alert, oriented and free of drug or alcohol intoxication with no complaints referable to the spine: most may be cleared clinically without the need for C-spine x-rays
2. significant trauma, but no strong evidence of spine or spinal cord injury: the em-

phasis here is in ruling-out a bony lesion and preventing injury
3. patients with neurologic deficit: the emphasis here is to define the skeletal injury and to take steps to prevent further cord injury and loss of function and minimize or reverse the present deficit. The pros and cons of the high-dose methylprednisolone protocol (*see page 704*) should be weighed if a neurologic deficit is identified

CLINICAL CRITERIA TO RULE-OUT CERVICAL SPINE INSTABILITY

To date, there has not been a case of a significant occult cervical spine injury[18, 19] in a trauma patient who met all of the criteria in *Table 25-5*[A]:

MANAGEMENT IN THE FIELD

1. immobilization prior to and during extrication from vehicle and transport to prevent active or passive movements of the spine. For possible C-spine injuries in football players, *see Table 25-6* for the National Athletic Trainers' Association (NATA) guidelines for helmet removal. When CPR is necessary it takes precedence. Caution with intubation (*see below*)
   A. log-roll patient to turn
   B. place patient on back-board
   C. sandbags on both sides of the head with a 3 inch strip of adhesive tape from one side of the back-board to the other across the forehead immobilizes the spine as well as a rigid orthosis[20] but allows movement of the jaw and access to the airway
   D. a rigid cervical collar (e.g. Philadelphia collar) may be used to supplement
2. maintain blood pressure (*see below* under *Hypotension*)
   A. pressors: treats the underlying problem (essentially a traumatic sympathectomy). Dopamine is the agent of choice, and is preferred over fluids (except as necessary to replace losses) (see *Cardiovascular agents for shock*, page 6 for pressors). ✖ Avoid phenylephrine (*see below*)
   B. fluids as necessary to replace losses
   C. military anti-shock trousers (MAST): immobilizes lower spine, compensates for lost muscle tone in cord injuries (prevents venous pooling)
3. maintain oxygenation (adequate FIO_2 and adequate ventilation)
   A. if no indication for intubation: use NC or face mask
   B. intubation
      1. indications: may be required for
         a. airway compromise
         b. hypopnea:
            i. from paralyzed intercostal muscles

Table 25-5 Clinical criteria for cervical spine stability

1. awake, alert, oriented (no mental status changes, including no alcohol or drug intoxication)
2. no neck pain (with no distracting pain)
3. no neurologic deficits

Table 25-6 NATA helmet removal guidelines*

- most injuries can be visualized with the helmet in place
- neurological exam can be done with the helmet in place
- the patient may be immobilized on a spine board with the helmet in place
- the facemask can be removed with special tools to access the airway
- hyperextension must be avoided following removal of the helmet and shoulder pads

✖ NB: do not remove the helmet in the field. In a controlled setting (usually after x-rays) the helmet and shoulder-pads are removed together as a unit to avoid neck flexion or extension

Possible indications for removal of helmet

- face mask cannot be removed in a reasonable amount of time
- airway cannot be established even with face mask removed
- life threatening hemorrhage under the helmet that can be controlled only by removal
- helmet & strap do not hold head securely so that immobilizing the helmet does not adequately immobilize the spine (e.g. poor fitting or damaged helmet)
- helmet prevents immobilization for transportation in an appropriate position
- certain situations where the patient is unstable (M.D. decision)

*   for more details, see http://www.nata.org

A. although reports of bony or ligamentous abnormalities have be described as possibly occurring in these patients, there has been no report of a patient who had neurologic injury as a result of these abnormalities

          ii.   from paralyzed diaphragm (phrenic nerve = C3, 4 & 5)
          iii. or from depressed LOC
   2.   caution with intubation with uncleared C-spine
       a.   use chin lift (not jaw thrust) without neck extension
       b.   nasotracheal intubation may avoid movement of C-spine but patient must have spontaneous respirations
       c.   avoided tracheostomy or cricothyroidotomy if possible (may compromise later anterior cervical spine surgical approaches)
   4.   brief <u>motor</u> exam to identify possible deficits (also to document delayed deterioration); ask patient to:
       A.   move arms
       B.   move hands
       C.   move legs
       D.   move toes

MANAGEMENT IN THE HOSPITAL

Basic phases of management with respect to the spine:
1. stabilization (medical & spinal), preliminary evaluation & treatment
2. evaluation of spinal stability
3. subsequent (definitive) treatment

PRACTICE PARAMETER 25-2 MANAGEMENT OF SCI IN THE HOSPITAL

Clinical Assessment

Options[21]: the ASIA international standards for neurological and functional assessment of spinal cord injury **(SCI)** (*see page 711*) is recommended

Functional outcome assessment

Guidelines[21]: the Functional Impairment Measure™ **(FIM™)** (*see page 901*) is recommended

Options[21]: the modified Barthel index (*see page 900*) is recommended

Critical care management

Options[22]: monitor patients with acute SCI (especially those with severe cervical level injuries) in an ICU or similar monitored setting

Options[22]: cardiac, hemodynamic & respiratory monitoring after acute SCI is recommended

Options[23]: hypotension (SBP < 90 mm Hg) should be avoided or corrected ASAP

Options[23]: maintain MAP at 85-90 mm Hg for the first 7 days after SCI to improve spinal cord perfusion

---

STABILIZATION AND INITIAL EVALUATION

1. immobilization: maintain backboard/head-strap (*see above*) to facilitate transfers to CT table, etc. Once studies are completed, remove patient from backboard by logrolling (early removal from board reduces risk of decubitus ulcers)
2. <u>hypotension</u> (spinal shock): maintain SBP ≥ 90 mm Hg. Spinal cord injuries cause hypotension by a combination of factors (*see page 698*) which may further injure spinal cord[24] or other organ systems
    A.   pressors if necessary: dopamine is agent of choice (✘ avoid phenylephrine: non-inotropic and possible reflex increase in vagal tone with bradycardia)
    B.   careful hydration (abnormal hemodynamics → propensity to pulmonary edema)
    C.   atropine for bradycardia associated with hypotension
3. oxygenation (*see above*)
4. NG tube to suction: prevents vomiting and aspiration, and decompresses abdomen which can interfere with respirations if distended (paralytic ileus is common, and usually lasts several days)
5. indwelling (Foley) urinary catheter: for I's & O's and to prevent distension from

urinary retention
6. DVT prophylaxis: *see below*
7. temperature regulation: vasomotor paralysis may produce poikilothermy (loss of temperature control), this should be treated as needed with cooling blankets
8. electrolytes: hypovolemia and hypotension cause increased plasma aldosterone which may lead to hypokalemia
9. more detailed neuro evaluation (see *ASIA (American Spinal Injury Association) motor scoring system*, page 711). Patients may be stratified using the ASIA impairment scale (see *Table 25-13*, page 713)
   A. focused history: key questions should center on:
      1. mechanism of injury (hyperflexion, extension, axial loading…)
      2. history suggestive of loss of consciousness
      3. history of weakness in the arms or legs following the trauma
      4. occurrence of numbness or tingling at any time following the injury
   B. palpation of the spine for point tenderness, a "step-off", or widened interspinous space
   C. motor level assessment
      1. skeletal muscle exam (can localize dermatome)
      2. rectal exam for voluntary anal sphincter contraction
   D. sensory level assessment
      1. sensation to pinprick (tests spinothalamic tract, can localize dermatome): be sure to test sensation in face also (spinal trigeminal tract can sometimes descend as low as ≈ C4)
      2. light (crude) touch: tests anterior cord (anterior spinothalamic tract)
      3. proprioception/joint position sense (tests posterior columns)
   E. evaluation of reflexes
      1. muscle stretch reflexes: usually absent initially in cord injury
      2. abdominal cutaneous reflexes
      3. cremasteric reflex
      4. sacral
         a. bulbocavernosus: *see footnote, page 712*
         b. anal-cutaneous reflex
   F. examine for signs of autonomic dysfunction
      1. altered patterns of perspiration (abdominal skin may have low coefficient of friction above lesion, and may seem rough below due to lack of perspiration)
      2. bowel or bladder incontinence
      3. priapism: persistent penile erection
10. radiographic evaluation: *see below*
11. medical management specific to spinal cord injury:
    A. methylprednisolone (*see below*)
    B. experimental/investigational drugs: none of these agents shown to have unequivocal benefit in man: naloxone, DMSO, Lazaroid®. Tirilazad mesylate (Freedox®) was less beneficial than methylprednisolone[25]

METHYLPREDNISOLONE

> ### PRACTICE PARAMETER 25-3 METHYLPREDNISOLONE IN SCI
>
> ★ Still highly controversial even among experts[26-28]. See *Critique* below
>
> **Options**: treatment with methylprednisolone for 24 or 48 hrs after SCI is an option that should be undertaken only with the knowledge that the evidence suggesting harmful side effects is more consistent than any demonstrated clinical benefit

It has been asserted that beneficial (sensory and motor) effects at 6 weeks, 6 months and 1 year are seen (for both complete and incomplete injuries) when methylprednisolone (**MP**) is administered as shown below, but only if given **within 8 hours** of injury (NB: outcome is possibly worse at 1 year if the drug is started after 8 hrs from injury)[29, 30].

Exclusionary criteria from the study (these patients were not studied, and no determination was made whether the drug was helpful or not, or safe or not):
1. cauda equina syndrome (*see page 305*)
2. gunshot wounds (**GSW**) to the spine: a retrospective study showed no benefit and increased risk of complications with steroids with GSW[31]
3. life-threatening morbidity

4. pregnancy
5. narcotic addiction
6. age < 13 years
7. patient on maintenance steroids

Administration

1. **concentration**: in the following protocol, all solutions are mixed as 62.5 mg/ml (e.g. by diluting 16 gm methylprednisolone with bacteriostatic water to 256 ml)
2. **bolus**: 30 mg/kg initial IV bolus over 15 minutes, infused as shown in *Eq 25-1* with an IV controller (this delivers 0.48 ml/kg of solution in 15 minutes):

$$\text{bolus rate (ml/hr)} = \text{patient s weight (kg)} \times 1.92 \quad \text{(for 15 minutes)}$$ **Eq 25-1**

3. followed by a 45 minute pause
4. **maintenance infusion**: then 5.4 mg/kg/hr continuous infusion as shown in *Eq 25-2* (infusion is maintained during any necessary surgery if possible)

$$\text{maintenance rate (ml/hr)} = \text{patient s weight (kg)} \times 0.0864 \quad \text{(for 23 or 47 hours*)}$$ **Eq 25-2**

* **duration** of maintenance infusion: when therapy is initiated ≤ 3 hrs after injury, the infusion is administered for 23 hrs. If therapy is started between 3 and 8 hrs of injury, there may be an incremental benefit in 47 hrs of infusion, with slightly higher risk of infection and pneumonia[25]

Critique

A metaanalysis[234] of the literature could not identify any study that replicated the results of the original studies. At 1 year the MP group only showed a slight sensory advantage over the placebo group. Furthermore, high-dose MP may cause acute corticosteroid myopathy[235] **(ACM)** which might indicate that some patients that improved after MP were actually recovering from their ACM. ACM and it's associated complications (prolonged ventilator dependency...) should be added to the list of potential complications of high-dose MP (hyperglycemia, pneumonia, sepsis).

DEEP-VEIN THROMBOSIS IN SPINAL CORD INJURIES

Also see *Thromboembolism in neurosurgery*, page 25. Incidence of DVT may be as high as 100% when ^{125}I-fibrinogen is used[32]. Overall mortality from DVT is 9% in SCI patients.

PRACTICE PARAMETER 25-4 DVT IN PATIENTS WITH CERVICAL SCI
Standards[33]: prophylactic treatment of thromboembolism in patients with severe motor deficits due to SCI. Choices include: • LMW heparin, rotating beds, adjusted dose heparin, or some combination of these measures • or, low-dose heparin + pneumatic compression stockings or electrical stimulation **Guidelines**[33]: ✗ <u>not</u> recommended: low-dose heparin used alone ✗ <u>not</u> recommended: oral anticoagulation alone **Options**[33]: • duplex doppler ultrasound, impedance plethysmography & venography are recommended as diagnostic tests for DVT in patients with SCI • vena cava interruption filters for patients who do not respond to, or are not candidates for, anticoagulation

PROPHYLAXIS

Study of 75 patients found titrating dose of SQ heparin q 12 hrs to a PTT of 1.5 times control resulted in lower incidence of thromboembolic events (DVT, PE) than "mini-dose" heparin (5000 U SQ q 12 hrs) (7% vs. 31%)[34]. Heparin can cause thrombosis, thrombocytopenia and chronic therapy may produce osteoporosis (see *heparin*, page 22).

RADIOGRAPHIC EVALUATION AND INITIAL C-SPINE IMMOBILIZATION

There is controversy regarding what constitutes a minimal radiographic evaluation of the cervical spine in multiple trauma patient. No imaging modality is 100% accurate.

PRACTICE PARAMETER 25-5 X-RAYS AND IMMOBILIZATION IN CERVICAL SCI

Asymptomatic trauma patients

Standards[35]: radiographic studies are <u>not</u> indicated in patients who have:
* no mental status changes (and no alcohol or drugs)
* no neck pain or tenderness (with no distracting pain)
* no neurologic deficits
* and who do not have significant associated injuries that detract from their general evaluation

Symptomatic trauma patients

Standards[36]
* 3 view C-spine x-rays (AP, lateral & odontoid) adequately demonstrating from the craniocervical junction down to the C7-T1 interspace
* supplement this with additional thin cut CT through areas of suspicion or areas not visualized on plain x-ray

C-spine immobilization

Options[36]
* C-spine immobilization in <u>awake</u> patients with neck pain or tenderness and normal C-spine x-rays (including indicated CT scans) may be discontinued after either
    A. normal & adequate dynamic flexion-extension C-spine x-rays
    B. or a normal cervical MRI is obtained within 48 hrs of injury
* C-spine immobilization in <u>obtunded</u> patients with normal C-spine x-rays (including indicated CT scans) may be discontinued after:
    A. normal & adequate dynamic flexion-extension C-spine x-rays performed under fluoroscopic guidance
    B. or a normal cervical MRI is obtained within 48 hrs of injury
    C. or at the discretion of the treating physician

Asymptomatic patients (as outlined above in *x-rays and immobilization in cervical SCI*) may be considered to have a stable cervical spine and <u>no</u> radiographic studies of the cervical spine are indicated. Factors associated with increased risk of failing to recognize spinal injuries include: decreased level of consciousness (due to injury or drugs/alcohol), multiple injuries, technically inadequate x-rays[37] (also, see *Delayed cervical instability*, page 743).

See *X-rays, C-Spine* on page 140 for normal vs. abnormal findings. *Table 25-7* lists some indicators that should alert the reviewer that there may be significant C-spine trauma (they do <u>not</u> indicate definite instability by themselves).

All patients with possible spine injuries should have the following studies:
1. cervical spine: must be cleared radiographically from the cranio-cervical junction down through and including the C7-T1 junction (incidence of pathology at C7-T1 junction may be as high as 9%[39]):
    A. lateral portable C-spine x-ray while in rigid collar: this study by itself will miss ≈ 15% of injuries[40]
    B. if all 7 cervical vertebra <u>AND</u> the C7-T1 junction are adequately visualized and are normal, and if the patient has no neck pain or tenderness and is neurologically intact[A], then remove the cervical collar and complete the remainder of the cervical spine series (AP and open-

Table 25-7 Radiographic signs of C-spine trauma (modified[38])

Soft tissues
• retropharyngeal space > 7 mm, or retrotracheal space > 14 mm (adult) or 22 mm (peds) (see *Table 5-8*, page 141 for details)
• displaced prevertebral fat stripe
• tracheal deviation & laryngeal dislocation

Vertebral alignment
• loss of lordosis
• acute kyphotic angulation
• torticollis
• widened interspinous space
• axial rotation of vertebra
• discontinuity in contour lines (*see page 140*)

Abnormal joints
• ADI: > 4 mm (adult) or > 5 mm (peds) (see *Table 5-7*, page 140 for details)
• narrowed or widened disc space
• widening of apophyseal joints

A. neurologically intact implies that patient is alert, not intoxicated, and able to report pain reliably

mouth odontoid (**OMO**) view). Lateral, AP, and OMO views together detect essentially all unstable fractures in intact[A] patients[41] (although the AP view rarely provides unique information[42]). In a severely injured patient, limitation to an AP and lateral view usually suffices for the <u>acute</u> (but not complete) evaluation[43]

    C. if the above studies are normal, but there is neck pain, tenderness or neurologic findings (there may be a spinal cord injury even with normal plain films), or if the patient is unable to reliably verbalize neck pain or cannot be examined for neurologic deficit, then further studies are indicated, which may include any of the following:

        1. **oblique views**[A]: demonstrates the neural foramina (may be blocked with a unilateral locked facet (*see page 737*)), and helps assess the integrity of the articular masses and lamina (the lamina should align like shingles on a roof)[43]

        2. flexion-extension views: *see below*

        3. CT scan: helpful in identifying bony injuries. However, CT cannot exclude significant soft-tissue or ligamentous injury[44]

        4. MRI: utility is limited to specific situations (*see page 708*) and the accuracy has not been determined

        5. polytomograms

        6. **pillar view**: demonstrates the cervical articular masses en face (reserved for cases of suspected articular mass fracture)[45]: the head is rotated to one side (requires that the upper cervical spine injury has been excluded by previous radiographs), the x-ray tube is off centered 2 cm from midline in the opposite direction and the beam is angled 25° caudad, centered at the superior margin of the thyroid cartilage

    D. if subluxation is present at any level and is ≤ **3.5 mm** and the patient is neurologically intact[A], obtain flexion-extension films (*see below*)

        1. if no pathologic movement, may discontinue cervical collar

        2. even if no instability is demonstrated, may need delayed films once pain and muscle spasms have resolved to reveal instability

    E. if <u>lower</u> C-spine (and/or cervical-thoracic junction) are not well visualized

        1. repeat lateral C-spine x-ray with caudal traction on the arms (if not contraindicated based on other injuries, e.g. to shoulders)

        2. if still not visualized, then obtain a "swimmer's" (Twining) view: the x-ray tube is positioned above the shoulder furthest from the film, and aimed towards the axilla closest to the film with the tube angled 10-15° toward the head while the arm is elevated above the head

        3. if still not visualized

           a. CT scan through non-visualized levels (CT is poor for evaluating alignment and for fractures in the horizontal plane, thin cuts with reconstructions may ameliorate this shortcoming)

           b. if CT not available and if patient is neurologically intact, keep patient in collar and obtain "non-emergent" midline sagittal plane laminograms (polytomograms)

    F. for questions regarding stability of the subaxial spine, see page 733

    G. patients with C-spine fractures or dislocations should have daily C-spine x-rays during initial traction or immobilization

2. thoracic and lumbosacral spine: AP and lateral x-rays for all trauma patients who:

    A. were thrown from a vehicle, or fell ≥ 6 feet to the ground

    B. complain of back pain

    C. are unconscious

    D. are unable to reliably describe back pain or have altered mental status preventing adequate exam

    E. have an unknown mechanism of injury, or other injuries that cast suspicion of spine injury

3. reminder: when abnormalities of questionable vintage are identified, a bone scan may be helpful to distinguish an old injury from an acute one (less useful in the elderly; in an adult, a bone scan will become "hot" within 24-48 hrs of injury, and will remain hot for up to a year; in the elderly, the scan may not become hot for 2-3 weeks and can remain so for over a year)

4. CT scan through area of bony abnormality or level of neurologic deficit (*see below*)

A. some authors include oblique views in a "minimal" evaluation[43], others do not[41]

FLEXION-EXTENSION CERVICAL SPINE X-RAYS

Purpose: to disclose occult instability.

It is possible to have a purely ligamentous injury involving the posterior ligamentous complex without any bony fracture (see *Hyperflexion sprain*, page 736). Lateral flexion-extension views help detect these injuries, and also evaluate other injuries (e.g. compression fracture) for stability. For patients with limited flexion due to paraspinal muscle spasm (sometimes resulting from pain), a rigid collar should be prescribed, and if the pain persists 2-3 weeks later[46] the flexion-extension films should be repeated.

✖ Contraindications

1. the patient must be cooperative and free of mental impairment (i.e. no head injury, street or prescription drugs, alcohol...)
2. there should not be any subluxation > **3.5 mm** at any level on cross-table C-spine x-rays (which is a marker for possible instability, *see page 736*)
3. patient must be neurologically intact (if there is any degree of spinal cord injury, proceed instead first with imaging studies, e.g. MRI)

Technique

The patient should be sitting, and is instructed to flex the head slowly, and to stop if it becomes painful. Serial x-rays are taken at 5-10° increments (or followed under fluoro with spot films at the end of movement), and if normal, the patient may be encouraged to flex further. This is repeated until evidence of instability is seen, or the patient cannot flex further because of pain or limitation of motion. The process is then repeated for extension.

Normal flexion-extension views demonstrate slight anterior subluxation distributed over all cervical levels with preservation of the normal contour lines (see *Figure 5-10*, page 141).

CT SCAN

Obtained through levels of abnormality identified on plain films or myelogram, or at level of neurologic deficit in patients with normal films. Thin cuts (1.5-3 mm) through the level of suspicion are required. Assesses bony anatomy in detail; with intrathecal contrast (i.e. after myelogram), also delineates any neural impingement. Usually non-emergent in patients with complete cord lesions or with no neurologic deficit.

EMERGENT MYELOGRAM OR MRI

Indications for emergent myelogram (usually employing water soluble contrast with CT to follow) (✖ Caution: pressure shifts from LP exacerbates deficit in 14% of patients with complete block[47]) or MRI in spinal cord injury:

1. incomplete lesion (to check for soft tissue compressing cord) with normal alignment
2. deterioration (worsening deficit or rising level) including after closed reduction
3. neurologic deficit not explained by radiographic findings, including:
   A. fracture level different from level of deficit
   B. no bony injury identified: further imaging is done to R/O soft tissue compression (disc herniation, hematoma...) that would require surgery

Cervical myelogram in patients with cervical spine injuries usually requires C1-2 puncture to achieve adequate dye concentration in the cervical region without dangerous extension of the neck or tilting of the patient. An MRI, if an option, is usually preferable.

TRACTION/REDUCTION OF CERVICAL SPINE INJURIES

See *PRACTICE PARAMETER 25-6* below.

Purpose

To reduce fracture-dislocations, maintain normal alignment and/or immobilize the cervical spine to prevent further spinal cord injury. Reduction decompresses the spinal cord and roots, and may facilitate bone healing.

The rapidity with which reduction should be done is controversial[4].

Contraindications

1. atlanto-occipital dislocation: *see page 717*
2. types IIA or III hangman's fracture: *see page 725*
3. skull defect at anticipated pin site: may necessitate alternate pin site
4. use with caution in pediatric age group (do not use if age ≤ 3 yrs)

Options[48]
- early closed reduction of C-spine fracture/dislocation injuries with cran-iocervical traction to restore anatomic alignment in awake patients
- ✖ not recommended: closed reduction in patients with an additional ros-tral injury
- patients with C-spine fracture-dislocation who cannot be examined dur-ing attempted closed reduction, or before open posterior reduction, should undergo cervical MRI before attempted reduction*. The pres-ence of a significant herniated disc in this setting is a relative indication for anterior decompression before reduction
- cervical MRI is also recommended for patients who fail attempts at closed reduction*

---

* NB: prereduction MRI will show disrupted or herniated discs in 33-50% of patients with facet sublux-ation. These findings do not seem to significantly influence outcome after closed-reduction in <u>awake</u> patients; ∴ the usefulness of prereduction MRI in this setting is uncertain

Application of tongs or halo ring

Choice of device: a number of cranial "tongs" are available. Crutchfield tongs re-quire predrilling holes in the skull. Gardner-Wells tongs are probably the most common tongs in use. If halo-vest immobilization is anticipated after acute stabilization, a halo ring may be used for the initial cervical traction, and then converted to vest traction later at an appropriate time (e.g. post-fusion).

Preparation: placed with patient in cart. Shave hair around proposed pin sites (*see below*). Betadine skin prep, then infiltrate local anesthetic. Optional: incise skin with #11 scalpel (prevents pins from driving in surface contaminants).

Gardner-Wells tongs: Pin sites: the pins are placed in the temporal ridge (above the temporalis muscle), **2-3 finger-breadths (3-4 cm) above pinna**. Place directly above external acoustic meatus for <u>neutral</u> position traction; 2-3 cm posterior for <u>flexion</u> (e.g. for locked facets); 2-3 cm anterior for <u>extension</u>. One pin has a central spring-loaded force-indicator. Tighten pins until the indicator protrudes 1 mm beyond the flat surface. Retighten pins daily until indicator protrudes 1 mm for 3 days only, then stop.

Halo ring: Many halo rings can be placed right from the start, and used for traction, and then later (e.g. after successful closed reduction, or post-op following reduction/fusion) converted to a halo-vest immobilizer. The usual sites for the pins are used. Tip: prior to penetrating forehead skin for anterior pins, have the patient close their eyes and hold them closed as the pin is advanced. This avoids the problem where the patients eyes are "pinned open".

Post-placement care: Transfer to a bed with ortho headboard with tongs in place. Tie rope to tongs/halo and feed through pulley in head of bed. Slight flexion or extension is achieved by changing the height of the pulley relative to the patients long axis.

X-rays: lateral C-spine x-rays <u>immediately</u> after application of traction and at reg-ular intervals and after every change in weights and every move from bed. Check align-ment and rule-out atlanto-occipital dislocation: the distance from the basion to the odontoid should be ≤ 5 mm in adults, and ≤ 10 mm in peds (due to incomplete ossification of the dens in children).

Weight: if there is no malalignment and traction is being used just to stabilize the injury and to compensate for ligamentous instability, use 5 lbs for the upper C-spine or 10 lbs for lower levels. To reduce locked facets, *see page 737*. May remove cervical collar once patient is in traction with adequate reduction or stabilization.

Pin care: clean (e.g. half strength hydrogen peroxide), then apply povidone-iodine ointment. Frequency: in hospital: q shift. At home following discharge: twice daily.

Reduction of locked facets
See page 737.

Complications
1. skull penetration by pins. May be due to:
   A. pins placed too tightly
   B. pins placed too low in thin squamous portion of temporal bone
   C. elderly patients, especially those with an osteoporotic skull

---

D. invasion of bone with tumor: e.g. multiple myeloma
E. fracture at pin site
2. reduction of cervical dislocations may be associated with neurologic deterioration which is usually due to retropulsed disc[49] and requires immediate investigation with myelogram/CT or MRI
3. overdistraction from excessive weight (especially with upper cervical spine injuries), may also endanger supporting tissues
4. caution with C1-C3 injury, especially with posterior element fracture (traction may pull fragments in towards canal)
5. infection:
    A. osteomyelitis in pin sites: risk is reduced with good pin care
    B. subdural empyema: rare[50, 51] (see page 223)

INDICATIONS FOR EMERGENCY DECOMPRESSIVE SURGERY

Caution: laminectomy in the face of acute spinal cord injury has been associated with neurologic deterioration in some cases. When emergency decompressive is indicated, it is usually combined with a stabilization procedure.

Modified recommendations of Schneider[52]

In patients with <u>complete</u> spinal cord lesions, no study has demonstrated improvement in neurologic outcome with either open decompression or closed reduction[53]. In general, surgery is reserved for <u>incomplete</u> lesions (possibly excluding central cord syndrome, see page 714) with extrinsic compression, who, following maximal possible reduction of subluxation show:
1. progression of neurologic signs
2. complete subarachnoid block by Queckenstedt test or radiographically (on myelography or MRI)
3. myelogram, CT, or MRI shows bone fragments or soft tissue elements (e.g. hematoma) in the spinal canal causing spinal cord compression
4. necessity for decompression of a vital cervical root
5. compound fracture or penetrating trauma of the spine
6. acute anterior spinal cord syndrome (see page 716)
7. non-reducible fracture-dislocations from locked facets causing spinal cord compression

Contraindications to emergent operation
1. <u>complete</u> spinal cord injury ≥ 24 hrs (no motor or sensory function below level of lesion)
2. medically unstable patient
3. central cord syndrome (controversial, see page 714)

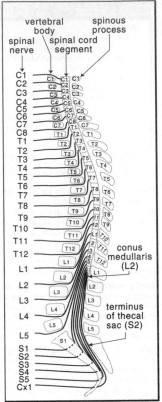

Figure 25-1 Relationship between spinal cord, nerve roots, and bony spine

---

25.4. Neurological assessment

Evaluation of the level of the lesion requires familiarity with the following concepts

---

about the relationship between the bony spinal canal and the spinal cord and nerves (*see Figure 25-1*).

1. since there are 8 pairs of cervical nerves and only 7 cervical vertebra
   A. cervical nerves 1 through 8 exit <u>above</u> the pedicles of their like-numbered vertebra
   B. thoracic, lumbar and sacral nerves exit <u>below</u> the pedicles of their like-numbered vertebra
2. due to disproportionately greater growth of the spinal column than the spinal cord during development, the following relationships of the spinal <u>cord</u> to the vertebral column exist:
   A. to determine which segment of the cord underlies a given vertebra:
      1. from T2 through T10: add 2 to the number of the spinous process
      2. for T11, T12 and L1, remember that these overlie the 11 lowest spinal segments (L1 through L5, S1 through S5, and Coxygeal-1)
   B. the conus medullaris in the adult lies at about L1 or L2 of the spine

ASIA (AMERICAN SPINAL INJURY ASSOCIATION) MOTOR SCORING SYSTEM

A system[54, 55] that may be rapidly applied to grade 10 key motor segments using the Royal Medical Research Council of Great Britain Grading Scale (*Table 20-1*, page 548) from 0-5 on the left and the right, for a total score of 100 possible points (*see Table 25-9*). NB: most muscles receive innervation from two adjacent spinal levels, the levels listed in *Table 25-9* are the <u>lower</u> of the two. The standard considers a segment intact if the motor grade is fair (≥ 3). For additional information, see www.asia-spinalinjury.org.

See *Table 20-3*, page 548 and *Table 20-5*, page 550 for detailed tables of motor innervation.

Table 25-9 Key muscles for motor level classification (EXTREMITIES)

RIGHT grade	Segment	Muscle	Action to test	LEFT grade
0-5	C5	biceps	flex elbow	0-5
0-5	C6	wrist extensors	cock up wrist	0-5
0-5	C7	triceps	extend elbow	0-5
0-5	C8	flexor digitorum profundus	flex middle distal phalanx	0-5
0-5	T1	hand intrinsics	abduct little finger	0-5
0-5	L2	iliopsoas	flex hip	0-5
0-5	L3	quadriceps	straighten knee	0-5
0-5	L4	tibialis anterior	dorsiflex foot	0-5
0-5	L5	EHL	dorsiflex big toe	0-5
0-5	S1	gastrocnemius	plantarflex foot	0-5
50		← TOTAL POSSIBLE POINTS →		50
GRAND TOTAL: 100				

Table 25-8 Key sensory landmarks

Level	Dermatome
C2	occipital protuberance
C3	supraclavicular fossa
C4	top of acromioclavicular joint
C5	Lateral side of antecubital fossa
C6	thumb, dorsal surface, proximal phalanx
C7	middle finger, dorsal surface, proximal phalanx
C8	little finger, dorsal surface, proximal phalanx
T1	medial (ulnar) side of antecubital fossa
T2	apex of axilla
T3	third intercostal space **(IS)**
T4	fourth IS (nipple line)
T5	fifth IS (midway between T6 & T8)
T6	sixth IS (xiphoid process)
T7	seventh IS (midway between T6 & T8)
T8	eighth IS (midway between T6 & T10)
T9	ninth IS (midway between T8 & T10)
T10	tenth IS (umbilicus)
T11	eleventh IS (midway between T10 & T12)
T12	inguinal ligament at mid-point
L1	half the distance between T12 & L2
L2	mid-anterior thigh
L3	medial femoral condyle
L4	medial malleolus
L5	dorsum of foot at 3rd metatarsal phalangeal joint
S1	lateral heel
S2	popliteal fossa in the mid-line
S3	ischial tuberosity
S4-5	perianal area (taken as 1 level)

Table 25-10   Axial muscle evaluation[56]

Level	Muscle	Action to test
C4	diaphragm	tidal volume (TV), FEV$_1$, and vital capacity (VC)
T2-9 T9-10 T11-12	intercostals upper abdominals lower abdominals	use sensory level, abdominal reflexes, & Beevor's sign (*see below*)

MORE DETAILED MOTOR EVALUATION

Table 25-11   Skeletal muscles and their major spinal innervation
(major contributing segment is shown in boldface)

Segment	Muscle	Action to test	Reflex
C1-4	neck muscles		
C3, 4, 5	diaphragm	inspiration, TV, FEV$_1$, VC	
C5, 6	deltoid	abduct arm > 90°	
C5, 6	biceps	elbow flexion	biceps
C6, 7	extensor carpi radialis	wrist extension	supinator
C7, 8	triceps, extensor digitorum	elbow and finger extension	triceps
C8, T1	flexor digitorum profundus	grasp (flex distal phalanges)	
C8, T1	hand intrinsics	abduct little finger, adduct thumb	
T2-9	intercostals*		
T9,10	upper abdominals*	Beevor's sign†	abdominal cutaneous reflex‡
T11,12	lower abdominals*		
L2, 3	iliopsoas, adductors	hip flexion	cremasteric reflex§
L3, 4	quadriceps	knee extension	infrapatellar (knee jerk)
L4, 5	medial hamstrings, tibialis anterior	ankle dorsiflexion	medial hamstrings
L5, S1	lateral hamstrings, posterior tibialis, peroneals	knee flexion	
L5, S1	extensor digitorum, EHL	great toe extension	
S1, 2	gastrocs, soleus	ankle plantarflexion	achilles (ankle jerk)
S2, 3	flex digitorum, flex hallucis		
S2, 3, 4	bladder, lower bowel, anal sphincter	clamp down during rectal exam	anal cutaneous reflexΔ, bulbo-cavernosus & priapism

*   also use sensory level to help evaluate these segments

†   **Beevor's sign**: used to assess abdominal musculature for level of lesion. Patient lifts head off of bed by flexing neck; if lower abdominal muscles (below ≈ T9) are weaker than upper abdominal musculature, then umbilicus moves cephalad. Not helpful if both upper and lower abdominals are weak

‡   the **abdominal cutaneous reflex**: scratching one quadrant of abdomen with sharp object causes contraction of underlying abdominal musculature, causing umbilicus to migrate toward that quadrant. Upper abdominal reflex: T8-9. Lower abdominal reflex: T10-12. This is a cortical reflex (i.e. reflex loop ascends to cortex, and then descends to abdominal muscles). The presence of this response indicates an incomplete lesion for cord injuries above the lower thoracic level

§   **cremasteric reflex**: L1-2 superficial reflex

Δ   **Anal-cutaneous reflex**: AKA anal wink. Normal reflex: mild noxious stimulus (e.g. pinprick) applied to skin in region of anus results in involuntary anal contraction.

Bulbocavernosus (BC) reflex: contraction of anal sphincter in response to pinching penile shaft, or in response to tug on Foley catheter is normal (must be differentiated from the movement of the catheter balloon). Presence of BC reflex used to be taken as an indication of an incomplete injury, but its presence alone is no longer considered to have a good prognosis for recovery.

Priapism: in presence of spine trauma, indicates injury to spinal cord resulting in loss of sympathetic tone → dominance of parasympathetic tone. A poor prognosticator for return of function

SENSORY LEVEL ASSESSMENT
(DERMATOMES & SENSORY NERVES)

ASIA standards[54]

28 key points identified in *Table 25-8* are scored separately for pinprick and light touch on the left & right side using the grading scale shown in *Table 25-12*, for a maximum possible total of 112 points for pinprick (left & right) and 112 points for light touch (left & right).

Points of note:
1. "C4 cape" AKA "bib" region across the upper chest: sensory segments "jump" from C4 to T2 with the intervening levels distributed exclusively on the UEs (see *Figure 3-7*, page 75). The point of transition is inconstant from person to person

Table 25-12 Sensory grading scale

Grade	Description
0	absent
1	impaired (partial or altered appreciation)
2	normal
NT	not testable

RECTAL EXAM

1. external anal sphincter is tested by insertion of the examiner's finger
   A. perceived sensation is recorded as present or absent. Any sensation felt by the patient indicates that the injury is sensory incomplete
   B. note resting sphincter tone and any voluntary sphincter contraction
2. bulbocavernosus reflex (**BC**): *see footnote, page 712*

ADDITIONAL EXAM

The following elements are considered optional but it is recommended that they be graded as absent, impaired or normal:
1. position sense: test index finger and great toe on both sides
2. awareness of deep pressure/deep pain

ASIA IMPAIRMENT SCALE

The ASIA impairment scale[54] is shown in *Table 25-13*, and is modified from the from the Frankel Neurological Performance scale[57].

Table 25-13 ASIA impairment scale

Class	Description
A	**Complete**: No motor or sensory function preserved in sacral segments S4-5
B	**Incomplete**: Sensory but no motor function preserved below the neurologic level (includes sacral segments S4-5)
C	**Incomplete**: Motor function preserved below the neurologic level (more than half of key muscles below the neurologic level have a muscle grade < 3)
D	**Incomplete**: Motor function preserved below the neurologic level (more than half of key muscles below the neurologic level have a muscle grade ≥ 3)
E	**Normal**: Sensory & motor function normal

25.5. Spinal cord injuries

25.5.1. Complete spinal cord injuries

See *page 698* for definition of complete vs. incomplete spinal cord injury.

In addition to loss of voluntary movement, sphincter control and sensation below the level of the injury, there may be priapism. Hypotension and bradycardia (spinal shock, *see page 698*) may also present.

BULBAR-CERVICAL DISSOCIATION

Results from spinal cord injury at or above ≈ C3 (includes SCI from atlanto-occipital and atlantoaxial dislocation). Bulbar-cervical dissociation produces immediate pulmonary and, often, cardiac arrest. Death results if CPR is not instituted within minutes. Patients are usually quadriplegic and ventilator dependent (phrenic nerve stimulation may eventually allow independence from ventilator).

25.5.2.   Incomplete spinal cord injuries

CENTRAL CORD SYNDROME

⚑ Key features
- disproportionately greater motor deficit in the upper extremities than lower
- usually results from hyperextension injury in the presence of osteophytic spurs
- surgical decompression is often employed on a non-urgent basis

Central cord syndrome (CCS) is the most common type of incomplete spinal cord injury syndrome. Usually seen following acute hyperextension injury in an older patient with pre-existing acquired stenosis as a result of bony hypertrophy (anterior spurs) and infolding of redundant ligamentum flavum (posteriorly), sometimes superimposed on congenital spinal stenosis. Translational movement of one vertebra on another may also contribute. A blow to the upper face or forehead is often disclosed on history, or is suggested on exam (e.g. lacerations or abrasions to face and/or forehead). This often occurs in relation to a motor vehicle accident or to a forward fall, often while intoxicated. Younger patients may also sustain CCS in sporting injuries (see *burning hands syndrome*, page 743). CCS may occur with or without cervical fracture or dislocation[58]. Also may occur in rheumatoid arthritis.

PATHOMECHANICS

Theory: the centermost region of the spinal cord is a vascular watershed zone which renders it more susceptible to injury from edema. Long tract fibers passing through the cervical spinal cord are somatotopically organized such that cervical fibers are located more medially than the fibers serving the lower extremities (see *Figure 3-6*, page 73).

PRESENTATION[59]

The clinical syndrome is somewhat similar to that seen in syringomyelia.
1. motor: weakness of upper extremities with lesser effect on lower extremities
2. sensory: varying degrees of disturbance below level of lesion may occur
3. myelopathic findings: sphincter dysfunction (usually urinary retention)

Hyperpathia to noxious and non-noxious stimuli is also common, especially in the proximal portions of the upper extremities, and is often delayed in onset and extremely distressing to the patient[60]. Lhermitte's sign occurs in ≈ 7% of cases.

NATURAL HISTORY

There is often an initial phase of improvement (characteristically: LEs recover first, bladder function next, UE strength then returns with finger movements last; sensory recovery has no pattern) followed by a plateau phase and then late deterioration[61]. 90% of patients are able to walk with assistance within 5 days[62]. Recovery is usually incomplete, and the amount of recovery is related to the severity of the injury and patient age[63].

If CCS results from hematomyelia with cord destruction (instead of cord contusion), then there may be extension (upward or downward).

EVALUATION

Findings: young patients tend to have disc protrusion, subluxation, dislocation or fractures[62]. Older patients tend to have multi-segmental canal narrowing due to osteophytic bars, discs, and inbuckling of ligamentum flavum[62].

C-spine x-rays: may demonstrate congenital narrowing, superimposed osteophytic spurs, traumatic fracture/dislocation. Occasionally, AP narrowing alone without spurs may be seen[58]. Plain x-rays will fail to demonstrate canal narrowing due to: thickening or inbuckling of ligamentum flavum, hypertrophy of facet joints, and poorly calcified spurs[58].

Cervical CT scan: also helpful in diagnosing fractures and osteophytic spurs. Not as good as MRI for assessing status of discs, spinal cord and nerves.

MRI: discloses compromise of anterior spinal canal by discs or osteophytes (when combined with plain C-spine x-rays, it increases the ability to differentiate osteophyte from traumatic disc herniation). Also good for evaluating ligamentum flavum. T2WI may show spinal cord edema acutely[64], and can detect hematomyelia. MRI is poor for identifying fractures.

TREATMENT

PRACTICE PARAMETER 25-7 ACUTE CENTRAL CORD INJURIES

Options[63]
- because of possible cardiac, pulmonary & BP disturbances, *many** of these patients *may* require management in an ICU or other monitored setting (for cardiac, hemodynamic & respiratory monitoring), *especially* patients with severe neurologic deficits
- maintain MAP 85-90 mm Hg (use BP augmentation if necessary) for the 1st week after injury to improve spinal cord perfusion
- early reduction of fracture-dislocation injuries is recommended
- surgical decompression, particularly for focal and anterior spinal cord compression that is approached anteriorly, *seems** to be of benefit in *selected* patients

* all italics added

The indications, timing and best treatment method for CCO remains controversial. Initial management options include the methylprednisolone spinal-cord injury protocol for patients seen within 8 hours of the time of injury (*see page 704*).

Indications for surgery:
1. continued compression of the spinal cord[65 (p 1010)] that correlates with the level of deficit with any of the following:
   A. persistent significant motor deficit following a varying period of recovery (see *Timing of surgery* below)
   B. deterioration of function
   C. continued significant dysesthetic pain
2. instability of the spine

Improvement has been shown in short and long-term follow-up with subacute decompression of the offending lesion[62]. Nonsurgical treatment results in a longer period of pain and weakness in many cases.

Timing of surgery: Classic teaching was that *early* surgery for this condition is contraindicated because this may worsen the deficit. In the absence of spinal instability, traditional management consisted of bed rest in a soft collar for ~ 3-4 weeks, with consideration for surgery after this time, or else gradual mobilization in the same collar for an additional 6 weeks. It is presently felt that there is no solid evidence that *early* decompressive surgery (without cord manipulation) is actually harmful, but there is also no evidence that it is helpful, either. There may be good justification for *early* surgery in the rare patient who is improving and then deteriorates[66], however, great restraint must be used in avoiding what would be an inappropriate operation in many patients[67]. Surgery may improve the rate and degree of recovery in selected patients[68]. Surgery has been recommended for patients with gross spinal instability or for patients with significant persistent cord compression (e.g. by osteophytic spurs) who fail to progress consistently after an initial period of improvement[64], often within 2-3 weeks following the trauma. Better results occur with decompression within the first few weeks or months rather than very late (e.g. ≥ 1-2 years)[65 (p 1010)].

Surgical considerations: The most rapid procedure to decompress the cord is often a multi-level laminectomy. This is frequently accompanied by dorsal migration of the spinal cord which may be seen on MRI[61]. With myelopathy, fused patients fare better than those that are just decompressed without fusion. Fusion may be accomplished posteriorly (e.g. with lateral mass plates) at the time of decompression, or anteriorly (e.g. multi-level discectomy, or corpectomy with strut graft and anterior cervical plating) at the same sitting as the laminectomy or at a later date.

PROGNOSIS
    In patients with cord contusion without hematomyelia, ≈ 50% will recover enough LE strength and sensation to ambulate independently, although typically with significant spasticity. Recovery of UE function is usually not as good, and fine motor control is usually poor. Bowel and bladder control often recovers. Elderly patients with this condition generally do not fare as well as younger patients, with or without surgical treatment (only 41% over age 50 become ambulatory, versus 97% for younger patients[69]).

ANTERIOR CORD SYNDROME
    AKA anterior spinal artery syndrome. Cord infarction in the territory supplied by the anterior spinal artery. Some say this is more common than central cord syndrome.
    May result from occlusion of the anterior spinal artery, or from anterior cord compression, e.g. by dislocated bone fragment, or by traumatic herniated disc.

Presentation
1. paraplegia, or (if higher than ≈ C7) quadriplegia
2. **dissociated sensory loss** below lesion:
    A. loss of pain and temperature sensation (spinothalamic tract lesion)
    B. preserved two-point discrimination, position sense, deep pressure sensation (posterior column function)[70]

Evaluation
    It is vital to differentiate a non-surgical condition (e.g. anterior spinal artery occlusion) from a surgical one (e.g. anterior bone fragment). This requires one or more of: myelography, CT, or MRI.

Prognosis
    The worst prognosis of the incomplete injuries. Only ≈ 10-20% recover functional motor control. Sensation may return enough to help prevent injuries (burns, decubitus ulcers…).

BROWN-SÉQUARD SYNDROME
    Spinal cord hemisection. Usually a result of penetrating trauma, it is seen in 2-4% of traumatic spinal cord injuries[71]. Also may occur with radiation myelopathy, cord compression by spinal epidural hematoma, large cervical disc herniation[72], spinal cord tumors, spinal AVMs and cervical spondylosis.

Classical form (rarely found in this pure form):
*   contralateral findings: **dissociated sensory loss**
    ♦   loss of pain and temperature sensation inferior to lesion beginning 1-2 segments below (spinothalamic tract lesion)
    ♦   preserved light (crude) touch due to redundant ipsilateral and contralateral paths (anterior spinothalamic tracts)
*   ipsilateral findings:
    ♦   loss of posterior column function (proprioception & vibratory sense)
    ♦   motor paralysis (due to corticospinal tract lesion) below lesion

Prognosis
    This syndrome has the best prognosis of any of the incomplete spinal cord injuries. ≈ 90% of patients with this condition will regain the ability to ambulate independently as well as anal and urinary sphincter control.

POSTERIOR CORD SYNDROME
    AKA contusio cervicalis posterior. Relatively rare. Produces pain and paresthesias (often with a burning quality) in the neck, upper arms, and torso. There may be mild paresis of the UEs. Long tract findings are minimal.

25.6.   Cervical spine fractures

Also see *C-Spine*, page 140 for cervical x-rays. One system of classifying cervical spine fractures identifies the following <u>subatlantal</u> injuries[73]:
1. hyperextension fracture-dislocations
    A. posterior fracture-dislocation of the dens
    B. traumatic spondylolisthesis of the axis (hangman's fracture, *see page 724*)
    C. hyperextension sprain (momentary dislocation) with fracture
    D. hyperextension fracture-dislocation with fractured articular pillar
    E. hyperextension fracture-dislocation with comminution of the vertebral arch
2. hyperflexion fracture-dislocations
    A. anterior fracture-dislocation of the dens (*see page 727*)
    B. hyperflexion sprain: rare. Occurs when posterior ligaments are disrupted but locking of articular facets does not occur (*see page 736*)
    C. locked articular facets with fracture (*see page 736*)
    D. "teardrop" fracture-dislocation (*see page 734*)

25.6.1.   Atlanto-occipital dislocation

Atlanto-occipital dislocation (**AOD**) AKA craniocervical junction dislocation. Disruption of the stability of the craniocervical junction. Probably underdiagnosed, may be present in ≈ 1% of patients with "cervical spine injuries"[74] (definition of cervical spine injuries not specified), found in 8-19% of fatal cervical spine injury autopsies[75, 76]. More than twice as common in pediatric age group as adults. Patients usually either have minimal neurological deficit or exhibit bulbar-cervical dissociation (**BCD**) (*see page 714*). Most mortality results from anoxia due to respiratory arrest as a result of BCD.

Classification[77] (*see Figure 25-2*)

Type I   anterior dislocation of occiput relative to the atlas
Type II   longitudinal dislocation (distraction)
Type III   posterior dislocation of occiput

Combinations (e.g. anterior-distracted AOD[78]) may also occur.

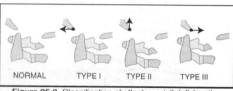

NORMAL   TYPE I   TYPE II   TYPE III

Figure 25-2 Classification of atlanto-occipital dislocation

PRACTICE PARAMETER 25-8 ATLANTO-OCCIPITAL DISLOCATION INJURIES

Diagnosis

Options[79]
- lateral C-spine x-ray
- if it is desired to employ a radiologic method of measurement, the BAI-BDI method (*see page 720*) is recommended
- upper cervical prevertebral soft-tissue swelling on an otherwise nondiagnostic plain lateral C-spine x-ray should prompt additional imaging
- if there is clinical suspicion of AOD, and plain x-rays are nondiagnostic, CT or MRI is recommended, especially for non-Type II dislocations

Treatment

Options[79]
- treatment with internal fixation & arthrodesis using one of a variety of methods
- ✖ CAUTION: traction may be used in the management of AOD, but it is associated with a 10% risk of neurologic deterioration

---

Ligaments of the occipito-atlanto-axial complex

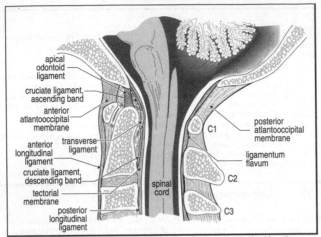

Figure 25-3 Sagittal view of the ligaments of the craniovertebral junction
Modified with permission from "*In Vitro* Cervical Spine Biomechanical Testing" BNI Quarterly, Vol.9, No. 4, 1993

Stability of this joint complex is primarily due to ligaments, with little contribution from bony articulations and joint capsules (*see Figure 25-3* through *Figure 25-5*):

1. ligaments that connect the atlas to the occiput:
   A. anterior atlanto-occipital membrane: cephalad extension of the anterior longitudinal ligament. Extends from anterior margin of foramen magnum **(FM)** to anterior arch of C1
   B. posterior atlantooccipital membrane: connects the posterior margin of the FM to posterior arch of C1
   C. the ascending band of the cruciate ligament

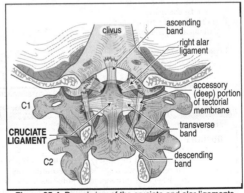

Figure 25-4 Dorsal view of the cruciate and alar ligaments
Viewed with tectorial membrane removed.
Modified with permission from "*In Vitro* Cervical Spine Biomechanical Testing" BNI Quarterly, Vol.9, No. 4, 1993

2. ligaments that connect the axis (viz. the odontoid) to the occiput:
   A. **tectorial membrane**: some authors distinguish 2 components
      1. superficial component: cephalad continuation of the posterior longitudinal ligament. A strong band connecting the dorsal surface of the dens to the ventral surface of the FM above, and dorsal surface of C2 & C3 bodies below
      2. accessory (deep) portion: located laterally, connects C2 to occipital condyles

B. alar ("check") ligaments[80]
  1. occipito-alar portion: connects side of the dens to occipital condyle
  2. atlanto-alar portion: connects side of the dens to the lateral mass of C1
C. apical odontoid ligament: connects tip of dens to the FM. Little mechanical strength
3. ligaments that connect the axis to the atlas:
A. **transverse (atlanto-axial) ligament**: the horizontal component of the **cruciate** ligament. Holds the dens to

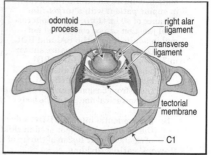
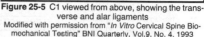

Figure 25-5 C1 viewed from above, showing the transverse and alar ligaments
Modified with permission from "*In Vitro* Cervical Spine Biomechanical Testing" BNI Quarterly, Vol.9, No. 4, 1993

the anterior atlas via a strap-like mechanism (*see Figure 25-5*). The strongest ligament of the spine[81]. Provides the majority of the strength
B. atlanto-alar portion of the alar ligaments (*see above*)
C. descending band of the cruciate ligament

The most important structures in maintaining atlanto-occipital stability are the tectorial membrane and the **alar ligaments**. Without these, the remaining cruciate ligament and apical dentate ligament are insufficient.

CLINICAL PRESENTATION
1. may be neurologically intact, therefore must be ruled-out in any major trauma
2. bulbar-cervical dissociation: *see page 714*
3. may have lower cranial nerve deficits (as well as VI palsies) ± cervical cord injury
4. worsening neurologic deficit with the application of cervical traction: check lateral C-spine films immediately after applying traction (*see page 709*)

RADIOGRAPHIC EVALUATION

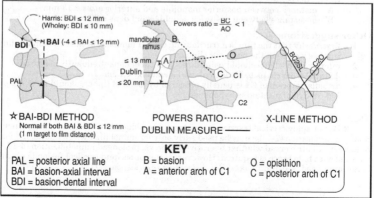

Figure 25-6 Measurements used to diagnose atlanto-occipital dislocation (AOD)
Numbers shown are corresponding normal values (*see text* for details and for peds)

Numerous measurements have been devised to radiographically quantitate this relationship. None are completely reliable[82]. Some better known methods (*see Figure 25-6*):

1. ★ BAI-BDI method: the recommended method[79]. Based on lateral radiograph in supine patient with a target-film distance of 40 in. (1 m), the occipitocervical junction can be considered normal in adults if both the BAI and BDI are ≤ **12 mm** (normal values are shown in *Table 25-14*)[83]. Both BAI & BDI should be measured in adults

Table 25-14   BAI-BDI normal values

Normal	BAI (mm)	BDI (mm)
Adult	-4 to +12*	2-15 (mean, 7.5 ± 4.3) Suggested cutoff: **12 mm**
Peds	0 to 12	unreliable in age < 13

*   even in flexion-extension, BAI ≤ 12 mm

   A. basion-axial interval **(BAI)** = distance from basion to rostral extension of posterior axial line **(PAL)** (the posterior cortical margin of the body of the axis). Better for <u>anterior</u> or <u>posterior</u> AOD
   B. basion-dental interval **(BDI)** = distance from basion to the closest point on the tip of the dens (not used in children < 13 years because of variable age of ossification & fusion of the tip of the odontoid). Better for <u>distracted</u> AOD
2. **Powers' ratio**[74]: dividing the distance **BC** (basion to posterior arch of atlas) by **AO** (opisthion to anterior arch of atlas) (*see Figure 25-6*). The interpretation is shown in *Table 25-15*. Applies only to <u>anterior</u> AOD (i.e. not for posterior or distracted AOD). Cannot be used with any fracture involving the atlas or the foramen magnum, or with congenital anatomic abnormalities. Requires identification of 4 reference points[A]

Table 25-15   Powers' ratio

Ratio BC/AO	Interpretation	Comment
< 0.9	normal	1 standard deviation below the lowest case of AOD
≥ 0.9 and < 1	"grey zone" (indeterminate)	included 7% of normals and no cases of AOD
≥ 1	AOD	encompassed all AOD cases

3. X-line (occipital-axial lines) method[84]: requires identification of 6 reference points[A]. 2 lines (75% sensitive[84]):
   A. C2O line drawn from the posteroinferior corner of axis body to the opisthion: should intersect tangentially
   B. BC2SL drawn from the basion to a point midway on the C2 spinolaminar line: should intersect tangentially with the posterosuperior dens
4. BDI (distance between the basion & dens), normal values:
   A. Harris[78, 83]: ≤ 12 mm (*see above*)
   B. Wholey measure[85]: ≤ 10 mm (50% sensitive[84])[B]
5. Dublin measure[86] (25% sensitive[84]):
   A. distance between posterior mandible and anterior atlas ≤ 13 mm
   B. or distance between posterior mandible and dens ≤ 20 mm

Other suggestions
1. first, verify that the film is a true lateral: check alignment of the two mandibular rami as well as of the posterior clinoids
2. inferior tip of clivus should point directly to tip of dens (frequently obscured)
3. distance from clivus to C1 articulation should be < 1 cm
4. articular process of C1 is usually obscured by mastoid tip (or, should meet occipital condyle if mastoid is hypoplastic)

TREATMENT
   ✖ Do not apply cervical traction in an attempt to reduce AOD because of risk of neurologic deterioration (2-4 lbs may be used early only for immobilization in adults, <u>not</u> for reduction). Controversial whether operative fusion vs. prolonged immobilization (4-12 months) with halo brace is required. However, posterior occipito-cervical fusion is usually recommended (see *atlanto-occipital dislocation injuries*, page 717).

A. requires identification of the opisthion which cannot be done in ~ 56% of lateral C-spine x-rays[83]
B. 6 ft target-film distance in a sitting patient[85] which is not practical in the E/R[78]

25.6.2. Occipital condyle fractures

❦ Key features:
- may present with lower cranial nerve deficits which may be delayed in onset (e.g. hypoglossal nerve palsy), mono-, para-, or quadriparesis or plegia
- rarely diagnosed on plain x-rays which are often reported as normal
- usually treated with cervical immobilization (collar)

Rare. Occipital condyle fractures (OCF) were first described in 1817 by Bell[87].

Classification[88]:
Type I   comminuted from impact: may occur from axial loading
Type II   extension of linear basilar skull fracture[89]
Type III avulsion of condyle fragment (traction injury): may occur during rotation, lateral bending, or a combination of mechanisms. Considered unstable by many authorities

PRACTICE PARAMETER 25-9 OCCIPITAL CONDYLE FRACTURES
Diagnosis
Guidelines[90]
• clinical suspicion should be raised by the presence of ≥ 1 of the following: blunt trauma with high-energy craniocervical injuries, altered consciousness, occipital pain or tenderness, impaired cervical movement, lower cranial nerve palsies, or retropharyngeal soft-tissue swelling
• CT is recommended for establishing the diagnosis
Options[90]: MRI is recommended to assess the integrity of the craniocervical ligaments
Treatment
Options[90]: external cervical immobilization

Treatment
Controversial. Lower cranial nerve deficits often develop in untreated cases of OCF, and may resolve or improve with external immobilization. Types I & II have been treated with or without external immobilization (cervical collar or, occasionally, halo) without obvious difference. External immobilization x 6-8 weeks is suggested for Type III fractures because of the higher risk of delayed deficits.

25.6.3. Atlantoaxial dislocation

Lower morbidity and mortality than atlanto-occipital dislocation[91]. May be either:
1. rotatory: (*see below*) usually seen in children after a fall or minor trauma
2. anterior: more ominous (*see below*)

ATLANTOAXIAL ROTATORY SUBLUXATION

Rotational deformity at the atlanto-axial junction is usually of short duration and easily corrected. Rarely, the atlantoaxial joint locks in rotation (AKA atlanto-axial rotatory *fixation*[92]). Usually seen in children. May occur spontaneously, with rheumatoid arthritis[93], with congenital dens anomalies, following major or minor trauma (including neck manipulation or even with neck rotation while yawning[92]), or with an infection of the head or neck including upper respiratory tract

Table 25-16 Classification (Fielding) and treatment of rotatory atlantoaxial subluxation

Type	Description		Treatment for Grisel's syndrome*[94]
	TL†	facet capsule	
I	intact	bilateral injury	soft collar
II	injured	unilateral injury	Philadelphia collar or SOMI
III	injured	bilateral injury	halo

*   6-8 weeks of immobilization, then check stability with flexion-extension x-rays. Fusion for residual instability

†   TL = transversse ligament

(known as **Grisel's syndrome**[94]: inflammation may cause mechanical and chemical injury to the facet capsules and/or transverse ligament (**TL**)). The classification scheme of Fielding[92] is shown in *Table 25-16*.

The dislocation may be at the occipito-atlantal and/or the atlanto-axial articulations[95]. The mechanism of the irreducibility is poorly understood. With an intact TL, rotation occurs without anterior displacement. If the TL is incompetent as a result of trauma or infection, there may also be anterior displacement with more potential for neurologic injury. Posterior displacement occurs only rarely[92].

The vertebral arteries (**VA**) may be compromised in excessive rotation, especially if it is combine with anterior displacement.

Clinical findings

Patients are usually young. Neurologic deficit is rare. Findings may include: neck pain, headache, torticollis (characteristic "**cock robin**" head position with ≈ 20° lateral tilt to one side, 20° rotation to the other, and slight (≈ 10°) flexion - *see page 370* for DDx), reduced range of motion, and facial flattening[92]. Although the patient cannot reduce the dislocation, they can increase it with head rotation towards the subluxed joint with potential injury to the high cervical cord.

Brainstem and cerebellar infarction and even death may occur with compromise of circulation through the VAs[96].

Radiographic evaluation

X-rays: findings may be confusing. Pathognomonic finding on AP C-spine x-ray in severe cases: frontal projection of C2 with simultaneous oblique projection of C1[97 (p 124)]. In less severe cases, the C1 lateral mass that is forward appears larger and closer to the midline than the other.

Asymmetry of the atlantoaxial joint is not correctable with head rotation, which may be demonstrated by persistence of asymmetry on open mouth odontoid views with the head in neutral position and then rotated 10-15° to each side.

The spinous process of the axis is tilted in one direction and rotated to the other (may occur in torticollis of any etiology).

CT scan: demonstrates rotation of the atlas[95].

MRI: may assess the competence of the transverse ligament.

Treatment

Treatment of Grisel's syndrome: appropriate antibiotics for causative pathogen with traction (*see below*) and then immobilization (*see Table 25-16*) for the subluxation.

Traction: The subluxation may be reduced with gentle traction (in children start with 7-8 lbs and gradually increase up to 15 lbs over several days, in adults start with 15 lbs and gradually increase up to 20). If the subluxation is present > 1 month, traction is less successful. Active left-right neck rotation is encouraged in traction.

If reducible, immobilization in traction or halo is maintained **x** 3 months[92] (range: 6-12 weeks).

Subluxation that cannot be reduced or that recurs following immobilization should be treated by surgical arthrodesis after 2-3 weeks of traction to obtain maximal reduction. The usual fusion is C1 to C2 (*see page 623*) unless other fractures or conditions are present[92]. Fusion may be performed even if the rotation between C1 & C2 is not completely reduced.

ANTERIOR ATLANTOAXIAL DISLOCATION[91]

One third of patients have neurologic deficit or die. May be due to:
1. incompetence of the odontoid process
   A. fracture
   B. congenital hypoplasia (e.g. Morquio syndrome, *see page 337*)
2. disruption (rupture) of the transverse (atlantal) ligament (**TL**) (see *Atlanto-dental interval (ADI)*, page 140). Attachment points of the TL may be weakened in rheumatoid arthritis. Isolated *traumatic* rupture of the transverse ligament is rare

Evaluation

CT & MRI are recommended to evaluate the TL.

Treatment

Fusion is recommended when the TL is disrupted or with irreducible subluxations. Odontoid fractures with an intact ligament are managed as outlined in that section (*see page 728).*

25.6.4. Atlas (C1) fractures

Acute C1 fractures account for 3-13% of cervical spine fractures[98]. 56% of 57 patients had isolated C1 fractures; 44% had combination C1-2 fractures; 9% had additional non-contiguous C-spine fractures. 21% had associated head injuries[98].

ISOLATED C1 (ATLAS) INJURIES

CLASSIFICATION[99]
Type I: fractures involving a single arch (31-45% of C1 fractures)
Type II: burst fracture (37-51%): the classic Jefferson fracture (*see below*)
Type III: lateral mass fractures of the atlas (13-37%)

Jefferson fracture
Named for Sir Geoffrey Jefferson. Classically described as a four-point (burst) fracture of the C1 ring[100], but also taken to include the more common three or two-point fractures[101], the latter through the C1 arches (thinnest portion). Usually from <u>axial</u> load (a "blow-out" fracture). 41% chance of an associated C2 fracture.

In pediatrics, it is critical to differentiate a C1 fracture from the normal synchondroses (*see page 142*), and from pseudospread of the atlas (*see page 701*). A fracture may also occur through the unfused synchondroses.

<u>Unstable</u>, usually no neurologic deficit if isolated (due to large canal diameter at this level, plus tendency for fragments to be forced <u>outwards</u>).

CLINICAL
Neurologic deficit is rare. 3 of 25 patients with Jefferson fractures sustained neurologic injuries (1 complete injury, 2 central cord syndromes) in one series.

EVALUATION
Complete C-spine series and thin section high-resolution CT from C1 through C3 to delineate details of C1 fracture and to assess for associated C2 injury. MRI is an option to assess the integrity of the transverse ligament.

Assessing integrity of transverse ligament
1. may be inferred indirectly from
   A. abnormal overhang of lateral masses on open-mouth odontoid view (see *"Rule of Spence"* below)
   B. atlantodental interval (**ADI**) > 3 mm (*see page 140*) is also a marker for TL disruption[102]
2. MRI may be able to image the ligament directly

"Rule of Spence": On AP or open-mouth odontoid x-ray, if the sum total overhang of both C1 lateral masses on C2 is **≥ 7 mm** (x + y in *Figure 5-9*, page 139), the transverse ligament is probably disrupted[103, 104] (when corrected for an 18% magnification factor, it has been suggested that the criteria be increased to **≥ 8.2 mm**[105]). Total overhang of C1 lateral masses on C2 was ≥ 7 mm in 16% of 32 patients with isolated C1 injury.

TREATMENT

PRACTICE PARAMETER 25-10 ISOLATED ATLAS FRACTURES
Treatment

Options[106]: for <u>isolated</u> atlas fractures:
 • if the transverse ligament is intact: cervical immobilization alone
 • if the transverse ligament is disrupted: either
     A. cervical immobilization alone
     B. or, surgical fixation and fusion

Treatment options are delineated in *Table 25-17*[106]. When external immobilization is employed, it is used for 8-16 weeks (mean = 12).

OUTCOME

In many series[98, 107], treatment without surgery results in satisfactory outcome.

Table 25-17   Treatment options for isolated C1 fractures

Fracture type	Treatment options
anterior or posterior arch	collar or SOMI

anterior AND posterior arch (burst)
   stable (TL* intact)
   unstable (TL disrupted)
	
	collar or SOMI, halo
	halo, C1-2 stabilization & fusion

lateral mass fractures
   comminuted fracture
   transverse process fracture
	
	collar or SOMI, halo
	collar or SOMI

*   abbreviations: TL = transverse ligament of the atlas

25.6.5.   Axis (C2) fractures

Acute fractures of the axis represent ≈ 20% of cervical spine fractures. Neurological injury is uncommon, and occurs in < 10% of cases. Most injuries may be treated by rigid immobilization.

CATEGORIES
1.   odontoid fractures (*see page 727*): type II is the most common injury of the axis
2.   hangman's fracture: *see below*
3.   miscellaneous C2 fractures: *see page 730*

HANGMAN'S FRACTURE

❢ Key features
* bilateral fracture through the pars interarticularis of C2 with traumatic subluxation of C2 on C3, most often from hyperextension + axial loading
* usually stable with no neurologic deficit
* most do well with non-halo immobilization **x** 8-14 weeks (exceptions: severe/unstable fractures (*see page 726*) or those that do not remain in alignment in brace)

AKA **traumatic spondylolisthesis of the axis**. The term "hangman's fracture" **(HF)** was coined by Schneider et al.[108] although the mechanism of most modern HFs (hyperextension and axial loading, from MVAs or diving accidents) differs from that sustained in judicial hangings (where submental placement of the knot results in hyperextension and *distraction*[109]). It is a bilateral fracture through the pars interarticularis (isthmus) of the pedicle of C2 (*see Figure 25-7*). There is often anterior subluxation of C2 on C3 (in pediatrics, consider pseudosubluxation in the differential diagnosis, *see page 701*). Usually <u>stable</u>. Deficit is rare. Nonunion is rare. 90% heal with immobilization only. Operative fusion is rarely needed. Fractures of C2 that do not go through the isthmus are not true hangman's fractures and may require different management (see *Miscellaneous C2 fractures*, page 730).

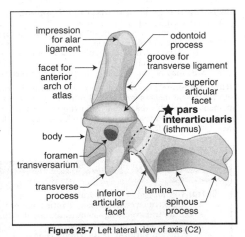

Figure 25-7 Left lateral view of axis (C2)

Labels: impression for alar ligament; facet for anterior arch of atlas; body; foramen transversarium; transverse process; inferior articular facet; odontoid process; groove for transverse ligament; superior articular facet; ★ **pars interarticularis** (isthmus); lamina; spinous process

CLASSIFICATION

Two different systems, that of Frances and that of Effendi are presented below. Not all fractures fit into one or both of these classification systems[116].

In a large series of axis fractures[115], the most common fracture pattern was Effendi Type I (72%) and Francis Grade I (65%); and there was a close correlation as follows:

Effendi Type I ≈ Francis Grade I
Effendi Type III ≈ Francis Grade IV

Grading system of Effendi et al.[110] (modified by Levine[111]): (*see Table 25-18*). Based on the mechanism of injury. Angulation is measured as the angle between the inferior endplate of C2 and that of C3.

Table 25-18   Classification of hangman's fractures (modified Effendi system)*

Type	Description	Radiographic Findings	Mechanism	Comment
I	vertical pars fx just posterior to the VB	≤ 3 mm subluxation of C2 on C3 & no angulation	axial loading & extension	Stable on flexion/extension x-rays. Neurologic deficit rare
I A	fx lines on each side are not parallel	fx line may not be visible on x-ray. Anterior C2 VB may be subluxed 2-3 mm anteriorly on C3 & the C2 VB may appear elongated. CT demonstrates the fx	may be hyperextension + lateral bending	"atypical hangman's fracture"[113]. Fx may pass thru foramen transversarium on one side. Spinal canal may be narrowed. 33% incidence of paralysis
II	vertical fx thru pars. Disruption of C2-3 disc & posterior longitudinal ligament	subluxation of C2 on C3 > 3 mm and/or angulation†. Slight anterior compression of C3 possible	axial loading & extension with rebound flexion	May lead to early instability. Neurologic deficit rare. Usually reduces with traction
IIA	oblique fx (usually anterior-inferior to posterior superior)	little subluxation (usually ≤ 3 mm) but more angulation (can be > 15°)	flexion distraction (posterior arch falls in tension)	Rare (< 10%). Unstable. ✖ Traction → increased angulation & widening of disc space
III	vertical pars fx. C2-3 facet capsules disrupted. Posterior arch of C3 is free floating. Anterior longitudinal ligament may be disrupted or stripped off C3	facets of C2/C3 may be subluxed or locked	unclear, may be flexion (capsule disruption) followed by compression (isthmus fracture)	Rare. Neurologic deficit may occur; may be fatal. Facet dislocation cannot be reduced closed. ✖ Traction may be dangerous (*see text*)

*   Effendi et al.[110], Levine and Edwards[111], Sonntag and Dickman[91] and Levine[112]
†   amount of angulation was not specified in original article

Grading system of Francis et al.[114]: Shown in *Table 25-19*. The methodology of measurements is depicted in *Figure 25-8*.

Table 25-19   Grading system of Francis for hangman's fracture*

Grade	Angulation θ	Displacement
I	< 11°	d < 3.5 mm
II	> 11°	
III	< 11°	d > 3.5 mm and
IV	> 11°	d/b < 0.5
V		disc disruption

*   see *Figure 25-8* for methodology

PRESENTATION

Most (≈ 95%) are neurologically intact, those few with deficits are usually minor (paresthesias, monoparesis...) and many recover within one month[114]. Almost all conscious patients will have cervical pain usually in the upper posterior cervical region, and occipital neuralgia is not uncommon[117]. There is a high incidence of associated head injury and there will be other associated C-spine injuries (e.g. C1 fracture (*see above*) or clay shoveler's fracture (*see page 733*)) in ≈ one third, with most occurring in the upper 3 cervical levels. There are usually external signs of injury to the face and head associated with the hyperextending and axial force.

EVALUATION

Plain lateral C-spine x-rays show the fracture in 95% of cases. Oblique films, polytomograms, and/or CT may be needed in the remainder. Most fractures pass through the pars or the transverse foramen[114], 7% go through the body of C2 (also see *Miscellaneous C2 fractures*, page 730). Instability can usually be identified as marked anterior displacement of C2 on C3 (guideline[114]: unstable if displacement exceeds 50% of the AP diameter of C3 vertebral body), excessive angulation of C2 on C3, or by excessive motion on flexion-extension films.

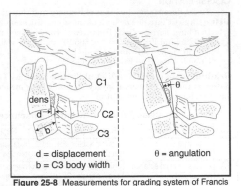

d = displacement
b = C3 body width

θ = angulation

Figure 25-8 Measurements for grading system of Francis

Patients suspected of having modified Effendi Type I fractures and are neurologically intact should have physician-supervised flexion-extension x-rays to rule out a reduced type II fracture.

The vertebral arteries should be evaluated (angiogram or MRA) in patients with stroke-like symptoms.

TREATMENT

PRACTICE PARAMETER 25-11 ISOLATED HANGMAN'S FRACTURE

Options[118]
- hangman's fractures may initially be managed with external immobilization in most cases (halo or collar)
- surgical stabilization should be considered in cases of:
  A. severe angulation of C2 on C3 (Effendi II, Francis II & IV)
  B. disruption of the C2-3 disc space (Effendi III, Francis V)
  C. or inability to establish or maintain alignment with external immobilization
---

Nonsurgical management produces adequate reduction in 97-100% and results in a fusion rate of 93-100% of cases[91, 119, 120] if the external immobilization is adequately maintained for 8-14 weeks[121] (average time for healing is ≈ 11.5 weeks[114]). Specific treatment depends on the reliability of the patient and the degree of stability as described below. Most cases do well with non-halo immobilization[120].

STABLE FRACTURES (EFFENDI TYPES I OR IA, OR FRANCIS GRADES I OR II)

Treat with immobilization (Philadelphia collar[122 (p 2326)] or cervicothoracic orthosis **(CTO)** (e.g. SOMI) is usually adequate) **x** 3 months[112]. Halo-vest may be needed in unreliable patients or for combination C1-C2 fractures. Schneider reported 50 cases of Type I fracture treated with non-halo fixation, only 1 was taken to surgery and was found to already be fused.

UNSTABLE FRACTURES

Effendi Type II

Reduce with gentle cervical traction (most reduce with ≤ 30 lbs[112]) with the head in slight extension (preferably in halo ring) under close monitoring to prevent "iatrogenic hanging" in cases with ligamentous instability[114].

Type II fractures with ≤ 5 mm of subluxation & angulation < 10°: once reduced, apply halo-vest and begin to mobilize (usually within 24 hrs of injury). Verify that immobilization is adequate in the halo with upright lateral C-spine x-ray, operate if inadequate. After 8-12 weeks, change to Philadelphia collar or CTO until fusion is definitely complete (usually 3-4 months).

Type II fractures with > 5 mm subluxation or ≥ 10° of angulation: Concerns:
1. risk of settling if immediately mobilized in halo-vest
2. healing with significant angulation may result in chronic pain
3. if not reduced, the gap may be too large for bony bridging using traction alone

Therefore surgical fusion in these patients is recommended.

Alternatively, traction can be maintained for ≈ 4 weeks and then reduction should be reassessed 1 hour after removing weight from traction, and if stable, again 24 hours after mobilizing in a vest. If unstable, return to traction and repeat trial at 5 & 6 weeks. If still unstable at 6 weeks, surgical fusion is recommended[112].

Effendi Type IIA

✖ Traction will accentuate the deformity[112]. Fractures should be reduced by immediate placement in halo vest (bypassing traction) with extension and <u>compression</u> applied. Halo-vest immobilization **x** 3 months produces ≈ 95% union rate.

Effendi Type III

✖ Reduction with traction may be dangerous with locked facets. ORIF is recommended[91]. MRI prior to surgery is recommended to assess the C2-3 disc.

SURGICAL TREATMENT

Indications

Few patients have indications for surgical treatment of HF, and include those with:
1. inability to reduce the fracture (includes most Effendi Type III & some Type II)
2. failure of external immobilization to prevent movement at fracture site
3. traumatic C2-3 disc herniation with compromise of the spinal cord[123]
4. established non-union: evidenced by movement on flexion-extension film[114], see *Flexion-extension cervical spine x-rays*, page 708 (all failures of nonoperative treatment had displacement > 4 mm[91])

Hangman's fractures likely to need surgery[115] are those with:
1. Effendi Type II or III
2. or Francis grade II, IV or V or if:
   A. anterior displacement of C2 VB > 50% of the AP diameter of the C3 VB
   B. or if angulation produces widening of either the anterior or posterior borders of the C2-3 disc space > the height of the normal C3-4 disc below

Surgical options
1. fusion techniques: both include C2 to C3 fusion
   A. posterior approach: requires inclusion of C1 (i.e. C1-3 wiring and fusion), and occasionally the occiput is incorporated
   B. anterior C2-3 discectomy[114] with fusion. Optional anterior plating via a transverse anterior cervical incision midway between the angle of the jaw and the thyroid cartilage[119, 123]
      1. preserves more motion by excluding C1
      2. this approach is also recommended for established non-union[114]
      3. also used when at least a partial reduction cannot be achieved
2. screw placement from posterior approach through the C2 pedicle across the fracture fragment[112]. The fracture must be reduced to employ this technique.

TREATMENT ENDPOINT

Plain x-rays should show trabeculation across the fracture site or interbody fusion of C2 to C3. Flexion-extension lateral radiographs should show no movement at the fracture site.

ODONTOID FRACTURES

Significant force is required to produce an odontoid fracture in a young individual, and is usually sustained in an MVA, a fall from a height, a skiing accident, etc. In patients > 70 years age, simple falls with head trauma may produce the fracture. Odontoid fractures comprise ≈10-15% of all cervical spine fractures[124]. They are easily missed on initial evaluation, especially since significant associated injuries are frequent and may mask symptoms. Pathologic fractures can also occur, e.g. with metastatic involvement (*see page 517*).

Flexion is the most common mechanism of injury, with resultant anterior displacement of C1 on C2 (atlantoaxial subluxation). Extension only occasionally produces odontoid fractures, usually associated with posterior displacement.

Signs and symptoms

The frequency of fatalities at the time of the accident resulting directly from odontoid fractures is unknown, it has been estimated as being between 25-40%[125]. 82% of patients with Type II fractures were neurologically intact, 8% had minor deficits of scalp or limb sensation, and 10% had significant deficit (monoparesis to quadriplegia)[126]. Type III fractures are rarely associated with neurologic injury.

Common symptoms are high posterior cervical pain, sometimes radiating in the distribution of the greater occipital nerve (occipital neuralgia). Almost all patients with high posterior cervical pain will also have paraspinal muscle spasm, reduced range of motion of the neck, and tenderness to palpation over the upper cervical spine. A very suggestive finding is the tendency to support the head with the hands when going between the upright and supine position. Paresthesias in the upper extremities and slight exaggeration of muscle stretch reflexes may also occur. Myelopathy may develop in patients with nonunion (*see page 729*).

Classification

The classification system of Anderson and D'Alonzo[127] is shown in *Figure 25-9* and *Table 25-20*.

Type I fractures are due to avulsion at the attachment of the alar ligament. They are very rare. Although long considered to be a stable injury, they may not occur as an isolated fracture and may be a manifestation of atlanto-occipital dislocation[128]. Also, it may be a marker for possible disruption of the transverse ligament[129] which may result in atlantoaxial instability.

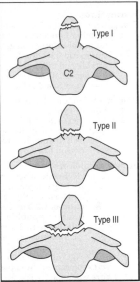

Figure 25-9 Major types of odontoid fractures (AP view)

Table 25-20   Classification of odontoid fractures

Type	Characteristics	Stability
I	through tip (above transverse ligament), rare	unstable*
II	through base of neck, the most common dens fracture (may be best seen on AP x-ray)	usually unstable
IIA	similar to type II, but with large bone chips at fracture site[130], comprise ≈ 3% of type II odontoid fractures. Diagnosed by plain radiographs and/or CT	usually unstable
III	through body of C2 (usually involves marrow space). May involve superior articular surface	usually stable

*   controversial, *see text*

Steele's rule of thirds: each of the following occupies one third of the area of the canal at the level of the atlas: dens, space, spinal cord[103].

TREATMENT

PRACTICE PARAMETER 25-12 ISOLATED ODONTOID FRACTURES

Guidelines[118]: isolated Type II odontoid fractures in adults ≥ 50 years age should be considered for surgical stabilization & fusion

Options[118]
- Type I, II & III fractures may be managed initially with external cervical immobilization
- Type II & III: consider surgical fixation for:
    A.   fracture displacement ≥ 5 mm
    B.   or Type IIA fracture (comminution)
    C.   or inability to maintain alignment with external immobilization

---

TYPE I

So rare that meaningful analysis is difficult. Due to possible associated atlanto-axial instability, surgical fusion may at times be necessary.

TYPE II

Treatment remains controversial. No agreement has been reached after many attempts to identify factors that will predict which type II fractures are most likely to heal with immobilization and which will require operative fusion. Critical review of the literature reveals a paucity of well designed studies. A wide range of nonunion rates with immobilization alone (5-60%) is quoted: **30%** is probably a reasonable estimate for overall nonunion rate, with 10% nonunion rate for those with displacement < 6 mm[131]. Possible key factors in predicting nonunion include:

1. degree of displacement: probably the most important factor
   A. some authors feel that displacement > 4 mm increases nonunion[127, 132]
   B. some authors use ≥ 6 mm as the critical value, citing a 70% nonunion rate[121] in these regardless of age or direction of displacement
2. age:
   A. children < 7 yrs old almost always heal with immobilization alone
   B. some feel that there is a critical age above which the nonunion rate increases, and the following ages have been cited: age > 40 yrs (possibly ≈ doubling the nonunion rate)[132], age > 55 yrs[133], age > 65 yrs[134], yet others do not support increasing age as a factor[131]

Indications for surgery

Given the above, there can be no hard and fast rules. The following is offered as a guideline (also, see *isolated odontoid fractures* above).

★ Surgical treatment (instead of external immobilization) is recommended for odontoid Type II fractures in patients ≥ 7 years age with any of the following:
1. displacement ≥ 5 mm
2. instability at the fracture site in the halo vest (*see below*)
3. age ≥ 50 years: increases nonunion rate (with halo) 21-fold[135]
4. nonunion (*see Table 25-22* for radiographic criteria) including firm fibrous union[136], especially if accompanied by myelopathy[117]
5. disruption of the transverse ligament: associated with delayed instability[137]

Surgical options

1. odontoid compression screw: appropriate for acute type II fractures (*see page 625*)
2. C1-2 arthrodesis: *see page 623* for options including wiring/fusion, transarticular screws, halifax clamps...

Immobilization

For those not meeting surgical indications above, 10-12 weeks of immobilization as suggested in *Table 25-21* is recommended.

Halo vest appears superior to a SOMI brace and is felt by some to be superior to a Philadelphia collar[131, 138] (there is no Class I medical evidence). If a halo is used, obtain supine and upright lateral C-spine x-rays in the halo. If there is movement at the fracture site, then surgical stabilization is recommended.

In patients who are poor surgical candidates, there is theoretical and anecdotal rationale to consider calcitonin therapy (*see page 749*) in conjunction with a rigid cervical orthosis[139].

Nonunion

The radiographic criteria for nonunion are shown in *Table 25-22*. The most common symptom of nonunion is continued high posterior cervical pain beyond the time that the

Table 25-21 Immobilization for odontoid fractures

Fracture Type	Option
Type I	collar, halo
Type II*	halo, collar*
Type IIA*	halo*
Type III*	collar, halo*

* consider surgery for these, use indicated brace when surgery not deemed appropriate

Table 25-22 Radiographic criteria of nonunion of odontoid fractures

1. defect in the dens with contiguous sclerosis of both fragments (vascular pseudarthrosis)
2. defect in the dens with contiguous resorption of both fragments (rarefying osteitis or atrophic pseudarthrosis)
3. defect in the dens with definite loss of cortical continuity
4. movement of dens fragment demonstrated on flexion-extension x-rays

brace is removed. Late myelopathy can develop in as many as 77% of mobile nonunions[125, 140] as a result of motion and soft tissue proliferation around the unstable fracture site.

TYPE IIA
Early surgery is recommended for all type IIA fractures[130].

TYPE III
≈ 90% heal with external immobilization (and analgesics) if adequately maintained for 8-14 weeks[121]. A halo-vest brace is probably best[138]. If a less rigid orthosis is used, monitor with frequent C-spine x-rays to rule-out nonunion.

SURGICAL TREATMENT
See *Atlantoaxial fusion (C1-2 arthrodesis)* on page 623 and *Anterior odontoid screw fixation* on page 625 for surgical options and operative details.

MISCELLANEOUS C2 FRACTURES

Comprise ≈ 20% of C2 fractures[91]. Includes fractures of spinous process, lamina, facets, lateral mass or C2 vertebral body. Fractures of spinous process or lamina may be treated with Philadelphia collar or cervicothoracic orthosis (CTO). Fractures which compromise the anterior or middle columns (i.e. fractures of facets, C2 body, or lateral mass) requires CTO or halo-vest if nondisplaced, or halo if displaced.

PRACTICE PARAMETER 25-13 FRACTURES OF THE AXIS BODY
Treatment
Options[118]: external immobilization is recommended for isolated axis body fractures

OS ODONTOIDEUM

A separate bone ossicle of variable size with smooth cortical borders separated from a foreshortened odontoid peg, occasionally may fuse with the clivus. May mimic Type 1 or 2 odontoid fracture. Etiology is debated with evidence to support both of the following (diagnosis & treatment do not depend on which etiologic theory is correct):
1. congenital: developmental anomaly (nonunion of dens to body of axis). However, does not follow known ossification centers, and has been demonstrated in 9 patients with previously normal odontoid processes[141]
2. acquired: postulated to represent an old nonunion fracture or injury to vascular supply of developing odontoid[141, 142]

True os odontoideum is rare. **Ossiculum terminale**: nonunion of the apex at the secondary ossification center, is more common.

Two anatomic types:
1. **orthotopic**: ossicle moves with the anterior arch of C1
2. **dystopic**: ossicle is functionally fused to the basion. May sublux anterior to the C1 arch

Presentation
Main groups identified in the literature[143]:
1. occipitocervical/neck pain
2. myelopathy: further subdivided[141]
   A. transient myelopathy: common following trauma
   B. static myelopathy
   C. progressive myelopathy
3. intracranial signs or symptoms: from vertebrobasilar ischemia
4. incidental finding

Most patients are neurologically intact and present with atlantoaxial instability which may be discovered incidentally. Many symptomatic and asymptomatic patients have been reported with no new problems over many years of follow-up[144]. Conversely, cases of precipitous spinal cord injury after seemingly minor trauma have been reported[145].

Σ The natural history is variable, and predictive factors for deterioration, especially in asymptomatic patients, have not been identified[146].

Evaluation

For diagnosis, see *os odontoideum* below.

It is critical to R/O C1-2 instability. However, myelopathy does not correlate with the degree of C1-2 instability. An AP canal diameter < 13 mm does correlate with the presence of myelopathy.

Treatment

Regardless of whether os odontoideum is congenital or an old non-union fracture, immobilization is unlikely to result in fusion. Therefore, when treatment is elected, surgery is required (usually atlantoaxial arthrodesis, *see page 623*).

PRACTICE PARAMETER 25-14 OS ODONTOIDEUM
Diagnosis
Options[146] • recommended: the following plain C-spine x-rays: AP, open-mouth odontoid, lateral (static & flexion-extension) • consider: tomography (CT or plain) and/or MRI of craniocervical junction
Management

Options[146]
• patients without neurologic signs or symptoms (even with C1-2 instability) may be followed with clinical & radiographic surveillance
• those with neurologic signs or symptoms and C1-2 instability
   A. may be managed with posterior C1-2 internal fixation and fusion
   B. options:
      1. posterior wiring & fusion. Post-op halo immobilization is recommended following these procedures
      2. C1-2 transarticular screw fixation and fusion: successful screw placement seems to obviate the need for post-op halo
• consider occipitocervical fusion with or without C1 laminectomy for patients with irreducible cervicomedullary compression and/or evidence of associated occipitoatlantal instability
• consider transoral decompression in patients with irreducible ventral cervicomedullary compression

25.6.6. Combination C1-2 injuries

Combination C1-2 injuries are relatively common and may imply more significant structural and mechanical injury than isolated C1 or C2 fractures. The frequency of C2 fractures in C1-2 combination injuries is shown in *Table 25-23*. 5-53% of patients with Type II or III odontoid fractures and 6-26% of hangman's fractures have an associated C1 fracture[147].

Table 25-23 Accompanying C2 injuries

Injury	%
Type II dens fracture	40%
Type III dens fracture	20%
hangman's fracture	12%
other	28%

TREATMENT

Treatment options[147] are summarized in *Table 25-24*.

PRACTICE PARAMETER 25-15 COMBINATION ATLAS & AXIS FRACTURES

Options[147]
• recommended: base treatment primarily on the type of C2 injury
• recommended: external immobilization of most C1-2 fractures
• consider surgical stabilization* for these situations†:
   A. C1-Type II odontoid combination fractures with an ADI ≥ 5 mm
   B. C1-hangman's combination fractures with C2-3 angulation ≥ 11°

* loss of integrity of the C1 ring may necessitate modification of the surgical technique

† these injuries are potentially unstable (see *Axis (C2) fractures* on page 724)

Only 1 nonunion (C1-Type II odontoid, treated initially with halo). No new neuro deficits.

Table 25-24 Treatment options for combination C1-C2 injuries

Injury	Treatment options
C1 + hangman's	
stable	collar, halo, surgery*
untable (C2-3 angulation ≥ 11°)	halo, surgery
C1 + Type II odontoid fracture	
stable (ADI* < 5 mm)	collar, halo, surgery
unstable (ADI ≥ 5 mm	halo, surgery
C1 + Type III odontoid fracture	halo
C1 + miscellaneous C2	collar, halo

* abbreviations: ADI = atlantodental interval; surgery = surgical fixation & fusion

25.6.7.   Subaxial (C3 through C7) injuries/fractures

SPINAL CORD INJURY WITHOUT RADIOGRAPHIC ABNORMALITY (SCIWORA)

PRACTICE PARAMETER 25-16 SCIWORA

Diagnosis

Options[148]
- recommended: plain C-spine x-rays and spinal CT through the suspected level of injury to R/O occult fractures
- MRI of the region of suspected injury may provide useful diagnostic information
- consider: plain x-rays of the entire spinal column
- ✖ not recommended: spinal angiography or myelography

Treatment

Options[148]
- recommended: external immobilization until stability is confirmed with flexion-extension x-rays
- consider: external immobilization of the injured spinal segment for up to 12 weeks
- consider: avoidance of "high-risk" activities for up to 6 months after SCIWORA

Prognosis

Options[148]
- MRI through the region of neurologic injury may provide useful information about neurologic outcome after SCIWORA

Although spinal cord injuries are uncommon in children, there is a subgroup of these in which no radiographic evidence of bony or ligamentous disruption can be demonstrated (including on dynamic flexion-extension x-rays). This is attributed to the normally increased elasticity of the spinous ligaments and paravertebral soft-tissue in the young population[149]. The age range of children with SCIWORA is 1.5-16 yrs, it has a much higher incidence in age ≤ 9 yrs[11]. The spinal cord may undergo contusion, transection, infarction, stretch injuries, or meningeal rupture. Additional etiologies include: blunt abdominal trauma with disruption of bloodflow from the aorta or segmental branches, traumatic disc herniation. There may be an increased risk of SCIWORA among young children with asymptomatic Chiari I malformation[150].

54% of children had a delay between injury (at which time some children experience transient numbness, paresthesias, Lhermitte's sign, or a feeling of total body weakness) and the onset of objective sensorimotor dysfunction ("latent period") ranging from 30 minutes to 4 days.

Radiographic evaluation

In addition to plain films and flexion-extension films (to identify overt instability which would require surgical fusion), should include MRI which may show increased signal within the spinal cord parenchyma on T2WI. There were no intraspinal space occupying lesions in 13 patients studied with myelography/CT[149].

Management

Surgical intervention, including laminectomy, has shown no benefit in the few cases where it has been tried[152].

Due to a 20% rate of repeat injury (some due to trivial trauma, and some without identifiable trauma) within 10 weeks of the original trauma when treated with only a rigid collar and restriction of contacts sports (both for 2 months), more aggressive measures have been recommended (*see Table 25-25*).

Table 25-25   Treatment protocol for SCIWORA
(modified[151])

- admit patient to hospital (helps emphasize seriousness of injury)
- BR with rigid cervical collar until flexion-extension films are normal
- MRI of cervical spine to document presence of spinal cord injury
- detailed discussion with patient and family about seriousness of injury and rationale for treatment outlined here
- immobilization in Guilford brace for 3 months*
- prohibition of contact and noncontact sports
- regular follow-up visits for monitoring condition and compliance
- liberalize activities at 3 months if flexion-extension films are normal

*   this represents a conservative recommendation, a less restrictive recommendation is immobilization for 1-3 weeks[152] (see *PRACTICE PARAMETER 25-16 SCIWORA*)

CLAY SHOVELER'S FRACTURE

Avulsion of spinous processes (usually C7) first described in Perth, Australia (pathomechanics: during the throwing phase of shovelling, clay may stick to the shovel jerking the trapezius and other muscles which are attached to cervical spinous processes)[153]. Can also occur with: whiplash injury[154], injuries that jerk the arms upwards (e.g. catching oneself in falling), neck hyperflexion, or a direct blow to the spinous process.

This fracture is stable, and by itself poses little risk. If the patient is intact, they should have further study (flexion-extension C-spine x-rays or CT scan through the affected level) to R/O other occult fractures. A rigid collar is used PRN pain.

FRACTURE CLASSIFICATION ON THE BASIS OF MECHANISM OF INJURY

A system adapted from the one of Allen et al.[155] divides cervical spine fracture/dislocations into 8 major groups based on the dominant loading force and neck position at the time of injury as shown in *Table 25-26*. Grades of severity within each group are described, and any of these fractures may also be associated with rotatory loads.

Table 25-26   Examples of types of cervical spine injuries*

Major load-ing force	Acting alone	With compression	With distraction
Flexion (734)	unilateral or bilateral facet dislocation (736)	• anterior VB fx. with kyphosis • disruption of inter-spinous ligament • teardrop fx. (734)	• torn posterior ligaments (may be occult) • dislocated or locked facets (736)
Extension† (738)	fractured spinous process and possibly lamina†	fracture through facet region† (including horizontilization of facet) (738)	disruption of ALL with retrolisthesis of superior vertebrae on inferior one†
Neutral position		burst fracture (734)	complete ligamentous disruption (very unstable)

*   abbreviations: ALL = anterior longitudinal ligament; VB = vertebral body; fx = fracture; numbers in parentheses are page numbers for that topic

†   in the presence of stenosis, any of the extension injuries may produce a central cord syndrome

Stability

Guidelines for determination of *biomechanical* instability (*see page 698*) of the subaxial cervical spine published by White and Panjabi[1 (p 314)] are shown in *Table 25-27*. In general, compromise of anterior elements produces more instability in extension, whereas compromise of the posterior elements produces more instability in flexion (important in patient transfers and immobilization). NB: certain conditions such as ankylosing spondylitis may cause an otherwise stable injury to be unstable (*see page 343*).

VERTICAL COMPRESSION INJURIES

In order to apply a purely compressive force to the cervical spine, reversal of the normal cervical lordosis is required, as may occur in a slightly flexed posture. Burst fractures are the most common result, with the possibility of retropulsion of bone into the spinal canal.

FLEXION INJURIES OF THE SUBAXIAL SPINE

Constitutes up to 15% of cervical spine trauma. Common causes include: MVAs, falls from a height, and diving into shallow water[157].

COMPRESSION FLEXION INJURIES
The classic diving injury is the prototypical example. Posterior element fractures occur in up to 50% of compression flexion injuries[158]. Although flexion-compression injuries do distract the posterior elements to some degree, most do not produce posterior ligamentous injuries. Subtypes include: teardrop fractures (*see below*), quadrangular fractures (*see page 735*).
Treatment: mild cervical compression fractures without neurologic deficit or retropulsion of bone into the spinal canal are usually treated with a rigid orthosis until x-rays show healing has occurred (usually 6-12 wks). Stability is assessed with flexion-extension views (*see page 708*) before discontinuing the brace. More severe compression fractures heal in a halo brace with ≈ 90% rate of ankylosing fusion.

Table 25-27 Guidelines for diagnosing clinical instability of the mid & lower C-spine[1]

Item	Points*
anterior elements† destroyed or unable to function	2
posterior elements† destroyed or unable to function	2
positive **stretch test**‡	2
spinal cord damage	2
nerve root damage	1
abnormal disc narrowing	1
developmentally narrow spinal canal, either • sagittal diameter < 13 mm, OR • Pavlov ratio§ < 0.8	1
dangerous loading anticipatedΔ	1
Radiographic criteria	
• neutral position x-rays	
sagittal plane displacement > 3.5 mm or 20%	2
relative sagittal plane angulation > 11°	2
OR	
• flexion-extension x-rays	
sagittal plane translation > 3.5 mm or 20%	2
sagittal plane rotation > 20°	2
Unstable if total ≥ 5	

* if there is inadequate information for any item, add half of the value for that item to the total

† in the C-spine, posterior elements = anatomic components posterior to the posterior longitudinal ligament

‡ stretch test: apply incremental cervical traction loads of 10 lbs q 5 mins up to 33% body wt. (65 lbs max). Check X-ray and neuro exam after each Δ. Positive if Δ in separation > 1.7 mm or Δ angle > 7.5° on x-ray or change in neuro exam. This test is contraindicated if obvious instability

§ **Pavlov ratio** = the ratio of (distance from the midlevel of the posterior VB to the closest point on the spinolaminar line) : (the AP diameter of the middle of the VB)

Δ e.g. heavy laborers, contact sports athletes, motorcyclists

---

PRACTICE PARAMETER 25-17 SUBAXIAL FRACTURE-DISLOCATIONS*

Options[156]
- initial treatment: closed or open reduction is recommended
- subsequent treatment: rigid external immobilization, anterior arthrodesis with plate fixation, or posterior arthrodesis with plate or rod fixation

* excluding facet dislocations, *see page 737* for those injuries

---

TEARDROP FRACTURES
Originally described by Schneider & Kahn[159]. Results from hyperflexion or axial loading at the vertex of the skull with the neck flexed (eliminating the normal cervical lordosis)[160] (often mistakenly attributed to hyperextension because of the retrolisthesis). There are varying degrees of severity. Pathologically, the injury consists of complete disruption of all of the ligaments, the facet joints and the intervertebral disk[161]. An important feature is displacement of the inferior margin of the fractured vertebral body

---

posteriorly into the spinal canal[159]. Usually unstable.

Seen in ≈ 5% of patients in a large series with x-ray evidence of cervical spine trauma[73]. Patients are often quadriplegic, although some may be intact and some may have anterior cervical cord syndrome (*see page 716*). Possible associated injuries and radiographic findings include[161, 162]:

1. a small chip of bone (the "teardrop") just beyond the anterior inferior edge of the involved vertebral body (**VB**) on lateral cervical spine film
2. often associated with a fracture through the sagittal plane of the VB which can almost always be seen on AP view. Thin cut CT scan is more sensitive
3. a large triangular fragment of the anterior inferior VB
4. other fractures through the vertebral body may also occur
5. the fractured vertebrae is usually displaced <u>posteriorly</u> on the vertebra below (easily appreciated on oblique x-rays, see *Figure 25-11*, page 737). However, cases without retrolisthesis are also described[158]
6. the fractured body is often wedged anteriorly (kyphosis), and may also be wedged laterally
7. disruption of the facet joints which may be appreciated as separation of the joints on lateral x-ray, often unmasked by cervical traction
8. prevertebral soft-tissue swelling (*see page 141*, for measurements)
9. narrowing of the intervertebral disc below the fracture (indicating disruption)

Distinguishing between teardrop fracture and avulsion fracture

Rationale: Teardrop fractures must be distinguished from a simple **avulsion fracture** of a small chip of bone which may also result in a small chip of bone off the anterior inferior VB, usually pulled off by traction of the anterior longitudinal ligament (**ALL**) in hyper<u>extension</u>. Although there may be disruption of the ALL in these cases, it does not usually cause instability.

Methodology: In a patient with a small bone chip off of the inferior anterior VB, a "teardrop" fracture needs to be ruled-out. Determine if the following criteria are met:

* neurologically intact (because of the need for cooperation, this includes mental status, and excludes the inebriated or concussed patient)
* size of bone fragment is small
* no malalignment of vertebral bodies
* no evidence of VB fracture in sagittal plane on AP C-spine x-rays or on CT
* no posterior element fracture on x-ray or CT
* no prevertebral soft tissue swelling at level of fragment (*see page 141*)
* and no loss of vertebral body height or disc space height

If the above criteria are met, obtain flexion-extension C-spine x-rays (see *Flexion-extension cervical spine x-rays*, page 708). If no abnormal movement, discharge patient in rigid collar (e.g. Philadelphia collar), and repeat the films in 4-7 days (i.e. after the pain has subsided to be certain that alignment is not being maintained by cervical muscle spasm from pain), D/C collar if 2nd set of films is normal.

If the patient does not meet the above criteria, treat them as an unstable fracture and obtain a CT scan through the fractured vertebra to evaluate for associated fractures (e.g. sagittal plane fracture that may not be apparent on plain x-ray).

MRI assesses the integrity of the disc and gives some information about the posterior ligaments.

Treatment of teardrop fracture

If the disc and ligaments are intact (determined by MRI) then an option is to employ a halo brace until the fragment is healed (perform flexion-extension x-rays after removing the halo to rule-out persistent instability). Alternatively, surgical stabilization may be performed, especially if ligamentous or disc injury is seen on MRI. When the injury is primarily posterior due to disruption of the posterior ligaments and facet joints, and if there is no anterior compromise of the spinal canal, then a posterior fusion suffices. Severe injuries with canal compromise often require a combined anterior decompression and fusion (performed first) followed by posterior fusion using either a modified Bohlman triple-wire technique or lateral mass plates.

QUADRANGULAR FRACTURES[163]

Four features:

1. oblique vertebral body (**VB**) fracture passing from anterior-superior cortical margin to inferior end plate
2. posterior subluxation of superior VB on the inferior VB

---

3. angular kyphosis
4. disruption of disc and anterior and posterior ligaments

Treatment: May require combined anterior and posterior fusion.

DISTRACTION FLEXION INJURIES

Ranges from hyperflexion sprain (mild, *see below*) to minor subluxation (moderate) to bilateral locked facets (severe, *see below*). Posterior ligaments are injured early and are usually evidenced by widening of the interspinous distance (*see page 142*).

HYPERFLEXION SPRAIN

A purely ligamentous injury that involves disruption of the posterior ligamentous complex without bony fracture. May be missed on plain lateral C-spine x-rays if they are obtained in normal alignment (requires flexion-extension views, see *Flexion-extension cervical spine x-rays*, page 708). Instability may be concealed when films are obtained shortly after the injury if spasm of the cervical paraspinal muscles splints the neck and prevents true flexion[164]. For patients with limited flexion, a rigid collar should be prescribed, and if the pain persists 1-2 weeks later the films should be repeated (including flexion-extension).

Radiographic signs of hyperflexion sprain[165] (x-rays may also be normal):
1. kyphotic angulation
2. anterior rotation and/or slight (1-3 mm) subluxation
3. anterior narrowing and posterior widening of the disc space
4. increased distance between the posterior cortex of the subluxed vertebral body and the anterior cortex of the articular masses of the subjacent vertebra
5. anterior and superior displacement of the superior facets (causing widening of the facet joint)
6. fanning (abnormal widening) of the interspinous space on lateral C-spine x-ray, or increased interspinous distance on AP (see *Interspinous distances*, page 142)

SUBLUXATION

Cadaver studies have shown that horizontal subluxation **> 3.5 mm** of one vertebral body on another, or > 11° of angulation of one vertebral body relative to the next indicates ligamentous instability[166, 167] (see *Table 25-27*, page 734). Thus, if subluxation of ≤ 3.5 mm on plain films is seen, and there is no neuro deficit, obtain flexion-extension films (see *Flexion-extension cervical spine x-rays*, page 708). If no abnormal movement, remove cervical collar.

LOCKED FACETS

Severe flexion injuries can result in **locked facets** (AKA "sprung" facets AKA "jumped" facets) with reversal of the normal "shingled" relationship between facets (normally the inferior facet of the level above is posterior to the superior facet of the level below). Involves disruption of facet capsule. Facets that have not completely locked but have had significant ligamentous disruption allowing distraction just short of the point of locking are known as **"perched facets"**.

Flexion + rotation → unilateral locked facets. Hyperflexion → bilateral locked facets.

Unilateral locked facets: 25% of patients are neurologically intact, 37% have root deficit, 22% have incomplete cord injuries, and 15% are complete quadriplegics[168].

Bilateral locked facets: Occurs with disruption of ligaments of apophyseal joints, ligamentum flavum, longitudinal and interspinous

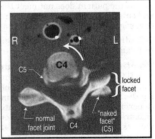

Figure 25-10 Locked facet (left C4-5). (CT scan). Note the rotation of the C4 vertebral body on C5 (curved arrow)

ligaments, and the anulus. Rare. Most common at C5-6 or C6-7. 65-87% have complete quadriplegia, 13-25% incomplete, ≤ 10% are intact. Adjacent fractures (VB, facet, lamina, pedicle...) occur in 40-60%[155, 169]. Nerve root deficits may also occur.

Diagnosis

C-spine x-rays: both unilateral **(ULF)** and bilateral locked facets **(BLF)** will produce subluxation (ULF → rotatory subluxation).

BLF: usually produces > 50% subluxation on lateral C-spine x-ray.

ULF:

1. AP: spinous processes above the subluxation rotate to the same side as the locked facet (with respect to those below)
2. lateral: **"bow-tie sign"** (visualization of left & right facets at the level of the injury instead of the normal superimposed position[168]). Subluxation may be seen. Disruption of the posterior ligamentous complex may produce widening of the interspace between spinous processes

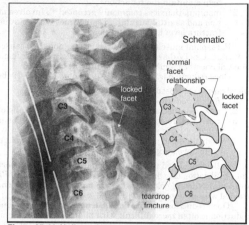

Figure 25-11 Unilateral locked facets (left C4 on C5) & C5 **teardrop fracture** (*see page 734*)
60° LAO C-spine x-ray on left, and schematic on right (sagittally oriented VB fracture through C5 seen on CT scan, not shown). Note the anterior subluxation of C4 on C5, and the slight retrolisthesis of C5 on C6

3. oblique (*see Figure 25-11*): may demonstrate the locked facet which will be seen blocking the neural foramen (use ≈ 60° LAO for left locked facet, 60° RAO for right)

CT: "naked facet sign": the articular surface of the facet will be seen with the appropriate articulating mate either absent or on the wrong side of the facet (*see Figure 25-10*). With ULF, CT also demonstrates the rotation of the level above anteriorly on the level below on the side of the locked facet.

MRI: the best test to rule-out traumatic disc herniation (found in 80% of BLF)[170], but if obtaining the MRI delays reduction or surgery, the potential benefit is controversial.

Treatment

PRACTICE PARAMETER 25-18 SUBAXIAL FACET DISLOCATIONS

Options[156]
- initial treatment: closed or open reduction is recommended
- subsequent treatment
  - A. rigid external immobilization, anterior arthrodesis with plate fixation, or posterior arthrodesis with plate or rod or interlaminar clamp fixation
  - B. prolonged bedrest in traction if the above treatment options are not available

---

Closed reduction of locked facets: Two methods:

1. traction: more commonly employed in the U.S. Initial weight (in lbs) ≈ **3 x cervical vertebral level**, increase in 5-10 lb increments usually at 10-15 minute intervals until desired alignment is attained (assess neurologic exam and lateral C-spine x-ray or fluoroscopy after each Δ to avoid overdistraction). Under most circumstances, **do not exceed 10 lbs per vertebral level** (some say 5 lbs/level). Stop if occipitocervical instability is demonstrated or if any disc space height exceeds 10 mm (overdistraction). With unilateral locked facets, one may add gentle manual torsion <u>towards</u> the side of the locked facets. With bilateral locked facets, one may add gentle manual posterior tension (e.g. with a rolled towel under the occiput). Once the facets are perched or distracted, gradual reduction of the

weights will usually result in reduction (placing the neck in slight extension may help maintain the reduction)

2. manipulation: less commonly accepted[168]. Involves manually applying axial traction and sagittal angulation sometimes with rotation and direct pressure at the fracture level under fluoroscopy

Paraspinal muscle relaxation (but not enough to cause obtundation) may assist in reduction. Use IV diazepam (Valium®) and/or narcotic (e.g. meperidine (Demerol®)). General anesthesia may be used in difficult cases.

Once reduction is achieved, the patient is left in 5-10 lbs of traction for stabilization.

Disadvantage of closed reduction
1. fails to reduce ≈ 25% of cases of BLF
2. risks overdistraction at higher levels or worsening of other fractures
3. risk of neurologic deterioration due to compression by traumatically herniated disc[169]
4. adds time and potentially pain to the patient's care, especially since many will go on to have surgical fusion anyway

Following closed reduction, the need for internal (operative) stabilization vs. external stabilization (i.e. bracing) may be addressed (see *Stabilization* below). Neurologic worsening following closed reduction may occur with disc herniation[171] and should be treated with prompt discectomy.

Open reduction and fixation is usually required if reduction is not achieved. Closed reduction is often more difficult with bilateral locked facets than with unilateral.

Open reduction of locked facets: Stabilization: Surgical fusion is commonly performed after successful closed reduction, failed closed reduction, or following open reduction.

If there are fracture fragments about the articular surfaces, there may be satisfactory healing with halo vest immobilization (for 3 months) once closed reduction is achieved[172]. Frequent x-rays are needed to rule-out redislocation[173]. Flexion-extension x-rays are obtained upon halo removal and surgery is required for continued instability. Up to 77% of patients with unilateral or bilateral facet dislocation (with or without facet fracture fragments) will have a poor anatomic result with halo vest alone (although late instability was uncommon), suggesting that surgery should be considered for all of these patients[174]. Surgical fusion is more clearly indicated in cases without facet fracture fragments (ligamentous instability alone may not heal) or if open reduction is required.

If surgery is indicated, an MRI should be done beforehand if possible. A posterior approach is preferred if there are no anterior masses (such as traumatic disc herniation or large osteophytic spurs), if subluxation of the bodies is > one third the VB width (suggesting severe posterior ligamentous injury), or for fractures of the posterior elements. A posterior approach is mandatory if there is an unreducible dislocation. Options for posterior approach: see *Choice of posterior technique*, page 740.

EXTENSION INJURIES OF THE SUBAXIAL SPINE

EXTENSION INJURY WITHOUT BONY INJURY

In the presence of cervical spondylosis, extension injuries can produce spinal cord injury without any evidence of bony injury. Injury patterns include central cord syndrome (*see page 714*) usually in the older adult, and SCIWORA (*see page 732*) usually in young children. Middle aged adults with hyperextension dislocations that reduce spontaneously immediately may present with spinal cord injury and no bony abnormality on x-ray, but there may be rupture of the anterior longitudinal ligament and/or intervertebral disc on MRI or autopsy. Extension forces may also be associated with carotid artery dissections (*see page 885*).

HORIZONTAL FACET OR SEPARATION FRACTURE OF THE ARTICULAR MASS

Extension combined with compression and rotation may produce fracture of one pedicle and one lamina which permits the detached articular mass to rotate forward to a more horizontal orientation[175] (horizontilization of the facet). May be associated with rupture of the ALL and fissure of the disc at one or two levels. Unstable. Neuro deficit is common.

25.6.8.   Treatment of subaxial cervical spine fractures

Management of some types of C-spine fractures is covered in the preceding sections. Also, see *subaxial fracture-dislocations*, page 734. For injuries not specifically addressed, general management principles are as follows[1]:

1. immobilize and reduce externally (if possible): may use traction x 0-7 days
2. determine if there is an indication for decompression as soon as practical (clinical conditions permitting), and decompress if needed. Although controversial, the following are generally accepted indications for acute decompression in patients *without* complete spinal cord injury:
   A. radiographic evidence of bone or foreign material in the spinal canal with associated spinal cord symptoms
   B. complete block on CT, myelogram or MRI
   C. clinical judgement: e.g. a progressive incomplete spinal cord injury where the surgeon believes that decompression would be beneficial
3. ascertain stability of the injury (*see page 733*)
   A. stable fractures: treat in non-halo orthosis for 1-6 weeks (*see page 741*)
   B. unstable fractures: all of the following choices are appropriate, with little evidence to recommend one scheme over another in most cases
      1. traction x 7 weeks, followed by orthosis x 8 weeks
      2. halo x 11 weeks, followed by orthosis x 4 weeks
      3. surgical fusion, followed by orthosis x 15 weeks
      4. surgical fusion with internal immobilization (plates, screws...) ± orthosis for short period of time (≈ several weeks)

SURGICAL TREATMENT

IN PATIENTS WITH COMPLETE SPINAL CORD LESIONS

Operating on a patient with a complete cord injury does not result in significant recovery of neurologic function[121]. However, aggressive non-surgical reduction of traumatic subluxation should be pursued.

The primary goal of surgery in this setting is spinal stabilization, allowing the patient to be placed in a sitting position for improved pulmonary function, for psychological benefit, and to allow initiation of rehabilitation. Although the spine will fuse spontaneously in many cases (taking ≈ 8-12 weeks), surgical stabilization expedites the mobilization process and reduces the risk of delayed kyphotic angulation deformity. Early surgery may lead to further neurological injury, and should be delayed until the patient has stabilized medically and neurologically. In most cases, performing surgery within 4-5 days (if the patient is otherwise stable) is probably early enough to help reduce pulmonary complications.

IN PATIENTS WITH INCOMPLETE LESIONS

Patients with incomplete cord injuries who have compromise of the spinal canal (by bone, disc, unreducible subluxation or hematoma) and either do not improve with nonoperative therapy or deteriorate neurologically should undergo surgical decompression and stabilization[121]. This may facilitate some further return of spinal cord function. An exception may be the central cord syndrome (*see page 714*).

ANTERIOR OR POSTERIOR?

The choice of technique depends to a large degree on the mechanism of injury, as the treatment should tend to counteract the instability, and ideally should not compromise structures that are still functioning. Instrumentation (wires/cables, plates, clamps...) immobilize the area of instability while bony fusion is occurring. In the absence of bony fusion, all mechanical devices will eventually fail, and so it becomes a "race" between fusion and instrument failure. Extensive injuries (including teardrop fractures (*see page 734*) and compression burst fractures) may require a combined anterior and posterior approach (staged, or in a single sitting; anterior decompression precedes posterior fusion).

Indications: The procedure of choice for most flexion injuries. Useful when there is minimal injury to the vertebral bodies and in the absence of anterior compression of the spinal cord and nerves. Including: posterior ligamentous instability, traumatic subluxation, unilateral or bilateral locked facets, simple wedge compression fractures.

The most common technique consists of open or closed reduction, followed by lateral mass plates/rods or wiring and fusion. Interlaminar Halifax clamps are an[176]. Although successes have been reported using methylmethacrylate[177], it does not bond to bone and weakens with age, and thus its use in the setting of traumatic injury is discouraged[178].

Choice of posterior technique: If the anterior column is capable of weight-bearing and the posterior elements are not damaged or absent, wiring and fusion provides adequate stability. If the anterior weight-bearing column is significantly damaged, or if there is absence or compromise of the lamina or spinous processes, then either a combined anterior-posterior approach is needed or posterior instrumentation (e.g. lateral mass screw-plate or rod fixation) with fusion is recommended[179].

ANTERIOR APPROACH

Indications:
1. fractured vertebral body with bone retropulsed into the spinal canal
2. most extension injuries
3. severe fractures of posterior elements that preclude posterior stabilization and fusion

Usually consists of:
1. corpectomy: decompresses the neural elements (if necessary) and removes fractured and structurally compromised bone

AND
2. strut graft fusion: replaces the involved body or bodies with either:
   A. bone (usually iliac crest, rib or fibula, either homologous or cadaveric)
   B. or titanium cage
3. usually accompanied with compression plates
4. usually followed with external immobilization

POSTERIOR CERVICAL PLATES (AKA LATERAL MASS PLATES OR RODS)

Indications and use:
1. for internal stabilization for fusion when the posterior elements are compromised
   A. in the presence of laminectomy[180]
   B. with laminar fractures
2. for posterior stabilization when the anterior weight-bearing column is damaged (in which case wiring alone does not provide adequate stabilization)[179]
3. for cervicothoracic instability[181]: avoids the need to split the sternum to gain anterior access to upper T-spine. NB: the C7-T1 junction is a difficult location for lateral mass plates because of the large forces at this level[182]

COMPLICATIONS OF SURGICAL TREATMENT
1. hardware problems
   A. wire failure
      1. improper wire gauge for type of fracture
      2. improper wire-handling
      3. inadequate post-operative immobilization
         a. improper brace selected
         b. poor patient compliance with immobilization device
   B. problems with plating
      1. screw pull-out or loosening
      2. fatigue fracture of plate
      3. screw injury: nerve root, spinal cord or vertebral artery
2. failure of graft to take
3. judgmental error
   A. failure to incorporate all unstable levels
   B. improper surgical approach

ANTERIOR CERVICAL FUSION

May be used in cases with traumatic subluxation of the cervical spine. Does not depend on integrity of posterior elements to achieve stability.

CERVICAL BRACING

COLLARS

Soft (sponge rubber) collar: does not immobilize the cervical spine to any significant degree. Its function is primarily to remind the patient to reduce neck movements.

Philadelphia collar: inadequate for stabilizing the upper and mid-cervical spine and for preventing rotation.

POSTER BRACES

Distinguished from cervicothoracic orthoses by the lack of straps under the axilla. Includes the four poster brace. Generally good for preventing flexion at midcervical levels.

CERVICOTHORACIC ORTHOSES

Cervicothoracic orthoses (**CTO**) incorporate some form of body vest to immobilize the cervical spine. The following are presented in increasing degree of immobilization.

Guilford brace: essentially a ring around the occiput and chin connected by two posts to anterior and posterior thoracic pads.

SOMI brace: acronym for Sternal Occipital Mandibular Immobilization. Good for bracing against flexion (especially upper cervical spine). Inadequate for hyper-extension type injuries because of weak occipital support. Has special forehead attachment to allow patient to eat comfortably without mandibular support.

"Yale brace": a sort of extended Philadelphia collar. The most effective CTO for bracing against flexion-extension and rotation. Major shortcoming is poor prevention of lateral flexion (only ~ 50% reduced).

HALO-VEST BRACE

Can immobilize the upper or lower cervical spine, not very good for mid-cervical spine. Unable to provide adequate distraction support following vertebral body resection when patient assumes upright position (i.e. it is not a portable cervical traction device).

FOLLOW-UP SCHEDULE

After initial management (surgical or nonsurgical) of cervical spine problems (stable or unstable) the follow-up schedule shown in *Table 25-28* is suggested to permit recognition of problems in time for treatment[1]. The schedule is initiated following removal of brace, cast, completion of bed rest and initial physical therapy.

Table 25-28 Follow-up schedule

1.	3 weeks
2.	6 weeks
3.	3 months
4.	6 months
5.	1 year

25.6.9. Sports related cervical spine injuries

Any of the previously described injuries can be sports related. This section considers injuries peculiar to sports. Also *see page 633* for sports-related head injuries.

Bailes et al.[183] classified sports-related spinal cord injuries (**SCI**) as shown in *Table 25-29*. Type II injuries include spinal concussion, spinal neuropraxia (*see below*), and the burning hands syndrome (*see below*), all in the absence of radiographic abnormalities and all with complete resolution of symptoms. Patients should be carefully evaluated, and return to competition should not be allowed in the presence of neurologic deficit, radiographically demon-

Table 25-29 Sports-related spinal cord injuries

Type	Description
I	permanent SCI
II	transient SCI without radiographic abnormality
III	radiologic abnormality without neurologic deficit

strated injury, certain congenital C-spine abnormalities, and possibly for "repeat offenders" (see *Return to play and pre-participation guidelines*, page 743). Type III injuries are the most common. Unstable injuries should be treated appropriately (*see page 739*).

Table 25-30 C-spine-related contraindications for participation in contact sports*

Condition†	C.I.‡
Congenital§	
1. odontoid abnormalities (serious injury may result from atlanto-axial instability)	
A. complete aplasia (rare)	absolute
B. hypoplasia (seen in conjunction with achondroplasia and spondyloepiphyseal dysplasia)	absolute
C. os odontoideum (probably of traumatic origin)	absolute
2. atlanto-occipital fusion (partial or complete fusion of atlas to occiput): sudden onset of symptoms & sudden death have been reported	absolute
3. Klippel-Feil anomaly (congenital fusion of 2 or more cervical vertebrae)Δ	
A. Type I: mass fusion of C-spine to upper T-spine	absolute
B. Type II: fusion of only 1 or 2 interspaces	
1. associated with limited ROM, occipitocervical anomalies, instability, disc disease or degenerative changes	absolute
2. associated with full ROM and none of the above	none
Acquired	
1. cervical spinal stenosis¶	
A. asymptomatic	none
B. with one episode of cord neuropraxia	relative
C. cord neuropraxia + MRI evidence of cord defect or edema	absolute
D. cord neuropraxia + ligamentous instability, symptoms or neurologic findings > 36 hrs, or multiple episodes	absolute
2. spear tackler's spine (*see text*)	absolute
3. spina bifida occulta: rare, incidental x-ray finding	none
Post-traumatic upper cervical spine	
1. atlantoaxial instability (ADI > 3 mm adults, > 4 mm peds)	absolute
2. atlantoaxial rotatory fixation (may be associated with disruption of transverse ligament)	absolute
3. fractures	
A. healed, pain-free, full ROM, & no neurologic findings with any of the following fractures: nondisplaced Jefferson fracture; odontoid fracture; or lateral mass fracture of axis	none
B. all others	absolute
4. post-surgical atlantoaxial fusion	absolute
Post-traumatic subaxial cervical spine	
1. ligamentous injuries: > 3.5 mm subluxation, or > 11° angulation on flexion-extension views	absolute
2. fractures	
A. healed, stable fractures listed here with normal exam: VB compression fracture without posterior involvement; spinous process fractures	none
B. VB fractures with sagittal component or posterior bony or ligamentous involvement	absolute
C. comminuted fracture with displacement into spinal canal	absolute
D. lateral mass fracture producing facet incongruity	absolute
3. intervertebral disc injury	
A. healed herniated disc treated conservatively	none
B. S/P ACDF with solid fusion, no symptoms, normal exam and full pain-free ROM	none
C. chronic herniated disc with pain, neuro findings or ↓ ROM, or acute herniated disc	absolute
4. S/P fusion	
A. stable one-level fusion	none
B. stable two-level fusion	relative
C. fusion > 2 levels	absolute

* organized contact sports[187]: boxing, football, ice hockey, lacrosse, rugby & wrestling

†   also *see page 633* for cranial-related (and craniocervical) conditions (e.g. Chiari I malformation…)

‡   C.I. = contraindications, classified as absolute, relative (i.e. uncertain) or none

§   congenital abnormalities may have particular relevance to *Special Olympics*

Δ   NB: Klippel-Feil may be associated with abnormalities in other organ systems (e.g. cardiac) which may impact on participation in contact sports (*see page 119*)

¶   Pavlov ratio (*see page 334*) has a low positive predictive value for injuries in contact sports and is therefore not a useful screening test (i.e. an asymptomatic Pavlov ratio < 0.8 is not a contraindication to participation)

FOOTBALL-RELATED CERVICAL SPINE INJURIES

Football players with suspected C-spine injury should not have their helmet removed in the field (*see page 702*). The following terms probably originated as locker-room jargon for various cervical spine-related injuries usually sustained in playing football. Medical definitions have subsequently been retro-fitted to them. As a result, the precise definitions may not be uniformly agreed upon. Although the semantics may differ, it is more important from a diagnostic and therapeutic standpoint to distinguish nerve root injuries, brachial plexus injuries, and spinal cord injuries.

1. **cervical cord neuropraxia**[184] **(CCN)**: sensory changes which may involve numbness, tingling or burning. May or may not be associated with motor symptoms of weakness or complete paralysis. Typically lasts < 15 mins (although may persist up to 48 hrs), involves all 4 extremities in 80%. Narrowing of the sagittal diameter of the cervical spinal canal is felt to be contributory. With resumption of contact activities, recurrence rate is ≈ 56%, with higher risks of recurrence among those with narrower canals. Evaluation should include cervical MRI. Torg[184] feels that uncomplicated cases of CCN (no spinal instability and no MRI evidence of cord defect or edema) have a low risk of permanent injury and does not recommend activity restrictions

2. **"stinger"** or **"burner"**: distinct from the burning hands syndrome. Unilateral. Burning dysesthetic pain radiating down one arm from the shoulder, sometimes associated with weakness involving the C5 or C6 nerve roots. Usually follows a tackle. May result from downward traction on the upper trunk of the brachial plexus or by direct nerve root compression in the neural foramina (not a SCI)

3. **burning hands syndrome**[185]: similar to a stinger, but bilateral. Represents a SCI (possibly a mild variant of a central cord syndrome, *see page 714*)

4. other neurologic injuries include: vascular injury to carotid or vertebral arteries. Usually related to intimal dissection (*see page 883*) following a direct blow to the neck or by extreme movements. Symptoms are those of a TIA or CVA

Spear tackler's spine

Rule changes in 1976 banned spearing (the practice of using the football helmet as a battering ram to tackle an opponent) and resulted in a reduction of the number of football-related occurrences of cervical spine fractures and quadriplegia[186].

Four characteristics of spear tackler's spine:
1. cervical spinal stenosis
2. loss of normal cervical lordosis
3. evidence of pre-existing traumatic abnormalities
4. documented spear-tackler's technique

Suggested management:

The athlete is removed from competition until the cervical lordosis returns and the player learns to use other tackling techniques.

RETURN TO PLAY AND PRE-PARTICIPATION GUIDELINES

Return to play **(RTP)** and pre-participation evaluation guidelines related to the cervical spine are shown in *Table 25-30* (modified[187]). These are just guidelines, and do not insure safety. Clinical judgement must always be employed.

25.6.10.   Delayed cervical instability

Definition (adapted[188]): cervical instability that is not recognized until beyond 20 days after the injury. The instability itself may be delayed, or the recognition may be delayed. Reasons for delayed cervical instability:
1. inadequate radiologic evaluation[37]
    A. incomplete studies (e.g. must see all the way to C7-T1 junction)
    B. suboptimal studies: motion artifact, incorrect positioning… Etiologies in-

clude: poor patient cooperation as a result of agitation/intoxication, portable films, poor technique...

2. abnormality missed on x-ray
   A. overlooked fracture, subluxation
   B. injury failed to be demonstrated despite sufficiently adequate x-rays[188A]
      1. type of fracture not demonstrated on the radiographs obtained
      2. patient positioning (e.g. supine) may reduce some malalignment
      3. spasm of cervical muscles may reduce and/or stabilize the injury
      4. microfractures
3. inadequate models: some findings may be judged to be stable using certain models, but in the long-run may be unstable (there is no perfect model for instability)

Further studies or repeat x-rays several weeks after the trauma should be considered in patients with neurologic deficit, persistent pain, significant degenerative changes when the original films were suboptimal, subluxations < 3 mm, or when surgery is contemplated[189].

25.6.11. Blunt vertebral artery injuries

> **PRACTICE PARAMETER 25-19** VERTEBRAL ARTERY INJURIES AFTER NONPENETRATING CERVICAL TRAUMA
>
> **Diagnosis**
>
> **Options**[190]: conventional angiography or MRA after nonpenetrating cervical trauma in patients who have complete SCI, fracture through the foramen transversarium, facet dislocation, and/or vertebral subluxation
>
> **Treatment**
>
> **Options**[190]
> - recommended: anticoagulation with IV heparin for vertebral artery injury **(VAI)** with evidence of posterior circulation stroke
> - recommended: either observation or treatment with anticoagulation in for VAI with evidence of posterior ischemia
> - recommended: observation for VAI with no evidence of posterior circulation ischemia

Vertebral artery injury **(VAI)** may be associated with blunt trauma and may produce vertebrobasilar insufficiency **(VBI)**. Fractures through the foramen transversarium, facet fracture-dislocation, or vertebral subluxation are frequently identified in patients with blunt VAI[191-193].

Mechanisms of injury
1. motor vehicle accident: the most common etiology

Treatment
Strokes were more frequent in patients with VAI who were not treated initially with IV heparin despite an asymptomatic VAI[193].

25.7. Thoracolumbar spine fractures

64% of spine fractures occur at the thoracolumbar **(TL)** junction, usually T12-L1. 70% of these occur without immediate neurologic injury.

THREE COLUMN MODEL

Denis' 3 column model of the spine (described below and illustrated in *Figure 25-12*) attempts to identify CT criteria of instability of thoracolumbar spine fractures[194]. This model has generally good predictive value, however, any attempt to create "rules" of in-

---

A. *see page 706* for recommendations of extent of radiologic workup

stability will have some inherent inaccuracy.

1. <u>anterior</u> column: composed of anterior half of disc and vertebral body (**VB**) (includes anterior anulus fibrosus (**AF**)) plus the anterior longitudinal ligament (**ALL**)
2. <u>middle</u> column: posterior half of disc and vertebral body (includes posterior wall of vertebral body and posterior AF) and posterior longitudinal ligament (**PLL**)
3. <u>posterior</u> column: posterior bony complex (posterior arch) with interposed posterior ligamentous complex (supraspinous and interspinous ligament, facet joints and capsule, and ligamentum flavum (**LF**)). Injury to this column alone does <u>not</u> cause instability

CLASSIFICATION INTO MAJOR & MINOR INJURIES

MINOR INJURIES

Involve only a part of a column and do not lead to acute instability (when not accompanied by major injures). Includes:

1. fracture of transverse process: usually neurologically intact except in two areas:
    A. L4-5 → lumbosacral plexus injuries (there may be associated renal injuries, check U/A for blood)
    B. T1-2 → brachial plexus injuries
2. fracture of articular process or pars interarticularis
3. isolated fractures of the spinous process: in the TL spine: these are usually due to direct trauma. Often difficult to detect on plain x-ray

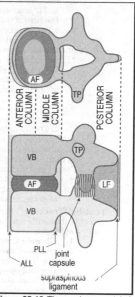

Figure 25-12 Three column model of the spine (TP = transverse process, see text for other abbreviations)
(Adapted from Spine, Denis F, Vol. 8, pp. 317-31, 1983, with permission)

MAJOR INJURIES

The McAfee classification describes 6 main types of fractures[195]. A simplified system with four categories follows (also *see Table 25-31*):

1. **compression fracture**: compression failure of anterior column. Middle column intact (unlike the 3 other major injuries below) acting as a fulcrum,
    A. 2 subtypes:
        1. lateral (rare)
        2. anterior: most common between T6-T8 and T12-L3
            a. lateral x-ray: wedging of the VB anteriorly, no loss of height of posterior VB, no subluxation
            b. CT: spinal canal intact. Disruption of anterior end-plate
    B. clinical: no neurologic deficit
2. **burst fracture**: pure axial load → compression of vertebral body → compression failure of anterior and middle columns. Occur mainly at TL junction, usually between T10 and L2
    A. 5 subtypes (L5 burst fractures may constitute a rare subtype, *see page 748*)
        1. fracture of both end-

Table 25-31 Column failure in the four major types of thoracolumbar spine injuries*

Fracture type	Column		
	Anterior	Middle	Posterior
compression	compression	intact	intact, or distraction if severe
burst	compression	compression	intact
seat-belt	intact or mild compression of 10-20% of anterior VB	distraction	
fracture-dislocation	compression, rotation, shear	distraction, rotation, shear	

* adapted[194] with permission

plates: seen in lower lumbar region (where axial load → increased extension, unlike T-spine where axial load → flexion)
2. fracture of superior end-plate: the most common burst fracture. Seen at TL junction. Mechanism = axial load + flexion
3. fracture of inferior end-plate: rare
4. burst rotation: usually midlumbar. Mechanism = axial load + rotation
5. burst lateral flexion: mechanism = axial load + lateral flexion
B. radiographic evaluation
1. lateral x-ray: cortical fracture of posterior VB wall, loss of posterior VB height, retropulsion of bone fragment from end plate(s) into canal
2. AP x-ray: increase of interpediculate distance (**IPD**), vertical fracture of lamina, splaying of facet joints: ↑ IPD indicates failure of _middle_ column.
3. CT: demonstrates break in posterior wall of VB with retropulsed bone in spinal canal (average: 50% obstruction of canal area), increase in IPD with splaying of posterior arch (including facets)
4. myelogram: large central defect
C. clinical: depends on level (thoracic cord more sensitive and less room in canal than conus region), the impact at the time of disruption, and the extent of canal obstruction
   • ≈ 50% intact at initial examination (half of these recalled leg numbness, tingling, and/or weakness initially after trauma that subsided)
   • of patients with deficits, only 5% had _complete_ paraplegia
3. **seat-belt fracture**[A]: flexion → compression of anterior column & distraction failure of both middle and posterior columns
A. 4 subtypes
1. **Chance fracture**: one level, through bone
2. one level, through ligaments
3. two level, through bone in middle column, through ligament in anterior and posterior columns
4. two level, through ligament in all 3 columns
B. radiographic evaluation
1. plain x-ray: ↑ interspinous distance, pars interarticularis fractures, and horizontal split of pedicles and transverse process. No subluxation
2. CT: poor for this type (most of fracture is in plane of axial CT cuts). May detect pars fracture
C. clinical: no neurologic deficit
4. **fracture-dislocation**: failure of all 3 columns due to compression, tension, rotation or shear → subluxation or dislocation
A. x-ray: occasionally, may be reduced when imaged. Look for other markers of significant trauma (multiple rib fractures, unilateral articular process fractures, spinous process fractures, horizontal laminar fractures)
B. 3 subtypes
1. flexion rotation: posterior and middle columns totally ruptured, anterior compressed → anterior wedging
   a. lateral x-ray: subluxation or dislocation. Preserved posterior VB wall. Increased interspinous distance
   b. CT: rotation and offset of VBs with ↓ canal diameter. Jumped facets
   c. clinical: 25% neurologically intact. 50% of those with deficits were complete paraplegics
2. shear: all 3 columns disrupted (including ALL)
   a. when trauma force directed posteriorly to anteriorly (more common) VB above shears forward fracturing the posterior arch (→ free floating lamina) and the superior facet of the inferior vertebra
   b. clinical: all 7 cases were complete paraplegics
3. flexion distraction
   a. radiographically resemble seat-belt type with addition of subluxation, or with compression of anterior column > 10-20%
   b. clinical: neurologic deficit (incomplete in 3 cases, complete in 1)

A. some call this a flexion-distraction fracture, but that term is also used for a subtype of fracture-dislocation

ASSOCIATED INJURIES

In addition to the above, associated injuries include: vertebral end-plate avulsion, ligamentous injuries, and hip and pelvic fractures.

STABILITY AND TREATMENT OF THORACOLUMBAR SPINE FRACTURES

Instability may be categorized as:
* 1st degree: mechanical instability
* 2nd degree: neurological instability
* 3rd degree: mechanical & neurological instability

Anterior column injury

Isolated anterior column injuries are usually stable and are treated as outlined in *Table 25-32*. The following exceptions may be <u>unstable</u> (1st degree) and often require surgery[194, 196]:

Table 25-32 Treatment of stable anterior or middle column thoracolumbar spine injuries

* treat initially with analgesics and recumbency (bed-rest) for comfort **x** 1-3 weeks
* diminution of pain is a good indication to commence mobilization with or without external immobilization (corset or Boston brace or TLSO **x** ≈ 12 weeks) depending on the degree of kyphosis
* vertebroplasty (± kyphoplasty) may be an option (*see page 750*)
* serial x-rays to rule-out progressive deformity

UNSTABLE

1. a single compression fracture with:
   A. loss of > 50% of height with angulation (particularly if the anterior part of the wedge comes to a point)
   B. kyphotic angulation > 40° (or > 25%) at one segment
   C. residual spinal canal ≤ 50% of normal
2. 3 or more contiguous compression fractures
3. neurologic deficit
4. disrupted posterior column or more than minimal middle column failure
5. progressive kyphosis: risk of progressive kyphosis is increased when loss of height of anterior vertebral body is > 75%. Risk is higher for lumbar compression fractures than thoracic

Middle column failure

<u>Unstable</u> (often requiring surgery) with the following exceptions which should be stable (stable injuries may be treated as outlined in *Table 25-32*):

STABLE

1. above T8 if the ribs and sternum are intact (provides anterior stabilization)
2. below L4 if the posterior elements are intact
3. Chance fracture (anterior column compression, middle column distraction)
4. anterior column disruption with <u>minimal</u> middle column failure

Posterior column disruption

Not <u>acutely</u> unstable unless accompanied by failure of the middle column (posterior longitudinal ligament and posterior anulus fibrosus). However, <u>chronic</u> instability with kyphotic deformity may develop (especially in children).

Seat-belt type injuries without neurologic deficit

No immediate danger of neurologic injury. Treat most with external immobilization in extension (e.g. Jewett hyperextension brace or molded TLSO).

Fracture-dislocation

Unstable. Treatment options:
1. surgical decompression and stabilization: usually needed in cases with
   A. compression with > 50% loss of height with angulation
   B. or, kyphotic angulation > 40° (or > 25%)
   C. or, neurologic deficit
   D. or, desire to shorten length of time of bedrest
2. prolonged bedrest: an option if none of the above are present

Burst fractures

Not all burst fractures are alike. Some burst fractures may eventually cause neurologic deficit (even if no deficit initially). Middle column fragments in canal endanger the neuro elements. Criteria have been proposed to differentiate mild burst fractures from severe ones. Recommendations[197]: surgical treatment for all patients with partial neurologic deficit, or those with angular deformity ≥ 20°, a residual canal diameter ≤ 50% of normal, or an anterior body height ≤ 50% of the posterior height.

L5 burst fractures: These fractures are extremely rare, and it is difficult for instrumentation to maintain alignment at this level[198]. Therefore, if neurologic deficit ia absent or mild, conservative treatment should be considered[198, 199]. Regardless of treatment, patients will probably lose ≈ 15° of lordosis between L4 and the sacrum. Permanent neurologic loss may occur[199].

Early reports of conservative management utilized ≈ 6-10 weeks of bed rest followed by mobilization in a brace. A more contemporary approach utilizes 10-14 days of bed rest. The patient should be fitted with a TLSO with a unilateral non-movable thigh cuff in 10° of flexion (on either side, to reduce motion at the fracture segment). Mobilization should be done very gradually as the pain allows. The brace should be worn ≈ 4-6 months, and serial x-rays should be performed to rule-out progressive deformity.

If surgical treatment is indicated, a posterior approach with fusion and fixation of L4-S1 may be performed utilizing pedicle screws.

SPINAL INSTRUMENTATION

With fragments inside the canal, it used to be thought that distraction alone would "pull" the fragments back into their normal position (**ligamentotaxis**). This requires an intact PLL (which is not the case with middle column failure), and even then is not assured[200]. Intraoperative ultrasound may demonstrate residual canal fragments[201], and if needed the fragments may be impacted anteriorly out of the canal, e.g. using Sypert spinal impactors.

Anterior instrumentation of the lower lumbar spine is difficult, and is usually not recommended below ≈ L4.

Wound infections

Postoperative wound infections with spinal instrumentation are usually due to *Staph. aureus*, and may respond to prolonged antibiotic administration without hardware removal[195]. Occasionally, removal of instrumentation and debridement must be employed in addition to antibiotics.

OSTEOPOROTIC SPINE FRACTURES

Osteoporosis is defined as a condition of skeletal fragility as a result of low bone mass, microarchitectural deterioration of bone, or both[202]. It is found primarily in elderly white females, and rarely occurs prior to menopause. Lifetime risk of symptomatic vertebral body **(VB)** osteoporotic compression fractures is 16% for women, and 5% for men. There are ≈ 700,000 VB compression fractures per year in the U.S.

These patients are often found to have significant VB compression fractures on plain films after presenting with back pain following a seemingly minor fall. CT often shows an impressive amount of bone retropulsed into the canal.

Risk factors

Factors that increase the risk of osteoporosis include:
1. weight < 58 kg
2. cigarette smoking[203]
3. low-trauma VB fracture in the patient or a first degree relative
4. drugs
   A. heavy alcohol consumption
   B. AEDs (especially phenytoin)
   C. warfarin
   D. steroid use:
      1. bone changes can be seen with 7.5 mg/d of prednisone for > 6 months
      2. VB fractures occur in 30-50% of patients on prolonged glucocorticoids
5. postmenopausal female
6. males undergoing androgen deprivation therapy (e.g. for prostate Ca). Orchiectomy or ≥ 9 doses of gonadotropin-releasing hormone agonists had a 1.5 fold increase in risk of all fractures[204]
7. physical inactivity
8. low calcium intake

Factors that protect against osteoporosis include impact exercise and excess body fat.

DIAGNOSTIC CONSIDERATIONS
Pre-fracture diagnosis
1. measuring bone fragility is not possible
2. the best correlate with bone fragility is radiographic measurement of bone mineral density **(BMD)**
   A. T-score: osteoporosis is defined as > 2.5 standard deviations **(SD)** below the mean for healthy young adults[205]
   B. Z-score: compared to mean value of normal subjects of same age and sex
      1. SD < -1 lowest 25%
      2. SD < -2 lowest 2.5%
3. patients with low-trauma fractures or fragility fractures are considered osteoporotic even if their BMD are greater than these cutoffs

DEXA scan (dual energy x-ray absorptiometry): the preferred way to measure BMD
1. proximal femur: BMD in this location is the best predictor for future fractures
2. LS spine: best location to assess response to treatment (need AP <u>and</u> lateral views, since AP often overestimates BMD)

Post-fracture considerations
1. other causes of pathologic fracture, especially neoplastic (e.g. multiple myeloma, metastatic breast cancer), should be ruled out
2. younger patients with osteoporosis require evaluation for a remediable cause of the osteoporosis (hyperthyroidism, steroid abuse, hyperparathyroidism, osteomalacia, Cushing's syndrome)

TREATMENT[206-209]

PREVENTION OF OSTEOPOROSIS
High calcium intake during childhood may increase peak bone mass. Weight-bearing exercise also helps. Also effective: estrogen (see below), biphosphonates (alendronate and risedronate), and raloxifene.

TREATING ESTABLISHED OSTEOPOROSIS
Drugs that increase bone formation include:
1. intermittent low-dose parathyroid hormone: still experimental
2. sodium fluoride: 75 mg/d increases bone mass but did <u>not</u> significantly reduce the fracture rate. 25 mg PO BID of a delayed-release formulation (Slow Fluoride®) reduced fracture rate but may make bone more fragile and could increase risk of hip fractures. Fluoride increases demand for Ca^{++}, therefore supplement with 800 mg/d Ca^{++} and 400 IU/d vitamin D. Not recommended for use > 2 yrs

Drugs that reduce bone resorption are less effective on cancellous bone (found mainly in the spine and at the end of long bones[207]). Medications include:
1. estrogen: cannot be used in men. May be more effective if started soon after menopause. Large prospective controlled studies are lacking[209]. Studies have shown increased vertebral bone mass by > 5% and decreased rate of vertebral fractures by 50%. Also reduces risk of CAD, but may increase risk of breast cancer (controversial[208]) and DVTs. In patients with an intact uterus, add progestin to reduce risk of endometrial cancer, either cyclically as medroxyprogesterone acetate 10 mg/day for 12-14 days/month, or continuously as 2.5 mg/day
2. calcium: current recommendations are for 1,000-1,500 mg/d for postmenopausal women[210] taken with meals
3. vitamin D or analogues: usually given with calcium therapy. Vitamin D 400-800 IU/d is usually sufficient. If urinary Ca^{++} remains low, high dose vitamin D (50,000 IU q 7-10 d) may be tried. Since high-dose formulations have been discontinued in the U.S., analogues such as calcifediol (Calderol®) 50 µg/d or calcitriol (Rocaltrol®) up to 0.25 µg/d may be tried with Ca^{++} supplement. With high dose vitamin D or analogues, monitor serum and urinary Ca^{++}
4. calcitonin: derived from a number of sources, salmon is one of the more common. Benefit in preventing fractures is less well established[209]
   A. parenteral salmon calcitonin (Calcimar®, Miacalcin®): indicated for patients for whom estrogen is contraindicated. Expensive ($1,500-3,000/yr) and must be given IM or sub-Q. 30-60% of patients develop antibodies to the drug which negates its effect. **Rx**: 0.5 ml (100 U) of calcitonin (given with

calcium supplements to prevent hyperparathyroidism) SQ q d

    B. intranasal forms (Miacalcin nasal spray): less potent. 200-400 IU/d given in one nostril (alternate nostrils daily) plus Ca^{++} 500 mg/d and vitamin D

5. biphosphonates: carbon-substituted analogues of pyrophosphate have a high affinity for bone and inhibit bone resorption by destroying osteoclasts. Not metabolized. Remain bound to bone for several weeks

    A. **etidronate** (Didronel®), a 1st generation drug. May reduce rate of VB fractures, not confirmed on F/U. Not FDA approved for osteoporosis. Possible increased risk of hip fractures due to inhibition of bone mineralization may not occur with 2nd & 3rd generation drugs listed below. **Rx** 400 mg PO daily **x** 2 wks followed by 11-13 weeks of Ca^{++} supplementation

    B. **alendronate** (Fosamax®): can cause esophageal ulcers. **Rx** Prevention: 5 mg PO daily; treatment 10 mg PO daily; taken upright with water on an empty stomach at least 30 minutes before eating or drinking anything else. Once weekly dosing of 35 mg for prevention and 70 mg for treatment[209, 211]. Taken concurrently with 1000-1500 mg/d Ca^{++} and 400/d IU of vitamin D

    C. **risedronate** (Actonel®): **Rx** Prevention or treatment: 5 mg PO daily, or 35 mg once/week[211] on an empty stomach (as for alendronate, *see above*)

    D. not FDA approved for osteoporosis: tiludronate (Skelid®), pamidronate (Aredia®) (some are used for Paget's disease, *see page 342*)

6. estrogen analogues:

    A. **tamoxifen** (Nolvadex®), an estrogen antagonist for breast tissue but an estrogen agonist for bone, has a partial agonist effect on uterus associated with an increased incidence of endometrial cancer

    B. **raloxifene** (Evista®): similar to tamoxifen but is an estrogen antagonist for uterus[212]. Decreases the effect of warfarin (Coumadin®).

        Rx: 60 mg PO q d. SUPPLIED: 60 mg tablets

TREATMENT OF OSTEOPOROTIC VERTEBRAL COMPRESSION FRACTURES

Patients rarely have neurologic deficit. They are also usually fragile elderly women who usually do not tolerate large surgical procedures well, and the rest of their bones are also osteoporotic which are poor for internal fixation.

Management consists primarily of analgesics and bed rest followed by progressive mobilization, often in an external brace (often not tolerated well). Surgery is rarely employed. In cases where pain control is difficult to obtain or where neural compression causes deficit, limited bony decompression may be considered. Percutaneous vertebroplasty (*see below*) is a newer option.

Typical time course of conservative treatment:

1. initially, severe pain may require hospital or subacute care facility admission for adequate pain control utilizing

    A. sufficient pain medication

    B. bed rest for about 7-10 days (DVT prophylaxis recommended)

2. begin physical therapy (**PT**) after ≈ 7-10 days as patient tolerates (prolonged bed rest can promote "disuse osteoporosis")

    A. pain control as patient is mobilized may be enhanced by a <u>lumbar brace</u> which may work by reducing movement which causes repetitive "microfractures"

    B. discharge from the hospital with lumbar brace for outpatient PT

3. pain subsides on the average after 4-6 weeks (range 2-12 weeks)

PERCUTANEOUS VERTEBROPLASTY (PVP)

Transpedicular injection of polymethylmethacrylate[A] (**PMMA**) into the compressed bone with the following goals:

1. to try and stabilize the bone: may prevent progression of kyphosis

2. to *shorten* the duration of pain (sometimes providing pain relief within minutes to hours). Mechanism of pain relief may be due to stabilization of bone, or due to heat released in exothermic curing of cement

Indications

1. painful osteoporotic compression fractures:

    A. usually do not treat fractures producing < 5-10% loss of height

---

A. NB: as of the time of this writing, PMMA is not FDA approved for treatment of spinal compression fractures, and there are no randomized controlled trials comparing PVP to conservative treatment

B. severe pain that interferes with patient activity
C. failure to adequately control pain with oral pain medication
D. ★ pain localized to fracture level
2. vertebral hemangiomas that cause vertebral collapse or neurologic deficit as a result of extension into the spinal canal (not for incidental hemangiomas): *see page 512*
3. osteolytic metastases and multiple myeloma[213]: pain relief and stabilization
4. pathologic compression fractures[214] from metastases: PVP does not give rapid pain relief as with osteoporotic compression fractures (it may actually be necessary to increase pain meds for 7-10 days post PVP)
5. pedicle screw salvage when pedicle fractures during pedicle screw placement

Contraindications
1. coagulopathy
2. completely healed fractures
3. active infections: sepsis, osteomyelitis, discitis and epidural abscess
4. spinal instability
5. focal neurologic exam: may indicate herniated disc, retropulsed fragment in canal. Get CT or MRI to rule these out
6. relative contraindications:
    A. fractures > 80% loss of VB height (technically challenging)
    B. acute burst fractures
    C. significant canal compromise from tumor or retropulsed bone
    D. partial or total destruction of the posterior VB wall: <u>not</u> an absolute contraindication

Complications
Complication = rate: 1-9%. Lowest when used to treat osteoporotic compression fractures, higher with vertebral hemangiomas, highest with pathological fractures
1. methacrylate leakage:
    A. into soft tissues: usually of little consequence
    B. into spinal canal: symptomatic spinal cord compression is very rare
    C. into neural foramen
    D. into disc space
    E. venous: can get into vena cava, case report of pulmonary embolism
2. radiculopathy: 5-7% incidence. Some cases may be due to heat released during cement curing. Often treated conservatively: steroids, pain meds, nerve block...
3. pedicle fracture
4. rib fracture
5. transverse process fracture
6. anterior penetration with needle: puncture of great vessels, pneumothorax...
7. increased incidence of future VB compression fractures at adjacent levels

Management of some associated developments
1. chest pain
    A. get rib x-rays
    B. VQ scan if indicated
2. patient starts coughing during injection: fairly common. May be reaction to rib pain or to odor of PMMA, may also indicate solvent in lungs. Stop injecting
3. back pain: take x-ray to rule-out new fracture or PMMA in veins
4. neurologic symptoms: get CT scan

Pre-procedure evaluation
1. plain x-rays: minimum requirement
2. **CT**: helps rule-out bony compromise of spinal canal which may indicate increased risk of leakage for PMMA into canal during procedure
3. **MRI**: not mandatory, may be helpful in some cases
    A. short tau inversion recovery (**STIR**) images demonstrate bone edema indicative of acute fractures (not as good for differentiating pathology)[215]
4. patients with multiple compression fractures: consider getting **bone scan** and perform PVP in the VB near the level of pain that lights up the most (↑ activity on bone scan correlates with strongly with good outcome from PVP)

Procedure
1. pain medication
    A. remember, this procedure is being done with the patient lying on their stomach and is usually being done in frail, elderly females who smoke.

Therefore use caution to avoid oversedation and respiratory compromise
B. sedation and pain medication
C. use of local anesthetic during needle placement
D. additional pain medication just prior to injection
2. use bi-plane fluoro (or alternate AP and lateral views) to get needle to enter medial aspect of pedicle and place tip ≈ 1/2 to 2/3 of the way through the VB
3. test inject with contrast (e.g. iohexol (Omnipaque 300) *see page 127*) (do digital subtraction study if equipment is available)
   A. a little venous enhancement is acceptable
   B. if you visualize vena cava
      1. do not pull needle back (the fistula has already been created)
      2. push needle in a little further, or
      3. push some gelfoam (soaked in contrast) through the needle, or
      4. inject a very small amount of PMMA under visualization and allow it to set to block the fistula
4. inject PMMA (that has been opacified with tantalum or barium-sulfate) under fluoroscopic visualization until:
   A. 3-5 cc injected (minimal compression fractures accept more cement, sometimes up to ≈ 8 cc). No correlation between amount of PMMA injected and pain relief[213]
   B. PMMA approaches posterior VB wall or enters disc space, vena cava, pedicle, or spinal canal

Post-procedure
1. PVP is likely to be an outpatient procedure in the future, but for now, most facilities admit overnight
2. watch for
   A. chest or back pain (may indicate rib fracture)
   B. fever: may be reaction to cement
   C. neurologic symptoms
3. activity
   A. gradual mobilization after ≈ 2 hours
   B. ± physical therapy
   C. ± short term use of external brace (most centers do not use)
4. institute medical treatment for osteoporosis: remember the patient with fragility fractures by definition has osteoporosis with risk of future fractures

25.8. Sacral fractures

Uncommon. Usually caused by shear forces. Identified in 17% of patients with pelvic fractures[216] (∴ keep in mind that neurologic deficits in patients with pelvic fractures may be due to associated sacral fractures).

The sacrum below S2 is not essential to ambulation or support of the spinal column, but may still be unstable since pressure to the area may occur when supine or sitting.

Neurologic injuries occur in 22-60%[216]. Three characteristic clinical presentations based on zone of involvement[216, 217] as shown in *Table 25-33*.

Treatment

In one series[218], all 35 fractures were treated without surgery, and only 1 patient with a complete cauda equina syndrome did not improve. Others feel that surgery may have a useful role[216]:
1. operative reduction and internal fixation of unstable fractures may aid in pain control and promote early ambulation
2. decompression and/or surgical reduction/fixation may possibly improve radicular or sphincter deficits

Some observations[216]:
1. reduction of the ala may promote L5 recovery with Zone I fractures
2. Zone II fractures with neurologic involvement may recover with or without surgical reduction and fixation
3. horizontal Zone III with severe deficit: controversial. Reduction & decompression does not ensure recovery, which may occur with nonoperative management

Table 25-33   Classification of sacral fractures

Zone I	Zone II	Zone III Vertical	Zone III Transverse
Zone I: Region of ala sparing the central canal and neural foramina. Occasionally associated with partial L5 root injury possibly as a result of entrapment of the L5 root between the upwardly migrated fracture fragment and the transverse process of the L5 vertebra	**Zone II**: Region of sacral foramina. A vertical fracture which may be associated with unilateral L5, S1 and/or S2 nerve root involvement (producing sciatica). Bladder dysfunction is rare	**Zone III**: Region of sacral canal. Frequently associated with sphincter dysfunction (occurs only with bilateral root injuries) and saddle anesthesia. Subdivided[216]:	

| | | **Vertical**: almost always associated with pelvic ring fracture | **Transverse** (horizontal): rare. Often due to a direct blow to the sacrum as in a fall from a great height. Marked displacement of fracture fragment can produce severe deficit* (bowel & bladder incontinence) |

* significant deficit is rare in fractures at or below S4

25.9.   Gunshot wounds to the spine

Most are due to assaults with handguns. Distribution: cervical 19-37%, thoracic 48-64%, and lumbosacral 10-29% (roughly proportional to lengths of each segment). Spinal cord injury due to civilian GSWs are primarily due to direct injury from the bullet (unlike military weapons which may create injury from shock waves and cavitation). Steroids are not indicated (*see page 704*).

Indications for surgery:
1. injury to the cauda equina (whether complete or incomplete) if nerve root compression is demonstrated[219]
2. neurologic deterioration: suggesting possibility of spinal epidural hematoma
3. compression of a nerve root
4. CSF leak
5. spinal instability: very rare with isolated GSW to the spine
6. to remove a copper jacketed bullet: copper can cause intense local reaction[220]
7. incomplete lesions: very controversial. Some series show improvement with surgery[221], others show no difference from unoperated patients
8. debridement to reduce the risk of infection: more important for <u>military</u> GSW where there is massive tissue injury, not an issue for most civilian GSW except in cases where the bullet has traversed GI or respiratory tract
9. vascular injuries
10. surgery for late complications:
    A. migrating bullet
    B. lead toxicity[222] (plumbism): absorption of lead from a bullet occurs only when it lodges in joints, bursae, or <u>disc space</u>. Findings include: anemia, encephalopathy, motor neuropathy, nephropathy, abdominal colic
    C. late spinal instability: especially after surgery

25.10.   Penetrating trauma to the neck

Most often, injuries to the soft-tissues of the neck fall into the purvey of general/trauma surgeons and/or vascular surgeons. However, depending on local practice patterns, neurosurgeons may participate in care of these injuries, or they may get involved by virtue of associated spinal injuries. Also, see *Gunshot wounds to the spine*, page 753.

Trauma surgeons have traditionally divided penetrating injuries of the neck into 3 zones[223], and although definitions vary, the following is a general scheme[224]:

Zone I: inferiorly from the head of the clavicle to include the thoracic outlet
Zone II: from the clavicle to the angle of the mandible
Zone III: from the angle of the mandible to the base of the skull

The mortality rate for penetrating injury to the neck is ≈ 15%, with most early deaths due either to asphyxiation from airway compromise, or exsanguination externally or into the chest or upper airways. Late death is usually due to cerebral ischemia or complications from spinal cord injury.

Vascular injuries: Venous injuries occur in ≈ 18% of penetrating neck wounds, and arterial injuries in ≈ 12%. Of the cervical arteries, the common carotid is most usually involved, followed by the ICA, the ECA, and then the vertebral artery. Outcome probably correlates most closely with neurologic condition on admission, regardless of treatment.

Vertebral artery (**VA**): the majority of injuries are penetrating. Due to the proximity of other vessels, the spinal cord and nerve roots, injuries are rarely isolated to the VA. 72% of documented VA injuries had no related physical findings on exam[225].

EVALUATION

Neurologic examination: global deficits may be due to shock or hypoxemia due to asphyxiation. Cerebral neurologic deficits are usually due to vascular injury with cerebral ischemia. Local findings may be related to cranial nerve injury. Unilateral UE deficits may be due to nerve root or brachial plexus involvement. Median or ulnar nerve dysfunction can occur from compression by a pseudoaneurysm of the proximal axillary artery. Spinal cord involvement may present with complete injury, or with an incomplete spinal cord injury syndrome (*see page 714*). Shock due to spinal cord injury is usually accompanied by bradycardia (*see page 698*), as opposed to the tachycardia seen with hypovolemic shock.

Cervical spine x-rays: assesses trajectory of injury and integrity C-spine.

Angiography: indicated in most cases if the patient is stable (especially for zone I or III injuries, and for zone II patients with no other indication for exploration, or for patients with penetration of the posterior triangle or wounds near the transverse processes where the VA may be injured). Patients actively hemorrhaging need to be taken to the OR without pre-op angiography. Angiographic abnormalities include:
1. extravassation of blood
    A. expanding hematoma into soft tissues: may compromise airway
    B. pseudoaneurysm
    C. AV fistula
    D. bleeding into airways
    E. external bleeding
2. intimal dissection, with
    A. occlusion, or
    B. luminal narrowing (including possible "string sign")
3. occlusion by soft tissue or bone

TREATMENT

Airway: stable patients without airway compromise should not have "prophylactic" intubation to protect the airway. Immediate intubation is indicated for hemodynamically unstable patients or for airway compromise. Options:
1. endotracheal: preferred
2. cricothyroidotomy: if endotracheal intubation cannot be performed (e.g. due to tracheal deviation or patient agitation) or if there is evidence of cervical spine injury and manipulation of the neck is contraindicated, then cricothyroidotomy is performed with placement of a #6 or 7 cuffed endotracheal tube (followed by a standard tracheostomy in the OR once the patient is stabilized)

3. awake nasotracheal: may be considered in the setting of possible spinal injury

Exploration: surgical exploration has been advocated for all wounds that pierce the platysma and enter the anterior triangles of the neck[226], however, 40-60% of these explorations will be negative. Although a selective approach may be based on angiography, false negatives have resulted in some authors recommending exploration of all zone II injuries[227].

Carotid artery: choices are primary repair, interposition grafting, or ligation. Patients in coma or those with severe strokes caused by vascular occlusion of the carotid artery are poor surgical candidates for vascular reconstruction due to a high mortality rate ≥ 40%[224], however the outcome with ligation is worse. Repair of injuries is recommended in patients with no or only minor neurologic deficit. ICA ligation is recommended for bleeding that cannot be controlled and was used for extravassation of dye at the base of the skull in 1 patient[228].

Vertebral artery: injuries are more often managed by ligation than by direct repair[229], especially when bleeding occurs during exploration. Less urgent conditions (e.g. AV fistula) requires knowledge of the patency of the contralateral VA and the ability to fill the ipsilateral PICA from retrograde flow through the BA before ligation can considered (arteriographic anomalies contraindicate ligation in 15% of cases). Proximal occlusion may be accomplished with an anterior approach after the sternocleidomastoid is detached from the sternum. The VA is the normally the first branch of the subclavian artery. Alternatively, endovascular techniques may be used, e.g. detachable balloons for proximal occlusion, or thrombogenic coils for pseudoaneurysms. Distal interruption may also be required, and this necessitates surgical exposure and ligation. Optimal management of a thrombosed injured VA in a foramen transversarium is unknown, and may require arterial bypass if ligation is not a viable option.

25.11. Chronic management of spinal cord injuries

Most of the following topics are treated elsewhere in this manual, but are pertinent to spinal cord injured **(SCI)** patients, and reference to the specific section is made.
1. autonomic hyperreflexia: *see below*
2. **ectopic bone**, includes **para-articular heterotopic ossification**: ossification of some joints that occurs in 15-20% of paralyzed patients
3. osteoporosis and pathologic fracture: *see page 748*
4. spasticity: *see page 367*
5. syringomyelia: *see page 349*
6. deep vein thrombosis: *see below* and also *page 25*
7. shoulder-hand syndrome: possibly sympathetically maintained

RESPIRATORY MANAGEMENT PROBLEMS IN SPINAL CORD INJURIES
In attempting to wean high level SCI patients from a ventilator, it may be helpful to change tube feedings to Pulmonaid® which lowers the CO_2 load.

Patients with cervical SCIs are more prone to pneumonia due to the fact that most of the effort in a normal cough originates in the abdominal muscles which are paralyzed.

AUTONOMIC HYPERREFLEXIA
🛈 Key features
- exaggerated autonomic response to normally innocuous stimuli
- occurs only in patients with spinal cord lesions <u>above</u> ≈ T6
- patients complain of pounding headache, flushing and diaphoresis above lesion
- can be life threatening, requires rapid control of hypertension and a search for an elimination of offending stimuli

AKA autonomic dysreflexia. Autonomic hyperreflexia[230, 231] **(AH)** is an exaggerated autonomic response (sympathetic usually dominates) secondary to stimuli that would only be mildly noxious under normal circumstances. It occurs in ≈ 30% of quadriplegic and high paraplegic patients (reported range is as high as 66-85%), but does <u>not</u> occur in patients with lesions below T6 (only patients with lesions above the origin of the splanchnic outflow are prone to develop AH, and the origin is usually T6 or below). It is rare in first 12-16 weeks post-injury.

During attacks, norepinephrine (NE) (but not epinephrine) is released. Hypersensitivity to NE may be partially due to subnormal resting levels of catecholamines. Homeostatic responses include vasodilatation (above the level of the injury) and bradycardia (however, sympathetic stimulation may also cause tachycardia).

Stimulus sources causing episodes of autonomic hyperreflexia:
1. bladder: 76% (distension 73%, UTI 3%, bladder stones…)
2. colorectal: 19% (fecal impaction 12%, administering enema or suppository 4%)
3. decubitus ulcers/skin infection: 4%
4. DVT
5. miscellaneous: tight clothing or leg bag straps, procedures such as cystoscopy or debriding decubitus ulcers, case report of suprapubic tube

PRESENTATION
- paroxysmal HTN: 90%
- anxiety
- diaphoresis
- piloerection
- pounding H/A
- ocular findings:
  - ◆ mydriasis
  - ◆ blurring of vision
  - ◆ lid retraction or lid lag
- erythema of face, neck and trunk: 25%
- pallor of skin below the lesion (due to vasoconstriction)
- pulse rate: tachycardia (38%) or mild elevation over baseline, bradycardia (10%)
- "splotches" over face and neck: 3%
- muscle fasciculations
- increased spasticity
- penile erection
- Horner's syndrome
- triad seen in 85%: cephalgia (H/A), hyperhidrosis, cutaneous vasodilatation

EVALUATION
In the appropriate setting (e.g. a quadriplegic patient with an acutely distended bladder), the symptoms are fairly diagnostic.

Many features are also common to pheochromocytoma. Studies of catecholamine levels have been inconsistent, however they can be mildly elevated in AH. The distinguishing feature of AH is the presence of hyperhidrosis and flushing of the face in the presence of pallor and vasoconstriction elsewhere on the body (which would be unusual for a pheochromocytoma).

TREATMENT
1. immediately elevate HOB (to decrease ICP), check BP q 5 min
2. treatment of choice: identify and eliminate the offending stimulus
   A. make sure bladder is empty (if catheterized check for kinks or sediment plugs). Caution: irrigating bladder may exacerbate AH (consider suprapubic aspiration)
   B. check bowels (avoid rectal exam, may exacerbate). Palpate abdomen or check abdominal x-ray (AH from this usually resolves spontaneously without manual disimpaction)
   C. check skin and toenails for ulceration or infection
   D. remove tight apparel
3. HTN that is extreme or that does not respond quickly may require treatment to prevent seizures and/or cerebral hemorrhage/hypertensive encephalopathy. Caution must be used to prevent hypotension following the episode. Agents used include: sublingual nifedipine[232] 10 mg SL, IV phentolamine (alpha cholinergic blocker, see page 469) or nitroprusside (Nipride®) (see page 4)
4. consider diazepam (Valium®) 2-5 mg IVP (@ < 5 mg/min). Relieves spasm of skeletal and smooth muscle (including bladder sphincter). Is also anxiolytic

PREVENTION
Good bowel/bladder and skin care are the best preventative measures.

Prophylaxis in patients with recurrent episodes

1. phenoxybenzamine (Dibenzyline®): an alpha blocker. Not helpful during the acute crisis. May not be as effective for alpha stimulation from sympathetic ganglia as with circulating catecholamines[233]. The patient may also develop hypotension after the sympathetic outflow subsides. Thus this is used only for resistant cases (note: will not affect sweating which is mediated by acetylcholine).

   Rx Adult: wide range quoted in literature: average 20-30 mg PO BID

2. beta-blockers: may be necessary in addition to α-blockers to avoid possible hypotension from ß$_2$ receptor stimulation (a theoretical concern)

3. phenazopyridine (Pyridium®): a topical anesthetic that is excreted in the urine. May decrease bladder wall irritation, however, the primary cause of irritation should be treated if possible.

   Rx Adult: 200 mg PO TID after meals. SUPPLIED: 100 mg, 200 mg tabs.

4. "radical measures" such as sympathectomy, pelvic or pudendal nerve section, cordotomy, or intrathecal alcohol injection have been advocated in the past, but are rarely necessary and may jeopardize reflex voiding

5. prophylactic treatment prior to procedures may employ use of anesthetics even in regions rendered anesthetic by the cord injury. Nifedipine 10 mg SL has also been used effective for AH during cystoscopy and prophylactically[232]

25.12. References

1. White A A, Panjabi M M: *The problem of clinical instability in the human spine: A systematic approach.* In **Clinical biomechanics of the spine**. J.B. Lippincott, Philadelphia, 2nd ed., 1990, Chapter 5: pp 277-378.
2. Waters R L, Adkins R H, Yakura J, *et al.*: Profiles of spinal cord injury and recovery after gunshot injury. **Clin Orthop** 267: 14-21, 1991.
3. Atkinson P P, Atkinson J L D: Spinal shock. **Mayo Clin Proc** 71: 384-9, 1996.
4. Chesnut R M: *Emergency management of spinal cord injury.* In **Neurotrauma**, Narayan R K, Wilberger J E, and Povlishock J T, (eds.). McGraw-Hill, New York, 1996: pp 1121-38.
5. Hirsch S A, Hirsch P J, Hiramoto H, *et al.*: Whiplash syndrome: Fact or fiction? **Orthop Clin North Am** 19: 791-5, 1988.
6. Riley L H, Long D, Riley Jr. L H: The science of whiplash. **Medicine (Baltimore)** 74: 298-9, 1995.
7. Spitzer W O, Skovron M L, Salmi L R, *et al.*: Scientific monograph of the Quebec task force on whiplash-associated disorders: Redefining "whiplash" and its management. **Spine** 20 (Suppl #8S): 1S-73S, 1995.
8. Radanov B P, Sturzenegger M, Di Stefano G: Long-term outcome after whiplash injury. **Medicine (Baltimore)** 74: 281-97, 1995.
9. Hamilton M G, Myles S T: Pediatric spinal injury: Review of 61 deaths. **J Neurosurg** 77: 705-8, 1992.
10. Section on Disorders of the Spine and Peripheral Nerves of the American Association of Neurological Surgeons and the Congress of Neurological Surgeons: Chapter 12: Management of pediatric cervical spine and spinal cord injuries. **Neurosurgery** 50 Supplement (3): Guidelines for the management of acute cervical spine and spinal cord injuries: S85-99, 2002.
11. Hamilton M G, Myles S T: Pediatric spinal injury: Review of 174 hospital admissions. **J Neurosurg** 77: 700-4, 1992.
12. Mandabach M, Ruge J R, Hahn Y S, *et al.*: Pediatric axis fractures: Early halo immobilization, management and outcome. **Pediatric Neurosurgery** 19: 225-32, 1993.
13. Garton H J L, Park P, Papadopoulos S M: Fracture dislocation of the neurocentral synchondroses of the axis. Case illustration. **J Neurosurg** (Spine 3) 96:

14. Suss R A, Zimmerman R D, Leeds N E: Pseudospread of the atlas: False sign of Jefferson fracture in young children. **AJR** 140: 1079-82, 1983.
15. Bailey D K: The normal cervical spine in infants and children. **Radiology** 59: 712-9, 1952.
16. Townsend E H, Rowe M L: Mobility of the upper cervical spine in health and disease. **Pediatrics** 10: 567-74, 1952.
17. Jacobson G, Bleeker H H: Pseudosubluxation of the axis in children. **Am J Roentgenol** 82: 472-81, 1959.
18. Bachulis B L, B L W, Hynes G D, *et al.*: Clinical indications for cervical spine radiographs in the traumatized patient. **Am J Surg** 153: 473-8, 1987.
19. Harris M B, Waguespack A M, Kronlage S: 'Clearing' cervical spine injuries in polytrauma patients: Is it really safe to remove the collar? **Orthopedics** 20: 903-7, 1997.
20. Podolsky S M, Daraff L J, Simon R R, *et al.*: Efficacy of cervical spine immobilization methods. **J Trauma** 23: 687-90, 1983.
21. Section on Disorders of the Spine and Peripheral Nerves of the American Association of Neurological Surgeons and the Congress of Neurological Surgeons: Chapter 3: Clinical assessment after acute cervical spinal cord injury. **Neurosurgery** 50 Supplement (3). Guidelines for the management of acute cervical spine and spinal cord injuries: S21-9, 2002.
22. Section on Disorders of the Spine and Peripheral Nerves of the American Association of Neurological Surgeons and the Congress of Neurological Surgeons: Chapter 7: Management of acute spinal cord injuries in an intensive care unit or other monitored setting. **Neurosurgery** 50 Supplement (3): Guidelines for the management of acute cervical spine and spinal cord injuries: S51-7, 2002.
23. Section on Disorders of the Spine and Peripheral Nerves of the American Association of Neurological Surgeons and the Congress of Neurological Surgeons: Chapter 8: Blood pressure management after acute spinal cord injury. **Neurosurgery** 50 Supplement (3): Guidelines for the management of acute cervical spine and spinal cord injuries: S58-62, 2002.
24. Meguro K, Tator C H: Effect of multiple trauma on mortality and neurological recovery after spinal cord

350, 2002.

or cauda equina injury. **Neurol Med Chir** 28: 34-41, 1988.

25. Bracken M B, Shepard M J, Holford T R, *et al.*: Administration of methylprednisolone for 24 or 48 hours or tirilazad mesylate for 48 hours in the treatment of acute spinal cord injury. **JAMA** 277: 1597-604, 1997.

26. Bracken M B, Members of the National Acute Spinal Cord Injury Study Group: Comments. **Neurosurgery** 50 Supplement (3): Guidelines for the management of acute cervical spine and spinal cord injuries: Sxiv-xx, 2002.

27. Hurlbert R J: Methylprednisolone for acute spinal cord injury: An inappropriate standard of care. **J Neurosurg** (Spine 1) 93: 1-7, 2000.

28. Section on Disorders of the Spine and Peripheral Nerves of the American Association of Neurological Surgeons and the Congress of Neurological Surgeons: Chapter 9: Pharmacological therapy after acute cervical spinal cord injury. **Neurosurgery** 50 Supplement (3): Guidelines for the management of acute cervical spine and spinal cord injuries: S63-72, 2002.

29. Bracken M B, Shepard M J, Collins W F, *et al.*: A randomized, controlled trial of methylprednisolone or naloxone in the treatment of acute spinal-cord injury. **N Engl J Med** 322: 1405-11, 1990.

30. Bracken M B, Shepard M J, Collins W F, *et al.*: Methylprednisolone or naloxone treatment after acute spinal cord injury: 1-year follow-up data. **J Neurosurg** 76: 23-31, 1992.

31. Heary R F, Vaccaro A R, Mesa J J, *et al.*: Steroids and gunshot wounds to the spine. **Neurosurgery** 41: 576-84, 1997.

32. Hamilton M G, Hull R D, Pineo G F: Venous thromboembolism in neurosurgery and neurology patients: A review. **Neurosurgery** 34: 280-96, 1994.

33. Section on Disorders of the Spine and Peripheral Nerves of the American Association of Neurological Surgeons and the Congress of Neurological Surgeons: Chapter 10: Deep venous thrombosis and thromboembolism in patients with cervical spinal cord injuries. **Neurosurgery** 50 Supplement (3): Guidelines for the management of acute cervical spine and spinal cord injuries: S73-80, 2002.

34. Green D, Lee M Y, Ito V Y, *et al.*: Fixed- vs adjusted-dose heparin in the prophylaxis of thromboembolism in spinal cord injury. **JAMA** 260: 1255-8, 1988.

35. Section on Disorders of the Spine and Peripheral Nerves of the American Association of Neurological Surgeons and the Congress of Neurological Surgeons: Chapter 4: Radiographic assessment of the cervical spine in asymptomatic trauma patients. **Neurosurgery** 50 Supplement (3): S30-5, 2002.

36. Section on Disorders of the Spine and Peripheral Nerves of the American Association of Neurological Surgeons and the Congress of Neurological Surgeons: Chapter 5: Radiographic assessment of the cervical spine in symptomatic trauma patients. **Neurosurgery** 50 Supplement (3): Guidelines for the management of acute cervical spine and spinal cord injuries: S36-43, 2002.

37. Walter J, Doris P, Shaffer M: Clinical presentation of patients with acute cervical spine injury. **Ann Emerg Med** 13: 512-5, 1984.

38. Clark W M, Gehweiler J A, Laib R: Twelve significant signs of cervical spine trauma. **Skeletal Radiol** 3: 201-5, 1979.

39. Nichols C G, Young D H, Schiller W R: Evaluation of cervicothoracic junction injury. **Ann Emerg Med** 16: 640-2, 1987.

40. Shaffer M, Doris P: Limitation of the cross table lateral view in detecting cervical spine injuries: A retrospective analysis. **Ann Emerg Med** 10: 508-13, 1981.

41. MacDonald R L, Schwartz M L, Mirich D, *et al.*: Di-

42. Holliman C, Mayer J, Cook R, *et al.*: Is the AP radiograph of the cervical spine necessary in evaluation of trauma? **Ann Emerg Med** 19: 483-4, 1990 (abstract).

43. Harris J H: Radiographic evaluation of spinal trauma. **Orthop Clin North Am** 17: 75-86, 1986.

44. Tehranzedeh J, Bonk T, Ansari A, *et al.*: Efficacy of limited CT for non-visualized lower cervical spine in patients with blunt trauma. **Skeletal Radiol** 23: 349-52, 1994.

45. Miller M D, Gehweiler J A, Martinez S, *et al.*: Significant new observations on cervical spine trauma. **AJR** 130: 659-63, 1978.

46. Wales L, Knopp R, Morishima M: Recommendations for evaluation of the acutely injured spine: A clinical radiographic algorithm. **Ann Emerg Med** 9: 422-8, 1980.

47. Hollis P H, Malis L I, Zappulla R A: Neurological deterioration after lumbar puncture below complete spinal subarachnoid block. **J Neurosurg** 64: 253-6, 1986.

48. Section on Disorders of the Spine and Peripheral Nerves of the American Association of Neurological Surgeons and the Congress of Neurological Surgeons: Chapter 6: Initial closed reduction of cervical spine fracture-dislocation injuries. **Neurosurgery** 50 Supplement (3): Guidelines for the management of acute cervical spine and spinal cord injuries: S44-50, 2002.

49. Robertson P A, Ryan M D: Neurological deterioration after reduction of cervical subluxation: Mechanical compression by disc material. **J Bone Joint Surg** 74B: 224-7, 1992.

50. Garfin S R, Botte M J, Triggs K J, *et al.*: Subdural abscess associated with halo-pin traction. **J Bone Joint Surg** 70A: 1338-40, 1988.

51. Dill S R, Cobbs C G, McDonald C K: Subdural empyema: Analysis of 32 cases and review. **Clin Inf Dis** 20: 372-86, 1995.

52. Schneider R C, Crosby E C, Russo R H, *et al.*: Traumatic spinal cord syndromes and their management. **Clin Neurosurg** 20: 424-92, 1972.

53. Wagner F C, Chehrazi B: Early decompression and neurological outcome in acute cervical spinal cord injuries. **J Neurosurg** 56: 699-705, 1982.

54. American Spinal Injury Association: **International standards for neurological classification of spinal cord injury, revised 2000.** 6th ed. American Spinal Injury Association, Chicago, IL, 2000.

55. Ditunno J F, Jr.: New spinal cord injury standards, 1992. **Paraplegia** 30 (2): 90-1, 1992.

56. Lucas J T, Ducker T B: Motor classification of spinal cord injuries with mobility, morbidity and recovery indices. **Am Surg** 45: 151-8, 1979.

57. Frankel H L, Hancock D O, Hyslop G, *et al.*: The value of postural reduction in the initial management of closed injuries of the spine with paraplegia and tetraplegia. Part I. **Paraplegia** 7: 179-92, 1969.

58. Epstein N, Epstein J A, Benjamin V, *et al.*: Traumatic myelopathy in patients with cervical spinal stenosis without fracture or dislocation: Methods of diagnosis, management, and prognosis. **Spine** 5: 489-96, 1980.

59. Schneider R C, Cherry G, Pantek H: The syndrome of acute central cervical spinal cord injury. **J Neurosurg** 11: 546-77, 1954.

60. Merriam W F, Taylor T K F, Ruff S J, *et al.*: A reappraisal of acute traumatic central cord syndrome. **J Bone Joint Surg** 68B: 708-13, 1986.

61. Levi L, Wolf A, Mirvis S, *et al.*: The significance of dorsal migration of the cord after extensive cervical laminectomy for patients with traumatic central cord syndrome. **J Spinal Disord** 8: 289-95, 1995.

62. Chen T Y, Lee S T, Lui T N, *et al.*: Efficacy of sur-

gical treatment in traumatic central cord syndrome. **Surg Neurol** 48: 435-40, 1997.

63. Section on Disorders of the Spine and Peripheral Nerves of the American Association of Neurological Surgeons and the Congress of Neurological Surgeons: Chapter 21: Management of acute central spinal cord injuries. **Neurosurgery** 50 Supplement (3): Guidelines for the management of acute cervical spine and spinal cord injuries: S166-72, 2002.

64. Massaro F, Lanotte M, Faccani G: Acute traumatic central cord syndrome. **Acta Neurol (Napoli)** 15: 97-105, 1993.

65. Rothman R H, Simeone F A, (eds.): **The spine**. 3rd ed., W.B. Saunders, Philadelphia, 1992.

66. Fox J L, Wener L, Drennan D C, *et al*.: Central spinal cord injury: Magnetic resonance imaging confirmation and operative considerations, **Neurosurgery** 22: 340-7, 1988.

67. Ducker T B: Comment on Fox J L, et al.: Central spinal cord injury: Magnetic resonance imaging confirmation and operative considerations. **Neurosurgery** 22: 346-7, 1988.

68. Bose B, Northrup B E, Osterholm J L, *et al*.: Reanalysis of central cervical cord injury management. **Neurosurgery** 15: 367-72, 1984.

69. Penrod I. E, Hegde S K, Ditunno J F: Age effect on prognosis for functional recovery in acute, traumatic central cord syndrome. **Arch Phys Med Rehabil** 71: 963-8, 1990.

70. Schneider R C: The syndrome of acute anterior spinal cord injury. **J Neurosurg** 12: 95-122, 1955.

71. Roth E J, Park T, Pang T, *et al*.: Traumatic cervical Brown-Sequard and Brown-Sequard plus syndromes: The spectrum of presentations and outcomes. **Paraplegia** 29: 582-9, 1991.

72. Kulliana C D, Duchin D E: Brown-Sequard syndrome produced by cervical disc herniation: Case report and literature review. **Surg Neurol** 45: 359-61, 1996.

73. Gehweiler J A, Clark W M, Schaaf R E, *et al*.: Cervical spine trauma: The common combined conditions. **Radiology** 130: 77, 1979.

74. Powers B, Miller M D, Kramer R S, *et al*.: Traumatic anterior atlanto-occipital dislocation. **Neurosurgery** 4: 12-7, 1979.

75. Alker G J, Leslie E V: High cervical spine and craniocervical junction injuries in fatal traffic accidents: A radiological study. **Orthop Clin North Am** 9: 1003-10, 1978.

76. Bucholz R W, Burkhead W Z, Graham W, *et al*.: Occult cervical spine injuries in fatal traffic accidents. **J Trauma** 19: 768-71, 1979.

77. Traynelis V C, Marano G D, Dunker R O, *et al*.: Traumatic atlanto-occipital dislocation. Case report. **J Neurosurg** 65: 863-70, 1986.

78. Harris J H, Jr., Carson G C, Wagner L K, *et al*.: Radiologic diagnosis of traumatic occipitovertebral dissociation: 2. Comparison of three methods of detecting occipitovertebral relationships on lateral radiographs of supine subjects. **AJR Am J Roentgenol** 162 (4): 887-92, 1994.

79. Section on Disorders of the Spine and Peripheral Nerves of the American Association of Neurological Surgeons and the Congress of Neurological Surgeons: Chapter 14: Diagnosis and management of traumatic atlanto-occipital dislocation injuries. **Neurosurgery** 50 Supplement (3): Guidelines for the management of acute cervical spine and spinal cord injuries: S105-13, 2002.

80. Dvorak J, Panjabi M M: Functional anatomy of the alar ligaments. **Spine** 12: 183-89, 1987.

81. Dickman C A, Crawford N R, Brantley A G U, *et al*.: *In vitro* cervical spine biomechanical testing. **BNI Quarterly** 9 (4): 17-26, 1993.

82. Przybylski G J, Clyde B L, Fitz C R: Craniocervical junction subarachnoid hemorrhage associated with atlanto-occipital dislocation. **Spine** 21 (15): 1761-8, 1996.

83. Harris J H, Carson G C, Wagner L K: Radiologic diagnosis of traumatic occipitovertebral dissociation: 1. Normal occipitovertebral relationships on lateral radiographs of supine subjects. **AJR Am J Roentgenol** 162 (4): 881-6, 1994.

84. Lee C, Woodring J H, Goldstein S J, *et al*.: Evaluation of traumatic atlantooccipital dislocations. **AJNR Am J Neuroradiol** 8 (1): 19-26, 1987.

85. Wholey M H, Bruwer A J, Baker H L: The lateral roentgenogram of the neck (with comments on the atlanto-odontoid-basion relationship). **Radiology** 71: 350-6, 1958.

86. Dublin A B, Marks W M, Weinstock D, *et al*.: Traumatic dislocation of the atlanto-occipital articulation (AOA) with short-term survival. With a radiographic method of measuring the AOA. **J Neurosurg** 52 (4): 541-6, 1980.

87. Bell C L: Surgical observations. **Middlesex Hosp J** 4: 469, 1817.

88. Anderson P A, Montesano P X: Morphology and treatment of occipital condyle fractures. **Spine** 13 (7): 731-6, 1988.

89. Jacoby C G: Fracture of the occipital condyle. **AJR Am J Roentgenol** 132 (3): 500, 1979 (letter).

90. Section on Disorders of the Spine and Peripheral Nerves of the American Association of Neurological Surgeons and the Congress of Neurological Surgeons: Chapter 15: Occipital condyle fractures. **Neurosurgery** 50 Supplement (3): Guidelines for the management of acute cervical spine and spinal cord injuries: S114-9, 2002.

91. Sonntag V K H, Dickman C A: *Treatment of upper cervical spine injuries*. In **Spinal trauma: Current evaluation and management**, Rea G L and Miller C A, (eds.), Neurosurgical topics. Committee A P. American Association of Neurological Surgeons, 1993: pp 25-74.

92. Fielding J W, Hawkins R J: Atlanto-axial rotatory fixation. (fixed rotatory subluxation of the atlanto-axial joint). **J Bone Joint Surg** 59A: 37-44, 1977.

93. Lourie H, Stewart W A: Spontaneous atlantoaxial dislocation: A complication of rheumatic disease. **N Engl J Med** 265: 677-81, 1961.

94. Wetzel F T, La Rocca H: Grisel's syndrome. **Clin Orthop** (240): 141-52, 1989.

95. Fielding J W, Stillwell W T, Chynn K Y, *et al*.: Use of computed tomography for the diagnosis of atlanto-axial rotatory fixation. **J Bone Joint Surg** 60A: 1102-4, 1978.

96. Schneider R C, Schemm G W: Vertebral artery insufficiency in acute and chronic spinal trauma. With special reference to the syndrome of acute central cervical spinal cord injury. **J Neurosurg** 18: 348-60, 1961.

97. Banna M: *Spinal fractures and dislocations*. In **Clinical radiology of the spine and the spinal cord**. Aspen Systems Corporation, Rockville, Maryland, 1985, Chapter 4: pp 102-59.

98. Hadley M N, Dickman C A, Browner C M, *et al*.: Acute traumatic atlas fractures: Management and long-term outcome. **Neurosurgery** 23: 31-5, 1988.

99. Landells C D, Van Peteghem P K: Fractures of the atlas: Classification, treatment and morbidity. **Spine** 13 (5): 450-2, 1988.

100. Papadopoulos S M: *Biomechanics of occipito-atlanto-axial trauma*. In **Spinal trauma: Current evaluation and management**, Rea G L and Miller C A, (eds.). Neurosurgical topics. Committee A P. American Association of Neurological Surgeons, 1993: pp 17-23.

101. Alker G J, Oh Y S, Leslie E V, *et al*.: Postmortem radiology of head and neck injuries in fatal traffic accidents. **Radiology** 114: 611-7, 1975.

102. Panjabi M M, Oda T, Crisco J J, 3rd, *et al*.: Experimental study of atlas injuries. I. Biomechanical analysis of their mechanisms and fracture patterns.

Spine 16 (10 Suppl): S460-5, 1991.

103. Spence K F, Decker S, Sell K W: Bursting atlantal fracture associated with rupture of the transverse ligament. **J Bone Joint Surg** 52A: 543-9, 1970.

104. Fielding J W, Cochran G B, Lawsing J F, 3rd, *et al.*: Tears of the transverse ligament of the atlas. A clinical and biomechanical study. **J Bone Joint Surg Am** 56 (8): 1683-91, 1974.

105. Heller J G, Viroslav S, Hudson T: Jefferson fractures: The role of magnification artifact in assessing transverse ligament integrity. **J Spinal Disord** 6 (5): 392-6, 1993.

106. Section on Disorders of the Spine and Peripheral Nerves of the American Association of Neurological Surgeons and the Congress of Neurological Surgeons: Chapter 16: Isolated fractures of the atlas in adults. **Neurosurgery** 50 Supplement (3): Guidelines for the management of acute cervical spine and spinal cord injuries: S120-4, 2002.

107. Levine A M, Edwards C C: Fractures of the atlas. **J Bone Joint Surg Am** 73 (5): 680-91, 1991.

108. Schneider R C, Livingston K E, Cave A J E, *et al.*: 'Hangman's fracture' of the cervical spine. **J Neurosurg** 22: 141-54, 1965.

109. Wood-Jones F: The ideal lesion produced by judicial hanging. **Lancet** 1: 53, 1913.

110. Effendi B, Roy D, Cornish B, *et al.*: Fractures of the ring of the axis: A classification based on the analysis of 131 cases. **J Bone Joint Surg** 63B: 319-27, 1981.

111. Levine A M, Edwards C C: The management of traumatic spondylolisthesis of the axis. **J Bone Joint Surg** 67A: 217-26, 1985.

112. Levine A M: *Traumatic spondylolisthesis of the axis: "Hangman's fracture"*. In **The cervical spine**, The Cervical Spine Research Society Editorial Committee, (ed.). Lippincott-Raven, Philadelphia, 3rd ed., 1998, Chapter 30: pp 429-48.

113. Starr J K, Eismont F J: Atypical hangman's fractures. **Spine** 18 (14): 1954-7, 1993.

114. Francis W R, Fielding J W, Hawkins R J, *et al.*: Traumatic spondylolisthesis of the axis. **J Bone Joint Surg** 63B: 313-8, 1981.

115. Greene K A, Dickman C A, Marciano F F, *et al.*: Acute axis fractures. Analysis of management and outcome in 340 consecutive cases. **Spine** 22: 1843-52, 1997.

116. Burke J T, Harris J H, Jr.: Acute injuries of the axis vertebra. **Skeletal Radiol** 18 (5): 335-46, 1989.

117. The Cervical Spine Research Society Editorial Committee, (ed.) **The cervical spine**. 2nd ed., J.B. Lippincott, Philadelphia, 1989.

118. Section on Disorders of the Spine and Peripheral Nerves of the American Association of Neurological Surgeons and the Congress of Neurological Surgeons: Chapter 17: Isolated fractures of the axis in adults. **Neurosurgery** 50 Supplement (3): Guidelines for the management of acute cervical spine and spinal cord injuries: S125-39, 2002.

119. Tuite G F, Papadopoulos S M, Sonntag V K H: Caspar plate fixation for the treatment of complex hangman's fractures. **Neurosurgery** 30: 761-5, 1992.

120. Coric D, Wilson J A, Kelly D L: Treatment of traumatic spondylolisthesis of the axis with nonrigid immobilization: A review of 64 cases. **J Neurosurg** 85: 550-4, 1996.

121. Sonntag V K H, Hadley M N: Nonoperative management of cervical spine injuries. **Clin Neurosurg** 34: 630-49, 1988.

122. Youmans J R, (ed.) **Neurological surgery**. 2nd ed., W. B. Saunders, Philadelphia, 1982.

123. Hadley M N: Comment on Tuite G F, et al.: Caspar plate fixation for the treatment of complex hangman's fractures. **Neurosurgery** 30: 761-5, 1992.

124. Husby J, Sorensen K H: Fracture of the odontoid process of the axis. **Acta Orthop Scand** 45: 182-92, 1974.

125. Crockard H A, Heilman A E, Stevens J M: Progressive myelopathy secondary to odontoid fractures: Clinical, radiological, and surgical features. **J Neurosurg** 78: 579-86, 1993.

126. Przybylski G J: Management of odontoid fractures. **Contemp Neurosurg** 20 (18): 1-6, 1998.

127. Anderson L D, D'Alonzo R T: Fractures of the odontoid process of the axis. **J Bone Joint Surg** 56A: 1663-74, 1974.

128. Scott E W, Haid R W, Peace D: Type I fractures of the odontoid process: Implications for atlanto-occipital instability: Case report. **J Neurosurg** 72: 488-92, 1990.

129. Naim-ur-Rahman, Jamjoom Z A, Jamjoom A B: Ruptured transverse ligament: An injury that is often forgotten. **Br J Neurosurg** 14: 375-7, 2000.

130. Hadley M N, Browner C M, Liu S S, *et al.*: New subtype of acute odontoid fractures (type IIA). **Neurosurgery** 22: 67-71, 1988.

131. Hadley M N, Dickman C A, Browner C M, *et al.*: Acute axis fractures: A review of 229 cases. **J Neurosurg** 71: 642-7, 1989.

132. Apuzzo M L J, Heiden J S, Weiss M H, *et al.*: Acute fractures of the odontoid process. An analysis of 45 cases. **J Neurosurg** 48: 85-91, 1978.

133. Ekong C E U, Schwartz M L, Tator C H, *et al.*: Odontoid fracture: Management with early mobilization using the halo device. **Neurosurgery** 9: 631-7, 1981.

134. Dunn M E, Seljeskog E L: Experience in the management of odontoid process injuries: An analysis of 128 cases. **Neurosurgery** 18: 306-10, 1986.

135. Lennarson P J, Mostafavi H, Traynelis V C, *et al.*: Management of type II dens fractures: A case-control study. **Spine** 25 (10): 1234-7, 2000.

136. Bohler J: Anterior stabilization for acute fractures and non-unions of the dens. **J Bone Joint Surg** 64: 18-28, 1982.

137. Dickman C A, Greene K A, Sonntag V K: Injuries involving the transverse atlantal ligament: Classification and treatment guidelines based upon experience with 39 injuries. **Neurosurgery** 38 (1): 44-50, 1996.

138. Polin R S, Szabo T, Bogaev C A, *et al.*: Nonoperative management of types II and III odontoid fractures: The Philadelphia collar versus the halo vest. **Neurosurgery** 38: 450-7, 1996.

139. Darakchiev B J, Bulas R V, Dunsker S: Use of calcitonin for the treatment of an odontoid fracture: Case report. **J Neurosurg** (Spine 1) 93: 157-60, 2000.

140. Paridis G R, Janes J M: Posttraumatic atlanto-axial instability: The fate of the odontoid process fracture in 46 cases. **J Trauma** 13: 359-67, 1973.

141. Fielding J W, Hensinger R N, Hawkins R J: Os odontoideum. **J Bone Joint Surg** 62A: 376-83, 1980.

142. Ricciardi J E, Kaufer H, Louis D S: Acquired os odontoideum following acute ligament injury. **J Bone Joint Surg** 58A: 410-2, 1976.

143. Clements W D, Mezue W, Mathew B: Os odontoideum: Congenital or acquired? That's not the question. **Injury** 26 (9): 640-2, 1995.

144. Spierings E L, Braakman R: The management of os odontoideum. Analysis of 37 cases. **J Bone Joint Surg Br** 64 (4): 422-8, 1982.

145. Menezes A H, Ryken T C: Craniovertebral abnormalities in down's syndrome. **Pediatr Neurosurg** 18 (1): 24-33, 1992.

146. Section on Disorders of the Spine and Peripheral Nerves of the American Association of Neurological Surgeons and the Congress of Neurological Surgeons: Chapter 19: Os odontoideum. **Neurosurgery** 50 Supplement (3): Guidelines for the management of acute cervical spine and spinal cord injuries: S148-55, 2002.

147. Section on Disorders of the Spine and Peripheral Nerves of the American Association of Neurologi-

cal Surgeons and the Congress of Neurological Surgeons: Chapter 18: Management of combination fractures of the atlas and axis in adults. **Neurosurgery** 50 Supplement (3): Guidelines for the management of acute cervical spine and spinal cord injuries: S140-7, 2002.

148. Section on Disorders of the Spine and Peripheral Nerves of the American Association of Neurological Surgeons and the Congress of Neurological Surgeons: Chapter 13: Spinal cord injury without radiographic abnormality. **Neurosurgery** 50 Supplement (3): Guidelines for the management of acute cervical spine and spinal cord injuries: S100-4, 2002.

149. Pang D, Wilberger J E: Spinal cord injury without radiographic abnormalities in children. **J Neurosurg** 57: 114-29, 1982.

150. Bondurant C P, Oró J J: Spinal cord injury without radiographic abnormality and Chiari malformation. **J Neurosurg** 79: 833-8, 1993.

151. Pollack I F, Pang D, Sclabassi R: Recurrent spinal cord injury without radiographic abnormalities in children. **J Neurosurg** 69: 177-82, 1988.

152. Madsen J R, Freiman T: Cervical spinal cord injury in children. **Contemp Neurosurg** 20 (26): 1-5, 1998

153. Hall R D M: Clay-shoveller's fracture. **J Bone Joint Surg** 22: 63-75, 1940.

154. Gershon-Cohen J, Budin E, Glauser F: Whiplash fractures of cervicodorsal spinous processes. **JAMA** 155: 560-1, 1954.

155. Allen B L, Ferguson R L, Lehmann T R, et al.: A mechanistic classification of closed, indirect fractures and dislocations of the lower cervical spine. **Spine** 7: 1-27, 1982.

156. Section on Disorders of the Spine and Peripheral Nerves of the American Association of Neurological Surgeons and the Congress of Neurological Surgeons: Chapter 20: Treatment of subaxial cervical spine injuries. **Neurosurgery** 50 Supplement (3): Guidelines for the management of acute cervical spine and spinal cord injuries: S156-65, 2002.

157. Abitbol J-J, Kostuik J P: *Flexion injuries to the lower cervical spine.* In **The cervical spine**, The Cervical Spine Research Society Editorial Committee, (ed.). Lippincott-Raven, Philadelphia, 3rd ed., 1998, Chapter 32: pp 457-64.

158. Fuentes J-M, Bloncourt J, Vlahovitch B, et al.: La tear drop fracture: Contribution à l'étude du mécanisme et des lésions ostéo-disco-ligamentaires. **Nirochirurgie** 29: 129-34, 1983 ([French]).

159. Schneider R C, Kahn E A, Arbor A: Chronic neurologic sequelae of acute trauma to the spine and spinal cord. The significance of acute flexion or teardrop cervical fracture-dislocation of the cervical spine. **J Bone Joint Surg** 38A, 1956.

160. Torg J S, Vegso J J, Sennett B: The national football head and neck injury registry: 14-year report of cervical quadriplegia (1971-1984). **Clin Sports Med** 6: 61-72, 1987.

161. Harris J H, Edeiken-Monroe B, Kopaniky D R: A practical classification of acute cervical spine injuries. **Orthop Clin North Am** 17: 15-30, 1986.

162. Gehweiler J A, Osborne R L: **The radiology of vertebral trauma.** W. B. Saunders, Philadelphia, 1980.

163. Favero K J, VanPeteghem P K: The quadrangular fragment fracture: Roentgenographic features and treatment protocol. **Clin Orthop** 239: 40-6, 1989.

164. Webb J K, Broughton R B K, McSweeney T, et al.: Hidden flexion injury of the cervical spine. **J Bone Joint Surg** 58B: 322-7, 1976.

165. Fazl M, LaFebvre J, Willinsky R A, et al.: Posttraumatic ligamentous disruption of the cervical spine, an easily overlooked diagnosis: Presentation of three cases. **Neurosurgery** 26: 674-7, 1990.

166. White A A, Johnson R M, Panjabi M M, et al.: Biomechanical analysis of clinical stability in the cervical spine. **Clin Orthop** 109: 85-96, 1975.

167. White A A, Southwick W O, Panjabi M M: Clinical instability in the lower cervical spine - A review of past and current concepts. **Spine** 1: 15-27, 1976.

168. Andreshak J L, Dekutoski M B: Management of unilateral facet dislocations: A review of the literature. **Orthopedics** 20: 917-26, 1997.

169. Payer M, Schmidt M H: Management of traumatic bilateral locked facets of the subaxial cervical spine. **Contemp Neurosurg** 27 (6): 1-4, 2005.

170. Rizzolo S J, Piazza M R, Cotler J M, et al.: Intervertebral disc injury complicating cervical spine trauma. **Spine** 16 (6 Suppl): S187-9, 1991.

171. Doran S E, Papadopoulos S M, Ducker T B, et al.: Magnetic resonance imaging documentation of coexistent traumatic locked facets of the cervical spine and disc herniation. **J Neurosurg** 79: 341-5, 1993.

172. Sonntag V K H: Management of bilateral locked facets of the cervical spine. **Neurosurgery** 8: 150-2, 1981.

173. Glasser J A, Whitehall R, Stamp W G, et al.: Complications associated with the halo vest. **J Neurosurg** 65: 76-9, 1986.

174. Sears W, Fazl M: Prediction of stability of cervical spine fracture managed in the halo vest and indications for surgical intervention. **J Neurosurg** 72: 426-32, 1990.

175. Roy-Camille R, Saillant G: Osteosynthese des fractures du rachis cervical. **Actual Chir Orthop Hop R Poincarré Mason, Paris** 8: 175-94, 1970.

176. Aldrich E F, Crow W N, Weber P B, et al.: Use of MR imaging-compatible Halifax interlaminar clamps for posterior cervical fusion. **J Neurosurg** 74: 185-9, 1991.

177. Branch C L, Kelly D L, Davis C H, et al.: Fixation of fractures of the lower cervical spine using methylmethacrylate and wire: Technique and results in 99 patients. **Neurosurgery** 25: 503-13, 1989.

178. Cooper P R: Comment on Branch C L, et al.: Fixation of fractures of the lower cervical spine using methylmethacrylate and wire. **Neurosurgery** 25: 512-3, 1989 (comment).

179. McGuire R A: *Cervical spine arthrodesis.* In **The cervical spine**, The Cervical Spine Research Society Editorial Committee, (ed.). Lippincott-Raven, Philadelphia, 3rd ed., 1998, Chapter 36: pp 499-508.

180. Fehlings M G, Cooper P R, Errico T J: Posterior plates in the management of cervical instability: Long-term results in 44 patients. **J Neurosurg** 81: 341-9, 1994.

181. Chapman J R, Anderson P A, Pepin C, et al.: Posterior instrumentation of the unstable cervicothoracic spine. **J Neurosurg** 84: 552-8, 1996.

182. An H S, Vaccaro A, Cotler J M, et al.: Spinal disorders at the cervicothoracic junction. **Spine** 19: 2557-64, 1994.

183. Bailes J E, Hadley M N, Quigley M R, et al.: Management of athletic injuries of the cervical spine and spinal cord. **Neurosurgery** 29: 491-7, 1991.

184. Torg J S, Corcoran T A, Thibault L F, et al.: Cervical cord neuropraxia: Classification, pathomechanics, morbidity, and management guidelines. **J Neurosurg** 87: 843-50, 1997.

185. Maroon J C: "Burning hands" in football spinal cord injuries. **JAMA** 238: 2049-51, 1977.

186. Cantu R C, Mueller F O: Catastrophic spine injuries in football. **J Spinal Disord** 3: 227-31, 1990.

187. Torg J S, Ramsey-Emrhein J A: Management guidelines for participation in collision activities with congenital, developmental, or post-injury lesions involving the cervical spine. **Clin Sports Med** 16: 501-31, 1997.

188. Herkowitz H N, Rothman R H: Subacute instability of the cervical spine. **Spine** 9: 348-57, 1984.

189. Delfini R, Dorizzi A, Facchinetti G, et al.: Delayed post-traumatic cervical instability. **Surg Neurol** 51: 588-95, 1999.

190. Section on Disorders of the Spine and Peripheral Nerves of the American Association of Neurological Surgeons and the Congress of Neurological Surgeons: Chapter 22: Management of vertebral artery injuries after nonpenetrating cervical trauma. **Neurosurgery** 50 Supplement (3): Guidelines for the management of acute cervical spine and spinal cord injuries: S173-8, 2002.

191. Louw J A, Mafoyane N A, Small B, *et al*.: Occlusion of the vertebral artery in cervical spine dislocations. **J Bone Joint Surg Br** 72 (4): 679-81, 1990.

192. Willis B K, Greiner F, Orrison W W, *et al*.: The incidence of vertebral artery injury after midcervical spine fracture or subluxation. **Neurosurgery** 34 (3): 435-41; discussion 441-2, 1994.

193. Biffl W L, Moore E E, Elliott J P, *et al*.: The devastating potential of blunt vertebral arterial injuries. **Ann Surg** 231 (5): 672-81, 2000.

194. Denis F: The three column spine and its significance in the classification of acute thoracolumbar spinal injuries. **Spine** 8: 817-31, 1983.

195. Chedid M K, Green C: A review of the management of lumbar fractures with focus on surgical decision-making and techniques. **Contemp Neurosurg** 21 (11): 1-5, 1999.

196. Hitchon P W, Jurf A A, Kernstine K, *et al*.: Management options in thoracolumbar fractures. **Contemp Neurosurg** 22 (21): 1-12, 2000.

197. Hitchon P W, Torner J C, Haddad S F, *et al*.: Management options in thoracolumbar burst fractures. **Surg Neurol** 49: 619-27, 1998.

198. Court-Brown C M, Gertzbein S D: The management of burst fractures of the fifth lumbar vertebrae. **Spine** 12: 308-12, 1987.

199. Frederickson B E, Yuan H A, Miller H: Burst fractures of the fifth lumbar vertebrae: A report of four cases. **J Bone Joint Surg** 64A: 1088-94, 1982.

200. Bose B, Osterholm J L, Northrup B E, *et al*.: Management of lumbar translocation injuries: Case reports. **Neurosurgery** 17: 958-61, 1985.

201. Blumenkopf B, Daniels T: Intraoperative ultrasonography (IOUS) in thoracolumbar fractures. **J Spinal Disord** 1: 86-93, 1988.

202. Consensus Development Conference: Prophylaxis and treatment of osteoporosis. **Am J Med** 90: 107-10, 1991.

203. Daniell H W: Osteoporosis of the slender smoker: Vertebral compression fracture and loss of metacarpal cortex in relation to postmenopausal cigarette smoking and lack of obesity. **Arch Int Med** 136: 298-304, 1976.

204. Shahinian V B, Kuo Y F, Freeman J L, *et al*.: Risk of fracture after androgen deprivation for prostate cancer. **N Engl J Med** 352 (2): 154-64, 2005.

205. Kanis J A, Melton J, Christiansen C, *et al*.: The diagnosis of osteoporosis. **J Bone Miner Res** 9: 1137-41, 1994.

206. Choice of drugs for postmenopausal osteoporosis. **Med Letter** 34: 101-2, 1992.

207. Riggs B L, Melton L J: The prevention and treatment of osteoporosis. **N Engl J Med** 327: 620-7, 1992.

208. Khosla S, Riggs B L: Treatment options for osteoporosis. **Mayo Clin Proc** 70: 978-82, 1995.

209. Drugs for prevention and treatment of postmenopausal osteoporosis. **Med Letter** 42: 97-100, 2000.

210. National Institutes of Health Consensus Development Conference: Optimum calcium intake. **JAMA** 272: 1942-8, 1994 (consensus conference).

211. Once-A-week risedronate *(Actonel)*. **Med Letter** 44 (1141): 87-8, 2002.

212. Raloxifene for postmenopausal osteoporosis. **Med Letter** 40: 29-30, 1998.

213. Cotten A, Dewatre F, Cortet B, *et al*.: Percutaneous

214. Fourney D R, Schomer D F, Nader R, *et al*.: Percutaneous vertebroplasty and kyphoplasty for painful vertebral body fractures in cancer patients. **J Neurosurg** 98 (1 Suppl): 21-30, 2003.

215. Bendok B R, Halpin R J, Rubin M N, *et al*.: Percutaneous vertebroplasty. **Contemp Neurosurg** 26 (8): 1-6, 2004.

216. Gibbons K J, Soloniuk D S, Razack N: Neurological injury and patterns of sacral fractures. **J Neurosurg** 72: 889-93, 1990.

217. Denis F, Davis S, Comfort T: Sacral fractures: An important problem. Retrospective analysis of 236 cases. **Clin Orthop** 227: 67-81, 1988.

218. Sabiston C P, Wing P C: Sacral fractures: Classification and neurologic implications. **J Trauma** 26: 1113-5, 1986.

219. Robertson D P, Simpson R K: Penetrating injuries restricted to the cauda equina: A retrospective review. **Neurosurgery** 31: 265-70, 1992.

220. Messer H D, Cereza P F: Copper jacketed bullets in the central nervous system. **Neuroradiology** 12: 121-9, 1976.

221. Benzel E C, Hadden T, Coleman J E: Civilian gunshot wounds to the spinal cord and cauda equina. **Neurosurgery** 20: 281-5, 1987.

222. Linden M A, Manton W I, Stewart R M, *et al*.: Lead poisoning from retained bullets. Pathogenesis, diagnosis, and management. **Ann Surg** 195: 305-13, 1982.

223. Monson D O, Saletta J D, Freeark R J: Carotid vertebral trauma. **J Trauma** 9: 987-9, 1969.

224. Perry M O: *Injuries of the brachiocephalic vessels*. In **Vasc surg**, Rutherford R B, (ed.). W.B. Saunders, Philadelphia, 4th ed., 1995, Vol. 1, Chapter 47: pp 705-13.

225. Reid J D S, Weigelt J A: Forty-three cases of vertebral artery trauma. **J Trauma** 28: 1007-12, 1988.

226. Fogelman M J, Stewart R D: Penetrating wounds of the neck. **Am J Surg** 91: 581-96, 1956.

227. Meyer J P, Barrett J A, Schuler J J, *et al*.: Mandatory versus selective exploration for penetrating neck trauma. A prospective assessment. **Arch Surg** 122: 592-7, 1987.

228. Ledgerwood A M, Mullins R J, Lucas C E: Primary repair vs ligation for carotid artery injuries. **Arch Surg** 115: 488-93, 1980.

229. Meier D E, Brink B E, Fry W J: Vertebral artery trauma: Acute recognition and treatment. **Arch Surg** 116: 236-9, 1981.

230. Erickson R P: Autonomic hyperreflexia: Pathophysiology and medical management. **Arch Phys Med Rehabil** 61: 431-40, 1980.

231. Kewalramani L S, Orth M S: Autonomic dysreflexia in traumatic myelopathy. **Am J Phys Med** 59: 1-21, 1980.

232. Dykstra D D, Sidi A A, Anderson L C: The effect of nifedipine on cyctoscopy-induced autonomic hyperreflexia in patients with high spinal cord injuries. **J Urol** 138: 1155-7, 1987.

233. Sizemore G W, Winternitz W W: Autonomic hyperreflexia - suppression with alpha-adrenergic blocking agents. **N Engl J Med** 282: 795, 1970.

234. Short D J, El Masry W S, Jones P W: High dose methylprednisolone in the management of acute spinal cord injury - a systematic review from a clinical perspective. **Spinal Cord** 38 (5): 273-86, 2000.

235. Qian T, Guo X, Levi A D, et al.: High-dose methylprednisolone may cause myopathy in acute spinal cord injury patients. **Spinal Cord** 43 (4): 199-203, 2005.

vertebroplasty for osteolytic metastases and myeloma: Effects of the percentage of lesion filling and the leakage of methyl methacrylate at clinical follow-up. **Radiology** 200: 525-30, 1996.

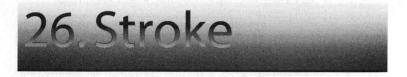

26. Stroke

Cerebrovascular accidents (**CVA**), AKA stroke. Also see *Occlusive cerebro-vascular disease*, page 869, *Intracerebral hemorrhage* on page 849, and *SAH and aneurysms* on page 781.

26.1. Strokes in general

CEREBRAL BLOOD FLOW (CBF) AND OXYGEN UTILIZATION

Table 26-1 shows typical CBF values and the corresponding neurophysiologic state. CBF < 20 is generally associated with ischemia and if prolonged will produce cell death[1]. However, this assumes normal metabolic rate and may be more applicable to *global* cerebral hypoperfusion[2]. The notion that there is a higher CBF threshold for loss of electrical excitability than that for cell death lead to the concept of the ischemic **penumbra** - cells that were nonfunctioning but still viable[1].

CBF is related to blood pressure as shown in *Eq 26-1*,

$$CBF = \frac{CPP}{CVR} = \frac{MAP - ICP}{CVR}$$

Eq 26-1

where CPP = cerebral perfusion pressure (*see page 647*), CVR = cerebrovascular resistance (*see below*), and MAP = mean arterial pressure.

Cerebrovascular resistance (CVR) is affected by the $PaCO_2$ such that there is a linear increase in CBF with increasing $PaCO_2$ within the range of 20-80 mm Hg.

CVR is also affected by changes in CPP which produce changes in blood vessel tone via a myogenic mechanism. In the range of CPP = 50-150 mm Hg the CVR of normal brain tissue varies linearly to maintain an almost constant CBF. This phenomenon is called (cerebral) **autoregulation**, which is altered in pathologic states.

Table 26-1 Effects of variations in CBF

CBF (ml per 100 gm tissue/min)	Condition
45-65	normal brain at rest
75-80	gray matter
20-30	white matter
16-18	EEG becomes flatline
15	physiologic paralysis
12	brainstem auditory evoked response (BSAER) changes
10	alterations in cell membrane transport (cell death; CVA)

The **cerebral metabolic rate of oxygen consumption ($CMRO_2$)** averages 3.0-3.8 ml/100 gm tissue/min. The ratio of CBF to $CMRO_2$ (the **coupling**[3] ratio) in the quiescent brain is 14-18. With focal cortical activity, local CBF increases ≈ 30% while $CMRO_2$ increases ≈ 5%[4]. $CMRO_2$ can be manipulated to some degree (*see page 806*).

ABRUPT ONSET OF NEW FOCAL DEFICIT

For a patient presenting to the E/R with the abrupt onset of a new focal cerebral deficit:
* 5% are seizure, tumor, or psychogenic
* 95% are vascular (i.e stroke):
  * 85% ischemic infarct: early angiography has shown that arterial occlusion can be demonstrated in 80% of these, regardless of subtype[5]
    * 41% unknown cause (may decrease with the use of early angiography)

- 21% lacune (small artery or arteriole cerebrovascular lesion)
- 16% cardiogenic embolus[6]
- atherosclerotic plaques in the aortic arch > 4 mm thick are a risk factor for recurrent CVAs and other vascular events (MI, peripheral embolism, and death from vascular causes)[7]
- 11% large artery cerebrovascular lesion
- 11% tandem arterial pathology
- ◆ 15-30% hemorrhagic[A]: ICH, SAH or SDH

Table 26-2 Outcome in CVAs

Outcome	%
died	23%
home	48%
nursing home	26%
transfer to rehabilitation unit	3%

OUTCOME

The 1980 statistics for disposition at time of discharge for ~ 1,800 CVAs is shown in *Table 26-2*.

26.1.1. Modifiable risk factors for stroke

1. hypertension: the most powerful & treatable risk factor. Both systolic & diastolic BP are independently correlated with risk of CVA[8]
2. cigarette smoking: relative risk values of 1.5-2.2[9-11]
3. blood lipids: lowering lipids may reduce the risk of some types of cerebrovascular disease
4. alcohol: heavy consumption is associated with increased risk of CVA, whereas moderate use may have no effect or may be slightly protective. The effects may be different for ischemic vs. hemorrhagic CVA[12]
5. antiplatelet therapy: reduces the risk of CVA and other vascular events in high-risk patients. The optimal dose is not known, the acceptable range is 30-1300 mg/d, with a recommended initial dose of 325 mg/d[13]

26.1.2. Evaluation

CAT SCAN (EMERGENT)

A noncontrast brain CT scan should be done ASAP to rule-out hemorrhage (intraparenchymal or SAH), hematoma, early signs of ischemia, old infarcts or injuries, and other lesions (e.g. tumor).

Emergent CT is more strongly indicated in the following situations:
1. if anticoagulation (e.g. heparin) or thrombolytic therapy is considered (to rule-out hemorrhage, massive infarction…)
2. if ICH suspected (e.g. if level of consciousness unusually depressed)
3. if surgical lesion possible (see *Emergency carotid endarterectomy*, page 879)

CAT scan findings with ischemic CVAs ("pale" infarcts)
NB: These principles do not apply to small lacunar infarcts, nor to hemorrhagic CVAs.

First 12-24 hrs: CT is normal in 8-69% of MCA CVAs[14]. Early findings may include:
1. hyperdense artery sign (*see below*)
2. focal low attenuation within the gray matter[B]
3. mass effect[B]
   A. effacement of the cerebral sulci (often subtle)[16]
   B. midline shift
4. loss of the gray-white interface[B]
5. attenuation of the lentiform nucleus
6. loss of the insular ribbon (hypodensity involving the insular region)

A. Intracerebral hemorrhage **(ICH)** should be suspected with smooth onset of symptoms over minutes to hours, presence of severe H/A, frequent vomiting, and when depression of level of consciousness is prominent (in contrast to ischemic infarct which typically has significant motor or sensory deficit with little or no impairment of consciousness except with massive or brainstem stroke); these features may be less prominent in lobar ICH. Also see *Intracerebral hemorrhage*, page 849

B. these findings are probably due to increased water content resulting from the following: cellular edema arising from altered cell permeability which produces a shift of sodium and water from the extracellular to the intracellular compartment, which also increases the extracellular osmotic pressure causing transudation of water from capillaries into the interstitium[15]

---

7. enhancement: occurs in only 33%. CVA becomes isodense (call "masking" effect) or hyperdense with normal brain, and, rarely, may be the only indication of infarction[16]

48 hrs: most CVAs can be seen as areas of low density by this time.

1-2 wks: CVAs are sharply demarcated.

3 wks: CVA approaches CSF density.

In 5-10% there may be a short window (at around day 7-10) where the CVA becomes isodense, called "fogging effect". IV contrast will usually demonstrate these.

Mass effect: common from day 1 to 25. Then atrophy is usually seen by ≈ 5 wks (2 wks at the earliest). Serial CT scans have shown that midline shift increases after ischemic CVA and reaches a maximum 2-4 days after the insult.

Calcifications: only ≈ 1-2% of CVAs calcify (in adults, it is probably a much smaller fraction than this; and in peds it is a higher percentage than this). Therefore, in an adult, calcifications almost rule-out a CVA (consider AVM, low grade tumor...).

Hyperdense artery sign: The cerebral vessel (usually the MCA) appears as a high density on unenhanced CT, indicating intra-arterial clot (thrombus or embolus)[17]. Seen in 12% of 50 patients scanned within 24 hrs of CVA, and in 34% of 23 <u>very</u> early CTs done to R/O hemorrhage. Sensitivity for MCA occlusion is low, but specificity is high (although it may also be seen with carotid dissection, or (usually bilaterally) with calcific atherosclerosis or high hematocrit[17]). Does <u>not</u> have independent prognostic significance[18].

Enhancement: CT enhancement with IV contrast in CVA:
1. many enhance by day 6, most by day 10, some will enhance up to 5 wks
2. **rule of 2's**: 2% enhance at 2 days, 2% enhance at 2 mos
3. **gyral enhancement**: AKA called "ribbon" enhancement. Common. Usually seen by 1 week (grey matter enhances > white). DDx includes inflammatory infiltrating lesions such as lymphoma, neurosarcoidosis... (due to breakdown of BBB)
4. as a rule of thumb: there should not be enhancement at the same time as there is mass effect

MRI

In patients able to cooperate, MRI is more sensitive than CT (especially between 8 and 24 hrs post-ictus), especially in brainstem or cerebellar infarction. Four types of MRI enhancement patterns have been described[19]:
1. intravascular enhancement: occurs in ≈ 75% of 1-3 day-old cortical infarcts, and is probably due to sluggish flow and vasodilatation (thus, it is not seen with complete occlusion). May indicate areas of brain at risk of infarction
2. meningeal enhancement: especially involving the dura. Seen in 35% of cortical CVAs 1-3 days old (not seen in deep cerebral or brainstem CVAs). No angiographic nor CT equivalent
3. transitional enhancement: above two types of enhancement coexist with early evidence of BBB breakdown; usually seen on days 3-6
4. parenchymal enhancement: classically appears as a cortical or subcortical gyral ribbon enhancement. May not be apparent for the first 1-2 days, and gradually approaches 100% by 1 week. Enhancement may eliminate "fogging effect" (as on CT) which may obscure some CVAs at ≈ 2 weeks on unenhanced T2WI

EMERGENCY CEREBRAL ANGIOGRAPHY (OR DVI)
1. early CVA in carotid distribution + history of amaurosis fugax or bruit or retinal emboli, etc. suggesting increasing carotid stenosis, thrombogenic ulcerated plaque, or carotid dissection
2. if diagnosis still questionable (e.g. aneurysm, vasculitis)
3. with rapid recovery, suggesting carotid TIA in face of increasing stenosis
4. <u>AVOID</u> angio if unstable or if severe disabling neuro deficit

Findings:
1. cutoff sign: vessel ends abruptly at the point of obstruction
2. string sign: narrow strand of contrast in a vessel with high grade stenosis
3. **"luxury perfusion"**: reactive hyperemia is a recognized response of cerebral tissue to injury (trauma, infarction, epileptogenic focus...). Luxury perfusion is blood flow in excess of demand due to abolition of CBF autoregulation due to acidosis[20]. On angiography it shows up as accelerated circulation adjacent to the infarct with a stain or blush and early venous drainage

NIH STROKE SCALE (NIHSS)

Administer in order shown. Record initial performance only (do not go back).

1a. Level of consciousness (LOC)

0   alert; keenly responsive
1   not alert, but arousable by minor stimulation to obey, answer or respond
2   not alert, requires repeated stimulation to attend, or is obtunded and requires strong painful stimulation to make movements (not stereotyped)
3   comatose: responds only with reflex motor (posturing) or autonomic effects, or is totally unresponsive, flaccid and areflexic

1b. Level of consciousness questions

Patient is asked the month and their age.

0   answers both questions correctly: must be correct (no credit for being close)
1   answers one question correctly, or cannot answer because of: ET tube, orotracheal trauma, severe dysarthria, language barrier, or any other problem not secondary to aphasia.
2   answers neither question correctly, or is: aphasic, stuporous, or does not comprehend the questions

1c. Level of consciousness commands

Patient is asked to open and close the eyes, and then to grip and release the non-paretic hand. Substitute another 1-step command if both hands cannot be used. Credit is given for an unequivocal attempt even if it cannot be completed due to weakness. If there is no response to commands, demonstrate (pantomime) the task. Record only first attempt.

0   performs both tasks correctly
1   performs one task correctly
2   performs neither task correctly

2. Best gaze

Test only horizontal eye movement. Use motion to attract attention of aphasic patients.

0   normal
1   partial gaze palsy (gaze abnormal in one or both eyes, but forced deviation or total gaze paresis are not present) or patient has an isolated cranial nerve III, IV or VI paresis
2   forced deviation or total gaze paresis not overcome by oculocephalic (Doll's eyes) maneuver (do not do caloric testing)

3. Visual

Visual fields (upper and lower quadrants) are tested by confrontation. May be scored as normal if patient looks at side of finger movement. Use ocular threat where consciousness or comprehension limits testing. Then test with double sided simultaneous stimulation (**DSSS**).

0   no visual loss
1   partial hemianopia (clear cut asymmetry), or extinction to DSSS
2   complete hemianopia
3   bilateral hemianopia (blind, including cortical blindness)

4. Facial palsy

Ask patient (or pantomime) to show their teeth, or raise eyebrows and close eyes. Use painful stimulus and grade grimace response in poorly responsive or non-comprehending patients.

0   normal symmetrical movement
1   minor paralysis (flattened nasolabial fold, asymmetry on smiling)
2   partial paralysis (total or near total paralysis of lower face)
3   complete paralysis of one or both sides (absent facial movement in upper and lower face)

5. Motor Arm (5a = left, 5b = right)

Instruct patient to hold the arms outstretched, palms down (at 90° if sitting, or 45° if supine). If consciousness or comprehension impaired, cue patient by actively lifting arms into position while verbally instructing patient to maintain position.

0   no drift (holds arm at 90° or 45° for full 10 seconds)
1   drift (holds limbs at 90° or 45° position, but drifts before full 10 seconds but does not hit bed or other support)
2   some effort against gravity (cannot get to or hold initial position, drifts down to bed)
3   no effort against gravity, limb falls
4   no movement
9   amputation or joint fusion: explain

6. Motor leg (6a = left, 6b = right)

While supine, instruct patient to maintain the non-paretic leg at 30°. If consciousness or comprehension impaired, cue patient by actively lifting leg into position while verbally instructing patient to maintain position. Then repeat in paretic leg.

0   no drift (holds leg at 30° full 5 seconds)
1   drift (leg falls before 5 seconds, but does not hit bed)
2   some effort against gravity (leg falls to bed by 5 seconds)
3   no effort against gravity (leg falls to

bed immediately)

4 no movement

9 amputation or joint fusion: explain

‾‾‾‾

7. Limb ataxia

(Looking for unilateral cerebellar lesion). Finger-nose-finger and heel-knee-shin tests are performed on both sides. Ataxia is scored only if clearly out of proportion to weakness. Ataxia is absent in the patient who cannot comprehend or is paralyzed.

0 absent

1 present in one limb

2 present in two limbs

9 amputation or joint fusion: explain

‾‾‾‾

8. Sensory

Test with pin. When consciousness or comprehension impaired, score sensation normal unless deficit clearly recognized (e.g. clear-cut asymmetry of grimace or withdrawal). Only hemisensory losses attributed to stroke are counted as abnormal.

0 normal, no sensory loss

1 mild to moderate sensory loss (pinprick dull or less sharp on the affected side, or loss of superficial pain to pinprick but patient aware of being touched)

2 severe to total (patient unaware of being touched in the face, arm and leg)

9. Best language

In addition to judging comprehension of commands in the preceding neurologic exam, the patient is asked to describe a standard picture, to name common items, and to read and interpret the standard text in the box below. The intubated patient should be asked to write.

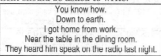

You know how.
Down to earth.
I got home from work.
Near the table in the dining room.
They heard him speak on the radio last night.

0 normal, no aphasia

1 mild to moderate aphasia (some loss of fluency, word finding errors, naming errors, paraphasias and/or impairment of communication by either comprehension or expression disability)

2 severe aphasia (great need for inference, questioning and guessing by listener; limited range of information can be exchanged)

3 mute or global aphasia (no usable speech or auditory comprehension) or patient in coma (item 1a = 3)

10. Dysarthria

Patient may be graded based on information already gleaned during evaluation. If patient is thought to be normal, have them read (or repeat) the standard text shown in this box.

MAMA
TIP-TOP
FIFTY-FIFTY
THANKS
HUCKLEBERRY
BASEBALL PLAYER
CATERPILLAR

0 normal speech

1 mild to moderate (slurs some words, can be understood with some difficulty)

2 severe (unintelligible slurred speech in the absence of, or out of proportion to any dysphasia, or is mute/anarthric)

9 intubated or other physical barrier

11. Extinction and inattention (formerly neglect)

Sufficient information to identify neglect may already be gleaned during evaluation. If the patient has severe visual loss preventing visual DSSS, and the cutaneous stimuli are normal, the score is normal. Scored as abnormal only if present.

0 normal, no sensory loss

1 visual, tactile, auditory, spatial or personal inattention or extinction to DSSS in one of the sensory modalities

2 profound hemi-inattention or hemi-inattention to more than one modality. Does not recognize own hand or orients to only one side of space.

A. Distal motor function (not part of NIHSS) (a = left arm, b = right)

Patients hand is held up at the forearm by the examiner, and is asked to extend the fingers as much as possible. If patient cannot do so, the examiner does it for them. Do not repeat the command.

0 normal (no finger flexion after 5 seconds)

1 at least some extension after 5 seconds (any finger movement is scored)

2 no voluntary extension after 5 seconds

26.1.3.   Management of RIND, TIA, or CVA

THROMBOLYTIC THERAPY

Plasminogen activators catalyze the conversion of plasminogen to the fibrinolytic compound plasmin. Available agents include streptokinase (Streptase®) and alteplase (recombinant tissue plasminogen activator (**rtPA**)) (Activase®) which is FDA approved for the IV treatment of acute ischemic CVA (*see below*). Streptokinase has been associated with a worse outcome at 3 months[21, 22] (even when given within 3 hours of onset of CVA the outcome was no better than placebo[21]). Activase converts more fibrin-bound and less circulating plasminogen to plasmin than does streptokinase.

TISSUE PLASMINOGEN ACTIVATOR

A randomized double-blind NINDS study of 624 patients with an ischemic stroke having a clearly defined time of onset and a CT scan prior to drug administration, found no significant reduction of deficit at 24 hrs in patients receiving alteplase as recommended (*see below*) initiated within **3 hrs** of the onset of symptoms. However, rtPA patients had improved neurologic outcome at 3 months (these patients were 30% more likely to have minimal or no disability)[23] which persisted at 6 and 12 mos[24] in all subgroups of *ischemic* stroke. The recurrent stroke rate in control and rtPA patients was similar (5%). In contrast, statistical benefit at 90 days could not be confirmed in the ECASS II study[25].

Exclusionary criteria:
1. intracerebral hemorrhage **(ICH)**: on admitting CT, or history of prior ICH
2. serious head trauma within past 3 months
3. SBP > 185 mm Hg, or DBP > 110 mm Hg
4. rapidly improving or minor symptoms
5. history of GI or urinary tract hemorrhage within past 21 days
6. arterial puncture at non-compressible site within past 7 days
7. patients on anticoagulants, or those receiving heparin within the past 48 hrs
8. PT > 15 seconds or platelet count < 100,000/mm³
9. seizure at onset of CVA
10. symptoms suggestive of SAH
11. major surgery within last 14 days
12. another CVA within past 3 months
13. blood glucose > 400 mg% or < 50 mg%

Exclusionary criteria added by manufacturer:
14. NIH stroke scale **(NIH-SS)** > 22
15. age > 77
16. CT scan evidence of early intracerebral ischemia

Additional ECASS II exclusionary criteria[25]:
1. unknown time of onset of symptoms
2. coma or severe stupor
3. hemiplegia + fixed eye deviation
4. seizure in the past 6 mos
5. CNS surgery within past 3 months

A large placebo-controlled European trial (ECASS) using 1.1 mg/kg rtPA given within 6 hrs of hemispheric ischemia found no benefit when analyzed according to intention to treat[26]. This supports the theory that the benefit to risk ratio may be lower with later initiation of treatment, higher doses, and/or inadequate control of BP.

Table 26-3   Management of HTN after administration of rtPA for acute CVA*

BP† (mm Hg)	Intervention
SBP 180-230 and/or DBP 110-120	labetalol 10 mg IV over 1-2 mins, repeat or double dose q 10-20 mins up to 150 mg. If labetalol contraindicated, use nifedipine 10 mg SL
SBP > 230 and/or DBP 121-140	as above, but if labetalol contraindicated or ineffective, use nitroprusside (*see page 4*)
DBP > 140	start nitroprusside 0.5-10 µg/kg/min (*see page 4*)

*   this scheme is not intended for use outside of NINDS/rtPA study

†   SBP = systolic blood pressure, DBP = diastolic BP

ICH following rtPA

There is an increased risk of *symptomatic* intracerebral hemorrhage **(ICH)** with the use of rtPA (NINDS study: 6.4% vs. 0.6% with placebo; ECASS II: 8.8% vs. 3.4%). In spite of this, the NINDS study found that mortality in the rtPA group was similar to controls at 3 mos (17% vs. 21%). The following factors were associated with an increased risk of symptomatic ICH (with only a 57% efficiency rate of predicting ICH): severity of NIH-SS score, or pre-treatment CT showing brain edema or mass effect. In one study, ICH did not influence outcome except in the rare instance when a massive hematoma occurred[27].

Outcomes were still better in the treated group, and the conclusion is that these patients are still reasonable candidates for rtPA[28].

Treatment protocol
Also, see *Exclusionary criteria*, page 768.

Rx alteplase (Activase®): initiated < 3 hrs from onset of deficit (NINDS protocol): 0.09 mg/kg IV bolus over 1-2 mins, followed by 0.81 mg/kg constant infusion over 60 minutes. The NINDS protocol[23] required that no anticoagulants nor antiplatelet drugs be given for 24 hrs after treatment, and BP was maintained as illustrated in *Table 26-3*. Some clinicians prefer starting heparin acutely after rtPA, however the NINDS investigators highly recommend getting a non-contrast CT first since there was a significant incidence of subclinical intracerebral hemorrhages.

MANAGEMENT OF PATIENTS NOT UNDERGOING THROMBOLYTIC THERAPY
These guidelines are for TIA, RIND, or CVA, but not SAH (for this, *see page 786*) nor intracerebral hemorrhage **(ICH)** (*see page 856*)[29]. The following guidelines for initial management should be maintained 48 hrs after last neuro deterioration.
1. frequent VS with crani checks (q 1 hr **x** 12 hrs, then q 2 hrs)
2. activity: bed rest
3. labs:
   A. routine: CBC + platelet count, electrolytes, PT/PTT, U/A, EKG, CXR, ABG
   B. "special" (when appropriate): RPR (to rule-out neurosyphilis), ESR (to rule-out giant cell arteritis), hepatic profile, cardiac profile
   C. at 24 hrs: CBC, platelet count, cardiac profile, lipid profile, EKG
4. O_2 at 2 L per NC; repeat ABG on 2 L O_2
5. monitor cardiac rhythm **x** 24 hrs (literature quotes 5-10% prevalence of EKG changes, and 2-3% acute MIs in patients with CVAs)
6. diet: NPO
7. nursing care
   A. indwelling Foley (urinary) catheter If consciousness impaired or if unable to use urinal or bedpan; intermittent catheterization q 4-6 hrs PRN no void if Foley not used
   B. accurate I's & O's; notify M.D. for urine output < 20 cc/hr **x** 2 hrs by Foley, or < 160 cc in 8 hrs if no Foley
8. IV fluids: NS or 1/2 NS at 75-125 cc/hr for most patients (to eliminate dehydration if present)
   A. avoid glucose: hyperglycemia may extend ischemic zone (penumbra)[30]. Although hyperglycemia may be a stress response and may not be neurotoxic[31], recommendations are to strive for normoglycemia[32]
   B. avoid overhydration in cases of ICH, CHF, or SBP > 180. It had been suggested that an optimal Hct for compromise between O_2 delivery and decreased viscosity was ≈ 33% and that fluid management should strive for this, however the early promise of this theory has not been borne out
9. treat CHF and arrhythmias (check CXR & EKG). MI or myocardial ischemia may present with neuro deficit, these patients should be admitted to CCU
10. avoid diuretics unless volume overloaded
11. blood pressure **(BP)** management:
    A. for patients presenting with HTN: management must take baseline BP into account: see *Hypertension in stroke patients* below for management
    B. for patients presenting with hypotension (SBP < 110 or DBP < 70):
       1. unless contraindicated (viz.: ICH, cerebellar infarct, or decreased cardiac output) give 250 cc NS over 1 hr, then 500 cc over 4 hrs, then 500 cc over 8 hrs
       2. if fluid ineffective or contraindicated: consider pressors
12. medications
    A. ASA 325 mg PO q d (unless hemorrhagic stroke proven or suspected)
    B. stool softener
13. see following sections for discussion of anticoagulation (*page 770*), steroids (*page 771*), and mannitol (*page 771*)

HYPERTENSION IN STROKE PATIENTS
HTN may actually be needed to maintain CBF in the face of elevated ICP, and it usually resolves spontaneously. Therefore treat HTN cautiously and slowly to avoid rap-

id reduction and overshooting the target. Avoid treating mild HTN. Indications to treat HTN emergently include:
1. acute LV failure (rare)
2. acute aortic dissection (rare)
3. acute hypertensive renal failure (rare)
4. neurologic complications of HTN
   A. hypertensive encephalopathy
   B. converting a massive pale (ischemic) infarct into a hemorrhagic infarct
   C. patients with ICH (some HTN is needed to maintain CBF, see *Initial management of ICH*, page 856)

Hypertension treatment algorithm (modified[29])

Recommended lower limits for treatment endpoints are shown in *Table 26-4*.

1. If DBP > 140 (malignant hypertension): ≈ 20-30% reduction is desirable. Sodium nitroprusside (Nipride®) IV drip or IV labetalol are agents of choice; arterial-line monitor recommended; sympatholytics (e.g. trimethaphan) contraindicated (they reduce CBF)

2. SBP > 230 or DBP 120-140 **x** 20 mins: labetalol (unless contraindicated, *see page 4*): start at 10 mg slow IVP over 2 mins, then double q 10 min (20, 40, 80, then 160 mg slow IVP) until controlled or total of 300 mg given. Maintenance: effective dose (from above) q 6-8 hrs PRN SBP > 180 or DBP > 110

3. SBP 180-230 or DBP 105-120: defer emergency treatment unless there is evidence of LV failure or if readings persist **x** 60 mins
   A. unless contraindicated (see *labetalol*, page 4) oral labetalol dosed as follows:
      1. for SBP > 210 or DBP > 110: 300 mg PO BID
      2. for SBP 180-210 or DBP 100-110: 200 mg PO BID
   B. if labetalol contraindicated:
      nifedipine start with 10 mg PO/SL, if still HTN after 1 hr, give 20 mg; then follow with 10-20 mg PO or SL q 6 hrs
   C. if monotherapy fails, or labetalol contraindicated, try either:
      • hydralazine (Apresoline®) 10 mg slow IVP q 6 hrs (SIDE EFFECTS: tachycardia, use with caution in ASHD)
      OR
      • captopril (Capoten®) 6.25 mg, 12.5 mg or 25 mg PO q 8 hrs

4. SBP < 180 or DBP < 105: antihypertensive therapy usually not indicated

Table 26-4 Guidelines for lower limits of treatment endpoints for HTN in strokes

	No prior history of HTN	Prior history of HTN
do not lower **SBP** below	160-170 mm Hg	180-185 mm Hg
do not lower **DBP** below	95-105 mm Hg	105-110 mm Hg

ANTICOAGULANTS

Heparin: To date, there has been only one prospective trial[33] utilizing heparin as it is administered in the U.S.[A], and there was no significant difference in outcome[34]. Recent megatrials[35] have shown that the recurrent stroke rate in the 7 days following a CVA was only 0.6-2.2% per week[33]. Effectiveness is unproven in strokes and TIAs except with cardiogenic brain embolism (see *Cardiogenic brain embolism*, page 773). Anticoagulation may also be hazardous[36], however the complication rate has not been assessed prospectively (small, nonrandomized studies have found symptomatic ICH in 1-8%, and other bleeding complications in 3-12%[33]). Conversion rate of pale → hemorrhagic CVA is 2-5% (dog studies suggest the risk is increased only when HTN not well controlled). **Conclusion**: the risk of heparin therapy for acute focal cerebral ischemia exceeds any proven benefit[33], and is not justified in most cases (especially when used just to placate the frustrated clinician)[37, 38]. The American Heart Association has recommended: "Until more data are available, the use of heparin remains a matter of preference of the treating physician"[33]. A small but significant reduction in recurrent stroke has been shown with ASA.

Warfarin: High-intensity warfarin therapy has proven helpful for the antiphospholipid antibody syndrome (**APLAS**) (*see page 775*).

For the rare indication for anticoagulation therapy:

A. continuous IV infusion of unfractionated heparin titrated to keep APTT 1.5-2.5 **x** control

1. first, R/O hemorrhage by CT before beginning therapy
2. ASA 325 mg PO q d in all patients with non-hemorrhagic CVA where anticoagulants or surgery not indicated
3. anticoagulants (heparin/warfarin):
   A. indications (rare)
      1. probably effective for cardiogenic emboli (see *Cardiogenic brain embolism* below)
      2. shown ineffective for stroke in evolution (neuro deficit that begins, recurs, fluctuates, or worsens while patient in hospital), crescendo TIA[A] or completed stroke
      3. unproven, but generally used for carotid dissection
   B. contraindicated with large cardiac embolism, large stroke (risk of hemorrhagic conversion), peptic-ulcer disease that has bled in past 6 mos, uncontrolled severe HTN
   C. start IV heparin and simultaneous warfarin (Coumadin®) (maintain heparin during first ≈ 3 days of warfarin because of initial hypercoagulability, see *Anticoagulation*, page 21 for target APTT and INR)
   D. stop warfarin after 6 months (benefits decline, risks rise)

DEXAMETHASONE (DECADRON®) AND STEROIDS
1. for steroid responsive vasculitis, e.g. giant cell arteritis (temporal arteritis)
2. if cerebellar infarct/bleed with mass effect suspected

MANNITOL
1. for cerebellar infarct/bleed, prior to surgery, or if mass effect
2. contraindicated in hypotension
3. initial dose: 50 to 100 gm

EMERGENCY SURGERY
1. herniation from subdural hematoma
2. suboccipital craniectomy for progressive neurologic deterioration due to brainstem compression from cerebellar hemorrhage/infarction (*see below*)
3. carotid endarterectomy for high grade carotid stenosis ipsilateral to fluctuating neuro deficit (see *Emergency carotid endarterectomy*, page 879)

CEREBELLAR INFARCTION

Relatively rare (seen on only 0.6% of all CTs obtained for any reason[40]). Cerebellar infarcts may be classified as involving the PICA distribution (cerebellar tonsil and/or inferior vermis), superior cerebellar artery distribution (superior hemisphere or superior vermis), or other indeterminate patterns[41].

Early findings
In most cases the onset is sudden, without premonitory symptoms[42]. The first 12 hrs after onset were characterized by lack of progression. Early findings are due to the intrinsic cerebellar lesion (ischemic infarction or hemorrhage):
1. symptoms
   A. dizziness or vertigo
   B. nausea/vomiting
   C. loss of balance, often with a fall and inability to get up
   D. headache (infrequent in one series[42])
2. signs
   A. truncal and appendicular ataxia
   B. nystagmus
   C. dysarthria

Later findings
Patients with cerebellar infarction may subsequently develop increased pressure within the posterior fossa (due to cerebellar edema or mass effect from clot), with brain-

---

A. in 74 patients with recent TIAs, elevating PTT 1.5-2.5 x normal with heparin did not reduce recurrent TIAs nor CVAs. Bleeding occurred in 9 (12.2%). Additional risk: hemorrhage from heparin induced thrombocytopenia[39]

stem compression (particularly posterior pons). Clinical findings generally increase between 12-96 hrs following onset.

80% of patients developing signs of brainstem compression will die, usually within hours to days. Surgical decompression (*see below*) should probably be done as soon as any of the following signs develop[A] if there is no response to medical therapy[43]. Findings proceed in the approximate following sequence if there is no intervention:

1. abducens (VI) nerve palsy
2. loss of ipsilateral gaze (compression of VI nucleus and lateral gaze center)
3. peripheral facial nerve paresis (compression of facial colliculus)
4. confusion and somnolence (may be partly due to developing hydrocephalus)
5. Babinski sign
6. hemiparesis
7. lethargy
8. small but reactive pupils
9. coma
10. posturing→ flaccidity
11. ataxic respirations

Imaging studies

CT scan: may be normal very early in these patients. There may be subtle findings of a tight posterior fossa: compression or obliteration of basal cisterns or 4th ventricle.

MRI: more sensitive, but may be difficult to obtain quickly, and is very difficult in a ventilated patient.

Suboccipital craniectomy for cerebellar infarction

Unlike the situation with *supra*tentorial masses causing herniation, there are several reports of patients in deep coma from direct brainstem compression who were operated upon quickly who made useful recovery[43-45]. Guidelines for patients with cerebellar *hemorrhage* appear on page 860.

Avoid using ventricular drainage alone as this may cause upward cerebellar herniation (*see page 160*) and does not relieve the direct brainstem compression.

26.1.3.1.   Malignant middle cerebral artery territory infarction

This label is applied to a distinct syndrome that occurs in up to 10% of stroke patients[46, 47], with a mortality of up to 80% (mostly due to severe postischemic cerebral edema → increased ICP → herniation)[47].

Patients usually present with findings of severe hemispheric CVA (hemiplegia, forced eye and head deviation) often with CT findings of major infarct within the first 12 hours. Most develop drowsiness shortly after admission. There is progressive deterioration during the first 2 days, and subsequent transtentorial herniation usually within 2-4 days of stroke. Fatalities are often associated with: severe drowsiness, dense hemiplegia, age > 45-50 yrs[48], early hypodensity involving > 50% of the MCA distribution on CT scan[49], midline shift > 8-10 mm, early sulci effacement and hyperdense MCA sign[48].

Neurosurgeons may be involved in caring for these patients because some reports have advocated aggressive therapies in these patients in an attempt to reduce morbidity and mortality. Options include:

1. conventional measures to control ICP (with or without ICP monitor): mortality is still high, and elevated ICP is not a common cause of initial deterioration
2. hemicraniectomy: *see below*
3. ✖ to date, the following treatments have not improved outcome: agents to lyse clot, hyperventilation, mannitol, or barbiturate coma

Hemicraniectomy for malignant MCA territory infarction

May reduce mortality to as low as 32% in nondominant hemisphere CVAs[50] (37% in all comers[51]) with surprising reduction of hemiplegia, and in dominant hemisphere CVAs, with only mild-moderate aphasia (better results occur with early surgery, especially if surgery is performed <u>before</u> any changes associated with herniation occur). Results need to be validated with a controlled study.

A. it is important to recognize a lateral medullary syndrome (**LMS**) (*see page 777*) which may often accompany a cerebellar infarct. With LMS, the signs are usually present from the onset (dysphagia, dysarthria, Horner's syndrome, ipsilateral facial numbness, crossed sensory loss...), and are not accompanied by a change in sensorium. There is no place for surgical decompression in LMS since it represents primary brainstem ischemia and not compression

Indications: No firm indications. Guidelines:
1. age < 70 years
2. more strongly considered in right hemisphere infarction than left
3. clinical and CT evidence of acute, complete ICA or MCA infarcts and direct signs of impending or complete severe hemispheric brain swelling (severe post-admission neurologic deterioration is the usual step that triggers surgical intervention)

Technique: See reference[52].

26.1.4. Cardiogenic brain embolism

About one stroke in six is cardioembolic. Emboli may be composed of fibrin-rich thrombi (e.g. mural thrombi due to segmental myocardial hypokinesis following MI or ventricular aneurysm), platelets (e.g. nonbacterial thrombotic endocarditis), calcified material (e.g. in aortic stenosis), or tumor particles (e.g. atrial myxoma).

Following acute myocardial infarction (AMI): 2.5% of patients will have a CVA within 1-2 weeks of an AMI (the period when most emboli occur). The risk is higher with anterior wall MI ($\approx$ 6%) vs. inferior wall MI ($\approx$ 1%).

Atrial fibrillation (A-fib): Nonrheumatic patients with A-fib have a 3-5 fold increased risk of stroke[53], with a 4.5% rate of stroke per year without treatment[54]. The incidence of A-fib in the U.S. is 2.2 million. About 75% of CVAs in patients with A-fib are due to left atrial thrombi[55]. Independent risk factors for CVA in patients with A-fib are: advanced age, prior embolism (CVA or TIA), HTN, DM, and echocardiographic evidence of left atrial enlargement or left ventricular dysfunction[53].

Prosthetic heart valves: Patients with mechanical prosthetic heart valves on long-term anticoagulation have an embolism rate of 3%/year for mitral and 1.5%/year for aortic valves. With bioprosthetic heart valves and no anticoagulation the risk is 2-4%/year.

Paradoxical embolism: Paradoxical embolism can occur with a patent foramen ovale which is present in 10-18% of the general population, but in up to 56% of young adults with unexplained CVA[56].

DIAGNOSIS

No specific neurologic features can distinguish these patients.

The diagnosis of cardiogenic brain embolism **(CBE)** as a cause of a stroke relies on demonstrating a potential cardiac source, the absence of cerebrovascular disease, and non-lacunar stroke.

Large areas of hemorrhagic transformation within an ischemic infarct may be more indicative of CBE due to thrombolysis of the clot and reperfusion of infarcted brain with subsequent hemorrhagic conversion. Hemorrhagic transformation most often occurs within 48 hrs of a CBE stroke, and is more common with larger strokes.

DETECTION OF CARDIAC SOURCE

Most centers rely on echocardiography (without transesophageal ability). Using restricted criteria (i.e. excluding mitral valve prolapse), about 10% of patients with ischemic CVA will have potential cardiac source detected by echo, and most of these patients have other manifestations of cardiac disease. In CVA patients without clinical heart disease, only 1.5% will have a positive echo; the yield is higher in younger patients without cerebrovascular disease[57].

EKG may detect atrial fibrillation which may be seen in 6-24% of ischemic strokes, and may be associated with a 5-fold increased risk of CVA (*see below*).

TREATMENT

CBE is essentially the only condition for which anticoagulation has been shown to significantly reduce the rate of further CVAs.

One must balance the risk of recurrent emboli (12% of patients with a cardioembolic CVA will have a second embolic CVA within 2 weeks) against that of converting a pale infarct into a hemorrhagic one. No study has shown a clear benefit of <u>early</u> anticoagulation.

Recommendations for anticoagulation:
1. if anticoagulation is to be used, it should not be instituted within the first 48 hrs of a probable CBE stroke
2. CT should be obtained after 48 hrs following a CBE stroke and before starting anticoagulation (to R/O hemorrhage)
3. anticoagulation should not be used in the face of large infarcts
4. start heparin and warfarin simultaneously. Continue heparin for 3 days into warfarin therapy (see *Anticoagulation*, page 21)
5. optimal range of oral anticoagulation to minimize subsequent embolism and/or hemorrhage has not been determined, but pending further data, an INR of 2-3 appears satisfactory
6. patients with asymptomatic A-fib have 66-86% reduction in stroke risk with warfarin (Coumadin®)[53, 58]. ASA is only about half as effective, but may be sufficient for those without associated risk factors (listed on page 773)[53]

26.2. CVA in young adults

Only 3% of ischemic CVAs **(ICVAs)** occur in patients < 40 yrs age[59]. Over 10% of ICVAs occur in patients ≤ 55 yrs[60]. Incidence: 10 per 100,000 persons age 35-44 yrs[61], 73 per 100,000 for age < 55 yrs[60].

ETIOLOGIES

The differential diagnosis is lengthy[59], with <u>trauma</u> being the most common cause of strokes (22%) in patients under 45 yrs[62]. Most of the rest are covered by the small number of etiologies listed below (excludes: trauma, post-op CVA, SAH, and intracerebral hemorrhage).
1. **atherosclerosis**: 20% (all 18 patients in one series had either ID-DM, or were males > 35 yrs with ≥ 1 risk factors (*see below*), most had TIAs earlier)
2. **embolism** with recognized source: 20%
   A. cardiac origin is the most common (see *Cardiogenic brain embolism* above), most have previously known cardiac disease:
      1. rheumatic heart disease
      2. prosthetic valve
      3. endocarditis
      4. mitral valve prolapse **(MVP)**: present in 5-10% of young adults, in 20-40% of young adults with CVA (although one series found MVP in only 2% of CVA in young adults[61])
      5. A-fib
      6. left-atrial myxoma
   B. fat embolism syndrome: neurologic manifestation is usually global neurologic dysfunction
   C. paradoxical embolism: ASD, pulmonary AVM including Osler-Weber-Rendu syndrome, patent foramen ovale (see *Cardiogenic brain embolism* above)
   D. amniotic fluid embolism: may occur typically in the post-partum period
3. **vasculopathy**: 10%
   A. inflammatory
      1. Takayasu's
      2. infective: TB, syphilis, ophthalmic zoster
      3. amphetamine abuse
      4. herpes zoster ophthalmicus **(HZO)**: usually presents with delayed contralateral hemiplegia with a mean of ≈ 8 weeks following HZO[63]
      5. mucormycosis: a nasal and orbital fungal infection primarily in diabetics and immunocompromised patients that causes an arteritis which may thrombose the orbital veins and ICA or ACA. Produces proptosis, ocular palsy, and hemiplegia
      6. associated with systemic disease
         a. SLE (lupus) (also *see below* under *Coagulopathy*)
         b. arteritis (especially periarteritis nodosa, *see page 61*): when confined to CNS is usually multifocal and progressive, but may mimic CVA early
         c. multiple sclerosis **(MS)**

       d.   cancer
       e.   rheumatoid arthritis
  B. non-inflammatory
     1. fibromuscular dysplasia: *see page 63*
     2. carotid or vertebral artery dissections (including posttraumatic)
     3. moyamoya disease: *see page 892*
     4. **homocystinuria**: a genetic defect in methionine metabolism that produces intimal thickening and fibrosis in almost all vessels with associated thromboembolic events (arterial and venous, including dural venous sinuses). Estimated risk of stroke is 10-16%. Patients have a Marfan's syndrome-like physical appearance, malar blotches, mental retardation, and elevated levels of urinary homocystine
     5. pseudoxanthoma elasticum
4. **coagulopathy**: 10%. The following are associated with hypercoagulable states
  A. SLE: lupus anticoagulant → prolonged PTT incompletely corrects with 50/50 mix. Collagen vascular disease only rarely presents initially with CVA
  B. polycythemia or thrombocytosis
  C. sickle cell disease
  D. TTP (thrombotic thrombocytopenic purpura)
  E. antithrombin III deficiency (controversial - not seen in large series of young adults with CVA)
  F. protein C or protein S deficiency (familial): protein C attenuates hemostatic reactions, homozygous deficiency is fatal in the neonatal period. Heterozygous deficiency is associated with thrombotic strokes. A rare complication during initial therapy with warfarin is a drop in protein C before other coagulation factors resulting in a hypercoagulable state
  G. **antiphospholipid-antibody syndrome (APLAS)**[64, 65]: causes venous and/or arterial thrombosis. The two best known antiphospholipid-antibodies are anticardiolipin antibodies (**ACLA**), and lupus anticoagulant (**LAC**). Once they become symptomatic, treatment is high-intensity warfarin therapy to an INR ≥ 3[66]. There is a dramatic increase in thrombotic events after discontinuing warfarin. Aspirin is useless
  H. following use of the drug 3,4-methylenedioxymethamphetamine (**MDMA**, known on the street as ecstasy)[67], possibly independent of the hypercoagulable state that occurs with hyperthermia when insufficient fluids are consumed in conjunction with use of the drug
5. **peripartum**: 5% (usually within 2 wks of parturition)
6. miscellaneous causes: 35%
  A. uncertain etiology
  B. oral contraceptives (**BCP**): associated with ninefold increased risk for CVA, many with prior migraine history
  C. venous thrombosis (including dural sinus thrombosis): incidence may be increased with use of BCP
  D. **migraine**[68]: widely accepted, but difficult to assess objectively (incidence of stroke in these patients may be same as general population). Rare. Usually occurs in women, with a benign long-term course; recurs in < 3%. Possible mechanisms include: vasospasm, platelet dysfunction and arteriopathy[69]. CVAs often occur during a migrainous attack[70] or shortly thereafter
  E. cocaine abuse[71]: stroke may result from vasoconstriction, or from HTN in the presence of aneurysms or AVMs (frank vasculitis occurs[72] but is rare with cocaine, unlike amphetamines); strokes with alkaloidal cocaine ("crack") are ≈ equally divided between ischemic and hemorrhagic

RISK FACTORS

    In a retrospective "neighborhood control" study of 201 Australian patients aged 15-55 (mean = 45.5) with first-time ICVAs, the following risk factors were identified[60]:
1. diabetes: odds ratio = 12
2. HTN: odds ratio = 6.8
3. current cigarette smoking: odds ratio = 2.5
4. long-term heavy alcohol consumption: odds ratio = 15 (heavy alcohol ingestion within 24 hrs preceding the CVA was not a risk factor)

1. history & physical exam directed at uncovering systemic disease (see above) and modifiable risk factors (see above)
2. cardiology workup including EKG and echocardiogram
3. bloodwork (include as appropriate): electrolytes, CBC, platelet count and/or function, ESR (elevation may suggest SLE, arteritis, atrial myxoma...), PT/PTT, VDRL (should be obtained in all young adults with stroke), fasting lipid profile, ANA, antithrombin III, protein C, PPD, sickle-cell screen, toxicology screen (blood and urine, to R/O drugs such as cocaine), SPEP, lupus anticoagulant, serum amino acid, tissue plasminogen-activator and -inhibitor
4. miscellaneous tests: U/A, CXR, CSF exam when indicated
5. cerebral angiography: not always necessary for patients with obvious systemic disease or strong evidence for cardiac embolism; may occasionally diagnose cerebral embolism if performed within 48 hrs of ictus

26.3.   Lacunar strokes

Small infarcts in deep noncortical cerebrum or brainstem (see Table 26-5) resulting from occlusion of penetrating branches of cerebral arteries. Size of infarcts ranges from 3-20 mm (CT detects larger ones; better sensitivity in white matter).

Small (3-7 mm) lacunes may be due to **lipohyalinosis** (vasculopathy due to HTN) of arteries < 200 microns (may also be cause of many ICHs); this vasculopathy is indicative of small vessel disease, unlikely to be prevented by carotid endarterectomy.

Table 26-5   Typical locations for lacunar strokes
(in descending frequency)

* putamen
* caudate
* thalamus
* pons
* internal capsule (IC)
* convolutional white matter

Clinically, diagnosis virtually excluded by: aphasia, apractagnosia, sensorimotor CVA, monoplegia, homonymous hemianopsia (**HH**), severe isolated memory impairment, stupor, coma, LOC, or seizures.

L'etat lacunaire: multiple lacunes → chronic progressive neuro decline with one or more episodes of hemiparesis; results in invalidism, dysarthria, small-step gait (marche á petits pas), imbalance, incontinence, pseudobulbar signs, dementia. Many signs and symptoms are possibly due to NPH (unrecognized originally).

LACUNAR SYNDROMES
Major syndromes (see reference[73] for others):
1. **pure sensory CVA or TIA**: (the most common lacunar manifestation) usually isolated unilateral numbness of face, arm, and leg. Only 10% of TIA go on to CVA. Lacune in sensory (posteroventral) thalamus → CT detection is poor. **Dejerine-Roussy** = rare thalamic pain syndrome that may develop late
2. **pure motor hemiparesis (PMH)**: (2nd most common) pure unilateral motor deficit of face, arm and leg with no sensory deficit, HH, etc.. Lacune in posterior limb of IC, or in lower basis pontis where corticospinal (**CS**) tracts coalesce, or rarely in mid-cerebral peduncle
3. **ataxic hemiparesis**: contralateral PMH + cerebellar ataxia of affected limbs (if they can move). Lacune in basis pontis at junction of upper third and lower two thirds → dysarthria, nystagmus and unidirectional toppling possible. Differential severity in face, arm and leg possible because CS fibers dispersed by nuclei pontis (unlike compact pyramids and peduncle)
   A. variant: dysarthria-clumsy hand syndrome: lesion in same location or genu of IC. May be mimicked by a cortical infarct, but latter will have numb lips
4. **PMH sparing the face**: lacune in medullary pyramid; at onset, there may be vertigo and nystagmus (approaching lateral medullary syndrome)
   A. variant: thalamic dementia: central region of one thalamus + adjacent subthalamus → abulia, memory impairment + partial Horner's (miosis + anhydrosis)
5. **mesencephalothalamic syndrome**: "top o' the basilar embolism". III palsy, **Parinaud's syndrome** & abulia, may have amnesia. Infarct typically butterfly shaped & bilateral

6. **Weber's syndrome**: Cr. N. III palsy with contralateral PMH (no sensory loss). Usually due to occlusion of interpeduncular branches of basilar artery → central midbrain infarction, disrupting cerebral peduncle and issuing fibers of III. May also be due to aneurysm of basilar bifurcation or BA-SCA junction
7. PMH with crossed VI palsy: lacune in paramedian inferior pons
8. cerebellar ataxia with crossed III palsy (<u>Claude</u> syndrome): lacune in dentatorubral tract (superior cerebellar peduncle)
9. **hemiballism**: classically, infarct or hemorrhage in subthalamic semilunar nucleus of Luys
10. lateral medullary syndrome: *see below*
11. **locked-in syndrome**: bilateral PMH from infarct at IC, pons, pyramid or (rarely) cerebral peduncles

LATERAL MEDULLARY SYNDROME

AKA **Wallenberg's syndrome**, AKA PICA syndrome. Classically attributed to PICA occlusion, but in 80-85% of cases the <u>vertebral artery</u> is also involved[74]. No cases have been reported arising from brainstem hemorrhage. Onset is usually acute. The findings are listed in *Table 26-6* (NB: <u>absence of pyramidal tract findings</u>, and <u>no change in sensorium</u>). The location of the lesion and medullary structures are shown in *Figure 26-1*.

Table 26-6 Findings in lateral medullary syndrome[75 (p 547)]

GENERALIZED symptoms	Responsible lesion
• vertigo, N/V, nystagmus, diplopia, oscillopsia	vestibular nucleii & connections
IPSILATERAL to lesion	**Responsible lesion**
• facial pain, paresthesias, & impaired sensation	descending tract and nucleus V over half of face
• ataxia of limbs	(restiform body?)
• Horner's syndrome	descending sympathetic tract
• dysphagia, diminished gag, hoarseness	exiting fibers of IX & X
• numbness of arm, trunk, or leg	cuneate & gracile nuclei
• hiccups	?
CONTRALATERAL to lesion	**Responsible lesion**
• impaired pain & temp sense over half of body	spinothalamic tract

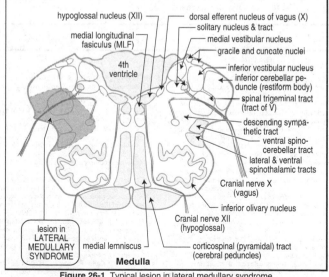

Figure 26-1 Typical lesion in lateral medullary syndrome

This is essentially the only location where a lesion will produce sensory loss on one side of the face (ipsilateral to the lesion) and contralateral sensory loss in the body. All in the absence of pyramidal tract findings (i.e. overt weakness).

These patients sometimes develop severe cerebellar swelling that responds to neurosurgical decompression (the tissue aspirates easily).

26.4. Miscellaneous CVA

See *Figure 3-9*, page 77 for the distribution territories of the major cerebral arteries.

"OCCLUSION" SYNDROMES

Recurrent medial striate artery (of Heubner): causes expressive aphasia + mild hemiparesis (UE > LE, proximal muscles weaker than distal).

Anterior choroidal artery (AChA) syndrome: The complete triad consists of contralateral hemiplegia, hemihypesthesia and homonymous hemianopsia, however, incomplete forms are more common[76]. Occlusion is usually due to small vessel disease and CT or MRI usually shows infarct in posterior limb of IC (just above temporal horn of lateral vent)[77] and white matter posterior and lateral to it. However, occlusion is sometimes tolerated fairly well, and ligation of this artery was actually utilized in treatment of Parkinsonism at times without ill effect[75 (p 540)] (see *Surgical treatment of Parkinson's disease*, page 365).

WATERSHED INFARCT

An ischemic infarction in a territory located at the periphery of two bordering arterial distributions due to a disturbance in flow in one or both of the arteries.

EMOTIONAL INCONTINENCE

AKA emotionalism or emotional lability[78]. Usually consists of uncontrollable fits of crying or laughter in response to minor events. Generally without emotional content. Described with a variety of lesions in the cortex, diencephalon, and brainstem, but usually involving systems controlling motor function (pyramidal or extrapyramidal fibers) and an interruption of a control system purportedly located at the base of the brainstem. May respond to SSRI therapy (e.g. paroxetine)[76].

26.5. References

1. - J, Siesjö B K, Symon L: Thresholds in cerebral ischemia - the ischemic penumbra. **Stroke** 12: 723-5, 1981.

2. Powers W J, Grubb R L, Darriet D, *et al.*: Cerebral blood flow and cerebral metabolic rate of oxygen requirements for cerebral function and viability in humans. **J Cereb Blood Flow Metab** 5: 600-8, 1985.

3. Raichle M E, Grubb R L, Gado M H, *et al.*: Correlation between regional cerebral blood flow and oxidative metabolism. In vivo studies in man. **Arch Neurol** 33: 523-6, 1976.

4. Henegar M M, Silbergeld D L: Pharmacology for neurosurgeons. Part II: Anesthetic agents, ICP management, corticosteroids, cerebral protectants. **Contemp Neurosurg** 18 (10): 1-6, 1996.

5. del Zoppo G J, Poeck K, Pessin M S, *et al.*: Recombinant tissue plasminogen activator in acute thrombotic and embolic stroke. **Ann Neurol** 32: 78-86, 1992.

6. Cerebral Embolism Task Force: Cardiogenic brain embolism. **Arch Neurol** 43: 71-84, 1986.

7. The French Study of Aortic Plaques in Stroke Group: Atherosclerotic disease of the aortic arch as a risk factor for recurrent ischemic stroke. **N Engl J Med** 334: 1216-21, 1996.

8. MacMahon S, Rodgers A: Blood pressure, antihypertensive treatment and stroke risk. **J Hypertens Suppl** 12 (10): S5-14, 1994.

9. Abbott R D, Yin Y, Reed D M, *et al.*: Risk of stroke in male cigarette smokers. **N Engl J Med** 315 (12): 717-20, 1986.

10. Colditz G A, Bonita R, Stampfer M J, *et al.*: Cigarette smoking and risk of stroke in middle-aged women. **N Engl J Med** 318 (15): 937-41, 1988.

11. Shinton R, Beevers G: Meta-analysis of relation between cigarette smoking and stroke. **Br Med J** 298: 789-94, 1989.

12. Biller J, Feinberg W M, Castaldo J E, *et al.*: Guidelines for carotid endarterectomy: A statement for healthcare professionals from a special writing group of the Stroke Council, American Heart Association. **Circulation** 97 (5): 501-9, 1998.

13. From the Ad Hoc Committee on Guidelines for the Management of Transient Ischemic Attacks of the Stroke Council of the American Heart Association: Guidelines for the management of transient ischemic attacks. **Stroke** 25: 1320-35, 1994.

14. Moulin T, Cattin F, Crépin-Leblond T, *et al.*: Early CT signs in acute middle cerebral artery infarction: Predictive value for subsequent infarct locations and

outcome. **Neurology** 47: 366-75, 1996.

15. Aarabi B, Long D M: Dynamics of cerebral edema. **J Neurosurg** 51: 779-84, 1979.

16. Wall S D, Brant-Zawadzki M, Jeffrey R B, *et al.*: High frequency CT findings within 24 hours after cerebral infarction. **AJR** 138: 307-11, 1982.

17. Tomsick T A, Brott T G, Olinger C P, *et al.*: Hyperdense middle cerebral artery: Incidence and quantitative significance. **Neuroradiology** 31: 312-5, 1989.

18. Manelfe C, Larrue V, von Kummer R, *et al.*: Association of hyperdense middle cerebral artery sign with clinical outcome in patients treated with plasminogen activator. **Stroke** 30: 769-72, 1999.

19. Elster A D, Moody D M: Early cerebral infarction: Gadopentetate dimeglumine enhancement. **Radiology** 177: 627-32, 1990.

20. Lassen N A: Control of cerebral circulation in health and disease. **Circ Res** 34: 749-60, 1974.

21. Donnan G A, Davis S M, Chambers B R, *et al.*: Streptokinase for acute ischemic stroke with relationship to time of administration. **JAMA** 276: 961-6, 1996.

22. The Multicenter Acute Stroke Trial - European Study Group: Thrombolytic therapy with streptokinase in acute ischemic stroke. **N Engl J Med** 335: 145-50, 1996.

23. The National Institute of Neurological Disorders and Stroke rt-PA Stroke Study Group: Tissue plasminogen activator for acute ischemic stroke. **N Engl J Med** 333: 1581-7, 1995.

24. Kwiatkowski T G, Libman R B, Frankel M, *et al.*: Effects of plasminogen activator for acute ischemic stroke at one year. **N Engl J Med** 340: 1781-7, 1999.

25. Hacke W, Kaste M, Fieschi C, *et al.*: Randomized double-blind placebo-controlled trial of thrombolytic therapy with intravenous alteplase in acute ischemic stroke (ECASS II). **Lancet** 352: 1245-51, 1998.

26. Hacke W, Kaste M, Fieschi C, *et al.*: Intravenous thrombolysis with recombinant tissue plasminogen activator for acute hemispheric stroke. The European cooperative acute stroke study (ECASS). **JAMA** 274: 1017-25, 1995.

27. Toni D, Fiorelli M, Bastianello S, *et al.*: Hemorrhagic transformation of brain infarct: Predictability in the first 5 hours from stroke onset and influence on clinical outcome. **Neurology** 46: 341-5, 1996.

28. The National Institute of Neurological Disorders and Stroke rt-PA Stroke Study Group: Intracerebral hemorrhage after intravenous t-PA therapy for ischemic stroke. **Stroke** 28: 2109-18, 1997.

29. Brott T, Reed R L: Intensive care for acute stroke in the community hospital setting: The first 24 hours. **Stroke** 20: 694-7, 1989.

30. Pulsinelli W A, Levy D E, Sigsbee B, *et al.*: Increased damage after ischemic stroke in patients with hyperglycemia with or without established diabetes mellitus. **Am J Med** 74: 540-4, 1983.

31. Tracey F, Crawford V L S, Lawson J T, *et al.*: Hyperglycemia and mortality from acute stroke. **Quart J Med** 86: 439-46, 1993.

32. Wass C T, Lanier W L: Glucose modulation of ischemic brain injury: Review and clinical recommendations. **Mayo Clin Proc** 71: 801-12, 1996.

33. Swanson R A: Intravenous heparin for acute stroke. What can we learn from the megatrials? **Neurology** 52: 1746-50, 1999.

34. Duke R J, Bloch R F, Turpie A G, *et al.*: Intravenous heparin for the prevention of stroke progression in acute partial stable stroke. **Ann Intern Med** 105: 825-8, 1986.

35. Barer D: Interpretation of IST and CAST stroke trials. **Lancet** 350: 440, 1997 (letter).

36. Genton E, Barnett H J M, Fields W S, *et al.*: Cerebral ischemia: The role of thrombosis and of anti-

37. Scheinberg P: Heparin anticoagulation. **Stroke** 20: 173-4, 1989.

38. Phillips S J: An alternative view of heparin anticoagulation in acute focal brain ischemia. **Stroke** 20: 295-8, 1989.

39. Ramirez-Lassepas M, Quiñones M R, Nino H H: Treatment of acute ischemic stroke: Open trial with continuous intravenous heparinization. **Arch Neurol** 43: 386-90, 1986.

40. Tomaszek D E, Rosner M J: Cerebellar infarction: Analysis of twenty-one cases. **Surg Neurol** 24: 223-6, 1985.

41. Hinshaw D, Thompson J, Haso A, *et al.*: Infarctions of the brain stem and cerebellum: A correlation of computer tomography and angiography. **Radiology** 137: 105-12, 1980.

42. Sypert G W, Alvord E C: Cerebellar infarction: A clinicopathological study. **Arch Neurol** 32: 357-63, 1975.

43. Heros R C: Surgical treatment of cerebellar infarction. **Stroke** 23: 937-8, 1992.

44. Heros R C: Cerebellar hemorrhage and infarction. **Stroke** 13: 106-9, 1982.

45. Chen H-J, Lee T-C, Wei C-P: Treatment of cerebellar infarction by decompressive suboccipital craniectomy. **Stroke** 23: 957-61, 1992.

46. Moulin D E, Lo R, Chiang J, *et al.*: Prognosis in middle cerebral artery occlusion. **Stroke** 16: 282-4, 1985.

47. Hacke W, Schwab S, Horn M, *et al.*: Malignant middle cerebral artery territory infarction: Clinical course and prognostic signs. **Arch Neurol** 53: 309-15, 1996.

48. Wijdicks E F M, Diringer M N: Middle cerebral artery territory infarction and early brain swelling: Progression and effect of age on outcome. **Mayo Clin Proc** 73: 829-36, 1998.

49. von Kummer R, Meyding-Lamadé U, Forsting M, *et al.*: Sensitivity and prognostic value of early CT in occlusion of the middle cerebral artery trunk. **AJNR** 15: 9-15, 1994.

50. Carter B S, Ogilvy C S, Candia G J, *et al.*: One-year outcome after decompressive surgery for massive nondominant hemispheric infarction. **Neurosurgery** 40: 1168-76, 1997.

51. Schwab S, Steiner T, Aschoff A, *et al.*: Early hemicraniectomy in patients with complete middle cerebral artery infarction. **Stroke** 29: 1888-93, 1998.

52. Delashaw J B, Broaddus W C, Kassell N F, *et al.*: Treatment of right hemispheric cerebral infarction by hemicraniectomy. **Stroke** 21: 874-81, 1990.

53. Blackshear J L, Kopecky S L, Litin S C, *et al.*: Management of atrial fibrillation in adults: Prevention of thromboembolism and symptomatic treatment. **Mayo Clin Proc** 71: 150-60, 1996.

54. Atrial Fibrillation Investigators: Risk factors for stroke and efficacy of antithrombotic therapy in atrial fibrillation: Analysis of pooled data from five randomized controlled trials. **Arch Intern Med** 154: 1449-57, 1994.

55. Hart R G, Helperin J L: Atrial fibrillation and stroke: Revisiting the dilemmas. **Stroke** 25: 1337-41, 1994.

56. Lechat P, Mas J L, Lascault G, *et al.*: Prevalence of patent foramen ovale in patients with stroke. **N Engl J Med** 318: 1148-52, 1988.

57. Cerebral Embolism Task Force: Cardiogenic brain embolism. **Arch Neurol** 46: 727-43, 1989.

58. Stroke Prevention in Atrial Fibrillation Study Group: Preliminary report of the stroke prevention in atrial fibrillation study. **N Engl J Med** 322: 863-8, 1990.

59. Hart R G, Miller V T: Cerebral infarction in young adults: A practical approach. **Stroke** 14: 110-4, 1983.

60. You R X, McNeil J J, O'Malley H M, *et al.*: Risk factors for stroke due to cerebral infarction in young

adults. **Stroke** 28: 1913-8, 1997.

61. Adams H P, Butler M J, Biller J, *et al.*: Nonhemor-
    rhagic cerebral infarction in young adults. **Arch
    Neurol** 43: 793-6, 1986.
62. Hilton-Jones D, Warlow C P: The causes of stroke
    in the young. **J Neurol** 232: 137-43, 1985.
63. Verghese A, Sugar A M: Herpes zoster ophthalmic-
    us and granulomatous angiitis: An ill-appreciated
    cause of stroke. **J Am Geriatr Soc** 34: 309-12,
    1986.
64. Toschi V, Motta A, Castelli C, *et al.*: High preva-
    lence of antiphosphatidylinositol antibodies in
    young patients with cerebral ischemia of undeter-
    mined cause. **Stroke** 29: 1759-64, 1998.
65. Tanne D, Triplett D A, Levine S R: Antiphospholip-
    id-protein antibodies and ischemic stroke: Not just
    cardiolipin anymore. **Stroke** 29: 1755-8, 1998 (edi-
    torial).
66. Khamashta M A, Cuadrado M J, Mujic F, *et al.*: The
    management of thrombosis in the antiphospholipid-
    antibody syndrome. **N Engl J Med** 332: 993-7,
    1995.
67. Milroy C M, Clark J C, Forrest A R: Pathology of
    deaths associated with "ecstasy" and "eve" misuse. **J
    Clin Pathol** 49: 149-53, 1996.
68. Welch K M A, Levine S R: Migraine-related stroke
    in the context of the international headache society
    classification of head pain. **Arch Neurol** 47: 458-
    62, 1990.
69. Rothrock J F, Walicke P, Swenson M R, *et al.*: Mi-
    grainous stroke. **Arch Neurol** 45: 63-7, 1988.
70. Spaccavento L J, Solomon G D: Migraine as an eti-
    ology of stroke in young adults. **Headache** 24: 19-
    22, 1984.
71. Levine S R, Brust J C M, Futrell N, *et al.*: Cere-
    brovascular complications of the use of the 'crack'
    form of alkaloidal cocaine. **N Engl J Med** 323: 699-
    704, 1990.
72. Kaye B R, Fainstat M: Cerebral vasculitis associated
    with cocaine abuse. **JAMA** 258: 2104-6, 1987.
73. Fisher C M: Lacunar strokes and infarcts: A review.
    Neurology (NY) 32: 871-6, 1982.
74. Fisher C M, Karnes W E, Kubik C S: Lateral med-
    ullary infarction: The pattern of vascular occlusion.
    J Neuropath Exp Neurol 29: 323-79, 1961.
75. Adams R D, Victor M: **Principles of neurology**.
    2nd ed. McGraw-Hill, New York, 1981.
76. Derex L, Ostrowsky K, Nighoghossian N, *et al.*: Se-
    vere pathological crying after left anterior choroidal
    artery infarction: Reversibility with paroxetine
    treatment. **Stroke** 28: 1464-6, 1997.
77. Helgason C, Caplan L R, Goodwin J, *et al.*: Anterior
    choroidal artery-territory infarction: Report of cases
    and review. **Arch Neurol** 43: 681-6, 1986.
78. House A, Dennis M, Molyneux A, *et al.*: Emotion-
    alism after stroke. **Br Med J** 289: 991-4, 1989.

27. Aneurysms

27.1.   Introduction to SAH

Etiologies
Etiologies of subarachnoid hemorrhage **(SAH)** include[1]:
- trauma: the most common cause of SAH[2, 3]
- "spontaneous SAH"
  - ruptured intracranial aneurysms: **75-80%** of spontaneous SAHs (*see page 799*)
  - cerebral AVMs: 4-5% of cases
  - certain vasculitides that involve the CNS (see *Vasculitis and vasculopathy*, page 58)
  - rarely due to tumor (many case reports[4-15])
  - cerebral artery dissection (may also be post-traumatic)
    - carotid artery (*see page 885*)
    - vertebral artery (*see page 886*) may cause intraventricular blood (especially 4th and third ventricle)
  - rupture of a small superficial artery
  - rupture of an infundibulum (*see page 784*)
  - coagulation disorders: iatrogenic or bleeding dyscrasias
  - dural sinus thrombosis
  - spinal AVM: usually cervical or upper thoracic (*see page 347*)
  - pretruncal nonaneurysmal SAH: *see page 823*
  - rarely reported with some drugs: e.g. cocaine (*see page 152*)
  - sickle cell disease
  - pituitary apoplexy: *see page 438*
  - no cause can be determined in 14-22% (see *SAH of unknown etiology*, page 822)

Incidence
Estimated annual rate of aneurysmal SAH in most western populations: 6-8 per 100,000 population[16, 17].

Outcome of aneurysmal SAH
- 10-15% of patients die before reaching medical care
- mortality is 10% within first few days
- 30-day mortality rate was 46% in one series[16], and in others over half the patients died within 2 weeks of their SAH[27]
- overall mortality is ≈ 45% (range: 32-67%)[28]
- about 8% die from progressive deterioration from the initial hemorrhage[18 (p 27)]
- among patients surviving the initial hemorrhage treated without surgery, rebleeding is the major cause of morbidity and mortality (*see page 789*), the risk is ≈ 15-20% within 2 weeks. The goal of early surgery (see *Timing of aneurysm surgery*, page 804) is to reduce this risk
- of those reaching neurosurgical care, vasospasm (*see page 791*) kills 7%, and causes severe deficit in another 7%[19]
- about ≈ 30% of survivors have moderate to severe disability[28]
- ≈ 66% of those who have successful aneurysm clipping never return to the same quality of life as before the SAH[28, 29]
- patients ≥ 70 yrs age fare worse for each neurologic grade[22]

Miscellaneous facts about SAH
- peak age for aneurysmal SAH is 55-60 years, ≈ 20% of cases occur between ages 15-45 yrs[20]
- 30% of aneurysmal SAHs occurs during sleep

- 50% of patients with aneurysms have warning symptoms, usually 6-20 days before SAH[21] (see *Presentation other than major rupture*, page 801)
- headache is lateralized in 30%, most to the side of the aneurysm
- SAH is complicated by intracerebral hemorrhage in 20-40%, by intraventricular hemorrhage in 13-28%, and by subdural blood in 2-5%
- soft evidence suggests that rupture incidence is higher in spring and autumn
- patients ≥ 70 yrs age have a higher proportion with a severe neurologic grade[22]

Risk factors for SAH[1]
- hypertension
- oral contraceptives
- substance abuse
  - ♦ cigarette smoking[23]
  - ♦ following cocaine abuse: *see page 152*
  - ♦ alcohol consumption[24]: controversial[25]
- diurnal variations in blood pressure[26]
- pregnancy and parturition (see *Pregnancy & intracranial hemorrhage*, page 825)
- slight increased risk during lumbar puncture and/or cerebral angiography in patient with cerebral aneurysm
- slight increased risk with advancing age[16]
- conditions with an increased incidence of cerebral aneurysms (*see page 801*)

CLINICAL FEATURES

SYMPTOMS OF SAH

Sudden onset of severe H/A (*see below*), usually with vomiting, syncope (apoplexy), neck pain (meningismus), and photophobia. If there is LOC, patient may subsequently recover consciousness[30]. Focal cranial nerve deficits may occur (e.g. third nerve palsy from aneurysmal compression, causing diplopia and/or ptosis). Low back pain may develop due to irritation of lumbar nerve roots by dependent blood.

Headache

The most common symptom, present in up to 97% of cases. Usually severe (classic description: "the worst headache of my life") and sudden in onset. They may clear and the patient may not seek medical attention (referred to as a **sentinel hemorrhage** or headache, or **warning headache**; they occur in 30-60% of patients presenting with SAH). If severe or accompanied by reduced level of consciousness, most patients present for medical evaluation. Patients with H/A due to minor hemorrhages will have blood on CT or LP. However, warning headaches may also occur without SAH and may be due to aneurysmal enlargement or to hemorrhage confined within the aneurysmal wall[31]. Warning H/A are usually sudden in onset, severe, and clear within 1 day.

Differential diagnosis of severe, acute, paroxysmal headache: 25% will have SAH[32]
1. subarachnoid hemorrhage, AKA "warning headache" or sentinel H/A (*see above*)
2. benign "**thunderclap headaches**" (**BTH**) or crash migraine[33]. Severe global headaches of abrupt onset that reach maximal intensity in < 1 minute, accompanied by vomiting in ≈ 50%. They may recur, and are presumably a form of vascular headache. Some may have transient focal symptoms. There are no clinical criteria that can reliably differentiate these from SAH[34]. There is no subarachnoid blood on CT and LP, which should probably be performed on at least the first presentation to R/O SAH. Earlier recommendations to angiogram these individuals[35] have since been tempered by experience[36, 37]
3. **benign orgasmic cephalgia**: a severe, throbbing, sometimes "explosive" H/A with onset just before or at the time of orgasm. In a series of 21 patients[38], neurologic exam was normal in all, and angiography done in 9 was normal. 9 had a history of migraine in the patient or a family member. No other symptoms developed in 18 patients followed for 2-7 yrs. Recommendations for evaluation are similar to that for thunderclap headaches above

SIGNS

Meningismus (*see below*), hypertension, focal neurologic deficit (e.g. oculomotor palsy, hemiparesis), obtundation or coma (*see below*), ocular hemorrhage (*see below*).

Meningismus
Nuchal rigidity (especially to flexion) often ensues in 6 to 24 hrs. Patients may have a positive **Kernig's sign** (flex thigh to 90° with knee bent, then straighten knee, positive sign if this causes pain in hamstrings) or **Brudzinski's sign** (flex patient's neck, involuntary hip flexion is a positive sign).

Coma following SAH
Coma may follow SAH because of any one or a combination of the following[39]:
1. increased ICP
2. damage to brain tissue from intraparenchymal hemorrhage (may also contribute to increased ICP)
3. hydrocephalus
4. diffuse ischemia (may be secondary to increased ICP)
5. seizure
6. low blood flow (reduced CBF) due to reduced cardiac output (*see page 789*)

Ocular hemorrhage
Three types of ocular hemorrhage (**OH**) may occur in association with SAH. They occur alone or in various combinations in 20-40% of patients with SAH[40].
1. subhyaloid (preretinal) hemorrhage: seen funduscopically in 11-33% of cases as bright red blood near the optic disc that obscures the underlying retinal vessels. May be associated with a higher mortality rate[41]
2. (intra)retinal hemorrhage: may surround the fovea
3. hemorrhage within the vitreous humor (**Terson's syndrome** or just **Terson syndrome**). Occurs in 4-27% of cases of aneurysmal SAH[42-44], usually bilateral. May occur with other causes of increased ICP including ruptured AVMs. Fundus copy reveals vitreous opacity. Often missed on initial examination. When sought, usually present on initial exam, however it may develop as late as 12 days post SAH, and may be associated with rebleeding[43]. The mortality rate may be higher in SAH patients with vitreous hemorrhage than in those without. Patients should be followed for complications of OH (elevated intraocular pressure, retinal membrane formation → retinal detachment, retinal folds[45]). Most cases clear spontaneously in 6-12 mos. Vitrectomy should be considered in patients whose vision fails to improve[44] or if more rapid improvement is desired[46]. The long-term prognosis for vision is good in ≈ 80% of cases with or without vitrectomy[46]

The pathomechanics of OH may be due to compression of the central retinal vein and the retinochoroidal anastamoses by elevated CSF pressure[44] causing venous hypertension and disruption of retinal veins.

LABORATORY/RADIOGRAPHIC FINDINGS

EVALUATION
Sequence of evaluation for a patient with suspected SAH:
1. tests to diagnose SAH
   A. non-contrast high-resolution CT scan: *see below*
   B. if CT is negative: LP in questionable cases (for findings, *see below*)
2. cerebral angiography in confirmed cases or if high degree of suspicion: (*see below*)
3. if angiogram is negative: see *SAH of unknown etiology*, page 822

CT SCAN
A good quality (e.g. no motion artifact) non-contrast high-resolution CT will detect SAH in ≥ 95% of cases if scanned within 48 hrs of SAH. Blood appears as high density (white) within subarachnoid spaces. CT also assesses the following:
1. ventricular size: hydrocephalus occurs acutely in 21% of aneurysmal ruptures[47] (also see *Hydrocephalus after SAH*, page 790)
2. hematoma: intracerebral hemorrhage or large amount of subdural blood with mass effect may need emergent evacuation
3. infarct
4. amount of blood in cisterns and fissures: important prognosticator for vasospasm (*see page 792*) and can identify pretruncal hemorrhage (*see page 823*)
5. with multiple aneurysms, CT may identify which aneurysm bled (*see page 819*)
6. can predict aneurysm location in ≈ 70% of cases
   A. blood predominantly within ventricles, especially 4th and third, suggests

lower posterior fossa source, such as PICA aneurysm or VA dissection
B. blood predominantly in anterior interhemispheric fissure suggests a-comm aneurysm
C. blood predominantly in sylvian fissure is compatible with p-comm or MCA aneurysm

LUMBAR PUNCTURE

The most sensitive test for SAH. However, false positives may occur, e.g. with traumatic taps (see *Differentiating SAH from traumatic tap*, page 173).

✖ Caution: lowering the CSF pressure may possibly precipitate rebleeding by increasing the transmural pressure (*see page 790*). Therefore remove only a small amount of CSF (several ml) and use a small (≤ 20 Ga) spinal needle.

Findings (also, see *Table 10-4*, page 172):
1. opening pressure: elevated
2. appearance:
   A. non-clotting bloody fluid that does not clear with sequential tubes
   B. **xanthochromia**: pink or yellow coloration of CSF supernatant due to heme pigments released by the breakdown of RBCs. The most reliable means of differentiating traumatic tap from SAH. Usually not apparent until 2-4 hours after the SAH. Is present in almost 100% at 12 hours after the bleed, and remains in 70% at 3 weeks, and is still detectable in 40% at 4 weeks. Spectrophotometry is more accurate than visual inspection
3. cell count: RBC count usually > 100,000 RBCs/mm³. Compare RBC count in first to last tube (should not drop significantly)
4. protein: elevated due to blood breakdown products
5. glucose: normal, or reduced (RBCs may metabolize some glucose with time)

MRI

Not sensitive acutely within the first 24-48 hrs[48] (too little met-Hb) especially with thin layers of blood, better after ≈ 4-7 days (excellent for subacute to remote SAH, > 10-20 days). May be helpful in determining which of multiple aneurysms bled[49] (*see page 819*) and in searching for evidence of remote hemorrhage (sensitivity of FLAIR images may be greater than that of CT scan).

CEREBRAL ANGIOGRAM

The "gold standard" for evaluation of cerebral aneurysms. Demonstrates source (usually aneurysm) in ≈ 80-85% (remainder are so-called "SAH of unknown etiology", *see page 822*). Shows if radiographic vasospasm is present (clinical vasospasm almost never occurs < 3 days following SAH, see *Vasospasm*, page 791).

General principles:
1. study the vessel of highest suspicion first (in case patient's condition should change, necessitating discontinuation of procedure)
2. continue to do complete 4 vessel angiogram (even if aneurysm(s) have been demonstrated) to rule out additional aneurysms and assess collateral circulation
3. if there is an aneurysm or suspicion of one, obtain additional views to help delineate the neck and orientation of the aneurysm (*see index for specific aneurysm*)
★ 4. if no aneurysm is seen, before an arteriogram can be considered negative, must:
   A. visualize both PICA origins: 1-2% of aneurysms occur at PICA origin. Both PICAs can usually be visualized with one VA injection if there is enough flow to reflux down the contralateral VA. Occasionally it is necessary to see more of the contralateral VA than what refluxes to PICA
   B. flow contrast through the ACoA: if both ACAs fill from one side, this is usually satisfactory. It may be necessary to perform a cross compression AP study with carotid injection (first, rule-out plaque in the carotid to be compressed), or use a higher injection rate to facilitate flow through the ACoA

Infundibulum

A funnel shaped initial segment of an artery, to be distinguished from an aneurysm. Found in 7-13% of otherwise normal arteriograms[51, 52], with a higher incidence in cases of multiple or familial aneurysms. Bilateral in 25%[52]. Most commonly found at the

Table 27-1 Criteria of an infundibulum

1. triangular in shape
2. mouth (widest portion) < 3 mm[50]
3. vessel at apex

origin of the p-comms. Criteria for differentiating from aneurysms are shown in *Table 27-1*. Although they may bleed[53-55], there is less risk of rupture than with a saccular aneurysm (no infundibulum < 3 mm in size bled[56] in the cooperative study). However, infundibula have been documented to progress to an aneurysm which may bleed[57].

Recommended treatment: at the time of surgery for another reason, consider treating an infundibulum with wrapping, or placing in an encircling clip, or sacrificing the artery if it can be done safely (infundibula lack a true neck).

MAGNETIC RESONANCE ANGIOGRAPHY (MRA)

The experience with MRA is evolving as investigators determine optimal acquisition protocols[58] and improvements are made in scanner hardware and software. Sensitivity is probably ≈ 86% for detecting intracranial aneurysms **(IAs)** > 3 mm diameter (compared to intra-arterial digital subtraction angio)[59, 60] although rates as high as 95% have been quoted[61]. The false positive rate is ≈ 16%[60]. There are a number of complicated parameters that affect MRA's ability to detect IAs including: size, rate and direction of blood flow in the aneurysm relative to the magnetic field, and thrombosis and calcification. At this time, MRA may be useful as a screening test in high-risk patients including first degree relatives of patients with IAs.

CT ANGIOGRAPHY (CTA)

Some centers have shown good results with CTA, reporting a sensitivity of 95% and specificity of 83% in detecting aneurysms a small as 2.2 mm[62]. CTA shows a 3-dimensional image[63] and demonstrates the relation to nearby bony structures.

27.2. Grading SAH

Two widely quoted grading scales are presented here.

HUNT AND HESS GRADE

See *Table 27-2* and *Table 27-3* for grading system. Grades 1 and 2 were operated upon as soon as an aneurysm was diagnosed. Grade ≥ 3 managed until the condition improved to Grade 2 or 1. Exception: life threatening hematoma or multiple bleeds (which were operated on regardless of grade).

Analysis of data from the International Cooperative Aneurysm Study revealed that with normal consciousness, Hunt and Hess **(H&H)** grades 1 and 2 had identical outcome, and that hemiparesis and/or aphasia had no effect on mortality.

Table 27-2 Hunt and Hess classification* of SAH[64]

Grade	Description
1	asymptomatic, or mild H/A and slight nuchal rigidity
2	Cr. N. palsy (e.g. III, VI), moderate to severe H/A, nuchal rigidity
3	mild focal deficit, lethargy, or confusion
4	stupor, moderate to severe hemiparesis, early decerebrate rigidity
5	deep coma, decerebrate rigidity, moribund appearance

Add one grade for serious systemic disease (e.g. HTN, DM, severe atherosclerosis, COPD) or severe vasospasm on arteriography.

*   original paper did not consider patient's age, site of aneurysm, or time since bleed; patients were graded on admission and pre-op

Table 27-3 Modified classification[65] adds the following

Grade	Description
0	unruptured aneurysm
1 a	no acute meningeal/brain reaction, but with fixed neuro deficit

Mortality:

Admission Hunt and Hess Grade 1 or 2: 20%.

Patients taken to O.R. (for any procedure) at H&H Grade 1 or 2: 14%.

Major cause of death in Grade 1 or 2 is rebleed.

Signs of meningeal irritation increases surgical risk.

WORLD FEDERATION OF NEUROLOGIC SURGEONS
(WFNS) GRADING OF SAH

Due to lack of data on the significance of features such as headache, nuchal rigidity, and major focal neurologic deficit, the WFNS Committee on a Universal SAH Grading Scale grading system was developed and is shown in *Table 27-4*. It uses the Glasgow Coma Scale **(GCS)** (see *Table 8-1*, page 154) to evaluate level of consciousness, and uses the presence or absence of major focal neurologic deficit to distinguish grade 2 from grade 3.

Table 27-4 WFNS SAH grade[66]

WFNS grade	GCS score*	Major focal deficit†
0‡		
1	15	–
2	13-14	–
3	13-14	+
4	7-12	+ or –
5	3-6	+ or –

*   GCS = Glasgow Coma Scale, see *Table 8-1*, page 154

†   aphasia, hemiparesis or hemiplegia (+ = present, – = absent)

‡   intact aneurysm

27.3.   Initial management of SAH

Initial management concerns

1. rebleeding: the major concern during the initial stabilization[67].
2. hydrocephalus: acute hydrocephalus is usually obstructive (due to blockage of CSF flow by blood clot). In later stages, hydrocephalus is usually communicating (due toxic effect of blood breakdown products on arachnoid granulations) (see *Hydrocephalus after SAH*, page 790)
3. delayed ischemic neurologic deficit **(DIND)**, usually attributed to vasospasm. Begins to be of concern several days following the SAH
4. hyponatremia with hypovolemia: *see page 788*
5. DVT and pulmonary embolism: *see page 25*
6. seizures: *see page 787*
7. determining source of bleeding: usually requires 4-vessel cerebral **angiography**. The timing of this takes into consideration the patients condition (unstable or pre-morbid patients are not candidates) and the possibility of early surgery (angiography is usually done as soon as possible if early surgery is contemplated)

MONITORS/TUBES

Also see *Admitting orders* below.

1. arterial-line: for patients who are hemodynamically unstable, stuporous or comatose, those with difficult to control hypertension, or those requiring frequent labs (e.g. ventilator patients)
2. intubate patients who are comatose or unable to protect airway (e.g. stridorous)
3. PA-catheter: indicated for
   A. Hunt and Hess **(H&H)** grade ≥ 3 (except good grade 3 patients)
   B. patients with possible CSW or SIADH
   C. hemodynamically unstable patients
4. cardiac rhythm monitor: arrhythmias may occur following SAH (*see page 789*)
5. **intraventricular catheter (IVC)** AKA ventriculostomy. Possible indications:
   A. patients developing acute hydrocephalus following SAH or in those with significant intraventricular blood (allows measurement of ICP as well as drainage of blood laden CSF). IVC causes symptomatic improvement in almost two-thirds[47]. May increase the risk of rebleeding (*see page 790*), however, the risk of untreated hydrocephalus is probably higher[68]
   B. H&H grade ≥ 3 (except good grade 3 patients). Some experts feel that if a high grade patient improves with an IVC that the prognosis may be more favorable. If ICP is elevated, management includes the use of mannitol (see *ICP treatment measures*, page 655). As an alternative to an IVC, consider serial LPs in these patients (lower ICP cautiously, *see page 784*)

ADMITTING ORDERS
1. admit to ICU (monitored bed)
2. VS with neuro checks q 1 hr
3. activity: BR with HOB at 30°. SAH precautions (i.e. low level of external stimulation, restricted visitation, no loud noises)
4. nursing
   A. strict I's & O's
   B. daily weights
   C. knee high TED hose (pneumatic compression boots **(PCB)** if available)
   D. indwelling Foley catheter if patient lethargic, incontinent, or unable to void
      in urinal or bedpan
5. diet:
   A. if preparing for early surgery: NPO
   B. if not considering for early surgery
      1. if alert: clear liquids
      2. if lethargic: NPO
6. IV fluids: early aggressive fluid therapy to head off cerebral salt wasting
   A. NS + 20 mEq KCl/L at ≈ 2 ml/kg/hr (typically 140-150 ml/hr) (see *Blood
      pressure and volume management* below)
   B. if Hct < 40%[69], give 500 ml of 5% albumin over 4 hrs upon admission
7. medications (avoid IM medications to reduce pain)
   A. prophylactic anticonvulsants
      1. seizure incidence: excluding seizures at the time of hemorrhage, ≈ 3%
         of patients with SAH have seizures during the acute illness[70]. 5% have
         a seizure in the immediate post-op period with or without SAH[71].
         10.5% incidence in 5 years follow-up (20% for MCA, 9% for PCA, and
         2.5% for ACA aneurysms)[72]
      2. use of prophylactic anticonvulsants is controversial[73], however, a gen-
         eralized seizure may be devastating in the presence of a tenuous an-
         eurysm, and thus AEDs are given by many authorities[74] at least for 1
         week post-op[71]
      3. phenytoin is the usual agent used, avoid IV if possible because of pain
         and phlebosclerosis (circumvented with fosphenytoin). Load with 17
         mg/kg, maintenance of 100 mg TID
      4. some prophylaxis is provided by barbiturates (e.g. phenobarbital)
         when given for sedation (*see below*) or burst suppression in the O.R.
   B. sedation (not oversedation): e.g. with propofol
   C. analgesics: fentanyl (unlike morphine, does not cause histamine release.
      Lowers ICP) 25-100 μg (0.5-2 ml) IVP, q 1-2 hrs PRN (avoid Demerol® be-
      cause it may lower seizure threshold)
   D. dexamethasone (Decadron®): may help with H/A and neck pain. Effect on
      edema controversial. Usually given pre-op prior to craniotomy
   E. stool softener in patients able to take PO (docussate 100 mg PO BID)
   F. anti-emetics: avoid phenothiazines which may lower seizure threshold. Use
      e.g. Zofran® (ondansetron) 4 mg IV over 2-5 minutes, may repeat in 4 & 8
      hours, and then q 8 hours for 1-2 days
   G. calcium channel blockers: nimodipine (Nimotop®) 60 mg PO/NG q 4 hrs ini-
      tiated within 96 hrs of SAH (see *Calcium channel blockers*, page 799)
   H. H₂ blockers (e.g. ranitidine) or proton pump inhibitors (e.g. Prevacid® (lan-
      soprazole) 30 mg p.o. or IV q d): to reduce risk of stress ulceration
   I. ✖ these agents impair coagulation and are contraindicated: ASA, dextran[75],
      heparin, and repeated administration of hetastarch (Hespan®)[76, 77] over a
      period of days
8. oxygenation
   A. in non-intubated patient: O₂ 2 L per NC PRN (based on ABG) if tolerated
   B. in ventilated patient: strive for normocarbia and pO₂ > 100 mm Hg
9. HTN: SBP 120-150 mm Hg by cuff is a guideline with unclipped aneurysm (see
   Blood pressure and volume management below)
10. labs
   A. ABG, electrolytes, CBC, PT/PTT on admission
   B. ABG, electrolytes, CBC q day (ABG q 6 hrs if patient unstable, electrolytes
      q 12 hrs if hyponatremia develops, see *Hyponatremia following SAH* below)
   C. serum and urine osmolality if urine output high or low (see *Syndrome of in-
      appropriate antidiuretic hormone secretion*, page 13)

D. follow Hct and (optional) serum fibrinogen (to assess viscosity, important for flow in vasospasm)
E. CXR daily until stable: patients with SAH are at risk for neurogenic pulmonary edema[78], *see page 7*
F. if available, transcranial doppler to monitor MCA velocities (*see page 793*)

BLOOD PRESSURE AND VOLUME MANAGEMENT

With an unsecured (unclipped) aneurysm, gentle volume expansion with slight hemodilution and mild elevation of blood pressure may help prevent or minimize the effects of vasospasm[79] and cerebral salt wasting. However, extreme hypertension must be avoided (to reduce risk of re-bleeding).

With a clipped aneurysm, aggressive volume expansion with hyperdynamic therapy is used (*see page 797*).

Initial blood pressure

Ideal blood pressure is controversial, and must take patient's baseline into consideration, **SBP ≈ 120-150** by cuff is a guideline.

If blood pressure is labile, labetalol should be used in conjunction with an arterial-line. Avoid hypotension as it may exacerbate ischemia.

Long acting drugs (e.g. ACE inhibitors such as Vasotec (*see page 4* for IV or *page 6* for PO)) should be started in patients requiring continued therapy. In patients who were normotensive prior to SAH with easily controlled HTN, Vasotec may be used PRN in conjunction with a beta blocker (e.g. labetalol, *see page 4*).

MANAGEMENT OF SPECIFIC PROBLEMS FOLLOWING SAH

HYPONATREMIA FOLLOWING SAH

Background

Hypovolemia and hyponatremia frequently follow SAH as a result of natriuresis and diuresis. Although hyponatremia had been attributed to a rise in ADH[80] (thought to produce SIADH with *hyper*volemia), the ADH increment is usually transient, lasting only ≈ 4 days and hypervolemia did not occur. Another theory is based on the fact that there is often a delayed peak in **atrial natriuretic factor (ANF)** (a 28-amino acid polypeptide) after an initial smaller rise[81] that was frequently followed by urinary loss of sodium (**cerebral salt wasting (CSW)**, *see page 14*) that mimics SIADH, and volume depletion. Although CSW has clearly been shown to be the cause of hyponatremia in the majority of these patients[82], there are still doubts that ANF is *the* operative natriuretic factor in SAH[83]. A rise in ANP and brain natriuretic peptide (**BNP**) after SAH is associated with the development of a negative fluid balance[84].

Routine labs are identical in SIADH and CSW[85], but the extracellular fluid volume (which is more difficult to measure) is low in CSW and is normal or elevated in SIADH (see *Table 1-7*, page 15 for a comparison of the two conditions). The neurologic effects of hyponatremia (*see page 12*) may mimic delayed ischemic neurologic deficit from vasospasm, and hyponatremic patients have about 3 times the incidence of delayed cerebral infarction after SAH than normonatremic patients[86].

Factors that may increase the risk of hyponatremia after SAH include: history of diabetes, CHF, cirrhosis, adrenal insufficiency, or the use of any of the following drugs: NSAIDs, acetaminophen, narcotics, thiazide diuretics[87].

Treatment

✖ Caution! Restricting fluids which is the treatment for SIADH may be hazardous in the case of CSW (which is more likely to occur after SAH than is SIADH) since dehydration increases blood viscosity which exacerbates ischemia from vasospasm[86].
• treat hypovolemia with infusions of crystalloid (e.g. NS), PRBCs, or colloids (avoid repeated administration of hetastarch, *see above*)
• treat the hyponatremia of CSW with supplemental PO salt intake, NS or hypertonic saline (rapid correction or over-correction carries the risk of central pontine myelinolysis (**CPM**), *see page 12*), or fludrocortisone acetate (0.2 mg IV or PO BID, risks include pulmonary edema, hypokalemia and HTN), *see page 15*
♦ one study used urea (Ureaphil®) 0.5 grams/kg (dissolve 40 gm in 100-150 ml NS) IV over 30-60 mins q 8 hrs[88] and used NS + 20 mEq KCl/L at 2

ml/kg/hr as the main IV until the hyponatremia was corrected (unlike mannitol, urea does not increase ADH secretion). They supplemented with colloids (viz. 250 ml of 5% albumin IV q 8-12 hrs **x** 72 hrs)

CARDIAC PROBLEMS FOLLOWING SAH

Arrhythmias & EKG changes: SAH may be associated with cardiac arrhythmias (some life-threatening) and EKG changes in over 50% of cases (including: broad or inverted T-waves, Q-T prolongation, S-T segment elevation or depression, U-waves, premature atrial or ventricular contraction, SVT, V-flutter or V-fib[89]). Occasionally, SAH may produce EKG abnormalities indistinguishable from an acute MI[90, 91]. Possible mechanism: hypothalamic ischemia causes increased sympathetic tone and resultant catecholamine surge producing subendocardial ischemia[92] or coronary artery vasospasm[93].

"Stunned myocardium": Reversible postischemic myocardial dysfunction[94]. Classically seen in patients following cardiac surgery, and recently attributed to a defect in troponin-I (TnI)[95]. Some patients may develop myocardial hypokinesis following SAH[93]. May appear compatible with an MI on echocardiography, yet, enzymes are negative and the condition reverses completely in most cases within about 5 days. However, ≈ 10% of these patients may progress on to an actual MI. The mechanism may be the same as that producing arrhythmias and EKG changes (*see above*).

Hypotension usually does not occur since the reduced cardiac output (**CO**) is generally offset by an increase in SVR. However, the reduced CO may impair the ability to tolerate barbiturates administered for cerebral protection during early surgery due to their myocardial suppressant effect. Inotropic agents such as dopamine may be effective in this situation. Intraoperative TEE monitoring may be a useful guide for titrating pressors. The reduced CO may also impede the use of hyperdynamic therapy for vasospasm.

REBLEEDING

Approximately 3000 North Americans die each year from rebleeding of ruptured cerebral aneurysms[96]. The maximal frequency of rebleeding is in the 1st day (4% on day 1), then 1.5% daily for 13 d. 15-20% rebleed within 14 d, 50% will rebleed within 6 months, thereafter the risk is ≈ 3%/yr[A] with a mortality rate of 2%/yr[97]. 50% of deaths occur in the 1st month. In a study of 33 patients who rebled, the highest risk of rebleeding occurred in the first 6 hours following SAH[67].

The rebleeding risk increases in patients with higher Hunt and Hess grades[67].

Pre-operative ventriculostomy (e.g. for acute post-SAH hydrocephalus) (*see page 790*) and possibly lumbar spinal drainage (*see page 806*) increase the risk of rebleeding.

The risk of rebleeding in SAH of unknown etiology and with AVMs, as well as the risk of bleeding with incidental multiple unruptured aneurysms, are all similar at ≈ 1%/yr (may actually be less in SAH of unknown etiology, *see page 822*)[98].

Prevention of rebleeding

The optimal method of preventing rebleeding appears to be early treatment (coiling or surgery). However, delays in surgical treatment still provide a window for rebleeding. Bed rest and hyperdynamic therapy do <u>not</u> prevent rebleeding[74].

Antifibrinolytic therapy: The role of clot lysis in <u>early</u> rebleeding is uncertain.

/ tranexamic acid (Cyklokapron®) \ / DRUG INFO \

Reduces the risk of early rebleeding[99].

Rx: 1 gm IV as soon as diagnosis of SAH is verified (if patient is to be transported to another facility for definitive care, the dose is given before the patient is transported), followed by 1 gm q 6 hours until the aneurysm is occluded; this treatment did not exceed 72 hours.

A. to understand the calculation of <u>cumulative</u> risk for aneurysmal rupture, *see page 836* (that discussion is related to AVMs but the same concepts pertain to aneurysms)

(EACA) an antifibrinolytic agent, competitively inhibits activation of plasminogen to plasmin. Existing plasmin is neutralized by endogenous antiplasmins. EACA does reduce the risk of rebleeding. However, the incidence of hydrocephalus and delayed ischemic deficits (vasospasm) are increased[100] with prolonged use. There may also be a lag of 24-48 hrs before effectiveness occurs[101]. Because of the increased rate of cerebral infarction, EACA was found not to reduce early mortality, and its use was discouraged.

Reevaluation in a non-randomized study[102] excluding grade IV and V patients, suggests that the problems with EACA may be minimized by use of an IV loading dose (to eliminate the lag-period to effectiveness) and by limiting the length of time of use to that time until the patient can undergo <u>early</u> surgery. Further study is needed.

Rx high-dose[102]: EACA 10 gm IV loading dose, followed by 48 gm/day continuous maintenance infusion. Maintenance dose is adjusted to serum EACA levels.

HYDROCEPHALUS AFTER SAH

ACUTE HYDROCEPHALUS

The frequency of hydrocephalus **(HCP)** on the initial CT after SAH depends on the defining criteria used, with a reported range of 9-67%[103]. A realistic range is ≈15-20% of SAH patients, with 30-60% of these showing no impairment of consciousness[103, 104]. 3% of those <u>without</u> HCP on initial CT develop HCP within 1 week[103].

Factors felt to contribute to acute HCP include: blood interfering with CSF flow through the Sylvian aqueduct, fourth ventricle outlet, or subarachnoid space, and/or with reabsorption at the arachnoid granulations.

Findings associated with acute HCP include[104]:
* increasing age
* admission CT findings: intraventricular blood, diffuse subarachnoid blood, and thick focal accumulation of subarachnoid blood (intraparenchymal blood did <u>not</u> correlate with chronic HCP, and patients with a normal CT had a low incidence)
* hypertension: on admission, prior to admission (by history), or post-op
* by location:
  ◆ posterior circulation aneurysms have a higher incidence of HCP
  ◆ MCA aneurysms correlate with low incidence of HCP
* miscellaneous: hyponatremia, patients who were not alert on admission, use of preoperative antifibrinolytic agents, and low Glasgow outcome score

Treatment

About half the patients with acute HCP and impaired consciousness improved spontaneously[103]. Patients in poor grade (H&H IV-V) with large ventricles may be symptomatic from the HCP and consideration should be given to ventriculostomy which caused improvement in ≈ 80% of patients in whom it was used[103]. There is probably an increased risk of aneurysmal rebleeding in patients undergoing ventriculostomy shortly after SAH[103, 105, 106] especially if performed early and if ICP is lowered precipitously. The mechanism is controversial, but may be due to an increase in the **transmural pressure** (the pressure across the aneurysm wall which equals the difference between arterial pressure and ICP).

When a ventriculostomy is used, it is recommended to keep ICP in the range of **15-25 mm Hg**[107] and to avoid rapid pressure reduction (unless absolutely necessary) to decrease the risk of IVC induced aneurysmal rebleeding.

CHRONIC HCP

Chronic HCP is due to pia-arachnoid adhesions or permanent impairment of the arachnoid granulations. Acute HCP does not inevitably lead to chronic HCP. 8-45% (reported range in literature[108]) of all ruptured aneurysm patients, and ≈ 50% of those with acute HCP following SAH need permanent CSF diversion. The presence of intraventricular blood increases this risk[108]. There is controversy as to whether the use of ventriculostomy for acute HCP increases[109] or possibly even decreases[108] the incidence of shunt dependency.

27.4. Vasospasm

Cerebral vasospasm is a condition that is most commonly seen following aneurysmal subarachnoid hemorrhage (SAH), but may also follow other intracranial hemorrhages (e.g. intraventricular hemorrhage from AVM[110], and SAH of unknown etiology), head trauma (with or without SAH)[111], brain surgery, lumbar puncture, hypothalamic injury, infection, and may be associated with preeclampsia (*see page 64*). Vasospasm has two not-necessarily reconcilable definitions (see *Definitions* below):
1. clinical vasospasm: *see below*
2. radiographic vasospasm: *see below*

27.4.1. Definitions

CLINICAL VASOSPASM
AKA **delayed ischemic neurologic deficit (DIND)**, AKA symptomatic vasospasm. A delayed focal ischemic neurologic deficit following SAH. Clinically characterized by confusion or decreased level of consciousness with focal neurologic deficit (speech or motor). The diagnosis is one of exclusion, and sometimes cannot be made with certainty. For clinical findings, *see page 791*.

RADIOGRAPHIC VASOSPASM (AKA ANGIOGRAPHIC VASOSPASM)
Arterial narrowing demonstrated on cerebral angiography, often with slowing of contrast filling. The diagnosis is solidified by previous or subsequent angiograms showing the same vessel(s) with normal caliber. Since only larger arteries may be visualized angiographically, the diagnosis is limited to narrowing of these vessels.

SYMPTOMATIC VASOSPASM
When the DIND corresponds to a region of vasospasm seen on angiogram, this is sometimes referred to as "symptomatic vasospasm".

27.4.2. Characteristics of cerebral vasospasm

Clinical findings
Findings usually develop gradually, and may progress or fluctuate. May include:
1. non-localizing findings
   A. new or increasing H/A
   B. alterations in level of consciousness (lethargy...)
   C. disorientation
   D. meningismus
2. focal neurological signs may occur including cranial nerve palsies and focal motor deficits. Also, symptoms may cluster into one of the following "syndromes" (vasospasm incidence is higher in the distribution of the ACA than in that of the MCA)
   A. **anterior cerebral artery (ACA) syndrome**: frontal lobe findings predominate (abulia, grasp/suck reflex, urinary incontinence, drowsiness, slowness, delayed responses, confusion, whispering). Bilateral anterior cerebral artery distribution infarcts are usually due to vasospasm following an ACoA aneurysm rupture
   B. **middle cerebral artery (MCA) syndrome**: hemiparesis, monoparesis, aphasia (or apractagnosia of non-dominant hemisphere - inability to use objects or perform skilled motor activities, due to lesions in the lower occipital or parietal lobes; subtypes: ideomotor apraxia and sensory apraxia)

Incidence
- radiographic cerebral vasospasm (CVS) is identified in 30-70% of arteriograms performed around the 7th day following SAH, whereas symptomatic CVS occurs in only 20-30% of patients with SAH[19]
- radiographic CVS may occur in the absence of clinical deficit, and vice-versa

Severity

- CVS is the most significant cause of morbidity and mortality in patients surviving SAH long enough to reach medical care, even exceeding direct effects of aneurysmal rupture as well as re-bleeding
- CVS ranges in severity from mild reversible dysfunction, to severe permanent deficits secondary to ischemic infarction in 7% of SAH patients, extensive enough to be fatal in 7% of SAHs[19]
- earlier onset of CVS is associated with greater deficit

Time course of vasospasm

- onset: almost never before day 3 post-SAH[112]
- maximal frequency of onset during days 6-8 post-SAH (however, rarely can occur as late as day 17)
- clinical CVS is almost always resolved by day 12 post-SAH. Once radiographic CVS is demonstrated, it usually resolves slowly over 3-4 weeks
- onset is usually insidious, but ≈ 10% have an abrupt and severe deterioration

Correlated findings

- blood clots are especially spasmogenic when in direct contact with the proximal 9 cm of the ACA and the MCA
- not all patients with SAH develop CVS, and CVS can follow other insults besides SAH (e.g head trauma without SAH)
- the Hunt and Hess grade on admission correlates with the risk of CVS (*see Table 27-5*)
- the amount of blood on CT correlates with the severity of CVS[113, 114] (*see Table 27-6*) (also holds true for traumatic SAH[3])
- higher incidence with increasing age of patient
- a history of active cigarette smoking is an independent risk factor[115]
- history of preexisting hypertension
- there is good but not perfect correlation between the site of major blood clots on CT, the focality of delayed ischemic neurological deficits, and the visualization of angiographic CVS in corresponding arteries
- pial enhancement on CT ≈ 3 days after SAH (with IV contrast administration) may correlate with higher risk of CVS (indicates increased permeability of BBB)[116], but this is controversial[117]
- for patients undergoing early surgery, if there is little SAH left on a CT done 24 hours post-op, there is little risk of vasospasm
- antifibrinolytic therapy reduces rebleeding, but increases the risk of hydrocephalus and vasospasm[100] (*see page 789*)
- angiographic dye can exacerbate CVS
- hypovolemia

Table 27-5 Correlation of DIND with Hunt and Hess grade

Hunt and Hess grade	% DIND (clinical vasospasm)
1	22%
2	33%
3	52%
4	53%
5	74%

Table 27-6 Grading system of Fisher[113]
(correlation between the amount of blood on CT and the risk of vasospasm)

Fisher group	Blood on CT*	No. of pts.	-- VASOSPASM --		Clinical vasospasm (DIND)
			Slight	Severe	
1	no subarachnoid blood detected	11	2	2†	0
2	diffuse or vertical layers‡ < 1 mm thick	7	3	0	0
3	localized clot and/or vertical layer‡ ≥ 1 mm	24	1	23	23
4	intracerebral or intraventricular clot with diffuse or no SAH§	5	2	0	0

* measurements made in the greatest longitudinal & transverse dimension on a printed EMI CT scan (no scaling to actual thickness) performed within 5 d of SAH in 47 patients; falx never contributed more than 1 mm thickness to interhemispheric blood

† may actually be 0 since 1 patient was scanned late and 1 developed spasm only peripherally

‡ "vertical layer" refers to blood within "vertical" subarachnoid spaces including interhemispheric fissure, insular cistern, ambient cistern

§ reflux of blood into ventricles frequently indicates obstruction of CSF circulation, and is associated with high incidence of hydrocephalus

27.4.3. Pathogenesis

Poorly understood. Risk of developing vasospasm is higher in cases where arterial blood at high pressure contacts the vessels at the base of the brain. Rarely occurs in the setting of intraparenchymal or intraventricular hemorrhage (e.g. from AVM) or in SAH with distribution limited to the cerebral convexity.

Pathological changes observed within the vessel wall are outlined in *Table 27-7*.

Table 27-7 Pathological changes in vasospasm

Time	Vessel layer	Pathologic change
day 1-8	adventitia	↑ inflammatory cells (lymphocytes, plasma cells, mast cells) and connective tissue
	media	muscle necrosis and corrugation of elastica
	intima	thickening with endothelial swelling and vacuolization, opening of interendothelial tight junctions[118, 119]
day 9-60	intima	proliferation of smooth muscle cells → progressive intimal thickening

In humans, CVS is a chronic condition with definite long-term changes in the morphology of the involved vessels. Endothelin 1 (ET1) appears to be a critical mediator and has been shown to cause potent and prolonged vasospasm[120].

27.4.4. Diagnosis of cerebral vasospasm

Diagnosis requires appropriate clinical criteria, and ruling-out other conditions that can produce delayed neurologic deterioration, as shown in *Table 27-8*.

ANCILLARY TESTS FOR VASOSPASM

In addition to angiographically demonstrating vasospasm:

* transcranial Doppler **(TCD)**: *see below*
* alterations in intracranial pulse wave[122]
* CTA: can demonstrate vasospasm[123]
* MRA: may be useful for management of vasospasm (not a practical alternative to conventional angiography)[124]
* continuous quantitatively analyzed EEG monitoring in the ICU:
   ◆ a decline of the percent of alpha activity (defined here as 6-14 Hz) called "relative alpha" **(RA)** from a mean of 0.45 to 0.17 predicted the onset of vasospasm earlier than TCD or angiographic changes[125]
   ◆ a decline of total EEG power (amplitude) was 91% sensitive for predicting vasospasm[126]
* alterations in cerebral blood flow **(CBF)**:
   ★ MRI: DWI and PWI may detect early ischemia (*see page 136*)
   ◆ xenon CT: may detect large global changes in CBF, but too insensitive to detect focal blood flow changes[127, 128]
   ◆ positron emission tomography **(PET)**[129] or SPECT scans (non-quantitative, and takes longer than xenon studies)

Table 27-8 Diagnosis of clinical vasospasm[121]

* delayed onset or persisting neuro deficit
* onset 4-20 days post-SAH
* deficit appropriate to involved arteries
* rule-out other causes of deterioration
   * rebleeding
   * hydrocephalus
   * cerebral edema
   * seizure
   * metabolic disturbances: hyponatremia...
   * hypoxia
   * sepsis
* ancillary tests (*see text*)
   * transcranial Doppler
   * CBF studies
   * SPECT
   * cerebral angiography

Table 27-9 Interpretation of transcranial doppler for vasospasm

Mean MCA velocity (cm/sec)	MCA:ICA (Lindegaard) ratio	Interpretation
< 120	< 3	normal
120-200*	3-6	mild vasospasm*
> 200	> 6	severe vasospasm

* velocities in this range are specific for vasospasm but are only ≈ 60% sensitive

Transcranial Doppler (TCD)

Narrowing of the arterial lumen as occurs in vasospasm elevates the blood flow velocity which may be detected with TCD[130-132]. Detectable changes may precede clinical symptoms by up to 24-48 hrs. Findings are often more helpful when baseline studies performed before vasospasm is likely to have begun are available.

Typical values are shown for the MCA in *Table 27-9*. Also, daily increases of > 50 cm/sec may suggest vasospasm. There is less correlation between velocities and vasospasm in the anterior cerebral arteries (ACA). Distinguishing vasospasm from hyperemia (which increases blood flow velocities in both the MCA and the ICA) is facilitated by using the ratio of these velocities (the so-called **Lindegaard ratio**) also shown in *Table 27-9*.

27.4.5.   Treatment for vasospasm

See *page 796* for management protocol.

Numerous treatments for cerebral arterial vasospasm have been evaluated. See the survey articles by Wilkins[133, 134] for an extensive list of agents and techniques studied. Vasospasm in humans does not respond to the large variety of drugs that reverse experimental vasospasm in animal models.

PREVENTION OF VASOSPASM

Vasospasm can often be mitigated by preventing post-SAH hypovolemia and anemia by employing hydration and blood transfusion. Although <u>early surgery</u> with aneurysm clipping does not prevent CVS (in fact, manipulation of vessels may increase the risk), it facilitates treatment of CVS by eliminating the risk of rebleeding (permitting safe use of hyperdynamic therapy) and removal of clot (*see below*) may reduce the incidence of CVS (see *Timing of aneurysm surgery*, page 804 for discussion of early surgery).

VASOSPASM TREATMENT OPTIONS

Treatment options fall into the following categories:
1. direct pharmacological arterial dilatation
    A. smooth muscle relaxants:
        1. calcium channel blockers*: did not succeed in counteracting vasospasm, but they may provide a neuroprotectant effect (*see page 799*)
        2. endothelin receptor antagonists†: ET_A antagonists (clazosentan) and $ET_{A/B}$ antagonists[135, 136]
    B. sympatholytics
    C. intra-arterial papaverine§[137, 138]: short-lived (*see below*)
    D. αICAM-1 inhibition† (antibody to intracellular adhesion molecule)
2. direct mechanical arterial dilatation: balloon angioplasty§ (*see below*)
3. indirect arterial dilatation: utilizing hyperdynamic therapy* (*see below*)
4. surgical treatment to dilate arteries: cervical sympathectomy‡ [139]
5. removal of potential vasospasmogenic agents
    A. removal of blood clot: does not completely prevent vasospasm
        1. mechanical removal at the time of aneurysm surgery[140, 141]
        2. subarachnoid irrigation with thrombolytic agents† at the time of surgery or post-op through cisternal catheters[142-145] (must be initiated within ≈ 48 hrs of clipping) or intrathecally[146]. Hazardous with incompletely clipped aneurysm[145]
    B. CSF drainage: via serial lumbar punctures, continuous ventricular drainage, or postoperative cisternal drainage[147]
6. protection of the CNS from ischemic injury:
    A. calcium channel blockers* (*see page 799*)
    B. NMDA (N-methyl-D-aspartate) receptor antagonists†
        1. Selfotel®: a selective competitive NMDA receptor antagonist (like PCP & ketamine), and like these agents, may cause hallucinations, paranoia, delerium... at all but the lowest doses[148]. Recently abandoned in studies for use in acute stroke due to an increase in brain-related deaths[149]. No benefit demonstrated in severe closed head injury[150]
        2. eliprodil
        3. cerestat
    C. free radical scavengers†
        1. tirilazad mesylate (Freedox®): a 21-aminosteroid. Improved outcome

was observed in males given 6 mg/kg/d[151] (females metabolize the drug at 3-4 **x** the rate as males, and a study with 15 μg/kg/d in females is planned). Overall the drug does not look as promising as it did initially

2. nicaraven[152]

7. improvement of the rheologic properties of intravascular blood to enhance perfusion of ischemic zones (also an endpoint of hyperdynamic therapy)* (*see page 798*)
   • includes: plasma, albumin, low molecular weight dextran‡, perfluorocarbons†, mannitol (*see page 806*)
   • the optimal hematocrit is controversial, but ≈ 30-35% is a good compromise between lowered viscosity without overly reducing O_2 carrying capacity (hemodilution is used to lower Hct; phlebotomy is not used)

8. extracranial-intracranial bypass around zone of vasospasm‡[153, 154]

* technique that is generally accepted for standard usage
§ technique that is accepted for use but not necessarily standard or available at all centers
† experimental or research technique with potential for future application
‡ technique not generally used or no longer accepted

Promising agents in trials

• **nicardipine prolonged release implants (NPRIs):** placed intra-op in the cisterns (where thick clots were located) decreased the incidence of vasospasm in patients with thick blood clots (Fisher Group 3, see *Table 27-6*, page 792)[155]
• **clazosentan** (AXV-034343): a selective endothelin IA receptor antagonist[156]: reduces frequency and severity of vasospasm

Vasodilatation by angioplasty

Catheter directed balloon angioplasty of vessels demonstrated to be in vasospasm[157, 158]: available only in centers with interventional neuroradiologists. Risks of the procedure: arterial occlusion, arterial rupture, displacement of aneurysm clip[159, 160], arterial dissection. Only feasible in large cerebral vessels (distal arteries not accessible). Clinical improvement occurs in ≈ 60-80%.

Criteria for transluminal balloon angioplasty (**TBA**):
1. failure of hyperdynamic therapy
2. ruptured aneurysm is repaired
3. optimal results when performed within 12 hours of onset of symptoms
4. may be done immediately post-clipping for vasospasm that was observed pre-op
5. controversial: asymptomatic vasospasm seen on the contralateral side during angioplasty for ipsilateral vasospasm. Some would balloon the asymptomatic side, but others cite the complication rate and would observe
6. ✖ cerebral infarction (CVA): a contraindication to TBA

Vasodilatation by intra-arterial drug injection

Vasodilatation by intra-arterial drug (**IAD**) injection may be considered the "poorman's" angioplasty since it could be performed by angiographers who are not interventional neuroradiologists. However, the effects are shorter-lived and less profound at their peak than with angioplasty. While IAD can be repeated, this requires multiple arterial catheterizations. IAD is still of value to help open up vessels to allow placement of the angioplasty balloon, and for vessels inaccessible to angioplasty balloons.

Agents used for vasodilatation:
1. papaverine: usually 200-300 mg infused over 30 mins. May exacerbate vasospasm in some cases[161], may produce thrombocytopenia[162], and unless carefully titrated, it can elevate ICP[163]. Largely abandoned because of limited success
2. verapamil: angiography of ICA is performed. If vasospasm is seen, 8 mg of verapamil is injected over 2 minutes (**Rx**: mix 2 vials of Verapamil (each vial is 5 mg in 2 cc) with 6 cc of NS to get 10 mg in 10 cc, inject 8 cc to give 8 mg). Then the other ICA is checked, and similarly injected if indicated. Can also be done in vertebral arteries. Takes 30 minutes for full effect. First ICA that was injected is then rechecked for improvement. Watch BP for hypotension

27.4.6. Vasospasm management "protocol"

Table 27-10 QUICK REFERENCE GUIDE:
Post-clipping management pertinent to vasospasm*

Condition	Management

No vasospasm
• clinically intact
• normal TCD
	1. hemodynamics:
	  A. normotension or 30% above baseline
	  B. keep SBP > 120 mm Hg
	  C. normal SVR (800-1200)
	2. IVF: NS 200 ml/hr

Subclinical vasospasm
• high TCDs (> 200 cm/sec) and/or radiographic evidence of vasospasm
• clinically intact
	1. monitors: PA catheter, A-line
	2. elderly and patients with CAD: EKG, cardiac echo & cardiac enzymes to assess left ventricle function
	3. monitor for signs/symptoms of adverse effects of triple-H therapy (chest pain, pulmonary rhonchi, EKG changes…)
	4. hemodynamics
	  A. maintain SBP 160-220 mm Hg. If pressors necessary:
	    1. dopamine + levophed§
	    2. add Neosynephrine§ if tachycardia > 140-150 BPM
	    3. if SBP still low: consider dobutamine§ if SVR > 800 and PCWP within desired parameters
	  B. keep SVR WNL
	  C. maintain PCWP 12-14 mm Hg
	5. fluids: monitor I's & O's and serum sodium
	  A. IVF: NS + Plasmanate 200-250 ml/hr (Δ to 1/2 NS if Na > 150)
	  B. begin DDAVP§ if UO > 200 ml/hr **x** 4 hrs
	6. hematocrit: keep Hct ≤ 33%

Clinical vasospasm • DIND • high TCDs and/or radiographic vasospasm	1. increase SBP to try and reverse DIND 2. increase PCWP to 18-21 mm Hg (monitor CXR for pulmonary edema) 3. refractory cases: consider cerebral angiography ± angioplasty (*see page 795*) or ± intraarterial verapamil (*see page 795*)

§ **TRIPLE-H THERAPY QUICK REFERENCE (Hypertension, Hypervolemia, Hemodilution)**

1. hypertension
   A. dopamine (*see page 7*)
      1. start at 2.5 µg/kg/min (renal dose)
      2. titrate up to 15-20 µg/kg/min
   B. levophed
      1. start at 1-2 µg/min
      2. titrate every 2-5 minutes: double the rate up to 64 µg/min, then increase by 10µg/min
   C. Neosynephrine (phenylephrine): does not exacerbate tachycardia
      1. start at 5 µg/min
      2. titrate every 2-5 minutes: double the rate up to 64 µg/min, then increase by 10µg/min up to a max of 10 µg/kg
   D. dobutamine: positive inotrope
      1. start at 5 µg/kg/min
      2. increase dose by 2.5 µg/kg/min up to a maximum of 20 µg/kg/min
2. hypervolemia
   A. fluids: normal saline ± plasmanate: 200-250 ml/hr
   B. DDAVP: antidiuretic (counteracts urinary loss of circulating fluid volume)
      1. 2-4 µg SQ q d in divided doses
      2. reduce or hold for volume overload or excessive hemodilution
3. hemodilution
   A. target hematocrit (Hct): ≤ 33%
   B. transfuse for Hct < 25%

* see text for details

ROUTINE MONITORING FOR ALL SAH PATIENTS
1. serial neuro exams
2. daily CBC with differential
3. transcranial Doppler monitoring (where available): usually Mon-Weds-Fri

Patients with clinical suspicion of vasospasm (DIND), or with TCD <u>increases</u> of > 50 cm/sec or with absolute velocities > 200:

1. move patient to the ICU and placed on triple-H therapy for 6 hours if this is not already instituted
2. option: perfusion CT or MRI (if available)
3. if no response to 6 hrs of triple-H therapy, or if perfusion CT suggests vasospasm, patient is taken to angiography to confirm presence of vasospasm and for interventional neuroradiologic treatment (intraarterial verapamil, angioplasty...)

When a patient develops signs suggestive of vasospasm:

1. diagnostic measures (primarily to rule-out other causes of deficit)
   A. STAT non-contrast CT to rule-out hydrocephalus, edema, infarct or rebleed
   B. STAT bloodwork
      1. electrolytes to rule-out hyponatremia[80]
      2. CBC to assess rheology and rule out sepsis or anemia
      3. ABG to rule out hypoxemia
   C. repeat transcranial doppler (**TCD**) if available to detect changes indicative of vasospasm
2. treatment measures
   A. insert ICP monitor if ICP felt to be problematic, treat elevated ICP with mannitol or CSF drainage before institution hyperdynamic therapy (**HDT**) (caution: the diuresis from mannitol works against hypervolemia; also, exercise caution in lowering ICP with unsecured aneurysm, *see page 790*)
   B. administer O_2 to keep pO_2 > 70 mm Hg
   C. activity: bed rest, HOB elevated to ≈ 30°
   D. TED hose and/or sequential compression boots
   E. A-line to monitor BP
   F. PA catheter to monitor PCWP and cardiac output when possible (central line to monitor CVP when PA catheter cannot be placed)
   G. monitoring labs:
      1. ABG and H/H daily
      2. serum and urine electrolytes and osmolalities q 12 hr (creatinine elevations may indicate peripheral ischemia from vasopressors)
      3. CXR daily
      4. frequent EKG
   H. strict I & O measurements
   I. continue calcium channel blockers (*see below*)
   J. initiate hyperdynamic (triple-H) therapy (*see below*)

HYPERDYNAMIC THERAPY (HDT) - "TRIPLE-H THERAPY"

AKA "triple-H" therapy (for: hypervolemia, hypertension and hemodilution)[164] or induced arterial hypertension. Elevating systemic blood pressure by expanding circulating blood volume has demonstrated benefit[165, 166], but may not reduce overall morbidity and mortality[167]. Inducing HTN may be risky with an unclipped ruptured aneurysm. In the case of multiple aneurysms, the risk of hemorrhage from a previously unruptured aneurysm appears low enough to justify volume expansion once the ruptured aneurysm has been clipped[168]. Initiating therapy before CVS is apparent may minimize morbidity from CVS[79, 169] (patients with SAH often develop hypovolemia early in their course[86, 170, 171], and once CVS is evident, changes have already occurred, some possibly irreversible).

PROTOCOL FOR HYPERDYNAMIC THERAPY (modified[165])

Monitors
- indwelling urinary catheter (Foley)
- A-line: essential
- PA catheter: highly recommended. Consider employing one with a pacing port in case this is needed to counteract reflex bradycardia. A catheter with continuous cardiac output (**cCO**) measuring capability is ideal, which avoids the need to inflate balloon periodically
- some centers monitor transcranial doppler (**TCD**)
- perfusion CT

Endpoints

- ✖ to avoid severe cerebral edema or hemorrhagic infarction, do not institute in patient who demonstrates massive edema or a large ischemic infarct coincident with the onset of DIND, especially within the first 6 days post-SAH[172]
- • use fluids, pressors… (see below) to increase SBP in 15% increments until neurologically improved or the following endpoints all reached
  - ◆ elevate CVP to 8-12 cm H$_2$O, or PCWP to 18-20 mm Hg^A
    (for unclipped aneurysms: CVP 6-10 cm H$_2$O, PCWP 6-10 mm Hg)
  - ◆ maximum BP in clipped aneurysms: SBP < 240 mm Hg, mean BP < 150
    (for unclipped aneurysm: SBP < 160)
  - ◆ reduction of elevated TCD readings back towards baseline
- • then allow BP to fall to level required to sustain acceptable neurologic function
- • if triple-H therapy fails, use endovascular techniques if available (see page 795)

Methods of inducing hyperdynamic therapy

Proceed to each step only if needed to meet above endpoints or reverse neurologic deficit.

1. volume expansion: goal is euvolemia or very slight hypervolemia
   A. primary IV fluid is crystalloid, usually isotonic (e.g. NS)
   B. blood (whole or PRBC) when Hct drops < 40%
   C. colloid: plasma fraction or 5% albumin (at 100 ml/hr) to maintain 40% Hct (if Hct is > 40%, use crystalloids[69])
   D. mannitol 20% at 0.25 gm/kg/hr as a drip may improve rheologic properties of blood in the microcirculation (avoid hypovolemia from resultant diuresis)
   E. ✖ avoid hetastarch (Hespan®) and dextran which impair coagulation (see page 787)
   F. replace urinary output (U.O.) with crystalloid (if Hct < 40%, then use 5% albumin, usually @ ≈ 20-25 ml/hr)
2. pressors: also see Hypotension (shock), page 6. A SBP of 100-220 may be required to reverse ischemic symptoms, and is generally safe with a clipped aneurysm in the absence of underlying ischemic heart disease
   A. dobutamine: a pure ß agonist. May improve blood flow in cerebral microcirculation at stable MAP. **Rx**: start at 5 µg/kg/min and titrate to maximize cardiac output (usually 5-18 µg/kg/min)
   B. dopamine may alternatively be used (see page 7)
   C. if symptoms not reversed after 30-60 mins, add phenylephrine, an alpha agonist. **Rx**: start at 2 µg/kg/min and titrate to maximize MAP (usually 2-15 µg/kg/min)
3. bradycardia (reflex vagal response) is treated with atropine 1 mg IM q 3-4 hrs to keep pulse 80-120 (or pace through PA catheter pacing port)
4. compensatory diuresis: replace U.O. with albumin (see above). Diuresis may be counteracted with vasopressin (Pitressin®). Caution needs to be exercised due to possible exacerbation of hyponatremia. Use either:
   - • aqueous vasopressin 5 U SQ titrate to urine output < 200 ml/hr
   OR
   - • vasopressin IV drip, start at 0.1 U/min and titrate up to 0.5 U/min to keep urine output < 200 ml/hr
5. fludrocortisone (Florinef®) 2 mg/d (NB: this dose is ≈ 10 times higher than the homeostatic dose for adrenal replacement therapy, see page 11) or desoxycortisone 20 mg/d in divided doses
6. digitalis if vascular congestion seen on CXR accompanied by decreased cardiac output or ABG deterioration

Complications of hyperdynamic therapy:
1. intracranial complications[172]
   A. may exacerbate cerebral edema and increase ICP
   B. may produce hemorrhagic infarction in an area of previous ischemia
2. extracranial complications
   A. pulmonary edema in 17%
   B. 3 rebleeds (1 fatal)
   C. dilutional hyponatremia in 3%
   D. MI in 2%
   E. complications of PA catheter[173]:

A. these CVPs and PCWPs are given as a guideline. It is best to determine what CVP or PCWP optimizes the individual patient's cardiac output, and then maintain that level

1. catheter related sepsis: 13%
2. subclavian vein thrombosis: 1.3%
3. pneumothorax: 1%
4. hemothorax: may be promoted by coagulopathy from dextran[172]

The above protocol was used in 58 patients with vasospasm (22 unsecured aneurysm, 2 SAH of unknown etiology) with the following results: neurological improvement occurred in 81%; temporary in 7%. No change was seen in 16%. 10% deteriorated.

CALCIUM CHANNEL BLOCKERS

Trials with calcium channel blockers
Calcium channel blockers **(CCB)** (AKA calcium antagonist) block the "slow-channel" of calcium influx which reduces the contraction of smooth and cardiac muscle, but does not affect skeletal muscle. It is thus theorized that the abnormal contraction of vascular smooth muscle that may contribute to vasospasm may be mitigated by the administration of CCBs.

CCBs may be more beneficial in neuroprotection than in preventing vasospasm. Their beneficial impact may derive from a number of possible effects:
1. increased red blood cell deformability (which improves blood rheology)
2. prevention of calcium entry into ischemic cells which may mediate the injury from cerebral infarction[174]
3. anti-platelet aggregating effect[175]
4. dilatation of collateral leptomeningeal arteries[176]

Agents presently available
1. **nimodipine** (Nimotop®): a CCB with preferential CNS action. Blocks dihydropyridine-sensitive (L-type) calcium channels. Does not alter radiographic vasospasm[177], and there is no statistically significant difference in mortality. However, outcome is improved[178].
   Rx: 60 mg PO or per NG (IV form not available in the U.S.) q 4 hrs (monitor BP)[177, 179, 180] initiated within 96 hrs of SAH. Dosage is halved for liver failure. Administer either for 21 days or until the patient is discharged home in good neurological condition, whichever occurs first[121]
2. **nicardipine** (Cardene®)[181]: initial trials with indicated a lower incidence of vasospasm in the highest dose group[182], however it has subsequently been shown to be no better than placebo in overall outcome (however, it may reduce the need for HDT). Given as an IV drip at 148 µg/kg/hr (high dose[182]: 0.15 mg/kg/hr)
3. miscellaneous: nifedipine (20 mg PO start TID and increase to QID), diltiazem, and others. Systemic effects usually limit dosage. Less widely used in the U.S. since nimodipine was approved by the FDA in 1989

Side effects of CCBs
Possible side effects include:
1. systemic hypotension: may be mitigated by administration of intravenous volume expansion
2. renal failure
3. pulmonary edema

27.5. Cerebral aneurysms

EPIDEMIOLOGY
Incidence difficult to estimate. Range of autopsy prevalence of aneurysms: 0.2-7.9% (variability depends on use of dissecting microscope, hospital referral and autopsy pattern, overall interest). Recent studies[183] indicate prevalence of **5%**. Ratio of ruptured:unruptured (incidental) aneurysm is 5:3 to 5:6 (rough estimate is 1:1, i.e. 50% of these aneurysms rupture)[184]. Only 2% of aneurysms present during childhood[185].

ETIOLOGY

The exact pathophysiology of the development of aneurysms is still controversial. In contrast to extracranial blood vessels, there is less elastic in the tunica media and adventitia of cerebral blood vessels, the media has less muscle, the adventitia is thinner, and the internal elastic lamina is more prominent[186, 187]. This, together with the fact that large cerebral blood vessels lie within the subarachnoid space with little supporting connective tissue[188 (p 1644)] may predispose to the development of aneurysms. Aneurysms tend to arise in areas where there is a curve in the parent artery, in the angle between it and a significant branching artery, and point in the direction that the parent artery would have continued had the curve not been present[189].

The etiology of aneurysms may be:
- congenital predisposition (e.g. defect in the muscular layer of the arterial wall, referred to as a **medial gap**)
- "atherosclerotic" or hypertensive: presumed etiology of most saccular aneurysms, probably interacts with congenital predisposition described above
- embolic: as in atrial myxoma
- infectious (so called "mycotic aneurysms", *see page 821*)
- traumatic (see *Traumatic aneurysms*, page 820)
- associated with other conditions (*see below*)

LOCATION

Saccular aneurysms, AKA **berry aneurysms** are usually located on major named cerebral arteries at the apex of branch points which is the site of maximum hemodynamic stress in a vessel[190]. More peripheral aneurysms do occur, but tend to be associated with infection (mycotic aneurysms) or trauma. **Fusiform aneurysms** are more common in the vertebrobasilar system. Dissecting aneurysms should be categorized with arterial dissection (*see page 883*).

Saccular aneurysms location:
- 85-95% in carotid system, with the following 3 most common locations:
  - ♦ ACoA (single most common): 30% (ACoA & ACA more common in males)
  - ♦ p-comm: 25%
  - ♦ middle cerebral artery (MCA): 20%
- 5-15% in posterior circulation (vertebro-basilar)
  - ♦ ≈ 10% on basilar artery: basilar bifurcation, AKA basilar tip, is the most common, followed by BA-SCA, BA-VA junction, AICA
  - ♦ ≈ 5% on vertebral artery: VA-PICA junction is the most common
- 20-30% of aneurysm patients have multiple aneurysms[191] (*see page 819*)

PRESENTATION OF ANEURYSMS

MAJOR RUPTURE

The most frequent presentation
1. most commonly produces SAH (*see page 781*), which may be accompanied by:
2. intracerebral hemorrhage: occurs in 20-40% (more common with aneurysms distal to the Circle of Willis, e.g. MCA aneurysms)
3. intraventricular hemorrhage: occurs in 13-28%[192] (*see below*)
4. subdural blood in 2-5%

Intraventricular hemorrhage

See page 938 for other etiologies of intraventricular hemorrhage **(IVH)**.

IVH occurs in 13-28% of ruptured aneurysms in clinical series (higher in autopsy series)[192]. The prognosis appears to be worse when IVH occurs (64% mortality)[192]. The size of the ventricles on admission was the most important prognosticator (large vents being worse). Patterns that may occur:
1. a-comm aneurysm: tends to produce IVH by rupture through the lamina terminalis into the anterior 3rd or lateral ventricles
2. distal basilar artery or carotid terminus aneurysms: may rupture through the floor of the 3rd ventricle
3. distal PICA aneurysms: may rupture directly into 4th ventricle through the foramen of Luschka[193]

May be thought of as possible "warning signs".
1. mass effect
    A. giant aneurysms: including brain stem compression producing hemiparesis and cranial neuropathies
    B. cranial neuropathy (average latency from symptom to SAH was 110 days[A]) including:
        1. non-pupil-sparing third nerve palsy produced by expanding by p-comm aneurysm (or, less commonly, basilar apex aneurysm)
        2. visual loss due to[194]
            a. compressive optic neuropathy with ophthalmic artery aneurysms: characteristically produces nasal quadrantanopsia
            b. chiasmal syndromes due to ophthalmic, a-comm, or basilar apex aneurysms
        3. facial pain syndromes in the ophthalmic or maxillary nerve distribution that may mimic trigeminal neuralgia can occur with intracavernous or supraclinoid aneurysms[194, 195]
    C. intra- or suprasellar aneurysm producing endocrine disturbance[196] due to pituitary gland or stalk compression
2. minor hemorrhage: warning or sentinel hemorrhage (see *Headache*, page 782). This group had the shortest latency (10 days) between symptom and SAH[A]
3. small infarcts or transient ischemia due to distal embolization (including amaurosis fugax, homonymous hemianopsia...)[194]: average latency from symptom to SAH was 21 days[A]
4. seizures: at surgery, an adjacent area of encephalomalacia may be found[194]. The seizures may arise as a result of localized gliosis and do not necessarily represent aneurysmal expansion as there is no data to indicate an increased risk of hemorrhage in this group
5. headache[194] without hemorrhage: abates after treatment in most cases
    A. acute: may be severe and "thunderclap" in nature[35], some describe as "worst headache of my life". Has been attributed to aneurysmal expansion, thrombosis, or intramural bleeding[31], all without rupture
    B. present for ≥ 2 weeks: unilateral in about half (often retro-orbital or periorbital), possibly due to irritation of overlying dura. Diffuse or bilateral in the other half, possibly due to mass effect → increased ICP
6. incidentally discovered (i.e. asymptomatic, e.g. those found on angiography, CT or MRI obtained for other reasons)

27.5.1. Conditions associated with aneurysms

*   autosomal dominant polycystic kidney disease: (*see below*)
*   fibromuscular dysplasia **(FMD)**: prevalence of aneurysms in renal FMD is 7%, in aortocranial FMD 21%
*   arteriovenous malformations **(AVM)** including moyamoya disease (see *AVMs and aneurysms*, page 837)
*   connective tissue disorders[197]: Ehlers-Danlos type IV (deficient collagen type III), Marfan's syndrome (*see page 883*), pseudoxanthoma elasticum
*   multiple other family members with intracranial aneurysms. **Familial intracranial aneurysm syndrome (FIA)**: 2 or more relatives, third degree or closer, harbor radiographically proven aneurysms (also, see *Familial aneurysms*, page 819)
*   coarctation of the aorta[198]
*   Osler-Weber-Rendu syndrome
*   atherosclerosis[25]
*   bacterial endocarditis

POLYCYSTIC KIDNEY DISEASE
Adult polycystic kidney disease is seen in 1 of every 500 autopsies, and approximate-

---

A. the average latency quoted for some of these symptoms comes from a retrospective study of patients presenting with SAH who were identified as having a warning symptom[21]

ly 500,000 people in the U.S. carry the mutant gene for autosomal dominant polycystic kidney disease **(ADPKD)**. Renal function is usually normal during the first few decades of life, with progressive chronic renal failure ensuing. HTN is a common sequelae. Transmission is autosomal dominant, with 100% penetrance by 80 yrs of age[199]. Cystic disease of other organs may occur (viz.: liver in ≈ 33%, and occasionally lung, pancreas)[200].

The reported prevalence of aneurysms with ADPKD varies widely, from 10-30%[201], with 15% being a reasonable estimate[202]. In addition to the increased incidence of aneurysms, there appears to be an increased risk of rupture[203]. As a result, patients with AD-PKD carry a 10-20 fold increased risk of SAH compared to the general population[204]. These aneurysms are rarely discovered before age 20 years. The average rate of rupture of incidental aneurysms is ≈ 2%/yr (see *Unruptured aneurysms*, page 816). Using these statistics, together with the life expectancy of patients with ADPKD, and other estimations (of operative morbidity and mortality, etc.), decision analysis has been used to recommend that arteriography <u>not</u> be routinely employed in patients older than 25 yrs[201]. However, patients with symptoms possibly due to unruptured aneurysms, and those with SAH, should undergo angiography and subsequent surgical repair of any aneurysms discovered (especially those > 1 cm diameter). A decision analysis study[202] determined that screening with <u>MRA</u> was beneficial compared to treating patients once they became symptomatic. In a young patient with ADPKD with either a history of aneurysms or a kindred of ADPKD with aneurysms, repeat screening may be effectively repeated every ≈ 2-3 years (in a kindred of ADPKD without aneurysms, every 5-20 yrs was recommended)[202].

27.6. Treatment options for aneurysms

The best treatment for an aneurysm depends on the condition of the patient, the anatomy of the aneurysm, the ability of the surgeon, and must be weighed against the natural history of the condition. When treatment is indicated, surgical "clipping" of the aneurysm at the neck to exclude it from the circulation is considered to be the optimal treatment for most ruptured aneurysms. For unruptured aneurysms, *see page 816*.

The ideal goal of surgical treatment is usually to place a clip across the neck of the aneurysm to exclude the aneurysm from the circulation (*see below*) without occluding normal vessels. When the aneurysm cannot be clipped because of the nature of the aneurysm, or poor medical condition of the patient, the options below may be considered.

Decisions regarding treatment options have to take into account the natural history of the aneurysm. This involves information related primarily to:
1. risk of bleeding into subarachnoid space
   A. for ruptured aneurysms: this is the risk of *rebleeding: see page 789*
   B. for unruptured aneurysms: *see page 816*
   C. for cavernous carotid artery aneurysms: this risk is low (*see page 818*)
2. **spontaneous thrombosis** of an aneurysm is a rare occurrence[205-207] (estimates in *autopsy* series is 9-13%[207]). However they may reappear[208, 209], and delayed rupture may occur sometimes even years later

Therapies that do not directly address the aneurysm
The hope here is that the aneurysm will not bleed and that it will thrombose (*see above*).
1. continue medical management initiated on admission: i.e. control of HTN, continue calcium-channel blockers, stool softeners...continue bed rest for ≈ 1 week then allow bedside commode
2. treatment options generally <u>not</u> used
   A. antifibrinolytic therapy (e.g. ε-aminocaproic acid **(EACA)**): ✖ NB: <u>NOT USED</u>. Reduces rebleeding, but increases the incidence of arterial vasospasm and hydrocephalus[100]
   B. serial LPs: an historical treatment[210], may increase the risk of aneurysmal rupture

Endovascular and other "nonsurgical" techniques to treat the aneurysm
1. trapping: effective treatment requires distal AND proximal arterial interruption by direct surgical means (ligation or occlusion with a clip), by placement of a detachable balloon[211], or some combination. May also incorporate vascular bypass (e.g. EC-IC bypass) to maintain flow distal to trapped segment[212]
2. proximal ligation (hunterian ligation): useful for giant aneurysms[213, 214]. For non-

giant aneurysms provides little benefit and adds the risk of thromboembolism (which may be reduced by occluding the CCA rather than the ICA[214]). This may elevate the risk of developing aneurysms in the contralateral circulation[215]

3. thrombosing aneurysm:
   A. with Guglielmi detachable coils (*see below*)
   B. balloon embolization: intra-aneurysmal placement of detachable balloon by interventional neuroradiologic technique[157]. Risks: possible subsequent aneurysm growth[216], hemorrhage during balloon inflation, embolization of thrombus[217], balloon deflation. Has effectively been superseded by coil embolization (*see below*)

Surgical treatment for aneurysms

1. placement of clip across the neck of the aneurysm: the "gold standard"
2. wrapping or coating the aneurysm: although this should never be the goal of surgery, situations may arise in which there is little else that can be done (e.g. fusiform basilar trunk aneurysms, aneurysms with significant branches arising from the dome, or part of the neck within the cavernous sinus)
   A. with muscle: the first method used to surgically treat an aneurysm[218] (the patient described died from rebleeding)
   B. with cotton or muslin: popularized by Gillingham[219]. Analysis of 60 patients showed that 8.5% rebled in ≤ 6 mos, and the annual rebleeding rate was 1.5% thereafter[220] (similar to natural history)
   C. with plastic resin or other polymer: may be slightly better than muscle or gauze[221]. One study with long follow-up found no protection from rebleeding during the first month, but thereafter the risk was slightly lower than the natural history[221]. Other studies show no difference from natural course[222]
   D. Teflon and fibrin glue: a recent entry[223]

GUGLIELMI DETACHABLE COILS (GDC)

Electrolytically detachable platinum coils placed either during open surgery or, more commonly, via endovascular techniques[224-226]. Goals:
1. to promote thrombosis of the aneurysmal sac to prevent (re)bleeding
2. to reduce symptoms of mass effect[227], if any

Available data: There has been no long-term prospective randomized trial to compare GDC to microsurgery (MS)[228, 229]. The largest trial to date, the International Subarachnoid Hemorrhage Aneurysm Trial (ISAT)[230] had the important shortcomings detailed in *Table 6-11*. Also, still unresolved: GDC vs. MS for *unruptured* aneurysms.

Results

Procedural morbidity rate of GDC (mostly aneurysmal rupture): ≈ 4%,; mortality = 1%[231].

Results may be reported as occlusion rates or in terms of recurrence of SAH. Depending on criteria and timing of follow-up, MS fares better than GDC with occlusion rates and prevention of recurrent SAH.

Results of ISAT study: at 1 year follow-up, there was an absolute reduction of risk of having a poor outcome of 7% with GDC (24%) than with MS (31%).

Treatment failures may be due to:
1. early failure
   A. intraprocedural rupture
   B. vasospasm preventing endovascular treatment (< 1.5%)
   C. failure to achieve initial obliteration: 39% are completely obliterat-

Table 6-11 Methodological short comings of ISAT

1. only 20% of 9559 patients presenting with SAH were randomized*
   - selection could introduce bias
   - more nonrandomized patients underwent MS than GDC
   - guidelines not provided for which patients to consider for GDC
2. most study centers were located in Europe, Australia & Canada
3. the expertise of the surgeons and the interventionalists were not reported and were not necessarily comparable
4. the following features are not entirely representative of SAH patients at large
   - 80% of patients were in good clinical condition (H&H grade 1 or 2)
   - 93% of aneurysms were ≤ 10 mm diameter
   - 97% were in the anterior circulation
5. rebleeding rate: after GDC (2.4%) or MS (1.0%) was high for both groups, and the difference could be more significant beyond the 1 year follow-up provided

---

* most SAH patients were referred specifically for MS or GDC. The only patients that were were randomized were those for whom a panel decided it was not clear which procedure would be superior. Outcomes were not provided for non-randomized patients

ed, 46% are ≥ 95% occluded, and 15% are < 95% occluded[232]. Of aneurysms not initially occluded[232]:
1. 46% progressively thrombosed
2. 26% showed stable neck remnants
3. 28% showed enlargement of residual neck
2. late failure
   A. failure of partially obliterated aneurysms to go on to thrombose
   B. coil compaction
   C. enlargement of residual neck
   D. recanalization of aneurysm: 1.8% risk[232]

Recurrent SAH following GDC placement
1. ISAT study: 0.16% at 1 year[230]
2. 5% incidence of SAH (rebleeding) within 6 months of treatment (high compared to MS) in one series of 75 patients with acutely ruptured aneurysms[233]
3. in another series of 141 coiled aneurysms[232] (42% incidental, 41% acutely ruptured): 1 patient rebled within 6 months (1.7% of the ruptured group)

Additional treatment: Data on long-term efficacy is lacking. At least 20% of patients with relatively short follow-up needed retreatment in one series[234]. In the ISAT study, more than 4 times as many patients undergoing GDC needed additional procedures than did the MS group[230].

Recommended indications
Favorable situations for GDC:
1. inaccessible ruptured aneurysms
2. may be considered in cases where there is a failure of attempted clipping, or with aneurysms that are technically difficult to clip (a category that is very vague and varies widely with the experience of the neurosurgeon[228])
3. elderly patients (> 75 yrs): there appears to be a significant reduction in morbidity with GDC compared to MS
4. aneurysm configuration[235]:
   A. dome-to-neck ratio (AKA fundus-to-neck ratio) ≥ 2
   B. and an absolute neck diameter < 5 mm

Poor candidates for GDC:
1. giant aneurysms (> 20 mm diameter)[233]
2. very small aneurysms[233]
3. aneurysms with wide necks[233] (including small aneurysms)

Controversial areas with GDC:
1. unruptured aneurysms

Patients with residual filling of the aneurysm should undergo surgical clipping since there is significant risk of rebleeding.

27.7.   Timing of aneurysm surgery

Controversy exists between so-called "early surgery" (generally, but not precisely defined as ≤ 48-96 hrs post SAH) and "late surgery" (usually ≥ 10-14 days post SAH). Also *see page 815* for timing issues related to basilar bifurcation aneurysms.

Early surgery advocated for the following reasons:
1. if successful, virtually eliminates the risk of rebleeding which occurs most frequently in the period immediately following SAH (see *Rebleeding*, page 789)
2. facilitates treatment of vasospasm which peaks in incidence between days 6-8 post SAH (never seen before day 3) by allowing induction of arterial hypertension and volume expansion without danger of aneurysmal rupture
3. allows lavage to remove potentially vasospasmogenic agents from contact with vessels (including use of thrombolytic agents, *see page 794*)
4. although operative mortality is higher, overall patient mortality is lower[236]

Arguments against early surgery, in favor of late surgery include:
1. inflammation and brain edema are most severe immediately following SAH
   A. this necessitates more brain retraction
   B. at the same time this softens the brain making retraction more difficult (re-

tractors have more tendency to lacerate the more friable brain)
2. the presence of solid clot that has not had time to lyse impedes surgery
3. the risk of intra-operative rupture is higher with early surgery
4. possible increased incidence of vasospasm following early surgery from mechanotrauma to vessels

Factors that favor choosing early surgery include:
1. good medical condition of patient
2. good neurologic condition of patient (Hunt and Hess **(H&H)** grade ≤ 3)
3. large amounts of subarachnoid blood, increasing the likelihood and severity of subsequent vasospasm (see *Table 27-6*, page 792). Having the aneurysm clipped permits use of hyperdynamic therapy for vasospasm (see *Hyperdynamic therapy (HDT)* - *"Triple-H therapy"*, page 797)
4. conditions that complicate management in face of unclipped aneurysm: e.g. unstable blood pressure; frequent and/or intractable seizures
5. large clot with mass effect associated with SAH
6. early rebleeding, especially multiple rebleeds
7. indications of imminent rebleeding: e.g. development of 3rd nerve palsy with p-comm aneurysm (traditionally regarded as an indication for urgent treatment[237, 238]), increase in aneurysm size on repeat angiography

Factors that favor choosing delayed surgery (10-14 days post SAH) include:
1. poor medical condition and/or advanced age of patient (age may not be a separate factor related to outcome, when patients are stratified by H&H grade[239])
2. poor neurologic condition of patient (H&H grade ≥ 4): controversial. Some say the risk of rebleeding and its mortality argues for early surgery even in bad grade patients[240] since denying surgery on clinical grounds may result in withholding treatment in some patients who would do well (54% of H&H grade IV and 24% of H&H grade V patients had favorable outcome in one series[239]). Some data show no difference in surgical complications in good and bad grade patients with anterior circulation aneurysms[241]
3. aneurysms difficult to clip because of large size, or difficult location necessitating a lax brain during surgery (e.g. difficult basilar bifurcation or mid-basilar artery aneurysms, giant aneurysms)
4. significant cerebral edema seen on CT
5. the presence of active vasospasm

Conclusions
    There is insufficient Class 1 data to make any firm conclusions. Therefore the following is based on trials that are non-randomized, etc.
1. there is an overall trend towards better outcome with early surgery than with later surgery, however, the advantage of early surgery (reduced rebleeding) is at least partially offset by the disadvantages of early surgery[242] (*see above*)
2. outcomes seem worse when surgery is performed between days 4-10 after SAH (the "vasospastic interval") than if performed early or late

27.8. General technical considerations of aneurysm surgery

The goal of aneurysm surgery is to prevent rupture or further enlargement of the aneurysm, while at the same time preserving all normal vessels and minimizing injury to brain tissue and cranial nerves. This is usually accomplished by excluding the aneurysm from the circulation with a clip across its neck. Placing the clip too low on the aneurysm neck may occlude the parent vessel, while too distal placement may leave a so-called "aneurysmal rest" which is not benign (*see below*).
    See *Intraoperative aneurysm rupture* below for general measures to reduce the risk of this complication during surgery.

Aneurysmal rest
    When a portion of the aneurysm neck is not occluded by a surgical clip, it is referred to as an aneurysmal rest. A "dog-ear" occurs when a clip is angled to leave part of the neck at one end, and obliterates the neck at the other. Rests are not innocuous, even if only 1-2 mm, because they may later expand and possibly rupture years later, especially

in younger patients[243]. The incidence of rebleeding was 3.7% in one study, with an annual risk of 0.4-0.8% during the observation period of 4-13 yrs[244]. Patients should be followed with serial angiography, and any increase in size should be treated by reoperation or endovascular techniques if possible.

SURGICAL EXPOSURE
To avoid excessive brain retraction, surgical exposure requires sufficient bony removal and adequate brain relaxation (*see below*).

BRAIN RELAXATION
More critical for ACoA and basilar tip than for easier to reach aneurysms such as p-comm or MCA.... Techniques include:
1. hyperventilation
2. CSF drainage: provides brain relaxation and a field dry of CSF, and removes blood & blood breakdown products. ✖ CSF drainage before opening the dura is associated with an increased risk of aneurysmal rebleeding (*see page 789*)
   A. ventriculostomy: risks include seizures, bleeding from catheter insertion, infection (ventriculitis, meningitis), possible increased risk of vasospasm
      1. placed pre-op in cases of acute post-SAH hydrocephalus (*see page 790*)
      2. placed intra-op
   B. lumbar spinal drainage (*see below*)
   C. intra-operative drainage of CSF from cisterns
3. diuretics: mannitol and/or furosemide. Although proof is lacking, lowering ICP by this or any means may theoretically increase the risk of rebleeding[245]

Lumbar spinal drainage
May be inserted with Touhy needle following induction of anesthesia (to minimize BP elevation), prior to final positioning. CSF is gradually withdrawn by the anesthesiologist only after the dura is opened (to minimize chances of intraoperative aneurysmal bleeding), usually a total of 30-50 cc are removed in ~ 10 cc aliquots.

Risks include[109]: aneurysmal rebleeding (≤ 0.3%), back pain (10%, may be chronic in 0.6%), catheter malfunction preventing CSF drainage (< 5%), catheter fracture or laceration resulting in retained catheter tip in the spinal subarachnoid space, post-op CSF fistula, spinal H/A (may be difficult to distinguish from post-craniotomy H/A), infection, neuropathy (from nerve root impingement with needle), epidural hematoma (spinal and/or intracranial).

CEREBRAL PROTECTION DURING SURGERY

PATHOPHYSIOLOGY OF CEREBRAL ISCHEMIA
The **cerebral metabolic rate of oxygen consumption (CMRO$_2$)** (*see page 763*) arises from neurons utilizing energy for two functions: 1) maintenance of cell integrity (homeostasis) which normally accounts for ~ 40% of energy consumption, and 2) conduction of electrical impulses. Occlusion of an artery produces a central core of ischemic tissue where the CMRO$_2$ is not met. The oxygen deficiency precludes aerobic glycolysis and oxidative phosphorylation. ATP production declines and cell homeostasis cannot be maintained, and within minutes irreversible cell death occurs; a so-called cerebral infarction. Surrounding this central core is the **penumbra**, where collateral flow (usually through leptomeningeal vessels) provides marginal oxygenation which may impair cellular function without immediate irreversible damage. Cells in the penumbra may remain viable for hours.

CEREBRAL PROTECTION BY INCREASING THE ISCHEMIC TOLERANCE OF THE CNS
1. drugs that mitigate the toxic effects of ischemia without reducing CMRO$_2$
   A. calcium channel blockers: nimodipine, nicardipine, flunarizine
   B. free radical scavengers: superoxide dismutase, dimethylthiourea, lazaroids, barbiturates, Vitamin C
   C. mannitol: although not a cerebral protectant *per se*, it may help re-establish blood flow to compromised parenchyma by improving the microvascular perfusion by transiently increasing CBV and decreasing blood viscosity
2. reduction of CMRO$_2$

A. by reducing the electrical activity of neurons: titrating these agents to a iso-electric EEG reduces $CMRO_2$ by up to a maximum of $\approx 50\%$
   1. barbiturates: in addition to reducing $CMRO_2$, they also redistribute blood flow to ischemic cortex, quench free radicals, and stabilize cell membranes. For dosing of thiopental, *see below*
   2. etomidate (*see below*) ⎱ shorter acting and less myocardial de-
   3. isoflurane (*see page 1*) ⎰ pression than with barbiturates
B. by reducing the maintenance energy of neurons: no drugs developed to date can accomplish this, only **hypothermia** has any effect on this. Below mild hypothermia, extracerebral effects must be monitored (*see page 658*)
   1. even **mild hypothermia** (core temperatures down to 33° C) has beneficial effects
   2. **moderate hypothermia**: 32.5-33° C has been used for head injury
   3. **deep hypothermia** to 18° C permits the brain to tolerate up to 1 hour of circulatory arrest
   4. **profound hypothermia** to < 10° C allows several hours of complete ischemia (the clinical usefulness of this has not been substantiated)

ADJUNCTIVE CEREBRAL PROTECTION TECHNIQUES USED IN ANEURYSM SURGERY
1. systemic hypotension
   A. usually used during final approach to aneurysm and during manipulation of aneurysm for clip application
   B. theoretical goals
      1. to reduce turgor of aneurysm facilitating clip closure, especially with atherosclerotic neck
      2. to decrease transmural pressure (*see page 790*) to reduce the risk of intraoperative rupture
   C. danger of hypoxic injury to other organs and brain (including areas of impaired autoregulation as well as normal areas). Because of this, some surgeons avoid this method
2. "focal" hypotension: using temporary aneurysm clips (especially designed with low closing force to avoid intimal injury) placed on parent vessel (small perforators will not tolerate temporary clips without injury)
   A. used in conjunction with methods of cerebral protection against ischemia
   B. may be combined with systemic <u>hypertension</u> to increase collateral flow
   C. the proximal ICA can tolerate an hour or more of occlusion in some cases, whereas the perforator bearing segments of the MCA and the basilar apex may tolerate clipping for only a few minutes
   D. in addition to the risk of ischemia, there is the risk of intravascular thrombosis and subsequent release of emboli upon removal of the clip
3. circulatory arrest, utilized in conjunction with deep hypothermia
   A. candidates include patients with large aneurysms that contain significant atherosclerosis and/or thrombosis that impedes clip closure and a dome that is adherent to vital neural structures

SYSTEMATIC APPROACH TO CEREBRAL PROTECTION[246]
The following factors may mandate the use of temporary clips (and associated techniques of cerebral protection): giant aneurysm, calcified neck, thin/fragile dome, adherence of dome to critical structures, vital arterial branches near the aneurysm neck, intraoperative rupture. Aside from giant aneurysms, most of these factors may be difficult to identify pre-op. Therefore, Solomon provides some degree of cerebral protection to all patients undergoing aneurysm surgery.
1. spontaneous cooling is permitted during surgery, which usually results in a body temperature of 34° C by the time that dissection around the aneurysm begins
2. if temporary clipping is utilized
   A. if a long segment of the ICA is being trapped, administer 5000 U IV heparin to prevent thrombosis and subsequent emboli
   B. < 5 mins temporary clip occlusion: no further intervention
   C. up to 10 or 15 mins occlusion: administer thiopental 5 mg/kg loading bolus, followed by drip infusion titrated to burst suppression on compressed spectral array EEG
   D. > 20 mins occlusion: not tolerated (except possibly ICA proximal to p-comm), terminate operation if possible and plan repeat operation utilizing
      1. deep hypothermic circulatory arrest (*see above*)

2. endovascular techniques
3. bypass grafting around the segment to be occluded

POSTOPERATIVE ANGIOGRAPHY

Due to the fact that unexpected findings (aneurysmal rest, unclipped aneurysm, or major vessel occlusion) were seen on 19% of post-op angiograms (the only predictive factor identified was a new post-op deficit, which signalled major vessel occlusion) the use of routine post-op angiography has been recommended[247].

SOME DRUGS USEFUL IN ANEURYSM SURGERY

papaverine — DRUG INFO

A smooth muscle relaxant. May work by blocking calcium channels. Used for topical application on arteries to reverse vasoconstriction resulting from manipulation (mechanical "vasospasm"), and more recently via intra-arterial injection[137, 138], with a case report of exacerbation of vasospasm with intra-arterial injection[161].

Usual concentration: 30 mg in 9 cc NS. Applied with Gelfoam® or cotton pledget soaked in this mixture; generally left in contact with vessels for ≈ 2 minutes. Can also apply solution directly to vessels with syringe and leave in contact with vessels.

etomidate (Amidate®) — DRUG INFO

A short acting hypnotic with GABA-like effects that suppresses neuronal electrical activity which reduces neuronal metabolism by as much as 50%. Inhibits release of excitatory neurotransmitters. May be useful for neuroprotection when temporary vessel occlusion is required. Less myocardial suppression and less prolongation of post-op anesthetic effect than with barbiturates[248]. ≈ 0.4-0.5 mg/kg causes burst suppression in less than 2 minutes in the majority of patients, with a maximum drop in BP of 5%. Consciousness is usually regained in 3-5 minutes due to redistribution. Additional doses in increments of 0.1 mg/kg may be given as electrical activity returns.

SIDE EFFECTS: may increase epileptiform activity (may be blocked with pre-op AEDs). In protracted doses, can reduce steroid synthesis by adrenocortical suppression precipitating hypoadrenalism, which may be offset by standard neurosurgical pre-op steroids.

propofol (Diprivan®) — DRUG INFO

May be used to achieve burst suppression without some of the side effects of etomidate[249], and with shorter duration of action than other barbiturates. Results are preliminary, further investigation is needed to demonstrate the degree of neuroprotection. High doses may produce hypotension, for neuroprotection doses of 170 µg/kg/min (if tolerated) are recommended[250]. May also be used as a continuous drip for sedation (see page 37), and for ICP management (see page 663). Reverses rapidly upon discontinuation (usually within 5-10 minutes).

SIDE EFFECTS: Reports of possible anaphylactic reaction with angioneurotic edema of the airways[251]. Case reports of metabolic acidosis.

27.8.1. Intraoperative aneurysm rupture

EPIDEMIOLOGY

Reported rates of intraoperative aneurysm rupture (**IAR**) range from ≈ 18% in the cooperative study (1963-1978)[252] to 40% in a more recent series[253]. Although rupture rate may be higher in early surgery than with late surgery[253], other series found no difference[254].

Morbidity and mortality for patients experiencing significant IAR is ≈ 30-35% (vs. ≈ 10% in the absence of this complication), although IAR may primarily affects outcome when it occurs during induction of anesthesia or opening of dura[253].

PREVENTION OF INTRAOPERATIVE RUPTURE

Presented as a list here to be incorporated into general operative techniques.

1. prevent hypertension from catecholamine response to pain:
    A. insure deep anesthesia during headholder pin placement and skin incision
    B. consider local anesthetic (without epinephrine) in headholder pin-sites and along incision line
2. minimize increases in transmural pressure: reduce MAP to slightly below baseline just prior to dural opening
3. reduce shearing forces on aneurysm during dissection by minimizing brain retraction:
    A. radical removal of sphenoid wing for circle of Willis aneurysms
    B. reduce brain volume by a number of mechanisms: diuretics (mannitol, furosemide), CSF drainage through lumbar subarachnoid drain at the time of dural incision, hyperventilation
4. reduce risk of large tear in aneurysm fundus or neck:
    A. utilize sharp dissection in exposing aneurysm and in removing clot from around aneurysm
    B. whenever possible, completely mobilize and inspect aneurysm before attempting clip application

DETAILS OF INTRAOPERATIVE RUPTURE

Rupture can occur during any of the three following stages of aneurysm surgery[255]:
A. initial exposure (predissection)
    1. rare. Brain can become surprisingly tight even when bleeding seems to be into open subarachnoid space. Usually carries poor prognosis
    2. possible causes:
        A. vibration from bone work: dubious
        B. increasing transmural pressure upon opening the dura
        C. hypertension from catecholamine response to pain (*see above*)
    3. management tactics:
        A. have anesthesiologist radically drop BP
        B. control bleeding (with anterior circulation aneurysms) by placing temporary clip across ICA as it exits from cavernous sinus, or if not possible then compress ICA in patient's neck through drapes
        C. if necessary to gain control, resect portions of frontal or temporal lobe
B. dissection of the aneurysm: accounts for the majority of IARs, two basic types:
    1. tears caused by blunt dissection
        A. tends to be profuse, proximal to the neck, and difficult to control
        B. do not attempt definitive clipping unless adequate exposure has been achieved (which is usually not the case with these tears)
        C. **temporary clipping**: this step is often necessary in this situation, after the temporary clip is in place return the MAP to normal and administer neuroprotective agent (e.g. etomidate, *see page 808*)
        D. once the temporary clip is in place, it is better to take a few extra moments to improve the exposure and apply a well placed permanent clip instead of hastily clipping and trying to restore circulation
        E. microsutures may need to be placed to close any portion of the tear that extends onto the parent vessel
    2. laceration by sharp dissection
        A. tend to be small, often distally on fundus, and usually easily controlled by a single suction
        B. may respond to gentle tamponade with a small cottonoid
        C. may shrink down with repeated low current strokes with the bipolar (avoid the temptation to use continuous high current)
C. clip application: bleeding at this point is usually due to either
    1. inadequate exposure of aneurysm: clip blade may penetrate unseen lobe of aneurysm; similar to tears caused by blunt dissection (*see above*). Bleeding worsens as clip blades become approximated
        A. prompt opening and removal of clip at the first hint of bleeding may minimize the extent of the tear
        B. utilize 2 suckers to determine if definitive clipping can be done, or what is more common, to allow temporary clipping (*see above*)
    2. poor technical clip application: tends to abate as clip blades become approximated; inspect the blade tips for the following:
        A. to be certain that they span the breadth of the neck. If not, a second longer

clip is usually applied parallel to the first, which may then be advanced
B. to verify that they are closely approximated. If not, tandem clips may be necessary, and sometimes multiple clips are needed

27.9. Aneurysm recurrence after treatment

Incompletely treated aneurysms may increase in size and or bleed. This includes aneurysm that are clipped or coiled where there is still aneurysm filling, or a persistent aneurysm rest or a neck (*see page 805*).

Additionally, even an aneurysm that has been completely obliterated may recur, and therefore one has to consider the *durability* of treatment. The risk of recurrence of a completely clipped aneurysm is ≈ 1.5% at 4.4 years[256].

27.10. Aneurysm type by location

27.10.1. Anterior communicating artery aneurysms

The single most common site of aneurysms presenting with SAH[257]. May present with diabetes insipidus (**DI**) or other hypothalamic dysfunction.

CT SCAN
SAH in these aneurysms results in blood in the anterior interhemispheric fissure in essentially all cases, and is associated with intracerebral hematoma in 63% of cases[258]. Intraventricular hematoma is seen in 79% of cases, with the blood entering the ventricles from the intracerebral hematoma in about one third of these. Acute hydrocephalus was present in 25% of patients (late hydrocephalus, a common sequelae of SAH, was not studied).

Frontal lobe infarcts occur in 20%, usually several days following SAH[258]. One of the few causes of the rare finding of bilateral ACA distribution infarcts is vasospasm following hemorrhage from rupture of an ACoA aneurysm. This results in prefrontal lobotomy-like findings of apathy and abulia.

ANGIOGRAPHIC CONSIDERATIONS
Essential to evaluate contralateral carotid, to determine if both ACAs fill the aneurysm. If the aneurysm fills with one side only, it is desirable to inject the other side while cross compressing the side that fills the aneurysm to see if collateral flow is present. Also, determine if either carotid fills both ACAs, or if each ACA fills from the ipsilateral carotid injection (may permit trapping).

If additional views are needed to better demonstrate aneurysm
Try oblique 25° away from injection side, center beam 3-4 cm above lateral aspect of ipsilateral orbital rim, orient x-ray tube in Towne's view. A submental vertex view may also visualize the area but the image may be degraded by the amount of interposed bone.

SURGICAL TREATMENT

Approaches
1. pterional approach: the usual approach (*see below*)
2. subfrontal approach: especially useful for aneurysms pointing superiorly when there is a large amount of frontal blood clot (allows clot removal during approach)
3. anterior interhemispheric approach[259]: ✖ contraindicated for anteriorly pointing aneurysms as the dome is approached first & proximal control cannot be obtained
4. transcallosal approach

PTERIONAL APPROACH

Side of craniotomy:

A right pterional craniotomy is used with the following exceptions (for which a left pterional crani is used):

1. large ACoA aneurysm pointing to right: left crani exposes neck before dome
2. dominant left A1 feeder to aneurysm (with no filling from right A1): left crani provides proximal control
3. additional left sided aneurysm

27.10.2. Distal anterior cerebral artery aneurysms

Aneurysms of the distal anterior cerebral artery **(DACA)** (i.e. the ACA distal to the ACoA) are usually located at the origin of the frontopolar artery, or at the bifurcation of the pericallosal and callosomarginal arteries at the genu of the corpus callosum. Aneurysms located more distally are usually posttraumatic, infectious (mycotic), or due to tumor embolus[260]. DACA aneurysms are often associated with intracerebral hematoma or interhemispheric subdural hematoma[261] since the subarachnoid space is limited here. Conservative treatment of DACA aneurysms is often associated with poor results. Unruptured DACA aneurysms have a higher incidence of bleeding than unruptured aneurysms in other locations. These aneurysms are fragile and adherent to the brain, which predisposes to frequent premature intraoperative rupture.

On arteriography, if both ACAs fill from a single sided carotid injection, it may be difficult to make the important determination as to which ACA feeds the aneurysm. Multiple aneurysms are commonly associated with DACA aneurysms.

TREATMENT

Mycotic aneurysms should be treated as outlined on page 821.

Aneurysms up to 1 cm from the ACoA may be approached through a standard pterional craniotomy with partial gyrus rectus resection.

Aneurysms > 1 cm distal to the ACoA up to the genu of the corpus callosum, including those of the pericallosal/callosomarginal bifurcation, may be approached surgically by a basal frontal interhemispheric approach[262] via a frontal craniotomy using a bicoronal skin incision. A right sided craniotomy is preferred in most instances (exception: aneurysm dome buried in the right cerebral hemisphere making retraction hazardous), but should cross to the contralateral side by a couple centimeters.

ACA aneurysms distal to the genu of the corpus callosum may also be approached by an interhemispheric approach.

Surgical complications: Prolonged retraction on the cingulate gyrus may produce akinetic mutism that is usually temporary. The pericallosal arteries are small in caliber and may be atherosclerotic, which together increases the risk of occlusion of the parent artery with the aneurysm clip.

27.10.3. Posterior communicating artery aneurysms

May occur at either end of p-comm; that is at the junction with the PCA, or more commonly at the junction with carotid (typically points laterally, posteriorly, and inferiorly). May impinge on the third nerve in either case and cause third nerve palsy (ptosis, mydriasis, "down and out" deviation) that, is not pupil sparing in 99% of cases.

ANGIOGRAPHIC CONSIDERATIONS

Vertebral artery **(VA)** injection is necessary to help evaluate the p-comm artery:

1. if the p-comm is patent: determine if there is a "fetal circulation" where the posterior circulation is fed only through the p-comm
2. determine if the aneurysm fills from VA injection

If additional views are needed to better demonstrate aneurysm

Try paraorbital oblique 55° away from injection side, center beam 1 cm posterior to inferior portion of lateral rim of ipsilateral orbit, orient x-ray tube 12° cephalad.

27.10.4. Carotid terminus (bifurcation) aneurysms

If additional views are needed to better demonstrate aneurysm
Try oblique 25° away from injection side, center beam 3-4 cm above lateral aspect of ipsilateral orbital rim, orient x-ray tube in Towne's view. Also may try submentovertex view.

27.10.5. Middle cerebral artery (MCA) aneurysms

The following considers MCA aneurysms of the "trifurcation" region.

SURGICAL TREATMENT

APPROACHES
1. trans-sylvian approach through a <u>pterional craniotomy</u>: the most common
2. superior temporal gyrus approach[263]:
    A. advantages: minimizes brain retraction, possible reduced vasospasm from manipulation of proximal vessels
    B. disadvantages: proximal control difficult, slightly larger bone flap, possible increased risk of seizures

27.10.6. Supraclinoid aneurysms[264]

Applied anatomy
The carotid artery exits the cavernous sinus and enters the subarachnoid space at the dural constriction known as the **carotid ring** (AKA clinoidal ring). The supraclinoid portion of the carotid artery may be divided into the following segments[265]:
1. **ophthalmic segment**: the largest portion of the supraclinoid ICA. Lies between the take-off of the ophthalmic artery and the posterior communicating artery (PCoA) origin. The proximal portion of this (including the origin of the ophthalmic artery) is often obscured by the anterior clinoid process. Branches include:
    A. ophthalmic artery: usually originates from the supracavernous ICA just after the ICA enters the subarachnoid space. Enters the optic canal positioned inferolateral to the optic nerve
    B. superior hypophyseal artery: the largest of several perforators supplying the dura of the cavernous sinus and the superior pituitary gland and stalk
2. communicating segment: from the PCoA origin to the origin of the anterior choroidal artery (AChA)
3. choroidal segment: from AChA origin to the terminal bifurcation of the ICA

27.10.6.1. Ophthalmic segment aneurysms[266]

Ophthalmic segment aneurysms **(OSAs)** include (NB: nomenclature varies among authors):
1. ophthalmic artery aneurysms:
2. superior hypophyseal artery aneurysms:
    A. paraclinoid variant: usually does not produce visual symptoms
    B. suprasellar variant: when giant, may mimic pituitary tumor on CT

PRESENTATION (EXCLUDING INCIDENTAL DISCOVERY)

OPHTHALMIC ARTERY ANEURYSMS
Arise from the ICA just distal to the origin of ophthalmic artery. They project dorsally or dorsomedially towards the lateral portion of the optic nerve.

Presentation:
- ≈ 45% present as SAH
- ≈ 45% present as visual field defect:
    A. as the aneurysm enlarges it impinges on the lateral portion of the optic nerve → temporal fiber compression → ipsilateral <u>monocular superior nasal quadrantanopsia</u>
    B. continued enlargement → upward displacement of the nerve against the **falciform ligament** (or fold) → superior fiber compression → monocular nasal inferior field cut
    C. in addition to near-complete loss of vision in the involved eye, compression of the optic nerve near the chiasm may produce a superior temporal quadrant defect in the <u>contralateral</u> eye (**junctional scotoma** AKA "pie in the sky" defect) (after they decussate, nasal retinal fibers course anteriorly for a short distance in the contralateral optic nerve, so-called **anterior knee of Wildbrand**)[267]
- ≈ 10% present as both

SUPERIOR HYPOPHYSEAL ARTERY ANEURYSMS

Originate in the small subarachnoid pocket medial to the ICA near the lateral aspect of the sella. The direction of enlargement is dictated by the size of this pocket and the height of the lateral sellar wall, resulting in two variants: paraclinoid & suprasellar.

Suprasellar variant may actually grow to a size large enough to compress pituitary stalk and cause hypopituitarism and "classic" chiasmal visual symptoms (bilateral temporal hemianopsia).

ANGIOGRAPHIC CONSIDERATIONS

A notch can often be observed in the in the anterior, superior, medial aspect of giant ophthalmic artery aneurysms due to the optic nerve[268].

If additional views are needed to better demonstrate aneurysm

Try oblique 25° away from injection side, center beam 3-4 cm above lateral aspect of ipsilateral orbital rim, orient x-ray tube in Towne's view. Try submentovertex view.

SURGICAL TREATMENT[264]

OPHTHALMIC ARTERY ANEURYSMS

If necessary, the ophthalmic artery may be sacrificed without worsening of vision in the vast majority. Clipping a contralateral ophthalmic artery aneurysm is not technically difficult, and is not uncommonly required as OSAs are often multiple.

The aneurysm arises from the superomedial aspect of the ICA just distal to the ophthalmic artery origin, and projects superiorly.

SUPERIOR HYPOPHYSEAL ARTERY ANEURYSMS

If necessary, the superior hypophyseal artery on one side may be clipped without demonstrable deleterious effect (due to bilateral supply to stalk and pituitary). Clipping a contralateral superior hypophyseal aneurysms is not really feasible.

27.10.7. Posterior circulation aneurysms

(See page 815 for *basilar tip* aneurysms). Clinical syndrome of SAH in the posterior fossa is indistinguishable from that due to anterior circulation aneurysms except for possible increased tendency towards respiratory arrest and subsequent neurogenic pulmonary edema[269]. Vasospasm following posterior fossa SAH may be more likely to cause midbrain symptoms than vasospasm due to SAH elsewhere.

HYDROCEPHALUS

In Yamaura's series[270], 12% of patients required external ventricular drainage **(EVD)** following posterior fossa SAH to remove bloody CSF causing hydrocephalus, and 20% eventually required permanent ventricular shunt.

27.10.7.1. Vertebral artery aneurysms

Traumatic vertebral artery aneurysms **(VAA)** (AKA dissecting aneurysms) are more common than non-traumatic VAAs. The following discussion concerns non-traumatic VAA.

Most VAAs arise at the VA-PICA junction. Other sites: VA-AICA, VA-BA.

ANGIOGRAPHIC CONSIDERATIONS

Angiography of VAA should assess the contralateral VA for patency in case of the need to trap the aneurysm. **Allcock test** (vertebral angiography with carotid compression) may be used to assess patency of circle of Willis. Test occlusion with a balloon catheter can determine if patient will tolerate occlusion (a double lumen balloon will even allow measurement of distal back pressure).

PICA ANEURYSMS

For PICA anatomy, see *Figure 3-11*, page 80. For arteriogram, see *Figure 5-5*, page 133.

Comprise ≈ 3% of cerebral aneurysms. 3 common sites:
1. VA at the VA-PICA junction[184]:
   A. saccular aneurysms: most commonly at the distal (superior) angle. An aneurysm in this location should be suspected with a CT showing blood predominantly in the 4th ventricle[193] (aneurysmal dome may adhere to foramen of Luschka; rupture fills the ventricles with little subarachnoid blood visible on CT). The level is as varied as the PICA origin, and ranges from as low as the foramen magnum to as high as the ponto-medullary junction. Most VA-PICA aneurysms lie in the anterolateral portion of the medullary cistern[271], anterior to the first dentate ligament[272]. However, the PICA origin may sometimes lie in the midline or across it
   B. fusiform aneurysms: usually the result of prior arterial dissection: *see page 886*
2. PICA aneurysms distal to the VA-PICA junction: tend to be fragile and often develop multiple hemorrhages in a relatively short period, ∴ should be treated promptly, even when discovered incidentally
3. fusiform VA aneurysms involving PICA

ANGIOGRAPHIC CONSIDERATIONS

If additional views are needed to better demonstrate aneurysm

Try paraorbital oblique 55° away from injection side, center beam on foramen magnum, orient x-ray tube 12° cephalad.

TREATMENT
Options:
1. direct aneurysmal clipping is the preferred treatment
2. endovascular coil embolization: not as effective as clipping for relief of symptoms due to brainstem or cranial nerve compression
3. choices for unclippable and uncoilable aneurysms (e.g. fusiform, giant, or dissecting aneurysms) include:
   A. proximal (hunterian) VA ligation[273] which must be <u>distal</u> to the PICA origin to prevent severe morbidity or mortality[274]
   B. balloon occlusion of the VA distal to the PICA origin
   C. midcervical VA balloon occlusion (allows collateral flow through suboccipital muscular branches)

27.10.7.2. Vertebrobasilar junction aneurysms

ANGIOGRAPHIC CONSIDERATIONS

If additional views are needed to better demonstrate aneurysm

Try oblique 15° away from injection side, center beam on foramen magnum, orient x-ray tube 25° Towne. Try submentovertex view.

SURGICAL APPROACHES
1. suboccipital approach: for most; performed in lateral oblique position
2. subtemporal-transtentorial approach if the vertebrobasilar junction is high; performed in supine position

27.10.7.3. AICA aneurysms

ANGIOGRAPHIC CONSIDERATIONS

If additional views are needed to better demonstrate aneurysm
Try AP or submentovertex view, center beam on nasion, orient x-ray tube 15° caudad.

27.10.8. Basilar bifurcation aneurysms

AKA **basilar tip aneurysms**. The most common posterior circulation aneurysm. Comprise ≈ 5% of intracranial aneurysms.

PRESENTATION
Most present with SAH indistinguishable from SAH due to anterior circulation aneurysmal rupture. Enlargement of the aneurysm prior to rupture may rarely compress the optic chiasm → bitemporal field cut (mimicking pituitary tumor), or occasionally may compress the third nerve as it exits from the interpeduncular fossa → oculomotor nerve palsy[269].

CT/MRI SCAN
May occasionally be seen on CT or MRI as round mass in region of suprasellar cistern. With SAH, tend to see blood in interpeduncular cistern with some reflux into 4th (and to a lesser extent, third and lateral) ventricle. Occasionally may mimic pretruncal nonaneurysmal SAH (see page 823).

ANGIOGRAPHY
Dome usually points superiorly. Should evaluate flow through posterior communicating arteries (may require Allcock test) in case trapping is required. Need to assess the height of the basilar bifurcation in relation to the dorsum sella (see Approaches below).

If additional views are needed to better demonstrate aneurysm
Try oblique 25° away from or towards injection side, center beam 3-4 cm above lateral aspect of ipsilateral superior orbital rim, orient x-ray tube 25° Towne. Try submentovertex view.

SURGICAL TREATMENT

TIMING
Initial experience tended to favor allowing basilar tip aneurysms to "cool-down" for ≈ 10-14 days after SAH before attempting surgery to permit cerebral edema to subside. More recently, early surgery for these aneurysms has been advocated as for anterior circulation aneurysms[275] (see *Timing of aneurysm surgery*, page 804). However, some surgeons still recommend waiting ≈ 1 week[276], and most would agree that if there are obvious technical difficulties because of size, configuration or location of the aneurysm, that early surgery may not be appropriate. Also, if during the craniotomy it becomes apparent that cerebral edema is impairing the exposure, the operation should be aborted and attempted again at a later date.

APPROACHES
1. right subtemporal craniotomy (classical approach of Drake): approached through the incisura or division of the tentorium. Most basilar tip aneurysms are probably best approached via pterional approach (see below) except for posteriorly pointing

aneurysms
- A. advantage:
  1. less distance to basilar tip
  2. may be better than pterional approach for aneurysms projecting posteriorly or posteroinferiorly[276]
- B. disadvantages:
  1. requires temporal lobe retraction (minimized with lumbar drainage, mannitol, and possibly zygomatic arch section[277])
  2. poor visualization of contralateral P1 segment and thalamoperforators
2. pterional approach (described by Yasargil): trans-Sylvian (*see below*)
- A. advantages:
  1. little or no retraction on temporal lobe (unlike subtemporal approach)
  2. better visualization of both P1 segments and thalamoperforators
  3. other aneurysms, e.g. of the anterior circulation, can be dealt with at the same sitting
- B. disadvantages:
  1. increases reach to aneurysm by ≈ 1 cm compared to subtemporal
  2. requires wide splitting of the sylvian fissure
  3. operating field is narrower than subtemporal approach
  4. perforators arising from the posterior aspect of P1 may not be visible
3. modified pterional craniotomy: may allow trans-sylvian *or* subtemporal approach[276]. The craniotomy is taken further posteriorly than a standard pterional craniotomy
4. orbitozygomatic approach: allows access to portions of the basilar artery below the bifurcation. May be augmented by removal of the top of the clivus

Optional resection of the temporal tip will increase exposure of either approach. Unlike most anterior circulation aneurysms, securing proximal control is very difficult.

If the basilar bifurcation is high above the dorsum sella, then more retraction is required on a subtemporal approach than for a normal bifurcation height (near the dorsum sella). A high bifurcation is dealt with on a trans-sylvian approach by opening the sylvian fissure more widely, or by a subfrontal approach through the third ventricle via the lamina terminalis[278]. A low bifurcation may require splitting the tentorium behind the 4th nerve.

PTERIONAL APPROACH[279]

Risks include: oculomotor palsy in ≈ 30% (most are minimal and temporary).

Approach is from the <u>right</u> unless:
1. additional left sided aneurysm (e.g. p-comm aneurysm) which could be treated simultaneously by a left sided approach
2. aneurysm points to the right
3. aneurysm is located to the left of midline (the operation is more difficult when the aneurysm is even just 2-3 mm contralateral to the craniotomy)[276]
4. patient has right hemiparesis or left oculomotor palsy

OUTCOME

If the aneurysm is not giant, then these may be as safe to clip as anterior circulation aneurysms. Overall mortality is 5%, and morbidity is 12% (mostly due to injury to perforating vessels)[29].

27.11.   Unruptured aneurysms

Unruptured intracranial aneurysms (**UIA**) includes **incidental aneurysms** (those that do not produce any symptoms and are discovered incidentally) and aneurysms that produce symptoms other than those due to hemorrhage (e.g. pupillary dilatation due to third nerve compression). UIA merit consideration for treatment since the outcome from SAH with or without surgery is poor even under the best of circumstances. About 65% of patients die from the first SAH[280], and even in patients with no neurologic deficit after aneurysm rupture, only 46% fully recover, and only 44% return to their former jobs[1]. Estimated prevalence of incidental aneurysms is 5-10% of the population[1].

PRESENTATION
See items other than "rupture" in *Presentation of aneurysms*, page 800.

NATURAL HISTORY
Risk of bleeding from UIA differs from aneurysms that have ruptured. True risk is not known with certainty. The largest, most detailed study to date is the ISUIA[281].

Spontaneous thrombosis of unruptured aneurysms may occur rarely (*see page 802*).

The natural history and treatment results are influenced by[282] (see *Surgical outcome* below):
1. patient factors:
   A. history of previous SAH from a separate aneurysm[281] significantly increases the risk of rupture of an UIA
   B. patient age
   C. concurrent medical conditions
2. aneurysm characteristics[281]
   A. aneurysm size: the most important predictor for future rupture (*see below*) except (for unknown reasons) in patients with prior SAH from another source
   B. location: p comm, vertebrobasilar/posterior cerebral, and basilar tip UIAs were more likely to rupture
   C. morphology
3. surgical capabilities
   A. experience of the surgical team
   B. possibly by ancillary services available

An estimate for UIA is ≈ 1% per year. The risk of bleeding in patients with multiple aneurysms was higher (6.8%) than for patients with single aneurysms (2.3%)[283].

Aneurysm size: Risk of rupture appears critically dependent on aneurysm diameter[284]. Estimated annual risk of rupture of aneurysms of diameter **< 10 mm** is **0.05%** (range: 0-4%)[183, 281]A and is lower than for diameters > **10 mm** which is 1% (range: 0.46-1.54%)[281, 285] (this seems paradoxical since the mean diameter of aneurysms on post-rupture angiograms is 7.5 mm; this may be due to a shrinkage of aneurysms following rupture). The rupture rate was 6% in the first year with giant (≥ 2.5 cm) UIAs. Furthermore, aneurysms are *not* static, and have been shown to increase in size on serial angiograms[286].

SURGICAL OUTCOME
There are no prospective randomized studies of treatment natural history vs. treatment options[282], and most data are either from personal series or are retrospective. Summary of 260 patients show no surgical mortality, and morbidity of 0-10.3% (6.5% major and 8% minor morbidity in the multicenter study)[1]. A recent study found surgical mortality of 2.3% at 30-days, and 3.8% at 1 year[281]. A meta-analysis found 2.6% case fatality[287].

Operative morbidity was mild in 5%, moderate to severe in 6%[287]. Morbidity also increased with aneurysm size (2.3% for diameter < 5 mm, 6.8% for 6-15 mm, and 14% for 16-25 mm)[281]. Morbidity also varied with location (4.8% for p-comm, 8.1% for MCA, 11.8% for ophthalmic, 15.5% for anterior communicating, and 16.8% for carotid bifurcation). Morbidity also increases with patient age (6.5% for age < 45 yrs, 14% for age 45-64, and 32% for age > 64)[281].

MANAGEMENT
To understand the calculation of *cumulative* risk for aneurysmal rupture, *see page 836* for a discussion of this issue related to AVMs which also pertains to aneurysms.

Decision analysis
Requires data about the natural history (*see above*), life expectancy, and morbidity and mortality of SAH and aneurysm surgery.

A. selection bias may play a role in lowering the apparent SAH rate as follows: enlarging aneurysms (which have increased risk of rupture) may produce symptoms and may be preferentially referred for surgery, and the inclusion of cavernous carotid aneurysms (which rarely cause SAH)

In one such study[288], using the values shown in *Table 27-12*, the result obtained was that a life expectancy of 12 more years is the break-even point, i.e. if the patient is not expected to live for 12 more years, then non-surgical management is a better choice than surgery (this result involves numerous assumptions and estimations; e.g. 5% "risk aversiveness" (intermediate), relates to patient's fears of immediate surgical risk vs. risk of rupture spread over many years). Another analysis of various scenarios for a 50 year old female found that treatment was cost effective for UIAs that were symptomatic, ≥ 10 mm diameter, or with a previous history of SAH[289].

Table 27-12 Data used in decision analysis of management of unruptured aneurysms[288]

	Typical value	Range
annual risk of rupture*	1%	0.5-2%
3 month mortality of SAH	55%	50-60%
serious morbidity after SAH	15%	10-20%
surgical morbidity & mortality	2% & 6%	4-10%

* this is an intermediate risk for aneurysms 6-10 mm diameter (NB: size may change; small aneurysms may grow)

Management recommendations based on aneurysm size

Numerous recommendations have been made for a critical size above which an unruptured aneurysm should be considered for surgery, and have included 3 mm[285], 5 mm[290], 7 mm[291], and 9 mm[183]. And again, the patient's expected longevity must be taken into account. One proposal is to promptly treat unruptured aneurysms ≥ 10 mm, to repair those measuring 7-9 mm in young and middle-aged patients, and to follow smaller aneurysms with serial angiography[292]. **Summary of the American Heart Association Stroke Council recommendations**

Table 27-13 summarizes factors favoring treatment made based on a review of the literature[282] (only level IV and V evidence was found, and therefore only grade C recommendations can be made (i.e. an array of potential actions, any of which could be considered appropriate)[293, 294]). Patients for whom expectant management is elected should have periodic CT, MRA or selective contrast angiography seeking changes in aneurysm size or configuration. Symptomatic large or giant aneurysms carry increased risk of treatment.

Table 27-13 Factors favoring treatment of UIAs

Factor	Features favoring treatment
patient age	young age (risk of SAH accumulates with time)
previous SAH	UIA in patient with previous SAH due to another aneurysm
aneurysm location	basilar apex
aneurysm size	small UIAs approaching 10 mm in size, and in particular UIAs ≥ 10 mm size
aneurysm configuration	UIAs with daughter aneurysm or other unique hemodynamic featrures
family history	family members with aneurysms of aneurysmal SAH
symptomatic aneurysms	development of new symptoms related to mass effect may indicate enlargment and urgent treatment is recommended
changes on follow-up studies	enlargment or change in configuration

In all treatment decisions, coexisting medical conditions must be taken into account.

UNRUPTURED CAVERNOUS CAROTID ARTERY ANEURYSMS

Most cavernous carotid artery aneurysms **(CCAAs)** develop on the horizontal segment of the artery.

Presentation:
1. CCAAs may be discovered incidentally
   A. on arteriography for other reason
   B. on MRI
   C. occasionally on CT
2. when symptomatic:
   A. usually present with:
      1. headache
      2. cavernous sinus syndrome (*see page 918*): primarily produces diplopia (due to ophthalmoplegia). Classically the third nerve palsy from enlarging CCAA will <u>not</u> produce a dilated pupil because the sympathet-

ics which dilate the pupil are also paralyzed[70 (p 1492)]

    3. those that expand through the carotid ring into the subarachnoid space may cause monocular blindness[264]

B. rarely, pain (retro-orbital or pain mimicking trigeminal neuralgia[194, 195]) or a carotid-cavernous fistula (**CCF**) are the sole manifestation

C. when CCAAs rupture, they usually produce a CCF

D. life threatening complications are rare, but may be more common with *giant* intracavernous aneurysms[295]. Manifestations include:
    1. SAH[295, 296]   } especially CCAAs
    2. arterial epistaxis from rupture into sphenoid sinus (usually with traumatic aneurysms, *see page 820*) } that straddle the carotid ring[A]
    3. emboli

Indications for treatment:
1. unruptured CCAAs: the natural history is not precisely known
    A. symptomatic: patients with intolerable pain or visual problems[297]
    B. giant aneurysms: especially those that straddle the clinoidal ring[A]
    C. aneurysms that enlarge on serial imaging
    D. controversial: incidental aneurysms in the distribution of a stenotic carotid artery for which carotid endarterectomy is indicated. There has been no evidence that doing the endarterectomy increases the risk of rupture, and, as indicated above, most ruptures are not life threatening and so the carotid disease should be treated according to it's own merits
2. ruptured CCAAs:
    A. emergent treatment for cases with epistaxis or SAH
    B. urgent treatment for CCFs with severe eye pain or threat to vision

Treatment options for CCAAs:
    Treatment of small incidental intracavernous CCAAs is not generally indicated[282].
    For other unruptured CCAAs, options include detachable coils in an attempt to thrombose the aneurysm (*see page 803*). This results in reduction of mass effect in ~ 50%. Open surgical treatment is rarely appropriate. Aneurysms that rupture and produce a carotid-cavernous fistula may be treated by detachable balloon occlusion (*see page 845*).

27.12.   Multiple aneurysms

    Multiple aneurysms are present in 15-33.5% of cases of SAH[1]. In one study of multiple factors, hypertension was found to be the most important one associated with multiplicity[299].
    When a patient presents with SAH and is found to have multiple aneurysms, the following may be clues as to which aneurysm has bled:
1. epicenter (center of greatest concentration) of blood on CT or MRI[49]
2. area of vasospasm on angiogram
3. irregularities in the shape of the aneurysm (so-called "Murphy's tit")
4. if none of the above help, then suspect the largest aneurysm

---

27.13.   Familial aneurysms

    The role of inheritance in the development of intracranial aneurysms (**IA**) is well established for disorders such as polycystic kidney disease, and connective tissue disorders such as Ehlers-Danlos type IV, Marfan's syndrome, and pseudoxanthoma elasticum (see *Conditions associated with aneurysms*, page 801).
    Additional cases of IAs in identical twins[300, 301] as well as familial aggregations of IAs without a recognized inherited disorder have also been reported but are felt to be rare (it has been estimated that < 2% of IAs are familial[302]). Most reported cases consist of only 2 family members with IAs, and these are most commonly siblings[303]. Analysis of case re-

---

A. subarachnoid extension of CCAAs may be indicated by "waisting" of the aneurysm on angiography[298]

ports reveals that when IAs occur in siblings they tend to occur at identical or mirror images sites, and in comparison to sporadic IAs, familial IAs tend to rupture at a smaller size and at a younger age, and that the incidence of anterior communicating artery aneurysms is lower[304]. It has been postulated that IAs occurring in siblings may represent a distinct population of IAs[305].

The indications and best method for investigation of asymptomatic relatives of a patient found to harbor an intracranial aneurysm are controversial. Negative studies (angiography, DSA, MRA...) do not guarantee that at a later date an aneurysm will not be discovered that either subsequently developed or expanded, or was simply not detected on the initial study[306-308]. Cerebral angiography is the most sensitive study, however, the risk and expense may not justify its use as a screening test in many cases. Furthermore, there is some evidence that aneurysms that rupture tend to do so shortly after their formation[183] which would reduce the value of screening.

Screening recommendations: first-degree relatives (especially siblings) are at higher risk of harboring IAs[309] and should undergo MRI and MRA screening. Findings suspicious for IA(s) require follow-up with four vessel arteriography to confirm suspected lesions (MRA has a high false-positive rate of ≈ 16%[60]) and to rule-out additional IAs.

27.14. Traumatic aneurysms

Traumatic aneurysms **(TAs)** comprise < 1% of intracranial aneurysms[310, 311]. Most are actually false aneurysms, AKA pseudoaneurysms (a rupture of all the vessel wall layers with the "wall" of the aneurysm being formed by surrounding cerebral structures[312]). They may occur rarely in childhood. The mechanism of injury usually falls into one of the following groups[313]:

1. those arising from penetrating trauma: usually from gunshot wounds, although penetration with a sharp object (which is less common) may be more prone to cause traumatic aneurysms[314]
2. those arising from closed head injury: more common. Theories of pathogenesis include traction injury to the vessel wall or entrapment within a fracture. Tend to occur either:
   A. peripherally
      1. distal anterior cerebral artery aneurysms: secondary to impact against the falcine edge
      2. distal cortical artery aneurysms: often associated with an overlying skull fracture, sometimes a growing skull fracture
   B. at the skull base, usually involving the ICA in one of the following sites:
      1. petrous portion
      2. cavernous carotid artery:
         a. aneurysm enlargement may cause a progressive cavernous sinus syndrome
         b. rupture may lead to a posttraumatic carotid-cavernous fistula (*see page 845*) or to massive epistaxis in the presence of a sphenoid sinus fracture[315-317]

         } virtually always associated with basal skull fractures

      3. supraclinoid carotid artery
3. iatrogenic: following surgery in or around the skull base, the sinuses, or orbits (including following transsphenoidal surgery[318])

Presentation

1. delayed intracranial hemorrhage (subdural, subarachnoid, intraventricular, or intraparenchymal): the most common presentation. TAs tend to have a high rate of rupture
2. recurrent epistaxis
3. progressive cranial nerve palsy
4. enlarging skull fracture
5. may be incidental finding on CT scan
6. severe headache

Treatment

Although cases have been reported with spontaneous resolution, direct treatment is usually recommended. ICA aneurysms at the skull base should undergo balloon trapping or balloon embolization. Peripheral lesions should be treated surgically with clipping of aneurysm neck, excision of the aneurysm, coiling, or wrapping if no other method is feasible.

27.15. Mycotic aneurysms

The name *"mycotic"* originated with Osler in whose time the term referred to any infectious process[319] rather than the current usage which infers a fungal etiology. Currently accepted terminology favors **infectious aneurysm** (or bacterial aneurysm). Infectious aneurysms can, however, also occur with fungal infections[320]. Tend to form in distal (often unnamed) vessels.

EPIDEMIOLOGY & PATHOPHYSIOLOGY
* comprise ≈ 4% of intracranial aneurysms
* occurs in 3-15% of patients with subacute bacterial endocarditis **(SBE)**
* most common location: distal MCA branches (75-80%)
* at least 20% have or develop multiple aneurysm
* increased frequency in immunocompromised patients (e.g. AIDS) and drug users
* most probably start in the adventitia (outer layer) and spread inward

EVALUATION
Blood cultures and LP may identify the infectious organism. *Table 27-14* shows typical pathogens recovered. Patients with suspected infectious aneurysm(s) should undergo echocardiography to look for signs of endocarditis.

Table 27-14 Pathogens implicated in mycotic aneurysms[321 (p 933-40)]

Organism	%	Comment
streptococcus	44%	*S. viridans* (classic cause of SBE)
staphylococcus	18%	*S. aureus* (cause of acute bacterial endocarditis)
miscellaneous	6%	(pseudomonas, enterococcus, corynebacter...)
multiple	5%	
no growth	12%	
no info	14%	
total	99%	

TREATMENT
These aneurysms usually have fusiform morphology and are usually very friable, therefore surgical treatment is difficult and/or risky. Most cases are treated acutely with antibiotics which are continued 4-6 weeks. Serial angiography (at 7-10 days and 1.5, 3, 6 and 12 months, even if aneurysms seem to be getting smaller, they may subsequently increase[322] and new ones may form) helps document effectiveness of medical therapy (serial MRA may be a viable alternative in some cases). Aneurysms may continue to shrink following completion of antibiotic therapy[323]. Delayed clipping may be more feasible; indications include:
* patients with SAH
* increasing size of aneurysm while on antibiotics[324] (controversial, some say not mandatory[323])
* failure of aneurysm to reduce in size after 4-6 weeks of antibiotics[324]

Patients with SBE requiring valve replacement should have bioprosthetic (i.e. tissue) valves instead of mechanical valves to eliminate the need for risky anticoagulation.

27.16. Giant aneurysms

Definition: > 2.5 cm (≈ 1 inch) diameter. Two types: saccular (probably an enlarged "berry" aneurysm) and fusiform. Comprise 3-5% of intracranial aneurysms; peak age of presentation 30-60 years; female:male ratio = 3:1. Drake's series of 174 giant aneurysms[325]: 35% presented as hemorrhage, with 10% showing some evidence of remote bleeding. The bleeding rate is unknown, but is probably less than the ≈ 2%/year for non-giant aneurysms.

May also present as TIAs (by reducing flow or by emboli) or as a mass. About one third have a neck amenable to clipping.

Drake contends that even after thorough radiographic evaluation, actual operative visualization is the only way to definitively assess the aneurysm and its branches.

Angiogram: Often underestimates the size of the lesion secondary to thrombosed regions of the aneurysm that do not fill with contrast. CT or MRI is required to visualize the thrombosed portion.

CT scan: Frequently have a significant amount of edema surrounding the aneurysm. May see contrast enhancement of the brain surrounding the aneurysm; probably due to increased vascularity secondary to inflammatory reaction to the aneurysm.

MRI scan: Turbulence within → complicated signal on T1WI. **Pulsation artifact** (linear distortion radiation through aneurysm) on MRI helps differentiate giant aneurysms from solid or cystic lesions.

TREATMENT
Options include:
1. direct surgical clipping: usually possible in only ≈ 50% of cases
2. vascular bypass of aneurysm with subsequent clipping
3. trapping
4. proximal arterial ligation (hunterian ligation)
    A. for vertebral-basilar aneurysms[213]: results in improvement of cranial nerve deficit in ≈ 95% of patients
5. wrapping: *see page 803*

27.17.   SAH of unknown etiology

Recent estimates of incidence: **7-10%**. This is a heterogeneous category, and a better term might be "angiogram-negative SAH" (*see page 784* for requirements to be met before considering an arteriogram to be negative). The quantity of blood on CT may predict the chances of an arteriogram disclosing a cerebral aneurysm[326-329].

Patients with angiogram-negative SAH tend to be younger, less hypertensive, and more commonly male than those with positive angiography[327].

Possible causes of SAH with a negative angiogram include:
1. aneurysm that fails to be demonstrated in initial angiogram
    A. inadequate angiography, causes include:
        1. incomplete angio: *see page 784*
            a. must see both PICA origins (1-2% of aneurysms occur here)
            b. need to cross-fill through the ACoA (*see page 784*)
        2. degradation of images due to
            a. poor patient cooperation (e.g. from agitation). Either sedate patient (use caution in non-intubated patients) or repeat the study at a later time when patient more cooperative
            b. poor quality equipment providing substandard images
    B. obliteration of aneurysm by the hemorrhage
    C. thrombosis of the aneurysm after SAH: *see page 802*
    D. aneurysm too small to be visualized[330]: although "microaneurysms" may be a source of SAH, their natural history and optimal treatment are unknown
    E. lack of filling of aneurysm due to vasospasm (of parent artery or of aneurysmal orifice)
2. nonaneurysmal SAH from source that fails to show up on angiography. *See page 781* for etiologies of SAH other than aneurysm (many of which may not be demonstrated on angiography), including:
    A. angiographically occult (or cryptic) vascular malformation: *see page 840*
    B. pretruncal nonaneurysmal SAH: *see below*

Risk of rebleeding
Overall rebleed rate is 0.5%/yr, which is lower than with aneurysmal SAH or rebleeding from AVMs. There is also a smaller risk of delayed cerebral ischemia (vasos-

pasm). Neurological outcome is likewise better.

MANAGEMENT

General measures

These patients are still at risk for the same complications of SAH as with aneurysmal SAH: vasospasm, hydrocephalus, hyponatremia, rebleeding, etc. (*see page 786*) and should be managed as any SAH (*see page 786*). Some subgroups may be at lower risk for complications and may be managed accordingly (e.g. see *Pretruncal nonaneurysmal SAH (PNSAH)* below).

Repeat angiography

Early (pre-CT) studies showed low yield (1.8-9.8%) of positive repeat angiogram after technically adequate negative study[331] with a range of 2-24% quoted more recently[330, 332, 333]. CT scan findings are helpful in the decision to repeat angiography[334]. 70% of cases with diffuse SAH and thick layering of blood in the anterior interhemispheric fissure were associated with an ACoA aneurysm that showed up on repeat angiography[328]. The absence of blood on CT (performed within 4 days of SAH), or thick blood in the perimesencephalic cisterns alone (*see below*) were unlikely to be associated with a missed aneurysm.

Recommendations regarding repeat angio:
1. repeat angio after 10-14 days (allows some spasm to resolve) if:
   A. technically adequate 4 vessel angiogram is negative, and evidence for SAH is strong
   B. original angio was incomplete or if there are suspicious findings
2. if CT localizes blood clot to particular area, place special attention to this area on repeat angio
3. do not repeat angio for classic pretruncal SAH (*see below*) or if no blood on CT

Other studies

1. imaging studies of the brain: MRI (with MRA if available) or CT (with angio-CT if available). This may visualize an aneurysm that fails to show up on angiography, and may identify other sources of SAH such as angiographically occult vascular malformation (*see page 840*), tumor…
2. tests to rule-out spinal AVM: a rare cause of intracerebral SAH (*see page 347*)
   A. spinal MRI: cervical, thoracic and lumbar
   B. spinal angiography: too difficult and risky to be justified in most cases of angio negative SAH. Consider in cases with high suspicion of spinal source

Surgical exploration

Advocated by some for cases of SAH with CT findings compatible with an aneurysmal source in which a suspicious area is demonstrated angiographically[330] with careful explanation to the patient and family of the possibility of negative operative findings.

27.18. Nonaneurysmal SAH

For etiologies of SAH other than aneurysm, *see page 781*.

Pretruncal nonaneurysmal SAH (PNSAH)

Nee perimesencephalic nonaneurysmal SAH[335], the suggestion to change the name to pretruncal nonaneurysmal SAH was proposed because improved neuroimaging techniques have shown the true anatomic localization of the blood to be in front of the brain stem (truncus cerebri) centered in front of the pons rather than perimesencephalic[336]. Blood often extends into the interpeduncular or premedullary cisterns.

A distinct entity considered to be a benign condition with good outcome and less risk of rebleeding and vasospasm than other patients with SAH of unknown etiology[337] (no **rebleeding** occurred in 37 patients with PNSAH and 45 months mean follow-up[338], nor in 169 patients with 8-51 months follow-up[333]; **vasospasm** has been reported in only 3 patients and may have been related to cerebral angiography rather than the PNSAH, and although it is low, the incidence of angiographic vasospasm may be higher than originally thought[339]).

The actual etiology has yet to be determined, but it may be secondary to rupture of a small perimesencephalic vein or capillary[339].

Presentation

Patients may present with severe paroxysmal H/A, meningismus, photophobia, and nausea. Loss of consciousness is rare. These patients are usually not critically ill (all were grade 1 or 2), however, complications such as hyponatremia or cardiac abnormalities may occur. Preretinal hemorrhages and sentinel H/A have not occurred. CT and/or MRI demonstrate characteristic findings (see below) although it may initially be missed on CT[339], and LP may yield bloody CSF. All have negative angiography.

Epidemiology

PNSAH has been reported to comprise 20-68% of cases of angiogram-negative SAH[337, 340] (depending on the timing of CT, adequacy of angiography, and the definition of PNSAH). However, the true incidence is probably more in the range of 50-75%[333].

The reported age range is 3-70 years (mean: 50 yrs)[333], 52-59% are male, and pre-existing HTN was present in 3-20% of patients.

Relevant anatomy

Posterior fossa cisterns:

The perimesencephalic cisterns include: interpeduncular, crural, ambient and quadrigeminal cisterns. The prepontine cistern lies immediately anterior to the pons.

Liliequist's membrane (LM)[341]:

Basically considered to separate the interpeduncular cistern from the chiasmatic cistern[342] (forming a competent barrier in only 10-30%). In further detail, the superior leaflet of LM (diencephalic membrane) separates the interpeduncular cistern from the chiasmatic cistern medially and from the carotid cisterns laterally[343, 344]. The inferior leaflet (the mesencephalic membrane) separates the interpeduncular from the prepontine cistern.

The diencephalic membrane is thicker and is more often competent, effectively isolating the chiasmatic cistern. However, the carotid cisterns often communicate with the crural cisterns and in turn with the interpeduncular cistern[344].

Thus, blood in the carotid or prepontine cistern is compatible with a low-pressure pretruncal source of bleeding, however, blood in the chiasmatic cistern should raise concern about aneurysmal rupture.

Diagnostic criteria

Without knowledge of the actual substrate of PNSAH, the following suggested diagnostic criteria must be viewed as empirical (adapted[333]):

1. CT or MRI scan performed ≤ 2 days from ictus meeting the criteria shown in *Table 27-15* (later scans render the diagnosis unreliable, e.g. washout could cause an aneurysmal SAH to fit the criteria). This criteria implies that blood should be contained inferior to Liliequist's membrane (LM) (i.e. perimesencephalic and/or prepontine cisterns). Extension into the suprasellar cistern is common. Significant amounts of blood penetrating LM to the chiasmatic, sylvian, or interhemispheric cisterns should be viewed with suspicion

2. a negative high-quality 4-vessel cerebral angiogram[346] (radiographic vasospasm is common, and does not preclude the diagnosis nor does it mandate repeat angiography). NB: ≈ 3% of patients with a ruptured basilar bifurcation aneurysm meet the criteria of *Table 27-15*[347], therefore an <u>initial</u> arteriogram is mandatory

3. appropriate clinical picture: no loss of consciousness, no sentinel H/A, SAH grade 1 or 2 (see *Grading SAH*, page 785). Variance from this should raise suspicion of alternate pathogenesis

Table 27-15 CT or MRI criteria for PNSAH[339, 345]

1. epicenter of hemorrhage immediately anterior to brain stem (interpeduncular or prepontine cistern)
2. there may be extension into anterior part of ambient cistern or basal part of the sylvian fissure
3. absence of complete filling of anterior interhemispheric fissure
4. no more than minute amounts of blood in lateral portion of sylvian fissure
5. absence of frank intraventricular hemorrhage (small amounts of blood sedimenting in the occipital horns of the lateral ventricles is permissible)

Repeat angiography

Controversial. Angiography carries ≈ 0.2-0.5% risk of permanent neurologic deficit in this population[333]. Most experts agree that repeat angiography is not indicated in patients meeting the criteria of PNSAH[332, 346] (although others recommend repeat angiography in all surgical candidates[330, 348]). One should probably repeat the study if any uncertainty exists or if there is a history of a condition associated with increased risk of cerebral aneurysms[339].

Treatment
Optimal treatment is not known with certainty. The low risk of rebleeding and delayed ischemia suggests that extreme measures are not indicated. The following recommendations are made[333, 339] (period not specified):
1. symptomatic treatment
2. cardiac monitoring
3. electrolyte monitoring for hyponatremia
4. follow patient clinically (and if appropriate, with repeat imaging studies) to rule-out hydrocephalus (transient ventricular enlargement is common, however, hydrocephalus requiring shunting is rare (only ≈ 1%)[333])
5. ✖ not recommended
   A. hyperdynamic therapy
   B. calcium channel blockers: use has not been investigated in PNSAH, but is probably not warranted due to low incidence of vasospasm
   C. activity restrictions (except in cases of increasing H/A with mobilization)
   D. anticonvulsants
   E. reduction of blood pressure below normal
   F. surgical exploration

27.19. Pregnancy & intracranial hemorrhage

Intracranial hemorrhage (subarachnoid or intraparenchymal) is a rare occurrence during pregnancy (estimated range of incidence: 0.01-0.05% of all pregnancies[349]) and yet is responsible for 5-12% of maternal deaths during pregnancy.

Intracranial hemorrhage of pregnancy (**ICHOP**) commonly occurs in the setting of eclampsia, and is more commonly intraparenchymal[350] and may be associated with loss of cerebrovascular autoregulation (*see page 64*). Symptoms of eclampsia with or without ICHOP include H/A, mental status changes, and seizures.

A literature review of 154 reported cases of ICHOP-related SAH revealed 77% were aneurysmal and 23% were from ruptured AVM (other series show the percentage of AVMs range from 21-48%). Mortality is ≈ 35% for aneurysmal and ≈ 28% for AVM hemorrhage (the latter being higher than in non-gravid patients). There is an increasing tendency for bleeding with advancing gestational age for both aneurysms and AVMs (earlier it had been asserted that this held true for aneurysms only[351]).

Patients with ICHOP having AVMs tend to be younger than those with aneurysm, paralleling the occurrence in the general population. One major oft-quoted study showed an increased risk of hemorrhage from AVMs during pregnancy[352] (citing an 87% hemorrhage rate), however another investigation disputes this assertion[353], and found the risk of hemorrhage to be 3.5% during the pregnancy in patients with no history of hemorrhage, or 5.8% in those with previous hemorrhage (however, this study may suffer from significant selection bias[354]). Literature review[349] found a risk of recurrent hemorrhage following ICHOP from aneurysm or AVM during the remainder of the pregnancy was 33-50%.

Management modifications for pregnant patients
1. neuroradiologic studies
   A. CAT scan: with shielding of the fetus, CAT scanning of the brain produces minimal radiation exposure
   B. MRI: generally accepted as having low potential for complications, however, the safety of gadopentetate dimeglumine (Magnevist®) has not been studied in human pregnancy
   C. angiography: with shielding of the fetus, radiation exposure is minimal. Iodinated contrast agents pose little risk to the fetus. The mother should be well hydrated during and after the study[349]
2. antiepileptic drugs: see *Pregnancy and antiepileptic drugs*, page 280
3. diuretics: the use of mannitol in pregnancy should be avoided to prevent fetal dehydration and maternal hypovolemia with uterine hypoperfusion

4. antihypertensives: nitroprusside should not be used in pregnancy
5. nimodipine is potentially teratogenic in animals, the effect on humans is unknown. It should be used only when the potential benefit justifies the risk

Neurosurgical management[349]

The currently recommended treatment of a ruptured aneurysm in the pregnant patient is surgical clipping. Treatment of hemorrhage from AVM is more controversial. A number of authors recommend basing the decision of treatment on neurosurgical rather than obstetrical considerations.

Obstetric management following ICHOP

Earlier recommendations were to perform C-section to avoid the hemodynamic stresses of labor and vaginal delivery, however, the risk of hemorrhage is not significantly different between vaginal delivery and C-section. Several reports have indicated that the fetal and maternal outcome is no different for vaginal delivery vs. C-section, and is probably more dependent on whether the offending lesion has been treated. C-section may be used for fetal salvage for a moribund mother in the third trimester. During vaginal delivery, the risk of rebleeding may be reduced by the use of caudal or epidural anesthesia, shortening the 2nd stage of labor, and low forceps delivery if necessary.

27.20. References

1. Wirth F P: Surgical treatment of incidental intracranial aneurysms. **Clin Neurosurg** 33: 125-35, 1986.
2. Greene K A, Marciano F F, Johnson B A, *et al*.: Impact of traumatic subarachnoid hemorrhage on outcome in nonpenetrating head injury. **J Neurosurg** 83: 445-52, 1995.
3. Taneda M, Kataoka K, Akai F, *et al*.: Traumatic subarachnoid hemorrhage as a predictable indicator of delayed ischemic symptoms. **J Neurosurg** 84: 762-8, 1996.
4. Dagi T F, Maccabe J J: Metastatic trophoblastic disease presenting as a subarachnoid hemorrhage. **Surg Neurol** 14: 175-84, 1980.
5. Memon M Y, Neal A, Imami R, *et al*.: Low grade glioma presenting as subarachnoid hemorrhage. **Neurosurgery** 14: 574-7, 1984.
6. Miller R H: Spontaneous subarachnoid hemorrhage: A presenting symptom of a tumor of the third ventricle. **Surg Clin N Amer** 41: 1043-8, 1961.
7. Glass B, Abbott K H: Subarachnoid hemorrhage consequent to intracranial tumors. **Arch Neurol Psych** 73: 369-79, 1955.
8. Gleeson R K, Butzer J F, Grin O D: Acoustic neurinoma presenting as subarachnoid hemorrhage. **J Neurosurg** 49: 602-4, 1978.
9. Yasargil M G, So S C: Cerebellopontine angle meningioma presenting as subarachnoid hemorrhage. **Surg Neurol** 6: 3-6, 1976.
10. Smith V R, Stein P S, MacCarty C S: Subarachnoid hemorrhage due to lateral ventricular meningiomas. **Surg Neurol** 4: 241-3, 1975.
11. Ernsting J: Choroid plexus papilloma causing spontaneous subarachnoid hemorrhage. **J Neurol Neurosurg Psychiatry** 18: 134-6, 1955.
12. Simonsen J: Fatal subarachnoid hemorrhage originating in an intracranial chordoma. **Acta Pathol Microbiol Scand** 59: 13-20, 1963.
13. Latchaw J P, Dohn D F, Hahn J F, *et al*.: Subarachnoid hemorrhage from an intracranial meningioma. **Neurosurgery** 9: 433-5, 1981.
14. Fortuna A, Palma L, Ferrante L, *et al*.: Repeated subarachnoid hemorrhage with vasospasm secondary to tuberculum sella meningioma. **J Neurosurg Sci** 21: 251-6, 1977.
15. Ellenbogen R G, Winston K R, Kupsky W J: Tumors of the choroid plexus in children. **Neurosurgery** 25: 327-35, 1989.
16. Broderick J P, Brott T G, Tomsick T, *et al*.: Intracerebral hemorrhage more than twice as common as subarachnoid hemorrhage. **J Neurosurg** 78: 188-91, 1993.
17. Linn F H H, Rinkel G J, Algra A, *et al*.: Incidence of subarachnoid hemorrhage: Role of region, year and CT scanning: A metaanalysis. **Stroke** 27: 625-9, 1996.
18. Sahs A L, Nibbelink D W, Torner J C, (eds.): **Aneurysmal subarachnoid hemorrhage: Report of the cooperative study**. Urban & Schwarzenberg, Baltimore-Munich, 1981: pp 370.
19. Kassell N F, Sasaki T, Colohan A R T, *et al*.: Cerebral vasospasm following aneurysmal subarachnoid hemorrhage. **Stroke** 16: 562-72, 1985.
20. Biller J, Toffol G J, Kassell N F, *et al*.: Spontaneous subarachnoid hemorrhage in young adults. **Neurosurgery** 21: 664-7, 1987.
21. Okawara S H: Warning signs prior to rupture of an intracranial aneurysm. **J Neurosurg** 38: 575-80, 1973.
22. Yamashita K, Kashiwagi S, Kato S, *et al*.: Cerebral aneurysms in the elderly in Yamaguchi, Japan. Analysis of the Yamaguchi data bank of cerebral aneurysm from 1985 to 1995. **Stroke** 28: 1926-31, 1997.
23. Bonita R: Cigarette smoking, hypertension and the risk of subarachnoid hemorrhage: A population-based case-control study. **Stroke** 17: 831-5, 1986.
24. Hillbom M, Kaste M: Does alcohol intoxication precipitate aneurysmal subarachnoid hemorrhage. **J Neurol Neurosurg Psychiatry** 44: 523-6, 1981.
25. Longstreth W T, Koepsell T D, Yerby M S, *et al*.: Risk factors for subarachnoid hemorrhage. **Stroke** 16: 377-85, 1985.
26. Tsementzis S A, Gill J S, Hitchcock E R, *et al*.: Diurnal variation of and activity during the onset of stroke. **Neurosurgery** 17: 901-4, 1985.
27. Sarti C, Tuomilehto J, Salomaa V, *et al*.: Epidemiology of subarachnoid hemorrhage in Finland from 1983 to 1985. **Stroke** 22: 848-53, 1991.
28. Hop J W, Rinkel G J, Algra A, *et al*.: Case-fatality rates and functional outcome after subarachnoid hemorrhage: A systematic review. **Stroke** 28: 660-4, 1997.
29. Drake C G: Management of cerebral aneurysm. **Stroke** 12: 273-83, 1981.
30. Mohr J P, Caplan L R, Melski J W, *et al*.: The Harvard cooperative stroke registry: A prospective

study. **Neurology** 28: 754-62, 1978.

31. Verweij R D, Wijdicks E F M, van Gijn J: Warning headache in aneurysmal subarachnoid hemorrhage: A case-control study. **Arch Neurol** 45: 1019-20, 1988.

32. Linn F H H, Wijdicks E F M, van der Graaf Y, *et al.*: Prospective study of sentinel headache in aneurysmal subarachnoid hemorrhage. **Lancet** 344: 590-3, 1994.

33. Fisher C M: Painful States: A neurological commentary. **Clin Neurosurg** 31: 32-5, 1984.

34. Linn F H H, Rinkel G J E, van Gijn J: Headache characteristics in subarachnoid hemorrhage and benign thunderclap headache. **J Neurol Neurosurg Psychiatry** 65: 791-3, 1998.

35. Day J W, Raskin N H: Thunderclap headache: Symptom of unruptured cerebral aneurysm. **Lancet** 2: 1247-8, 1986.

36. Wijdicks E F M, Kerkhoff H, van Gijn J: Long-term follow-up of 71 patients with thunderclap headache mimicking subarachnoid hemorrhage. **Lancet** 2: 68-70, 1988.

37. Markus H S: A prospective follow-up of thunderclap headache mimicking subarachnoid hemorrhage. **J Neurol Neurosurg Psychiatry** 54: 1117-8, 1991.

38. Lance J W: Headaches related to sexual activity. **J Neurol Neurosurg Psychiatry** 39: 1226-30, 1976.

39. Ogilvy C S, Rordorf G: *Mechanisms and treatment of coma after subarachnoid hemorrhage*. In **Subarachnoid hemorrhage: Pathophysiology and management**, Bederson J B, (ed.). Neurosurgical topics. Committee A P. American Association of Neurological Surgeons, Park Ridge, IL, 1997, Chapter 9: pp 157-71.

40. Manschot W A: Subarachnoid hemorrhage. Intraocular symptoms and their pathogenesis. **Am J Ophthalmol** 38: 501-5, 1954.

41. Tsementzis S A, Williams A: Ophthalmological signs and prognosis in patients with a subarachnoid hemorrhage. **Neurochirurgia** 27: 133-5, 1984.

42. Vanderlinden R G, Chisholm L D: Vitreous hemorrhages and sudden increased intracranial pressure. **J Neurosurg** 41: 167-76, 1974.

43. Pfausler B, Belcl R, Metzler R, *et al.*: Terson's syndrome in spontaneous subarachnoid hemorrhage: A prospective study in 60 consecutive patients. **J Neurosurg** 85: 392-4, 1996.

44. Garfinkle A M, Danys I R, Nicolle D A, *et al.*: Terson's syndrome: A reversible cause of blindness following subarachnoid hemorrhage. **J Neurosurg** 76: 766-71, 1992.

45. Keithahn M A Z, Bennett S R, Cameron D, *et al.*: Retinal folds in Terson syndrome. **Ophthalmology** 100: 1187-90, 1993.

46. Schultz P N, Sobol W M, Weingeist T A: Long-term visual outcome in Terson syndrome. **Ophthalmology** 98: 1814-9, 1991.

47. Milhorat T H: Acute hydrocephalus after aneurysmal subarachnoid hemorrhage. **Neurosurgery** 20: 15-20, 1987.

48. Consensus Conference: Magnetic resonance imaging. **JAMA** 259: 2132-8, 1988.

49. Hackney D B, Lesnick J E, Zimmerman R A, *et al.*: MR identification of bleeding site in subarachnoid hemorrhage with multiple intracranial aneurysms. **J Comput Assist Tomogr** 10: 878-80, 1986.

50. Yoshimoto T, Suzuki J: Surgical treatment of an aneurysm on the funnel-shaped bulge of the posterior communicating artery. **J Neurosurg** 41: 377-9, 1974.

51. Saltzman G F: Infundibular widening of the posterior communicating artery studied by carotid angiography. **Acta Radiol** 51: 415-21, 1959.

52. Wollschlaeger G, Wollschlaeger P B, Lucas F V, *et al.*: Experience and results with post-mortem cerebral angiography performed as routine procedure of the autopsy. **Am J Roentgenol Radium Ther Nucl Med** 101: 68-87, 1967.

53. Archer C R, Silbert S: Infundibula may be clinically significant. **Neuroradiology** 152: 247-51, 1978.

54. Trasi S, Vincent L M, Zingesser L H: Development of aneurysm from infundibulum of posterior communicating artery with documentation of prior hemorrhage. **AJNR** 2: 368-70, 1981.

55. Leblanc R, Worsley K J, Melanson D, *et al.*: Angiographic screening and elective surgery of familial cerebral aneurysms. **Neurosurgery** 35: 9-18, 1994.

56. Locksley H B: Report on the cooperative study of intracranial aneurysms and subarachnoid hemorrhage: Section V - part II: Natural history of subarachnoid hemorrhage, intracranial aneurysms, and arteriovenous malformations - based on 6368 cases in the cooperative study. **J Neurosurg** 25: 321-68, 1966.

57. Marshman L A G, Ward P J, Walter P H, *et al.*: The progression of an infundibulum to aneurysm formation and rupture: Case report and literature review. **Neurosurgery** 43: 1445-9, 1998.

58. Ronkainen A, Puranen M, Hernesniemi J, *et al.*: Intracranial aneurysms: MR angiographic screening in 400 asymptomatic individuals with increased familial risk. **Radiology** 195: 35-40, 1995.

59. Ross J S, Masaryk T J, Modic M T, *et al.*: Intracranial aneurysms: Evaluation by MR angiography. **AJNR** 11: 449-56, 1990.

60. Ronkainen A, Hernesniemi J, Puranen L, *et al.*: Familial intracranial aneurysms. **Lancet** 349: 380-4, 1997.

61. Atlas S W: MR angiography in neurologic disease. **Radiology** 193: 1-16, 1994.

62. Hsiang J N K, Liang E Y, Lam J M K, *et al.*: The role of computed tomographic angiography in the diagnosis of intracranial aneurysms and emergent aneurysm clipping. **Neurosurgery** 38: 481-7, 1996.

63. Dorsch N W C, Young N, Kingston R J, *et al.*: Early experience with spiral CT in the diagnosis of intracranial aneurysms. **Neurosurgery** 36: 230-8, 1995.

64. Hunt W E, Hess R M: Surgical risk as related to time of intervention in the repair of intracranial aneurysms. **J Neurosurg** 28: 14-20, 1968.

65. Hunt W E, Kosnik E J: Timing and perioperative care in intracranial aneurysm surgery. **Clin Neurosurg** 21: 79-89, 1974.

66. Drake C G: Report of world federation of neurological surgeons committee on a universal subarachnoid hemorrhage grading scale. **J Neurosurg** 68: 985-6, 1988.

67. Inagawa T, Kamiya K, Ogasawara H, *et al.*: Rebleeding of ruptured intracranial aneurysms in the actue stage. **Surg Neurol** 28: 93-9, 1987.

68. Redekop G, Ferguson G: *Intracranial aneurysms*. In **Neurovascular surgery**, Carter L P, Spetzler R F, and Hamilton M G, (eds.). McGraw-Hill, New York, 1995, Chapter 32: pp 625-48.

69. Vermeulen L C, Ratko T A, Erstad B L, *et al.*: The university hospital consortium guidelines for the use of albumin, nonprotein colloid, and crystalloid solutions. **Arch Intern Med** 155: 373-9, 1995.

70. Wilkins R H, Rengachary S S, (eds.): **Neurosurgery**. McGraw-Hill, New York, 1985.

71. Baker C J, Prestigiacomo C J, Solomon R A: Short-term perioperative anticonvulsant prophylaxis for the surgical treatment of low-risk patients with intracranial aneurysms. **Neurosurgery** 37: 863-71, 1995.

72. Richardson A E, Uttley D: Prevention of postoperative epilepsy. **Lancet** 1: 650, 1980.

73. Deuchsman C J, Haines S J: Anticonvulsant prophylaxis in neurological surgery. **Neurosurgery** 17: 510-7, 1985.

74. Biller J, Godersky J C, Adams H P: Management of aneurysmal subarachnoid hemorrhage. **Stroke** 19: 1300-5, 1988.

75. Nearman H S, Herman M L: Toxic effects of colloids in the intensive care unit. **Crit Care Med** 7: 713-23, 1991.

76. Bianchine J R: Intracranial bleeding during treatment with hydroxyethyl starch - letter in reply. **New Engl J Med** 317: 965, 1987..

77. Trumble E R, Muizelaar J P, Myseros J S: Coagulopathy with the use of hetastarch in the treatment of vasospasm. **J Neurosurg** 82: 44-7, 1995.

78. Ciongoli A K, Poser C M: Pulmonary edema secondary to subarachnoid hemorrhage. **Neurology (NY)** 22: 867-70, 1972.

79. Solomon R A, Fink M E, Lennihan L: Prophylactic volume expansion therapy for the prevention of delayed cerebral ischemia after early aneurysm surgery. **Arch Neurol** 45: 325-32, 1988.

80. Wise B L: SIADH after spontaneous subarachnoid hemorrhage: A reversible cause of clinical deterioration. **Neurosurgery** 3: 412-4, 1978.

81. Wijdicks E F M, Ropper A H, Hunnicutt E J, et al.: Atrial natriuretic factor and salt wasting after aneurysmal subarachnoid hemorrhage. **Stroke** 22: 1519-24, 1991.

82. Harrigan M R: Cerebral salt wasting syndrome: A review. **Neurosurgery** 38: 152-60, 1996.

83. Kröll M, Juhler M, Lindholm J: Hyponatremia in acute brain disease. **J Int Med** 232: 291-7, 1992.

84. Wijdicks E F M, Schievink W I, Burnett J C: Natriuretic peptide system and endothelin in aneurysmal subarachnoid hemorrhage. **J Neurosurg** 87: 275-80, 1997.

85. Nelson P B, Seif S M, Maroon J C, et al.: Hyponatremia in intracranial disease. Perhaps not the syndrome of inappropriate secretion of antidiuretic hormone (SIADH). **J Neurosurg** 55: 938-41, 1981.

86. Wijdicks E F M, Vermeulen M, Hijdra A, et al.: Hyponatremia and cerebral infarction in patients with ruptured intracranial aneurysms: Is fluid restriction harmful? **Ann Neurol** 17: 137-40, 1985.

87. Harbaugh R E: Aneurysmal subarachnoid hemorrhage and hyponatremia. **Contemp Neurosurg** 15: 1-5, 1993.

88. Reeder R F, Harbaugh R E: Administration of intravenous urea and normal saline for the treatment of hyponatremia in neurosurgical patients. **J Neurosurg** 70: 201-6, 1989.

89. Harries A D: Subarachnoid hemorhage and the electrocardiogram: A review. **Postgrad Med J** 57: 294-6, 1981.

90. Beard E F, Robertson J W, Robertson R C L: Spontaneous subarachnoid hemorhage simulating acute myocardial infarction. **Am Heart J** 58: 755-9, 1959.

91. Gascon P, Ley T J, Toltzis R J, et al.: Spontaneous subarachnoid hemorhage simulating acute transmural myocardial infarction. **Am Heart J** 105: 511-3, 1983.

92. Marion D W, Segal R, Thompson M E: Subarachnoid hemorrhage and the heart. **Neurosurgery** 18: 101-6, 1986.

93. Yuki K, Kodama Y, Onda J, et al.: Coronary vasospasm following subarachnoid hemorrhage as a cause of stunned myocardium. **J Neurosurg** 75: 308-11, 1991.

94. Braunwald E, Kloner R A: The stunned myocardium: Prolonged postischemic ventricular dysfunction. **Circulation** 66: 1146-9, 1982.

95. Murphy A M, Kögler H, Georgakopoulos D, et al.: Transgenic mouse model of stunned myocardium. **Science** 389: 491-5, 2000.

96. Kassell N F, Drake C G: Review of the management of saccular aneurysms. **Neurol Clin** 1: 73-86, 1983.

97. Winn H R, Richardson A E, Jane J A: The long-term prognosis in untreated cerebral aneurysms. I. The incidence of late hemorrhage in cerebral aneurysm: A 10-year evaluation of 364 patients. **Ann Neurol** 1: 358-70, 1977.

98. Jane J A, Kassell N F, Torner J C, et al.: The natural history of aneurysms and AVMs. **J Neurosurg** 62: 321-3, 1985.

99. Hillman J, Fridriksson S, Nilsson O, et al.: Immediate administration of tranexamic acid and reduced incidence of early rebleeding after aneurysmal subarachnoid hemorrhage: A prospective randomized study. **J Neurosurg** 97 (4): 771-8, 2002.

100. Kassell N F, Torner J C, Adams H P: Antifibrinolytic therapy in the acute period following aneurysmal subarachnoid hemorrhage: Preliminary observations from the cooperative aneurysm study. **J Neurosurg** 61: 225-30, 1984.

101. Glick R, Green D, Ts'ao C-H, et al.: High dose ε-aminocaproic acid prolongs the bleeding time and increases rebleeding and intraoperative hemorrhage in patients with subarachnoid hemorrhage. **Neurosurgery** 9: 398-401, 1981.

102. Leipzig T J, Redelman K, Horner T G: Reducing the risk of rebleeding before early aneurysm surgery: A possible role for antifibrinolytic therapy. **J Neurosurg** 86: 220-5, 1997.

103. Hasan D, Vermeulen M, Wijdicks E F M, et al.: Management problems in acute hydrocephalus after subarchnoid hemorrhage. **Stroke** 20: 747-53, 1989.

104. Graff-Radford N, Torner J, Adams H P, et al.: Factors associated with hydrocephalus after subarachnoid hemorrhage. **Arch Neurol** 46: 744-52, 1989.

105. Kusske J A, Turner P T, Ojemann G A, et al.: Ventriculostomy for the treatment of acute hydrocephalus following subarachnoid hemorrhage. **J Neurosurg** 38: 591-5, 1973.

106. van Gijn J, Hijdra A, Wijdicks E F M, et al.: Acute hydrocephalus after aneurysmal subarachnoid hemorrhage. **J Neurosurg** 63: 355-62, 1985.

107. Voldby B, Enevoldsen E M: Intracranial pressure changes following aneurysm rupture. 3. Recurrent hemorrhage. **J Neurosurg** 56: 784-9, 1982.

108. Auer L M, Mokry M: Disturbed cerebrospinal fluid circulation after subarachnoid hemorrhage and acute aneurysm surgery. **Neurosurgery** 26: 804-9, 1990.

109. Connolly E S, Kader A A, Frazzini V I, et al.: The safety of intraoperative lumbar subarachnoid drainage for acutely ruptured intracranial aneurysm: Technical note. **Surg Neurol** 48: 338-44, 1997.

110. Maeda K, Kurita H, Nakamura T, et al.: Occurrence of severe vasospasm following intraventricular hemorrhage from an arteriovenous malformation. **J Neurosurg** 87: 436-9, 1997.

111. Martin N A, Doberstein C, Zane C, et al.: Posttraumatic cerebral arterial spasm: Transcranial Doppler ultrasound, cerebral blood flow, and angiographic findings. **J Neurosurg** 77: 575-83, 1992.

112. Weir B, Grace M, Hansen J, et al.: Time course of vasospasm in man. **J Neurosurg** 48: 173-8, 1978.

113. Fisher C M, Kistler J P, Davis J M: Relation of cerebral vasospasm to subarachnoid hemorrhage visualized by CT scanning. **Neurosurgery** 6: 1-9, 1980.

114. Kistler J P, Crowell R M, Davis K R, et al.: The relation of cerebral vasospasm to the extent and location of subarachnoid blood visualized by CT. **Neurology** 33: 424-6, 1983.

115. Lasner T M, Weil R J, Riina H A, et al.: Cigarette smoking-induced increase in the risk of symptomatic vasospasm after aneurysmal subarachnoid hemorrhage. **J Neurosurg** 87: 381-4, 1997.

116. Fox J L, Ko J P: Cerebral vasospasm: A clinical observation. **Surg Neurol** 10: 269, 1978.

117. Davis J M, Davis K R, Crowell R M: Subarachnoid hemorrhage secondary to ruptured intracranial aneurysm: Prognostic significance of cranial CT. **AJNR** 1: 17-21, 1980.

118. Sasaki T, Kassell N F, Zuccarello M, et al.: Barrier disruption in the major cerebral arteries during the acute stage after experimental subarachnoid hemorrhage. **Neurosurgery** 19: 177-84, 1986.

119. Sasaki T, Kassell N F, Yamashita M, et al.: Barrier

disruption in the major cerebral arteries following experimental subarachnoid hemorrhage. **J Neurosurg** 63: 433-40, 1985.

120. Yanagisawa M, Kurihara H, Kimura S, *et al*.: A novel potent vasoconstrictor peptide produced by vascular endothelial cells. **Nature** 332 (6163): 411-5, 1988.

121. Findlay J M: Current management of cerebral vasospasm. **Contemp Neurosurg** 19 (24): 1-6, 1997.

122. Cardoso E R, Reddy K, Bose D: Effect of subarachnoid hemorrhage on intracranial pulse waves in cats. **J Neurosurg** 69: 712-8, 1988.

123. Ochi R P, Vieco P T, Gross C E: CT angiography of cerebral vasospasm with conventional angiographic comparison. **AJNR Am J Neuroradiol** 18 (2): 265-9, 1997.

124. Tamatani S, Sasaki O, Takeuchi S, *et al*.: Detection of delayed cerebral vasospasm, after rupture of intracranial aneurysms, by magnetic resonance angiography. **Neurosurgery** 40 (4): 748-53; discussion 753-4, 1997.

125. Vespa P M, Nuwer M R, Juhász C, *et al*.: Early detection of vasospasm after acute subarachnoid hemorrhage using continuous EEG ICU monitoring. **EEG Clin Neurophys** 103: 607-15, 1997.

126. Labar D R, Fisch B J, Pedley T A, *et al*.: Quantitative EEG monitoring for patients with subarachnoid hemorrhage. **EEG Clin Neurophys** 78: 325-32, 1991.

127. Weir B, Menon D, Overton T: Regional cerebral blood flow in patients with aneurysms: Estimation by xenon 133 inhalation. **Can J Neurol Sci** 5: 301-5, 1978.

128. Knuckney N W, Fox R A, Surveyor I, *et al*.: Early cerebral blood flow and CT in predicting ischemia after cerebral aneurysm rupture. **J Neurosurg** 62: 850-5, 1985.

129. Powers W J, Grubb R L, Baker R P, *et al*.: Regional cerebral blood flow and metabolism in reversible ischemia due to vasospasm: Determination by positron emission tomography. **J Neurosurg** 62: 539-46, 1985.

130. Seiler R W, Grolimund P, Aaslid R, *et al*.: Cerebral vasospasm evaluated by transcranial ultrasound correlated with clinical grade and CT-visualized subarachnoid hemorrhage. **J Neurosurg** 64: 594-600, 1986.

131. Lindegaard K F, Nornes H, Bakke S J, *et al*.: Cerebral vasospasm after subarachnoid hemorrhage investigated by means of transcranial Doppler ultrasound. **Acta Neurochir** 42: 81-4, 1988.

132. Sekhar L N, Wechsler L R, Yonas H, *et al*.: Value of transcranial Doppler examination in the diagnosis of cerebral vasospasm after subarachnoid hemorrhage. **Neurosurgery** 22. 813-21, 1988.

133. Wilkins R H: Attempted prevention or treatment of intracranial arterial spasm: A survey. **Neurosurgery** 6: 198-210, 1980.

134. Wilkins R H: Attempts at prevention or treatment of intracranial arterial spasm: An update. **Neurosurgery** 18: 808-25, 1986.

135. Foley P L, Caner H H, Kassell N F, *et al*.: Reversal of subarachnoid hemorrhage-induced vasoconstriction with an endothelin receptor antagonists. **Neurosurgery** 34: 108-13, 1994.

136. Zuccarello M, Soattin G B, Lewis A I, *et al*.: Prevention of subarachnoid hemorrhage-induced cerebral vasospasm by oral administration of endothelin receptor antagonists. **J Neurosurg** 84: 503-7, 1996.

137. Kaku Y, Yonekawa Y, Tsukahara T, *et al*.: Superselective intra-arterial infusion of papaverine for the treatment of cerebral vasospasm after subarachnoid hemorrhage. **J Neurosurg** 77: 842-7, 1992.

138. Kassell N F, Helm G, Simmons N, *et al*.: Treatment of cerebral vasospasm with intra-arterial papaverine. **J Neurosurg** 77: 848-52, 1992.

139. Hori S, Suzuki J: Early intracranial operations for ruptured aneurysms. **Acta Neurochir** 46: 93-104, 1979.

140. Mitzukami M, Kawase T, Tazawa T: Prevention of vasospasm by early operation with removal of subarachnoid blood. **Neurosurgery** 10: 301-6, 1982.

141. Nosko M, Weir B K A, Lunt A, *et al*.: Effect of clot removal at 24 hours on chronic vasospasm after subarachnoid hemorrhage in the primate model. **J Neurosurg** 66: 416-22, 1987.

142. Findlay J M, Weir B K A, Steinke D, *et al*.: Effect of intrathecal thrombolytic therapy on subarachnoid clot and chronic vasospasm in a primate. **J Neurosurg** 69: 723-35, 1988.

143. Findlay J M, Weir B K A, Kanamaru K, *et al*.: Intrathecal fibrinolytic therapy after subarachnoid hemorrhage: Dosage study in a primate model and review of literature. **Can J Neurol Sci** 16: 28-40, 1989.

144. Findlay J M, Weir B K A, Gordon P, *et al*.: Safety and efficacy of intrathecal thrombolytic therapy in a primate model of cerebral vasospasm. **Neurosurgery** 24: 491-8, 1989.

145. Findlay J M, Kassell N F, Weir B K A, *et al*.: A randomized trial of intraoperative, intracisternal tissue plasminogen activator for the prevention of vasospasm. **Neurosurgery** 37: 168-78, 1995.

146. Mizoi K, Yoshimoto T, Fujiwara S, *et al*.: Prevention of vasospasm by clot removal and intrathecal bolus injection of tissue-type plasminogen activator: Preliminary report. **Neurosurgery** 28: 807-13, 1991.

147. Ito U, Tomita H, Yamazaki S, *et al*.: Enhanced cisternal drainage and cerebral vasospasm in early aneurysm surgery. **Acta Neurochir** 80: 18-23, 1986.

148. Grotta J, Clark W, Coull B, *et al*.: Safety and tolerability of the glutamate antagonist CGS 19755 (selfotel) in patients with acute ischemic stroke. Results of a phase IIa randomized trial. **Stroke** 26: 602-5, 1996.

149. Davis S M, Albers G W, Diener H-C, *et al*: Termination of acute stroke studies involving selfotel treatment. **Lancet** 349: 32, 1997.

150. Morris G F, Bullock R, Marshall S B, *et al*.: Failure of the competitive N-methyl-D-aspartate antagonist selfotel (CGS 19755) in the treatment of severe head injury: Results of two phase III clinical trials. **J Neurosurg** 91: 737-43, 1999.

151. Kassell N F, Haley E C, Apperson-Hansen C, *et al*.: Randomized, double-blind, vehicle-controlled trial of tirilazad mesylate in patients with aneurysmal subarachnoid hemorrhage: A cooperative study in Europe, Australia, and New Zealand. **J Neurosurg** 84: 221-8, 1996.

152. Asano T, Takakura K, Sano K, *et al*.: Effects of a hydroxyl radical scavenger on delayed ischemic neurological deficits following aneurysmal subarachnoid hemorrhage: Results of a multicenter, placebo-controlled double-blind trial. **J Neurosurg** 84: 792-803, 1996.

153. Benzel E C, Kesterson L: Extracranial-intracranial bypass surgery for the management of vasospasm after subarachnoid hemorrhage. **Surg Neurol** 30: 231-4, 1988.

154. Batjer H, Samson D: Use of extracranial-intracranial bypass in the management of symptomatic vasospasm. **Neurosurgery** 19: 235-46, 1986.

155. Kasuya H, Onda H, Sasahara A, *et al*.: Application of nicardipine prolonged-release implants: Analysis of 97 consecutive patients with acute subarachnoid hemorrhage. **Neurosurgery** 56 (5): 895-902; discussion 895-902, 2005.

156. Vajkoczy P, Meyer B, Weidauer S, *et al*.: Clazosentan (axv-034343), a selective endothelin A receptor antagonist, in the prevention of a cerebral vasospasm following severe aneurysmal subarachnoid hemorrhage: Results of a randomized, double-blind, placebo-controlled, multicenter phase IIa study. **J**

Neurosurg 103: 9-17, 2005.
157. Hieshima G B, Higashida R T, Wapenski J, *et al.*: Balloon embolization of a large distal basilar artery aneurysm: Case report. **J Neurosurg** 65: 413-6, 1986.
158. Zubkov Y N, Nikiforov B M, Shustin V A: Balloon catheter technique for dilatation of constricted cerebral after aneurysmal subarachnoid hemorrhage. **Acta Neurochir** 70: 65-79, 1984.
159. Newell D W, Eskridge J M, Mayberg M R, *et al.*: Angioplasty for the treatment of symptomatic vasospasm following subarachnoid hemorrhage. **J Neurosurg** 71: 654-60, 1989.
160. Linskey M E, Horton J A, Rao G R, *et al.*: Fatal rupture of the intracranial carotid artery during transluminal angioplasty for vasospasm induced by subarachnoid hemorrhage. **J Neurosurg** 74: 985-90, 1991.
161. Clyde B L, Firlik A D, Kaufmann A M, *et al.*: Paradoxical aggravation of vasospasm with papaverine infusion following aneurysmal subarachnoid hemorrhage. Case report. **J Neurosurg** 84: 690-5, 1996.
162. Miller J A, Cross D T, Moran C J, *et al.*: Severe thrombocytopenia following intraarterial papaverine administration for treatment of vasospasm. **J Neurosurg** 83: 435-7, 1995.
163. McAuliffe W, Townsend M, Eskridge J M, *et al.*: Intracranial pressure changes induced during papaverine infusion for treatment of vasospasm. **J Neurosurg** 83: 430-4, 1995.
164. Origitano T C, Wascher T M, Reichman O H, *et al.*: Sustained increased cerebral blood flow with prophylactic hypertensive hypervolemic hemodilution ("triple-H" therapy) after subarachnoid hemorrhage. **Neurosurgery** 27: 729-40, 1990.
165. Kassell N F, Peerless S J, Durward Q J, *et al.*: Treatment of ischemic deficits from vasospasm with intravascular volume expansion and induced arterial hypertension. **Neurosurgery** 11: 337-43, 1982.
166. Awad I A, Carter L P, Spetzler R F, *et al.*: Clinical vasospasm after subarachnoid hemorrhage: Response to hypervolemic hemodilution and arterial hypertension. **Stroke** 18: 365-72, 1987.
167. Medlock M D, Dulebohn S C, Elwood P W: Prophylactic hypervolemia without calcium channel blockers in early aneurysm surgery. **Neurosurgery** 30: 12-6, 1992.
168. Swift D M, Solomon R A: Unruptured aneurysms and postoperative volume expansion. **J Neurosurg** 77: 908-10, 1992.
169. Solomon R A, Fink M E, Lennihan L: Early aneurysm surgery and prophylactic hypervolemic hypertensive therapy for the treatment of aneurysmal subarachnoid hemorrhage. **Neurosurgery** 23: 699-704, 1988.
170. Maroon J C, Nelson P B: Hypovolemia in patients with subarachnoid hemorrhage: Therapeutic implications. **Neurosurgery** 4: 223-6, 1979.
171. Wijdicks E F M, Vermeulen M, ten Haaf J A, *et al.*: Volume depletion and natriuresis in patients with a ruptured intracranial aneurysm. **Ann Neurol** 18: 211-6, 1985.
172. Shimoda M, Oda S, Tsugane R, *et al.*: Intracranial complications of hypervoemic therapy in patients with a delayed ischemic deficit attributed to vasospasm. **J Neurosurg** 78: 423-9, 1993.
173. Rosenwasser R H, Jallo J I, Getch C C, *et al.*: Complications of Swan-Ganz catheterization for hemodynamic monitoring in patients with subarachnoid hemorrhage. **Neurosurgery** 37: 872-6, 1995.
174. Schanne F A X, Kane A B, Young E E, *et al.*: Calcium dependence of toxic cell death. A final common pathway. **Science** 206: 700-2, 1979.
175. Dale J, Landmark K H, Myhre E: The effects of nifedipine, a calcium channel antagonist, on platelet function. **Am Heart J** 105: 103-5, 1983.
176. Auer L M: Pial arterial vasodilatation by intrave-

nous nimodipine in cats. **Drug Research** 31: 1423-5, 1981.
177. Allen G S, Ahn H S, Preziosi T J, *et al.*: Cerebral arterial spasm - A controlled trial of nimodipine in patients with subarachnoid hemorrhage. **N Engl J Med** 308: 619-24, 1983.
178. Barker F G, Ogilvy C S: Efficacy of prophylactic nimodipine for delayed ischemic deficit after subarachnoid hemorrhage: A metaanalysis. **J Neurosurg** 84: 405-14, 1996.
179. Petruk K C, West M, Mohr G, *et al.*: Nimodipine treatment in poor-grade aneurysm patients: Results of a multicenter double-blind placebo controlled trial. **J Neurosurg** 68: 505-17, 1988.
180. Ohman J, Heiskanen O: Effect of nimodipine on the outcome of patients after aneurysmal subarachnoid hemorrhage and surgery. **J Neurosurg** 69: 683-6, 1988.
181. Flamm E S: In **Intracranial aneurysms: Surgical timing and techniques**, Kikuchi H and Fukushima T, (eds.). Nishimura, New York, 1986: pp 216-29.
182. Haley E C, Kassell N F, Torner J C, *et al.*: A randomized controlled trial of high-dose intravenous nicardipine in aneurysmal subarachnoid hemorrhage: A report of the cooperative aneurysm study. **J Neurosurg** 78: 537-47, 1993.
183. Wiebers D O, Whisnant J P, Sundt T M, *et al.*: The significance of unruptured intracranial saccular aneurysms. **J Neurosurg** 66: 23-9, 1987.
184. Fox J L: **Intracranial aneurysms**. Springer-Verlag, New York, 1983.
185. Almeida G M, Pindaro J, Plese P, *et al.*: Intracranial arterial aneurysms in infancy and childhood. **Childs Brain** 3: 193-9, 1977.
186. Fang H: *A comparison of blood vessels of the brain and peripheral blood vessels*. In **Cerebral vascular diseases**, Wright I S and Millikan C H, (eds.). Grune and Stratton, New York, 1958: pp 17-22.
187. Wilkinson I M S: The vertebral artery: Extracranial and intracranial structure. **Arch Neurol** 27: 392-6, 1972.
188. Youmans J R, (ed.) **Neurological surgery**. 3rd ed., W. B. Saunders, Philadelphia, 1990.
189. Rhoton A L: Anatomy of saccular aneurysms. **Surg Neurol** 14: 59-66, 1981.
190. Ferguson G G: Physical factors in the initiation, growth, and rupture of human intracranial saccular aneurysms. **J Neurosurg** 37: 666-77, 1972.
191. Nehls D G, Flom R A, Carter L P, *et al.*: Multiple intracranial aneurysms: Determining the site of rupture. **J Neurosurg** 63: 342-8, 1985.
192. Mohr G, Ferguson G, Khan M, *et al.*: Intraventricular hemorrhage from ruptured aneurysm: Retrospective analysis of 91 cases. **J Neurosurg** 58: 482-7, 1983.
193. Yeh H S, Tomsick T A, Tew J M: Intraventricular hemorrhage due to aneurysms of the distal posterior inferior cerebellar artery. **J Neurosurg** 62: 772-5, 1985.
194. Raps E C, Galetta S L, Solomon R A, *et al.*: The clinical spectrum of unruptured intracranial aneurysms. **Arch Neurol** 50: 265-8, 1993.
195. Sano H, Jain V K, Kato Y, *et al.*: Bilateral giant intracavernous aneurysms: Technique of unilateral operation. **Surg Neurol** 29: 35-8, 1988.
196. White J C, Ballantine H T: Intrasellar aneurysms simulating hypophyseal tumors. **J Neurosurg** 18: 34-50, 1961.
197. ter Berg H W M, Bijlsma J B, Viega P J A, *et al.*: Familial association of intracranial aneurysms and multiple congenital anomalies. **Arch Neurol** 43: 30-3, 1986.
198. Bigelow N H: The association of polycystic kidneys with intracranial aneurysms and other related disorders. **Am J Med Sci** 225: 485-94, 1953.
199. Beeson P B, McDermott W, (eds.): **Cecil's textbook of medicine**. 15th ed., W. B. Saunders, Philadel-

phia, 1979.

200. Peebles B R: Polycystic disease of the kidneys and intracranial aneurysms. **Glasgow Med J** 32: 333-48, 1951.

201. Levey A S, Pauker S G, Kassirer J P: Occult intracranial aneurysms in polycystic kidney disease: When is cerebral angiography indicated? **N Engl J Med** 308: 986-94, 1983.

202. Butler W E, Barker F G, Crowell R M: Patients with polycystic kidney disease would benefit from routine magnetic resonance angiographic screening for intracerebral aneurysms: A decision analysis. **Neurosurgery** 38: 506-16, 1996.

203. Schievink W I, Prendergast V, Zabramski J M: Rupture of a previously documented small asymptomatic intracranial aneurysm in a patient with autosomal dominant polycystic kidney disease. **J Neurosurg** 89: 479-82, 1998.

204. Schievink W I, Torres V E, Piepgras D G, et al.: Saccular intracranial aneurysms in autosomal dominant polycystic kidney disease. **J Am Soc Nephrol** 3: 88-95, 1992.

205. Davila S, Oliver B, Molet J, et al.: Spontaneous thrombosis of an intracranial aneurysm. **Surg Neurol** 22: 29-32, 1984.

206. Kumar S, Rao V R K, Mandalam K R, et al.: Disappearance of a cerebral aneurysm: An unusual angiographic event. **Clin Neurol Neurosurg** 93: 151-3, 1991.

207. Sobel D F, Dalessio D, Copeland B, et al.: Cerebral aneurysm thrombosis, shrinkage, then disappearance after subarachnoid hemorrhage. **Surg Neurol** 45: 133-7, 1996.

208. Spetzler R F, Winestock D, Newton H T, et al.: Disappearance and reappearance of cerebral aneurysm in serial arteriograms: Case report. **J Neurosurg** 41: 508-10, 1974.

209. Atkinson J L D, Lane J I, Colbassani H J, et al.: Spontaneous thrombosis of posterior cerebral artery aneurysm with angiographic reappearance. **J Neurosurg** 79: 434-7, 1993.

210. Aring C D: Treatment of aneurysmal subarachnoid hemorrhage. **Arch Neurol** 47: 450-1, 1990.

211. Fox A J, Vinuela F, Pelz D M, et al.: Use of detachable balloons for proximal artery occlusion in the treatment of unclippable cerebral aneurysm. **J Neurosurg** 66: 40-6, 1987.

212. Bey L, Connolly S, Duong H, et al.: Treatment of inoperable carotid aneurysms with endovascular carotid occlusion after extracranial-intracranial bypass surgery. **Neurosurgery** 41: 1225-34, 1997.

213. Drake C G: Ligation of the vertebral (unilateral or bilateral) or basilar artery in the treatment of large intracranial aneurysms. **J Neurosurg** 43: 255-74, 1975.

214. Swearingen B, Heros R C: Common carotid occlusion for unclippable carotid aneurysms: An old but still effective operation. **Neurosurgery** 21: 288-95, 1987.

215. Drapkin A J, Rose W S: Serial development of 'de novo' aneurysms after carotid ligation: Case report. **Surg Neurol** 38: 302-8, 1992.

216. Kwan E S K, Heilman C B, Shucart W A, et al.: Enlargement of basilar artery aneurysms following balloon occlusion - "water-hammer effect": Report of two cases. **J Neurosurg** 75: 963-8, 1991.

217. Kurokawa Y, Abiko S, Okamura T, et al.: Direct surgery for giant aneurysm exhibiting progressive enlargement after intraaneurysmal balloon embolization. **Surg Neurol** 38: 19-25, 1992.

218. Dott N M: Intracranial aneurysms: Cerebral arteriography, surgical treatment. **Trans Med Chir Soc Edin** 40: 219-34, 1933.

219. Gillingham F J: The management of ruptured intracranial aneurysms. Hunterian lecture. **Ann R Coll Surg Engl** 23: 89-117, 1958.

220. Todd N V, Tocher J L, Jones P A, et al.: Outcome

following aneurysm wrapping: A 10-year follow-up review of clipped and wrapped aneurysms. **J Neurosurg** 70: 841-6, 1989.

221. Cossu M, Pau A, Turtas S, et al.: Subsequent bleeding from ruptured intracranial aneurysms treated by wrapping or coating: A review of the long-term results in 47 cases. **Neurosurgery** 32: 344-7, 1993.

222. Minakawa T, Koike T, Fujii Y, et al.: Long term results of ruptured aneurysms treated by coating. **Neurosurgery** 21: 660-3, 1987.

223. Pellissou-Guyotat J, Deruty R, Mottolese C, et al.: The use of teflon as wrapping material in aneurysm surgery. **Neurol Res** 16: 224-7, 1994.

224. Guglielmi G, Viñuela F, Dion J, et al.: Electrothrombosis of saccular aneurysms via endovascular approach. Part 2: Preliminary clinical experience. **J Neurosurg** 75: 8-14, 1991.

225. Guglielmi G, Viñuela F, Duckwiler G, et al.: Endovascular treatment of posterior circulation aneurysms by electrothrombosis using electrically detachable coils. **J Neurosurg** 77: 515-24, 1992.

226. McDougall C G, Halbach V V, Dowd C F, et al.: Endovascular treatment of basilar tip aneurysms using electrolytically detachable coils. **J Neurosurg** 84: 393-9, 1996.

227. Halbach V V, Higashida R T, Dowd C F, et al.: The efficacy of endosaccular aneurysm occlusion in alleviating neurological deficits produced by mass effect. **J Neurosurg** 80: 659-6, 1994.

228. McDougall C G, Spetzler R F: Cerebral aneurysms: Clip or coil? **Surg Neurol** 50: 395-7, 1998.

229. Johnston S C, Dudley R A, Gress D R, et al.: Surgical and endovascular treatment of unruptured cerebral aneurysms at university hospitals. **Neurology** 52: 1799-1805, 1999.

230. International Subarachnoid Hemorrhage Aneurysm Trial (ISAT) Collaborative Group: International subarachnoid hemorrhage aneurysm trial (ISAT) of neurosurgical clipping versus endovascular coiling in 2143 patients with ruptured intracranial aneurysms: A randomized trial. **Lancet** 360: 1267-74, 2002.

231. Brilstra E H, Rinkel G J E, van der Graaf Y, et al.: Treatment of intracranial aneurysms by embolization with coils: A systemic review. **Stroke** 30: 470-6, 1999.

232. Thornton J, Debrun G M, Aletich V A, et al.: Follow-up angiography of intracranial aneurysms treated with endovascular placement of Guglielmi detachable coils. **Neurosurgery** 50 (2): 239-49; discussion 249-50, 2002.

233. Raymond J, Roy D: Safety and efficacy of endovascular treatment of acutely ruptured aneurysms. **Neurosurgery** 41: 1235-46, 1997.

234. Zubillaga A, Guglielmi G, Viñuela F, et al.: Endovascular occlusion of intracranial aneurysms with electrically detachable coils: Correlation of aneurysm neck size and treatment results. **AJNR** 15: 815-20, 1994.

235. Debrun G M, Aletich V A, Kehrli P, et al.: Selection of cerebral aneurysms for treatment using Guglielmi detachable coils: The preliminary university of illinois at chicago experience. **Neurosurgery** 43 (6): 1281-95; discussion 1296-7, 1998.

236. Milhorat T H, Krauthem M: Results of early and delayed operations for ruptured intracranial aneurysms in two series of 100 consecutive patients. **Surg Neurol** 26: 123-8, 1986.

237. Leivo S, Hernesniemi J, Luukkonen M, et al.: Early surgery improves the cure of aneurysm-induced oculomotor palsy. **Surg Neurol** 45: 430-4, 1996.

238. Feely M, Kapoor S: Third nerve palsy due to posterior communicating artery aneurysm: The importance of early surgery. **J Neurol Neurosurg Psychiatry** 50: 1051-2, 1987.

239. Le Roux P D, Elliott J P, Newell D W, et al.: Predicting outcome in poor-grade patients with subarach-

noid hemorrhage: A retrospective review of 159 aggressively managed cases. **J Neurosurg** 85: 39-49, 1996.

240. Disney L, Weir B, Grace M, *et al*.: Factors influencing the outcome of aneurysm rupture in poor grade patients: A prospective series. **Neurosurgery** 23: 1-9, 1988.

241. Le Roux P D, Elliot J P, Newell D W, *et al*.: The incidence of surgical complications is similar in good and poor grade patients undergoing repair of ruptured anterior circulation aneurysms: A retrospective review of 355 patients. **Neurosurgery** 38: 887-97, 1996.

242. Kassell N F, Torner J C, Jane J A, *et al*.: The international cooperative study on the timing of aneurysm surgery. Part 2: Surgical results. **J Neurosurg** 73: 37-47, 1990.

243. Lin T, Fox A J, Drake C G: Regrowth of aneurysm sacs from residual neck following aneurysm clipping. **J Neurosurg** 70: 556-60, 1989.

244. Feuerberg I, Lindquist M, Steiner L: Natural history of postoperative aneurysm rests. **J Neurosurg** 66: 30-4, 1987.

245. Rosenorn J, Westergaard L, Hansen P H: Mannitol-induced rebleeding from intracranial aneurysm: Case report. **J Neurosurg** 59: 529-30, 1983.

246. Solomon R A: Methods of cerebral protection during aneurysm surgery. **Contemp Neurosurg** 16 (3): 1-6, 1995.

247. Macdonald R L, Wallace C, Kestle J R W: Role of angiography following aneurysm surgery. **J Neurosurg** 79: 826-32, 1993.

248. Batjer H H, Frankfurt A I, Purdy P D, *et al*.: Use of etomidate, temporary arterial occlusion, and intraoperative angiography in surgical treatment of large and giant cerebral aneurysms. **J Neurosurg** 68: 234-40, 1988.

249. Ravussin P, de Tribolet N: Total intravenous anesthesia with propofol for burst suppression in cerebral aneurysm surgery: Preliminary report of 42 patients. **Neurosurgery** 32: 236-40, 1993.

250. Batjer H H, Samson D S, Bowman M: Comment on Ravussin R and de Tribolet N: Total intravenous anesthesia with propofol for burst suppression in cerebral aneurysm surgery: Preliminary report of 42 patients. **Neurosurgery** 32: 240, 1993.

251. Couldwell W T, Gianotta S L, Zelman V, *et al*.: Life-threatening reactions to propofol. **Neurosurgery** 33: 1116-7, 1993 (letter).

252. Graf C J, Nibbelink D W: *Randomized treatment study: Intracranial surgery*. In **Aneurysmal subarachnoid hemorrhage - report of the cooperative study**, Sahs A L and Nibbelink D W, (eds.). Urban and Schwarzenburg, Baltimore, 1981: pp 145-202.

253. Schramm J, Cedzich C: Outcome and management of intraoperative aneurysm rupture. **Surg Neurol** 40: 26-30, 1993.

254. Kassell N F, Boarini D J, Adams H P, *et al*.: Overall management of ruptured aneurysm: Comparison of early and later operation. **Neurosurgery** 9: 120-8, 1981.

255. Batjer H, Samson D S: Management of intraoperative aneurysm rupture. **Clin Neurosurg** 36: 275-88, 1988.

256. David C A, Vishteh A G, Spetzler R F, *et al*.: Late angiographic follow-up review of surgically treated aneurysms. **J Neurosurg** 91: 396-401, 1999.

257. Locksley H B: Report on the cooperative study of intracranial aneurysms and subarachnoid hemorrhage: Section V. **J Neurosurg** 25: 219-39, 1966.

258. Yock D H, Larson D A: CT of hemorrhage from anterior communicating artery aneurysms, with angiographic correlation. **Radiology** 134: 399-407, 1980.

259. Yeh H, Tew J M: Anterior interhemispheric approach to aneurysms of the anterior communicating artery. **Surg Neurol** 23: 98-100, 1985.

260. Olmsted W W, McGee T P: The pathogenesis of peripheral aneurysms of the central nervous system: A subject review from the AFIP. **Radiology** 123: 661-6, 1977.

261. Fein J M, Rovit R L: Interhemispheric subdural hematoma secondary to hemorrhage from a callosomarginal artery aneurysm. **Neuroradiology** 1: 183-6, 1970.

262. Becker D H, Newton T H: Distal anterior cerebral artery aneurysm. **Neurosurgery** 4: 495-503, 1979.

263. Heros R C, Ojemann R G, Crowell R M: Superior temporal gyrus approach to middle cerebral artery aneurysms: Technique and results. **Neurosurgery** 10: 308-13, 1982.

264. Day A L: Clinicoanatomic features of supraclinoid aneurysms. **Clin Neurosurg** 36: 256-74, 1988.

265. Gibo H, Lenkey C, Rhoton A L: Microsurgical anatomy of the supraclinoid portion of the internal carotid artery. **J Neurosurg** 55: 560-74, 1981.

266. Day A L: Aneurysms of the ophthalmic segment: A clinical and anatomical analysis. **J Neurosurg** 72: 677-91, 1990.

267. Berson E L, Freeman M I, Gay A J: Visual field defects in giant suprasellar aneurysms of internal carotid. **Arch Ophthalmol** 76: 52-8, 1966.

268. Heros R C, Nelson P B, Ojemann R G, *et al*.: Large and giant paraclinoid aneurysms: Surgical techniques, complications, and results. **Neurosurgery** 12: 153-63, 1983.

269. Drake C G: The treatment of aneurysms of the posterior circulation. **Clin Neurosurg** 26: 96-144, 1979.

270. Yamaura A: Surgical management of posterior circulation aneurysms - part I. **Contemporary Neurosurg** 7: 1-6, 1985.

271. Hammon W M, Kempe L G: The posterior fossa approach to aneurysms of the vertebral and basilar arteries. **J Neurosurg** 37: 339-47, 1972.

272. Drake C G: The surgical treatment of vertebral-basilar aneurysms. **Clin Neurosurg** 16: 114-69, 1969.

273. Friedman A H, Drake C G: Subarachnoid hemorrhage from intracraniai dissecting aneurysm. **J Neurosurg** 60: 325-34, 1984.

274. Yamada K, Hayakawa T, Ushio Y, *et al*.: Therapeutic occlusion of the vertebral artery for unclippable vertebral aneurysm. **Neurosurgery** 15: 834-8, 1984.

275. Peerless S J, Hernesniemi J A, Gutman F B, *et al*.: Early surgery for ruptured vertebrobasilar aneurysms. **J Neurosurg** 80: 643-9, 1994.

276. Chyatte D, Philips M: Surgical approaches for basilar artery aneurysms. **Contemp Neurosurg** 13 (17): 1-6, 1991.

277. Pitelli S D, Almeida G G M, Nakagawa E J, *et al*.: Basilar aneurysm surgery: The subtemporal approach with section of the zygomatic arch. **Neurosurgery** 18: 125-8, 1986.

278. Canbolt A, Önal Ç, Kiris T: A high-position basilar top aneurysm apprached via third ventricle: Case report. **Surg Neurol** 39: 196-9, 1993.

279. Yasargil M G, Antic J, Laciga R, *et al*.: Microsurgical pterional approach to aneurysms of the basilar bifurcation. **Surg Neurol** 6: 83, 1976.

280. Tew J M: *Guidelines for management and surgical treatment of intracranial aneurysms*. In **Controversies in neurology**, Thompson R A and Green J R, (eds.). Raven Press, New York, 1983: pp 139-54.

281. The International Study Group of Unruptured Intracranial Aneurysms Investigators (ISUIA): Unruptured intracranial aneurysms - risk of rupture and risks of surgical intervention. **N Engl J Med** 339: 1725-33, 1998.

282. Bederson J B, Awad I A, Wiebers D O, *et al*.: Recommendations for the management of patients with unruptured intracranial aneurysms. A statement for healthcare professionals from the Stroke Council of the American Heart Association. **Circulation** 102: 2300-8, 2000.

283. Yasui N, Suzuki A, Nishimura H, *et al.*: Long-term follow-up study of unruptured intracranial aneurysms. **Neurosurgery** 40: 1155-60, 1997.

284. Juvela S, Porras M, Heiskanen O: Natural history of unruptured intracranial aneurysms: A long-term follow-up study. **J Neurosurg** 79: 174-82, 1993.

285. Solomon R A, Correll J W: Rupture of a previously documented asymptomatic aneurysm enhances the argument for prophylactic surgical intervention. **Surg Neurol** 30: 321-23, 1988.

286. Barth A, de Tribolet N: Growth of small saccular aneurysms to giant aneurysms: Presentation of three cases. **Surg Neurol** 41: 277-80, 1994.

287. Raaymakers T W, Rinkel G J, Limburg M, *et al.*: Mortality and morbidity of surgery for unruptured intracranial aneurysms: A meta-analysis. **Stroke** 29: 1531-8, 1998.

288. van Crevel H, Habbema J D F, Braakman R: Decision analysis of the management of incidental intracranial saccular aneurysms. **Neurology** 36: 1335-9, 1986.

289. Johnston S C, Gress D R, Kahn J G: Which unruptured cerebral aneurysms should be treated? A cost-utility analysis. **Neurology** 52: 1806-15, 1999.

290. Ausman J I, Diaz F G, Malik G M, *et al.*: Management of cerebral aneurysms: Further facts and additional myths. **Surg Neurol** 32: 21-35, 1989.

291. Ojemann R G: Management of the unruptured intracranial aneurysm. **N Engl J Med** 304: 725-6, 1981.

292. Piepgras D G: Management of incidental intracranial aneurysms. **Clin Neurosurg** 35: 511-8, 1989.

293. Cook D J, Guyatt G H, Laupacis A, *et al.*: Rules of evidence and clinical recommendations on the use of antithrombotic agents. **Chest** 102: 305S-11S, 1992.

294. Cook D J, Sackett D L: Rules of evidence and clinical recommendations on the use of antithrombotic agents. **Chest** 105: 647, 1994 (errata).

295. Hamada H, Endo S, Fukuda O, *et al.*: Giant aneurysm in the cavernous sinus causing subarachnoid hemorrhage 13 years after detection: A case report. **Surg Neurol** 45: 143-6, 1996.

296. Lee A G, Mawad M E, Baskin D S: Fatal subarachnoid hemorrhage from the rupture of a totally intracavernous carotid artery aneurysm: Case report. **Neurosurgery** 38: 596-9, 1996.

297. Kupersmith M J, Hurst R, Berenstein A, *et al.*: The benign course of cavernous carotid artery aneurysms. **J Neurosurg** 77: 690-3, 1992.

298. White J A, Horowitz M B, Samson D: Dural waisting as a sign of subarachnoid extension of cavernous carotid aneurysms: A follow-up case report. **Surg Neurol** 52: 607-10, 1999.

299. Ostergaard J R, Hog E: Incidence of multiple intracranial aneurysms. **J Neurosurg** 63: 49-55, 1985.

300. Fairhurn B: "Twin" intracranial aneurysms causing subarachnoid hemorrhage in identical twins. **Br Med J** 1: 210-11, 1973.

301. Schon F, Marshall J: Subarachnoid hemorrhage in identical twins. **J Neurol Neurosurg Psychiatry** 47: 81-3, 1984.

302. Toglia I U, Samii A R: Familial intracranial aneurysms. **Dis Nerv Syst** 33: 611-3, 1972.

303. Norrgard O, Angquist K-A, Fodstad H, *et al.*: Intracranial aneurysms and heredity. **Neurosurgery** 20: 236-9, 1987.

304. Lozano A M, Leblanc R: Familial intracranial aneurysms. **J Neurosurg** 66: 522-8, 1987.

305. Andrews R J: Intracranial aneurysms: Characteristics of aneurysms in siblings. **N Engl J Med** 279: 115, 1977 (letter).

306. Brisman R, Abbassioun K: Familial intracranial aneurysms. **J Neurosurg** 34: 678-82, 1971.

307. Schievink W I, Limburg M, Dreisen J J R, *et al.*: Screening for unruptured familial intracranial aneurysms: Subarachnoid hemorrhage 2 years after angiography negative for aneurysms. **Neurosurgery** 29: 434-8, 1991.

308. Vanninen R L, Hernesniemi J A, Puranen M I, *et al.*: Magnetic resonance angiographic screening for asymptomatic intracranial aneurysms: The problem of false negatives: Technical case report. **Neurosurgery** 38: 838-41, 1996.

309. Schievink W I, Schaid D J, Michels V V, *et al.*: Familial aneurysmal subarachnoid hemorrhage: A community-based study. **J Neurosurg** 83: 426-9, 1995.

310. Benoit B G, Wortzman G: Traumatic cerebral aneurysms: Clinical features and natural history. **J Neurol Neurosurg Psychiatry** 36: 127-38, 1973.

311. Parkinson D, West M: Traumatic intracranial aneurysms. **J Neurosurg** 52: 11-20, 1980.

312. Morard M, de Tribolet N: Traumatic aneurysm of the posterior inferior cerebellar artery: Case report. **Neurosurgery** 29: 438-41, 1991.

313. Buckingham M J, Crone K R, Ball W S, *et al.*: Traumatic intracranial aneurysms in childhood: Two cases and a review of the literature. **Neurosurgery** 22: 398-408, 1988.

314. Kieck C F, de Villiers J C: Vascular lesions due to transcranial stab wounds. **J Neurosurg** 60: 42-6, 1984.

315. Handa J, Handa H: Severe epistaxis caused by traumatic aneurysm of cavernous carotid artery. **Surg Neurol** 5: 241-3, 1976.

316. Maurer J J, Mills M, German W J: Triad of unilateral blindness, orbital fractures and massive epistaxis after head injury. **J Neurosurg** 18: 937-49, 1961.

317. Ding M X: Traumatic aneurysm of the intracavernous part of the internal carotid artery presenting with epistaxis. Case report. **Surg Neurol** 30: 65-7, 1988.

318. Ahuja A, Guterkman L R, Hopkins L N: Carotid cavernous fistula and false aneurysm of the cavernous carotid artery: Complications of transsphenoidal surgery. **Neurosurgery** 31: 774-9, 1992.

319. Bohmfalk G L, Story J L, Wissinger J P, *et al.*: Bacterial intracranial aneurysm. **J Neurosurg** 48: 369-82, 1978.

320. Horten B C, Abbott G F, Porro R S: Fungal aneurysms of intracranial vessels. **Arch Neurol** 33: 577-9, 1976.

321. Schmidek H H, Sweet W H, (eds.): **Operative neurosurgical techniques.** 1st ed., Grune and Stratton, New York, 1982.

322. Pootrakul A, Carter L P: Bacterial intracranial aneurysm: Importance of sequential angiography. **Surg Neurol** 17: 429-31, 1982.

323. Morawetz R B, Karp R B: Evolution and resolution of intracranial bacterial (mycotic) aneurysms. **Neurosurgery** 15: 43-9, 1984.

324. Bingham W F: Treatment of mycotic intracranial aneurysms. **J Neurosurg** 46: 428-37, 1977.

325. Drake C G: Giant intracranial aneurysms: Experience with surgical treatment in 174 patients. **Clin Neurosurg** 26: 12-95, 1979.

326. Hayward R D, O'Reilly G V A: Intracerebral hemorrhage: Accuracy of computerized transverse axial scanning in predicting the underlying etiology. **Lancet** 1: 1-6, 1976.

327. Cioffi F, Pasqualin A, Cavazzani P, *et al.*: Subarachnoid hemorrhage of unknown origin: Clinical and tomographical aspects. **Acta Neurochir** 97: 31-9, 1989.

328. Iwanaga H, Wakai S, Ochiai C, *et al.*: Ruptured cerebral aneurysms missed by initial angiographic study. **Neurosurgery** 27: 45-51, 1990.

329. Farres M T, Ferraz-Leite H, Schindler E, *et al.*: Spontaneous subarachnoid hemorrhage with negative angiography: CT findings. **J Comput Assist Tomogr** 16: 534-7, 1992.

330. Tatter S B, Crowell R M, Ogilvy C S: Aneurysmal and microaneurysmal 'angiogram negative' subarachnoid hemorrhage. **Neurosurgery** 37: 48-55, 1995.

331. Nishioka H, Torner J C, Graf C J, *et al.*: Cooperative study of intracranial aneurysms and subarachnoid hemorrhage: III. Subarachnoid hemorrhage of undetermined etiology. **Arch Neurol** 41: 1147-51, 1984.

332. Kaim A, Proske M, Kirsch E, *et al.*: Value of repeat-angiography in cases of unexplained subarachnoid hemorrhage (SAH). **Acta Neurol Scand** 93: 366-73, 1996.

333. Schwartz T H, Solomon R A: Perimesencephalic nonaneurysmal subarachnoid hemorrhage: Review of the literature. **Neurosurgery** 39: 433-40, 1996.

334. Rinkel G J E, van Gijn J, Wijdicks E F M: Subarachnoid hemorrhage without detectable aneurysm: A review of the causes. **Stroke** 24: 1403-9, 1993.

335. van Gijn J, van Dongen K J, Vermeulen M, *et al.*: Perimesencephalic hemorrhage. A nonaneurysmal and benign form of subarachnoid hemorrhage. **Neurology** 35: 493-7, 1985.

336. Schievink W I, Wijdicks E F M: Pretruncal subarachnoid hemorrhage: An anatomically correct description of the perimesencephalic subarachnoid hemorrhage. **Stroke** 28: 2572, 1997 (letter).

337. van Calenbergh F, Plets C, Goffin J, *et al.*: Nonaneurysmal subarachnoid hemorrhage: Prevalence of perimesencephalic hemorrhage in a consecutive series. **Surg Neurol** 39: 320-3, 1993.

338. Rinkel G J E, Wijdicks E F M, Vermeulen M, *et al.*: Outcome in perimesencephalic (nonaneurysmal) subarachnoid hemorrhage: A follow-up study in 37 patients. **Neurology** 40: 1130-2, 1990.

339. Wijdicks E F M, Schievink W I, Miller G M: Pretruncal nonaneurysmal subarachnoid hemorrhage. **Mayo Clin Proc** 73: 745-52, 1998.

340. Rinkel G J E, Wijdicks E F M, Hasan D, *et al.*: Outcome in patients with subarachnoid hemorrhage and negative angiography according to pattern of hemorrhage on computed tomography. **Lancet** 338: 964-8, 1991.

341. Liliequist B: The subarachnoid cisterns: An anatomic and roentgenologic study. **Acta Radiol (Stockh)** 185 (Suppl 1): 1-108, 1959.

342. Yasargil M G: **Microneurosurgery**. Thieme-Stratton Inc., New York, 1985.

343. Matsuno H, Rhoton A L, Peace D: Microsurgical anatomy of the posterior fossa cisterns. **Neurosurgery** 23: 58-80, 1988.

344. Brasil A V B, Schneider F L: Anatomy of Liliequist's membrane. **Neurosurgery** 32: 956-61, 1993.

345. Rinkel G J E, Wijdicks E F M, Vermeulen M, *et al.*: Nonaneurysmal perimesencephalic subarachnoid hemorrhage: CT and MR patterns that differ from aneurysmal rupture. **AJNR** 12: 829-34, 1991.

346. Adams H P, Gordon D L: Nonaneurysmal subarachnoid hemorrhage. **Ann Neurol** 29: 461-2, 1991.

347. Pinto A N, Ferro J M, Canhao P, *et al.*: How often is a perimesencephalic subarachnoid hemorrhage CT pattern caused by ruptured aneurysms? **Acta Neurochir** 124: 79-81, 1993.

348. Cloft H J, Kallmes D F, Dion J E: A second look at the second-look angiogram in cases of subarachnoid hemorrhage. **Radiology** 205: 323-4, 1997.

349. Dias M S, Sekhar L N: Intracranial hemorrhage from aneurysms and arteriovenous malformations during pregnancy and the puerperium. **Neurosurgery** 27: 855-66, 1990.

350. Crawford S, Varner M W, Digre K B, *et al.*: Cranial magnetic resonance imaging in eclampsia. **Obstet Gynecol** 70: 474-7, 1987.

351. Robinson J L, Hall C J, Sedzimir C B: Subarachnoid hemorrhage in pregnancy. **J Neurosurg** 36: 27-33, 1972.

352. Robinson J L, Hall C S, Sedzimir C B: Arteriovenous malformations, aneurysms, and pregnancy. **J Neurosurg** 41: 63-70, 1974.

353. Horton J C, Chambers W A, Lyons S L, *et al.*: Pregnancy and the risk of hemorrhage from cerebral arteriovenous malformations. **Neurosurgery** 27: 867-72, 1990.

354. Wiebers D O: Comment on Horton J C, et al.: Pregnancy and the risk of hemorrhage from cerebral arteriovenous malformations. **Neurosurgery** 27: 821-2, 1990.

28. Vascular malformations

This designation encompasses a number of non-neoplastic vascular lesions of the CNS. The four types described by McCormick in 1966 are[1]:
1. arteriovenous malformations **(AVMs)**: *see below*
2. venous angioma (*see page 839*)
3. cavernous malformation (*see page 841*) } also see *Angiographically occult vascular malformations*, page 840
4. capillary telangiectasia (*see page 840*) }

A possible fifth category is **direct fistula** AKA arteriovenous fistula (AV- fistula, not AVM): very rare. Single or multiple dilated arterioles that connect directly to a vein without a nidus. These are high-flow, high-pressure. Low incidence of hemorrhage. Usually amenable to interventional neuroradiological procedures. Examples include:
1. vein of Galen malformation (aneurysm): *see page 844*
2. dural AVM: *see page 843*
3. carotid-cavernous fistula: *see page 845*

28.1. Arteriovenous malformation

❢ Key features:
  • dilated arteries and veins with dysplastic vessels, no capillary bed and no intervening neural parenchyma
  • in adulthood, AVMs are medium-to-high pressure and high-flow
  • usually presents with hemorrhage, less often with seizures
  • these are congenital lesions with a lifelong risk of bleeding of ≈ 2-4% per year
  • demonstrable on angiography, MRI, or CT (especially with contrast)
  • main treatment options: stereotactic radiosurgery (usually for deep lesions < 3 cm dia) or surgical excision

DESCRIPTION
An abnormal collection of blood vessels wherein arterial blood flows directly into draining veins without the normal interposed capillary beds. There is no brain parenchyma contained within the nidus. AVMs are congenital lesions, that tend to enlarge somewhat with age and often progress from low flow lesions at birth to medium-to-high-flow high-pressure lesions in adulthood. AVMs appear grossly as a "tangle" of vessels, often with a fairly well circumscribed center (nidus), and draining "red veins" (veins containing oxygenated blood). Some classify parenchymal AVMs (as opposed to e.g. dural AVMs) as:
1. pial
2. subcortical
3. paraventricular
4. combined

EPIDEMIOLOGY
Prevalence: probably slightly greater than the usually quoted 0.14%.
Slight male preponderance. Congenital (therefore risk of hemorrhage is lifelong).
15-20% of patients with Osler-Weber-Rendu syndrome (hereditary hemorrhagic telangiectasia) have cerebral AVMs.

Comparison to aneurysms[2]
AVM:aneurysm ratio in U.S. is 1:5.3 (pre-CT era data). The average age of patients diagnosed with AVMs is ≈ 33 yrs, which is ≈ 10 yrs younger than aneurysms[3]. 64% of AVMs are diagnosed before age 40 (c.f. 26% for aneurysms).

PRESENTATION

1. hemorrhage (most common)[4]: 50% (61% quoted elsewhere[2], compared to 92% for aneurysms) (*see below*)
2. seizures
3. mass effect: e.g. trigeminal neuralgia due to CPA AVM
4. ischemia: by steal
5. H/A: rare. AVMs may occasionally be associated with migraines
6. bruit: especially with dural AVMs (*see page 843*)
7. increased ICP
8. findings limited almost exclusively to peds, usually with large midline AVMs that drain into an enlarged vein of Galen ("vein of Galen malformation", *see page 844*):
   A. hydrocephalus with macrocephaly: due to compression of Sylvian aqueduct by enlarged vein of Galen or to increased venous pressure
   B. congestive heart failure with cardiomegaly
   C. prominence of forehead veins (due to increased venous pressure)

HEMORRHAGE

Peak age for hemorrhage is between 15-20 yrs[2]. **10% mortality, 30-50% morbidity**[5] (neurological deficit) from each bleed. For a discussion of hemorrhage during pregnancy, see *Pregnancy & intracranial hemorrhage*, page 825.

1. 82% have a significant intraparenchymal component[6]
2. subarachnoid hemorrhage: *see page 781*
3. intraventricular hemorrhage
4. spontaneous subdural hematoma: *see page 676*

Hemorrhage related to AVM size

Small AVMs tend to present more often as hemorrhage than do large ones[7,8]. It was postulated that larger AVMs presented as seizure more often simply because their size made them more likely to involve the cortex. However, small AVMs are now thought to have much higher pressure in the feeding arteries[8]. Conclusion: small AVMs are more lethal than larger ones.

Annual and lifetime risk of hemorrhage and recurrent hemorrhage

The average risk of hemorrhage from an AVM is ≈ 2-4% per year[9] (reminder: risk varies by AVM size, *see above*). The risk of bleeding over the remainder of one's life is given by *Eq 28-1*[A].

$$\text{risk of bleeding (at least once)} = 1 - (\text{annual risk of not bleeding})^{\text{expected years of remaining life}} \quad \textbf{Eq 28-1}$$

For example, if a 3% annual risk of bleeding is used as an average, and the life expectancy is 25 years, the result is as illustrated in *Eq 28-2*.

$$\begin{bmatrix} \text{risk of bleeding (at least once in 25 years)} \\ \text{(assuming 3\% annual risk of bleeding)} \end{bmatrix} = 1 - 0.97^{25} = 0.53 = 53\% \quad \textbf{Eq 28-2}$$

Table 28-1 shows the risk for various ages using *Eq 28-1* (longevity is taken from insurance life-tables).

A study of 166 <u>symptomatic</u> AVMS with long average follow-up (mean: 23.7 yrs)[3] found the risk of major bleeding was constant at **4% per year**, independent of whether the AVM presented with or without hemorrhage. The mean time between presentation and hemorrhage was 7.7 yrs. The mortality rate was 1% per year, and the combined major morbidity and mortality rate was 2.7% per year.

Older studies may suffer from smaller numbers[7] or short follow-up (mean: 6.5 yrs)[2,4]. These studies suggested a higher risk of (re)bleeding depending on whether the initial presentation was hemorrhage (≈ 3.7% per year) vs. seizure (1-2% per year).

The hemorrhage risk may be higher in peds or with p-fossa AVMs[9].

Rebleeding: Reported rebleeding rate in the first year after hemorrhage was 6% in one series[10], 18% in another series[11] which declined to 2% per year after 10 years, and in another large series[3] the annual rate was 4% and did not vary regardless of presentation.

A. this analysis includes a number of assumptions including: a constant risk of rebleeding even early after an initial bleed, no change in risk during the lifetime (which may not be true e.g. in pregnancy), no difference in risk for various AVM locations or age groups

SEIZURES

The younger the patient at the time of diagnosis, the higher the risk of developing convulsions. 20 yr risk: age 10-19 → 44% risk; age 20-29 → 31%; age 30-60 → 6%. Patients presenting with hemorrhage have 22% risk of developing epilepsy in 20 yrs. No AVM found incidentally or presenting with neuro deficit developed seizures[7].

AVMs AND ANEURYSMS

7% of patients with AVMs have aneurysms. 75% of these are located on major feeding artery (probably from increased flow)[7]. These aneurysms may be classified into 1 of 5 types shown in *Table 28-2*. Aneurysms also may form within the nidus or on draining veins. When treating tandem AVMs and aneurysms, the symptomatic one is usually treated first (when feasible, both may be treated at the same operation)[12]. If it is not clear which bled, the odds are that it was the aneurysm. Although a significant number (≈ 66%) of related aneurysms will regress following removal of the AVM, this does not always occur. In one series, none of the 9 associated aneurysms ruptured or enlarged following AVM removal[12]

Table 28-1   Lifetime risk of hemorrhage*

Age at presentation	Estimated years to live†	Lifetime risk of hemorrhage		
		For 1% annual risk‡	For 2% annual risk	For 3% annual risk
0	76	53%	78%	90%
15	62	46%	71%	85%
25	52	41%	65%	79%
35	43	35%	58%	73%
45	34	29%	50%	64%
55	25	22%	40%	53%
65	18	16%	30%	42%
75	11	10%	20%	28%
85	6	5.8%	11%	17%

*   modified from reference[9]

†   based on 1992 Preliminary Life tables prepared by Metropolitan Life Insurance Company

‡   1% annual risk is also presented because it may be appropriate for incidental aneurysms (*see page 816*)

EVALUATION

MRI

1. flow void on T1WI or T2WI
2. feeding arteries
3. draining veins
4. increased intensity on partial flip-angle (to differentiate signal dropout on T1WI or T2WI from calcium)
5. if there is significant edema around the lesion on MRI, it may be a tumor that has bled rather than an AVM
6. gradient echo sequences help demonstrate surrounding hemosiderin which suggests a previous significant hemorrhage
7. a complete ring of low density (due to hemosiderin) surrounding the lesion suggests AVM over neoplasm

Table 28-2   Categories of aneurysms associated with AVMs*[12]

Type	Aneurysm location
I	proximal on ipsilateral major artery feeding AVM
IA	proximal on major artery related but contralateral to AVM
II	distal on superficial feeding artery
III	proximal or distal on deep feeding artery ("bizarre")
IV	on artery unrelated to AVM

*   excludes intra-nidal and venous aneurysms

ANGIOGRAPHY

1. tangle of vessels
2. large feeding artery
3. large draining veins

Not all AVMs show up on angiography (see *Angiographically occult vascular malformations*, page 840), and even fewer cavernous malformations and venous angiomas do.

GRADING

Spetzler-Martin grade of AVMs

Grade = sum of points from *Table 28-3*, ranges from 1 to 5. A separate grade 6 is reserved for untreatable lesions (by any means: surgery, SRS...), resection of these would

---

almost unavoidably be associated with disabling deficit or death.

Outcome based on Spetzler-Martin grade: 100 consecutive cases operated by Spetzler had the outcomes shown in *Table 28-4* (no deaths).

TREATMENT

Options and some pros and cons of each include:
1. surgery: the treatment of choice for AVMs. When surgical risk is unacceptably high, alternative procedures may be an option
   A. pros: eliminates risk of bleeding almost immediately. Seizure control improves
   B. cons: invasive, risk of surgery, cost (high initial cost of treatment may be offset by effectiveness or may be increased by complications)
2. radiation treatment
   A. conventional radiation: effective in ≈ 20% or less of cases[14,15]. Therefore not considered effective therapy
   B. stereotactic radiosurgery (**SRS**): accepted for some small (≤ 2.5-3 cm nidus), deep AVMs (see *Stereotactic radiosurgery*, page 537)
      1. pros: done as an outpatient, non-invasive, gradual reduction of AVM flow, no recovery period
      2. cons: takes 1-3 years to work (during that time there is a risk of bleeding), limited to smaller lesions
3. endovascular techniques: e.g. embolization (*see below*)
   A. pros: facilitates surgery and possibly SRS
   B. cons: usually inadequate by itself to permanently obliterate AVMs, induces acute hemodynamic changes, may require multiple procedures

Considerations to take into account in managing AVMs:
1. associated aneurysms: on feeding vessels, draining veins or intra-nidal
2. flow: high or low
3. age of patient
4. history of previous hemorrhage
5. size and compactness of nidus
6. availability of interventional neuroradiologist
7. general medical condition of the patient

Table 28-3 Spetzler-Martin AVM grading system[13]

Graded feature	Points
size*	
small (< 3 cm)	1
medium (3-6 cm)	2
large (> 6 cm)	3
eloquence of adjacent brain	
non-eloquent†	0
eloquent†	1
pattern of venous drainage‡	
superficial only	0
deep	1

* largest diameter of nidus on non-magnified angiogram (is related to and therefore implicitly includes other factors relating to difficulty of AVM excision, e.g. number of feeding arteries, degree of steal, etc.)

† eloquent brain: sensorimotor, language and visual cortex; hypothalamus and thalamus; internal capsule; brain stem; cerebellar peduncles; deep cerebellar nuclei

‡ considered superficial if all drainage is through cortical venous system; considered deep if any or all is through deep veins (e.g. internal cerebral veins, basal veins, or pre-central cerebellar vein)

Table 28-4 Surgical outcome by Spetzler-Martin grade

Grade	No.	No deficit		Minor deficit*		Major deficit†	
1	23	23	(100%)	0		0	
2	21	20	(95%)	1	(5%)	0	
3	25	21	(84%)	3	(12%)	1	(4%)
4	15	11	(73%)	3	(20%)	1	(7%)
5	16	11	(69%)	3	(19%)	2	(12%)

* minor deficit: mild brainstem deficit, mild aphasia, mild ataxia

† major deficit: hemiparesis, increased aphasia, homonymous hemianopsia

EMBOLIZATION

Used as an initial procedure, embolization facilitates surgery[16] and possibly SRS. It is usually inadequate by itself to treat conventional AVMs (may recanalize later), however, is useful as the primary treatment of direct fistulas (*see page 835*). May also be appropriate treatment for vein of Galen aneurysms and pial fistulas.

Agents
1. N-butyl cyanoacrylate (NBCA): investigational
2. isobutyl-2-cyanoacrylate: no longer available
3. solid particles: not appropriate for AVMs. If particles are small, they pass through to the venous system. If too large, they block some feeders, but other vessels will eventually parasitize (the goal is embolization of the nidus, not the feeders)

Timing and technical considerations before definitive treatment
When used before surgery, wait 3-30 days before operating (if symptoms develop, wait for patient to recover).

When used before SRS, wait ≈ 30 days (the immediate post-embolization angio usually looks better, and might result in parts of the AVM being left out of the desired isocenter). Avoid using radio-opaque material in the embolization mixture because this can render CT almost unusable for SRS treatment planning.

Risks
Berenstein's analysis of his series (1985-90) yielded the risks shown in *Table 28-5*.

Long term obliteration
When complete obliteration of the AVM by embolization used alone persists on arteriography at 6 months, it will remain so on the 2 year arteriogram. If there is AVM still visible at 6 months, it will not progress on its own to obliteration at 2 years.

Table 28-5 Risks of AVM embolization

risk	%
death*	1-2%
severe deficit	1.5%
mild deficit	9%
transient deficit	11%
1st time hemorrhage after embolization	3%
rehemorrhage after embolization	7%
new seizure	3%

* 0.5% in older series

SURGICAL TREATMENT

Medical management: Before direct surgical treatment, patient should ideally be pre-treated with propranolol 20 mg PO QID for 3 days to minimize post-op normal perfusion pressure breakthrough (postulated cause of postoperative bleeding and edema[17], *see below*). Labetalol has also been used perioperatively to keep MAP 70-80 mm Hg[18].

Basic tenets of AVM surgery

Postoperative deterioration
May be due to any of the following:
1. **normal perfusion pressure breakthrough**[17]: characterized by post-op swelling or hemorrhage. Thought to be due to loss of autoregulation, although this theory has been challenged[19]. Risk may be reduced by pre-op medication (*see above*)
2. **occlusive hyperemia**[20]: in the immediate post-op period probably due to obstruction of venous outflow from adjacent normal brain, in a delayed presentation may be due to delayed thrombosis of draining vein or dural sinus[21]. Risk may be elevated by keeping the patient "dry" post-op
3. rebleeding from a retained nidus of AVM
4. seizures

28.2. Venous angiomas

❢ Key features:
- usually demonstrable on angiography as a starburst (etc.) pattern
- represents the venous drainage of the area, and intervening brain is present, therefore treatment is rarely indicated
- seizures rare, hemorrhage even more rare
- low-flow, low-pressure

AKA venous malformation or venous anomaly. A tuft of medullary veins that converge into an enlarged central trunk that drains either to the deep or superficial venous system. The veins lack large amounts of smooth muscle and elastic. No abnormal arteries are found. There is neural parenchyma between the vessels. Most common in regions supplied by the MCA[22] or in the region of the vein of Galen. They may be associated with a cavernous malformation (*see page 841*). Occasionally may be angiographically occult, however, they classically produce a distinct **caput medusae** (other descriptive terms include: a hydra, spokes of a wheel, a spider, an umbrella, a mushroom, or a sunburst)[23 (p 1471)]. Non hereditary.

These are low-flow and low-pressure. Most are clinically silent, but rarely seizures and even less frequently hemorrhage may occur.

TREATMENT
In general, these should not be treated as they are the venous drainage of the brain in that vicinity. Surgery is indicated only for documented bleeding or for intractable seizures definitely attributed to the lesion.

28.3. Angiographically occult vascular malformations

Terminology is controversial.

Recommendation: use the term "**angiographically occult** (or **cryptic**) **vascular malformations**" (**AOVM**) to refer to cerebrovascular malformations that are not demonstrable on technically satisfactory cerebral angiography (i.e. good quality cut-films, with subtraction views, and the following as appropriate: magnification, angiotomography, rapid serial angiograms or delayed films)[24]. Many lesions have large patent vessels at surgery in spite of negative angiography[25]. Other imaging modalities (i.e. CT, MRI) may be able to reveal these lesions. Although often used interchangeably, the term "occult malformation" (omitting the word "angiographically") is suggested for use with lesions that also do not appear on other imaging modalities.

The reasons for a vascular lesion being angiographically cryptic include:
1. lesion that have hemorrhaged
    A. the bleeding may obliterate the lesion: difficult to substantiate[26]
    B. the clot may compress the lesion[26] which may re-open as clot dissolves
2. sluggish flow
3. small size of the abnormal vessels
4. may require very late angiographic films to visualize due to late filling

EPIDEMIOLOGY
Incidence of AOVM has been estimated as ≈ 10% of cerebrovascular malformations[22]. AOVMs were found at necropsy in 21 (4.5%) of 461 patients with spontaneous intracranial hemorrhage (**ICH**)[27], but refinements in angiography have occurred since this 1954 report.

The average age at diagnosis in one literature review[24] was 28 yrs.

PRESENTATION
AOVM most often present with seizures or H/A. Less commonly they may present with progressive neurologic symptoms (usually as a result of spontaneous ICH)[28]. They may also be discovered incidentally.

The natural history of this group of lesions is not accurately known.

HISTOLOGICAL TYPES OF AOVM
No difference in presentation, CT appearance, or surgical prognosis was found among the following subtypes[29] (the first 4 are the classic pathologic subtypes). The prevalence of each of these lesions[29, 30] is shown in *Table 28-6*.

1. **arteriovenous malformation (AVM)**: the most common AOVM (*see page 835*)
2. **venous angiomas**: most of these are not angiographically occult (*see above*)
3. **cavernous malformations**: thin walled sinusoids without interstitial cerebral parenchyma[22] (only rarely demonstrable angiographically[28]) (*see below*)
4. **capillary telangiectasia**: the least well understood AOVM. Slightly enlarged capillaries with low flow. Cannot be imaged on any radiographic study. Usually incidentally found at necropsy without clinical significance (risk of hemorrhage is

Table 28-6 Prevalence of subtypes of AOVM

Type	%
AVM	44-60%
cavernous angioma	19-31%
telangiectasias	4-12%
venous angioma	9-10%

very low, except possibly in brain stem). Has intervening neural tissue[22] (unlike cavernous malformations). Usually solitary, but may be multiple when seen as a part of a syndrome: Osler-Weber-Rendu (see below), Louis -Barr (ataxia telangiectasia), Myburn-Mason, Sturge-Weber. Should not be treated

5. mixed or unclassified angiomas: 11% of AOVM[29]

Osler-Weber-Rendu syndrome

AKA hereditary hemorrhagic telangiectasia **(HHT)**, a rare autosomal dominant genetic disorder of blood vessels affecting ≈ 1 in 5,000 people. 95% have recurrent epistaxis. Cerebrovascular malformations **(CVM)** include: telangiectasias, AVMs (the most common CVM, seen in 5-13% of HHT patients[31]), venous angiomas and aneurysms. Patients are also prone to pulmonary arteriovenous fistulas with associated risk of paradoxical cerebral embolism which predisposes to embolic stroke and cerebral abscess formation (see page 217).

IMAGING

CT: May show a well demarcated homogeneous or mottled high density[28] (high density due to hematoma, calcification, thrombosis, hemosiderin deposition, alterations in BBB, and/or increased blood volume[24]) with some form of contrast enhancement (around or within lesion) in 17 of 24 patients[28]. Surrounding edema or mass effect is rare (except in cases that have recently hemorrhaged).

MRI: May demonstrate previous hemorrhage(s)[32], (may be important when the presence of multiple occurrences affects therapeutic choices). T2WI finding: reticulated core of increased and decreased intensity, a prominent surrounding rim of reduced intensity may be present (due to hemosiderin laden macrophages from previous hemorrhages). GRASS image demonstrates flow related enhancement in ≈ 60% of cases, which allows signal dropout from flowing blood on other sequences to be differentiated from that due to calcium (and thus, bone) or air (limitations: hemosiderin causes signal dropout, and slow in-plane flow does not enhance)[33].

TREATMENT

Surgery is indicated mainly for evacuation of hematoma or diagnosis, especially when favorably located. Also consider surgery for recurrent hemorrhages (rupture has been reported even after normal angiography) or medically intractable seizures. Stereotactic radiosurgery has not had a satisfactorily high enough benefit to risk ratio even in symptomatic venous angiomas to justify its use[34].

28.3.1. Cavernous malformation

⚐ Key features:
- usually <u>not</u> demonstrable on angiography (see above), but may show up on MRI (flow void and/or previous hemorrhage) or CT (especially with contrast)
- usually presents with seizures, rarely with hemorrhage
- no intervening neural parenchyma, no arteries
- low-flow
- treatment is controversial: surgery may be best for symptomatic accessible lesions, radiosurgery may reduce risk of rebleeding for inaccessible ones

AKA **cavernous hemangioma, cavernoma, cavernous angioma**, and angioma. A well circumscribed, benign vascular hamartoma consisting of irregular thick and thin walled sinusoidal vascular channels located within the brain but lacking intervening neural parenchyma, large feeding arteries, or large draining veins. Usually 1-5 cm in size. Multiple in 50% of cases[35]. May hemorrhage, calcify, or thrombose. Rarely occur in the spinal cord[36]. Caverns are filled with blood in various stages of thrombus formation/organization/dissolution. Commonly associated with venous angiomas (see page 839), capillary telangiectasias may be found adjacent to lesions. Stain positive for angiogenesis factor[37]. Lesions may arise de novo[38], and may grow (although slower than hemangioblastomas), shrink, or remain unchanged with time[39].

PATHOLOGY

Gross appearance resembles a mulberry (facetiously but descriptively called a "hemorrhoid of the brain"). Light microscopy: stains for von Willebrand's factor. Smooth muscle layer is absent (except for some tiny portions). EM: shows abnormal gapping of the tight junctions between endothelial cells[40] (may permit leakage of blood).

Cerebral cavernous malformations (CM) comprise 5-13% of CNS vascular malformations, and develop in 0.02-0.13% of the population (based on large autopsy[41] and MRI series[42]). Most are supratentorial, but 10-23% are located in the posterior fossa with a predilection for the pons[43]. Rarely, may occur in spinal cord. XRT may be a risk factor[44] especially for spinal CMs (e.g. following craniospinal XRT[45] for medulloblastoma).

Two types: sporadic and hereditary. The latter may be inherited in a Mendelian autosomal dominant pattern with variable expressivity[46]. More common in Hispanic Americans[47]. Multiple lesions are more common in the familial form[42]. Genetics: there appears to be at least 3 gene loci (7q, 7p & 3q)[48]. There is 1 case report of spontaneous mutation.

PRESENTATION/NATURAL HISTORY

Seizures (60%), progressive neurologic deficit (50%), hemorrhage[A] (20%) (usually intraparenchymal), hydrocephalus, or as in incidental finding (over 50% in one series).

Hemorrhage: Risk is not well delineated. Even the definition of hemorrhage is controversial since, by definition, all CMs have surrounding hemosiderin indicative of small leaks. Risk of significant hemorrhage is much less than with AVM. CMs are prone to recurrent small hemorrhages that are rarely devastating. Overall hemorrhage rate is ≈ 2.6-3.1%/yr (appears higher in females 4.2%/yr than males 0.9%/yr)[42]. Controversial if hemorrhage increases the risk of future bleeding: it did not in one study[42] whereas another study[49] found only a 0.6%/yr risk of bleeding in lesions without prior hemorrhage. Pregnancy and parturition are not known to be risk factors for hemorrhage[46].

Σ | The bleeding rate is variable and the definition controversial, ∴ it is difficult to assign a risk of hemorrhage for any individual patient.

Seizures: The rate of new-seizure onset is 2.4%/yr[42].

EVALUATION

CT: May miss many small, and even some large lesions.

MRI: T2WI MRI is the most sensitive test. Findings are similar to AOVM in general (mixed signal core with low signal rim) (*see above*). The diagnosis is strongly suggested by finding multiple lesions with these characteristics and a positive family history[35]. A venous malformation may be seen adjacent to solitary CMs, but not with multiple lesions[50]. MRI appearance is nearly pathognomonic, and angiography is not necessary in classically appearing cases.

Angiography: Does not demonstrate lesion.

TREATMENT/MANAGEMENT
Options:
1. observe
2. surgical excision
3. stereotactic radiosurgery[51-54]

No randomized prospective study has been done. Determining treatment response is difficult since no imaging study can prove elimination of the lesion. Therefore it has been suggested that *recurrent hemorrhage rate* be followed as an endpoint.

Recommendations

Incidental lesions: Asymptomatic, incidentally discovered CMs should be managed expectantly. ✖ Since the radiographic appearance is almost pathognomonic, biopsy or excision solely to verify the diagnosis is rarely appropriate.

Surgery: Indications for surgery:
1. accessible lesions with
   A. focal deficit
   B. or symptomatic hemorrhage
   C. or seizures:

A. here, hemorrhage is defined as symptomatic, radiologically proven extralesional bleeding

1. <u>new onset</u> seizures: there is a suggestion that removing CMs before "kindling" (*see page 258*) occurs may have a better chance of preventing future seizures
2. difficult to manage seizures

2. less accessible lesions that repeatedly bleed with progressive neurologic deterioration may be considered for excision, even in delicate regions such as the brain stem[55-57] or spinal cord

Stereotactic radiosurgery (SRS): SRS was initially thought to be ineffective, but non-controlled studies have shown a possible reduction in recurrent *hemorrhage rate* with SRS following a 2 year latency period[54]. Side effects with SRS are not insignificant.

Σ | SRS may be considered for inaccessible lesions that meet other treatment criteria, but at this time is best reserved for patients enrolled in research protocols.

Familial considerations: First degree relatives of patients with more than one family member having a cavernous angioma should have contrast CT or preferably MRI screening and appropriate genetic counselling.

PROGNOSIS
When CMs can be completely removed, the risk of further growth or hemorrhage is essentially permanently eliminated[58] (however, recurrence of symptoms has been reported after partial and even seemingly-complete removal[57, 59]).
For CMs treated surgically, patients need to be aware that post-op neurologic worsening is very common, especially with brainstem CMs[60]. Worsening may be transient[61], but may take months to resolve.

28.4. Dural AVM

AKA dural arteriovenous fistula. Vascular abnormalities in which an arteriovenous shunt is contained within the leaflets of the dura mater, exclusively supplied by branches of the carotid or vertebral arteries before they penetrate the dura[62]. These are not true AVMs in the usual sense, and may qualify more as direct fistulas (*see page 835*).
Usually found adjacent to dural venous sinuses. The transverse (lateral) sinus is the most common[63] (63% of cases) with a slight left-sided predominance[64], with the epicenter of these almost invariably at the junction of the transverse and sigmoid sinuses. Dural AVMs (**DAVM**) also may arise in the tentorium.

Classified on the basis of the feeding arteries:
1. pure pial
2. mixed pial and dural
3. pure dural

EPIDEMIOLOGY
DAVMs comprise 10-15% of all intracranial AVMs[64]. 61-66% occur in females, and patients are usually in their 40's or 50's. They occur rarely in children, and when they do they tend to be complex and bilateral.

ETIOLOGY
Evidence supports the fact that DAVMs of the transverse-sigmoid sinus junction are not congenital but are acquired lesions, resulting from collateral revascularization following thrombosis of a venous sinus[65] (often sigmoid sinus occlusion, possibly from chronic infection or trauma).
The occipital artery is the dominant feeder in most cases.

Table 28-7 Clinical findings in 27 patients with dural AVMs[65]

Sign/symptom	No. (%)
pulsatile tinnitus	25 (92%)
occipital bruit	24 (89%)
headache	11 (41%)
visual impairment	9 (33%)
papilledema	7 (26%)

PRESENTATION
Common findings are listed in *Table 28-7*. Visual impairment included obscuration, and two patients that were blind from chronically elevated ICP. The risk of bleeding is less than with parenchymal AVMs. DAVMs may also be asymptomatic.

Indications:
1. neurologic dysfunction
2. hemorrhage
3. refractory symptoms

Endovascular embolization

May be performed transarterial or transvenous. Glue, coils, or a combination may be used.

Surgery

Preoperative embolization by an interventional neuroradiologist will usually facilitate surgical treatment[66]. The literature is rife with warnings about rapid blood loss that frequently occurs during surgery for these lesions (including just incising the scalp), with one report of 8 units lost in 4 minutes following elevation of the bone flap[65]. Thus, the use of the crainiotome is discouraged, as a sinus or venous laceration could produce a fatal hemorrhage. Contingencies for the rapid administration of blood products must be made (large bore central lines).

Stereotactic radiosurgery

May be used post-embolization[67]. Pan et al[68] reported a complete obliteration rate of 58% of transverse/sigmoid fistulae treated with only radiosurgery (1650-1900 cGy) or with radiosurgery after surgery/embolization had failed to produce complete obliteration. 71% of the patients were cured of their symptoms.

Radiosurgery represents an important adjunct to the treatment of DAVF. However, it should be reserved for benign DAVF that have failed other treatments. Aggressive DAVF require urgent and complete obliteration that cannot be provided by radiosurgery

---

28.5.   Vein of Galen malformation

Enlargement of the great cerebral vein of Galen (**VOG**) may occur in "vein of Galen *malformations*" (some refer to these as vein of Galen aneurysms) (congenital) or secondarily to high flow from adjacent deep parenchymatous AVMs or pial fistulae. Parenchymatous AVMs can be distinguished from true VOG malformations by retrograde filling of the of the internal cerebral veins in the former[69].

True VOG malformations are predictably fed from the medial and lateral choroidal, circumferential, mesencephalic, anterior choroidal, pericallosal and meningeal arteries[69, 70]. Agenesis of the straight sinus may be an associated finding.

Presentation

Newborns tend to present with congestive heart failure in first few weeks of life (due to high blood flow)[71] and a cranial bruit. Hydrocephalus may result from obstruction of the sylvian aqueduct by the enlarged VOG, or it may be caused by the increased venous pressure (which can also produce prominence of the scalp veins[72]).

Parenchymatous AVMs are usually diagnosed later in life due to neurological manifestations[73] including focal neurologic deficit and hemorrhage.

Classification

Classified based on the location of the fistula[74, 75]:
1. pure internal fistulae: single or multiple
2. fistulae between thalamoperforators and the VOG
3. mixed form: the most common
4. plexiform AVMs

Natural history

Untreated VOG malformations have a poor prognosis, with neonates having nearly 100% mortality, and 1-12 month olds having ≈ 60% mortality, 7% major morbidity, and 21% being normal[76].

Parenchymatous AVMs behave similar to other AVMs.

Treatment

Vein of Galen malformations: Pediatric patients are often in poor medical condition, limiting the efficacy of operative treatment. Treatment options for these include embolization of the main feeding arteries. Prognosis is poor. Those presenting with hydrocephalus from aqueductal obstruction often do so at the end of the first year of life. Neurosurgical excision may be considered here, and the prognosis is better.

Parenchymatous AVM with enlarged VOG: The AVM is treated by the same methods as other AVMs (embolization, resection or radiosurgery).

28.6. Carotid-cavernous fistula

Carotid-cavernous fistula (**CCF**) may be divided into post-traumatic and spontaneous.
1. traumatic (including iatrogenic): occur in 0.2% of patients with craniocerebral trauma. May also occur following percutaneous trigeminal rhizotomy[77]
2. spontaneous. Subclassified into 4 groups[78]:
    A. direct high-flow shunts between the internal carotid artery and cavernous sinus: frequently due to ruptured cavernous sinus ICA aneurysm
    B. dural shunts (low flow) between meningeal branches of the internal carotid artery and the cavernous sinus
    C. dural shunts (low flow) between meningeal branches of the external carotid artery and the cavernous sinus
    D. dural shunts (low flow) between meningeal branches of both the internal and external carotid artery and the cavernous sinus

PRESENTATION
1. orbital and/or retro-orbital pain
2. chemosis (arteriolization of conjunctiva)
3. pulsatile proptosis
4. ocular and/or cranial bruit
5. deterioration of visual acuity: may be due to hypoxic retinopathy as a result of reduced arterial pressure and increased venous pressure and increased intraocular pressure
6. diplopia: abducens (VI) palsy is the most common
7. ophthalmoplegia (usually unilateral, but may present initially as bilateral or may progress to bilateral)
8. rarely: SAH

TREATMENT
Even if normal ocular motility cannot be achieved in affected eye, preservation of vision is desirable because:
1. for some motility abnormalities, surgical treatment may reduce diplopia
2. patient may be provided with frosted eyeglass lens which will eliminate diplopia but will maintain peripheral vision
3. in the rare event of injury to contralateral eye (trauma, central retinal artery occlusion...) there would be "reserve" vision in the eye with reduced motility (with loss of the other eye, there would not be diplopia)

Approximately 50% of low flow CCF spontaneously thrombose, therefore one may observe these as long as visual acuity is stable and intra-ocular pressure is < ≈ 25. High flow lesions or those associated with progressive visual deterioration require treatment, usually in the form of balloon embolization by an interventional neuroradiologist.

BALLOON EMBOLIZATION
A detachable latex balloon is inflated in an attempt to reduce flow completely or sufficiently to allow thrombosis.

Routes available include:
1. transarterial through internal carotid
    A. balloon is placed within the fistula itself, preserving the parent (carotid) artery: the best option[79]. Usually possible only if aneurysm neck is narrow
    B. if this fails (e.g. wide aneurysm neck), two balloons may be placed on either side of fistula to trap it (sacrifices carotid artery, therefore test occlusion must be done first to determine if patient can tolerate this). Also a danger

of embolization with this
2. transarterial through external carotid: useful only for dural fistulas
3. transvenous:
   A. traversing heart to enter jugular vein, then through petrosal sinus to cavernous sinus. Lower success rate (≈ 20%) than transarterial route
   B. via superior ophthalmic vein: entered where supra-optic vein enters orbit to become superior ophthalmic vein. If possible, it is best to wait for vein to become arterialized by the higher flow pressure. Reports of "disasters" due to injury to the fragile vein performed before arteriolization took place may have been due to more primitive balloon catheters that were standard before current commercially produced versions were available (softer than original). Must avoid lacerating vein inside orbit, and avoid distal ligation of vein without proximal occlusion (shunts even more blood into eye)

28.7. References

1. McCormick W F: The pathology of vascular ('arteriovenous') malformations. **J Neurosurg** 24: 807-16, 1966.
2. Perret G, Nishioka H: Report on the cooperative study of intracranial aneurysms and subarachnoid hemorrhage: Arteriovenous malformations. **J Neurosurg** 25: 467-90, 1966.
3. Ondra S L, Troupp H, George E D, et al.: The natural history of symptomatic arteriovenous malformations of the brain: A 24-year follow-up assessment. **J Neurosurg** 73: 387-91, 1990.
4. Drake C G: Cerebral AVMs: Considerations for and experience with surgical treatment in 166 cases. **Clin Neurosurg** 26: 145-208, 1979.
5. Hartmann A, Mast H, Mohr J P, et al.: Morbidity of intracranial hemorrhage in patients with cerebral arteriovenous malformation. **Stroke** 29: 931-4, 1998.
6. Morgan M, Sekhon L, Rahman Z, et al.: Morbidity of intracranial hemorrhage in patients with cerebral arteriovenous malformation. **Stroke** 29: 2001, 1998 (letter).
7. Crawford P M, West C R, Chadwick D W, et al.: Arteriovenous malformations of the brain: Natural history in unoperated patients. **J Neurol Neurosurg Psychiatry** 49: 1-10, 1986.
8. Spetzler R F, Hargraves R W, McCormick P W, et al.: Relationship of perfusion pressure and size to risk of hemorrhage from arteriovenous malformations. **J Neurosurg** 76: 918-23, 1992.
9. Kondziolka D, McLaughlin M R, Kestle J R W: Simple risk predictions for arteriovenous malformation hemorrhage. **Neurosurgery** 37: 851-5, 1995.
10. Graf C J, Perret G E, Torner J C: Bleeding from cerebral arteriovenous malformations as part of their natural history. **J Neurosurg** 58: 331-7, 1983.
11. Fults D, Kelly D L: Natural history of arteriovenous malformations of the brain: A clinical study. **Neurosurgery** 15: 658-62, 1984.
12. Cunha M J, Stein B M, Solomon R A, et al.: The treatment of associated intracranial aneurysms and arteriovenous malformations. **J Neurosurg** 77: 853-9, 1992.
13. Spetzler R F, Martin N A: A proposed grading system for arteriovenous malformations. **J Neurosurg** 65: 476-83, 1986.
14. Laing R W, Childs J, Brada M: Failure of conventionally fractionated radiotherapy to decrease the risk of hemorrhage in inoperable arteriovenous malformations. **Neurosurgery** 30: 872-6, 1992.
15. Redekop G J, Elisevich K V, Gaspar L E, et al.: Conventional radiation therapy of intracranial arteriovenous malformations: Long-term results. **J Neurosurg** 79: 413-22, 1993.
16. Jafar J J, Davis A J, Berenstein A, et al.: The effect of embolization with N-butyl cyanoacrylate prior to

surgical resection of cerebral arteriovenous malformations. **J Neurosurg** 78: 60-9, 1993.
17. Spetzler R F, Wilson C B, Weinstein P, et al.: Normal perfusion pressure breakthrough theory. **Clin Neurosurg** 25: 651-72, 1978.
18. Orlowski J P, Shiesley D, Vidt D G, et al.: Labetalol to control blood pressure after cerebrovascular surgery. **Crit Care Med** 16: 765-8, 1988.
19. Young W L, Kader A, Prohovnik I, et al.: Pressure autoregulation is intact after arteriovenous malformation resection. **Neurosurgery** 32: 491-7, 1993.
20. al-Rodhan N R F, Sundt T M, Piepgras D G, et al.: Occlusive hyperemia: A theory for the hemodynamic complications following resection of intracerebral arteriovenous malformations. **J Neurosurg** 78: 167-75, 1993.
21. Wilson C B, Hieshima G: Occlusive hyperemia: A new way to think about an old problem. **J Neurosurg** 78: 165-6, 1993.
22. Steiger H J, Tew J M: Hemorrhage and epilepsy in cryptic cerebrovascular malformations. **Arch Neurol** 41: 722-4, 1984.
23. Wilkins R H, Rengachary S S, (eds.): **Neurosurgery**. McGraw-Hill, New York, 1985.
24. Cohen H C M, Tucker W S, Humphreys R P, et al.: Angiographically cryptic histologically verified cerebrovascular malformations. **Neurosurgery** 10: 704-14, 1982.
25. Shuey H M, Day A L, Quisling R G, et al.: Angiographically cryptic cerebrovascular malformations. **Neurosurgery** 5: 476-9, 1979.
26. Ropper A H, Davis K R: Lobar cerebral hemorrhages: Acute clinical syndromes in 26 cases. **Ann Neurol** 8: 141-7, 1980.
27. Russell D S: The pathology of spontaneous intracranial hemorrhage. **Proc R Soc Med** 47: 689-93, 1954.
28. Bitoh S, Hasegawa H, Fujiwara M, et al.: Angiographically occult vascular malformations causing intracranial hemorrhage. **Surg Neurol** 17: 35-42, 1982.
29. Lobato R D, Perez C, Rivas J J, et al.: Clinical, radiological, and pathological spectrum of angiographically occult intractranial vascular malformations. **J Neurosurg** 68: 518-31, 1988.
30. Rigamonti D, Hsu F P K, Huhn S: *Angiographically occult vascular malformations*. In **Neurovascular surgery**, Carter L P, Spetzler R F, and Hamilton M G, (eds.). McGraw-Hill, New York, 1995, Chapter 27: pp 521-40.
31. Willemse R B, Mager J J, Westermann C J, et al.: Bleeding risk of cerebrovascular malformations in hereditary hemorrhagic telangiectasia. **J Neurosurg** 92 (5): 779-84, 2000.
32. Lemme-Plaghos L, Kucharczyk W, Brant-Zawalski M, et al.: MRI of angiographically occult vascular

malformations. **AJNR** 7: 217-22, 1986.

33. Needell W M, Maravilla K R: MR flow imaging in vascular malformations using gradient recalled acquisition. **AJNR** 9: 637-42, 1988.

34. Lindquist C, Guo W-Y, Kerlsson B, *et al.*: Radiosurgery for venous angiomas. **J Neurosurg** 78: 531-6, 1993.

35. Rigamonti D, Drayer B P, Johnson P C, *et al.*: The MRI appearance of cavernous malformations (angiomas). **J Neurosurg** 67: 518-24, 1987.

36. Cosgrove G R, Bertrand G, Fontaine S, *et al.*: Cavernous angiomas of the spinal cord. **J Neurosurg** 68: 31-6, 1988.

37. Uranishi R, Baev N I, Ng P Y, *et al.*: Expression of endothelial cell angiogenesis receptors in human cerebrovascular malformations. **Neurosurgery** 48 (2): 359-67; discussion 367-8, 2001.

38. Detwiler P W, Porter R W, Zabramski J M, *et al.*: De novo formation of a central nervous system cavernous malformation: Implications for predicting risk of hemorrhage. Case report and review of the literature. **J Neurosurg** 87 (4): 629-32, 1997.

39. Clatterbuck R E, Moriarity J L, Elmaci I, *et al.*: Dynamic nature of cavernous malformations: A prospective magnetic resonance imaging study with volumetric analysis. **J Neurosurg** 93 (6): 981-6, 2000.

40. Wong J H, Awad I A, Kim J H: Ultrastructural pathological features of cerebrovascular malformations: A preliminary report. **Neurosurgery** 46 (6): 1454-9, 2000.

41. Simard J M, Garcia-Bengochea, Ballinger W E, *et al.*: Cavernous angioma: A review of 126 collected and 12 new clinical cases. **Neurosurgery** 18: 162-72, 1986.

42. Moriarity J L, Wetzel M, Clatterbuck R E, *et al.*: The natural history of cavernous malformations: A prospective study of 68 patients. **Neurosurgery** 44: 1166-73, 1999.

43. Kashiwagi S, van Loveren H R, Tew J M, *et al.*: Diagnosis and treatment of vascular brain-stem malformations. **J Neurosurg** 72: 27-34, 1990.

44. Detwiler P W, Porter R W, Zabramski J M, *et al.*: Radiation-induced cavernous malformation. **J Neurosurg** 89 (1): 167-9, 1998.

45. Maraire J N, Abdulrauf S I, Berger S, *et al.*: De novo development of a cavernous malformation of the spinal cord following spinal axis radiation. Case report. **J Neurosurg** 90 (4 Suppl): 234-8, 1999.

46. Hayman L A, Evans R A, Ferrell R F, *et al.*: Familial cavernous angiomas: Natural history and genetic study over a 5-year period. **Am J Med Genet** 11: 147-60, 1982.

47. Gunel M, Awad I A, Finberg K, *et al.*: A founder mutation as a cause of cerebral cavernous malformation in Hispanic Americans. **N Engl J Med** 334 (15): 946-51, 1996.

48. Gunel M, Awad I A, Finberg K, *et al.*: Genetic heterogeneity of inherited cerebral cavernous malformation. **Neurosurgery** 38 (6): 1265-71, 1996.

49. Kondziolka D, Lunsford L D, Kestle J R W: The natural history of cerebral cavernous malformations. **J Neurosurg** 83: 820-4, 1995.

50. Abdulrauf S I, Kaynar M Y, Awad I A: A comparison of the clinical profile of cavernous malformations with and without associated venous malformations. **Neurosurgery** 44 (1): 41-6; discussion 46-7, 1999.

51. Kondziolka D, Lunsford L D, Flickinger J C, *et al.*: Reduction of hemorrhage risk after stereotactic radiosurgery for cavernous malformations. **J Neurosurg** 83: 825-31, 1995.

52. Porter R W, Detwiler P W, Han P P, *et al.*: Stereotactic radiosurgery for cavernous malformations: Kjellberg's experience with proton beam therapy in 98 cases at the Harvard cyclotron. **Neurosurgery** 44 (2): 424-5, 1999.

53. Zhang N, Pan L, Wang B J, *et al.*: Gamma knife radiosurgery for cavernous hemangiomas. **J Neurosurg** 93 (Suppl 3): 74-7, 2000.

54. Pollock B E, Garces Y I, Stafford S L, *et al.*: Stereotactic radiosurgery for cavernous malformations. **J Neurosurg** 93 (6): 987-91, 2000.

55. Bicknell J M: Familial cavernous angioma of the brain stem dominantly inherited in hispanics. **Neurosurgery** 24: 102-5, 1989.

56. Ondra S L, Doty J R, Mahla M E, *et al.*: Surgical excision of a cavernous hemangioma of the rostral brain stem: Case report. **Neurosurgery** 23: 490-3, 1988.

57. Zimmerman R S, Spetzler R F, Lee K S, *et al.*: Cavernous malformations of the brain stem. **J Neurosurg** 75: 32-9, 1991.

58. Wascher T M, Spetzler R F: *Cavernous malformations of the brain stem*. In **Neurovascular surgery**, Carter L P, Spetzler R F, and Hamilton M G, (eds.). McGraw-Hill, New York, 1995, Chapter 28: pp 541-55.

59. Bertalanffy H, Gilsbach J M, Eggert H R, *et al.*: Microsurgery of deep-seated cavernous angiomas: Report of 26 cases. **Acta Neurochir** 108: 91-9, 1991.

60. Weil S M, Tew J M, Jr.: Surgical management of brain stem vascular malformations. **Acta Neurochir (Wien)** 105 (1-2): 14-23, 1990.

61. Bartolomei J, Wecht D A, Chaloupka J, *et al.*: Occipital lobe vascular malformations: Prevalence of visual field deficits and prognosis after therapeutic intervention. **Neurosurgery** 43 (3): 415-21; discussion 421-3, 1998.

62. Malik G M, Pearce J E, Ausman J I: Dural arteriovenous malformations and intracranial hemorrhage. **Neurosurgery** 15: 332-9, 1984.

63. Graeb D A, Dolman C L: Radiological and pathological aspects of dural arteriovenous fistulae. **J Neurosurg** 64: 962-7, 1986.

64. Arnautovic K I, Krisht A F: Transverse-sigmoid sinus dural arteriovenous malformations. **Contemp Neurosurg** 21 (15): 1-6, 2000.

65. Sundt T M, Piepgras D G: The surgical approach to arteriovenous malformations of the lateral and sigmoid dural sinuses. **J Neurosurg** 59: 32-9, 1983.

66. Barnwell S L, Halbach V V, Higashida R T, *et al.*: Complex dural arteriovenous fistulas: Results of combined endovascular and neurosurgical treatment in 16 patients. **J Neurosurg** 71: 352-8, 1989.

67. Lewis A I, Tomsick T A, Tew J M: Management of tentorial dural arteriovenous malformations. Transarterial embolization combined with stereotactic radiation or surgery. **J Neurosurg** 81. 851-9, 1994.

68. Pan D H, Chung W Y, Guo W Y, *et al.*: Stereotactic radiosurgery for the treatment of dural arteriovenous fistulas involving the transverse-sigmoid sinus. **J Neurosurg** 96 (5): 823-9, 2002.

69. Khayata M H, Casaco A, Wakhloo A K, *et al.*: Vein of Galen malformations: Intravascular techniques. In **Neurovascular surgery**, Carter L P, Spetzler R F, and Hamilton M G, (eds.). McGraw-Hill, New York, 1995, Chapter 55: pp 1029-39.

70. Lasjaunias P, Rodesch G, Pruvost P, *et al.*: Treatment of vein of Galen aneurysmal malformation. **J Neurosurg** 70: 746-50, 1989.

71. Cummings G R: Circulation in neonates with intracranial arteriovenous fistula and cardiac failure. **Am J Cardiol** 45: 1019-24, 1980.

72. Strassburg H M: Macrocephaly is not always due to hydrocephalus. **J Child Neurol** 4 (Suppl): S32-40, 1989.

73. Clarisse J, Dobbelaere P, Rey C, *et al.*: Aneurysms of the great vein of Galen. Radiological-anatomical study of 22 cases. **J Neuroradiol** 5: 91-102, 1978.

74. Yasargil M G: *AVM of the brain, clinical considerations, general and specific operative techniques, surgical results, nonoperated cases, cavernous and venous angiomas, neuroanesthesia*. In **Micron-**

---

eurosurgery. Georg Thieme, Stuttgart, 1988, Vol. IIIb: pp 317-96.

75. Litvak J, Yahr M D, Ransohoff J: Aneurysms of the great vein of Galen and mid-line cerebral arterio-venous anomalies. **J Neurosurg** 17: 945-54, 1960.

76. Johnston I H, Whittle I R, Besser M, *et al.*: Vein of Galen malformation: Diagnosis and management. **Neurosurgery** 20: 747-58, 1987.

77. Kuether T A, O'Neill O R, Nesbit G M, *et al.*: Direct carotid cavernous fistula after trigeminal balloon microcompression gangliolysis: Case report. **Neurosurgery** 39: 853-6, 1996.

78. Barrow D L, Spector R H, Braun I F, *et al.*: Classi-fication and treatment of spontaneous carotid-cav-ernous fistulas. **J Neurosurg** 62: 248-56, 1985.

79. Lewis A I, Tomsick T A, Tew J M, *et al.*: Long-term results in direct carotid-cavernous fistulas after treatment with detachable balloons. **J Neurosurg** 84: 400-4, 1996.

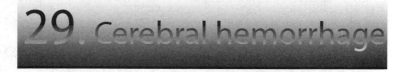

29. Cerebral hemorrhage

Intracerebral hemorrhage **(ICH)** is a hemorrhage within the brain parenchyma. Formerly commonly referred to as **"hypertensive hemorrhage"**, but hypertension is a debatable etiology (see *Hypertension as a cause?*, page 853).

29.1. Intracerebral hemorrhage in <u>adults</u>

❦ Key features
  • the second most common form of stroke (15-30% of strokes), but the most deadly
  • unlike ischemic infarct: smooth progressive onset over minutes to hours, often with severe headache, vomiting and alterations in level of consciousness
  • unenhanced CT scan of the brain is the initial diagnostic study of choice
  • the volume of the hematoma correlates highly with morbidity and mortality
  • the clot enlarges in at least 33% of cases within the first 3 hours of onset
  • angiography is recommended (as long as it doesn't delay emergent treatment) <u>except</u> for patients > 45 yrs of age with preexisting hypertension <u>and</u> ICH in thalamus, putamen or posterior fossa
  ❢ treatment
    ◆ rFVIIa given IV within 4 hours of onset limits the volume of the ICH
    ◆ the usefulness of surgery is still controversial, but seems limited to some cerebellar hemorrhages and select supratentorial hemorrhages that come within 1 cm of the cortical surface

EPIDEMIOLOGY

INCIDENCE
The second most common form of stroke (≈ 15-30% of all strokes, and the most deadly. Approximately 12-15 cases per 100,000/yr. Approximately twice the incidence as SAH[1]. Onset is usually during activity (rarely during sleep), which may be related to elevation of BP or increased CBF (see *Etiologies* below).

Risk factors
The following are epidemiologic risk factors, also see *Etiologies*, page 850 for others.
  1. age: the incidence increases significantly after age 55 years and doubles with each decade of age until age > 80 yrs where incidence is 25 times that during previous decade. Relative risk for age > 70 yrs is 7
  2. gender: more common in men
  3. race: in the U.S., ICH affects blacks more than whites. May be related to higher prevalence of HTN in blacks. Incidence may also be higher in orientals[2]
  4. previous CVA (any type) increases risk to 23:1
  5. alcohol consumption[2, 3]:
     A. recent use: moderate or heavy alcohol consumption both within the 24 hours and the week preceding the ICH were risk factors for ICH[4] as shown in *Table 29-1*
     B. chronic use: one study suggests that consuming > 3 drinks a day increases the risk of ICH by ≈ 7 times[5 (p 15)]
     C. ICH in patients with high ethanol con-

Table 29-1 Relative risk of ICH with EtOH consumption

Period prior to ICH	Amount* (g EtOH)	Relative risk
24 hours	41-120	4.6
	> 120	11.3
1 week	1-150	2.0
	151-300	4.3
	> 300	6.5

* 1 standard drink = 12 g EtOH

sumption were more commonly lobar[6]

6. cigarette smoking: does not increase the risk of ICH[7, 8]
7. street drugs: cocaine, amphetamines, phencyclidine[9]
8. liver dysfunction: hemostasis may be impaired on the basis of thrombocytopenia, reduced coagulation factors, and hyperfibrinolysis[10]

LOCATIONS OF HEMORRHAGE

Common sites of ICH are shown in *Table 29-2*. Common arterial feeders of ICHs:

- lenticulostriates: the source of putaminal hemorrhages (possibly secondary to microaneurysms of Charcot-Bouchard, *see below*)
- thalamoperforators
- paramedian branches of BA

Table 29-2   Common sites for ICH (modified[11])

%	Location
50%	striate body (basal ganglia); putamen most common; also includes: lenticular nucleus, internal capsule, globus pallidus
15%	thalamus
10-15%	pons (≈90% of these are hypertensive)
10%	cerebellum
10-20%	cerebral white matter
1-6%	brain stem

Lobar hemorrhage

Incorporates primary hemorrhages into the occipital, temporal, frontal and parietal lobes (including ICH arising from cortex and subcortical white matter), as opposed to hemorrhage of deep structures (e.g. basal ganglion, thalamus, and infratentorial structures)[12]. Accounts for 10-32% of nontraumatic ICHs[12]. With large hemorrhages, it may be difficult to make a distinction between lobar and deep ICH.

Lobar hemorrhages are more likely to be associated with structural abnormalities than deep hemorrhages (*see below*). They may also be more common in patients with high alcohol consumption (*see above*). Lobar hemorrhages may also have a more benign outcome than ganglionic-thalamic hemorrhages[12].

Etiologies: Although many causes of ICH can produce lobar hemorrhages (*see below* for a detailed list), those that are more likely to produce lobar hemorrhages include:
1. extension of a deep hemorrhage
2. cerebral amyloid angiopathy: the most common cause of lobar ICH in elderly normotensive patients (*see page 853*)
3. trauma
4. hemorrhagic transformation of an ischemic infarct: *see below*
5. tumor: *see page 854*. Multiple lobar hemorrhages may occur with metastases
6. cerebrovascular malformation (especially AVM): *see page 835*
7. rupture of an aneurysm: *see below* for circumstances likely to produce this
8. idiopathic

Internal capsule

There may be prognostic significance with regard to contralateral motor function if the hemorrhage is medial to and/or extending through the internal capsule (**IC**), or lateral to the IC and merely compressing it, making the clot more accessible to surgical treatment without damaging the IC.

ETIOLOGIES

History check list

Based on information in this section, the following check-list is presented to assist in the gathering of historical information important in evaluating the adult with ICH:
❑ 1. hypertension
❑ 2. drugs:
    A. sympathomimetics:
        1. amphetamines, cocaine
        2. appetite suppressants or nasal decongestants (phenylpropanolamine, pseudoephedrine)
    B. dietary supplements: especially ephedra alkaloids (ma huang)
    C. anticoagulants: warfarin in particular
    D. birth control pills: questionable association
    E. aspirin use
❑ 3. history of alcohol abuse

❏ 4. coagulopathies
❏ 5. leukemia
❏ 6. previous stroke
❏ 7. history of known vascular abnormalities (AVM, venous angioma…)
❏ 8. tumor: known history of cancer, especially those that tend to go to brain (lung, breast, GI, renal, melanoma…)
❏ 9. recent surgery: especially carotid endarterectomy, procedures requiring heparin…
❏ 10. recent childbirth and/or eclampsia or preeclampsia
❏ 11. history of recent trauma

ETIOLOGIES

1. "hypertension" (debatable as a cause or effect, see below) but is a risk factor
   A. acute hypertension (HTN): as may occur in eclampsia (see below) or with use of certain drugs (e.g. cocaine, phenylpropanolamine…, see page 852)
   B. chronic HTN: possibly causes degenerative changes within blood vessels
2. possibly associated with acutely increased CBF (globally or focally)[13], especially to areas previously rendered ischemic:
   A. following carotid endarterectomy[14, 15]
   B. following repair of congenital heart defects in children[16]
   C. previous CVA (embolic[17] or otherwise): hemorrhagic transformation may occur in up to 43% of CVAs during the first month[18]. May follow dislodgment or recanalization of an arterial occlusion, although it has been demonstrated with persistent occlusion[19]. May occur as early as ≤ 24 hrs after a CVA in patients with a negative CT done within 6 hours[20]. Two types[18, 21]:
      - type 1: diffuse or multifocal. Heterogeneous or mottled appearance within the boundaries of the CVA. Less hyperdense than primary ICH
      - type 2: extensive hematoma. Probably unifocal source. As hyperdense as primary ICH and may extend outside the original CVA boundaries. Unlike type 1, classically associated with anticoagulation therapy, and tends to occur in initial few days after CVA and is often associated with clinical worsening. May be difficult to distinguish from primary ICH, and may be frequently misdiagnosed as such[20]
   D. migraine: during[22] or following[23] a migraine attack (probably an exceedingly rare event)
   E. following surgery to remove an AVM: "normal perfusion pressure breakthrough". Some cases may be due to incomplete AVM excision
   F. physical factors: following strenuous physical exertion[24], exposure to cold[25]…
3. vascular anomalies
   A. AVM: rupture (see Arteriovenous malformation, page 835)
   B. aneurysm rupture
      1. saccular ("berry") aneurysms:
         a. aneurysms of the circle of Willis (COW): ICH may be more likely with aneurysms that have become adherent to brain surface by fibrosis from inflammation or previous hemorrhages. May produce ICH when they rupture instead of the usual SAH
         b. aneurysms distal to the COW (e.g. MCA aneurysms)
      2. microaneurysms of Charcot-Bouchard: see below
   C. venous angioma rupture
4. "arteriopathies"
   A. amyloid angiopathy: usually → repeated lobar hemorrhages (see below)
   B. fibrinoid necrosis[26, 27] (sometimes seen in cases of amyloid angiopathy)
   C. lipohyalinosis: subintimal lipid-rich hyaline material[28]
   D. cerebral arteritis (including necrotizing angiitis)
5. brain tumor (primary or met): see Hemorrhagic brain tumors below
6. coagulation or clotting disorders
   A. iatrogenic
      1. patients receiving anticoagulation therapy: see page 854
      2. thrombolytic therapy:
         a. for acute ischemic CVA: incidence of symptomatic ICH within 36 hrs of treatment with rtPA is 6.4% (vs. 0.6% in the placebo treated group)[29] (see page 768)

b. for acute MI or other thrombosis: incidence is ≈ 0.36-2%[30-32]. Risk is increased with higher doses than the recommended 100 mg of alteplase (Activase®, recombinant tissue plasminogen activator (**rt-PA**))[33], in older patients, in those with anterior MI or higher Killip class, and with bolus administration (vs. infusion)[34]. When heparin was used adjunctively, higher doses were associated with higher risk of ICH[35]. ICH is thought to occur in those patients with some preexisting underlying vascular abnormality[36]. Immediate coronary angioplasty is safer than rt-PA when available[32]

   3. one ASA qod was associated with increased risk of ICH[37], with a rate of 0.2-0.8% per year[38]

  B. leukemia
  C. thrombocytopenia:
    1. thrombotic thrombocytopenic purpura
    2. aplastic anemia

7. CNS infection:
  A. especially fungal, which attack blood vessels
  B. granulomas
  C. herpes simplex encephalitis: may initially produce low density lesions that progress to hemorrhagic ones

8. venous or dural sinus thrombosis: *see page 888*

9. drug related
  A. substance abuse
    1. alcohol: > 3 drinks/day increases the risk of ICH ≈ 7-fold (*see page 849*)
    2. drug abuse: especially sympathomimetics (cocaine[39, 40], amphetamine[41]
  B. drugs that raise BP:
    1. alpha-adrenergic agonists (sympathomimetics): phenylpropanolamine[42, 43] (may also cause ischemic CVA, *see page 775*) which was removed from OTC nasal decongestants and appetite suppressants, but other OTC alpha agonists (including phenylephrine, ephedrine[44], and pseudoephedrine[45]) are also problematic[46]
    2. ephedra alkaloids: sold as a dietary supplement (ma huang) to suppress appetite and increase energy. Associated in <u>case reports</u> with HTN, SAH, ICH, seizures and death[47]

10. post-traumatic: often in a delayed fashion[48, 49] (see *Hemorrhagic contusion*, page 669)

11. pregnancy related: the risk of ICH in pregnancy and puerperium (up to 6 weeks post partum) is ≈ 1 in 9,500 births[50]
  A. most commonly associated with eclampsia or preeclampsia: the mortality of eclampsia is ≈ 6% with ICH being the most frequent direct cause[51] (also see *Pregnancy & intracranial hemorrhage*, page 825)
  B. postpartum ICH (median 8 days, range 3-35 days) in the absence of eclampsia has been reported[52]; when associated with vasculopathy the term **postpartum cerebral angiopathy** has been used
  C. vascular findings:
    1. some cases associated with isolated cerebral vasculopathy in the absence of systemic vasculitis[53]
    2. some cases demonstrate vasospasm
    3. some cases show findings (e.g. patchy enhancement in occipital lobes) suggestive of cerebrovascular dysautoregulation (*see page 64*)
    4. some cases show no vascular-related abnormalities

12. post-operative:
  A. following carotid endarterectomy (*see above*)
  B. following craniotomy:
    1. at site of craniotomy[54]: risk factors identified
      a. especially within residual astrocytoma after subtotal resection
      b. following craniotomy for AVM (*see above*)
    2. at site remote from craniotomy. In a series of 37 patients, unlike hematomas at craniotomy site, the following were identified as <u>not</u> being related to risk of hemorrhage: HTN, coagulopathy, CSF drainage, underlying occult lesion
      a. following drainage of chronic SDH: *see page 675*
      b. cerebellar hemorrhage

      i.   following pterional craniotomy (this author incriminated possibly rapid overdrainage of CSF)[55]
     ii.   following temporal lobectomy[56]
13. idiopathic[12]

HYPERTENSION AS A CAUSE?

Hypertension **(HTN)** is controversial as cause of ICH since the incidence of both ICH and HTN increases with age (66% of patients > 65 yrs have HTN). The relative risk for ICH with HTN is 3.9-5.4, depending on the definition of HTN used[57]. Many patients with ICH are dramatically hypertensive on presentation, however, acute elevations of ICP from the hemorrhage may actually precipitate HTN (part of Cushing's triad, see *Table 24-17*, page 649). HTN is probably a risk factor primarily for pontine/cerebellar ICH and is probably not a factor in at least 35% of basal ganglion hemorrhages.

MICROANEURYSMS OF CHARCOT-BOUCHARD

AKA miliary aneurysms[58]. Occur primarily at bifurcation of small (< 300 µm) perforating branches of lateral lenticulostriate arteries in basal ganglia, more common in hypertensive patients[59]. Possibly the origin of some "hypertensive" ganglionic (putaminal) hemorrhages[60], but this is controversial.

(CEREBRAL) AMYLOID ANGIOPATHY

Cerebral amyloid angiopathy **(CAA)** AKA **congophilic angiopathy**. Pathologic deposition of beta amyloid protein (appears as birefringent "apple-green" under polarized light when stained with congo red) within the media of small meningeal and cortical vessels (especially those in white matter) without evidence of systemic amyloidosis[61]. Some vessels may show fibrinoid necrosis of vessel wall[62, 63].

Should be suspected in patients with recurrent hemorrhages (uncommon with "hypertensive hemorrhages"[64]) that are lobar in location (*see page 850*). **Gradient-echo MRI** may identify petechial hemorrhages or hemosiderin deposits from small cortical hemorrhages which may be associated with CAA[65]. Less likely in the case of basal ganglion or brain stem hemorrhages[12].

Incidence increases with age: CAA is present in ≈ 50% of those over 70 years of age[66], however, most do not hemorrhage. CAA is probably responsible for ≈ 10% of cases of ICH. May be associated with genetic factors (including the apolipoprotein E ε4 allele[67]), and may be more prevalent in patients with Down's syndrome. Although they are distinct diseases, there is some overlap between CAA and Alzheimer's disease; the amyloid in CAA is identical to that found in senile plaques of Alzheimer's disease. CAA may increase the risk of ICH by potentiating plasminogen[68] (may be of special relevance to patients receiving tissue plasminogen activator **(t-PA)** to treat MI or CVA).

Table 29-3 Criteria for the diagnosis of CAA[69]

Definite CAA	Full postmortem exam showing all 3 of the following:
	  A. lobar, cortical, or corticosubcortical hemorrhage
	  B. severe CAA
	  C. absence of another diagnostic lesion

Probable CAA with supporting pathological evidence	Clinical data & pathological tissue showing all 3 of the following:
	  A. lobar, cortical, or corticosubcortical hemorrhage
	  B. some degree of vascular amyloid deposition in specimen
	  C. absence of another diagnostic lesion

Probable CAA	Clinical data and MRI findings showing all 3 of the following:
	  A. age ≥ 60 yrs
	  B. multiple hemorrhages restricted to the lobar, cortical, or corticosubcortical region
	  C. absence of another cause of hemorrhage*

Possible CAA	Clinical data and MRI findings:
	  A. age ≥ 60 yrs
	  B. single lobar, cortical, or corticosubcortical hemorrhage without another cause*, or multiple hemorrhages with a possible but not a definite cause* or with some hemorrhages in an atypical location (e.g. brain stem)

* e.g. excessive anticoagulation (INR > 3.0), head trauma, ischemic CVA, CNS tumor, cerebrovascular malformation, vasculitis or blood dyscrasia

Patients with CAA may present with a TIA-like prodrome (*see below*).

Among patients with lobar hemorrhage, those with the apoE ε4 allele typically have their first hemorrhage > 5 yrs earlier than noncarriers (73 ± 8 yrs vs./ 79 ± 7 yrs)[67].

Diagnostic tests are useful mainly to rule-out other conditions. The definitive diagnosis of CAA requires pathologic evaluation of brain tissue. Criteria for the diagnosis of CAA are shown in *Table 29-3*[69].

HEMORRHAGIC BRAIN TUMORS

Although any brain tumor can hemorrhage, tumoral ICH is usually associated with malignancies. Tumors can also produce SAH(*see page 781*) or subdural hematomas.

Malignant tumors most commonly associated with ICH:
1. glioblastoma multiforme
2. lymphoma
3. metastatic tumors
   A. melanoma[70, 71]: ≈ 40% hemorrhage
   B. choriocarcinoma[70, 72, 73]: ≈ 60% hemorrhage
   C. renal cell carcinoma
   D. bronchogenic carcinoma: although only ≈ 9% hemorrhage, this tumor is such a frequent source of cerebral mets that it therefore is a more common source of tumoral ICH

Malignant tumors that hemorrhage less commonly include:
1. medulloblastoma[74-77] (most commonly in children)
2. gliomas[78, 79]

Some benign brain tumors that have been associated with ICH include:
1. meningiomas have been associated with intratumoral, subdural, and nearby parenchymal hemorrhage[80-83]. Tendency to bleed is similar for angioblastic variety as for other highly vascular meningiomas
2. pituitary adenoma (see *Pituitary apoplexy*, page 438)
3. oligodendroglioma (relatively benign): rarely presents with hemorrhage[84], classically after years of causing seizures
4. hemangioblastoma[85]
5. acoustic neuroma[86-88]
6. cerebellar astrocytoma[89]

ANTICOAGULATION PRECEDING ICH

10% of patients on warfarin develop a significant bleeding complication per year, including ICH (65% mortality in this group). The risk of ICH in patients treated with warfarin for A-fib varies between 0-0.3% per year[38] (historically, this was as high as ≈ 1.8% in older studies[90] from the 1960's and 70's), but when an elderly subgroup (mean age 80 yrs) was analyzed, this rate was 1.8% per year[38]. ICH was the only cause of fatal bleeding complications of warfarin therapy in one series where the cumulative risk of a fatal hemorrhage was 1% at 1 year and 2% at 3 yrs[91].

The risk of hemorrhagic complications was increased with the length and also the variability of the PT, and during the first three months of anticoagulation[91]. Patients with cerebral amyloid angiopathy (**CAA**) (*see above*) are also at increased risk of ICH following administration of antiplatelet drugs or anticoagulants[69].

CLINICAL

In general, the neurologic deficit with ICH is characterized by a smooth progressive onset over minutes to hours, unlike embolic/ischemic CVA where deficit is maximal at onset. With ICH, severe headache, vomiting and alterations in level of consciousness may be more common (H/A may not be more prevalent than in embolic CVA, but it is often a first and prominent symptom[12]).

Prodrome

TIA-like symptoms may precede lobar hemorrhages[92, 93] in patients with CAA, and may occur in up to ≈ 50% of patients for whom a complete history is obtainable. Unlike typical TIAs, these usually consist of numbness, tingling or weakness (involving the area where the hemorrhage will subsequently occur) that gradually spreads in a manner reminiscent of a Jacksonian-march and may spill-over vascular territories (probably an electrical phenomenon rather than an ischemic event). This is suggestive of but not pathognomonic for the subsequent development of lobar ICH.

Putaminal hemorrhage

The most common site for ICH. Smooth gradual deterioration in 62% (maximal deficit at onset in 30%); never fluctuating. Contralateral hemiparesis, may progress to hemiplegia or even coma or death. H/A in 14% at onset. No H/A at any time in 72%. Papilledema and **subhyaloid preretinal hemorrhage** are rare.

Thalamic hemorrhage

Classically, contralateral hemisensory loss. Also hemiparesis when internal capsule involved. Extension into upper brain stem → vertical gaze palsy, retraction nystagmus, skew deviation, loss of convergence, ptosis, miosis, anisocoria, ± unreactive pupils. H/A in 20-40%. Motor deficit similar to putaminal hemorrhage, but contralateral sensory deficit widespread and striking. Hydrocephalus may occur from compression of CSF pathways.

In 41 patients, when hemorrhage > 3.3 cm on CT, all died. Smaller hematomas usually caused permanent disability.

Cerebellar hemorrhage

May include any combination of the following:
1. symptoms of increased ICP (lethargy, N/V, HTN with bradycardia...) due to hydrocephalus from compression of the 4th ventricle → obstruction of CSF
2. direct of brain stem compression may produce:
   A. facial palsy: due to pressure on the facial colliculus
   B. these patients classically become comatose without first having hemiparesis, unlike many supratentorial etiologies
3. hydrocephalus may also occur with extension of the hemorrhage into the ventricular system

'Lobar hemorrhage

Syndromes associated with hemorrhage in the 4 cerebral lobes[12] (≈ 50% have H/A):
1. frontal lobe (the most distinctive of the syndromes): frontal H/A with contralateral hemiparesis, usually in the arm with mild leg and facial weakness
2. parietal lobe: contralateral hemisensory deficit and mild hemiparesis
3. occipital lobe: ipsilateral eye pain and contralateral homonymous hemianopsia, some may spare superior quadrant
4. temporal lobe: on dominant side, produces fluent dysphasia with poor auditory comprehension but relatively good repetition

Deterioration after the initial hemorrhage is usually due to any combination of the following:
1. rebleeding: *see below*
2. edema: *see below*
3. hydrocephalus: higher risk with intraventricular extension or posterior fossa ICH
4. seizures

Rebleeding or extension of bleed

Early rebleeding: Rebleeding (more so in basal ganglion hemorrhages than in lobar hemorrhages) has been documented during the first hour by "ultra-early" scanning and repeating CT scans. Rebleeding is usually accompanied by clinical deterioration[94]. The incidence of hematoma enlargement decreases with time, 33-38% in 1-3 hours[95], 16% in 3-6 hrs, and 14% between 24 hrs of onset and a second CT within 24 hrs of the first[96]. Patients with enlarging hematomas were more likely to have larger hematomas and/or coagulopathy, and had a worse outcome[96]. Rebleeding may still occur following surgical evacuation of clot even with satisfactory intraoperative hemostasis. Hemostatic agents (e.g. NovoSeven®) may reduce this risk, *see page 857*.

Late rebleeding: Quoted rates for late rebleeding from ICH range from 1.8–5.3% (depending on length of follow-up)[97]. Diastolic BP was significantly higher in the group with recurrent hemorrhage, with a 10%/yr risk for DBP > 90 mm Hg vs. < 1.5% for DBP ≤ 90 (mean F/U of 67 months)[97]. Other risk factors include diabetes and tobacco and alcohol abuse[98]. Recurrent hemorrhages may indicate underlying vascular malformations or amyloid angiopathy (lobar rebleeding is likely to be due to amyloid angiopathy[98]).

Edema

Edema and ischemic necrosis around the hemorrhage may cause delayed deterioration[26]. Although necrosis from mass effect of the clot contributes a small part to the edema, experiments indicate that by itself, the mass effect is insufficient to account for the amount of edema that occurs. It is believed that an edemogenic toxin is released from the clot. Experiments with various components of blood clots has disclosed that thrombin in concentrations that could be released from the clot causes increased permeability of the blood-brain-barrier, and is also a potent vasoconstrictor. This is the leading suspect as the major cause of delayed edema and deterioration. Also see *Cerebral edema*, page 85.

EVALUATION

CT SCAN
CT scan is rapid, and easily demonstrates blood as high density within the brain parenchyma immediately after hemorrhage. Although mass effect is common, the tendency for the hemorrhage to dissect through brain tissue often results in less mass effect than would be anticipated from the size of the clot.

Clot volume carries prognostic significance (*see page 859*). It can be measured volumetrically by CT, or it can be approximated by a **modified ellipsoid volume** as shown in *Eq 29-1*, where A, B and C are the diameters of the clot in each of the 3 dimensions.

$$\text{modified ellipsoid volume} \approx \frac{A \times B \times C}{2} \qquad \text{Eq 29-1}$$

On the average, the size of the clot decreases ≈ 0.75 mm/day, and the density decreases by ≈ 2 CT units/day, with little change for 1st 2 wks.

MRI
Usually <u>not</u> the procedure of choice for initial study. Does not show blood well within the first few hours. Difficult to ventilate or access patient during the study. Slower and more expensive than CT. May be useful later, e.g. to help diagnose cerebral amyloid angiopathy **(CAA)** (*see page 853*).

The appearance of ICH on MRI is very complicated. It is highly dependent on the age of the clot[99] with 5 stages identified (*see Table 29-4*).

Table 29-4 Variation of MRI appearance of ICH with time since hemorrhage*[99]

Stage	Age	Condition of hemoglobin	T1WI	T2WI
hyper-acute	< 24 hrs	oxy-Hgb (intracellular)	iso	sl. ↑
acute	1-3 d	deoxy-Hgb (intracellular)	sl. ↓	very ↓
subacute • early	> 3 d	met-Hgb (intracellular)	very ↑	very ↓
• late	> 7 d	met-Hgb (extracellular†)	very ↑	very ↑
chronic • center	> 14 d	hemichromes‡ (extracellular)	iso	sl. ↑
• rim		hemosiderin (intracellular)	sl. ↓	very ↓

*   Abbreviations: oxy-Hgb = oxyhemoglobin, deoxy-Hgb = deoxy-hemoglobin, met-Hgb =methemoglobin, iso = iso-intense to brain, ↓ = hypo-intense, ↑ = hyperintense, sl = slightly
†   when the RBCs lyse, the Hgb becomes extracellular
‡   diamagnetic (non-paramagnetic) heme derivatives

CEREBRAL ANGIOGRAPHY
For making the diagnosis of the ICH itself, angiography cannot reliably differentiate the mass effect from an ICH from that due to an ischemic infarct or tumor[100]. May demonstrate AVMs and aneurysms when they are associated with the ICH. The yield may be increased by delaying the study[12]. May demonstrate vascular blush in some cases of tumor. Normal arteriography cannot eliminate cerebral amyloid angiopathy[101].

For indications for cerebral angiography in ICH, *see below*.

ICH SCORE
The system of Hemphill et al.[102] assigns points based on 5 features as indicated in *Table 29-5*. The points are then summed for the "ICH score". The associated 30 day mortality is also tabulated.

INITIAL MANAGEMENT OF ICH
There is not uniform agreement on almost all aspects of the management of ICH from the optimal BP to the indications for surgery. The following is offered as a guide.

1. HTN: controversial. Issues: HTN may contribute to further bleeding, especially within the first hour[94]. However, some HTN may be needed to maintain perfusion[A]. Some say reduce MAP to pre-morbid level if known, or by ≈ 20% if unknown

Σ **Treat HTN. Suggested target BP ≈ 140/90. Avoid overcorrection (hypotension)**

2. intubate if stuporous or comatose
3. anticonvulsants (optional): e.g. phenytoin (load with 17 mg/kg slow IV over 1 hour, follow with 100 mg q 8 hrs, see *phenytoin (PHT) (Dilantin®)*, page 271)
4. hemostatic issues:
   A. check PT, PTT & platelet count (**PC**)
      1. correct coagulopathies (see *Correction of coagulopathies or reversal of anticoagulants*, page 24)
      2. platelets
         a. thrombocytopenia: although platelet transfusions are generally recommended only for PC < 50K, ICH is so serious that a suggestion is to keep PC > 75K
         b. patients on platelet inhibiting drugs (e.g. aspirin or Plavix®) should receive platelets
         c. when needed: start with 6 units of platelets (see *Platelets* on page 19)
   B. bleeding time: not generally helpful
   C. ★ hemostatic agents: NovoSeven® (recombinant activated coagulation factor VII (**rFVIIa**)) given IV within 4 hours of onset[104] reduces risk of clot enlargement on CT, and 90 day morbidity & mortality, with a small increase in thromboembolic complications (MI, CVA…). For details, *see below*. **Rx** studied: 40, 80 & 160 µg/kg IV over 1-2 minutes
5. steroids: controversial. No benefit from dexamethasone in ICH, with significantly more complications (primarily infectious, GI bleeding and diabetogenic)[105]. Consider use if significant peri-hemorrhage edema on imaging (suggested dosage[106]: 4 mg dexamethasone IV q 6 hrs, tapered over 7-14 days)
6. treat intracranial hypertension presumptively: mannitol and/or furosemide as tolerated, also helps with HTN (for more, see *ICP treatment measures*, page 655) If significant problems from suspected increased ICP, consider ICP monitor
7. follow electrolytes and osmolarity
   A. aggressively treat hyperglycemia (insulin drip if problematic)
   B. watch for SIADH
8. **angiography**: primarily to R/O underlying vascular malformation, but also to R/O aneurysm (a less common cause of ICH), and tumor (which is usually better diagnosed on contrast CT or MRI)
   A. if urgent surgery is indicated (e.g. for herniation), the delay in obtaining an angiogram may be detrimental and it may be best deferred to post-op
   B. ★ indications: angiography is recommended except for patients > 45 yrs of age with preexisting hypertension and ICH in thalamus, putamen or posterior fossa due to a 0% yield out of 29 patients in this group[107] and low yield in all patients with isolated deep ICH[108]

Table 29-5 ICH score[102]

Feature	Finding	Points
GCS (Glasgow Coma Scale score)	3-4	2
	5-12	1
	13-15	0
Age*	≥ 80 years	1
	< 80	0
Location	infratentorial	1
	supratentorial	0
ICH volume†	≥ 30 cc	1
	< 30 cc	0
Intraventricular blood	yes	1
	no	0
"ICH Score" = Total Points		0-6

* possible bias since treatment decisions in elderly patients may have differed from younger patients

† to estimate volume *see Eq 29-1*

ICH Score	30 day mortality	
0	0%	(26 pts)
1	13%	(32 pts)
2	26%	(27 pts)
3	72%	(32 pts)
4	97%	(29 pts)
5	100%	(6 pts)
6	≈ 100%*	(0 pts)

* no pt. in the study had a score of 6, but it is expected this would be associated with mortality

---

A. a study of 8 ICHs showed autoregulation was maintained, but with an elevated lower limit. However, CBF fell when MAP was lowered (using Arfonad) below the usual MAP, which averaged 80% of the admission MAP (admission HTN followed the ICH)[103]

1. patients > 45 yrs with HTN and a <u>lobar</u> ICH: angiography had a 10% yield[107], with the ratio of AVM:aneurysm ≈ 4.3:1
2. patients with intraventricular hemorrhage (without parenchymal hematoma): the yield of angiography was ≈ 65%[107], primarily AVM

C. an underlying lesion may be obliterated by ICH, especially acutely. If initial angio is negative, repeat after CT shows resorption of clot (≈ in 2-3 mos). If still negative, follow CT or MRI q 4–6 mos for ≈ 1 year to R/O tumor[26]. Delaying the initial angiogram for several weeks may increase the yield and is also an option[12]

D. MRI/MRA has ≈ 90% sensitivity for detecting structural abnormalities in this setting, and so a negative study cannot completely exclude this[107]

E. the yield of angiography in ICH would be expected to be lower in patients at increased risk of ICH: patients on warfarin, chronic alcoholics, patients with amyloid angiopathy…

NovoSeven® (recombinant activated coagulation factor VII (rFVIIa))

At the site of a tissue factor bearing cell, rFVIIa forms a complex with tissue factor resulting in thrombin production. It also converts factor X to its active form, Xa on the surface of activated platelets resulting in a "thrombin burst" at the site of damage[109]. Half life: 2.6 hrs. Expensive (≈ $10,000 per dose).

FDA approved to treat bleeding in patients with various bleeding diatheses (including hemophiliacs with antibodies to factor VIII or IX). Has been studied "off label" for ICH[104] in doses of 40, 80 & 160 µg/kg. There was a dose-related reduction in mean increase of ICH volume at 24 hrs, and thrombotic complications also increased

ANTICOAGULATION FOLLOWING ICH

Patients with ICH who require anticoagulation pose a management dilemma. In the case of embolic disease, the fear of extending an ICH or of converting it to a hematoma has traditionally outweighed the possible benefit of protection from further embolization. However, an anecdotal (retrospective uncontrolled) report of 12 such patients found no incidence of increased intracranial bleeding with either continued anticoagulation (6 patients) or resumption of anticoagulation after an hiatus (several days in 4 patients, 5 days in 1, and 14 days in 1)[110]. In another study[111] none of 35 patients who had resumption of warfarin had recurrent intracranial hemorrhage (ICH, SAH or subdural hematoma). While this does not prove that anticoagulation is safe after intracranial hemorrhage, it does demonstrate that if there is a strong indication for anticoagulation, and if there is not an acceptable alternative (e.g. Greenfield filter for DVT), that anticoagulation following in this setting is not always met with disastrous results.

The probability of having an ischemic stroke at 30 days following cessation of warfarin for a median of 10 days are approximately 2.9% for patients who had originally been treated with warfarin for prosthetic heart valves, 2.6% for those treated for atrial fibrillation, and 4.8% for those treated for cardioembolic stroke[111] ᴬ (see *Cardiogenic brain embolism*, page 773 for more details).

Recommendation

1-2 weeks off anticoagulation with **mechanical heart valves** (to observe ICH, or to evacuate a SDH or clip an aneurysm)[111, 114]. Patients requiring hemodialysis after ICH may have heparin-free dialysis.

SURGICAL TREATMENT

INDICATIONS

Amazingly, after continued attempts to penetrate this dilemma, considerable controversy persists regarding indications for surgery. Surgery may lower morbidity from rebleeding (especially if aneurysm or AVM are identified as the cause of the ICH), edema, or necrosis from mass effect of hematoma (unproven), but rarely causes neurologic improvement. Metaanalysis[115] yielded inconclusive results.

Randomized prospective studies (RPS) in the current CT/surgical era

One RPS[116] found lower mortality for patients with GCS 7-10 treated surgically ᴮ. However, survivors in this group were all severely disabled (none were independent).

A. these numbers may be gross underestimates as many patients died within 2 weeks, and follow-up imaging was scant[112]. Another study[113] showed a much higher rate of 20%

Another[106] found no benefit from surgery for <u>putaminal</u> hemorrhages, also with poor outcomes in all patients.

International STICH[117]: enrolled 1,033 patient, but had possible selection bias (the responsible neurosurgeon had to be uncertain of the benefits of medical vs. surgical treatment), "early surgery" had a somewhat long median time to treatment of 30 hours, and 26% of medically treated patients crossed over and had surgery at a mean of 60 hours. Given these limitations, the conclusion was that for supratentorial ICH there was no benefit of early surgery (although there may have been some benefit in the subgroup that a hematoma within 1 cm of the cortical surface). This trial may be viewed as a comparison of early vs. delayed surgery in patients subjectively judged to need surgery by the investigator.

A pilot study to investigate minimally invasive procedures (stereotactic instillation of tPA and then aspiration of the clot) is planned.

Conclusion

The decision to operate therefore must be individualized based on patient's neurologic condition, size and location of hematoma, patient's age, and the patient's and the family's wishes concerning "heroic" measures in the face of catastrophic illness.

Guidelines for considering surgery vs. medical management

(for separate indications for surgery for <u>cerebellar</u> hemorrhage, *see below*)

1. **NON-SURGICAL**: factors that favor medical management
    A. minimally symptomatic lesions: e.g. alert patient with subtle hemiparesis (especially patients with GCS > 10[116])
    B. situations with little chance of good outcome
        1. high ICH score (*see page 856*), which overlaps with the following
        2. massive hemorrhage with significant neuronal destruction (*see below*)
        3. large hemorrhage in dominant hemisphere
        4. poor neurologic condition: e.g. comatose with posturing (i.e. GCS ≤ 5), loss of brain stem function (fixed pupils, posturing...)
        5. ≈ age > 75 yrs: do not do well with surgery for this
    C. severe coagulopathy or other significant underlying medical disorder(s): in the event of herniation, rapid decompression may be considered in spite of the risks
    D. basal ganglion (putaminal) or thalamic hemorrhage: surgery is no better than medical management, and both have little to offer[106, 118] (*see below*)
2. **SURGICAL**: factors that favor rapid surgical removal of the blood clot
    A. lesions with marked mass effect, edema, or midline shift on imaging (removal is considered due to the potential for herniation)
    B. lesions where the symptoms (e.g. hemiparesis/plegia, aphasia, or sometimes just confusion or agitation...) appear to be due to increased ICP or to mass effect from the clot or surrounding edema. Symptoms attributable directly to brain injury from the hemorrhage are unlikely to be reversed by surgical evacuation
    C. **volume**: surgery for <u>moderate volume</u> hematomas (i.e. ≈ 10-30 cc) (see *Eq 29-1*, page 856) may be more appropriate than with:
        1. ✖ small clot (< 10 cc): mass effect is usually not significant
        2. ✖ large clot
            a. > 30 cc: associated with poor outcome (only 1 of 71 patients could function independently at 30 days[119])
            b. massive hemorrhage
                i. > 60 cc with GCS ≤ 8: 91% 30-day mortality[119]
                ii. > 85 cc (the volume of a sphere with a diameter of 5.5 cm): no patient survived, regardless of treatment in one series[120]
    D. persistent elevated ICP in spite of therapy (failure of medical management). Evacuating clot definitely lowers ICP, but the effect on outcome is uncertain
    E. rapid deterioration (especially with signs of brain stem compression) regardless of location
    F. favorable location, for example:
        1. lobar (as opposed to deep hemispheric): in spite of optimistic results in a non-randomized study done in 1983 indicating good outcomes in patients with deep hemorrhages treated with early surgery[60], a more re-

---

B. note: only 20% of these patients were operated on < 8 hrs from the bleed, and the mean time for all patients to operation was 14.5 hours (range: 6-48 hrs), which may be long

cent randomized study failed to confirm this benefit[106]
2. cerebellar: *see below*
3. external capsule
4. non-dominant hemisphere
G. young patient (especially age ≤ 50 yrs): they tolerate surgery better than elderly patients, and, unlike elderly patients with brain atrophy, they also have less room in the head to accommodate the mass effect of clot + edema
H. early intervention following hemorrhage: surgery after 24 hrs from onset of symptoms or deterioration is felt to be of little benefit[116]

Surgical indications for cerebellar hemorrhage: Recommendations[121]:
1. patients with a Glasgow Coma Scale **(GCS)** score ≥ 14 and hematoma < 4 cm diameter: treat conservatively
2. patients with GCS ≤ 13 or with a hematoma ≥ 4 cm: surgical evacuation
3. patients with absent brain stem reflexes and flaccid quadriplegia: intensive therapy is not indicated[A]
4. ventricular catheter for patients with hydrocephalus and no coagulopathy (caution: do not overdrain to avoid upward cerebellar herniation, *see page 160*). Most cases with hydrocephalus also require evacuation of the clot

VENTRICULOSTOMY *(IVC)* AKA EXTERNAL VENTRICULAR DRAINAGE *(EVD)*
May be used in patients with intraventricular extension of blood causing acute obstruction of the third ventricular outlet. In these cases, the IVC is usually placed in the lateral ventricle contralateral to the hemorrhage (to avoid putting the catheter directly in clot, which may obstruct the inlets). The prognosis for patients with a significant volume of intraventricular blood is poor. It may be difficult to maintain the patency of the catheter due to occlusion by clot, tissue plasminogen activator may help (*see below*).

Tissue plasminogen activator (rt-PA)
Intraventricular rt-PA may help lyse clot and maintain catheter patency or reopen a clotted catheter. No well-designed randomized study has been done; but anecdotal evidence suggests it is relatively safe. In cases of suspected aneurysm, AVM or other vascular malformation, it cannot be used until the source of bleeding has been corrected[123, 124].

Rx: 2-5 mg of rt-PA[123, 125, 126] in NS is administered through an intraventricular catheter **(IVC)**. The IVC is closed for 2 hours after injection[126]. Some centers have repeated the procedure daily up to 4 days PRN.

OUTCOME
Thalamic hemorrhages that tend to destroy the internal capsule **(IC)** are more likely to produce hemiplegia than hemorrhages lateral to the IC that compress but do not disrupt the IC.

Mortality: The chief cause of death is cerebral herniation[105], occurring mainly during the first week and mostly in patients with initial Glasgow Coma Scale scores ≤ 7. The in-hospital death rate decreased overall during the 1980s but increased for patients ≥ 65 years of age[127].

Quoted mortality rates vary widely, and depend on size and location of clot, age and medical condition of the patient, and etiology of the hemorrhage. Overall, the 30-day mortality rate is ≈ 44% for ICH[1], which is similar to that for SAH (≈ 46%). Patients with lobar hemorrhages (*see page 850*) tend to fare better than deep ICH (basal ganglion, thalamus...) with only ≈ 11% mortality in 26 patients[12].

A. some authors contend that the loss of brain stem reflexes from direct compression may not be irreversible[122], and that cerebellar hemorrhage represents a surgical emergency (and that the above criteria would thus deny potentially helpful surgery to some, *see page 772* for a discussion of cerebellar infarction and decompression)

29.2.   ICH in young adults

In a review of 72 patients age 15-45 yrs suffering nontraumatic ICH[128], a presumed cause was found in 76% (see Table 29-6). 3 patients had labor or post-partum hemorrhages (see page 852 and also Pregnancy & intracranial hemorrhage on page 825).

AVM: lobar hemorrhages in this age group are highly suggestive of AVM. Of 40 lobar hemorrhages, 37.5% were determined to be from AVMs[128].

Herpes simplex encephalitis: may produce hemorrhagic changes on CT, especially in the temporal lobes (see Herpes simplex encephalitis, page 225).

Drug abuse: especially with sympathomimetics such as cocaine (see page 852) should also be considered in young adults.

Leukemia: ICH may the initial presentation of leukemia in a young adult (may be due to metastases (chloroma) or to thrombocytopenia).

Table 29-6 Causes of spontaneous ICH in young adults[128]

Etiology	%
ruptured AVM	29.1%
arterial hypertension	15.3%
ruptured saccular aneurysm	9.7%
sympathomimetic drug abuse	6.9%
tumor*	4.2%
acute EtOH intoxication	2.8%
pre-eclampsia/eclampsia	2.8%
superior sagittal sinus thrombosis	1.4%
moyamoya	1.4%
cryoglobulinemia	1.4%
undetermined	23.6%

*   hemangioma, ependymoma, metastatic choriocarcinoma... (see Hemorrhagic brain tumors, page 854)

OUTCOME
Overall in-hospital survival (including those treated medically) was 87.5%.

29.3.   Intracerebral hemorrhage in the newborn

Occurs primarily in premature infants. AKA subependymal hemorrhage **(SEH)**, AKA germinal matrix hemorrhage **(GMH)**, AKA intraventricular hemorrhage **(IVH)** (IVH arises from extension of SEH through ependymal lining of ventricle and occurs in 80% of cases of SEH[129]).

ETIOLOGY

The highly vascular germinal matrix is part of the primordial tissue of the developing brain. It is located just beneath the ependymal lining of the lateral ventricles, and involutes around gestational weeks #32-34 which is normally prior to parturition. Thus, the matrix may persist out of utero in premature infants. A disproportionate amount of the total CBF perfuses the periventricular circulation through these capillaries which are immature and fragile and have impaired autoregulation[130, 131]. Most SEH/IVHs arise from matrix capillaries in the region of the head of the caudate nucleus, however, in preemies < 28 weeks gestation, hemorrhage may originate in the region of the body of the caudate, and in mature infants from the choroid plexus[129].

RISK FACTORS FOR SEH

Increased cerebral perfusion pressure **(CPP)** with the associated increased cerebral blood flow **(CBF)** are the common denominators for most risk factors for SEH. The elevated pressure may cause the hemorrhage by rupturing the fragile vessels of the germinal matrix, possibly already damaged by previous insults of high or fluctuating CBF.

Risk factors for SEH include[132]:
1. those associated primarily with increased CBF or CPP:
    A.   asphyxia: including hypercapnia (see below)
    B.   volume expansion
    C.   seizures
    D.   pneumothorax

E. cyanotic heart disease (including PDA)
F. infants being mechanically ventilated having RDS and fluctuating CBF velocity documented by Doppler flow meter[133]
2. extracorporeal membrane oxygenation (**ECMO**): due to heparinization in addition to increased CPP
3. maternal cocaine abuse[134]

Asphyxia is one of the most potent causes of increased CBF and is thus a major risk factor for SEH in the premature infant because:
1. hypertension occurs in asphyxia, and, since cerebral autoregulation is impaired in the premature infant, CBF increases with MAP
2. hypercapnia increases CBF
3. blood is shunted to the brain ("diving reflex")
4. elevated venous pressure due to myocardial failure from ischemia

EPIDEMIOLOGY

INCIDENCE
Depends on the method used for detection and the population being evaluated. Many SEHs are asymptomatic. Realistic incidence: **40-45%** of preemies < 1500 gm birth weight or < 35 weeks gestation (reported range varies from 35-90%). It is most common in infants < 32 weeks gestation.
ICH was found by CT in 43% (20/46) of preemies with birth-weight < 1500 gm; fatality among infants with IVH was 55%, without IVH 23%[135].
In one series, ultrasound (**U/S**) detected SEH in 90% of 113 preemies < 34 weeks gestation[136] (49% were grade III or IV, *see Table 29-7* for grading).

A substantial number occur within 6 hours of birth, 50% occur within 24 hours, and the majority (over 90%) occur in the first 72 hrs of life[137, 138]. Progression of hemorrhage has been documented in 10-20% of infants[138].

PREVENTION
Numerous studies have been conducted to find a method of directly reducing the incidence of SEH among premature infants. Many are controversial.
Measures used to treat other medical complications probably have more benefit indirectly in reducing SEH than those aimed directly at reducing SEH. In general, it is the sicker preemies that tend to have SEH. General measures include:
• indomethacin: increases arterial oxygenation by reducing patent ductus arteriosus (**PDA**) (although one study found no higher incidence of SEH with PDA[139]) and lowers CBF
• using surfactant to reduce RDS
• minimizing external stimulation (some centers use fentanyl drips)

CLINICAL
The most commonly used grading system of Papile et al. based on CT or U/S findings is shown in *Table 29-7*. SEH may present acutely, subacutely, or may be discovered incidentally e.g. as an accompaniment to hydrocephalus.

ACUTE PRESENTATION
SEH is usually heralded by a sudden neurologic deterioration.

It may be suspected clinically by:
• stupor
• changes in muscle tone or activity: usually decerebrate or decorticate posturing, sometimes flaccid paralysis
• seizures: actual seizures are rare in preemies
• tense fontanelle
• hypotension
• respiratory and cardiac irregularities ("**A's and B's**": apnea & bradycardia)

Table 29-7 Grading subependymal hemorrhage[135]

Grade	Description
I	subependymal
II	IVH without ventricular dilatation
III	IVH with ventricular dilatation
IV	IVH with parenchymal hemorrhage

- unreactive pupils and/or loss of extraocular muscle movements
- Hct drop > 10%
- elevated CSF protein and/or blood (latter usually not helpful)

SUBACUTE PRESENTATION
Usually smaller or more slowly developing hemorrhages, clinically may present as irritability, reduced motor activity, abnormal eye movements.

ASYMPTOMATIC HEMORRHAGE
Many ICHs will be clinically unsuspected, usually with smaller hemorrhages. These have a 78% 6-month survival, vs. 20% for those showing signs. Retrospectively, these SEHs may have been suggested by a fall in Hct or delays in neurologic development.

HYDROCEPHALUS
20-50% of infants with SEH will develop either transient or progressive hydrocephalus **(HCP)**. Grades III and IV are more often associated with progressive ventricular dilatation than are lower grades (however, HCP may develop even after low grade SEH[140]). Younger gestational age infants may be at lower risk.

Post SEH hydrocephalus usually occurs 1-3 weeks after the hemorrhage. Probably caused by cellular debris and/or the toxic effects of blood breakdown products on the arachnoid granulations (communicating HCP), or by an adhesive arachnoiditis in the posterior fossa or rarely by compression or blockage of critical pathways, e.g. at the sylvian aqueduct (obstructive HCP). In a case of HCP following intra-uterine SEH, aqueductal gliosis was found at autopsy[141].

Possible presentations
Abnormally increasing OFC (crossing percentile curves faster than body weight), lethargy, apnea and bradycardia, vomiting. There is progressive dilatation of the ventricular system on serial U/S or CT; if LP is done the OP is often > 120-140 mm CSF.

DIAGNOSIS

Ultrasound (U/S)
Performed through the open fontanelles[136]. Accuracy ≈ 88% (91% sensitivity, 85% specificity)[142]. U/S is invaluable because:
- it demonstrates the size of the ventricles, the location and size of the hematoma, and the thickness of the cortical mantle
- it may be brought to the infant's bedside (obviating transportation)
- it is non-invasive
- it is not adversely affected by occasional infant movements (eliminating the need for sedation)
- it does not expose the patient to radiation (radiation effects on the lens and other structures from serial CTs in the newborn is unknown)
- it may be followed serially with relative ease

CT scan
Sometimes necessary when U/S is not readily available, or in complicated cases where anatomy is difficult to deduce from U/S images.

TREATMENT
General measures are directed at optimizing CPP without further excessive elevation of CBF by carefully maintaining normal MAP and normalizing pCO_2, and by treating ventriculomegaly as outlined below.

While daily LPs can control the deleterious effects of posthemorrhagic HCP, they do not reduce the frequency of long-term HCP (requiring permanent shunting). Ventricular size must be monitored with serial U/S.

Ventriculomegaly
When detected, need to differentiate the following:
- transient ventriculomegaly: occurs in the first few days after SEH. This may not cause elevated ICP. As implied, it is self limited
- progressive ventriculomegaly: occurs in 20-50% of cases
- "hydrocephalus ex vacuo": due to loss of brain tissue or maldevelopment. Is not

progressive on serial U/S. OFCs may fall below normal due to lack of growing brain as stimulus for head growth

MEDICAL TREATMENT
- osmotic agents: isosorbide, glycerol. Effects are short-lived
- acetazolamide: a carbonic anhydrase inhibitor, slows production of CSF. Can cause electrolyte disturbances (see *acetazolamide (Diamox®)*, page 277)
- furosemide: decreases ICP by increasing serum osmolarity and by reducing CSF production. Can cause electrolyte disturbances

SURGICAL/INTERVENTIONAL TREATMENT
Due to poor operative results, surgical evacuation of an intracerebral hemorrhage in the newborn is not indicated with the possible exception of a posterior fossa hemorrhage causing brain stem compression that does not respond to medical treatment[143]. Supportive measures are usually in order.

For hemorrhages with intraventricular extension and communicating hydrocephalus (the usual type of HCP that occurs with SEH), management with **serial lumbar punctures**[144] is well accepted. Infants < 800 gm may not tolerate LPs because of desaturation when laying on their side, or the LP itself may be difficult. In these patients, consider 1-2 ventricular taps to at least obtain fluid for analysis (in some cases nothing further needs to be done).

Serial ventricular taps may be a viable short-term option for those infants who cannot tolerate LPs or in whom there is obstruction to CSF flow in the lumbar subarachnoid space (e.g. due to spinal subdural hematoma from previous LP). However it is not desirable for long-term use because of repeated trauma to brain (risk of porencephaly) and risk of intracerebral, intraventricular, or subdural hemorrhage.

If repeated taps are likely (i.e. large hemorrhage, or rapid recurrence of intracranial hypertension as determined by palpation of fullness of anterior fontanelle (**AF**) following several taps) the acceptable options include:
- continuing serial LPs
- placement of a ventricular catheter connected to a subcutaneous reservoir under the scalp for serial percutaneous taps. The favored option. May be converted to VP shunt if and when appropriate. Not recommended in infants < 1100 gms due to very high infection rate
- external ventricular drainage (**EVD**): similar to reservoir, but with possibility of inadvertent dislodgment (13%) and possibly higher rate of infection (6%)
- early VP shunting: high infection rate, peritoneal cavity not suitable in many cases, e.g. due to necrotizing enterocolitis (**NEC**), paucity of subcutaneous tissue through which to pass shunt tube... Not recommended for infants < 2500 gms

Serial taps (via ventricular reservoir or LP)
8-10 cc of fluid are removed initially, and this is repeated daily (or more often if AF become very tense before 24 hours elapse) for several days, and then usually varies from 5-10 cc qod to 15 cc TID depending on response. The frequency and volume of the taps are modified based on:
- fullness of AF: attempt to keep AF from becoming tense
- appearance of ventricles on serial U/S: strive to prevent progressive enlargement, reduction in size can usually be achieved
- follow OFC: should not cross percentile curves (need to differentiate from the so-called "**catch-up phase**" of brain growth which may occur once the infant overcomes their overall medical problems and is able to adequately utilize nutrition[145, 146]; serial U/S will show rapid brain growth without progressive ventriculomegaly in cases of catch-up brain growth)
- CSF protein concentration: controversial. Diminishes with serial taps. Some feel that as long as it is ≥ 100 mg/dl it is unlikely that significant spontaneous resorption will occur and continued serial taps will probably be needed
- NB: removal of this volume of fluid may cause electrolyte disturbances, primarily hyponatremia; follow serum electrolytes on regular basis

Follow with serial U/S on day 3-5, and then weekly for several weeks, and then biweekly. A baseline CT scan is often obtained when the patient is stable, and may be repeated PRN, e.g. if OFC crosses percentile curves.

Insertion of VP shunt or conversion of sub-Q reservoir to VP shunt
Indications and requirements:
1. symptomatic hydrocephalus (see *Hydrocephalus*, page 863) and/or progressive

ventriculomegaly
2. infant is extubated (and thus off ventilator)
3. infant weighs ≥ 2500 grams
4. no evidence of NEC (might create problems with peritoneal end of catheter)
5. CSF protein ideally < 100 mg/dl (because of concerns about plugging of the shunt, or causing ileus or malabsorption of the fluid[A], and also to see if patient will start reabsorbing CSF on their own)

Technical recommendations:
1. do not tap reservoir for at least 24 hrs before inserting a new ventricular catheter (allows ventricles to expand to facilitate catheterization)
2. obtain U/S the day prior to conversion
3. use a low or very-low pressure system (if CSF protein is high, consider a valveless system), upgrade later in infancy if necessary
4. avoid placing shunt hardware in areas on which these debilitated infants tend to lay (to prevent skin breakdown with hardware exposure)

OUTCOME

Short-term
Preemies with SEH have higher mortality than matched preemies without SEH.

The incidence of mortality and progression of hemorrhage is higher the earlier the hemorrhage occurs. The more severe the hemorrhage, the higher the mortality and the higher the risk of HCP (*see Table 29-8*).

Table 29-8 Short-term outcome of SEH (≈ 250 cases[129])

Severity of hemorrhage	Deaths (%)	Progressive hydrocephalus (%)
mild	0	0-10
moderate	5-15	15-25
severe	50-65	65-100

Long-term
The effect of low grade SEH on long-term neurodevelopment has not been studied well. Most investigators feel that higher grades of SEH are associated with greater degrees of handicaps than matched controls.

In one study of 12 infants with Grade II SEH treated with serial LPs and in the 7 with progressive ventriculomegaly with VP shunt followed for a mean of 4.5 years found all were ambulatory and 75% had IQ within normal range[148].

29.4. References

1. Broderick J P, Brott T G, Tomsick T, et al.. Intracerebral hemorrhage more than twice as common as subarachnoid hemorrhage. J Neurosurg 78: 188-91, 1993.
2. Gorelick P B, Kelly M A: Ethanol. In **Intracerebral hemorrhage**, Feldman E, (ed.). Futura Publishing Co., Armonk, New York, 1994, Chapter 9: pp 195-208.
3. Camargo C A: Moderate alcohol consumption and stroke: The epidemiological evidence. Stroke 20: 1611-26, 1989.
4. Juvela S, Hillbom M, Palomäki H: Risk factors for spontaneous intracerebral hemorrhage. Stroke 26: 1558-64, 1995.
5. Feldman E, (ed.) **Intracerebral hemorrhage**. Futura Publishing Co., Armonk, NY, 1994.
6. Monforte R, Estruch R, Graus F, et al.: High ethanol consumption as risk factor for intracerebral hemorrhage in young and middle-aged people. Stroke 21: 1529-32, 1990.
7. Shinton R, Beevers G: Meta-analysis of relation between cigarette smoking and stroke. Br Med J 298: 789-94, 1989.
8. Fogelholm R, Murros K: Cigarette smoking and risk of primary intracerebral hemorrhage: A population-
based case-control study. Acta Neurol Scand 87: 367-70, 1993.
9. Gorelick P B: Stroke from alcohol and drug abuse. A current social peril. Postgrad Med 88: 171-8, 1990.
10. Niizuma H, Shimizu Y, Nakasato N, et al.: Influence of liver dysfunction on volume of putaminal hemorrhage. Stroke 19: 987-90, 1988.
11. Schmidek H H, Sweet W H, (eds.): **Operative neurosurgical techniques**. 1st ed., Grune and Stratton, New York, 1982.
12. Ropper A H, Davis K R: Lobar cerebral hemorrhages: Acute clinical syndromes in 26 cases. Ann Neurol 8: 141-7, 1980.
13. Caplan L: Intracerebral hemorrhage revisited. Neurology 38: 624-7, 1988 (editorial).
14. Caplan L R, Skillman J, Ojemann R, et al.: Intracerebral hemorrhage following carotid endarterectomy: A hypertensive complication. Stroke 9: 457-60, 1979.
15. Bernstein M, Fleming J F R, Deck J H N: Cerebral hyperperfusion after carotid endarterectomy: A cause of cerebral hemorrhage. Neurosurgery 15: 50-6, 1984.
16. Humphreys R P, Hoffman H J, Mustard W T, et al.:

A. which was not seen with high protein fluid shunted from the subdural space[147]

Cerebral hemorrhage following heart surgery. **J Neurosurg** 43: 671-5, 1975.

17. Fisher C M, Adams R D: Observations on brain embolism with special reference to the mechanism of hemorrhagic infarction. **J Neuropathol Exp Neurol** 10: 92-3, 1951.

18. Hornig C R, Dorndorf W, Agnoli A L: Hemorrhagic cerebral infarction: A prospective study. **Stroke** 17: 179-85, 1986.

19. Okada Y, Yamaguchi T, Minematsu K, et al.: Hemorrhagic transformation in cerebral embolism. **Stroke** 20: 598-603, 1989.

20. Bogousslavsky J, Regli F, Uske A, et al.: Early spontaneous hematoma in cerebral infarct: Is primary cerebral hemorrhage overdiagnosed? **Neurology** 41: 837-40, 1991.

21. Cerebral Embolism Study Group: Cardioembolic stroke, early anticoagulation, and brain hemorrhage. **Arch Intern Med** 147: 626-30, 1987.

22. Raabe A, Krug U: Migraine associated bilateral intracerebral hemorrhages. **Clin Neurol Neurosurg** 101: 193-5, 1999.

23. Cole A, Aube M: Late-onset migraine with intracerebral hemorrhage: A recognizable syndrome. **Neurology** 37S1: 238, 1987 (abstract).

24. Lee K-C, Clough C: Intracerebral hemorrhage after break dancing. **N Engl J Med** 323: 615-6, 1990 (letter).

25. Caplan L R, Neely S, Gorelick P: Cold-related intracerebral hemorrhage. **Arch Neurol** 41: 227, 1984.

26. Ojemann R G, Heros R C: Spontaneous brain hemorrhage. **Stroke** 14: 468-75, 1983.

27. Rosenblum W I: Miliary aneurysms and 'fibrinoid' degeneration of cerebral blood vessels. **Hum Pathol** 8: 133-9, 1977.

28. Fisher C M: Pathological observations in hypertensive cerebral hemorrhage. **J Neuropathol Exp Neurol** 30: 536-50, 1971.

29. The National Institute of Neurological Disorders and Stroke rt-PA Stroke Study Group: Tissue plasminogen activator for acute ischemic stroke. **N Engl J Med** 333: 1581-7, 1995.

30. Aldrich M S, Sherman S A, Greenberg H S: Cerebrovascular complications of streptokinase infusion. **JAMA** 253: 1777-9, 1985.

31. Maggioni A P, Franzosi M G, Santoro E, et al.: The risk of stroke in patients with acute myocardial infarction after thrombolytic and antithrombotic treatment. **N Engl J Med** 327: 1-6, 1992.

32. Grines C L, Browne K F, Marco J, et al.: A comparison of immediate angioplasty with thrombolytic therapy for acute myocardial infarction. **N Engl J Med** 328: 673-9, 1993.

33. Public Health Service: Approval of thrombolytic agents. **FDA Drug Bull** 18: 6-7, 1988.

34. Mehta S R, Eikelboom J W, Yusuf S: Risk of intracranial hemorrhage with bolus versus infusion thrombolytic therapy: A meta-analysis. **Lancet** 356: 449-54, 2000.

35. Tenecteplase (TNKase) for thrombolysis. **Med Letter** 42: 106-8, 2000.

36. DaSilva V F, Bormanis J: Intracerebral hemorrhage after combined anticoagulant-thrombolytic therapy for myocardial infarction: Two case reports and a short review. **Neurosurgery** 30: 943-5, 1992.

37. The Steering Committee of the Physician's Health Study Group: Preliminary report: Findings from the aspirin component of the ongoing physician's health study. **N Engl J Med** 318: 262-4, 1988.

38. Blackshear J L, Kopecky S L, Litin S C, et al.: Management of atrial fibrillation in adults: Prevention of thromboembolism and symptomatic treatment. **Mayo Clin Proc** 71: 150-60, 1996.

39. Lowenstein D H, Collins S D, Massa S M, et al.: The neurologic complications of cocaine abuse. **Neurology** 37S1: 195, 1987 (abstract).

40. Levine S: Cocaine and stroke. Current concepts of cerebrovascular disease. **Stroke** 22: 25-9, 1987.

41. Harrington H, Heller A, Dawson D, et al.: Intracerebral hemorrhage and oral amphetamines. **Arch Neurol** 40: 503-7, 1983.

42. Kase C S, Foster T E, Reed J E, et al.: Intracerebral hemorrhage and phenylpropanolamine use. **Neurology** 37: 399-404, 1987.

43. Kernan W N, Viscoli C M, Brass L M, et al.: Phenylpropanolamine and the risk of hemorrhagic stroke. **N Engl J Med** 343: 1826-32, 2000.

44. Bruno A, Nolte K B, Chapin J: Stroke associated with ephedrine use. **Neurology** 43: 1313-6, 1993.

45. Stoessl A J, Young G B, Feasby T E: Intracerebral hemorrhage and angiographic beading following ingestion of catechoaminergics. **Stroke** 16: 734-6, 1985.

46. Phenylpropanolamine and other OTC alpha-adrenergic agonists. **Med Letter** 42: 113, 2000.

47. Haller C A, Benowitz N L: Adverse cardiovascular and central nervous system events associated with dietary supplements containing ephedra alkaloids. **N Engl J Med** 343: 1833-8, 2000.

48. Gudeman S K, Kishore P R, Miller J D, et al.: The genesis and significance of delayed traumatic intracerebral hematoma. **Neurosurgery** 5: 309-13, 1979.

49. Young H A, Gleave J R W, Schmidek H H, et al.: Delayed traumatic intracerebral hematoma: Report of 15 cases operatively treated. **Neurosurgery** 14: 22-5, 1984.

50. Wang K C, Chen C P, Yang Y C, et al.: Stroke complicating pregnancy and the puerperium. **Zhonghua Yi Xue Za Zhi (Taipei)** 62 (1): 13-9, 1999.

51. Salerni A, Wald S, Flannagan M: Relationships among cortical ischemia, infarction, and hemorrhage in eclampsia. **Neurosurgery** 22: 408-10, 1988.

52. Witlin A G, Mattar F, Sibai B M: Postpartum stroke: A twenty-year experience. **Am J Obstet Gynecol** 183 (1): 83-8, 2000.

53. Geocadin R G, Razumovsky A Y, Wityk R J, et al.: Intracerebral hemorrhage and postpartum cerebral vasculopathy. **J Neurol Sci** 205 (1): 29-34, 2002.

54. Kalfas I H, Little J R: Postoperative hemorrhage: A survey of 4992 intracranial procedures. **Neurosurgery** 23: 343-7, 1988.

55. Papanastassiou V, Kerr R, Adams C: Contralateral cerebellar hemorrhagic infarction after pterional craniotomy: Report of five cases and review of the literature. **Neurosurgery** 39: 841-52, 1996.

56. Toczek M T, Morrell M J, Silverberg G A, et al.: Cerebellar hemorrhage complicating temporal lobectomy: Report of four cases. **J Neurosurg** 85: 718-22, 1996.

57. Brott T, Thalinger K, Hertzberg V: Hypertension as a risk factor for spontaneous intracerebral hemorrhage. **Stroke** 17: 1078-83, 1986.

58. Wakai S, Nagai M: Histological verification of microaneurysms as a cause of cerebral hemorrhage in surgical specimens. **J Neurol Neurosurg Psychiatry** 52: 595-9, 1989.

59. Newton T H, Potts D G, (eds.): **Radiology of the skull and brain.** C. V. Mosby, Saint Louis, 1971.

60. Kaneko M, Tanaka K, Shimada T, et al.: Long-term evaluation of ultra-early operation for hypertensive intracerebral hemorrhage in 100 cases. **J Neurosurg** 58: 838-42, 1983.

61. Gilles C, Brucher J M, Khoubesserian P, et al.: Cerebral amyloid angiopathy as a cause of multiple intracerebral hemorrhages. **Neurology** 34: 730-5, 1984.

62. Mandybur T I: Cerebral amyloid angiopathy: The vascular pathology and complications. **J Neuropathol Exp Neurol** 45: 79-90, 1986.

63. Vonsattel J P, Myers R H, Hedley-White E T, et al.: Cerebral amyloid angiopathy without and with cerebral hemorrhages: A comparative histological study. **Ann Neurol** 30: 637-49, 1991.

64. Kase C S: *Cerebral amyloid angiopathy*. In **Intracerebral hemorrhage**, Kase C S and Caplan L R, (eds.). Butterworth-Heinemann, Boston, 1994: pp 179-200.

65. Greenberg S M, Briggs M E, Hyman B T, *et al*.: Apolipoprotein E ε4 is associated with the presence and earlier onset of hemorrhage in cerebral amyloid angiopathy. **Stroke** 27: 1333-7, 1996.

66. Vinters H V, Gilbert J J: Amyloid angiopathy: Its incidence and complications in the aging brain. **Stroke** 12: 118, 1981 (abstract).

67. Greenberg S M, Rebeck G W, Vonsattel J P V, *et al*.: Apolipoprotein E ε4 and cerebral hemorrhage associated with amyloid angiopathy. **Ann Neurol** 38: 254-9, 1995.

68. Kingston I B, Castro M J, Anderson S: In vitro stimulation of tissue-type plasminogen activator by Alzheimer amyloid beta-peptide analogues. **Nature Med** 1: 138-42, 1995.

69. Greenberg S M, Edgar M A: Cerebral hemorrhage in a 69-year old woman receiving warfarin. Case records of the Massachusetts general hospital. Case 22-1996. **N Engl J Med** 335: 189-6, 1996.

70. Scott M: Spontaneous intracerebral hematoma caused by cerebral neoplasms. **J Neurosurg** 42: 338-42, 1975.

71. Dublin A B, Norman D. Fluid-fluid level in cystic cerebral metastatic melanoma. **J Comput Assist Tomogr** 3: 650-2, 1979.

72. Acosta-Sison H: Extensive cerebral hemorrhage caused by the rupture of a cerebral blood vessel due to a chorionepithelioma embolus. **Am J Ob Gyn** 71: 1119, 1956.

73. Weir B, MacDonald N, Mielke B: Intracranial vascular complications of choriocarcinoma. **Neurosurgery** 2: 138, 1978.

74. Weinstein Z R, Downey E F: Spontaneous hemorrhage in medulloblastomas. **AJNR** 4: 986-8, 1983.

75. McCormick W F, Ugajin K: Fatal hemorrhage into a medulloblastoma. **J Neurosurg** 26: 78-81, 1967.

76. Chugani H T, Rosemblat A M, Lavenstein B L, *et al*.: Childhood medulloblastoma presenting with hemorrhage. **Childs Brain** 11: 135-40, 1984.

77. Zee C S, Segall H D, Miller C, *et al*.: Less common CT features of medulloblastoma. **Radiology** 144: 97-102, 1982.

78. Oldberg E: Hemorrhage into gliomas. **Arch Neurol Psych** 30: 1061-73, 1933.

79. Richardson R R, Siqueira E B, Cerullo L J: Malignant glioma: Its initial presentation as intracranial hemorrhage. **Acta Neurochir** 46: 77-84, 1979.

80. Nakao S, Sato S, Ban S, *et al*.: Massive intracerebral hemorrhage caused by angioblastic meningioma. **Surg Neurol** 7: 245-7, 1977.

81. Modesti L M, Binet E F, Collins G H: Meningiomas causing spontaneous intracranial hematomas. **J Neurosurg** 45: 437-41, 1976.

82. Goran A, Ciminello V J, Fisher R G: Hemorrhage into meningiomas. **Arch Neurol** 13: 65-9, 1965.

83. Cabezudo-Artero, Areito-Cebrecos, Vaquero-Crespo J: Hemorrhage associated with meningioma. **J Neurol Neurosurg Psych** 44: 456, 1981 (letter).

84. Little J R, Dial B, Belanger G, *et al*.: Brain hemorrhage from intracranial tumor. **Stroke** 10: 283-8, 1979.

85. Wakai S, Inoh S, Ueda Y, *et al*.: Hemangioblastoma presenting with intraparenchymatous hemorrhage. **J Neurosurg** 61: 956-60, 1984.

86. McCoyd K, Barron K D, Cassidy R J: Acoustic neurinoma presenting as subarachnoid hemorrhage. **J Neurosurg** 41: 391-3, 1974.

87. Gleeson R K, Butzer J F, Grin O D: Acoustic neurinoma presenting as subarachnoid hemorrhage. **J Neurosurg** 49: 602-4, 1978.

88. Yonemitsu T, Niizuna H, Kodama N, *et al*.: Acoustic neurinoma presenting as subarachnoid hemorrhage. **Surg Neurol** 20: 125-30, 1983.

89. Vincent F M, Bartone J R, Jones M Z: Cerebellar astrocytoma presenting as a cerebellar hemorrhage in a child. **Neurology** 30: 91-3, 1980.

90. Kawamata T, Takeshita M, Kubo O, *et al*.: Management of intracranial hemorrhage associated with anticoagulant therapy. **Surg Neurol** 44: 438-43, 1995.

91. Fihn S D, McDonell M, Martin D, *et al*.: Risk factors for complications of chronic anticoagulation: A multicenter study. **Ann Intern Med** 118: 511-20, 1993.

92. Smith D B, Hitchcock M, Philpot P J: Cerebral amyloid angiopathy presenting as transient ischemic attacks: Case report. **J Neurosurg** 63: 963-4, 1985.

93. Greenberg S M, Vonsattel J P, Stakes J W, *et al*.: The clinical spectrum of cerebral amyloid angiopathy: Presentations without lobar hemorrhage. **Neurology** 43: 2073-9, 1993.

94. Broderick J P, Brott T G, Tomsick T, *et al*.: Ultra-early evaluation of intracerebral hemorrhage. **J Neurosurg** 72: 195-9, 1990.

95. Brott T, Broderick J, Kothari R, *et al*.: Early hemorrhage growth in patients with intracerebral hemorrhage. **Stroke** 28 (1): 1-5, 1997.

96. Fujii Y, Tanaka R, Takeuchi S, *et al*.: Hematoma enlargement in spontaneous intracerebral hemorrhage. **J Neurosurg** 80: 51-7, 1994.

97. Arakawa S, Saku Y, Ibayashi S, *et al*.: Blood pressure control and recurrence of hypertensive brain hemorrhage. **Stroke** 29: 1806-9, 1998.

98. Gonzalez-Duarte A, Cantu C, Ruiz-Sandoval J L, *et al*.: Recurrent primary cerebral hemorrhage: Frequency, mechanisms, and prognosis. **Stroke** 29: 1802-5, 1998.

99. Bradley W G: MR appearance of hemorrhage in the brain. **Radiology** 189: 15-26, 1993.

100. Taveras J M, Gilson J M, Davis D O, *et al*.: Angiography in cerebral infarction. **Radiology** 93: 549-58, 1969.

101. Toffol G J, Biller J, Adams H P, *et al*.: The predicted value of arteriography in nontraumatic intracerebral hemorrhage. **Stroke** 17: 881-3, 1986.

102. Hemphill J C, 3rd, Bonovich D C, Besmertis L, *et al*.: The ich score: A simple, reliable grading scale for intracerebral hemorrhage. **Stroke** 32 (4): 891-7, 2001.

103. Kaneko T, Sawada T, Niimi T, *et al*.: Lower limit of blood pressure in treatment of acute hypertensive intracranial hemorrhage. **J Cereb Blood Flow Metab** 3S1: S51-2, 1983.

104. Mayer S A, Brun N C, Begtrup K, *et al*.: Recombinant activated factor VII for acute intracerebral hemorrhage. **N Engl J Med** 352 (8): 777-85, 2005.

105. Poungvarin N, Bhoopat W, Viriyavejakul A, *et al*.: Effects of dexamethasone in primary supratentorial intracerebral hemorrhage. **N Engl J Med** 316: 1229-33, 1987.

106. Batjer H H, Reisch J S, Plaizier L J, *et al*.: Failure of surgery to improve outcome in hypertensive putaminal hemorrhage: A prospective randomized trial. **Arch Neurol** 47: 1103-6, 1990.

107. Zhu X L, Chan M S Y, Poon W S: Spontaneous intracranial hemorrhage: Which patients need diagnostic cerebral angiography? A prospective study of 206 cases and review of the literature. **Stroke** 28: 1406-9, 1997.

108. Laissy J P, Normand G, Monroc M, *et al*.: Spontaneous intracerebral hematomas from vascualr causes: Predictive value of CT compared with angiography. **Neuroradiology** 33: 291-5, 1991.

109. Hoffman M, Monroe D M, 3rd: A cell-based model of hemostasis. **Thromb Haemost** 85 (6): 958-65, 2001.

110. Pessin M S, Estol C J, Lafranchise F, *et al*.: Safety of anticoagulation after hemorrhagic infarction. **Neurology** 43: 1298-1303, 1993.

111. Phan T G, Koh M, Wijdicks E F: Safety of discontinuation of anticoagulation in patients with intra-

cranial hemorrhage at high thromboembolic risk. **Arch Neurol** 57: 1710-3, 2000.

112. Hacke W: The dilemma of reinstituting anticoagulation for patients with cardioembolic sources and intracranial hemorrhage: How wide is the strait between skylla and karybdis? **Arch Neurol** 57: 1682-4, 2000 (editorial).

113. Bertram M, Bonsanto M, Hacke W, *et al.*: Managing the therapeutic dilemma: Patients with spontaneous intracerebral hemorrhage and urgent need for anticoagulation. **J Neurol** 247: 209-14, 2000.

114. Wijdicks E F, Schievink W I, Brown R D, *et al.*: The dilemma of discontinuation of anticoagulation therapy for patients with intracranial hemorrhage and mechanical heart valves. **Neurosurgery** 42: 769-73, 1998.

115. Hankey G J, Hon C: Surgery for primary intracerebral hemorrhage: Is it safe and effective? A systematic review of case series and randomized trials. **Stroke** 28: 2126-32, 1997.

116. Juvela S, Heiskanen O, Poranen A, *et al.*: The treatment of spontaneous intracerebral hemorrhage: A prospective randomized trial of surgical and conservative treatment. **J Neurosurg** 70: 755-8, 1989.

117. Mendelow A D, Gregson B A, Fernandes H M, *et al.*: Early surgery versus initial conservative treatment in patients with spontaneous supratentorial intracerebral haematomas in the international surgical trial in intracerebral haemorrhage (stich): A randomised trial. **Lancet** 365 (9457): 387-97, 2005.

118. Waga S, Miyazaki M, Okada M, *et al.*: Hypertensive putaminal hemorrhage: Analysis of 182 patients. **Surg Neurol** 26: 159-66, 1986.

119. Broderick J P, Brott T G, Duldner J E, *et al.*: Volume of intracerebral hemorrhage. A powerful and easy-to-use predictor of 30-day mortality. **Stroke** 24 (7): 987-93, 1993.

120. Volpin L, Cervellini P, Colombo F, *et al.*: Spontaneous intracerebral hematomas: A new proposal about the usefulness and limits of surgical treatment. **Neurosurgery** 15: 663-6, 1984.

121. Kobayashi S, Sato A, Kageyama Y, *et al.*: Treatment of hypertensive cerebellar hemorrhage - surgical or conservative management. **Neurosurgery** 34: 246-51, 1994.

122. Heros R C: Surgical treatment of cerebellar infarction. **Stroke** 23: 937-8, 1992.

123. Findlay J M, Grace M G A, Weir B K A: Treatment of intraventricular hemorrhage with tissue plasminogen activator. **Neurosurgery** 32: 941-7, 1993.

124. Engelhard H H, Andrews C O, Slavin K V, *et al.*: Current management of intraventricular hemorrhage. **Surg Neurol** 60 (1): 15-21; discussion 21-2, 2003.

125. Grabb P A: Traumatic intraventricular hemorrhage treated with intraventricular recombinant-tissue plasminogen activator: Technical case report. **Neurosurgery** 43: 966-9, 1998.

126. Rohde V, Schaller C, Hassler W E: Intraventricular recombinant tissue plasminogen activator for lysis of intraventricular hemorrhage. **J Neurol Neurosurg Psychiatry** 58: 447-51, 1995.

127. Chyatte D, Easley K, Brass L M: Increasing hospital admission rates for intracerebral hemorrhage during the last decade. **J Stroke Cerebrovasc Dis** 6: 354-60, 1997.

128. Toffol G J, Biller J, Adams H P: Nontraumatic intracerebral hemorrhage in young adults. **Arch Neurol** 44: 483-5, 1987.

129. Volpe J J: Neonatal intraventricular hemorrhage. **N Engl J Med** 304: 886-91, 1981.

130. Lou H C, Lassen N A, Friis-Hansen B: Impaired autoregulation of cerebral blood flow in the distressed newborn infant. **J Pediatr** 94: 118-21, 1979.

131. Milligan D W A: Failure of autoregulation and intraventricular hemorrhage in preterm infants. **Lancet** 1: 896-8, 1980.

132. Dykes F D, Lazzara A, Ahmann P, *et al.*: Intraventricular hemorrhage: A prospective evaluation of etiopathologies. **Pediatrics** 66: 42-9, 1980.

133. Perlman J M, McMenamin J B, Volpe J J: Fluctuating cerebral blood-flow velocity in respiratory distress syndrome. **N Engl J Med** 309: 204-9, 1983.

134. Volpe J J: Effect of cocaine use on the fetus. **N Engl J Med** 327: 399-407, 1992.

135. Papile L A, Burstein J, Burstein R, *et al.*: Incidence and evolution of subependymal and intraventricular hemorrhage: A study of infants with birth weights less than 1,500 gm. **J Pediatr** 92: 529-34, 1978.

136. Bejar R, Curbelo V, Coen R W, *et al.*: Diagnosis and follow-up of intraventricular and intracerebral hemorrhages by ultrasound studies of infant's brain through the fontanelles and sutures. **Pediatrics** 66: 661-73, 1980.

137. Tsiantos A, Victorin L, Relier J P, *et al.*: Intracranial hemorrhage in the prematurely born infant. **J Pediatr** 85: 854-9, 1974.

138. Perlman J M, Volpe J J: Cerebral blood flow velocity in relation to intraventricular hemorrhage in the premature newborn infant. **J Pediatr** 100: 956-9, 1982.

139. Ment L R, Duncan C C, Ehrenkranz R A, *et al.*: Intraventricular hemorrhage in the preterm neonate: Timing and cerebral blood flow changes. **J Pediatr** 104: 419-25, 1984.

140. Fishman M A, Dutton R Y, Okumura S: Progressive ventriculomegaly following minor intracranial hemorrhage in premature infants. **Dev Med Child Neurol** 26: 725-31, 1984.

141. Hill A, Rozdilsky B: Congenital hydrocephalus secondary to intra-uterine germinal matrix/intraventricular hemorrhage. **Dev Med Child Neurol** 26: 509-27, 1984.

142. Trounce J Q, Fagan D, Levene M I: Intraventricular hemorrhage and periventricular leucomalacia: Ultrasound and autopsy correlation. **Arch Dis Child** 61: 1203-7, 1983.

143. Rom S, Serfontein G L, Humphreys R P: Intracerebellar hematoma in the neonate. **J Pediatr** 93: 486-8, 1978.

144. Kreusser K L, Tarby T J, Kovnar E, *et al.*: Serial lumbar punctures for at least temporary amelioration of neonatal posthemorrhagic hydrocephalus. **Pediatrics** 75: 719, 1985.

145. Bridgers S L, Ment L R: Absence of hydrocephalus despite disproportionately increasing head size after the neonatal period in preterm infants with known intraventricular hemorrhage. **Childs Brain** 8: 423-6, 1981.

146. Sher P K, Brown S A: A longitudinal study of head growth in preterm infants: II. Differentiation between 'catch-up' head-growth and early infantile hydrocephalus. **Dev Med Child Neurol** 17: 711-8, 1975.

147. Aoki N, Miztani H, Masuzawa H: Unilateral subdural-peritoneal shunting for bilateral chronic subdural hematomas in infancy. **J Neurosurg** 63: 134-7, 1985.

148. Krishnamoorthy K, Kuehnle K J, Todres I D, *et al.*: Neurodevelopmental outcome of survivors with posthemorrhagic hydrocephalus. **Ann Neurol** 15: 201-4, 1984.

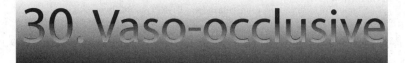

30. Vaso-occlusive

DEFINITIONS

TIA	(transient ischemic attack): a focal neurologic deficit that lasts ≤ 24 hours (by definition), but in up to 70% lasts only ≤ 10 minutes[1]; of patients with a deficit persisting > 60 minutes, only 14% will resolve within 24 hrs[2]; 90% of patients with TIAs will have had reversal within 4 hrs of onset
RIND	(reversible ischemic neurologic deficit): a focal deficit lasting ≥ 24 hrs but less than 1 week; comprised only 2.5% of 1343 patients admitted with TIA, RIND or CVA[2]
CVA	(cerebrovascular accident): AKA stroke (sometimes called completed stroke). A permanent (i.e. irreversible) neurologic deficit caused by inadequate perfusion of a region of brain or brain stem

30.1. Atherosclerotic cerebrovascular disease

30.1.1. Carotid artery

Atherosclerotic plaques begin to form in the carotid artery at 20 yrs of age. In the extracranial cerebral circulation, they typically start on the back wall of the common carotid artery (**CCA**). As they enlarge, they encroach on the lumen of the ICA. Calcified hard plaques may not change with time. The risk of CVA correlates with the degree of stenosis and the presence of ulcerations, and is also increased in hypercoagulable states and with increased blood viscosity.

PRESENTATION

Carotid artery lesions are considered symptomatic if there is one or more lateralizing ischemic episodes appropriate to the distribution of the lesion (a lesion is considered to be asymptomatic if the patient only has non-specific visual complaints, dizziness, or syncope not associated with TIA or stroke[3]). The majority (80%) of carotid atherothrombotic strokes occur without warning symptoms[4]. Symptomatic carotid disease may present as a TIA, RIND or CVA with any of the following findings:
* retinal insufficiency or infarction (central retinal artery is a branch of the ophthalmic artery): ipsilateral monocular blindness
    A. may be temporary: **amaurosis fugax**, AKA transient monocular blindness (**TMB**). Four types:
        Type I: embolic. Described "like a black curtain coming down". Complete loss of vision, usually lasts 1-2 minutes
        Type II: flow related. Retinal hypoperfusion → desaturation of color, usually described as a graying of vision
        Type III: vasospastic. May occur with migraines
        Type IV: miscellaneous. May occur with anticardiolipin antibodies
    B. blindness may be permanent
* middle cerebral artery symptoms:
    A. contralateral motor or sensory TIA (arm and face worse than leg) with hyperreflexia and upgoing toe
    B. language deficits if dominant hemisphere involved

EVALUATION

Check CBC with platelet count, fibrinogen, PT/PTT (to R/O hypercoagulable state). Funduscopic exam may show **Hollenhorst plaques** (cholesterol crystal emboli).

EVALUATION OF EXTENT OF DISEASE

Classification of patients based on the hemodynamics and also the embolic propensity of carotid lesions has thus far been too complex to be utilized in large studies. The tests described below place a great deal of emphasis on the greatest degree of stenosis which is probably an oversimplification.

Carotid artery ulcerations

Classified as shown in *Table 30-1*. Ulcerative lesions may provide no warning (i.e. TIA) before infarction. Large (Type B) or complex (Type C) ulcerations have a natural history similar to that of severe stenosis[6].

Table 30-1 Classification of carotid ulcerations[5, 6]

Type	Description	Annual stroke rate
A	small, smooth, shallow	0.5%
B	large, deep	0.5-4.5%
C	complex, cavitated	5-7%

ANGIOGRAPHY

The "gold standard" test is an intra-arterial angiogram. It is invasive, and too costly and risky (1-2% risk of CVA in this population in good hands[7]) to be used as a screening test. Also, unlike duplex doppler and MRA, it does not provide any information about the thickness of the plaque. Different definitions of the degree of stenosis are employed, *Table 30-2* compares the definitions used by the NASCET study[8] to that of the ECST[9]. For both, **N** is the linear diameter of the carotid artery at the site of greatest narrowing. The studies differ in the denominator, the NASCET uses **D** which is the diameter of the normal artery <u>distal</u> to the carotid bulb (taken at the first point at which the arterial walls become parallel), whereas the ECST uses **B** which is the estimated carotid bulb diameter.

For example, using the NASCET definition, the degree of stenosis is shown in *Eq 30-1*.

Table 30-2 Comparison of NASCET and ECST measurements of ICA stenosis*

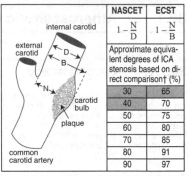

	NASCET	ECST
	$1 - \dfrac{N}{D}$	$1 - \dfrac{N}{B}$
	Approximate equivalent degrees of ICA stenosis based on direct comparison† (%)	
	30	65
	40	70
	50	75
	60	80
	70	85
	80	91
	90	97

*   adapted from Donnan G A, Davis S M, Chambers B R, et al.: Surgery for the Prevention of Stroke. Lancet 351: 1372, 1998, with permission

†   shaded boxes indicate degrees of stenosis for which surgery was NOT of clear benefit for *symptomatic* stenosis (*see page 874*)

$$\text{\% stenosis (NASCET)} = \left(1 - \frac{N}{D}\right) \times 100 \qquad \textbf{Eq 30-1}$$

The relationship between the degree of narrowing based on the NASCET definition vs. that of the ECST has also been estimated by equation[10] as shown in *Eq 30-2*.

$$\text{\% stenosis (by ECST)} = 0.6 \times \text{\% stenosis (by NASCET)} + 40\% \qquad \textbf{Eq 30-2}$$

DUPLEX DOPPLER ULTRASOUND

B-mode image evaluates the artery in cross-sectional plane, and spectrum analysis shows blood flow. Performs poorly with a "string sign". Cannot scan above the angle of the mandible. Lower frequencies give greater depth of penetration, but signal definition is sacrificed (used in transcranial doppler).

MAGNETIC RESONANCE ANGIOGRAPHY (MRA)

May obviate the need for angiography in some cases of carotid stenosis, specifically in symptomatic patients with a focal "gap" of signal intensity loss with distal reappearance of signal[11, 12]. Sometimes overestimates the degree of stenosis[13].

DIGITAL INTRAVENOUS ANGIOGRAM

Sometimes abbreviated: DIVA. Intravenous contrast is injected, and then digital processing techniques are used to produce a "subtraction" image to visualize blood vessels. Resolution is poor, and the dye load administered is much higher than with intra-arterial injection (regardless of whether cut-film angiography or digital subtraction techniques are used) angiography[14].

OCULAR PNEUMOPLETHYSMOGRAPHY

Ocular pneumoplethysmography **(OPG)** is considered abnormal if[15]:
- asymmetry ≥ 5 mm Hg in the ophthalmic systolic pressures **(OSP)**
- ratio of OSP to brachial systolic pressure **(BSP)** falls ≥ 1 mm below a regression line defined by *Eq 30-3*

$$\boxed{OSP = 38.94 + (0.4216 \times BSP)}$$ Eq 30-3

TREATMENT

Treatment alternatives are primarily between the following.
1. "best medical management": *see below*
2. carotid endarterectomy: *see page 874*
3. endovascular techniques: *see page 878*
   A. percutaneous angioplasty and retrograde open balloon angioplasty for carotid[16] and vertebrobasilar[17] stenosis
   B. angioplasty combined with stenting

MEDICAL TREATMENT

What constitutes "best medical management" has not been precisely determined, and recommendations are constantly changing. Some or all of the following are utilized:
- antiplatelet therapy:
  - ◆ usually aspirin **(ASA)** *(see below)*
  - ◆ ticlopidine may be used when ASA cannot be *(see below)*
  - ◆ no benefit from dipyridamole (Persantine®)
- antihypertensive therapy as appropriate
- good control of diabetes if present
- patients with asymptomatic A-fib should be treated with anticoagulation (see *Cardiogenic brain embolism*, page 773)
- antilipid therapy if needed
- intervention to help patients to quit smoking

Antiplatelet therapy

/ aspirin ⟍ ⟋ DRUG INFO ⟍

Irreversibly inhibits cyclooxygenase preventing synthesis of vascular prostacyclin (a vasodilator and platelet inhibitor) and platelet thromboxane A_2 (a vasoconstrictor and platelet activator). Platelets, lacking cellular organelles, cannot resynthesize cyclooxygenase whereas the vascular tissues do so rapidly[18]. NB: < 1000 mg ASA per day probably does not help with high grade stenosis where there is perfusion failure or flow failure. Some (but not all) studies show less effectiveness in women[19], and no large study has shown that ASA prevents a second stroke in patients that have already had one.

Rx: For angina, a bolus dose of 160-325 mg PO is followed by maintenance doses of 80-160 mg/d (lower doses appear to be as effective as higher doses)[20]. Optimal dose for cerebrovascular ischemia continues to be debated. 325 mg PO qd reduces risk of stroke following TIA by 25-30%. Daily doses of 81 or 325 mg when compared to higher doses were associated with a lower rate of CVA, MI and death (6.2% vs. 8.4%) following carotid endarterectomy[21].

/ ticlopidine (Ticlid®) ⟍ ⟋ DRUG INFO ⟍

A thienopyridine antiplatelet drug that may be more effective than ASA in preventing strokes[22] and reversible ischemic events[23]. Ticlopidine interferes with platelet membrane function by inhibiting ADP-induced platelet fibrinogen binding and release of platelet granule contents, as well as subsequent platelet-platelet interactions. Produces a time and dose dependent irreversible inhibition of platelet aggregation and prolongation of bleeding time. Takes ≈ 10 days for benefits to become apparent[20]. Use of clopidogrel is recommended over ticlopidine (*see below*).

SIDE EFFECTS: Significant neutropenia (absolute neutrophil count **(ANC)** < 1200/mm³) or agranulocytosis sometimes with thrombocytopenia occurs in ≈ 2.4%. Neutropenia usually ensues within 90 days of initiating therapy, and normalizes with discontinuation of the drug in 1-3 weeks. Therefore it is reserved for patients intolerant of ASA or for whom ASA has not been approved (viz.: previous thrombotic CVA, TIA in women[24]...).

Contraindicated in hemapoietic disorders (neutropenia, thrombocytopenia...), hemostatic disorders or active pathological bleeding, or with severe hepatic dysfunction.

Rx: 250 mg PO BID. Prior to initiating therapy, check CBC + platelet count. If ANC > 1200/mm³, initiate ticlopidine therapy. For ANC 450-1200, weigh risk vs. benefits, and if decision is made to initiate therapy, do so cautiously. For ANC < 450 therapy is contraindicated. Check CBC q 2 weeks **x** 3 months, and thereafter only if signs or symptoms of infection appear.

clopidogrel (Plavix®)　　　　　　DRUG INFO

Another thienopyridine (*see above*), with a lower incidence of severe neutropenia (0.04%) than ticlopidine (0.8%) and is close to that of ASA (≈ 0.02%)[25]. Only needs to be taken once a day. Requires several days to reach maximal effect (∴ a loading dose is used after an <u>acute</u> event, e.g. MI). Takes ≈ 5 days off the drug for platelet inhibition to reverse.

Rx: 75 mg PO qd (loading dose: 225 mg (3 pills) the first day of therapy if being prescribed following an acute event). SUPPLIED: 75 mg film-coated tablet.

aspirin/ER-dipyridamole (Aggrenox®)　　　　　DRUG INFO

37% risk reduction for stroke, probably more effective than aspirin or clopidogrel.
SIDE EFFECTS: H/A with initial therapy.
Rx: 1 capsule PO BID. SUPPLIED: aspirin 25 mg/extended-release dipyridamole 200 mg capsules.

30.1.1.1.　Asymptomatic carotid artery stenosis

❢ Key features
- natural history: reveals low stroke rate (2%/yr) half of which are not disabling
- large randomized trials have revealed moderate surgical benefit versus medical management for asymptomatic stenosis >60%
- selection criteria depend on patient's age, gender and comorbidities (and therefore life expectancy), and on perioperative complication rate

PRACTICE PARAMETER 30-1 ASYMPTOMATIC CAROTID STENOSIS*
For patients with a surgical risk < 3% and life expectancy ≥ 5 yrs
Standards[26]: carotid endarterectomy **(CEA)** is beneficial for: asymptomatic stenosis ≥ 60%   **Guidelines**[26]: unilateral CEA + simultaneous CABG for: stenosis > 60%   **Options**[26]: unilateral CEA for: stenosis > 50% with B or C ulcer (*see page 870*)
For patients with a surgical risk 3-5%
Guidelines[26]: ipsilateral CEA for: stenosis > 75% with contralateral ICA stenosis 75-100%   **Options**[26]:   • ipsilateral CEA for: stenosis > 75% irrespective of contralateral stenosis   • unilateral CEA + CABG for: bilateral asymptomatic carotid stenosis > 70% + CABG required   • ipsilateral CEA for: unilateral carotid stenosis > 70% & CABG required
For patients with a surgical risk 5-10%

NATURAL HISTORY

Stroke rate with an asymptomatic carotid bruit is **2%/yr** on either side, the ipsilateral CVA rate is 0.1-0.4%/yr, whereas it is 0.7-6%/yr when the bruit is accompanied by ipsilateral stenosis[27] (47% of patients with stenosis ≥ 80% on duplex scan developed ipsilateral CVA, TIA or carotid occlusion within 36 mos, usually within 6 mos[28]).

In the Asymptomatic Carotid Surgery Trial (**ACST**)[29], the stroke rate in the medically treated patients was **2.4%/yr** (similar to earlier studies[7, 30, 31]), with ≈ half of the CVAs being fatal or disabling. Mortality rate is 4%/yr (mostly from MI, which has a frequency ≈ 4-5 times higher than that of CVA). This is in contrast to annual stroke rates of 13%, 12% and 5% for patients with symptomatic carotid stenosis, and symptomatic and asymptomatic atrial fibrillation, respectively[8, 32, 33].

When asymptomatic hemodynamically significant bruits (as determined by positive ocular pneumoplethysmography (**OPG**)) were compared to those with normal OPGs, the annual total event rate (CVA + TIA) went from 2.3% to 5.2%, with 56% of all events ipsilateral to the abnormal OPG (3.5 yrs follow-up in 640 patients)[15].

SURGERY VS. MEDICAL MANAGEMENT: THE STUDIES

ACST[29]

Σ The largest multicenter randomized trial to date[29] revealed a moderate benefit for immediate CEA vs. medical management in patients age < 75 with asymptomatic stenosis ≥ 60%.

Details: 3,120 patients with ≥ 60% stenosis by duplex ultrasound were randomized to immediate CEA (50% had CEA within 1 month, 88% within 1 year) or medical therapy at the discretion of the treating physician. Mean follow-up: 3.4 years. Exclusion criteria included: poor surgical risk, prior ipsilateral CEA, and probable cardiac emboli. Surgeons were required to have a perioperative morbidity and mortality rate of < 6%.

Net five-year risk for all stroke or perioperative stroke or death: 6.4% in the CEA group, vs. 11.8% in the medical group (p<0.0001). Fatal or disabling stroke: 3.5 vs. 6.1. Fatal stroke alone: 2.1 vs. 4.2%. Although men and women benefited, men benefited more. CEA did not demonstrate a statistically significant benefit for patients over the age of 75. Statistical benefit was not seen in the immediate CEA group until nearly two years after surgery, despite a relatively low perioperative morbidity and mortality rate of 3.1%, (in contrast to patients with *symptomatic* stenosis (NASCET[31]) where benefit was seen much earlier).

ACAS[7]

Σ Large trial that randomized patients in good health with asymptomatic stenosis* ≥ 60% to CEA plus aspirin, or aspirin alone[7] found a reduced 5-year risk of ipsilateral stroke if CEA was performed with <3% perioperative morbidity and mortality and is added to aggressive management of modifiable risk factors.

* calculated in the same manner as the NASCET study

Details: CEA reduced 5-year stroke risk 66% in males, 17% in females (not statistically significant), and 53% overall. CEA did not significantly protect against *major* CVA or death (P = 0.16) (half of the CVAs were not disabling), and was somewhat protective against *any* stroke or death (P = 0.08). Excluded patients (age > 79 yrs, unstable CAD, uncontrolled HTN) may have been higher risk. Surgeons were carefully selected and the surgical morbidity (1.5%) and mortality (0.1%) was very low. Surprisingly, ≈ half of the total morbidity (1.2%) was related to angiography. The implication is that for a generally healthy white male with ACAS > 60%, management with CEA (when performed by a surgeon with a low complication rate, as described) reduces his annual risk of all strokes from 0.5% to 0.17% (the reduction of risk for severe stroke is less). The benefit from CEA is realized within less than one year after the CEA. This is in contrast to the ACST trial (*see above*) and is most likely due to the lower perioperative event rate. The risk from mortality from other causes (including MI) is ≈ 3.9% per year. Combined CVA and death rates in community hospitals[34] while improved over the last 20 yrs, remains higher at ≈ 6.3% than at centers used in this study.

Veteran's Administration Cooperative Study (VACS)[31]
CEA reduces ipsilateral neurologic events, but did not reduce the rate of ipsilateral CVAs nor death (most deaths were secondary to MI). This trial did not include women.

CASANOVA study[35]
No difference in outcome between CEA vs. aspirin (new CVA or death), but an unusual protocol lessened it's statistical validity[36].

30.1.1.2. Carotid endarterectomy

INDICATIONS
Table 30-3 shows the status of current studies for the surgical treatment of carotid stenosis (NB: some of the results may be contradictory).

The North American Symptomatic Carotid Endarterectomy Trial[8] (**NASCET**) found that for patients with a hemispheric or retinal TIA or a mild (non-disabling) CVA within 120 days and ipsilateral high-grade stenosis (> 70%), that carotid endarterectomy (**CEA**) reduced the rate of fatal and non-fatal CVAs (by 17% at 18 months) and death from any cause (by 7% at 18 months) when compared to best medical management[A]. Results were twice as good for patients with stenosis from 90-99% than for those with 70-79%. NB: for differences in techniques for measuring stenosis between NASCET and ECST, see *Table 30-2*, page 870.

For asymptomatic patients, *see page 872*.

Unresolved controversies
Include:
1. progressive CVA ("stroke in evolution"): see *Emergency carotid endarterectomy*, page 879
2. abrupt occlusion: see *Emergency carotid endarterectomy*, page 879
3. tandem lesions (e.g. carotid siphon and bifurcation)
4. progressive retinal ischemia

TIMING WITH RESPECT TO ACUTE CVA
Many acutely presenting neurologic deficits are not due to a lesion in the carotid artery (e.g. intracerebral hemorrhage, cardiogenic emboli). Those that *are* due to carotid disease do not fare well with surgery (see *Emergency carotid endarterectomy*, page 879).

Although the general trend is to wait 4-6 weeks after a completed stroke before doing a carotid endarterectomy, the data from Sundt (*see below*) indicates that a CVA is a risk factor for a complication only if it occurred within 7 days pre-op.

Table 30-3 Summary of study findings for carotid endarterectomy (CEA)*
(modified[37])

Stenosis	Relevant study	Recommendation	Risk reduction†
Symptomatic Narrowing			
70-99%	NASCET[8]	CEA	16.5 @ 2 yrs
> 60%	ECST[9]	CEA	11.6 @ 3 yrs
50-69%	NASCET[38]	CEA‡	10.1 @ 5 yrs
< 30%	NASCET[38]	BMM	0.8 @ 5 yrs
< 40%	ECST[39]	BMM	CEA worse @ 3 yrs
Asymptomatic Narrowing (*see page 872*)			
> 60%	ACAS[7], ACST§	CEA‡	6.3 @ 5 yrs
> 50%	VACS	± CEAΔ	
< 90%	CASANOVA	BMMΔ	

* abbreviations: NASCET = North American Symptomatic Carotid Endarterectomy Trial; ECST = European Carotid Surgery Trial; CASANOVA = Carotid Artery Stenosis with Asymptomatic Narrowing Operation Versus Aspirin; ACAS = Asymptomatic Carotid Atherosclerosis Study; ACST = Asymptomatic Carotid Atherosclerosis Study; VACS = Veteran's Administration Cooperative Study; CEA = carotid endarterectomy; BMM = best medical management

† reduction in risk of all nonfatal CVAs and death from any cause with CEA vs. BMM

‡ surgery moderately beneficial (requires low complication rate)

§ the overall health of the patient is critical

Δ results equivocal, *see text page 874*

A. when surgery was performed with perioperative risk of stroke or death of 5.8%

PRE-OP RISK FACTORS

Sundt identified the following pre-op factors that increase the risk of carotid endarterectomy (original figures[40], later modified[41 (p 226-30)]):

- medical risk factors: angina, MI within 6 mos, CHF, severe HTN (> 180/110), COPD, age > 70, severe obesity
- neurologic risk factors: progressing neuro deficit, resolved deficit < 24 hrs pre-op, generalized cerebral ischemia, recent CVA < 7 days pre-op, deficits from multiple CVAs, frequent TIAs not controlled by anti-coagulants (crescendo TIAs)
- angiographic risk factors: contralateral ICA occlusion, siphon stenosis, plaque extending > 3 cm distally in the ICA or > 5 cm proximally in CCA, carotid bifurcation at level of C2 with short/thick neck, soft thrombus propagating from ulcerated lesion

Based on above risk factors in 1,935 endarterectomies, 4 grades defined with the risks of morbidity and mortality (excludes minor complications not causing permanent morbidity) shown in *Table 30-4*:

Table 30-4   Morbidity and mortality from carotid endarterectomy (Sundt[41])

Grade	Risk factors*	Risk (in 1,935 operations)
I	Neurologically stable; no medical or angiographic risks; with unilateral or bilateral ulcerative-stenotic carotid disease.	< 1% risk (5 RIND, 6 CVA)
II	Neurologically stable; no medical risks, but with angiographic risks (contralateral ICA occlusion most common).	1.8% risk (6 RIND, 7 CVA)
III	Neurologically stable; medical risks, with or without angiographic risks.	4% risk (9 fatal MIs, 10 RIND, 10 CVAs (1 fatal))
IV	Neurologically unstable, with or without medical or angiographic risks.	8.5% risk (27 CVAs (8 fatal), 14 RIND, 2 fatal MIs)

*   see text for definition of medical, angiographic, and neurologic risk factors

Original paper (342 operations) included in non-permanent morbidity 5 patients who developed seizures associated with periodic lateralizing epileptiform discharges **(PLEDs)** post-op that were initially difficult to control, but did not require long-term anticonvulsants **(AEDs)**. All 5 had high-grade stenosis and a small pre-op CVA, and reactive hyperemia post-endarterectomy. Sundt recommends pre-op AEDs in these patients. Sundt cautions that although the risk of CVA is highest in Grade 4, some of the most dramatic results occurred in this group.

PATIENT MANAGEMENT

PERIOPERATIVE MANAGEMENT

PRE-OP MANAGEMENT (CAROTID ENDARTERECTOMY)
1. ASA 325 mg TID for at least 2 days, preferably 5 days pre-op[42] (NB: patients should be kept on their ASA for surgery, and if not on ASA they should be started, in order to reduce risks of MI and TIA[43])

POST-OP MANAGEMENT (CAROTID ENDARTERECTOMY)
1. patient monitored in ICU with A-line
2. keep patient well hydrated (run IVF ≥ 100 cc/hr for most adults)
3. SBP ideally 110 - 150 mm Hg (higher pressures are permitted in patients with chronic severe HTN)
   - A. BP frequently labile in 1st 24 hrs post-op, may be due to "new" pressure in carotid bulb; to prevent rebound hyper- or hypo-tension, avoid long acting agents
   - B. hypotension
     1. check EKG - R/O cardiogenic shock
     2. if mild, start with fluids (crystalloid or colloid)
     3. phenylephrine (Neo-Synephrine®) for resistant hypotension
   - C. hypertension: nitroprusside (Nipride®) is the agent of choice; be prepared to reduce dose quickly in anticipation of hypotension
4. avoid ASA and dipyridamole for 24-48 hrs post-op (causes oozing); may start

these 24-72 hrs post op (note: ASA 325 mg + dipyridamole 75 mg TID have been shown not to reduce the rate of restenosis after endarterectomy[44])
5. optional:
   A. 10 minutes after closing arteriotomy, reverse half of heparin with protamine
   B. LMD 40 at 40 ml/hr x 24 hrs post-op: inhibits platelets

POST-OP CHECK (CAROTID ENDARTERECTOMY)
In addition to routine, the following should be checked:
❑ 1. change in neurologic status due to cerebral dysfunction, including:
   A. pronator drift (R/O new hemiparesis)
   B. signs of dysphasia (especially for left sided surgery)
   C. mimetic muscle symmetry (assesses facial nerve function)
❑ 2. pupil diameter and reaction (R/O CVA, Horner's syndrome)
❑ 3. STA pulses (R/O external carotid occlusion)
❑ 4. tongue deviation (R/O hypoglossal nerve injury)
❑ 5. symmetry of lips (R/O weakness of lower lip depressors due to retraction of marginal mandibular branch of facial nerve against mandible, usually resolves in 6-12 wks, must differentiate from central VII palsy due to CVA)
❑ 6. check for hoarseness (R/O recurrent laryngeal nerve injury)
❑ 7. assess for hematoma in operative site: note any tracheal deviation, dysphagia

POST-OP COMPLICATIONS (CAROTID ENDARTERECTOMY)
To justify CEA, the absolute upper limit of (significant) complication rate is 5% (in practice, however, this should be ≤ 3%).
1. overall mortality[45]: 2.3%
2. disruption of arteriotomy closure: rare, but emergent (see below)
   A. evidenced by:
      1. swelling of neck: rupture may produce a pseudoaneurysm
      2. tracheal deviation (visible, palpable, or on CXR)
      3. symptoms: dysphagia, air hunger or worsening hoarseness, difficulty swallowing
   B. dangers:
      1. asphyxiation: most immediate danger
      2. stroke
      3. exsanguination (unlikely, unless skin closure is also disrupted)
   C. late (often delayed weeks to months): false aneurysm[46]. Risk = 0.33%. Presents as neck mass. Risk is increased with wound infection and possibly with patch graft as compared to endarterectomy alone[46-48]
3. stroke (cerebral infarction) intra-op or post-op rate[45]: 5%
   A. embolic (the most common cause of minor post-op neurologic deficit): source may be denuded media of endarterectomy
   B. intracerebral hemorrhagic (ICH) (breakthrough bleeding): occurs in < 0.6%[49]. Related to cerebral hyperperfusion in most[50, 51](see below). Usually occurs within first 2 weeks, often in basal ganglion 3-4 days post-op with hypertensive episode. Patients at greatest risk are those with severe stenosis and limited hemispheric collateral flow
   C. post-op ICA occlusion
      1. most common cause of major post-op CVAs, but may be asymptomatic
      2. risk is reduced by attention to technical details at surgery[41 (p 249)]
      3. some may be due to hypercoagulable state induced by heparin (predictable in patients whose platelet count drops while on heparin. No known therapy for this condition[41 (p 249-50)]
      4. the endarterectomized surface is highly thrombogenic for 4 hrs following endarterectomy (Sundt recommends not reversing heparin)
      5. in Sundt's series using patch graft[41 (p 229)]: 0.8% incidence, associated with major CVA in 33% and minor CVA in 20%
      6. occlusion rate with primary closure: 4% in Sundt's experience, 2-5% in literature[41 (p 249)]
4. post-op TIAs: most due to ICA occlusion. Some may be due to microemboli. Hyperperfusion syndrome produces a 1% incidence of post-op TIAs[41 (p 229)]
5. seizures[52]: usually focal in onset with possible generalization, most occur late (post-op day 5-13) with an incidence of ≈ 0.4%[49] to 1%[53]. May be due to cerebral

hyperperfusion[49], emboli[54], and/or intracerebral hemorrhage. Usually difficult to control initially, lorazepam and phenytoin are recommended (*see page 266*)

6. late restenosis: identifiable restenosis occurs in ≈ 25% by 1 yr, and half of these restenoses reduce luminal diameters by > 50%[55]. Restenosis within 2 yrs is usually due to fibrous hyperplasia, after 2 yrs it is typically due to atherosclerosis[56]

7. **cerebral hyperfusion syndrome** (AKA normal pressure hyperperfusion breakthrough): classically thought to result from return of blood flow to an area that has lost autoregulation due to chronic cerebral ischemia typically from high-grade stenosis. Controversial[51]. Usually presents as ipsilateral vascular H/A or eye pain that subsides within several days[57] or with seizures (± PLEDs on EEG, more common with Halothane®, due to petechial hemorrhages[49]). May cause ICH[58]. Most complications occur several days post-op

8. hoarseness: the most common cause is laryngeal edema and not superior nor recurrent laryngeal nerve injury

9. cranial nerve injury:
   A. hypoglossal nerve → tongue deviation towards the side of injury: incidence ≈ 1% (with mobilizing XII to allow displacement). Unilateral injury may cause speaking, chewing and swallowing difficulties. Bilateral injuries can cause upper airway obstruction[59]. The presence of a unilateral palsy is a contraindication to doing contralateral endarterectomy until the first side recovers. May last as long as four months
   B. vagus or recurrent laryngeal nerve → unilateral vocal cord paralysis: 1% risk
   C. mandibular branch of facial nerve → loss of ipsilateral lip depressor

10. headache[49]

11. hypertension[60, 61]: may develop 5-7 days post-op. Longstanding HTN may occur as a result of the loss of the carotid sinus baroreceptor reflex

COMPLICATION MANAGEMENT

1. post-op TIAs
   A. if TIA occurs in recovery room, emergency CT (to R/O hemorrhage) and then angiogram recommended to assess for ICA or CCA occlusion (vs. emboli)
   B. if TIA occurs later, consider emergent OPG; if abnormal → emergent surgery (if neurologically intact, pre-op angiogram is appropriate)[41]

2. fixed post-op deficit in distribution of endarterectomized carotid
   A. if deficit occurs immediately post-op (i.e. in PACU), recommend immediate re-exploration without delay for CT or angiogram[62] (case reports of no deficit when flow re-established in ≤ 45 mins). For later onset, workup is indicated. Technical considerations for emergency re-operation[41 (p 255)]:
      1. isolate the 3 arteries (CCA, ECA, & ICA)
      2. occlude CCA 1st, then ECA, and ICA last (to minimize emboli)
      3. open arteriotomy, check backflow; if none, pass a No. 4 Fogarty catheter into ICA, gently inflate and withdraw (avoid intimal tears)
      4. if good backflow established, close with vein patch graft
      5. remove tortuous vessel loops and kinks before closing
   B. immediate management (unless ICH or SDH are likely) includes
      1. fluids (e.g. Plasmanate®) to improve rheology and to elevate BP
      2. pressors (e.g. phenylephrine) to elevate SBP to ≈ 180 mm Hg
      3. oxygen
      4. heparinization (may be controversial)
   C. theoretical benefits of radiographic evaluation include:
      1. CT: identifies ICH or SDH that might require treatment other than re-exploration of the surgical site, elevating BP, etc.
      2. angiogram: identifies whether ICA is occluded, or if deficit is from another cause (e.g. emboli from endarterectomy site) that would not benefit from re-exploration

3. disruption of arteriotomy closure, management
   A. **OPEN WOUND** - if there is any stridor, it is critical to do this before trying to intubate (although ideally performed in O.R., the delay may be decisive). Evacuate clot (start with a sterile gloved finger) and stop bleeding, preferably without traumatizing the artery, a DeBakey clamp is optimal
   B. **INTUBATION** - high priority, may be difficult or impossible if trachea is deviated (open wound immediately). Preferably done by anesthesiologist in controlled setting (i.e. O.R.) unless there is acute airway obstruction

C. call O.R. and have them prepare set-up for endarterectomy, and take patient to O.R.

Anesthesia and monitoring
Most (but not all) surgeons monitor some parameter of neurologic function during carotid endarterectomy, and will alter technique (e.g. insert a vascular shunt) if there is evidence of hemodynamic intolerance of carotid clamping (only occurs in ≈ 1-4%).
1. local/regional anesthesia: permits "clinical" monitoring of patient's neurologic function[63, 64]. Disadvantages: patient movement during procedure (often exacerbated by sedation and alterations in CBF), lack of cerebral protection from anesthetic and adjunctive agents. The only prospective randomized study found no difference between local and general anesthesia[65]
2. general anesthesia, possibly including barbiturates (thiopental boluses of 125-250 mg until 15-30 second burst suppression on EEG, followed by small bolus injections or constant infusion to maintain burst suppression[42])
    A. EEG monitoring
    B. SSEP monitoring
    C. measurement of distal stump pressure after CCA occlusion (unreliable), e.g. using a shunt if stump pressure < 25 mm Hg

30.1.1.3. Carotid angioplasty

Initial concerns about dislodging debris which may embolize[66], recurrent stenosis[67], and lack of long-term follow-up has slowed the widespread acceptance of percutaneous transluminal angioplasty[68] **(PTA)** for carotid stenosis.

Indications: Still evolving. Since CVA rate is higher with PTA than with CEA, only certain situations appear appropriate for PTA, possibly including the following
1. symptomatic elderly (≥ 75 yrs age) with prohibitive surgical risk (this population is at high risk regardless of therapy chosen)
2. recurrent stenosis
3. radiation induced stenosis
4. critically ill patients with evolving CVAs who require thrombolytics

Risks include:
1. distal cerebral embolism: risk is not as high as was initially feared, but is still higher than with surgery
2. subintimal dissection: concerns lead to the use of stents
3. restenosis due to intimal hyperplasia induced by small subintimal hemorrhages
4. stroke:
    A. incidence during procedure: 5% for minor, and 1% for major stroke
    B. 30 day risk: all strokes and death = 9.3%, major stroke and death = 2.8%
    C. incidence of minor stroke is ≈10 **x** higher than with CEA, for major stroke it is ≈ the same
5. bradycardia: often controlled with atropine, sometimes requires temporary or even permanent pacemaker
6. complications from puncture site and/or IV contrast: retroperitoneal hematoma, distal LE ischemia and renal failure

Questions that arise regarding PTA:
1. is widening the vessel enough to reduce the risk of emboli, or is it necessary to remove the atherosclerotic plaque (as is done with carotid endarterectomy)?
2. does the disruption of the vessel wall and subsequent healing from PTA alone prevent further emboli, or is stenting necessary

Technique[69]
1. medications
    A. ASA 325 mg PO qd for at least 2 days prior to and on the day of the procedure
    B. ticlopidine 250 mg PO BID starting the day of the procedure
    C. heparin 5000 U given intra-arterially during the procedure
    D. atropine 1 mg IV during balloon inflation PRN bradycardia which occurs in > 30% of cases (from balloon distension of carotid sinus)

2. balloon catheter insertion is performed via femoral artery access
3. stenting is used for larger diameter vessels
4. initial balloon inflation is performed, and if a stent is placed, the balloon is reinflated after the stent is positioned

30.1.1.4. Emergency carotid endarterectomy

Rationale: animal studies have shown that several hours of reduced cerebral blood flow can be tolerated without permanent infarction. After a fixed mild to moderate deficit, some authors advocate waiting 4-6 wks before considering surgery; in this time period, there is a 21% incidence of recurrent CVA.

Emergency endarterectomy may be indicated to restore function, to treat high risk angiographic findings, or both. After retrospective analysis of 64 emergency endarterectomies[70] the guidelines given below were suggested. However, the efficacy of immediate surgical removal of obstruction is controversial and unproven. In one early study, over 50% of patients suffered fatal intracranial hemorrhage within 72 hours of emergency carotid endarterectomy.

INITIAL MANAGEMENT OF PATIENT PRESENTING WITH ACUTE NEURO DEFICIT
1. obtain history directed at determining presence of previous CVA and other serious medical illness
2. baseline neurological assessment including evaluation of STA pulses and carotid bruits
3. during evaluation: close control of BP. O_2 per NC. Labs + EKG (*see Management of RIND, TIA, or CVA*, page 768). Consider hemodilution with LMD
4. CT to R/O ICH or infarction (early CVA will not be visible)
5. when carotid disease is suspected, and CT negative for ICH or acute infarct, emergency angiography is performed

INDICATIONS FOR EMERGENCY CAROTID ENDARTERECTOMY
In patients with acute neurological deficits, the need for rapid decision making does not allow differentiating between TIA, stroke in evolution and acute stroke, nor in assessing the stability or fluctuating nature of the deficit.

For the following discussion, the definitions used in pre-op neurological assessment are shown in *Table 30-5*.

Table 30-5   Definitions for pre-op neuro assessment

Indications
1. sudden onset of a neurological deficit with the loss of a previously noted carotid bruit (ipsilateral to appropriate area of deficit)
   * angiography not necessary
   * take immediately to O.R.
   * very good prognosis
2. sudden onset of a deficit from proven carotid artery occlusion during angiography
   * take immediately to O.R.
   * good prognosis if no MCA embolus
3. presence of TIAs or an acute spontaneous mild or moderate neurological deficits with one of the following angiographic findings[A]
   A. severe stenosis (lumen dia < 1.5 mm) in proximal ICA with marked delay in flow
   B. stenosis in proximal ICA and presence of intraluminal filling defect
      * caution: surgical morbidity may be high
      * only about half of these will be thrombus, the rest will be atheromatous material
   C. complete ICA occlusion (also see *Totally occluded carotid* below)

Descriptor	Definition
intact	history of TIAs only
mild deficit	only slight impairment of normal activity
moderate deficit	significantly impairs function, but allows activities of daily living (**ADLs**) (aphasic patients have at least moderate deficit)
severe deficit	major loss of neurologic function that would significantly impair ADLs

---

A. some patients with severe deficits may benefit, but this is difficult to evaluate. Recommendation: if there is a significantly reduced level of consciousness and an infarct demonstrated on CT, then revascularization is unlikely to be of benefit and has high mortality. Emergency surgery may be of benefit in severe deficit if patient is alert and CT normal

4. **crescendo TIAs**: TIAs that abruptly increase in frequency to ≥ several per day (controversial)

Contraindications
Patients with depressed levels of consciousness or acute fixed deficits.

SURGICAL MANAGEMENT
1. for emergency surgery, it is essential that blood pressure be stable
2. in patients with complete occlusion, ICA is not occluded intra-op (to avoid breaking up thrombus, if present)
3. if thrombus present
    *   attempt spontaneous extrusion using back pressure
    *   if this fails, attempt to remove with smoothened suction catheter
    *   if this fails, pass balloon embolectomy catheter as far as base of skull (caution: avoid injury to distal ICA that could cause CCF)
    *   obtain intra-op angiogram unless thrombus emerges and backflow is excellent
    *   plicate ICA (avoid creating a blind pouch at origin) if there is good backflow or if satisfactory angiography cannot be obtained

Table 30-6 Surgical results

Presenting deficit	Same or improved	Deaths
intact or mild	92%	0
moderate	80%	1 (7%)
severe	77%	3 (13%)

SURGICAL RESULTS
Highest correlation was with presenting neurologic status (*see Table 30-6*).

30.1.1.5. Totally occluded carotid

PRESENTATION
3 patterns of CVA with carotid artery occlusion:
1. stump emboli: produces cortical infarcts. Emboli usually go up the external carotid (higher flow, and reverse flow that may occur through ICA initially prevents emboli from ICA). Later, ICA emboli may occur.
2. whole hemisphere CVA
3. watershed infarct

In symptomatic patients[71]: hemiparetic TIA 53%, dysphasic TIA 34%, fixed neuro deficit 21%, crescendo TIAs 21%, amaurosis fugax 17%, acute hemiplegia 6%. One series had 27% asymptomatic[72]. Patients may have the so-called "slow carotid stroke" of carotid occlusion which is a stuttering progressive stroke.

MRI
With watershed type of CVA: MRI may show so-called "string of pearls" sign (small areas of intraparenchymal increased density on DWI).

NATURAL HISTORY[70]
Patients with mild deficit and angiographically proven ICA occlusion have a stroke rate (in two series) of 3 or 5% per year (2 or 3.3% related to occluded side). In patients with acute ICA occlusion and profound neurological deficit, 2-12% make good recovery, 40-69% will have profound deficit, and 16-55% will have died by the time of follow-up.

SURGERY
Options include: endarterectomy, Fogarty balloon catheter embolectomy (utilizing a No. 2 French catheter with 0.2 ml balloon gently passed 10-12 cm up ICA from small arteriotomy made distal to atheromatous plaque[73]), extracranial-intracranial bypass. Restored patency rate is inversely related to suspected duration of occlusion. Chronically occluded ICA has poor patency rate and little gain from re-opening.

Determining the exact time of occlusion is frequently impossible. One must often rely on clinical grounds, therefore an occasional chronic occlusion will be included.

Retrograde filling of ICA to petrous or cavernous segment from ECA (e.g. via ophthalmic) or from contralateral ICA is a good sign of operability[71].

32% (15/47 cases) immediate surgical failures (no or minimal back bleeding), at least 3 deaths. Among immediate successes no CVAs and no TIAs. If operated < 2 days reported patency rate 70-100%, from 3-7 days 50-100%, 8-14 days 27-58%, 15-30 days 4-61%, over 1 month (2 series) 20-50%.

GUIDELINES
Emergency operations for acute neuro deficit associated with total occlusion should not be performed after about 2 hrs. Extremely poor neuro status (lethargy/coma) is a contraindication to surgery. For a stable patient with persistent mild/moderate deficit: delay operation 1-3 wks, heparinize if hemorrhagic infarct is ruled out. Patients without persistent neuro deficit: operate ASAP.

30.1.2. Vertebrobasilar insufficiency

CLINICAL

DIAGNOSTIC CRITERIA
Table 30-7 shows a mnemonic of the symptoms of vertebrobasilar insufficiency (**VBI**).

Clinical diagnosis of VBI
Requires 2 or more of the following:
* motor or sensory symptoms or both, occurring bilaterally in the same event
* diplopia: ischemia of upper brainstem (midbrain) near ocular nuclei
* dysarthria: ischemia of lower brainstem
⦁ homonymous hemianopsia: ischemia of occipital cortex (NB: this is binocular, in contrast to amaurosis fugax which is monocular)

Table 30-7 Mnemonic: "The 5 D's of VBI"
• "drop attack"
• diplopia
• dysarthria
• defect (visual)
• dizziness

VBI may be suspected in a patient with transient episodes of "dizziness" (vertigo that is otherwise unexplained, e.g. absence of orthostatic hypotension) that is initiated by positional changes. VBI may sometimes be due to occlusion of the VA at the C1-C2 level with head turning (see *Bow hunter's stroke* below). May be seen in os odontoideum (*see page 730*).

SYMPTOM COMPLEXES
Predicting site of lesion based only on clinical evaluation is very unreliable. Atheromatous and stenotic lesions occur most frequently at VA origin.

VBI symptoms may be due to:
1. hemodynamic insufficiency (may be the most common etiology), including:
   * **subclavian steal**: reversed flow in VA due to proximal stenosis of subclavian artery
   * stenosis of both VAs or of one VA where the other is hypofunctional (e.g. hypoplastic, occluded, or terminates in PICA) causing reduced distal flow in face of inadequate collaterals (see *Bow hunter's stroke* below)
2. embolism from ulcerations
3. atherosclerotic occlusion of brainstem perforators

NATURAL HISTORY
No clinical study accurately defines the natural history. The estimated stroke rate is 22-35% over 5 years, or 4.5-7% per year[74] (one study estimating 35% stroke rate in 5 years did not use angiography).
Risk of CVA after first VBI-TIA has been estimated as 22% for first year[75].

EVALUATION
Adequate investigation requires selective four-vessel angiography.

Anticoagulation is the mainstay of medical management. Alternatives include anti-platelet drugs such as ASA (efficacy of either remains unproven[14, 74]).

Surgical treatment includes:
* vertebral endarterectomy
* transposition of VA to ICA (with or without carotid endarterectomy, with or without saphenous vein patch graft) or to thyrocervical trunk or to subclavian artery[76]
* bypass grafting (e.g. occipital artery to PICA)
* C1-2 posterior arthrodesis (*see page 623*) may prevent potentially life-threatening CVA in cases of os odontoideum (*see page 731*)

BOW HUNTER'S STROKE

Bow hunter's stroke (**BHS**): defined as hemodynamic VBI induced by intermittent VA occlusion resulting from head rotation[77] (ischemic sequelae range from TIA to completed stroke). May occur with forced (e.g. with chiropractic neck manipulation[78]) or voluntary[79] head rotation.

Occlusion usually involves the VA <u>contralateral</u> to the direction of rotation, and usually occurs at the C1-C2 junction (due to the immobility of the VA at this location)[80]. However, other sites have also been reported[81, 82].

VA occlusion does not produce symptoms in most individuals due to collateral flow through the contralateral VA or through the circle of Willis, or both. Symptomatic occlusion usually involves the dominant VA[83], however, may also occur with non-dominant VA[79]). Most cases of BHS occur in patients with an **isolated posterior circulation** (incompetent posterior communicating arteries).

BHS has also been postulated as one possible cause of SIDS[84].

Contributing factors:
1. external VA compression[82]
   A. spondylotic bone spurs: particularly in the foramen transversarium[85]
   B. tumors
   C. fibrous bands (e.g. proximal to entrance of VA into C6 foramen transversarium[81])
   D. infectious processes
   E. trauma
2. tethering of the VA
   A. at the transverse foramina of C1 & C2
   B. along the sulcus arteriosus proximal to where the VA enters the dura
3. defect in odontoid process[86]
4. atherosclerotic vascular disease

Diagnosis
BHS should be suspected in patient with symptoms of VBI precipitated by head movement. This may be very difficult to differentiate from vertigo and nausea due to vestibular dysfunction (rotation of the body keeping the head motionless might be helpful[87]).

Dynamic cerebral angiography (DCA): ✖ NB: significant consequences can be precipitated during DCA in patients with BHS[80]. The involved VA shows loss of flow as the head is rotated from the neutral position to the contralateral side. Carotid injections demonstrate patency of P-comms and the presence of any persistent fetal anastamoses.

Treatment
Options include:
1. anticoagulation[87]
2. cervical collar: to remind patient not to turn their head
3. for compression at C1-2 (*see Table 30-8* for a comparison):
   A. C1-2 fusion: *see page 623*
   B. VA decompression: C1 "hemilaminectomy" via a posterior approach[89]
4. for compression at other sites:
   elimination of the source of compression where possible (e.g. sectioning of offend-

Table 30-8 Comparison of surgical treatment for BHS at C1-2

Procedure	Advantages	Disadvantages
C1-2 fusion	high success rate in eliminating symptoms	loss of 50-70% of neck rotation with possible discomfort
VA decompression	no loss of motion	33% continue to have symptoms[88]

ing fibrous band[81], removal of osteophytic spurs[85]...)

Management recommendations: For compression at C1-2, it is suggested that VA decompression be performed as the initial treatment. This should be followed by DCA to verify maintenance of patency with head turning. Patients who fail clinically or on DCA should undergo C1-2 fusion[80]. Patients need to know pros and cons of each option.

30.2.   Cerebral arterial dissections

❧ Key features
* hemorrhage into the medial layer of an artery
* may be spontaneous or post-traumatic, may be intracranial or extracranial
* may present with pain (usually ipsilateral H/A), Horner's syndrome (in carotid dissections), TIA/CVA, or SAH
* extracranial dissections are usually treated medically (anticoagulation), intracranial dissections with SAH are treated surgically

NOMENCLATURE

Some confusion has arisen because of inconsistent terminology in the literature. Although by no means standard, Yamaura[90] has suggested the following:

dissection	extravassation of blood between the intima and media, creating luminal narrowing or occlusion
dissecting aneurysm	dissection of blood between the media and adventitia, or at the media, causing aneurysmal dilatation, which may rupture into the subarachnoid space
pseudoaneurysm	rupture of artery with subsequent encapsulation of the extravascular hematoma, may or may not produce luminal narrowing

PATHOPHYSIOLOGY

The lesion common to all dissections is hemorrhage outside of the vascular lumen due to pathological trans-intimal extravassation of blood from the true lumen into the vessel wall. The hematoma may either dissect the internal elastic membrane from the intima[91] causing narrowing of the true lumen, or it may dissect into the subadventitial plane producing an adventitial outpouching from the vessel wall. Rupture through the vessel wall producing SAH occurs occasionally.

Subintimal dissection is more common with intracranial dissections, whereas extracranial vessels (including the aorta) usually dissect at the media or between media and adventitia.

"Spontaneous" dissections have been associated with a large number of conditions, oftentimes the association is unproven. These conditions include:
* fibromuscular dysplasia **(FMD)**: found in ≈ 15% of cases[92]
* cystic medial necrosis (or degeneration): originally thought to be a common finding, now thought to perhaps be linked to a higher likelihood of <u>fatal</u> dissection
* saccular aneurysm
* Marfan's syndrome: autosomal dominant inherited disorder of connective tissue. Phenotypic manifestations are due to production of abnormal fibrillin
* atherosclerosis: only rarely implicated as an etiology. More likely to be a factor with subintimal dissection of *extra*cranial arteries
* Takayasu's disease
* medial degeneration
* syphilitic arteritis (more common in the past, associated with 60% of dissections before 1950)
* polycystic kidney disease: associated with a higher incidence of cerebral aneurysms (*see page 801*)
* variant periarteritis nodosa
* allergic arteritis
* homocystinuria
* moyamoya disease[93] (*see page 892*)
* strenuous physical activity

Post-traumatic dissections may be secondary to minor injuries to already susceptible vessels, e.g. in a patient with fibromuscular dysplasia. Iatrogenic injuries today are most commonly due to angiography catheters.

EPIDEMIOLOGY

Occurs primarily in middle aged patients, with a mean age of ≈ 45 yrs (average age of traumatic dissections is slightly younger). More frequent in men[90, 92]. Incidence is unknown, since often times the condition produces mild, transient symptoms. Increased awareness of the condition has resulted in an increased rate of diagnosis. ICA dissection accounted for 2.5% of first strokes in one series[94].

The largest reported series[90] (literature review + new cases) of 260 cases found the incidence by location shown in *Table 30-9*. The vertebral artery was the most common intracranial site. Previously, the carotid has been cited as the most common site. This change may be due to the recent increased recognition of arterial dissections as a source of SAH (and vertebral dissections most often present as SAH). Multiple dissections occur in ≈ 10% (the most common: bilateral vertebrobasilar lesions).

Table 30-9 Spontaneous intracranial dissections by site

Location	Left	Right	Total
vertebral	122	82	204
basilar	35		35
internal carotid	17	13	30
middle cerebral	16	10	26
anterior cerebral	10	3	13
posterior cerebral	7	9	16
PICA	4	10	14
Total	176	127	338

CLINICAL

Cerebral arterial dissections may cause symptoms by:
- embolization secondary to:
  - ♦ platelet aggregation stimulated by the exposed surfaces
  - ♦ dislodged thrombus (formation of which is enhanced by reduced flow)
- reduced distal flow secondary to:
  - ♦ thrombosis due to reduced flow
  - ♦ occlusion of the true lumen by the expansion of the mural hematoma
- subarachnoid hemorrhage (atypical presentation, may be more common with posterior circulation dissection than with anterior circulation)[95]

The most common presentation in patients < 30 yrs of age was due to carotid dissection without SAH. In patients > 30 yrs, vertebrobasilar artery **(VBA)** dissection with SAH was the most common[90].

Headache, usually severe, often predates neurologic deficit by days or weeks. See following sections (carotid *page 885*, and vertebrobasilar *page 886*) for specifics.

EVALUATION

Angiography

The definitive diagnostic study. However, diagnosis is often delayed because errors in interpretation are frequent and include misinterpreting the dissection as:
1. an unusual saccular aneurysm (the most common error)
2. atherosclerotic lesions: with dissections, the location is unusual, the lesion may be isolated, the age is usually younger, and the stenosis is smooth
3. vasospasm following SAH: however, the narrowing with vasospasm is delayed in onset vs. the changes with dissection which are present from the beginning

Angiographic findings may include:
1. luminal stenosis: irregular stenosis over long segments of the artery often with focal areas of near total stenosis (**"string sign"**)
2. fusiform dilation with proximal or distal narrowing (string and pearl sign)
3. occlusion: artery usually tapers to a point
4. intimal flap: when seen, usually found at proximal end of dissection
5. may see proximal beading ("string of beads" configuration, indicative of FMD)
6. **"double lumen sign"**: true vessel lumen and a intramural false lumen with an intimal flap. Usually with retention of contrast within the false lumen well into the venous phase. The only pathognomonic sign
7. wavy "ripple" appearance
8. severe kinking (frequently bilateral). With VBA lesions: dolichoectasia

A characteristic of arterial dissections is that they often change configuration on repeat angiography[96] (some resolve, and some worsen).

MRI

Arteriogram is the gold standard test, but MRI (more than MRA) is catching up. Crescent sign: bright signal in wall of carotid on T2WI axial images (hematoma in vessel wall).

May visualize intimal flap and distinguish a dissection from a fusiform aneurysm. Role of MRA is yet to be determined.

CT

More useful for evaluating brain for infarction. Dissection can sometimes be visualized directly[97].

OUTCOME

An early review of the literature found an 83% mortality within a few weeks of presentation with vertebrobasilar artery **(VBA)** dissection[98]. A later report tempered that grim prognosis[99].

Based on a review of 260 cases[90], an overall mortality of 26% was found. 70% had a favorable outcome (based on Glasgow Outcome scale), 5% poor. Mortality was higher in carotid lesions (49%) than VBA lesions (22%). Mortality was 24% in the SAH group, and 29% in non-SAH cases.

30.2.1. Carotid dissection

See *Cerebral arterial dissections* above for general information. Post-traumatic is much more common than spontaneous.

SPONTANEOUS

Some cases considered "spontaneous" may actually be due to trivial trauma, including violent coughing, nose blowing, and simple neck turning. Usually seen in young women.

In spontaneous dissection, the most common initial symptom is ipsilateral headache. Most of these (60%) are orbital or periorbital, but they may also be auricular or mastoid (39%), frontal (36%), temporal (27%). May also produce sudden onset of severe pain over carotid artery **(carotidynia)**[48].

Incomplete Horner's syndrome **(oculosympathetic palsy)**: ptosis and miosis without anhidrosis (due to involvement of plexus around the ICA, sparing the ECA plexus which innervates facial sweat glands) may occur. Bruits may be heard by the examiner or by the patient. These and other clinical features are shown in *Table 30-10*.

May be a cause of infantile and childhood hemiplegia and hemiparesis[100].

Table 30-10 Clinical features of spontaneous ICA dissection[92]

Feature	%
focal cerebral ischemia	76%
headache	59%
oculosympathetic palsy	30%
bruit	25%
amaurosis fugax	10%
neck pain	9%
syncope	4%
scalp tenderness	2%
neck swelling	2%

POSTTRAUMATIC

Hyperextension with lateral rotation is a common mechanism of injury, and is thought to stretch the ICA over the transverse processes of the upper cervical spine. Usually seen following MVAs, other traumatic etiologies include: chiropractic manipulation, attempted strangulation[101], and following cerebral angiography. Initially, there may be no neurologic sequelae, however, progressive thrombosis, intramural hemorrhage or embolic phenomenon may develop in a delayed fashion. The distribution of time delays following trauma to time of presentation are shown in *Table 30-11* (the majority are evident within the 1st 24 hours).

In posttraumatic dissection, ischemic symptoms are the most common[92].

Table 30-11 Time to presentation after non-penetrating trauma

Time	%
0-1 hours	6-10% of cases
1-24 hours	57-73%
after 24 hours	17-35%

EVALUATION

Most dissections start ≈ 2 cm distal to the ICA origin. See section under *Cerebral arterial dissections*. on page 884 for radiographic findings.

TREATMENT

Optimal treatment has not been determined. For cases not presenting with bleeding, anticoagulate with IV heparin **x** 1-2 wks then warfarin (Coumadin®) an additional 4-12 wks (rationale: most heal with canalization in 6 wks). Repeat angiography may be helpful to evaluate the artery before discontinuing therapy. Anticoagulation risks include extension of the medial hemorrhage (with possible SAH), and intracerebral hemorrhage (conversion of pale infarct to hemorrhagic).

If symptoms due to emboli persist, may need surgical intervention. The decision to operate must be made with extreme caution, the vessel wall is usually thin and friable, and the dissection often extends up to the skull base. Options include:
1. repair with autogenous interposition vein graft
2. EC-IC bypass (requires immediate high-flow type, therefore saphenous vein graft commonly employed) followed by ICA ligation
3. carotid ligation (alone) may rarely be indicated

OUTCOME

Natural history is not well known. Many patients with minor symptoms may not present and presumably do well. In one series, 75% of patients returned to normal, 16% had a minor deficit, and 8% had a major deficit or died[102].

30.2.2.   Vertebrobasilar system artery dissection

VERTEBRAL ARTERY DISSECTIONS

See *Cerebral arterial dissections* on page 883 for general information. Less common than carotid dissection (16th case of extracranial dissection in literature reported in 1987[103]). Extracranial lesions outnumber intracranial.

Traumatic dissections tend to occur where the artery crosses bony prominences, e.g. at the C1-2 junction. Spontaneous dissections tend to be intracranial and commonly occur on the <u>dominant</u> VA.

SPONTANEOUS

Has been associated with FMD, migraine, and oral contraceptives[103]. Unrecognized or forgotten trauma or sudden head motion may have occurred in some cases reported as spontaneous. Commonly occurs in young adults (mean age: 48 yrs). With spontaneous dissections, 36% of patients have dissections at other sites, 21% of cases have bilateral VA dissections[104].

Dissecting aneurysms of the VA (possibly a distinct entity) are also described[105-107]. They tend to be fusiform, and may be amenable to clipping, and were associated with vertebral dissections in 5 of 7 cases reported in one series[108]. As of 1984, only ≈ 50 cases of dissecting aneurysms were published[108].

POST-TRAUMATIC

Can follow neck manipulation[109] (including chiropractic or similar, which comprise 11 of 15 case reports reviewed by Caplan, et al.[110]), automobile accidents, sudden head turning or direct blows to the back of the neck[110].

PRESENTATION

In spontaneous extradural dissections, neck pain is a prominent early finding in most patients, and is commonly located over the occiput and posterior cervical region.

Generalized severe headache is also common. TIAs or stroke (usually lateral medullary syndrome[111] (*see page 777*) or cerebellar infarction, especially in patients with occlusion of the third or fourth portion of the VA[110]). None of 5 patients developed new neurologic symptoms after the original stroke in an average of 21 months follow-up[110]. In 3 of these 5, VA dissection was bilateral.

Dissecting aneurysms may present with altered consciousness, and may cause SAH (seen in 6 of 30 cases of vertebrobasilar complex dissections)[108]. Rebleeding occurs in 24-30% of those cases presenting with SAH[104], making these lesions treacherous, with a very high mortality[112, 113].

Traumatic extradural dissections or pseudoaneurysms may have a similar presentation, but can also produce massive external hemorrhage or neck hematomas[104].

EVALUATION

See section under *Cerebral arterial dissections.* on page 884.

Angiography

Diagnosis by angiography may be difficult in many cases (the most common misdiagnosis is ruptured saccular aneurysm of unusual shape[114]).

In post-traumatic dissections most common finding is irregular stenosis of horizontal loops of distal extracranial VAs as they pass behind C1, often bilateral.

In 14 of 15 post-traumatic VA dissections, the lesion was located posterior to the atlas (distal extracranial 3rd segment), the single exception being a patient with direct trauma causing proximal VA involvement. This predilection is possibly explained by the fact that the first and third portions of the VA are movable, whereas the second and fourth are relatively immobilized by bone.

TREATMENT

Except for cases presenting with hemorrhage or large ischemic stroke, medical therapy should be started emergently, and consists of anticoagulation, with heparin acutely, followed by oral agents (e.g.Coumadin) probably for a total of 6 months.

Indications for surgery:

Surgical therapy is required for dissections presenting with SAH (due to their propensity to rebleed) and is recommended for most intradural dissections. For extradural lesions it is indicated for dissections that progress (angiographically) or for persistent symptoms in spite of adequate medical therapy.

At the time of surgery, the site of dissection may be recognized by fusiform or tubular enlargement of the artery with discoloration due to blood within the arterial wall (the discoloration has been described as black, bluish, purple, purple red, or brown[114]).

Surgical treatment of intradural dissection includes the following options:
1. non-clippable aneurysms may be candidates for Hunterian occlusion of the VA proximal to the BA (either by microsurgical technique, or by endovascular techniques which may not be as precise). Some may not tolerate clipping the dominant VA, especially if the contralateral VA is hypoplastic. Conversely, some may tolerate bilateral VA occlusion[115]). Balloon test occlusion[104] is recommended
   A. if the dissection involves the PICA origin, then clip proximal to dissection. PICA then fills from retrograde flow, and the reversal of flow across the site of dissection should push the intima back against the wall
   B. if the dissection is proximal to PICA and doesn't involve PICA, then trap the aneurysm between clips. PICA fills by retrograde flow
   C. if the aneurysm begins distal to the PICA origin, occlude the VA[95] distal to the PICA takeoff[116]
2. combining VA clipping (*see above*) with vascular bypass, options:
   A. side-to-side PICA-PICA anastamosis
   B. transplantation of the PICA origin to the VA outside the aneurysm
   C. occipital artery-to-PICA bypass
3. resection accompanied by autogenous interposition vein graft
4. endovascular techniques (balloons, coils, angioplasty...[104])
5. non occlusive external techniques
   A. clipping with specially designed clips for fusiform aneurysms (e.g. Sundt-Kees clip)
   B. wrapping: of dubious benefit

Basilar artery dissections tend to present with brain stem infarction and more rarely with SAH[113]. The prognosis is generally regarded as poor.

30.3. Extracranial-intracranial (EC/IC) bypass

Includes but not limited to superficial temporal artery-middle cerebral artery (STA-MCA) bypass. Results of the international cooperative EC/IC bypass study group[117]: 1377 patients with recent hemispheric CVA, retinal infarct or TIA with narrowing or occlusion of ipsilateral ICA or MCA. Randomized to medical (714 patients) (325 mg ASA QID) or STA-MCA bypass (663 patients), followed 55.8 mos mean. Perioperative (includes pre-op randomization period averaging 9 days until 30 days post-op) fatal stroke rate was 1.1%, non-fatal major stroke 4.5% (30 day post-op figures, 0.6% and 2.5%). Medical group 39 day major (fatal & non-fatal) stroke rate 1.3% → excess 3.2% major stroke rate in bypassed patients, with 96% patency rate at an average of 32 days post bypass. No subgroup was identified with any benefit from bypass. Two groups did worse (viz: severe MCA stenosis, and those with ischemic symptoms and occluded ICA).

30.4. Cerebrovascular venous thrombosis

Cerebrovascular venous thrombosis (CVVT) includes dural sinus thrombosis (DST) and cortical venous thrombosis.

ETIOLOGIES

Many conditions have been incriminated with CVVT. Some common ones are listed below (see reference[118 (p 1301)] for extensive list):
1. infection
   A. usually local, e.g. otitis media[119, 120] (leading to the now obsolete term otitic hydrocephalus), sinusitis, peritonsillar abscess, paranasal sinusitis[121]
   B. meningitis
2. pregnancy & puerperium: see below
3. birth control pills (BCP) (oral contraceptives)[122]
4. dehydration and cachexia (marantic thrombosis): includes burns and cachexia of neoplastic disease
5. cardiac disease (including CHF)
6. ulcerative colitis (UC): 1% of UC patients have some thrombotic complication (not necessarily intracranial), and this is the cause of ≈ 33% of deaths (usually pulmonary embolism)
7. periarteritis nodosa
8. sickle cell trait
9. trauma (including closed head injury): see below
10. iatrogenic: e.g. S/P radical neck surgery[123], transvenous pacemaker placement, post-craniotomy
11. malignancy: including myeloproliferative disorders
12. hypercoagulable state (AKA thrombophilia)
    A. protein C deficiency or resistance to activated protein C
    B. antithrombin III deficiency
    C. protein S deficiency
    D. antiphospholipid antibodies: associated with a variety of clinical syndromes including ischemic CVA, DVTs, thrombocytopenia, systemic lupus erythematosus (see page 775)
    E. paroxysmal nocturnal hemoglobinuria (PNH)
    F. plasminogen deficiency
    G. systemic lupus erythematosus[124]
13. diabetes mellitus: especially with ketoacidosis
14. homocystinuria: see page 775

15. Behçet's syndrome[125]: *see page 62*
16. rarely associated with lumbar puncture[126]

In the absence of factors such as BCP use, CVVT is highly suggestive of myeloproliferative disorder.

Pregnancy/puerperium
Highest risk is in first 2 wks post-partum. One series[127] found no case of CVVT occurred later than 16 days post-partum. Incidence ≈ 1/10,000 births.

Trauma
A rare sequelae of closed head injury[128]. CVVT occurs in ≈ 10% of combat injuries involving the brain. May occur in absence of skull fracture. CVVT should be suspected in patients with fractures or missiles crossing sinus.

FREQUENCY OF INVOLVEMENT OF DURAL SINUSES AND OTHER VEINS
1. sinuses
   A. superior sagittal sinus (SSS) and left transverse sinus (TS) (70% each)
   B. multiple sinuses in 71%
   C. inferior sagittal sinus: rare, first case report in 1997[129]
   D. straight sinus[130]
2. superficial cortical veins
3. deep venous system (e.g. internal cerebral vein)
4. cavernous sinus[131, 132]: rare. Thrombophlebitis of the cavernous sinus may be caused by sphenoid sinusitis

PATHOPHYSIOLOGY
Venous thrombosis reduces venous outflow from the brain and diminishes effective blood flow to the involved area. This venous engorgement causes white matter edema. The increased venous pressure may also lead to infarction and/or hemorrhage. These processes may all elevate ICP. Thus, clinical findings may be due to elevated ICP, and focal findings may be due to edema and/or hemorrhage. Cerebral infarction in this setting is called venous infarction.

CLINICAL
Clinical presentations of DST are shown in *Table 30-12*. There are no pathognomonic findings. Many signs and symptoms are due to elevated ICP. May present as a syndrome clinically indistinguishable from idiopathic intracranial hypertension (pseudotumor cerebri) (*see page 493*).

There is a high association of concurrent thromboembolic disease in other organs.

The anterior 1/3 of the SSS may occlude often without sequelae. Posterior to this, venous infarction is more likely to develop. Midportion SSS occlusion usually → increased muscle tone ranging from spastic hemi- or quadri-paresis to decerebration. Posterior SSS thrombosis → field cuts or cortical blindness, or massive CVA with cerebral edema and death. Occlusion of the TS

Table 30-12   Presentation of dural sinus thrombosis

Sign/symptom	Series A*	Series B*
H/A	100%	74%
N/V	75%	–
seizures	70%	29%
hemiparesis	70%	34%
papilledema	70%	45%
blurred vision	60%	–
altered consciousness	35%	26%

*   series A: 20 young females[127]; series B: 38 cases from France[133]

may occur without deficit unless the contralateral TS is hypoplastic, in which cases presentation is similar to posterior SSS occlusion.

SSS occlusion alone will not cause cranial nerve findings except perhaps for visual obscuration and abducens (VI) nerve palsy from elevated of ICP. Thrombosis in the jugular bulb may compress the nerves in the jugular foramen pars nervosa causing hoarseness, aphonia, difficulty swallowing and breathlessness (see *Vernet's syndrome*, page 86)[134].

DIAGNOSIS OF DST
Although angiography was often considered the "gold standard", MRI is probably

more accurate. Angiography is often used as a confirmatory test[135].

CT SCAN

Non-contrast CT

May be normal in 10-20% of cases of DST. Findings include:
1. hyperdense sinuses and veins (high density clots in cortical veins produce the **cord sign** which is pathognomonic for cerebral venous thrombosis; seen in only 2/30 patients)
2. petechial "flame" hemorrhages (intraparenchymal): seen in 20% (suspect sinus thrombosis with intracerebral hemorrhages in unusual locations for aneurysm or "hypertensive" hemorrhage)
3. small ventricles: seen in 50%
4. thrombosis of superior sagittal sinus may produce a triangular-shaped high density within the sinus (some refer to this as the **delta sign**, but this causes confusion with the "empty delta sign", *see below*) (there is also confusion when an apparent "empty delta sign" is seen <u>without</u> contrast, this may occur when there is blood surrounding the SSS, e.g. following subarachnoid hemorrhage, this has been called a "false delta sign" or **pseudodelta sign**[136])
5. white matter edema
6. above changes occurring <u>bilaterally</u>

IV contrast CT

Findings of DST include:
1. with <u>contrast</u>, the dura around the sinus may enhance and become denser than clot in 35% of cases[137]. Near the Torcular herophili this produces what has been called the **empty delta sign**[138], but sometimes this, too, is called the **delta sign**
2. gyral enhancement occurs in 32%
3. dense deep (white matter) veins (collateral flow)
4. intense tentorial enhancement (common)

MRI

Currently the mainstay of diagnosis and follow-up (demonstrates both vascular and parenchymal changes). Clearly differentiates occluded sinus from congenital absence. Shows cerebral edema and non-acute hemorrhagic changes to better advantage than CT. Also may help estimate age of clots (*see Table 30-13*). MR-angiography may increase the utility.

Table 30-13 MRI appearance of thrombosed sinuses at various stages

Age of clot in sinus	— Appearance of clotted sinus —	
	T1WI	T2WI
acute	iso-intense	decreased (black): can mimic flow void
subacute	increased (1st)	increased (2nd)
late (> 10 d, recanalized)	black (flow void)	black (flow void)

ANGIOGRAPHY FOR DST

Accuracy close to MRI. MRI has some advantages over angiography (e.g. on angiography a hypoplastic transverse sinus may not visualize, or non-opacified blood entering a sinus may mimic a filling defect).

Findings include:
1. non-filling of segments of sinuses, or filling defects
2. prolonged circulation time: in 50% of cases (may need delayed films to see veins)
3. stumps and abnormal collateral pathways

LP

OP usually increased. CSF bloody or xanthochromic.

BLOODWORK

To detect predisposing conditions when the etiology is unknown. Some tests that may be useful include evaluation for thrombophilia (protein C and S levels, antiphospholipid antibodies) as well as tests for specific predisposing conditions (CBC, Factor II level, serum homocystine level, paroxysmal nocturnal hemoglobinuria (PNH) panel, leukocyte alkaline phosphatase).

May be used in diagnosis of superior sagittal sinus thrombosis in the neonate[139].

TREATMENT

Should be aggressive because recoverability of brain is probably greater than with arterial occlusive stroke. Management is complicated because measures that counteract thrombosis (e.g. anticoagulation) tend to increase the risk of hemorrhagic infarct (the risk of which is already increased), and measures that lower ICP tend to increase blood viscosity → increased coagulability.

Specific measures
1. correct underlying abnormality when possible (e.g. antibiotics for infection)
2. **heparin** (systemic): (*see page 22* for dosing) especially if patient is in DIC. Several studies show a lower mortality rate with heparin than without[140-142]. It remains the best treatment even when there is evidence of intracerebral hemorrhage with the attendant risk of increasing the size of the hemorrhage[135]. There is no consensus on duration of treatment or if warfarin should be used afterwards. Success rate may be higher if administered before patient becomes moribund
3. avoid steroids (reduces fibrinolysis, increases coagulation)
4. control HTN
5. anticonvulsants to control seizures
6. monitor ICP if patient continues to deteriorate: ventriculostomy preferred, but caution must be used if patient is on heparin
   A. hydrate aggressively as ICP tolerates
   B. measures to lower ICP: in general, order is almost reverse of that for traumatic intracranial hypertension because diuretics → hypertonicity → ↑ viscosity → ↑ coagulation
      a. elevate HOB
      b. hyperventilation
      c. drain CSF
      d. pentobarbital coma
      e. use hyperosmotic and/or loop diuretics last. Replace fluid loss with isotonic IV fluids to prevent dehydration (i.e. goal is hypertonic euvolemia)
7. thrombolytic therapy: either systemically or infused directly into clotted sinus[135, 143], may be followed with heparin
   A. urokinase[130, 143] or streptokinase
   B. intravenous **tissue plasminogen activator (tPA)**: promising animal evidence[144], not yet reported in humans
8. when above measures fail, either
   A. decompressive craniectomy (± decompressive lobectomy): this decreases ICP, but may not improve outcome
   OR
   B. direct "attack" on clotted sinus: direct surgical treatment when deficit progresses in spite of above measures, or ICP not manageable (i.e. failure of medical therapy) (*see below*)
9. visual loss with papilledema may be treated with optic nerve sheath fenestration/decompression[145]
10. long-term treatment after resolution of acute phase with heparin and/or warfarin x 3-6 months

DIRECT SURGICAL TREATMENT FOR DST

Rarely indicated. Thrombectomy and sinus reconstruction are technically possible, but rethrombosis is common. Surgery may be indicated for abscess requiring excision.

Surgical technique for direct treatment of SSS thrombosis

PROGNOSIS

Mortality: approximately 30% (range: 5-70%) (10% in French series[133]).

Poor prognosticators: coma, extremes of age (infancy or elderly), rapid neurologic deterioration, focal signs.

30.5.   Moyamoya disease

Progressive spontaneous occlusion of one or usually both ICAs (at the level of the siphon) and their major branches, with secondary formation of anastamotic collateral capillary network at the base of the brain which fancifully resembles "moyamoya", the Japanese word for "puff of smoke"[146]. With progression, involvement includes the proximal MCAs and ACAs and on rare occasion the vertebrobasilar system. Associated aneurysms (*see below*) and rarely AVMs[147, 148] may be observed.

Eventually the dilated capillary (moyamoya) vessels disappear with the development of collaterals from the ECA (meningeal collaterals are called **"rete mirabile"**).

Pathophysiology

Etiology: The etiology is not known, although the immune system may be involved.

Pathology: The main trunks of involved intracranial skull base arteries are narrowed due to thickened intima (lipid deposits occur without evidence of inflammation). The internal elastic lamina may be thinned or duplicated. There are areas of focal fibrin deposition and thinning of the vessel wall, particularly the media and adventitia. Similar vascular changes may also occur in the heart, kidney and other organs, suggesting it may be a systemic vascular disease.

Associated aneurysms

Intracranial aneurysms are frequently associated with moyamoya disease (**MMD**). This may be a result of the increased flow through dilated collaterals, or it may be that patients with moyamoya may also have a congenital defect in the arterial wall that predisposes them to aneurysms. 3 usual sites of aneurysms in the Circle of Willis, 2) in peripheral portions of cerebral arteries, e.g. posterior/anterior choroidal, Heubner's, and 3) within moyamoya vessels. The frequency of aneurysms in the vertebrobasilar system is ≈ 62% which is much higher than in the general population[149]. Aneurysmal SAH may be the actual cause of some hemorrhages that were erroneously attributed to moyamoya vessels.

EPIDEMIOLOGY

Risk factors: A history of inflammation in the head & neck region has been implicated.

Demographics: Incidence in Japan is higher (< 1/100,000/yr) than in North America. Two peaks (may not be same disease): juvenile, age < 10 yrs (mean 3); adult, 3rd & 4th decade. Slight female predominance. Some evidence for familial tendency (some Asian families have an incidence as high as 7%), genetics not determined. Associated with some HLA antigens (B40 in juvenile form; B54(20) in adult). May also seen in association with:
* neurofibromatosis type 1
* tuberous sclerosis
* history of cerebral inflammatory disease, including meningitis (especially tubercular meningitis)
* sickle cell anemia
* retinitis pigmentosa
* atherosclerosis
* fibromuscular dysplasia
* pseudoxanthoma elasticum
* Down's syndrome
* Fanconi's anemia
* following radiation therapy for skull base glioma in children[150]
* head trauma

Natural history

Prognosis of untreated MMD is poor, with 73% rate of major deficit or death within 2 years of diagnosis in children, and similarly poor outlook in adults[151].

PRESENTATION

Juvenile form: Ischemic presentation more common (81%); includes TIAs (41%) which may alternate sides (alternating hemiplegia is a suggestive clinical finding), RINDs, or infarct (40%). Neurologic events are often provoked by straining or by hyperventilation (e.g. during crying or blowing a wind instrument) which is thought to produce hypocapnea with reactive vasoconstriction. May also present with seizures, progressive cognitive decline, or involuntary movements. Pathological process remains active through age 10 yrs, then stabilizes.

Adult form: Hemorrhage has been described as being more common (60%). Rupture of the fragile moyamoya vessels produces bleeding in the basal ganglia (BG), thalamus or ventricles (from the ventricular wall) in 70-80% of hemorrhages. SAH may occur, usually due to rupture of associated aneurysms (*see above*). In the pre-CT era, the most common form of hemorrhage was thought to be SAH from the rupture of moyamoya vessels, but most cases were probably intraventricular blood or SAH from associated aneurysms[152].

EVALUATION

ANGIOGRAPHY

In addition to helping to establish the diagnosis, angiography also identifies suitable vessels for anastamotic procedures. The complication rate is higher than with atherosclerotic occlusive disease. Avoid dehydration prior to and hypotension during the procedure. Six angiographic stages of MMD are described in *Table 30-14*[153] that tend to progress up until adolescence and stabilize by age 20.

There are no internationally accepted diagnostic criteria. Characteristic findings include:

Table 30-14 Six angiographic stages of MMD[153]

Stage	Finding
1	stenosis of suprasellar ICA, usually bilateral
2	development of moyamoya vessels at base of brain
3	increasing ICA stenosis & prominence of moyamoya vessels (most cases diagnosed at this stage)
4	entire circle of Willis and PCAs occluded, extracranial collaterals start to appear, moyamoya vessels begin to diminish
5	further progression of stage 4
6	complete absence of moyamoya vessels and major cerebral arteries

- stenosis/occlusion starting at termination of ICA and at origins of ACA and MCA
- abnormal vascular network in region of BG (intraparenchymal anastamosis)
- above findings are bilateral and usually symmetrical (if unilateral, the diagnosis is considered questionable[154])
- transdural anastomosis (**rete mirabile**), AKA "vault moyamoya". Contributing arteries: anterior falcial, middle meningeal, ethmoidal, occipital, tentorial, STA
- moyamoya collaterals may also form from internal maxillary artery via ethmoid sinus to forebrain in frontobasal region

EEG

Non-specific in the adult. Juvenile cases: high-voltage slow waves may be seen at rest, predominantly in the occipital and frontal lobes. Hyperventilation produces a normal buildup of monophasic slow waves (delta-bursts) that return to normal 20-60 seconds after hyperventilation. In > 50% of cases, after or sometimes continuous with buildup is a second phase of slow waves (this characteristic finding is called "**rebuild-up**") which are more irregular and slower than the earlier waves, and usually normalize in ≤ 10 minutes[155].

CT

Up to 40% of ischemic cases have normal CT. Low density areas (**LDAs**) may be seen, usually confined to cortex and subcortically (unlike atherosclerotic disease or acute infantile hemiplegia which tend to have LDAs in BG as well). LDAs tend to be multiple and bilateral, especially in the PCA distribution (poor collaterals), and are more common in children.

MRI AND MRA

MRA usually discloses the stenosis or occlusion of the ICA. Moyamoya vessels appear as flow voids on MRI and a fine network of vessels on MRA, and are demonstrated better in children than adults. Parenchymal ischemic changes are commonly shown, usually in watershed areas.

CBF is decreased in children with MMD, but relatively normal in adults. There is a shift of CBF from the frontal to the occipital lobes[156] probably reflecting the increasing dependency of CBF on the posterior circulation. Children with MMD have impaired autoregulation of CBF to blood pressure and CO_2 (with more impairment of vasodilatation in response to hypercapnia or hypotension than vasoconstriction in response to hypocapnia or hypertension)[157].

Xenon (Xe-133) CT can identify areas of low perfusion. Repeating the study after an acetazolamide challenge (which causes vasodilatation) evaluates reserve capacity of CBF and can identify areas of "steal" which are at high risk of future infarction.

TREATMENT

No medical or surgical treatment has been proven effective in reducing the rate of hemorrhage in the adult with MMD.

MEDICAL TREATMENT

Medical treatment with platelet inhibitors, anticoagulants, calcium channel blockers or other drugs has not proven to be of benefit [151]. Steroids may be considered for involuntary movements and acutely during recurrent TIAs.

SURGICAL TREATMENT

Patients with mass effect from clot may be candidates for urgent decompression. Revascularization procedures, however, should be performed when the patient is stable under nonemergent conditions.

Indications for revascularization procedures: Patients with MMD who have:
1. symptoms due to ischemia
2. previous hemorrhage
3. progressive neurologic deficits: cognitive decline, progressive seizures…

Surgical options: Various methods to revascularize the ischemic brain, include:
1. direct revascularization procedures: results are superior to indirect revascularization procedures[158, 159] if a donor and recipient vessel of sufficient caliber (≥ 1 mm outer dia) can be identified (may be difficult in the pediatric age group who are the most likely to benefit[160]). Otherwise, indirect revascularization procedures (*see below*) are options
   * STA-MCA bypass[161]: the procedure of choice
2. indirect revascularization procedures (may be combined with STA-MCA bypass):
   A. encephalomyosynangiosis (**EMS**): laying the temporalis muscle on the surface of the brain (may cause problems with muscle contractions during talking and chewing, and neural impulses on surface of brain)
   B. encephaloduroarteriosynangiosis (**EDAS**)[162, 163]: suturing the STA with a galeal cuff to a linear defect created in the dura. Variations on this technique include splitting the dura[164]
   C. omental transposition[165]: either as a pedicle graft or as a vascularized free flap. Felt to have higher potential to revascularize ischemic tissue than above procedures, but there is greater risk of mass effect from the thickness of the omentum
3. the above indirect revascularization procedures improve blood flow in the MCA distribution, but not ACA circulation. This may be rectified by:
   A. simple placement of frontal burr holes with opening of the underlying dura and arachnoid[166]
   B. "ribbon EDAS" where a pedicle of galea is inserted into the interhemispheric fissure on both sides[167]
4. stellate ganglionectomy and perivascular sympathectomy: unproven that this increases CBF permanently

Postoperatively following STA-MAC bypass procedures:
1. avoid hypertension: may cause bleeding at anastamotic site and in areas of increased perfusion within the brain
2. avoid hypotension: may result in graft occlusion
3. aspirin is started on the post-op day #1
4. watch for evidence of CSF leak
5. monitor coag studies and correct abnormalities

6. cerebral arteriogram is recommended 2-6 months post-op

PROGNOSIS

The mortality rate in adults ($\approx 10\%$) is higher than for juveniles ($\approx 4.3\%$)[154]. The cause of death was bleeding in 56% of 9 children and 63% of 30 adults. With treatment the prognosis is good in 58%[152].

30.6. References

1. Werdelin L, Juhler M: The course of transient ischemic attacks. **Neurology** 38: 677-80, 1988.
2. Levy D E: How transient are transient ischemic attacks? **Neurology** 38: 674-7, 1988.
3. Moneta G L, Taylor D C, Nicholls S C, et al.: Operative versus nonoperative management of asymptomatic high-grade internal carotid artery stenosis. **Stroke** 18: 1005-10, 1987.
4. Kistler J P, Furie K L: Carotid endarterectomy revisited. **N Engl J Med** 342: 1743-5, 2000.
5. Moore W S, Boren C, Malone J M, et al.: Natural history of nonstenotic, asymptomatic ulcerative lesions of the carotid artery. **Arch Surg** 113: 1352-9, 1978.
6. Martin N A, Hadley M N, Spetzler R F, et al.: Management of asymptomatic carotid atherosclerosis. **Neurosurgery** 18: 505-12, 1986.
7. The Executive Committee for the Asymptomatic Carotid Atherosclerosis Study: Endarterectomy for asymptomatic carotid artery stenosis. **JAMA** 273: 1421-8, 1995.
8. The North American Symptomatic Carotid Endarterectomy Trial: Beneficial effect of carotid endarterectomy in symptomatic patients with high-grade carotid stenosis. **N Engl J Med** 325: 445-53, 1991.
9. The European Carotid Surgery Trialists' Collaborative Group: Randomized trial of endartectomy for recently symptomatic carotid stenosis: Final results of the MRC European carotid surgery trial (ECST). **Lancet** 351: 1379-87, 1998.
10. Rothwell P M, Gibson R J, Slattery J, et al.: Equivalence of measurements of carotid stenosis: A comparison of three methods on 1001 angiograms. **Stroke** 25: 2435-39, 1994.
11. Anson J A, Heiserman J E, Drayer B P, et al.: Surgical decisions on the basis of magnetic resonance angiography of the carotid arteries. **Neurosurgery** 32: 335-43, 1993.
12. Heiserman J E, Zabramski J M, Drayer B P, et al.: Clinical significance of the flow gap in carotid magnetic resonance angiography. **J Neurosurg** 85: 384-7, 1996.
13. Anderson C M, Saloner D, Lee R E, et al.: Assessment of carotid artery stenosis by MR angiography: Comparison with x-ray angiography and color-coded Doppler ultrasound. **AJNR** 13: 989-1003, 1992.
14. Ausman J I, Shrontz C E, Pearce J E, et al.: Vertebrobasilar insufficiency: A review. **Arch Neurol** 42: 803-8, 1985.
15. Meissner I, Wiebers D O, Whisnant J P, et al.: The natural history of asymptomatic carotid artery occlusive lesions. **JAMA** 258: 2704-7, 1987.
16. Tsai F Y, Matovich V, Heishima G, et al.: Percutaneous transluminal angioplasty of the carotid artery. **AJNR** 7: 349-58, 1986.
17. Higashida R T, Hieshima G B, Tsai F Y, et al.: Transluminal angioplasty of the vertebral and basilar artery. **AJNR** 8: 745-9, 1987.
18. Weksler B B, Pett S B, Alonso D, et al.: Differential inhibition by aspirin of vascular and platelet prostaglandin synthesis in atherosclerotic patients. **N Engl J Med** 308: 800-5, 1983.
19. Grotta J C: Current medical and surgical therapy for cerebrovascular disease. **N Engl J Med** 317: 1505-16, 1987.
20. Théroux P, Fuster V: Acute coronary syndromes: Unstable angina and non-Q-wave myocardial infarction. **Circulation** 97: 1195-1206, 1998.
21. Taylor D W, Barnett H J M, Haynes R B, et al.: Low-dose and high-dose acetylsalicylic acid for patients undergoing carotid endarterectomy: A randomized controlled trial. **Lancet** 353: 2179-84, 1999.
22. Hass W K, Easton J D, Adams H P, et al.: A randomized trial comparing ticlopidine hydrochloride with aspirin for the prevention of stroke in high-risk patients. **N Engl J Med** 321: 501-7, 1989.
23. Bellavance A: Efficacy of ticlopidine and aspirin for prevention of reversible cerebrovascular ischemic events: The ticlopidine aspirin stroke study (TASS). **Stroke** 24: 1452-7, 1993.
24. Harbison L A: Stroke prevention in women: Role of aspirin versus ticlopidine. **Am J Med** 91: 288-92, 1991.
25. Clopidogrel for reduction of atherosclerotic events. **Med Letter** 40: 59-60, 1998.
26. Biller J, Feinberg W M, Castaldo J E, et al.: Guidelines for carotid endarterectomy: A statement for healthcare professionals from a Special Writing Group of the Stroke Council, American Heart Association. **Circulation** 97 (5): 501-9, 1998.
27. Bogousslavsky J, Despland P-A, Regli F: Asymptomatic tight stenosis of the internal carotid artery. **Neurology** 36: 861-3, 1986.
28. Roederer G O, Langlois Y E, Jager K A, et al.: The natural history of carotid arterial disease in asymptomatic patients with cervical bruits. **Stroke** 15: 605-13, 1984.
29. Halliday A, Mansfield A, Marro J, et al.: Prevention of disabling and fatal strokes by successful carotid endarterectomy in patients without recent neurological symptoms. Randomised controlled trial. **Lancet** 363 (9420): 1491-502, 2004.
30. Norris J W, Zhu C Z, Bornstein N M, et al.: Vascular risks of asymptomatic carotid stenosis. **Stroke** 22: 1485-90, 1991.
31. Hobson R W, Weiss D G, Fields W S, et al.: Efficacy of carotid endarterectomy for asymptomatic carotid stenosis. **N Engl J Med** 328: 221-7, 1993.
32. EAFT (European Atrial Fibrillation Trial) Study Group: Secondary prevention in non-rheumatic atrial fibrillation after transient ischemic attack or minor stroke. **Lancet** 342: 1255-62, 1993.
33. Albers G W: Atrial fibrillation and stroke. **Arch Intern Med** 154: 1443-8, 1994.
34. Mattos M A, Modi J R, Mansour M A, et al.: Evolution of carotid endarterectomy in two community hospitals: Springfield revisited - seventeen years and 2243 operations later. **J Vasc Surg** 21: 719-28, 1995.
35. CASANOVA Study Group: Carotid surgery versus medical therapy in asymptomatic carotid stenosis. **Stroke** 22: 1229-35, 1991.

36. Mayberg M R, Winn H R: Endarterectomy for asymptomatic carotid artery stenosis. Resolving the controversy. **JAMA** 273: 1459-61, 1995.

37. Chassin M R: Appropriate use of carotid endarterectomy. **N Engl J Med** 339: 1468-71, 1998 (editorial).

38. Barnett H J M, Taylor W, Eliasziw M, *et al.*: Benefit of carotid endarterectomy in patients with symptomatic moderate or severe stenosis. **N Engl J Med** 339: 1415-25, 1998.

39. The European Carotid Surgery Trialists' Collaborative Group: Endartectomy for moderate symptomatic carotid stenosis: Interim results of the MRC European carotid surgery trial. **Lancet** 347: 1591-3, 1996.

40. Sundt T M, Sandok B A, Whisnant J P: Carotid endarterectomy: Complications and preoperative assessment of risk. **Mayo Clin Proced** 50: 301-6, 1975.

41. Sundt T M: **Occlusive cerebrovascular disease.** W. B. Saunders, Philadelphia, 1987.

42. Spetzler R F, Martin N, Hadley M N, *et al.*: Microsurgical endarterectomy under barbiturate protection: A prospective study. **J Neurosurg** 65: 63-73, 1986.

43. Mayo Asymptomatic Carotid Endarterectomy Study Group: Results of a randomized controlled trial of carotid endarterectomy for asymptomatic carotid stenosis. **Mayo Clin Proc** 67: 513-8, 1992.

44. Harker L A, Bernstein E F, Dilley R B, *et al.*: Failure of aspirin plus dipyridamole to prevent restenosis after carotid endarterectomy. **Ann Int Med** 116: 731-6, 1992.

45. Brott T G, Labutta R J, Kempczinski R F: Changing patterns in the practice of carotid endarterectomy in a large metropolitan area. **JAMA** 255: 2609-12, 1986.

46. Branch C L, Davis C H: False aneurysm complicating carotid endarterectomy. **Neurosurgery** 19: 421-5, 1986.

47. McCollum C H, Wheeler W G, Noon G P, *et al.*: Aneurysms of the extracranial carotid artery. **Am J Surg** 137: 196-200, 1979.

48. Welling R E, Taha A, Goel T, *et al.*: Extracranial carotid artery aneurysms. **Surgery** 93: 319-23, 1983.

49. Reigel M M, Hollier L H, Sundt T M, *et al.*: Cerebral hyperperfusion syndrome: A cause of neurologic dysfunction after carotid endarterectomy. **J Vasc Surg** 5: 628-34, 1987.

50. Piepgras D G, Morgan M K, Sundt T M, *et al.*: Intracerebral hemorrhage after carotid endarterectomy. **J Neurosurg** 68: 532-6, 1988.

51. Ascher E, Markevich N, Schutzer R W, *et al.*: Cerebral hyperperfusion syndrome after carotid endarterectomy: Predictive factors and hemodynamic changes. **J Vasc Surg** 37 (4): 769-77, 2003.

52. Kieburtz K, Ricotta J J, Moxley R T: Seizures following carotid endarterectomy. **Arch Neurol** 47: 568-70, 1990.

53. Sundt T M, Sharbrough F W, Piepgras D G, *et al.*: Correlation of cerebral blood flow and electroencephalographic changes during carotid endarterectomy. **Mayo Clin Proc** 56: 533-43, 1981.

54. Wilkinson J T, Adams H P, Wright C B: Convulsions after carotid endarterectomy. **JAMA** 244: 1827-8, 1980.

55. Bernstein E F, Humber P B, Collins G M, *et al.*: Life expectancy and late stroke following carotid endartectomy. **Ann Surg** 198: 80-6, 1983.

56. Callow A D: Recurrent stenosis after carotid endarterectomy. **Arch Surg** 117: 1082-5, 1982.

57. Dolan J G, Mushlin A I: Hypertension, vascular headaches, and seizures after carotid endarterectomy. **Arch Intern Med** 144: 1489-91, 1984.

58. Caplan L R, Skillman J, Ojemann R, *et al.*: Intracerebral hemorrhage following carotid endarterectomy: A hypertensive complication. **Stroke** 9: 457-60, 1979.

59. Imparato A M, Bracco A, Kim G E, *et al.*: The hypoglossal nerve in carotid arterial reconstructions. **Stroke** 3: 576-8, 1972.

60. Skydell J L, Machleder H I, Baker J D, *et al.*: Incidence and mechanism of postcarotid endarterectomy hypertension. **Arch Surg** 122: 1153-5, 1987.

61. Lehv M S, Salzman E W, Silen W: Hypertension complicating carotid endarterectomy. **Stroke** 1: 307-13, 1970.

62. Baker W H: *Management of stroke during and after carotid surgery.* In **Cerebrovascular insufficiency**, Bergan J J and Yao J S T, (eds.). Grune and Stratton, New York, 1983: pp 481-95.

63. Zuccarello M, Yeh H-S, Tew J M: Morbidity and mortality of carotid endarterectomy under local anesthesia: A retrospective study. **Neurosurgery** 23: 445-50, 1988.

64. Lee K S, Courtland C H, McWhorter J M: Low morbidity and mortality of carotid endarterectomy performed with regional anesthesia. **J Neurosurg** 69: 483-7, 1988.

65. Forssell C, Takolander R, Bergqvist D, *et al.*: Local versus general anesthesia in carotid surgery. A prospective randomized study. **Eur J Vasc Surg** 3: 503-9, 1989.

66. DeMonte F, Peerless S J, Rankin R N: Carotid transluminal angioplasty with evidence of distal embolization: Case report. **J Neurosurg** 70: 138-41, 1989.

67. Culicchia F, Spetzler R F, Flom R A: Failure of transluminal angioplasty in the treatment of myointimal hyperplasia of the internal carotid artery: Case report. **Neurosurgery** 28: 148-51, 1991.

68. Smith R R, Moore T S, Russell W F: Transluminal angioplasty of the cerebral circulation. **Clin Neurosurg** 31: 117-34, 1983.

69. Fisher W S, Jordan W D: Carotid angioplasty. **Contemp Neurosurg** 19 (22): 1-6, 1997.

70. Walters B B, Ojemann R G, Heros R C: Emergency carotid endarterectomy. **J Neurosurg** 66: 817-23, 1987.

71. Hafner C D, Tew J M: Surgical management of the totally occluded internal carotid artery. **Surgery** 89: 710-7, 1981.

72. Satiani B, Burns J, Vasko J S: Surgical and nonsurgical treatment of total carotid artery occlusion. **Am J Surg** 149: 362-7, 1985.

73. McCormick P W, Spetzler R F, Bailes J E, *et al.*: Thromboendarterectomy of the symptomatic occluded internal carotid artery. **J Neurosurg** 76: 752-8, 1992.

74. Hopkins L N, Martin N A, Hadley M N, *et al.*: Vertebrobasilar insufficiency, part 2: Microsurgical treatment of intracranial vertebrobasilar disease. **J Neurosurg** 66: 662-74, 1987.

75. Robertson J T: Current management of vertebral basilar occlusive disease. **Clin Neurosurg** 31: 165-87, 1983.

76. Diaz F G, Ausman J I, de los Reyes R A, *et al.*: Surgical reconstruction of the proximal vertebral artery. **J Neurosurg** 61: 874-81, 1984.

77. Fox M W, Piepgras D G, Bartleson J D: Anterolateral decompression of the atlantoaxial vertebral artery for symptomatic positional occlusion of the vertebral artery. **J Neurosurg** 83: 737-40, 1995.

78. Pratt-Thomas H R, Berger K E: Cerebellar and spinal injuries after chiropractic manipulation. **JAMA** 133: 600-3, 1947.

79. Matsuyama T, Morimoto T, Sakaki T: Bow hunter's stroke caused by a nondominant vertebral artery occlusion: Case report. **Neurosurgery** 41: 1393-5, 1997.

80. Lemole G M, Henn J S, Spetzler R F, *et al.*: Bow hunter's stroke. **BNI Quarterly** 17: 4-10, 2001.

81. Mapstone T, Spetzler R F: Vertebrobasilar insufficiency secondary to vertebral artery occlusion from a fibrous band. Case report. **J Neurosurg** 56: 581-3,

1982.

82. George B, Laurian C: Impairment of vertebral artery flow caused by extrinsic lesions. **Neurosurgery** 24: 206-14, 1989.

83. Kuether T A, Nesbit G M, Clark W M, *et al.*: Rotational vertebral artery occlusion: A mechanism of vertebrobasilar insufficiency. **Neurosurgery** 41: 427-33, 1997.

84. Pamphlett R, Raisanen J, Kum-Jew S: Vertebral artery compression resulting from head movement: A possible cause of the sudden infant death syndrome. **Pediatrics** 103 (2): 460-8, 1999.

85. Okawara S, Nibbelink D: Vertebral artery occlusion following hyperextension and rotation of the head. **Stroke** 5 (5): 640-2, 1974.

86. Ford F R: Syncope, vertigo and disturbances of vision resulting from intermittent obstruction of vertebral arteries due to defect in odontoid process and excessive mobility of second cervical vertebra. **Bull Johns Hopkins Hosp** 91: 168-73, 1952.

87. Tatlow W F T, Bammer H G: Syndrome of vertebral artery compression. **Neurology** 7: 331-40, 1957.

88. Matsuyama T, Morimoto T, Sakaki T: Comparison of C1-2 posterior fusion and decompression of the vertebral artery in the treatment of bow hunter's stroke. **J Neurosurg** 86 (4): 619-23, 1997.

89. Shimizu T, Waga S, Kojima T, *et al.*: Decompression of the vertebral artery for bow-hunter's stroke. Case report. **J Neurosurg** 69 (1): 127-31, 1988.

90. Yamaura A: Nontraumatic intracranial arterial dissection: Natural history, diagnosis, and treatment. **Contemp Neurosurg** 16 (5): 1-6, 1994.

91. Goldstein S J: Dissecting hematoma of the cervical vertebral artery: Case report. **J Neurosurg** 56: 451-4, 1982.

92. Anson J, Crowell R M: Cervicocranial arterial dissection. **Neurosurgery** 29: 89-96, 1991.

93. Yamashita M, Tanaka K, Matsuo T, *et al.*: Cerebral dissecting aneurysms in patients with moyamoya disease. **J Neurosurg** 58: 120-5, 1983.

94. Bogousslavsky J, Despland P A, Regli F: Spontaneous carotid dissection with acute stroke. **Arch Neurol** 44: 137-40, 1987.

95. Friedman A H, Drake C G: Subarachnoid hemorrhage from intracranial dissecting aneurysm. **J Neurosurg** 60: 325-34, 1984.

96. Kitanaka C, Tanaki J-I, Kuwahara M, *et al.*: Nonsurgical treatment of unruptured intracranial vertebral artery dissection with serial follow-up angiography. **J Neurosurg** 80: 667-74, 1994.

97. Hodge C, Leeson M, Cacayorin E, *et al.*: Computed tomographic evaluation of extracranial carotid artery disease. **Neurosurgery** 21: 167-76, 1987.

98. Berger M S, Wilson C B: Intracranial dissecting aneurysms of the posterior circulation. Report of six cases and review of the literature. **J Neurosurg** 61: 882-94, 1984.

99. Pozzati E, Padovani R, Fabrizi A, *et al.*: Benign arterial dissection of the posterior circulation. **J Neurosurg** 75: 69-72, 1991.

100. Chang V, Newcastle N B, Harwood-Nash D C F, *et al.*: Bilateral dissecting aneurysms of the intracranial internal carotid arteries in an 8-year-old boy. **Neurology** 25: 573-9, 1975.

101. Biller J, Hingtgen W L, Adams H P, *et al.*: Cervicocephalic arterial dissections: A ten-year experience. **Arch Neurol** 43: 1234-8, 1986.

102. Hart R G, Easton J D: Dissections of cervical and cerebral arteries. **Neurol Clin North Am** 1: 255-82, 1983.

103. Leys D, Lesoin F, Pruvo J P, *et al.*: Bilateral spontaneous dissection of extracranial vertebral arteries. **J Neurol** 234: 237-40, 1987.

104. Halbach V V, Higashida R T, Dowd C F, *et al.*: Endovascular treatment of vertebral artery dissections and pseudoaneurysms. **J Neurosurg** 79: 183-91, 1993.

105. Miyazaki S, Yamaura A, Kamata K, *et al.*: A dissecting aneurysm of the vertebral artery. **Surg Neurol** 21: 171-4, 1984.

106. Hugenholtz H, Pokrupa R, Montpetit V J A, *et al.*: Spontaneous dissecting aneurysm of the extracranial vertebral artery. **Neurosurgery** 10: 96-100, 1982.

107. Senter H J, Sarwar M: Nontraumatic dissecting aneurysm of the vertebral artery. **J Neurosurg** 56: 128-30, 1982.

108. Shimoji T, Bando K, Nakajima K, *et al.*: Dissecting aneurysm of the vertebral artery. **J Neurosurg** 61: 1038-46, 1984.

109. Mas J L, Henin D, Bousser M G, *et al.*: Dissecting aneurysm of the vertebral artery and cervical manipulation: A case report with autopsy. **Neurology** 39: 512-5, 1989.

110. Caplan L R, Zarins C K, Hemmati M: Spontaneous dissection of the extracranial vertebral arteries. **Stroke** 16: 1030-8, 1985.

111. Okuchi K, Watabe Y, Hiramatsu K, *et al.*: [Dissecting aneurysm of the vertebral artery as a cause of Wallenberg's syndrome]. **No Shinkei Geka** 18: 721-7, 1990 (Japan).

112. Aoki N, Sakai T: Rebleeding from intracranial dissecting aneurysm in the vertebral artery. **Stroke** 21: 1628-31, 1990.

113. Pozzati E, Andreoli A, Limoni P, *et al.*: Dissecting aneurysms of the vertebrobasilar system: Study of 16 cases. **Surg Neurol** 41: 119-24, 1994.

114. Yamaura A, Watanabe Y, Saeki N: Dissecting aneurysms of the intracranial vertebral artery. **J Neurosurg** 72: 183-8, 1990.

115. Six E G, Stringer W L, Cowley A R, *et al.*: Posttraumatic bilateral vertebral artery occlusion. Case report. **J Neurosurg** 54: 814-7, 1981.

116. Yamada K, Hayakawa T, Ushio Y, *et al.*: Therapeutic occlusion of the vertebral artery for unclippable vertebral aneurysm. **Neurosurgery** 15: 834-8, 1984.

117. EC/IC Study Group: Failure of EC-IC arterial bypass to reduce the risk of ischemic stroke. **N Engl J Med** 313: 1191-200, 1985.

118. Wilkins R H, Rengachary S S, (eds.): **Neurosurgery**. McGraw-Hill, New York, 1985.

119. Symonds C P: Otitic hydrocephalus. **Brain** 54: 55-71, 1931.

120. Garcia R D J, Baker A S, Cunningham M J, *et al.*: Lateral sinus thrombosis associated with otitis media and mastoiditis in children. **Pediatr Infect Dis J** 14: 617-23, 1995.

121. Dolan R W, Chowdry K: Diagnosis and treatment of intracranial complications of paranasal sinus infections. **J Oral Maxillofac Surg** 53: 1080-7, 1995.

122. Shende M C, Lourie H: Sagittal sinus thrombosis related to oral contraceptives: Case report. **J Neurosurg** 33: 714-7, 1970.

123. Mahasin Z Z, Saleem M, Gangopadhyay K: Transverse sinus thrombosis and venous infarction of the brain following unilateral radical neck dissection. **J Laryngol Otol** 112: 88-91, 1998.

124. Flusser D, Abu-Shakra M, Baumgarten-Kleiner A, *et al.*: Superior sagittal sinus thrombosis in a patient with systemic lupus erythematosus. **Lupus** 5: 334-6, 1996.

125. Bousser M G: Cerebral vein thrombosis in Bechet's syndrome. **Arch Neurol** 39: 322, 1982.

126. Wilder-Smith E, Kothbauer-Margreiter I, Lämmle B, *et al.*: Dural puncture and activated protein C resistance: Risk factors for cerebral venous sinus thrombosis. **J Neurol Neurosurg Psychiatry** 63: 351-6, 1997.

127. Estanol B, Rodriguez A, Conte G, *et al.*: Intracranial venous thrombosis in young women. **Stroke** 10: 680-4, 1979.

128. Ferrera P C, Pauze D R, Chan L: Sagittal sinus thrombosis after closed head injury. **Am J Emerg Med** 16: 382-5, 1998.

129. Elsherbiny S M, Grunewald R A, Powell T: Isolated

inferior sagittal sinus thrombosis: A case report. **Neuroradiology** 39: 411-3, 1997.

130. Gerszten P C, Welch W C, Spearman M P, et al.: Isolated deep cerebral venous thrombosis treated by direct endovascular thrombolysis. **Surg Neurol** 48: 261-6, 1997.

131. Sofferman R A: Cavernous sinus thrombosis secondary to sphenoid sinusitis. **Laryngoscope** 93: 797-800, 1983.

132. Kriss T C, Kriss V M, Warf B C: Cavernous sinus thrombophlebitis: Case report. **Neurosurgery** 39: 385-9, 1996.

133. Bousser M G, Chiras J, Bories J, et al.: Cerebral venous thrombosis - A review of 38 cases. **Stroke** 16: 199-213, 1985.

134. Kalbag R M: Cerebral venous thrombosis. In **The cerebral venous system and its disorders**, Kapp J P and Schmidek H H, (eds.). Grune and Stratton, Orlando, 1984: pp 505-36.

135. Perkin G D: Cerebral venous thrombosis: Developments in imaging and treatment. **J Neurol Neurosurg Psychiatry** 59: 1-3, 1995.

136. Yeakley J W, Mayer J S, Patchell L L, et al.: The pseudodelta sign in acute head trauma. **J Neurosurg** 69: 867-8, 1988.

137. Rao K C V G, Knipp H C, Wagner E J: CT findings in cerebral sinus and venous thrombosis. **Radiology** 140: 391-8, 1981.

138. Virapongse C, Cazenave C, Quisling R, et al.: The empty delta sign: Frequency and significance in 76 cases of dural sinus thrombosis. **Radiology** 162: 779-85, 1987.

139. Lam A H: Doppler imaging of superior sagittal sinus thrombosis. **J Ultrasound Med** 14: 41-6, 1995.

140. Levine S R, Twyman R E, Gilman S: The role of anticoagulation in cavernous sinus thrombosis. **Neurology** 38: 517-22, 1988.

141. Villringer A, Garner C, Meister W, et al.: High-dose heparin treatment in cerebral sinus thrombosis. **Stroke** 19: 135, 1988 (abstract).

142. Einhäupl K M, Villringer A, Meister W, et al.: Heparin treatment in sinus venous thrombosis. **Lancet** 338: 597-600, 1991.

143. Horowitz M, Purdy P, Unwin H, et al.: Treatment of dural sinus thrombosis using selective catheterization and urokinase. **Ann Neurol** 38: 58-67, 1995.

144. Alexander L F, Tamamoto Y, Ayoubi S, et al.: Efficacy of tissue plasminogen activator in the lysis of thrombosis of the cerebral venous sinus. **Neurosurgery** 26: 559-64, 1990.

145. Horton J C, Seiff S R, Pitts L H, et al.: Decompression of the optic nerve sheath for vision-threatening papilledema caused by dural sinus occlusion. **Neurosurgery** 31: 203-12, 1992.

146. Yonekawa Y, Handa H, Okuno T: In **Stroke: Pathophysiology, diagnosis and management**, Barnett H J M and Mohr J P, (eds.). Churchill Livingston, New York, 1986: pp 805-29.

147. Kayama T, Suzuki S, Sakurai Y, et al.: A case of moyamoya disease accompanied by an arteriovenous malformation. **Neurosurgery** 18: 465-8, 1986.

148. Lichtor T, Mullan S: Arteriovenous malformation in moyamoya syndrome: Report of three cases. **J Neurosurg** 67: 603-8, 1987.

149. Kwak R, Ito S, Yamamoto N, et al.: Significance of

intracranial aneurysms associated with moyamoya disease (part I): Differences between intracranial aneurysms associated with moyamoya disease and usual saccular aneurysms - review of the literature. **Neurol Med Chir** 24: 97-103, 1984.

150. Rajakulasingam K, Cerullo L J, Raimondi A J: Childhood moyamoya syndrome: Postradiation pathogenesis. **Childs Brain** 5: 467-75, 1979.

151. Chang S D, Steinberg G K: Surgical management of moyamoya disease. **Contemp Neurosurg** 22 (10): 1-9, 2000.

152. Ueki K, Meyer F B, Mellinger J F: Moyamoya disease: The disorder and surgical treatment. **Mayo Clin Proc** 69: 749-57, 1994.

153. Suzuki J, Takaku A: Cerebrovascular "moyamoya" disease: Disease showing abnormal net-like vessels in base of brain. **Arch Neurol** 20: 288-99, 1969.

154. Nishimoto A: Moyamoya disease. **Neurol Med Chir** 19: 221-8, 1979.

155. Kodama N, Aoki Y, Hiraga H, et al.: Electroencephalographic findings in children with moyamoya disease. **Arch Neurol** 36: 16-9, 1979.

156. Ogawa A, Yoshimoto T, Suzuki J, et al.: Cerebral blood flow in moyamoya disease. Part 1. Correlation with age and regional distribution. **Acta Neurochir** 105: 30-4, 1990.

157. Ogawa A, Nakamura N, Yoshimoto T, et al.: Cerebral blood flow in moyamoya disease. Part 2. Autoregulation and CO_2 response. **Acta Neurochir** 105: 107-11, 1990.

158. Matsushima Y, Inoue T, Suzuki S O, et al.: Surgical treatment of moyamoya disease in pediatric patients - comparison between the results of indirect and direct vascularization. **Neurosurgery** 31: 401-5, 1992.

159. Ishikawa T, Houkin K, Kamiyama H, et al.: Effects of surgical revascularization on outcome of patients with pediatric moyamoya disease. **Stroke** 28: 1170-3, 1997.

160. Fabi A Y, Meyer F B: Moyamoya disease. **Contemp Neurosurg** 19 (15): 1-6, 1997.

161. Karasawa J, Kikuchi H, Furuse S, et al.: Treatment of moyamoya disease with STA-MCA anastamosis. **J Neurosurg** 49: 679-88, 1978.

162. Matsushima Y, Fukai N, Tanaka K, et al.: A new surgical treatment of moyamoya disease in children: A preliminary report. **Surg Neurol** 15: 313-20, 1980.

163. Matsushima Y, Inaba Y: Moyamoya disease in children and its surgical treatment. **Childs Brain** 11: 155-70, 1984.

164. Kashiwagi S, Kato S, Yasuhara S, et al.: Use of split dura for revascularization if ischemic hemispheres in moyamoya disease. **J Neurosurg** 85: 380-3, 1996.

165. Karasawa J, Kikuchi H, Kawamura J, et al.: Intracranial transplantation of the omentum for cerebrovascular moyamoya disease: A two-year follow-up study. **Surg Neurol** 14: 444-9, 1980.

166. Endo M, Kawano N, Miyasaka Y, et al.: Cranial burr hole for revascularization in moyamoya disease. **J Neurosurg** 71: 180-5, 1989.

167. Kinugasa K, Mandai S, Tokunaga K, et al.: Ribbon encephalo-duro-arterio-myo-synangiosis for moyamoya disease. **Surg Neurol** 41: 455-61, 1994.

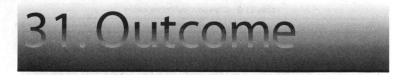

31. Outcome

CANCER

The **Karnofsky scale** (*Table 31-1*) is often used for grading functional status in patients with cancer.

Table 31-1   Karnofsky performance status scale (modified[1, 2])

Score	Criteria	General category
100	normal: no complaints, no evidence of disease	Able to carry on normal activity and work. No special care is needed
90	able to carry on normal activity: minor signs or symptoms	
80	normal activity with effort: some signs or symptoms	
70	cares for self: unable to carry on normal activity or to do active work	Unable to work. Able to live at home, care for most personal needs. Variable assistance is required
60	requires occasional assistance: cares for most of needs	
50	requires considerable assistance and frequent care	
40	disabled: requires special care and assistance	Unable to care for self. Requires equivalent of institutional or hospital care. Disease may be rapidly progressing
30	severely disabled: hospitalized; death not imminent	
20	very sick: hospitalized; active supportive care needed	
10	moribund: fatal processes are progressing rapidly	
0	dead	

HEAD INJURY

The **Ranchos Los Amigos scale** (*Table 31-2*) is often used in rating patient disability following head injury. The **Glasgow outcome scale** (*Table 31-3*) is frequently employed in outcome assessment.

Table 31-2   Ranchos Los Amigos cognitive scale

Level	Meaning
I	No response to pain, touch, sight or sound.
II	Generalized reflex responses to pain.
III	Localized response. Blinks to strong light, turns towards/away from sound, responds to physical discomfort, inconsistent responses to commands.
IV	**Confused - Agitated** Alert, very active, agitated, aggressive, or bizarre behaviors. Performs motor activities but behavior is non-purposeful, extremely short attention span.
V	**Confused - Non agitated** Gross attention to environment, easily distracted, requires continual redirection, difficulty learning new tasks, agitated by excess stimulation. May converse socially but with inappropriate verbalizations.
VI	**Confused - Appropriate** Inconsistent orientation to time and place. Retention span and recent memory impaired. Begins to recall past, consistently follows simple commands, goal directed behavior with assistance.
VII	**Automatic - Appropriate** Performs daily routine in highly familiar environment in a non-confused but automatic "robot-like" fashion. Skills deteriorate in unfamiliar environment. Lacks realistic planning for future.
VIII	**Purposeful - Appropriate**

Table 31-3   Glasgow outcome scale[3]

Score	Meaning
5	good recovery – resumption of normal life despite minor deficits ("return to work" not reliable)
4	moderate disability (disabled but independent) – travel by public transportation, can work in sheltered setting (exceeds mere ability to perform "activities of daily living")
3	severe disability (conscious but disabled) – dependent for daily support (may be institutionalized – but this is not a criteria)
2	persistent vegetative state – unresponsive & speechless; after 2-3 weeks, may open eyes & have sleep/wake cycles
1	death – most deaths ascribable to primary head injury occur within 48 hrs

CEREBROVASCULAR EVENTS

Several outcome grading scales have come to be favored for use following CVAs or SAH. Each emphasizes different aspects of outcome. The Barthel Index (*see below*) places weight on activities of daily living (**ADLs**), while others, such as the **modified Rankin scale**[4] (*Table 31-4*) assess levels of independence and includes a comparison to *previous* activity levels. While it does measure functional status, the modified Rankin is not sensitive to subtle neurologic deficits such as dysphasia or visual field defects.

Table 31-4   The modified* Rankin scale

Grade	Description
0	no symptoms at all
1	no significant disability despite symptoms: able to carry out all usual duties & activities
2	slight disability: unable to carry out all previous activities. Able to look after own affairs without assistance
3	moderate disability: requiring some help, but able to walk without assistance
4	moderately severe disability: unable to walk without assistance, and unable to attend to own bodily needs without assistance
5	severe disability: bedridden, incontinent, and requiring constant nursing care and attention

*   the original Rankin scale[5]: did not have Grade 0, Grade 1 did not include the words "despite symptoms" and "& activities", and it defined Grade 2 as "unable to carry out *some* of previous activities…"

Table 31-5   The Barthel index

Item	Original Barthel Index			Modified Barthel Index				
	Unable to perform task	Needs assistance	Fully independent	CODE 1 Unable to perform task	CODE 2 Attempts task but unsafe	CODE 3 Moderate help required	CODE 4 Minimal help required	CODE 5 Fully independent
Personal hygiene	0	0	5	0	1	3	4	5
Self bathing	0	0	5	0	1	3	4	5
Feeding	0	5	10	0	2	5	8	10
Toilet	0	5	10	0	2	5	8	10
Stair climbing	0	5	10	0	2	5	8	10
Dressing	0	5	10	0	2	5	8	10
Bowel control	0	5	10	0	2	5	8	10
Bladder control	0	5	10	0	2	5	8	10
Ambulation	0	5-10	15	0	3	8	12	15
Wheelchair*	0	0	5	0	1	3	4	5
Chair/bed transfers	0	5-10	15	0	3	8	12	15
TOTAL (range)	0	→ →	100	0	→ → → → →			100

*   score only if unable to walk and patient trained in wheelchair management

Barthel index: The original Barthel index[6, 7] assigns one of three scores to 10 ratable ADLs, and then the individual scores are summed (*see Table 31-5*). The modified Barthel index **(MBI)** with a 5-step scoring system also shown in *Table 31-5* appears to have greater sensitivity[8]. The total ranges from 0 to 100 (a score of 100 implies functional independence, not necessarily normality).

Of all the factors, independence in bathing was the most difficult. Abilities on the Barthel index tend to return in a fairly consistent order, and so most patients with the same score will have similar patterns of disability.

SPINAL CORD INJURY

Functional Independence Measure[M9-11] **(FIM™):** developed to provide uniform evaluation of disability for spinal cord injuries. Rates 18 items shown in *Table 31-6* (13 motor, 5 cognitive) on the 7 level scale shown in *Table 31-7*.

The FIM™ has high internal consistency and is a good indicator of burden of care[12, 13].

Table 31-7 The 7 FIM™ rating levels of disability

Degree of dependency	Level of function	Score
No helper	Complete independence	7
	Modified independence	6
Modified dependenc on a helper	Supervision	5
	Minimal assist (≥ 75% independent)	4
	Moderate assist (≥ 50% independent)	3
Complete dependenc on a helper	Maximal assist (≥ 25% independence)	2
	Total assist (< 25% independence)	1

Table 31-6 The Functional Independence Measure™ (FIM)

Classification	Item
Motor	
Self-care	1. Eating
	2. Grooming
	3. Bathing
	4. Dressing - upper body
	5. Dressing - lower body
	6. Toileting
Sphincter control	7. Bladder management
	8. Bowel management
Mobility	9. Bed, chair, wheelchair
	10. Toilet
	11. Tub, shower
Locomotion	12. Walk or wheelchair
	13. Stairs
Cognitive	
Communication	14. Comprehension
	15. Expression
Social cognition	16. Social interaction
	17. Problem solving
	18. Memory

31.1. References

1. Karnofsky D A, Burchenal J H: In **Evaluation of chemotherapy agents**, Macleod C M, (ed.). Columbia University Press, New York, 1949: pp 191-205.
2. Karnofsky D, Burchenal J H, Armistead G C, *et al.*: Triethylene melamine in the treatment of neoplastic disease. **Arch Intern Med** 87: 477-516, 1951.
3. Jennett B, Bond M: Assessment of outcome after severe brain damage: A practical scale. **Lancet** i: 480-4, 1975.
4. UK-TIA Study Group: The UK-TIA aspirin trial: Interim results. **Br Med J** 296: 316-20, 1988.
5. Rankin J: Cerebral vascular accidents in patients over the age of 60. 2. Prognosis. **Scott Med J** 2: 200-15, 1957.
6. Mahoney F I, Barthel D W: Functional evaluation: The Barthel index. **Maryland State Med J** 14: 61-5, 1965.
7. Wade D T, Hewer R L: Functional abilities after stroke: Measurement, natural history and prognosis. **J Neurol Neurosurg Psychiatry** 50: 177-82, 1987.
8. Shah S, Vanclay F, Cooper D. Improving the sensitivity of the Barthel index for stroke rehabilitation. **J Clin Epidemiol** 42 (8): 703-9, 1989.
9. Forer S, Granger C, et al.: **Functional independence measure**. The Buffalo General Hospital, State University of New York at Buffalo, Buffalo, NY, 1987.
10. Ditunno J F, Jr.: New spinal cord injury standards, 1992. **Paraplegia** 30 (2): 90-1, 1992.
11. Ditunno J F, Jr.: Functional assessment measures in CNS trauma. **J Neurotrauma** 9 Suppl 1: S301-5, 1992.
12. Dodds T A, Martin D P, Stolov W C, *et al.*: A validation of the functional independence measurement and its performance among rehabilitation inpatients. **Arch Phys Med Rehabil** 74 (5): 531-6, 1993.
13. Linacre J M, Heinemann A W, Wright B D, *et al.*: The structure and stability of the functional independence measure. **Arch Phys Med Rehabil** 75 (2): 127-32, 1994.

32. DDx

This section contains differential diagnoses[A] **(DDx)** grouped either by signs and symptoms (*see below*), or by location (starting on page 922). DDx that are better covered elsewhere in a section devoted primarily to that topic are listed in *Table 32-1*.

Table 32-1   Differential diagnoses covered outside this chapter
(followed by page number where the item may be found)

abducens palsy - 586	gyral enhancement - 765	sarcoidosis - 57
anisocoria - 582	hydrocephalus - 184	seizures
ankylosing spondylitis - 343	lateral disc herniation - 311	new onset, adult - 258
bladder dysfunction - 90	Meniere's disease - 592	new onset, peds - 259
brachial plexopathy - 554	meralgia paresthetica - 574	nonepileptic - 262
carpal tunnel syndrome - 566	multiple sclerosis - 49	status epilepticus - 264
cervical stenosis - *see below* & 333	ophthalmoplegia	schizencephaly - 112
chordomas - 465	painful - 586	spinal cord tumors - 506
coma - 155	painless - 587	spinal epidural abscess - 241
Creutzfeldt-Jakob disease - 229	papilledema - 581	synovial cyst (spinal) - 313
dementia - 44	Parinaud's syndrome - 86	thoracic outlet syndrome - 576
diabetes insipidus - 16	Parkinson's disease - 47	torticollis - 370
dizziness - 590	pineal region tumors - 476	trigeminal neuralgia - 379
extra-axial fluid (peds) - 678	pneumocephalus - 667	urinary retention - 91
facial nerve palsy (Bell's palsy) - 594	pseudotumor cerebri - 496	vertigo - 590
giant cell arteritis - 58	retinal hemorrhage - 689	

32.1.   Differential diagnosis (DDx) by signs and symptoms

32.1.1.   Myelopathy

Items marked with a dagger (†) may present as a spinal epidural mass.
1. congenital
   A. (Arnold)-Chiari malformation: Type I often presents in early adulthood (*see page 333*)
   B. tethered cord: often may not present until after some trauma
   C. syringomyelia: may be congenital or post-traumatic in quadriplegics, usually presents with a central cord syndrome (see *Syringomyelia*, page 349) or progressive myelopathy
   D. neurenteric cyst: *see page 98*
   E. cord compression that occurs with some mucopolysaccharidoses: e.g. Morquio syndrome (due to atlanto-axial subluxation), Hurler's syndrome
2. acquired
   A. cervical or thoracic spinal stenosis: often degenerative disease superimposed on congenitally narrow canal (congenital narrowing is frequent in achondroplastic dwarfs)

A. in general usage, the term *differential diagnosis* sometimes refers to conditions that may mimic the one under consideration, however, it may also denote possible *etiologies* of a particular condition or finding. No attempt is made herein to consistently distinguish between these two similar usages of the term, although whenever possible, the word *etiologies* is employed where appropriate

B. traumatic: including spinal shock, hematomyelia, spinal epidural hematoma (see *vascular* below), barotrauma, electrical injuries, compression by bone fracture†. May follow minor trauma in the setting of spinal stenosis

C. herniated intervertebral disc†: myelopathy more common in thoracic region, radiculopathy more common in cervical region (long tract signs are rare with herniated cervical disc)

D. kyphosis

E. extramedullary hematopoeisis†: hypertrophy of marrow → cord compression. Primarily in chronic anemias (e.g. thalassemia major) (*see page 27*)

F. bony compression secondary to incompetence of odontoid process or transverse atlantal ligament†. May be congenital, traumatic (*see page 727*), neoplastic, or inflammatory (especially rheumatoid arthritis)

G. epidural lipomatosis†: hypertrophy of epidural fat that may be secondary to Cushing's disease or prolonged exogenous steroid therapy [1], associated with obesity[2], or may be idiopathic[3]

H. ossification of the posterior longitudinal ligament (**OPLL**)[4] (*see page 345*)

I. arachnoiditis ossificans: a rare condition (only ≈ 43 case reports[5]) involving calcification of the arachnoid membrane. In the T-spine, may occur as ossified plaques or in a cylindrical form surrounding the spinal cord. May be difficult to detect on MRI and myelography. Plain unenhanced CT may be optimal for diagnosis

J. vertebral Paget's disease† (*see page 342*)

K. idiopathic spinal cord herniation[6]: rare. Thoracic spinal cord herniates through an anterior dural defect producing a Brown-Séquard syndrome or spastic paraparesis

3. neoplastic
   A. spine/spinal cord tumors (*see page 506* for details)†
      1. extradural (55%):
         a. primary tumors (rare) include: neurofibromas, chordomas, osteoid osteoma, aneurysmal bone cyst, vertebral hemangioma[1]
         b. if age > 40 yrs, suspect extradural lymphoma (primary or secondary) or leukemic deposits (chloroma), especially with pre-existing diagnosis of hematopoietic or lymphatic disorder
         c. epidural metastases become increasingly common after age 50 yrs. Occurs in up to 10% of cancer patients. 5-10% of malignancies present initially with cord compression. Also *see page 516*.
      2. intradural-extramedullary (40%): meningiomas, neurofibromas
      3. intradural-intramedullary: primary cord tumors (ependymoma, astrocytoma) and rarely intramedullary mets (*see page 508*)
   B. carcinomatous meningitis: neurologic deficit usually cannot be localized to a single level (*see page 491*)
   C. paraneoplastic syndrome: including effects on spinal cord or on peripheral nerves

4. vascular
   A. hematoma/hemorrhage
      1. spinal epidural hematoma†: usually associated with anticoagulation therapy[8] (*see page 353* and *page 23*)
         a. traumatic: following LP or epidural anesthesia (*see page 23*)
         b. spontaneous[9]: rare. Includes hemorrhage from spinal cord AVM (*see page 347*) or from vertebral hemangioma (*see page 512*)
      2. spinal subarachnoid hemorrhage: as in spinal epidural hematoma (*see above*), this may also be post-traumatic (e.g. following LP[10, 11]) or secondary to spinal cord AVM
      3. spinal subdural hematoma
      4. hematomyelia
   B. spinal cord infarction: uncommon with the elimination of syphilitic endarteritis. Most often in the territory of the anterior spinal artery, sparing posterior columns. Most commonly ≈ T4 level (watershed zone)
      1. atherosclerosis of radicular artery in elderly patient with hypotension is now the major cause of this rare condition
      2. clamping aorta during surgery (e.g. for abdominal aortic aneurysm)
      3. hypotension (relative or absolute) during surgery in the sitting position in the presence of spinal stenosis[12]. May be improved by avoiding absolute hypotension, using awake fiber-optic intubation and positioning, intraoperative SSEP monitoring and inducing hypertension if

changes occur with positioning, avoidance of sitting position, and avoiding hyperflexion, hyperextension and traction
4. aortic dissection
5. embolization of spinal arteries
C. spinal cord AVM (*see page 347*)†: 10-20% present as sudden onset of myelopathy usually in patients < 30 yrs[13], myelopathy may be secondary to:
1. mass effect from AVM: spinal AVMs account for < 5% of lesions presenting as cord "tumors"
2. rupture → SAH, hematomyelia, or epidural hematoma
3. watershed infarction due to "steal"
4. spontaneous thrombosis (necrotizing myelopathy of **Foix-Alajouanine** disease[14]): presents as spastic → flaccid paraplegia, with ascending sensory level
D. radiation myelopathy: due to microvascular occlusion (*see page 536*)
E. secondary to iodinated contrast material used for mesenteric or aortic angiography. Especially when angiogrammed in presence of hypotension, where cardiac output is shunted away from viscera and into spinal radicular arteries. Treatment: place patient sitting, remove ≥ 100 ml of CSF via LP and replace with equal amount of saline over 30 mins[15]
5. autoimmune
A. demyelinating: acute (idiopathic) **transverse myelitis (ATM)** (*see page 55*). Peak incidence during first 2 decades of life. Abrupt onset of LE weakness, sensory loss, back pain, and sphincter disturbance indistinguishable from spinal cord compression. Thoracic region most common. CT, MRI and myelogram all normal. CSF → pleocytosis and hyperproteinemia
B. multiple sclerosis **(MS)**: is diagnosed in only 7% of patients presenting as acute transverse myelopathy. Although more common in young adults, MS can occur at any time in life. Myelopathy of MS is usually insidious, and is usually incomplete (i.e. some sparing). Affects myelin, thus sparing gray matter. Abdominal cutaneous reflexes are almost always absent in MS
C. **Devic syndrome** (neuromyelitis optica): a variant of MS characterized by acute bilateral optic neuritis and transverse myelitis. In some cases spinal cord edema may become so severe as to cause complete block on myelography. More common in Asia and India than U.S. or Europe
D. post-viral (or post-vaccination): may be etiology of auto-immune process (i.e. transverse myelitis). Viral prodrome present in ≈ 37% of cases of ATM. Viral infection is usually most damaging to gray matter (e.g. poliomyelitis)
6. metabolic/toxic
A. (subacute) **combined system disease (CSD)** (AKA subacute combined columnal degeneration): due to vitamin B_{12} (cyanocobalamin) deficiency
1. dietary deficiency of B_{12}
2. **pernicious anemia**: malabsorption of B_{12} in the distal ileum due to lack of secretion of intrinsic factor (a small polypeptide) by gastric parietal cells[16])
3. other gastric disorders: low gastric pH e.g. in Zollinger-Ellison syndrome can inhibit attachment of intrinsic factor to ileal receptors

Onset is gradual and uniform. Begins with symmetrical paresthesias in feet or hands (posterior column involvement) → leg stiffness, weakness, and proprioceptive deficits with unsteadiness that is worse in the dark → spasticity → paraplegia → bowel and bladder dysfunction. Dementia (confusion, memory impairment, irritability...) occurs in advanced cases due to cerebral white matter changes. Visual disturbances with or without optic atrophy may be due to optic nerve demyelination. Serum B_{12} level is the most sensitive test. Most (but not all) patients will have a <u>macrocytic</u> anemia (folic acid deficiency also produces megaloblastic anemia, however, even in CSD, folic acid corrects the anemia, but <u>not</u> the neurologic deficits which may actually worsen). <u>Schilling test</u> determines the cause of the B_{12} deficiency even if B_{12} injections have already been given. Treatment is with B_{12} injections or large doses of oral preparations[17]
4. B_{12} levels that are WNL does not R/O B_{12} deficiency, if there are neurologic symptoms then malonic acid or other markers of B_{12} deficiency such as methylmalonic acid (also check homocysteine to R/O folate deficiency)

T2WI MRI may demonstrate increased signal within the white matter of the spinal cord, predominantly in the posterior columns but may also be seen in spinothalamic tracts

  B. toxins: local anesthetics used for spinal anesthesia rarely cause myelopathy
7. infectious
  A. (para) spinal abscess (AKA spinal epidural abscess) or epidural empyema†: often history of staphylococcus infection, usually a skin furuncle. Vertebral osteomyelitis often accompanies[18]. Produces local tenderness, back pain, fever, elevated ESR (see page 240)
  B. vertebral osteitis/osteomyelitis† (see page 243)
  C. pyogenic discitis†: spontaneous or following procedures (see page 245)
  D. AIDS related myelopathy: similar to B_{12} deficiency. Results in spastic weakness & ataxia. Can cause vacuolization of spinal cord. "**Tropical (spastic) paraparesis of AIDS**" also seen in HTLV-I infection[19]
  E. tuberculosis: Pott's disease, see *Tuberculous vertebral osteomyelitis:*, page 245
  F. spinal meningitis with pachymeningitis
  G. viral: herpes varicella-zoster rarely causes necrotizing myelopathy. Herpes simplex type 2 may cause ascending myelitis. Cytomegalovirus may cause transverse myelitis
  H. syphilitic involvement: may cause tabes dorsalis, syphilitic meningomyelitis, or spinal vascular syphilis. Diagnosed by serum and CSF serology
  I. parasitic cysts†
8. peripheral neuromuscular disorder
  A. Guillain-Barré syndrome: rapidly ascending weakness (mimics cord compression) with areflexia and near normal sensation (see page 53). Chronic immune demyelinating polyradiculoneuropathy (CIDP) is a similar syndrome that may progress over a longer period of time (see page 54)
  B. myopathies: including steroid myopathy (usually affects proximal > distal muscles)
9. degenerative
  A. **amyotrophic lateral sclerosis (ALS)**: slight spasticity of LEs (extreme spasticity is rare), atrophic weakness of the hands and forearms, fasciculations in the UEs, absence of sensory changes (including lack of pain), sphincter control usually preserved (see page 52)
  B. some forms of Creutzfeldt-Jakob disease (CJD) with predominant initial muscle wasting may mimic spinal cord disease or ALS (see page 229)

† items with dagger may also present as a spinal epidural mass

32.1.2.   Sciatica

Definition: pain in the distribution of the sciatic nerve. The sciatic nerve is comprised of components of nerve roots of L4-S3. The nerve passes out of the pelvis through the greater sciatic foramen along the back of the thigh. In the lower third of the thigh it divides into the tibial and common peroneal nerves.

The most common cause of sciatica is radiculopathy due to a herniated lumbar disc[20]. The differential diagnosis is similar to that for myelopathy (see above) but also includes:
1. congenital
  A. meningeal cyst (perineural cyst) (see *Spinal meningeal cysts*, page 348)
  B. conjoined nerve root: initially dismissed as a possible cause of radiculopathy, but current thinking recognizes that these may be symptomatic possibly by tethering
2. acquired
  A. spinal stenosis/spondylosis/spondylolysis/spondylolisthesis
  B. juxtafacet cyst: includes synovial cyst and ganglion cyst[21]: detection is increasing with the use of MRI (see page 313)
  C. nerve root sheath cyst: may arise near axilla of nerve root and cause compression of adjacent roots
  D. arachnoiditis ossificans: rare (see page 903). In the lumbar region may occur as columnar, cylindrical, or irregularly shaped masses[22]. May produce low back pain, radiculopathy, or cauda equina syndrome
  E. heterotopic ossification around the hip[23]

F. injection injuries from misplaced IM injections
G. compartment syndrome of the posterior thigh
H. injury complicating total hip arthroplasty[24]
I. radiation injury following treatment of nearby tumors

3. infectious
   A. discitis: usually causes excruciating pain with any movement (*see page 245*)
   B. Lyme disease: *see page 234*
   C. herpes zoster: a rare cause of radiculopathy[25]. Lumbosacral dermatomes are involved in ≈ 10-15% of zoster cases. Pain is usually independent of position. Typical herpetic skin lesions usually follow onset of pain by 3-5 days. 1-5% develop motor weakness (usually in arms or trunk). Sacral zoster can cause detrusor paralysis, producing urinary retention. 55% of those with motor symptoms have good recovery, 30% have fair to good recovery

4. neoplastic:
   A. spine tumors: multiple myeloma (*see page 514*), metastases (*see page 516*)...
   B. bone or soft-tissue tumors along the course of the sciatic nerve: may result in erroneous laminectomy for herniated lumbar disc[26]. Pain is usually <u>insidious</u> in onset, and <u>not positional</u> (*see below*)
      1. intra-abdominal or pelvic neoplasm
      2. tumors of the thigh
      3. tumors in the popliteal fossa or calf

5. inflammatory:
   A. pseudoradiculopathy of trochanteric bursitis. Rarely extends to the posterior thigh or as far distally as the knee (*see page 326*)
   B. myositis ossificans of the biceps femoris muscle[27]

6. vascular: sciatica may be mimicked by intermittent (i.e. vascular) claudication

7. referred pain of nonspinal origin: not dermatomal. Nerve root tensions signs (*see page 302*) are usually negative. Includes:
   A. pyelonephritis
   B. renolithiasis including ureteral obstruction
   C. cholecystitis
   D. appendicitis
   E. endometritis/endometriosis
   F. posterior perforating duodenal ulcer
   G. inguinal hernia, especially if incarcerated
   H. aortic dissection: *see page 907*

8. **piriformis syndrome**: sciatic nerve entrapment by the piriformis muscle. Produces pain in the sciatic distribution and weakness of external rotation and abduction of the hip. Symptoms are exacerbated by Freidberg's test (forced internal rotation of the hip with thigh extension)

9. more peripheral involvement (i.e. neuropathy) that may be confused with radiculopathy. Including:
   A. femoral neuropathy mistaken for L4 radiculopathy (*see below*)
   B. proximal sacral plexus lesion mistaken for S1 radiculopathy (*see below*)
   C. diabetic neuropathy (*see page 555*) including diabetic amyotrophy
   D. tumors (*see below*)

EXTRASPINAL TUMORS CAUSING SCIATICA

★ **Pain characteristics**: pain is almost always insidious in onset[26]. It may be intermittent initially, but eventually all patients develop pain that is constant, progressive and unaffected by position or rest[26]. Significant night pain is described in ≈ 80%.

Straight leg raising was positive in most, but in more than half the pain was localized to a specific point along the course of the nerve, distal to the sciatic notch[26]. Conservative treatment brings either no or only temporary relief.

Approximately 20% will have a previous history of tumor (usually neurofibromatosis or previous malignancy). Malignancies include[26]: metastatic lesions, primary bone sarcomas (chondrosarcoma...), soft-tissue sarcomas (liposarcoma...). Benign tumors include lipoma, neurofibroma, schwannoma, aneurysmal bone cyst of the sacrum, giant cell tumor of the sacrum (*see page 516*), tenosynovial giant cell tumor.

In two-thirds of cases, a detailed medical history and physical exam allowed localization and even determining the nature (bone tumor vs. soft-tissue) of the lesion[26]. Radiographs that show the entire pelvis and the proximal femur will demonstrate almost all tumors in these locations[26, 28].

Sciatica may result from nerve root involvement within the spinal canal (e.g. with lumbar disc herniation). Clinically this produces a nerve root syndrome (see *Nerve root syndromes*, page 304). Spinal imaging studies (MRI, myelogram/CT) will usually detect nerve root compression here. More peripheral involvement may be difficult to image.

L4 involvement

Femoral neuropathy is often mistakenly identified as an L4 radiculopathy. Distinguishing features are shown in *Table 32-2*.

L5 involvement

Peroneal nerve palsy may be mistaken for L5 radiculopathy (see *Foot drop*, page 909).

S1 involvement

Outside the spinal canal, S1 can also be involved as it enters the sacral plexus, e.g. by a pelvic tumor. In plexus lesions, EMG will show sparing of the paraspinal muscles (these nerves exit in

Table 32-2 Distinguishing femoral neuropathy from L4 radiculopathy

Feature	Femoral neuropathy	L4 radiculopathy
Sensory loss		
distribution (see *Figure 3-7*, page 75)	anterior thigh	dermatome from ≈ knee to medial malleolus, spares anterior thigh
Muscle weakness		
iliopsoas	weak	normal
thigh adductors	normal (innervated by obturator nerve)	may be weak
quadriceps	weak	weak

the region of the neural foramen) and the gluteus maximus and medius (superior and inferior gluteal nerves take-off just distal to the paraspinal nerves).

32.1.3.   Low back pain

The following considers primarily low back pain **(LBP)** without radiculopathy or myelopathy, although some overlap occurs. Trauma is usually obvious and is not discussed. See *Sciatica* on page 905 for differential diagnosis of that and also *Low back pain and radiculopathy* on page 289 for evaluation.

ACUTE LOW BACK PAIN

Similar to list for myelopathy (*see page 902*). Most cases are non-specific (e.g. **lumbosacral sprain**), only 10-20% can be given a precise pathoanatomical diagnosis[30]:
1. patients writhing in pain should be evaluated for an intraabdominal or vascular condition (e.g. pain of aortic dissection is typically described as a "tearing" pain): patients with neurogenic LBP tend to remain as still as possible, possibly needing to change positions at intervals
2. unrelenting pain at rest:
    A. spinal tumor (intradural or extradural) (*see page 506*)
        1. primary or metastatic spine tumor: suspected in patients with pain duration > 1 month, unrelieved by bed rest, failure to improve with conservative therapy, unexplained weight loss, age > 50 yrs[31]
        2. nocturnal back pain relieved by aspirin is suggestive of osteoid osteoma or benign osteoblastoma[32] (*see page 511*)
    B. infection (especially in IV drug abusers, diabetics, post spinal surgery, immunosuppressed patients, or those with pyelonephritis or UTI post-GU surgery). Fever is somewhat insensitive for spinal infections. Spine tenderness to percussion has 86% sensitivity with bacterial infections, but a low specificity of 60%[31]. Types of infections include:
        1. discitis
        2. spinal epidural abscess: should be considered in patients with back pain, fever, spine tenderness, or skin infection (furuncle)
        3. vertebral osteomyelitis
    C. inflammatory:
        1. **sacroiliitis**: pelvic x-rays may show sclerosis of one or both sacroiliac joints
            a. bilateral & symmetric
                i. **ankylosing spondylitis** (*see page 343*): morning back stiffness, no relief at rest, improvement with exercise[33]

Usually seen in males with symptom onset before age 40 yrs. Positive **Patrick's test** (*see page 303*) and pain on compressing the pelvis with the patient in the lateral decubitus position

    ii. Reiter syndrome: a reactive arthritis (usually 1-3 weeks following certain bacterial infections) with involvement of at least one other non-joint area (urethritis, uveitis/conjunctivitis, skin lesions, mucosal ulcerations…). 75% are HLA-B27 positive

    iii. may occur in Crohn's disease

  b. bilateral & asymmetric

    i. psoriatic arthritis

    ii. rheumatoid arthritis: adult & juvenile forms

  c. unilateral

    i. gout

    ii. osteoarthritis

    iii. infection

3. evolving neurologic deficit (**cauda equina syndrome**: perineal anesthesia, urinary incontinence or urgency or retention, progressive weakness) all require emergent diagnostic evaluation to rule-out treatable conditions such as:

  A. spinal epidural abscess: *see page 240*

  B. spinal epidural hematoma: *see page 353*

  C. spinal tumor (intradural or extradural): *see page 506*

  D. massive central disc herniation: *see page 305*

4. pathologic fracture: acute pain in patients at risk for osteoporosis or with known Ca should prompt evaluation for pathologic fractures

  A. lumbar compression fracture: see *Osteoporotic spine fractures*, page 748

  B. sacral insufficiency fracture[34]: especially in rheumatoid arthritis patients on chronic steroids, often with no antecedent history of trauma. May cause back pain and/or radiculopathy. Often missed on plain films, best seen on CT, but may also be detected on bone scan

5. coccydynia: pain and tenderness around the coccyx (*see page 353*)

6. tears in the annulus fibrosus ("annular tears")[35] (NB: also present in 40% of asymptomatic patients between 50-60 yrs age, and 75% between 60-70 yrs[36])

7. rarely following subarachnoid hemorrhage (**SAH**) due to irritation of lumbar nerve roots and dura: usually accompanied by other signs of SAH (*see page 782*)

8. myalgia: may be a side-effect of "statins" (drugs used to lower serum concentration of LDL cholesterol), sometimes with accompanying weakness and rarely with severe rhabdomyolysis and myoglobinuria leading to renal failure (risk may be increased with renal or hepatic dysfunction, advanced age, hypothyroidism, or serious infection)[37]

SUBACUTE LOW BACK PAIN

10% have LBP that persists > 6 weeks.

Differential diagnosis

Includes causes of acute LBP (above) and also:

1. continued pain at rest should prompt evaluation for spinal osteomyelitis (especially with fever and elevated ESR) or neoplasm if not already done

2. plain spine x-rays may show possibly causative conditions, although many or all of the following may also be seen in <u>asymptomatic</u> patients

  A. spondylolisthesis (*see page 324*)

  B. spinal osteophytes

  C. lumbar stenosis

  D. **Schmorl's node** or **nodule**: disc herniation through cartilaginous endplate into vertebral body (NB: may also be seen in 19% of asymptomatic patients[38]) (*see page 313*)

CHRONIC LOW BACK PAIN

After 3 months, only ≈ 5% of patients will continue to have persistent symptoms. A structural diagnosis is possible in only ≈ 50% of these patients. These patients account for 85% of the cost in lost work and compensation[30]. Differential diagnosis includes caus-

es of acute and subacute LBP listed above, as well as:
1. degenerative conditions
   A. degenerative spondylolisthesis (*see page 324*)
   B. spinal stenosis (affecting the spinal canal)
   C. lateral recess syndrome
2. spondyloarthropathies
   A. ankylosing spondylitis: look for erosive changes adjacent to SI joint and positive test for HLA-B27 antigen
   B. Paget's disease of the spine: vertebral involvement is very common in a patients with Paget's disease
3. psychological overlay: including secondary gain (financial, emotional...)

32.1.4.   Foot drop

❦ Key features:
- weak anterior tibialis (foot extension) innervated by deep peroneal nerve (L4, 5)
- most common etiologies: L4/L5 radiculopathy, common peroneal nerve palsy
- in a patient with foot drop, check posterior tibialis (foot inversion) and gluteus medius (internal rotation of flexed hip) - both are <u>spared</u> in peroneal nerve palsy and both should be involved with radiculopathy

Weakness of the anterior tibialis (primarily L4 and to a lesser extent L5), often accompanied by a weak extensor digitorum longus and extensor hallucis longus (primarily L5 with some S1 contribution), all of which are innervated by the <u>deep peroneal nerve</u>.

 With common peroneal nerve (**CPN**) palsy, there is <u>sparing</u> of posterior tibialis (foot inversion, innervated by posterior tibial nerve) and gluteus medius (internal rotation of the thigh with the hip flexed, innervated by superior gluteal nerve, primarily L5 with some L4, the takeoff is shortly after the roots exit from neural foramen). With L4 or L5 root lesions these muscles will also be weak, *see Table 32-4*.

One must also distinguish foot drop from a **flail foot** which results from paralysis of dorsiflexors <u>and</u> plantarflexors, e.g. in sciatic nerve dysfunction as can occur during surgery for hip fracture/dislocation[39] or injection injuries (IM injections should be give

Table 32-3   Localization of lesion with foot drop

Lesion	Motor deficit*					Sensory changes
	anterior tibialis (**L4**, 5 ankle dorsiflexion)	peroneus longus/brevis (**L5**, S1 foot eversion)	tibialis posterior (**L4**, 5 foot inversion)	biceps femoris (**L5**, S1, 2 knee flexion)	gastrocnemius (**S1**, 2 plantarflexion)	
deep peroneal nerve	x					minimal, or great toe web space
superficial peroneal nerve		x				lateral distal leg and dorsum of foot
common peroneal nerve (CPN)	x	x				all of the above
L4 or L5 radiculopathy	x	x	x			dermatomal (see *Figure 3-7*, page 75)
peroneal division of sciatic nerve†	x	x	x	x		as with common peroneal
main trunk of sciatic nerve	x	x	x	x	x	lateral distal leg and entire foot

*   **x** denotes that the indicated muscle is involved (i.e. weak)
†   see footnote *2 under *Table 32-4*

superiorly and laterally to a line drawn between the posterior superior iliac spine and the greater trochanter of the hip). NB: the peroneal division of the sciatic nerve tends to be more vulnerable to injury than the tibial division.

Etiologies of foot drop:
1. peripheral nerve palsies (more common) (*see Table 32-3* and *Table 32-4*)
   A. peroneal nerve injury (*also see Common peroneal nerve palsy*, page 575):
   may involve:
      1. deep peroneal nerve: isolated foot drop with minimal sensory loss (except possibly in great toe web space)

2. superficial peroneal nerve: weakness of peroneus longus and brevis (foot eversion) with <u>no</u> foot drop. Sensory loss: lateral aspect of lower half of leg and foot

3. common peroneal nerve: combination of above (i.e. foot drop + weak foot eversion, with sparing of tibialis posterior (foot inversion); sensory loss: lateral aspect of lower half of leg and foot)

Table 32-4 Physical exam to localize the lesion in a patient with LE weakness

Item to check	Rationale	Findings: exam
muscles innervated by the **obturator nerve**	involvement indicates lesion includes more than sciatic nerve/L5 root (e.g. paravertebral mass, cauda equina lesion if bilateral findings)	weakness of thigh adductors (**L2, L3**): adduct thigh while supine with knee extended
muscles innervated by the **femoral nerve**	(same as above)	weakness of quadriceps femoris (L2, **L3, L4**): extend knee
muscles innervated by **L5 branches** that exit the lumbar plexus very close to the neural foramina	involvement indicates very proximal lesion (e.g. nerve root or very proximal (paravertebral) lumbar plexus)*1	weakness of: 1. gluteus medius (**L4, L5**, S1): internally rotate thigh 2. gluteus maximus (**L5, S1**, 2): dig heel into bed while supine
L5 innervated muscles (via **sciatic nerve**) proximal to the takeoff of the common peroneal nerve*2	if muscles listed above are intact, involvement of muscles to the right localizes the lesion to sciatic nerve above mid thigh (e.g. injury to sciatic nerve at the greater sciatic notch)	1. slight weakness of biceps femoris (lateral hamstrings) (L5, **S1**, 2): flex the knee (with thigh flexed) 2. gastrocnemius weakness (foot plantarflexion) (this + foot drop = flail foot) unless injury only to peroneal division of sciatic nerve*2
muscles innervated by **tibial nerve**	sparing of these with foot drop indicates lesion distal to takeoff of common peroneal nerve (foot drop with weak foot inversion may be L4 or 5 radiculopathy)	weakness of tibialis posterior (**L4, L5**): invert foot (foot should be plantarflexed to eliminate anterior tibialis)
muscles innervated by **superficial peroneal nerve**	preservation of these localizes the lesion to the deep peroneal nerve	weakness of the peroneus longus and brevis (L5, S1): evert the foot

Abbreviations
CPN = common peroneal nerve
DPN = deep peroneal nerve
IGN = inferior gluteal nerve
SGN = superior gluteal nerve

*1 Note: EMG can differentiate root lesion from proximal plexus lesion by detecting involvement of paraspinal muscles which occurs in root but not in plexus lesions since dorsal rami exit proximal to plexus

*2 the peroneal division of the sciatic nerve is more vulnerable to injury than the tibial division for several reasons. It is thus not unusual to see isolated peroneal nerve injuries above the knee e.g. from hip dislocation or fractures, stab wounds, injection injuries…

B. L5 radiculopathy: (or, less commonly, L4). The most common cause is HLD, but can also occur with sacral ala fracture (*see page 753*)
  ♦ results in pain and/or sensory changes in L5 (or L4) dermatome
  ♦ weakness with radiculopathy tends to be more pronounced in distal muscles (e.g. anterior tibialis) than in proximal (e.g. gluteus maximus)
  ♦ a <u>painless</u> foot drop is more likely to be due to a peroneal neuropathy than to radiculopathy
C. lumbar plexus injury
D. lumbosacral plexus neuropathy: *see page 555*
E. injury to lateral trunk of sciatic nerve
F. peripheral neuropathy: weakness tends to be greater distally, producing

wrist or foot drop. Classic example: Charcot-Marie-Tooth (*see page 554*), findings tend to be rather dramatic in spite of the fact that it doesn't seem to bother the patient very much

2. central nervous system causes
   A. cortical lesion (UMN): parasagittal lesions in region of motor strip (sensation will be spared if the lesion does not extend posteriorly to the sensory cortex)[40]. There may be a Babinski sign or hyperactive Achilles reflex (so-called "spastic foot drop"). Usually painless
   B. spinal cord injury
3. non-neurogenic causes
   A. muscular dystrophy
   B. a painless foot-drop with an upgoing toe (Babinski): early ALS may present with this. Also, a cortical lesion may be suspected (*see above*)

Laboratory evaluation:
1. bloodwork: glucose, ESR
2. EMG: can help differentiate L5 radiculopathy from peroneal nerve palsy or from plexus lesion (*see Table 32-4*) (takes ≈ 3 weeks after onset to become positive) and can help diagnose motor neuron disease

32.1.5. Weakness/atrophy of the hands/UEs

Hand/UE weakness or atrophy with relatively preserved function in the LEs.
1. cervical spondylosis: often causes sensory disturbance (*see page 331*)
2. cervical radiculopathy: *see page 318*
3. amyotrophic lateral sclerosis (**ALS**): no sensory involvement. One of the few causes of clinically prominent fasciculations (*see page 52* for details of ALS, *see page 905* for other distinguishing features)
4. spinal cord pathology
   A. central cord syndrome: typically causes more involvement (weakness, sensory disturbance) in the UE than the LE (*see page 714*)
   B. syringomyelia: usually burning dysesthesias of the hands with dissociated sensory loss (*see page 349*)
5. brachial plexus injury: *see page 561*
6. brachial plexus neuropathy: *see page 554*
7. peripheral nerve problems, including
   A. carpal tunnel syndrome: *see page 565*
   B. ulnar neuropathy: *see page 569*
   C. other peripheral nerve entrapment syndromes: *see page 563*
8. foramen magnum lesions (*see page 924*): can cause **cruciate paralysis** with atrophy of the hands due to pressure on the pyramidal decussation
9. thoracic outlet syndrome: *see page 576*
10. botulism: *see page 916*

32.1.6. Radiculopathy, upper extremity (cervical)

See *Weakness/atrophy of the hands/UEs* above. In addition to those items:
1. primary shoulder pathology: characteristically, pain is aggravated by active and/or passive shoulder movement. In general, shoulder pathology does not produce pain referred to the neck
   A. rotator cuff tear
   B. bicipital tendonitis: tenderness over biceps tendon
   C. subacromial bursitis: there may be tenderness over the AC joint
   D. adhesive capsulitis
   E. impingement syndrome: the "empty can test" is usually positive (each arm held out in front, 30° lateral to straight forward, thumbs pointing down, as in emptying out a soda can. Examiner pushes down on the patient's hands while the patient resists. Test is positive if it reproduces pain)
2. shoulder pain is very common in polymyalgia rheumatica (*see page 61*), typically worsens with movement
3. interscapular pain: a common location for referred pain with cervical radiculopathy, may also occur with cholecystitis or some shoulder pathologies
4. MI: some cases of cervical radiculopathy (especially left C6) may present with

symptoms that are suggestive of an acute myocardial infarction
5. reflex sympathetic dystrophy: may be difficult to distinguish from cervical radiculopathy. Stellate ganglion blocks may help[41]

32.1.7.   Neck pain (cervical pain)

This section deals primarily with axial neck-pain without radicular features. For radicular features, see *Radiculopathy, upper extremity (cervical) above.*
1. cervical spondylosis (including facet arthritis)
2. cervical sprain: including whiplash associated disorder
3. fracture of the cervical spine: with upper cervical spine fractures (e.g. odontoid), patients characteristically hold their head in their hands, especially when going from recumbent to upright position
   A. traumatic
   B. pathologic (tumor invasion, rheumatoid arthritis)
4. occipital neuralgia: *see page 563*
5. herniated cervical disc:
   A. lateral herniated disc: if symptomatic, tends to produce more radicular symptoms in the UE than actual neck pain
   B. central disc herniation: if symptomatic, tends to produce myelopathy, does not produce any neck pain whatsoever in many cases
6. abnormalities of the craniocervical junction:
   A. Chiari 1 malformation: *see page 104*
   B. atlantoaxial subluxation
7. **fibromyalgia**: idiopathic chronic pain syndrome characterized by widespread nonarticular musculoskeletal pain, nodularity and stiffness[42, 43] without pathologic inflammation. Possible link to neuroendocrine dysfunction[44]. Afflicts 2% of the population[43], female:male ratio is 7:1. No diagnostic laboratory study. May be associated with psychiatric illness and multiple non-specific somatic complaints including malaise, fatigue, impaired sleep, GI complaints and cognitive impairment
8. Eagle's syndrome: elongation of the styloid process. Surgical resection can ameliorate the pain. Two variants:
   A. typical variant: history of tonsillectomy. Pharyngeal pain, dysphagia and otalgia
   B. second variant: AKA carotid artery-styloid process syndrome. Carotidynia radiating into ipsilateral eye and vertex

32.1.8.   Lhermitte's sign

Really a symptom. Electrical shock-like sensation radiating down the spine usually provoked by neck flexion (shocks radiating up the spine are sometimes referred to as re-verse Lhermitte's sign). Classically attributed to dysfunction of the posterior columns.

Etiologies:
1. multiple sclerosis (MS): *see page 50*
2. cervical spondylosis
3. subacute combined degeneration: check for vitamin B_{12} deficiency (*see page 904*)
4. cervical cord tumor
5. cervical disc herniation
6. radiation myelopathy: *see page 536*
7. Chiari type I malformation: *see page 104*
8. central cord syndrome: *see page 714*
9. SCIWORA (spinal cord injury without radiographic abnormality): *see page 732*

32.1.9.   Burning hands/feet

1. spinal cord syndromes:
   A. central cord syndrome (**CCS**): *see page 714*
   B. burning hands syndrome: a possible variant of CCS, described in football-related cervical spine injury (*see page 743*)
   C. numb-clumsy hand syndrome: seen in cervical myelopathy (*see page 333*)

2. complex regional pain syndrome **(CRPS)** AKA reflex sympathetic dystrophy: *see page 396*
3. peripheral neuropathy
   A. diabetic amyotrophy AKA Bruns-Garland syndrome: *see page 556*
4. **erythermalgia** AKA erythromelalgia: rare disorder characterized by erythema, edema, increased skin temperature, and burning pain of the hands and/or feet. Usually refractory to medical management, some success reported with epidural bipuvicaine[45], lidocaine patches[46], or cold soaks
   A. primary erythermalgia: etiology is idiopathic
   B. secondary erythermalgia: associated with autoimmune and rheumatologic factors
5. vascular:
   A. occlusive arterial disease: atherosclerosis, Raynaud's syndrome
   B. venous insufficiency

32.1.10. Muscle pain/tenderness

1. fibromyalgia: *see above*
2. myopathy
3. "statin" myopathy

32.1.11. Acute paraplegia or quadriplegia

Entities causing **spinal cord compression** usually present as: paraplegia or -paresis (or quadriplegia/paresis), urinary retention (may require checking post-void residual to detect), and impaired sensation below level of compression. May develop over hours or days. Reflexes may be hyper- or hypo-active. There may or may not be a Babinski sign. Excluding trauma, the most common cause is compression by tumor or bone.

Etiologies
Some overlap with myelopathy. For items with asterisk, see *Myelopathy*, page 902:
1. in infancy (may produce "floppy infant syndrome")
   A. **Werdnig-Hoffmann** disease, AKA spinal muscular atrophy: congenital degeneration of anterior horn cells. Only rarely evident at birth (where it presents as a paucity of movement), produces weakness, areflexia, and tongue fasciculations with normal sensation. Progresses over the first year or two to quadriplegia
   B. spinal cord injury during parturition: a rare sequela of breech delivery
   C. congenital myopathies: e.g. infantile acid maltase deficiency (Pompe disease)
   D. infantile botulism: ileus, hypotonia, weakness, mydriasis, *Claustridium botulinum* bacteria and toxin in feces
2. traumatic spinal cord injury
   A. major trauma: diagnosis is usually evident
   B. minor trauma: may cause cord injury in setting of spinal stenosis, may → central cord syndrome (see *Central cord syndrome*, page 714)
   C. atlantoaxial dislocation: from major trauma or due to instability from tumor or rheumatoid arthritis (*see page 338*)
3. congenital
   A. extradural spinal cord compression by bone secondary to cervical hemivertebra (symptoms not present at birth, may develop decades later, occasionally after minor trauma)
   B. cervical stenosis (usually with superimposed spondylosis): quadriplegia or central cord syndrome may follow minor trauma (see *page 714*)
   C. achondroplastic dwarfism: spinal stenosis (animal model: dachshund)
   D. syringomyelia: usually presents with central cord syndrome
4. metabolic
   A. combined system disease*
   B. thallium poisoning: usually causes sensory and autonomic symptoms, quadriplegia and dysarthria may be seen in severe cases
   C. central pontine myelinolysis: *see page 12*
5. infectious
   A. epidural spinal infection (abscess or empyema)*

B. post-viral (or post-vaccination): may be a transverse myelitis*
6. peripheral neuromuscular disorder*
    A. Guillain-Barré syndrome
    B. myopathies
7. neoplastic*: spinal cord tumors
8. autoimmune*
9. vascular
    A. acute pontomedullary infarction: age usually > 50 yrs. Patient is quadriplegic, alert, with bulbar palsies (eye movement abnormalities, impaired gag and speech)
    B. spinal cord infarction*: including AVM, radiation myelopathy...
10. miscellaneous compressive*: including epidural hematoma, bony compression, epidural lipomatosis
11. functional: hysteria, malingering
12. bilateral cerebral hemisphere lesion (involving both motor strips): e.g. post-cerebral irradiation or parasagittal lesion. Will not have sensory level

* for items with asterisk, see *Myelopathy*, page 902 for details

32.1.12.　Hemiparesis or hemiplegia

May be produced by anything that interrupts the corticospinal tract from its origin in the pyramidal cells of Betz in the motor strip down to the cervical spine. This results an upper motor neuron paralysis (see *Table 20-2*, page 548) which should also produce long tract findings, including Babinski sign ipsilateral to hemiplegia. Etiologies include:
1. lesions of the cerebral hemisphere in the region of the contralateral motor strip. Large lesions may also involve sensory cortex producing reduced sensation ipsilateral to the hemiparesis
    A. tumor (neoplasm): primary or metastatic
    B. traumatic: epidural or subdural hematoma, hemorrhagic contusion of the brain, compression by depressed skull fracture
    C. vascular:
        1. infarction
            a. ischemic: embolic, low flow (due to atherosclerosis, arterial dissection...)
            b. hemorrhagic: intracerebral hemorrhage, aneurysmal SAH...
        2. TIA
        3. RIND
    D. infection: cerebritis, abscess
2. lesions of the contralateral internal capsule: produces pure motor hemiplegia without sensory loss. Most common etiology is ischemic lacunar infarct
3. lesions of the brainstem: ischemic infarct, hemorrhage, tumor
4. lesions of cervicomedullary junction: foramen magnum lesions (*see page 924*)
5. unilateral spinal cord lesions above ≈ C5 producing a Brown-Séquard syndrome with sensory loss to pain and temperature *contralateral* to the weakness (*see page 716*). Etiologies include: trauma, large herniated cervical disc[29]
6. hypoglycemia can sometimes be associated with hemiparesis that clears after administration of glucose

32.1.13.　Syncope and apoplexy

Syncope may be defined as one or more episodes of brief loss of consciousness (**LOC**) with prompt recovery (this term is considered by many to signify a vasovagal episode). The uncommonly used term **lipothymia** may be less likely to imply an etiology. Prevalence may be as high as ≈ 50% (higher in the elderly). **Apoplexy** is traditionally considered a form of hemorrhage, usually intracerebral. The recovery from apoplexy would therefore usually be slower than for syncope.

Etiologies (adapted[47, 48])
1. vascular: a few myotonic jerks may be seen in cerebral ischemia
    A. cerebrovascular
        1. subarachnoid hemorrhage (most commonly aneurysmal)
        2. intracerebral hemorrhage

3. brain stem infarction
4. pituitary apoplexy (rare): *see page 438*
5. vertebrobasilar insufficiency (**VBI**): *see page 881*
6. rarely with migraine

B. cardiovascular
1. Stokes-Adams attacks: disorder of AV-node conduction in the heart resulting in syncope with bradycardia
2. carotid sinus syncope: minimal stimulation (e.g. tight shirt collar, syncope while shaving...) causes reflex bradycardia with hypotension, more common in patients with carotid vascular disease. Bedside carotid massage with ECG and BP monitor may diagnose[48]
3. cardiac standstill: seen rarely in patients with glossopharyngeal neuralgia (*see page 386*)
4. vasodepressor syncope (the common **faint**), AKA vasovagal response, and recently AKA **neurocardiogenic syncope**[49]: the most common cause of transient LOC. Hypotension usually with any of the following autonomic manifestations: pallor, nausea, heavy perspiration, pupillary dilatation, bradycardia, hyperventilation, salivation. Usually benign. Most common in age < 35 yrs
5. orthostatic hypotension: drop in SBP ≥ 25 mm Hg on standing
6. triggered syncope: includes micturition, tussive syncope, weight lifting syncope... (most involve elevation of intrathoracic pressure)

2. infectious
A. meningitis
B. encephalitis
3. seizure: in general, there are involuntary movements and confusion afterwards, lasts at least several minutes. **Todd's paralysis** may follow and usually resolves slowly over a period of a few hours (*see page 258*). There may be irritative special-sense phenomena (visual, auditory, or olfactory hallucinations)
A. generalized
D. complex partial
C. akinetic seizure
D. drop attack (loss of posture without LOC): seen in Lennox-Gastaut
4. metabolic: hypoglycemia (may produce seizure, usually generalized)
5. miscellaneous
A. intermittent ventricular obstruction: the classic example is a colloid cyst of the third ventricle, but this mechanism is questionable (*see page 457*)
B. narcoleptic cataplexy: narcolepsy is characterized by somnolence and sudden attacks of weakness (cataplexy) when awake. Easy arousal and lack of post-ictal drowsiness distinguishes cataplexy from a seizure
C. psychogenic
6. intracranial hypotension: usually with CSF shunt when upright (*see page 197*)
7. unknown: in ≈ 40% of cases no cause can be diagnosed

32.1.14.   Encephalopathy

Many etiologies are similar to that for coma (*see page 155*). EEG may be helpful in distinguishing some etiologies (*see page 145*).
1. a rare cause may be (spontaneous) intracranial hypotension (*see page 178*)
2. hypertensive encephalopathy from malignant hypertension

32.1.15.   Transient neurologic deficit

For apoplexy, etc., see *Syncope and apoplexy*, page 914.

The first three etiologies listed below cover most cases of transient neurologic deficit:
1. **transient ischemic attack (TIA)**: temporary neurologic dysfunction as a result of ischemia. Maximum deficit usually at onset. By definition, lasts ≤ 24 hrs, however most TIAs resolve within 20 minutes (*see page 869*)
2. **migraine**: unlike TIA, tends to progress in a march-like fashion over several minutes. May or may not be followed by headache (see *Migraine*, page 45)
3. **seizure**: may be followed by a Todd's paralysis (*see page 258*)
4. TIA-like syndrome

A. "tumor TIA": a transient deficit in a patient with a tumor, may be clinically indistinguishable from an ischemic TIA

B. TIA-like symptoms may occur as a prodrome to a lobar intracerebral hemorrhage[50, 51] in cases of cerebral amyloid angiopathy (**CAA**). Unlike typical TIAs, these usually consist of numbness, tingling or weakness that gradually spreads in a manner reminiscent of a Jacksonian-march and may cross-over vascular territories (*see page 854*). Caution: antiplatelet drugs and anticoagulation may increase the risk of hemorrhage in patients with CAA (*see page 853*)

C. chronic subdural hematoma: may cause recurrent TIA-like symptoms of the involved hemisphere[52] (including transient aphasia, hemisensory or motor abnormalities). The duration of symptoms tends to be longer than the typical TIA[52]. Postulated mechanisms include:
1. electrical basis: the possibility of epileptic activity due has not been supported in the literature; however, spreading depression of Leao has been considered[53]
2. impairment of venous outflow by compression of surface veins
3. compromised regional cerebral perfusion by indirect shifting of the anterior and posterior cerebral arteries[54]
4. transient elevations of ICP → variations in cerebral perfusion pressure

32.1.16. Diplopia

1. cranial nerve palsy of any one or combination of III, IV, or VI
   A. for multiple cranial nerve palsies, see *Multiple cranial nerve palsies (cranial neuropathies)* below
   B. VI palsy: can occur with increased intracranial pressure, e.g. in idiopathic intracranial hypertension (pseudotumor cerebri) (*see page 493*), sphenoid sinusitis… (*see page 586* for other causes of abducens palsy)
2. intraorbital mass compressing extraocular muscles
   A. orbital pseudotumor: *see page 587*
   B. meningioma
3. Graves' disease: hyperthyroidism + ophthalmopathy (*see page 929*)
4. myasthenia gravis
5. giant cell arteritis: *see page 58*
6. botulism: due to toxin from *Claustridium botulinum* (in adults: ingested or in wound). N/V, abdominal cramps, and diarrhea often precede neurologic symptoms. Neurologic involvement is typically symmetric. Dry mouth & cranial nerves palsies (diplopia, ptosis, loss of accommodation and pupillary light reflex) are followed by descending weakness. Bulbar paresis (dysarthria, dysphagia, dysphonia, flaccid facial muscles) follows. Muscles of the trunk/extremities and respiration progressively weaken in a descending fashion. Sensory disturbances are absent. Sensorium usually remains clear

32.1.17. Anosmia

1. severe upper respiratory infection with damage to the neuroepithelium: the most common cause
2. head trauma: second most common cause, occurs in 7-15% of patients with significant head trauma
3. nasal and sinus disease: third most common cause
4. may also be associated with Alzheimer's disease
5. olfactory sense diminishes with age: ≈ 50% of patients 65-85 years of age have some loss of sense of smell
6. intracranial neoplasms: olfactory groove meningioma (see *Foster-Kennedy syndrome*, page 85), esthesioneuroblastoma (*see page 938*)
7. metabolic abnormalities: vitamin deficiency
8. physical blockage of nasal passages: polyps…
9. endocrine abnormalities: diabetes…

32.1.18. Multiple cranial nerve palsies (cranial neuropathies)

The differential diagnosis is legion. The following is a framework (modified[55]):
1. congenital
   A. **Möbius syndrome**: AKA congenital facial diplegia. Facial plegia is complete in ≈ 35% (in rest, affects upper face more than lower face, unlike central or peripheral facial palsy), associated with abducens palsy in 70%, external ophthalmoplegia in 25%, ptosis in 10%, lingual palsy in 18%
   B. congenital facial diplegia may be part of facioscapulohumeral or myotonic muscular dystrophy
2. infectious
   A. chronic meningitis:
      1. spirochetal, fungal, mycoplasma, viral (including AIDS)
      2. mycobacterial AKA tuberculous (**TB**) meningitis: 6th nerve involved first and most frequently. CSF shows lymphocytic pleocytosis and hypoglycorrhachia. Smears are usually negative and multiple cultures are needed to diagnose
   B. Lyme disease: facial nerve weakness (Bell's palsy) is common, sometimes bilateral. Other cranial nerve involvement is rare (*see page 234*)
   C. neurosyphilis: rare nowadays except with AIDS. Diagnosed by serologic testing
   D. fungal infection
      1. cryptococcal meningitis: CSF analysis for cryptococcal antigen and India ink prep can detect (*see page 239*)
      2. aspergillosis: may extend to the orbit from sinuses and involve cranial nerves
      3. mucormycosis (phycomycosis): produces cavernous sinus syndrome, usually occurs in diabetics (*see page 586*)
   E. cysticercosis: especially with basal form (see *Neurocysticercosis*, page 236)
3. traumatic: especially with basal skull fractures. Lower cranial nerve palsies may occur (sometimes delayed in onset) with occipital condyle fractures (*see page 721*) or atlanto-occipital dislocation (*see page 719*)
4. neoplastic (brain stem compression and intrinsic lesions usually also produce long tract findings early). Also see *Jugular foramen syndromes*, page 86
   A. chordoma: *see page 465*
   B. sphenoid-ridge meningioma
   C. neoplasms of the temporal bone (often in conjunction with chronic otitis media and otalgia): adenoid cystic carcinoma, adenocarcinoma, mucoepidermoid carcinoma
   D. glomus jugulare tumors: often affects nerves IX, X, and XI. May cause pulsatile tinnitus (see *Paraganglioma*, page 467)
   E. carcinomatous meningitis: CSF pleocytosis and elevated protein. Palsies are painless or associated with diffuse headache. Sensory palsies are common, resulting in deafness and blindness (*see page 491*)
   F. invasive pituitary adenomas involving the cavernous sinus (*see page 442*): extraocular cranial neuropathies tend to develop after visual field deficits in these tumors, and are less common when compared to other intracavernous solid tumors[56]
   G. primary CNS lymphoma: *see page 461*
   H. multiple myeloma involving the skull base: *see page 514*
   I. intrinsic brain stem tumors: gliomas, ependymoma, metastases...
5. vascular
   A. aneurysm: intracranial or cavernous sinus (*see page 801*)
   B. stroke: brain stem CVA usually also produces long tract findings (e.g. Weber's syndrome, Millard-Gubler syndrome..., *see page 86*)
   C. vasculitis: Wegener's granulomatosis usually affects eighth nerve in addition to others
6. granulomatous
   A. sarcoidosis: ≈ 5% have CNS involvement, usually as fluctuating single or multiple cranial neuropathies (facial nerve is most common, and may be indistinguishable from Bell's palsy). CSF pleocytosis is common (*see page 56*)
7. inflammatory

8. neuropathies
    A. Guillain-Barré syndrome: cranial nerve involvement includes facial diple-
       gia, oropharyngeal paresis. Also causes peripheral neuropathy with proxi-
       mal muscle weakness > distal (see page 53)
    B. **idiopathic cranial polyneuropathy**: subacute onset of constant facial
       pain, usually retro-orbital. Frequently precedes sudden onset of cranial-
       nerve palsies usually involving III, IV & VI, less frequently V, VII, and low-
       er nerves (IX through XII). Olfactory and auditory nerves usually spared.
       Acute and chronic inflammation of unknown etiology similar to Tolosa-
       Hunt and orbital pseudotumor. Steroids reduce pain and expedite recovery
9. entrapment in abnormal bone
    A. **hyperostosis cranialis interna**: a rare autosomal dominant abnormality
       of the bone of the base of the skull causing recurrent facial palsy and other
       cranial nerve palsies[57]
    B. osteopetrosis: see below
    C. Paget's disease (see page 340) involving the skull: 8th nerve involvement
       (deafness) is most common. Optic nerve atrophy, and palsies of oculomotor,
       facial, IX, XI, olfactory nerves and others may also occur[58]
    D. fibrous dysplasia: see page 483

CAVERNOUS SINUS SYNDROME

Multiple cranial nerve palsies (involving any of the cavernous sinus cranial nerves:
III, IV, V1, V2, VI) which primarily produce diplopia (due to ophthalmoplegia). Classically the third nerve palsy (e.g. from an enlarging cavernous carotid artery aneurysm) will
not produce a dilated pupil because the sympathetics which dilate the pupil are also
paralyzed[59 (p 1492)]. Facial pain or altered facial sensation may occur.

For a list of lesions that may produce cavernous sinus syndrome, see page 929.

OSTEOPETROSIS

AKA "marble bone disease" (there is also some confusion with the term osteosclerosis; *osteosclerosis fragilis generalisata* is the obsolete term for osteopetrosis). A rare
group of genetic disorders of defective osteoclastic resorption of bone resulting in increased bone density, may be transmitted either as autosomal dominant or recessive[60].
The dominant form is usually benign and is seen in adults and adolescents. The recessive
("malignant") form is often associated with consanguinity, and is similar to hyperostosis
cranialis interna (see above), but in addition to the proclivity for the skull, also involves
ribs, clavicles, long bones, and pelvis (long-bone involvement results in destruction of
marrow and subsequent anemia). Cranial nerves involved primarily include optic (optic
atrophy and blindness are the most common neurologic manifestation), facial, and vesti-
bulo-acoustic (with deafness), trigeminal nerve may also be involved. There may also be
extensive intracranial calcifications, hydrocephalus, intracranial hemorrhage and seizures.

Bilateral optic nerve decompression via a supraorbital approach may improve or
stabilize vision[60].

32.1.19.   Binocular blindness

1. bilateral occipital lobe dysfunction
    A. bilateral posterior cerebral artery flow impairment
        1. top of the basilar syndrome
        2. increased intracranial pressure
            a. hydrocephalus with shunt malfunction
            b. pseudotumor cerebri (idiopathic intracranial hypertension): see
               page 493
            c. cryptococcal meningitis: decreased visual acuity (see page 239)
    B. trauma: bilateral occipital lobe injury (e.g. contrecoup injury)
2. seizures: epileptic blindness
3. migraine: cortical spreading depression
4. posterior ischemic optic neuropathy: usually in the setting of shock
5. bilateral vitreous hemorrhage: e.g. with SAH (Terson's syndrome)
6. functional: conversion reaction, hysterical blindness...

32.1.20. Monocular blindness

Due to a lesion anterior to the optic chiasm.
1. Amaurosis fugax: often described as a "shade coming down" over one eye
    A. TIA: usually due to occlusion of the retinal artery (*see page 869*)
    B. giant cell arteritis (GCA): usually due to ischemia of optic nerve or tracts
        (less commonly due to retinal artery occlusion)[61] (*see page 59*)
2. trauma: optic nerve injury
3. ruptured carotid cavernous aneurysm: resultant carotid cavernous fistula increases intraocular pressure by impeding venous return
4. intraorbital pathology: tumors
5. injury within the globe: retinal detachment, ocular trauma
6. unilateral vitreous hemorrhage: e.g. with SAH (Terson's syndrome)

32.1.21. Exophthalmos

Also spelled exophthalmus. AKA proptosis (of the eye).

Pulsatile
1. carotid cavernous fistula **(CCF)** (*see page 845*)
2. transmitted intracranial pulsation due to defect in orbital roof
    A. seen unilaterally e.g. in neurofibromatosis type 1 (*see page 502*)
    B. post-op following procedures that remove orbital roof or wall
3. vascular tumors

Non-pulsatile
1. tumor
    A   intraorbital tumor
        1. optic glioma (*see page 420*)
        2. optic sheath neuroma
        3. lymphoma
        4. optic sheath **meningioma**[62]
        5. orbital involvement with **multiple myeloma**: see page 514
        6. orbital invasion by invasive **pituitary adenoma**: see page 442
    B. due to hyperostosis from a sphenoid ridge meningioma
2. Grave's disease (hyperthyroidism + proptosis): usually bilateral (*see page 929*)
3. infection: orbital cellulitis (usually has concomitant sinusitis)
4. inflammatory: orbital pseudotumor
5. hemorrhage
    A. traumatic
    B. spontaneous
6. 3rd nerve palsy: up to 3 mm proptosis from relaxation of the rectus muscles
7. cavernous sinus occlusion (may affect both eyes)
    A. cavernous sinus thrombosis (*see page 889*)
    B. cavernous sinus tumor
8. pseudo-exophthalmos
    A. congenital macrophthalmos (bull's eye)
    B. lid retraction: e.g. in Grave's disease (*see page 929*)
    C. coronal craniosynostosis can cause a "relative" proptosis (*see page 100*)

32.1.22. Pathologic lid retraction

1. hyperthyroidism
2. psychiatric: schizophrenia...
3. steroids
4. Parinaud's syndrome: *see page 86*

32.1.23. Macrocephaly

Macrocephaly means increased size of the head[63]. Although sometimes used synonymously, some contend that the term **macrocrania** by convention refers to a head circumference > 98th percentile[64 (pp 203)]. Also, not to be confused with *macrencephaly* AKA *megalencephaly* (*see below*).

1. with ventricular enlargement
    A. (hydrostatic) hydrocephalus **(HCP)** (*see page 183* for etiologies)
        1. communicating
        2. obstructive
    B. hydranencephaly: *see page 180*
    C. constitutional ventriculomegaly: ventricular enlargement of no known etiology with normal neurologic function
    D. hydrocephalus ex vacuo: loss of cerebral tissue (more often associated with microcephaly, e.g. with TORCH infections)
    E. vein of Galen aneurysms: *see below*
2. with normal or mildly enlarged ventricles
    A. "external hydrocephalus": prominent subarachnoid spaces and basal cisterns (see *External hydrocephalus (AKA benign external hydrocephalus)*, page 181)
    B. subdural fluid
        1. hematoma
        2. hygroma
        3. effusion (benign and symptomatic, *see page 678*)
    C. cerebral edema: some consider this to be a form of pseudotumor cerebri[63]
        1. toxic: e.g. lead encephalopathy (from chronic lead poisoning)
        2. endocrine: hypoparathyroidism, galactosemia, hypophosphatasia, hypervitaminosis A, adrenal insufficiency...
    D. familial (hereditary) macrocrania
    E. idiopathic
    F. megalencephaly (AKA macrencephaly): an enlarged brain (*see page 113*)
    G. neurocutaneous syndromes: usually due to increased volume of brain tissue (megalencephaly, *see above*)[63]. Seen especially in neurofibromatosis and congenital hypermelanosis (Ito's syndrome). Less common in tuberous sclerosis and Sturge-Weber. Also seen in the rare hemimegalencephaly syndrome
    H. arachnoid cyst (AKA subependymal or subarachnoid cyst)[63]: a duplication of the ependyma or arachnoid layer filled with CSF. Usually reach maximal size by 1 month of age and do not enlarge further. Treatment is required in ≈ 30% due to rapid enlargement or growth beyond first month. Cyst may be shunted or fenestrated. Prognosis with true arachnoid cyst is generally good (unlike porencephalic cyst) if no increased ICP or progressive macrocephaly during 1st year of life
    I. arteriovenous malformation: especially vein of Galen "aneurysm" (*see page 844*). Auscultate for cranial bruit. With vein of Galen aneurysms, macrocephaly may be due to HCP from obstruction of the sylvian aqueduct[63]. With other malformations, macrocrania may be due to increased pressure in venous system without HCP
    J. brain tumors without hydrocephalus: brain tumors are rare in infancy, and most cause obstructive HCP. Tumors that occasionally present without HCP includes astrocytomas. May also be seen in the rare diencephalic syndrome (tumor of anterior hypothalamus, *see page 420*)
    K. "gigantism syndromes"
        1. Soto's syndrome: associated with advanced bone age on x-ray, and multiple dysplastic features of face, skin and bones
        2. exomphalomacroglossia-gigantism **(EMG)** syndrome: hypoglycemia (from abnormalities in islets of Langerhans), large birth weight, large umbilicus or umbilical hernia and macroglossia
    L. "craniocerebral disproportion"[63](*see page 678*): may be the same as benign extra-axial fluid of infancy
    M. achondroplastic dwarf: cranial structures are enlarged but the skull base is small, giving rise to a prominent forehead and an OFC ≥ 97th percentile for age
    N. Canavan's disease: AKA spongy degeneration of the brain, an autosomal recessive disease of infancy prevalent among Ashkenazi Jews. Produces symmetrical low attenuation of hemispheric white matter on CT[65] and macrocephaly
    O. neurometabolic diseases: usually due to deposition of metabolic substances

in the brain. Seen in Tay-Sachs gangliosidosis, Krabbe disease...
3. due to thickening of the skull
    A. anemia: e.g. thalassemia
    B. skull dysplasia: e.g. osteopetrosis (*see page 918*)

32.1.24.   Tinnitus

May be either subjective (heard only by patient) or objective (e.g. cranial bruit, can be heard by examiner as well, usually with a stethoscope). Objective tinnitus is almost always due to vascular turbulence (from increased flow or partial obstruction).

Pulsatile
Almost exclusively vascular lesions.
1. pulse synchronous:
    A. carotid cavernous fistula (*see page 845*)
    B. cerebral AVM: especially dural AVM (*see page 843*)
    C. glomus jugulare tumor (*see page 468*)
    D. cerebral aneurysm: especially giant aneurysm with turbulent flow
    E. hypertension
    F. hyperthyroidism
    G. idiopathic intracranial hypertension (pseudotumor cerebri): *see page 493*
    H. transmitted bruit: from heart (e.g. aortic stenosis), carotid artery
2. non pulse-synchronous: asymmetrical enlargement of sigmoid sinus and jugular vein may produce a low grade hum

Non-pulsatile
1. occlusion of external ear: cerumen, foreign body
2. middle ear infection (otitis media)
3. otosclerosis
4. stapedial muscle spasms as occurs in hemifacial spasm
5. CP-angle tumors: including acoustic neuroma (*see page 429*)
6. Meniere's disease
7. labyrinthitis
8. drugs
    A. salicylates: aspirin, bismuth subsalicylate (Pepto Bismol®)
    B. quinine
    C. aminoglycoside toxicity: streptomycin, tobramycin (tinnitus precedes hearing loss)

32.1.25.   Facial sensory changes

1. circumoral paresthesias
    A. hypocalcemia
    B. syringobulbia
2. unilateral facial sensory changes
    A. large acoustic neuroma
    B. trigeminal nerve neuroma
    C. compression of the spinal trigeminal tract (large compressive lesions may cause bilateral alteration of facial sensation) that chiefly manifests in diminution of pain and temperature sense with little effect on touch sense[66]. The tract usually extends as far down as ≈ C2 (although it may occasionally extend down to C4)

32.1.26.   Language disturbance

1. aphasia:
    A. injury to speech cortex (Wernicke's or Broca's area) or to subcortical association fibers
    B. transitory aphasia following a seizure (see *Todd's paralysis*, page 258)
    C. primary progressive aphasia of adulthood: idiopathic & degenerative
2. **akinetic mutism**: seen with bilateral frontal lobe dysfunction (e.g. with bilateral

ACA distribution infarction due to vasospasm from a-comm aneurysm rupture or with large bilateral frontal lesions; may actually be abulia) or with bilateral cingulate gyrus lesions
3. muteness of cerebellar origin[67, 68]
4. following transcallosal surgery: as a result of bilateral cingulate gyrus retraction or thalamic injury together with section of the midportion of the corpus callosum[69]

32.1.27. Swallowing difficulties

1. mechanical: the term globus describes a sensation of a lump in the throat
   A. ossification of the anterior longitudinal ligament (OALL): *see page 346*
      1. as part of diffuse idiopathic skeletal hyperostosis (DISH): *see page 346*
   B. post-op following ACDF
      1. it is normal to have a little post-op swelling and fullness
      2. may be increased with multiple levels and with anterior cervical platings
      3. as a complication from post-op hematoma
2. neurologic

32.2. Differential diagnosis (DDx) by location

32.2.1. Cerebellopontine angle (CPA) lesions

Acoustic neuroma, meningioma, and epidermoid account for most. For those lesions that may be cystic, *see below*.
1. **acoustic neuroma**: (80-90% of CPA lesions) ⎱ *see below* for features to differen-
2. **meningioma**: (5-10%) ⎰ tiate these two lesions
3. ectodermal inclusion tumors (*see page 474*)
   A. **epidermoid** (cholesteatoma): (5-7%)
   B. dermoid
4. metastases
5. neuroma from cranial nerves other than VIII (also *see below*)
   A. trigeminal neuroma: expands towards Meckel's cave
   B. facial nerve neuroma[70]: may arise in any portion of the VII nerve, with a predilection for the geniculate ganglion[71]. Hearing loss may be sensorineural from VIII nerve compression from tumors arising in the proximal portion of VII (cisternal or IAC segment), or it may be conductive from erosion of the ossicles by tumors arising in the second (tympanic, or horizontal) segment of VII. Facial palsy (peripheral) may also develop, usually late[70] (*see page 594*)
   C. neurinoma of lowest 4 cranial nerves (IX, X, XI, XII)
6. arachnoid cyst
7. neurenteric cyst: 6 reported cases as of 1998[72] (*see page 98*)
8. cholesterol granuloma (distinct from epidermoid): *see page 475*
9. aneurysm
10. dolichobasilar ectasia
11. extensions of:
    A. brain stem or cerebellar glioma
    B. pituitary adenoma
    C. craniopharyngioma
    D. chordoma & tumors of skull base
    E. fourth ventricle tumors (ependymoma, medulloblastoma)
    F. choroid plexus papilloma: from 4th ventricle through foramen of Luschka
    G. glomus jugulare tumor
    H. primary tumors of temporal bone (e.g. sarcoma or carcinoma)

Differentiating neuromas of V, VII and VIII cranial nerves
All 3 may present in the CPA and may cross from posterior fossa to middle fossa, but they do so in different manners. Acoustic neuromas show "transhiatal" extension by

passing through the tentorial hiatus medially. Most trigeminal neuromas show "transapicopetrosal" extension by crossing into the middle fossa via the petrous apex (although some show transhiatal extension). When facial neuromas cross, they tend to spread across the midpetrosal bone, which is characteristic for facial neuromas[70]. When a facial neuroma enlarges the IAC, unlike an acoustic neuroma, it tends to erode the anterosuperior aspect of the IAC.

Differentiating acoustic neuroma from meningioma
* acoustic neuroma (AN): progressive unilateral hearing loss, usually with tinnitus. Progression results in unsteadiness, with true vertigo being rare. Facial nerve usually unaffected by stretching, thus facial nerve signs and symptoms are usually late. Trigeminal nerve involvement may occur with tumors > 3 cm (check corneal reflex), with tic douloureux-like symptoms being unusual. Rarely calcified
* meningiomas: may be similar to ANs, with some exceptions that follow. Since they often arise from the superior anterior edge of the IAC, early facial nerve involvement is more common, and hearing loss is usually late. The following are more common than with ANs: tic-like pain, calcification and bony hypertrophy (vs. ANs which enlarge the IAC).

Cystic lesions of the CPA
The following CPA lesions may be cystic or may have a cystic component[72]:
1. neurenteric cyst
2. epidermoid cyst
3. choroidal cyst
4. arachnoid cyst
5. cystic schwannoma
6. cholesterol granuloma: may appear cystic

32.2.2. Posterior fossa lesions

The following addresses intra-axial p-fossa tumors (for extra-axial tumors, see *Cerebellopontine angle (CPA) lesions* above).

ADULT

Single lesion
1. rule of thumb: "the differential diagnosis of a solitary lesion in an adult p-fossa is metastasis, metastasis, metastasis, until proven otherwise"
2. **hemangioblastoma**: (*see page 459*) the most common PRIMARY intra-axial p-fossa tumor in adults (7-12% of p-fossa tumors). Very vascular nodule, often has cyst. Almost all p-fossa tumors are relatively avascular on angiography except these (look for serpentine signal voids especially in the periphery of the lesion on MRI[73], much less common in cavernous hemangioma)
3. pilocytic astrocytoma: solid or cystic, tends to occur in younger adults (*see page 419*)
4. brainstem glioma: an isolated glioblastoma multiforme in the posterior fossa of an adult is a reportable rarity
5. abscess
6. cavernous hemangioma
7. hemorrhage
8. infarction

Multiple lesions
1. metastases
2. hemangioblastoma (possibly as part of von Hippel-Lindau): *see page 459*
3. abscesses
4. cavernous hemangiomas

PEDIATRIC

Also see *Pediatric brain tumors*, page 480.

4 types account for ≈ 95% of infratentorial tumors in patients ≤ 18 yrs age[74]. The 3 most common are equal in incidence[64]:
1. PNET (including **medulloblastoma**): 27%. Most start at fastigium (roof of 4th ventricle), and most are solid

---

2. **cerebellar (pilocytic) astrocytoma**: 27%. Most start in cerebellar hemisphere
3. **brainstem gliomas**: 28%
4. ependymoma
5. choroid plexus papilloma
6. metastasis: neuroblastoma, rhabdomyosarcoma, Wilm's tumor…

32.2.3.   Foramen magnum lesions

1. extra-axial tumors: for more details of <u>tumors</u> (i.e. neoplasms only) *see page 492*
   A. meningioma
   B. chordoma (*see page 464*): a mass behind the dens compressing the spinal cord is a chordoma until proven otherwise
   C. neurilemmoma
   D. epidermoid
   E. chondroma
   F. chondrosarcoma
   G. metastases
2. non-neoplastic
   A. aneurysms or ectasia of the vertebral artery
   B. odontoid process in cases of cranial migration of the odontoid (*see page 139*)
   C. pannus from involvement of the odontoid with rheumatoid arthritis or old nonunion of fracture
   D. synovial cyst of the quadrate ligament of the odontoid[75]

32.2.4.   Atlantoaxial subluxation

1. incompetence of the transverse ligament: results in increased atlanto-dental interval (**ADI**)
   A. rheumatoid arthritis: erosion of insertion points of the ligament
   B. traumatic avulsion of the insertion points of the ligament
2. incompetence of the odontoid process: normal ADI
   A. odontoid fractures: *see page 727*
   B. erosion of the odontoid due to rheumatoid arthritis: *see page 338*
   C. neoplastic erosion of the odontoid:
      1. metastases to the upper cervical spine (*see page 517*)
      2. other tumors of the axis (*see below*)
   D. Morquio syndrome: hypoplasia of the dens (*see page 337*)
   E. congenital absence/dysplasia of the odontoid
   F. following transoral odontoidectomy: (*see page 613*)
   G. local infection

32.2.5.   Axis (C2) vertebra lesions

1. tumors: rare tumors with a wide variety of possible identities. For more details, *see page 506*. Some factors pertinent to this location[76]:
   A. primary bone
      1. chondroma
      2. chondrosarcoma: rare in the craniovertebral junction. Lobulated tumors with calcified areas
      3. chordoma
      4. osteochondroma (chondroma)
      5. osteoblastoma: *see page 511*
      6. osteoid osteoma: *see page 511*
      7. giant-cell tumors of bone: typically arise in adolescence. Lytic with bony collapse[77]
   B. metastatic: including
      1. breast cancer
      2. prostate cancer
      3. malignant melanoma
      4. paraganglioma
   C. miscellaneous

1. plasmacytoma
2. multiple myeloma
3. eosinophilic granuloma: osteolytic defect with progressive vertebral collapse. Occasionally occur in C2[78]
4. Ewing's sarcoma: malignant. Peak incidence during 2nd decade of life
5. aneurysmal bone cyst[79]
2. infection: osteomyelitis of the axis
3. pannus from old nonunion of fracture or from rheumatoid arthritis

32.2.6.   Multiple intracranial lesions on CT or MRI

1. neoplastic
   A. primary
      1. multicentric gliomas (≈ 6% of gliomas are multicentric, more common in neurofibromatosis, see *Multiple gliomas*, page 413)
      2. tuberous sclerosis (including giant cell astrocytomas); (usually periventricular)
      3. multiple meningiomas
      4. lymphoma
      5. PNET
      6. multiple neuromas (usually in neurofibromatosis, including bilateral acoustic neuromas)
   B. metastatic: usually cortical or subcortical, surrounded by prominent vasogenic edema. *See page 484.* More common tumors include:
      1. lung
      2. breast
      3. melanoma: may be higher density than brain on unenhanced CT
      4. renal cell
      5. gastrointestinal tumors
      6. genitourinary tract tumors
      7. choriocarcinoma
      8. testicular
      9. atrial myxoma
      10. leukemia
2. infection: mostly abscess or cerebritis. Most commonly due to:
   A. pyogenic bacteria
   B. toxoplasmosis: common in AIDS patients (*see page 230*)
   C. cryptococcus
   D. mycoplasma
   E. coccidiomycosis
   F. echinococcus
   G. schistosomiasis
   H. paragonimiasis
   I. aspergillosis
   J. candidiasis
   K. herpes simplex encephalitis (**HSE**): usually temporal lobe (*see page 225*)
3. inflammatory
   A. demyelinating disease
      1. MS: usually in white matter, periventricular, with little mass effect
      2. progressive multifocal leukoencephalopathy (**PML**): usually white matter
   B. gummas
   C. granulomas
   D. amyloidosis
   E. sarcoidosis
   F. vasculitis or arteritis
   G. collagen vascular disease, including:
      1. periarteritis nodosa (**PAN**) (*see page 61*)
      2. systemic lupus erythematosus (**SLE**)
      3. granulomatous arteritis
4. vascular
   A. multiple aneurysms (congenital or atherosclerotic)
   B. multiple hemorrhages, e.g. associated with DIC or other coagulopathies (including anticoagulant therapy)

C. venous infarctions (especially in dural sinus thrombosis, *see page 888*)
D. moyamoya disease (*see page 892*)
E. subacute hypertension (as in malignant HTN, eclampsia...) → symmetric confluent lesions with mild mass effect and patchy enhancement usually in occipital subcortical white matter (*see page 64*)
F. multiple strokes
1. lacunar strokes (l'etat lacunaire)
2. multiple emboli (e.g. in atrial fibrillation, mitral valve prolapse, SBE, air emboli)
3. sickle cell disease
5. hematomas and contusions
A. traumatic (multiple hemorrhagic contusions, multiple SDH)
B. "hypertensive" hemorrhages (amyloid angiopathy, etc.)
6. intracranial calcifications (*see page 933*)
7. miscellaneous
A. radiation necrosis
B. foreign bodies (e.g. post gunshot wound)
C. periventricular low densities
1. Binswanger's disease
2. transependymal absorption of CSF (e.g. in active hydrocephalus)

EVALUATION
Deciding which of the following tests are needed to evaluate a patient with multiple intracranial lesions must be individualized for the appropriate clinical setting.
1. cardiac echo: to R/O SBE that could shed septic emboli
2. "metastatic workup" (see *Metastatic workup*, page 488) including:
A. chest x-ray: to R/O primary bronchogenic Ca or pulmonary metastases of another Ca, but also to R/O pulmonary abscess that could shed septic emboli. Chest CT may be needed in cases of positive CXR or if CXR is negative and there is high suspicion of lungs as source of primary
B. abdominal CT: has largely replaced lower GI (barium enema) and IVP
C. mammogram in women

32.2.7. Ring-enhancing lesions on CT/MRI

First three account for most cases in adults:
1. **astrocytoma** (usually malignant astrocytoma, viz. glioblastoma multiforme)
2. **metastases**: (especially lung)
3. **abscess** (including toxoplasmosis abscess[80]): pyogenic abscesses are often (but not always) associated with fever and rapidly progressing neurologic deficit. May see visible growth over several days on serial imaging
4. others
A. lymphoma (primary brain lymphoma or metastatic systemic lymphoma): wall is thicker than abscess[81]. Incidence is increasing (*see page 461*)
B. radiation necrosis
C. resolving hematoma with capsule: ✖ NB: a ring enhancing lesion on <u>MRI</u> can occur with a resolving intracerebral hematoma and can mimic tumor (on a T1 gradient echo sequence, an continuous ring suggests hematoma, an interrupted ring suggests malignancy)
D. cysticercosis cyst (see *Neurocysticercosis*, page 236)
E. trauma
F. infarct

32.2.8. Leukoencephalopathy

Disease largely confined to the white matter. Many causes are demyelinating diseases.
1. anoxia/ischemia
2. intoxication: cyanide, organic solvents, carbon monoxide
3. vitamin deficiencies: B_{12} with subacute combined degeneration
4. infectious, especially viral:
A. progressive multifocal leukoencephalopathy (**PML**) (*see page 231*)
B. herpes varicella-zoster leukoencephalitis (*see page 227*)

C. HIV infection (AIDS): perivascular pattern of demyelination
D. cytomegalovirus infection
E. Creutzfeldt-Jakob disease: small and perivascular demyelination
5. metabolic derangements: hyponatremia, excessively rapid correction of hyponatremia (causing central pontine myelinolysis, *see page 12*)
6. hereditary: metachromatic leukodystrophy, adult-onset Schilder's disease
7. leuko-araiosis (*see page 936*)
8. multiple myeloma (*see page 515*)

32.2.9. Corpus callosum

1. lymphoma
2. MS plaque
3. tumefactive demyelinating lesions: *see page 51*
4. lipoma

32.2.10. Sellar and parasellar lesions

Includes suprasellar, intrasellar, and parasellar lesions that may cause enlarged, eroded or destroyed sella turcica. The considerations in adults (adenoma is the most common enhancing pituitary lesion) are different than for children (adenomas are rare, craniopharyngioma and germinoma are more common). Includes (modified[82]):
1. pituitary tumor
   A. adenoma
      1. microadenoma: *see page 438*
      2. macroadenoma
      3. invasive pituitary adenoma: *see page 442*
   B. carcinoma or carcinosarcoma
   C. pituitary "pseudotumor":
      1. thyrotroph hyperplasia due to hypothyroidism[83] causing chronic pituitary stimulation by TRH *see page 445*
      2. pituitary enlargement may occur in intracranial hypotension (*see page 178*)
2. vascular lesions
   A. aneurysm: ACoA, ICA (cavernous carotid or suprasellar variant of superior hypophyseal artery aneurysm, *see page 812*), ophthalmic, basilar bifurcation. Giant aneurysms may produce mass effect
   B. carotid cavernous fistula (CCF): *see page 845*
3. juxtasellar or suprasellar tumors or masses
   A. craniopharyngioma: in this region, these account for 20% of tumors in adult, 54% in peds
   B. meningioma (parasellar, tuberculum sellae, or diaphragm sella): to differentiate tuberculum sellae meningioma from pituitary macroadenoma on MRI, 3 characteristics of meningioma are: 1) bright homogeneous enhancement with gadolinium (c.f. heterogeneous, poor enhancement with macroadenoma), 2) suprasellar epicenter (vs. sellar), 3) tapered extension of intracranial dural base[84] (dural tail). Also, the sella is usually not enlarged, and even large suprasellar meningiomas rarely produce endocrine disturbances[85]
   C. pituitary tumor with extrasellar extension: tends to push carotids laterally (unlike meningioma which may encase carotid), more symmetric than meningioma
   D. germ cell tumors (GCT): choriocarcinoma, germinoma, teratoma, embryonal carcinoma, endodermal sinus tumor. Suprasellar GCTs are more common in females (c.f. pineal region GCT). Triad of a suprasellar GCT: diabetes insipidus, visual deficit and panhypopituitarism[86], may also present with obstructive hydrocephalus
   E. hypothalamic glioma
   F. chiasmal (optic) glioma
   G. metastasis
   H. parasitic infections: cysticercosis
   I. epidermoid cyst

J. suprasellar arachnoid cyst: see *Arachnoid cysts*, page 94
4. inflammatory
   A. lymphoid adenohypophysitis, AKA lymphocytic adenohypophysitis, AKA lymphocytic hypophysitis. A rare inflammatory disease of the pituitary gland, but increasingly recognized as a possible cause of hypopituitarism. Most cases occur in women (only 5 cases reported in men) often within 1 yr postpartum[87]. May be confused with dysgerminoma histologically[88, 89]. Probably an autoimmune disease that produces inflammation of the pituitary stalk with lymphocytic infiltrate. Difficult to distinguish radiographically from adenoma. Distinctive feature: tends to selectively affect a single pituitary hormone. May also cause DI[87]. Usually self limited, some treat with steroids
   B. pituitary granuloma[90]
5. empty sella syndrome:
   A. primary: *see page 499*
   B. secondary: following pituitary tumor resection (*see page 499*)

32.2.11. Intracranial cysts

Modified[91]:
1. arachnoid cysts: see *Arachnoid cysts*, page 94
2. low density tumor
3. chronic subdural hematoma or hygroma
4. suprasellar cyst from dilated third ventricle
5. interhemispheric cyst from porencephaly
6. posterior fossa cyst from Dandy-Walker malformation (*see page 110*)
7. enlarged cisterna-magna
8. old infarct: if it communicates with ventricle it is called a porencephalic cyst
9. cysts associated with isodense tumors:
   A. ganglioma
   B. cerebellar hemangioblastoma
   C. cystic astrocytoma
10. infectious
    A. cysticercosis: see *Neurocysticercosis*, page 236
    B. hydatid cyst: see *Echinococcosis*, page 238

MIDLINE CAVITIES

Three potential supratentorial midline cavities in the center of the brain and differentiating features are shown in *Table 32-5*.

Table 32-5   Features of midline brain cavities[92]

Cavity	Anatomy	Frequency	Clinical significance
cavum septum pellucidum **(CSP)** *(see text)*	located between leaflets of septum pellucidum	100% of preemies, 97% of newborns, 10% of adults	no known association with pathologic conditions
cavum vergae	directly posterior to, and often communicating with CSP	relatively uncommon	possible association with neurologic abnormalities*
cavum velum interpositum	due to separation of crura of fornix between thalami above the 3rd ventricle	present in 60% of children < 1 yr age, and in 30% between 1 and 10 yrs	no known association with pathologic conditions

*   including developmental delay, macrocephaly, Apert's syndrome, abnormal EEG

Cavum septum pellucidum (CSP)

AKA fifth ventricle, among others. A variable slit-like fluid-filled space between the leaflets of the left and right septum pellucidum. The compartment is usually isolated, although some communicate with third ventricle. The CSP is part of normal development, and persists until shortly after birth. Thus, it is present in ≈ all preemies. It is found in ≈ 10% of the adult population, usually representing an asymptomatic developmental anomaly. However, it is also commonly seen in boxers suffering from chronic traumatic encephalopathy (*see page 683*).

32.2.12.   Orbital lesions

4 compartments of the orbit: ocular (AKA globe, AKA bulbar), optic nerve sheath, intraconal, and extraconal. CT remains a strong imaging modality within the orbit (less susceptible to motion artifact than MRI, images bony structures to good advantage).
1. neoplastic
   A. cavernous hemangioma: the most common <u>benign</u> primary intra-orbital neoplasm. Choroidal hemangioma is seen in Sturge-Weber syndrome
   B. fibrohistiocytoma
   C. hemangiopericytoma

   } discrete tumors that may occur adjacent to but not envelope the optic nerve sheath

   D. capillary hemangioma: produces infantile proptosis; regresses spontaneously
   E. lymphangioma: produces infantile proptosis; does <u>not</u> regress
   F. melanoma: the most common primary ocular malignancy of adulthood
   G. retinoblastoma: congenital, malignant primary retinal tumor. 40% are bilateral, 90% are calcified (often a key differentiating feature; does not portend benignity as with other lesions). CT may show retinal detachment
   H. lymphoma of the orbit: causes painless proptosis. The 3rd most common cause of proptosis
   I. primary optic nerve tumors
      1. optic glioma
      2. optic nerve sheath meningioma
2. congenital
   A. Coats disease: telangiectatic vascular malformation of retina which leaks a lipid exudate causing retinal detachment. May mimic retinoblastoma. Vitreous is hyperintense on MRI on T1WI and T2WI due to lipid
   B. persistent hyperplastic primary vitreous
   C. retinopathy of prematurity (retrolental fibroplasia)
3. infectious
   A. toxocara endophthalmitis
4. inflammatory/collagen vascular disease: usually bilateral
   A. scleritis
   B. pseudotumor of the orbit: the most common intraconal lesion. Usually unilateral (*see page 587*)
   C. sarcoidosis: usually affects the conjunctiva and lacrimal gland and spares connective tissues and intraorbital muscles
   D. Sjögren's syndrome
5. vascular
   A. enlargement of the superior orbital vein: may occur in thrombosis of cavernous sinus or in carotid-cavernous fistula
   B. dural AVM
6. miscellaneous
   A. drusen: degenerated retinal pigment cells in the posterior globe that may resemble calcified masses on CT
   B. thyroid ophthalmopathy: Graves' disease (hyperthyroidism & swelling of EOMs → <u>painless</u> proptosis). 80% of cases are bilateral. The ophthalmopathy is independent of the level of thyroid hormone (possibly an autoimmune process). NB: a swollen inferior rectus muscle may resemble an orbital tumor if seen only on lower CT cut through the orbit
   C. EOM enlargement with steroid use or occasionally with obesity
   D. fibrous dysplasia

32.2.13.   Cavernous sinus lesions

Modified[93]:
1. primary tumors/lesions (rare)
   A. meningiomas[94]
   B. neurinomas
   C. aneurysms of the cavernous carotid artery

2. tumors from adjacent areas that may extend into cavernous sinus:
   A. meningiomas
   B. neurinomas
   C. chordomas
   D. chondromas
   E. chondrosarcomas
   F. pituitary tumors[95]
   G. nasopharyngeal carcinomas
   H. esthesioneuroblastomas
   I. nasopharyngeal angiofibromas
   J. metastatic tumors
3. inflammation: e.g. Tolosa-Hunt (*see page 587*)
4. infection: mucormycosis (phycomycosis). Usually in diabetics (*see page 586*)

32.2.14. Skull lesions

The most common <u>benign</u> tumors of skull are osteoma and hemangioma. Osteogenic sarcoma is the most common <u>malignancy</u>. *See page 480* for specific skull tumors.

EVALUATING ROENTGENOGRAPHIC SKULL LUCENCIES
There is enough overlap of features to prevent any systematic means of determining the etiology of all or even most radiographic skull lucencies. The following features should be noted for any lucency, some are more helpful than others (modified[96]):
1. multiplicity (single or multiple?): except for multiple venous lakes, the presence of 6 or more defects is usually indicative of a malignancy
2. origin (intradiploic, full thickness, inner or outer table only):
   A. most vault lesions originate intradiploically, so limitation to this space may merely signify early recognition of a lesion
   B. expansion of the diploë with bulging of one or both tables almost always signifies a benign lesion
   C. full thickness lesions affecting both tables congruently usually indicates malignancy, whereas non-congruent erosion is more common with benign lesions
3. edges (smooth or ragged):
   A. smooth edges, whether regular, distinct or indistinct have no predictive value
   B. irregular margins (especially ragged undermined edges) are more suggestive of infection (osteomyelitis) or malignancy
   C. sharply demarcated, full thickness punched out defects suggest myeloma
4. presence of peripheral **sclerosis**: circumferential bony sclerosis suggests benignity (may indicate slow expansion and longstanding nature). The ring of sclerosis is generally narrow except in fibrous dysplasia
5. presence or absence of peripheral vascular channels: presence is highly suggestive of benign lesions (seen in ≈ 66% of venous lakes and ≈ 50% of hemangiomas)
6. pattern within the lucency:
   A. hemangiomas classically show honeycomb or trabecular pattern (seen in ≈ 50% of cases) or sunburst pattern (seen in ≈ 11% of cases)
   B. fibrous dysplasia may show well defined islands of bone, or a grossly mottled appearance with randomly arranged cystic and dense areas
7. location on the cranial vault (high or low?): poor correlation with benign vs. malignant lesions
8. pain: eosinophilic granulomas are often <u>tender</u>

Remember: skull lesions may have an intracranial component. CT scanning is good for assessing bone (MRI is poor for this), however, CT may miss small intracranial lesions tucked within the convexity of the calvaria due to bone hardening artifact (MRI has better sensitivity in this type of an area).

Nuclear bone scan may be a helpful adjunctive test (see specific lesion for findings).

Biopsy: indicated for questionable skull lesions. If the bone has not been destroyed by soft tissue, biopsy may be accomplished with a Craig needle, and the specimen may need decalcification by the pathologist before histologic evaluation can be completed.

RADIOLUCENT LESION OR BONE DEFECT IN SKULL
• congenital or developmental
   A. epidermoid (cholesteatoma): <u>sclerotic</u> edge
   B. encephalocele, meningoencephalocele, dermal sinus
   C. **fibrous dysplasia**: *see page 483*. A benign condition in which normal bone is replaced by fibrous connective tissue. Tends to occur higher in calvaria. 3

types.
1. cystic: widening of the diplöe usually with thinning of the outer table and little involvement of the inner table. Typically involves calvaria
2. sclerotic: usually involves skull base (especially sphenoid bone) and facial bones
3. mixed: appearance is similar to cystic type with patches of increased density within the lucent lesions
D. hemangioma or AVM of bone or scalp
E. pacchionian depression
F. Albright's syndrome
G. congenital foramina: "holes" in skull traversed by emissary veins
H. parietal thinning: usually a bilateral process
I. frontal fenestrae
J. venous lakes
K. cerebral herniations: AKA occipital pacchionian granulations
• traumatic
A. surgical defect: burr hole, craniectomy
B. fracture
C. post-traumatic leptomeningeal cyst (see page 668)
D. following trauma in children[97]
• inflammatory
A. osteomyelitis: including tuberculosis[98]
B. sarcoidosis
C. syphilis
• neoplastic
A. hemangioma: fine, honeycombed matrix. Classic x-ray finding: "starburst" appearance due to radiating bone spicules (may occur in as few as ≈ 11% of cases[96])
B. intracranial tumor with erosion
C. lymphoma, leukemia
D. meningioma
E. metastasis: usually hot on bone scan
F. multiple myeloma, plasmacytoma: see page 514. Usually cool on bone scan
G. sarcoma or fibrosarcoma of bone
H. skin tumor with invasion (rodent ulcer)
I. neuroblastoma
J. lipoma
K. epidermoid (may also be considered congenital, thus also see above)
• miscellaneous
A. histiocytosis X (eosinophilic granuloma is the mildest form): perfectly round non-sclerotic punched out lesion, generally multiple, tender (see page 482)
B. Paget's disease (when seen as a zone of osteolysis without osteoblastic sclerosis on skull films, this is defined as **osteoporosis circumscripta**). Usually "hot" on bone scan
C. aneurysmal bone cyst: rare. Arises in diplöe and expands both tables which become thin but remain intact
D. brown tumor of hyperparathyroidism

DIFFUSE INCREASED DENSITY, HYPEROSTOSIS, OR CALVARIAL THICKENING

• common
1. anemia (sickle cell, iron deficiency, thalassemia, hereditary spherocytosis)
2. fibrous dysplasia, leontiasis ossea
3. hyperostosis interna generalisata
4. osteoblastic metastases (especially prostate, breast)
5. Paget's disease (begins with lytic zone and diploic thickening)
6. treated hydrocephalus

• uncommon
1. chronic phenytoin therapy
2. Engelman's disease (progressive diaphyseal dysplasia)
3. fluorosis
4. hypervitaminosis D
5. hypoparathyroidism, pseudohypoparathyroidism
6. meningioma
7. osteogenesis imperfecta
8. osteopetrosis (see page 918)
9. secondary polycythemia
10. syphilitic osteitis
11. tuberous sclerosis

- common
  1. congenital hemolytic anemia (e.g. thalassemia, sickle cell, hereditary spherocytosis, pyruvate kinase deficiency)
- uncommon
  1. hemangioma
  2. cyanotic congenital heart disease (with secondary polycythemia)
  3. iron deficiency anemia
  4. metastases: especially neuroblastoma, thyroid carcinoma
  5. multiple myeloma
  6. meningioma
  7. osteosarcoma
  8. polycythemia vera

Diffuse demineralization or destruction of the skull
(including "salt and pepper skull")

- common
  1. hyperparathyroidism, primary or secondary
  2. metastatic carcinoma or neuroblastoma
  3. multiple myeloma
  4. osteoporosis
- uncommon
  1. Paget's disease (osteoporosis circumscripta)

Focal increased density of skull base

- common
  1. fibrous dysplasia
  2. meningioma
- uncommon
  1. mastoiditis
  2. nasopharyngeal carcinoma
  3. osteoblastic metastasis
  4. osteoma of the outer table or diploe
  5. chondroma
  6. sarcoma of bone (e.g. osteosarcoma, chondrosarcoma)
  7. sphenoid sinusitis

Generalized increased density of skull base

- common
  1. fibrous dysplasia
  2. Paget's disease
- uncommon
  1. severe anemia (e.g. thalassemia, sickle cell)
  2. Engelman's disease (progressive diaphyseal dysplasia)
  3. fluorosis
  4. hyperparathyroidism, primary or secondary (treated)
  5. hypervitaminosis D
  6. idiopathic hypercalcemia
  7. meningioma
  8. osteopetrosis (_see page 918_)

Localized increased density or hyperostosis of the calvaria

- common
  1. anatomic variation (e.g. sutural sclerosis)
  2. fibrous dysplasia
  3. osteoma (_see page 481_)
  4. meningioma
  5. hyperostosis frontalis interna (_see page 483_)
  6. osteoblastic metastases (especially: prostate, breast)
  7. Paget's disease (begins with lytic zone and diploic thickening)
  8. cephalhematoma
  9. depressed skull fracture
- uncommon
  1. osteosarcoma
  2. chronic osteomyelitis, tuberculosis
  3. tuberous sclerosis
  4. radiation necrosis

32.2.15.   Combined intracranial/extracranial lesions

Lesion causing mass outside skull with intracranial component.
1. intra-axial: rule of thumb - "there is no intra-axial lesion that grows out of skull"
2. extra-axial:
   A. meningioma

1. may arise in diploe, grows outward and inward
2. intracranial meningioma can grow through bone by destroying it
3. intracranial meningioma can induce hyperostosis that causes extracranial mass
   B. metastatic disease (e.g. GI carcinoma, and especially prostate Ca)
   C. bone (skull) lesion:
   1. hemangioma
   2. epidermoid
   3. fibrous dysplasia (rare)
   4. giant cell tumor (rare)
   5. Ewing's sarcoma (rare in skull)
   6. aneurysmal bone cyst (5% occur in skull, occipital bone most common)

32.2.16. Intracranial calcifications

Often due to deposition of calcium in the media of medium-sized blood vessels without compromise of the lumen. Usually asymptomatic. Considered abnormal when
present to a significant enough degree to be visible on plain x-ray in a young person.

SINGLE INTRACRANIAL CALCIFICATIONS
1. physiologic
   A. choroid plexus: calcifications usually bilateral (*see below*)
   B. arachnoid granulation
   C. diaphragma sella
   D. dural (falcine, tentorial, sagittal sinus)
   E. habenular commisure
   F. petroclinoid or interclinoid ligaments
   G. pineal
2. infection
   A. cysticercosis cyst: single or multiple (see *Neurocysticercosis*, page 236)
   B. encephalitis, meningitis, cerebral abscess (acute and healed)
   C. granuloma (torulosis and other fungi)
   D. hydatid cyst
   E. tuberculoma
   F. paragonimiasis
   G. rubella
   H. syphilitic gumma
3. vascular
   A. aneurysm, including:
   1. vein of Galen aneurysm
   2. giant aneurysm
   B. arteriosclerosis (especially carotid artery in siphon region)
   C. hemangioma, AVM, Sturge-Weber syndrome
4. neoplastic: calcifications usually suggest a more benign process
   A. meningioma (*see page 126*)
   B. craniopharyngioma
   C. choroid plexus papilloma
   D. ependymoma
   E. glioma (especially oligodendroglioma, also astrocytoma)
   F. ganglioglioma
   G. lipoma of corpus callosum
   H. pinealoma
   I. hamartoma of tuber cinerium
5. miscellaneous
   A. hematoma: ICH, EDH or SDH. Calcifications usually only when chronic
   B. idiopathic
   C. tuberous sclerosis (*see page 504*)

MULTIPLE INTRACRANIAL CALCIFICATIONS
* common
   A. choroid plexus: the most common site for physiologic calcification (in lateral
      ventricles where it is usually bilateral and symmetric; rare in 3rd & 4th
      ventricles). Increases in frequency and extent with age (prevalence: 75% by

5th decade). Rare under age 3. Under age 10, consider possible choroid plexus papilloma. Involvement in the temporal horns is often associated with neurofibromatosis

B. basal ganglia **(BG)**: slight bilateral BG calcifications on CT are common, especially in the elderly. Considered a normal radiographic variant by some. They may be idiopathic, secondary to conditions such as hypoparathyroidism or long-term anticonvulsant use, or part of rare conditions such as Fahr's disease (*see below*). BG calcifications > 0.5 cm dia are possibly association with cognitive impairment and a high prevalence of psychiatric symptoms[99]

- uncommon
    - A. Fahr's disease: progressive idiopathic calcification of medial portions of basal ganglia, sulcal depths of cerebral cortex, and dentate nuclei[100]
    - B. hemangioma, AVM, Sturge-Weber syndrome, von Hippel-Lindau disease
    - C. basal cell nevus syndrome (falx, tentorium)
    - D. Gorlin's syndrome. Associated findings: mandibular cysts, rib and vertebral deformities, short metacarpals. Medulloblastoma seen in several patients
    - E. cytomegalic inclusion disease
    - F. encephalitis (e.g. measles, chickenpox, neonatal herpes simplex)
    - G. hematomas (SDH or EDH, chronic)
    - H. neurofibromatosis (choroid plexi)
    - I. toxoplasmosis
    - J. tuberculomas; tuberculous meningitis (treated)
    - K. tuberous sclerosis
    - L. hypoparathyroidism (including post-thyroidectomy cases[101]) and pseudohypoparathyroidism
    - M. multiple tumors (e.g. meningiomas, gliomas, metastases)
    - N. cysticercosis cyst: may be single or multiple (see *Neurocysticercosis*, page 236)

32.2.17. Intraventricular lesions

Intraventricular tumors represent only ≈ 10% of CNS neoplasms. A clue to differentiating a tumor located within the ventricle from an intraparenchymal tumor invaginating into the ventricle is a "cap" of CSF surrounding an intraventricular tumor on CT or MRI. The following is from a series of 73 patients with an intraventricular lesion on CT seen at UCSF[102].

1. **astrocytoma**: 15 patients (20%). The most common lesion. Hydrocephalus **(HCP)** present in 73%; hyperdense on non-contrast CT **(NCCT)** in 77%. Locations in descending order of frequency:
    - frontal horn (7)
    - third ventricle (4)
    - atrium (AKA trigone) (3)
    - fourth ventricle (1)
2. **colloid cyst**: 10 patients (14%). Only seen in third ventricle at foramen of Monro. 50% hyperdense on NCCT, 9 of 10 enhance (*see page 457*). DDx includes xanthogranuloma
3. **meningioma**: 9 patients (12%). 8 in atrium, 1 in frontal horn. All hyperdense with dense uniform enhancement. 4 calcified. 5 of 6 had dense tumor blush on angiogram, most supplied from anterior choroidal artery, posterior choroidal less common. Thought to arise from arachnoidal cells within the choroid plexus
4. **ependymoma**: 7 patients (10%). 4 in 4th ventricle, 3 in body of lateral ventricle
5. **craniopharyngioma**: 5 patients (7%). All in 3rd ventricle. All with punctate calcification. Squamous epithelial rests in region of lamina terminalis are felt to give rise to this uncommon variety of craniopharyngioma
6. **medulloblastoma**: 4 patients (5%). All filled 4th ventricle. All hyperdense with homogeneous enhancement
7. **cysticercosis**: 4 patients (5%). 2 in 4th ventricle, anterior 3rd in 1, panventricular in 1 (NB: incidence related to geographic location), *see page 236*
8. **choroid plexus papilloma**: 4 patients (5%). 2 in lateral ventricle (1 bilateral), 1 in 4th, 1 in 3rd. Non-obstructive HCP in 3 (possible CSF overproduction). Intense blush on angiogram
9. **epidermoid**: 3 patients. All in 4th ventricle. All hypodense with no enhancement. The most common 4th ventricular low density lesion in the U.S.

10. **dermoid**: 2 patients. 1 in 4th ventricle, 1 in frontal horn. Both had free floating fat in ventricles suggestive of cyst rupture. Tendency to form in midline
11. **choroid plexus carcinoma**: 2 patients. Both in atrium of lateral ventricle. Both extended into adjacent brain parenchyma with edema and shift. Intense blush on angio. NB: very rare lesion
12. **subependymoma**: 2 patients. 1 in 4th ventricle, 1 in frontal horn. Both isodense with minimal enhancement. Most commonly in floor of 4th ventricle near obex
13. **ependymal cyst**: 2 patients. Both in lateral ventricle. Absence of communication demonstrated by metrizamide cisternography
14. **arachnoid cyst**: 1 patient. Lateral ventricle.Absence of communication demonstrated by metrizamide cisternography
15. **arteriovenous malformation (AVM)**: 2 patients
16. **teratoma:** 1 patient. Located in anterior 3rd ventricle. Partially calcified with foci of fat density. Marked enhancement

Other intraventricular tumors
1. central neurocytoma: *see page 425*
2. metastases: breast and lung reported[103]

FEATURES TO HELP IDENTIFY TYPE OF INTRAVENTRICULAR TUMOR

By location within ventricular system
Table 32-6 shows the breakdown of tumor type by location within the ventricular system.

Table 32-6 Type of intraventricular tumors by location[102]
(numbers are patients out of 73*)

3rd ventricle		4th ventricle		Atrium		Body		Frontal horn	
colloid cyst	10	medulloblast.	4	meningioma	8	ependymoma	3	astrocytoma	7
craniopharyng	5	ependymoma	4	astrocytoma	3	ch. plexus papil.†	1	meningioma	1
astrocytoma	4	epidermoid	3	ch. plexus papil.	1	ch. plexus carc.	1	subependym.	1
teratoma	1	cysticercosis	2	ch. plexus carc.	1	ependym. cyst	1	dermoid	1
ch. plexus papil.	1	astrocytoma	1	arachnoid cyst	1	AVM	1		
cysticercosis	1	subependym.	1	ependym. cyst	1				
dermoid	1								
ch. plexus carc.	1								
AVM	1								

*   1 patient had cysticercosis diffusely throughout ventricles
†   1 patient with bilateral lateral ventricle papillomas

By location and age within lateral ventricle[104]
See *Table 32-7*.

This study excluded tumors that were clearly arising in the third ventricle or were predominantly parenchymal with intraventricular extension.

The teratoma and both PNETs occurred in age < 1 year, and all showed calcifications. Only one CPP occurred above age 5 years.

In adults > 30 years age, the only tumors found in the trigone were meningiomas. Subependymomas were the only nonenhancing

Table 32-7 Lateral ventricle tumor type by location & age

Age (yrs)	Location within lateral ventricle*		
	Foramen of Monro region	Trigone	Body
0-5	0	8 CPP	2 PNETs 1 teratoma
6-30	5 SGCAs 2 pilocytic astrocytomas 1 CPP 1 meningioma 1 oligodendroglioma	1 ependymoma 1 oligodendroglioma	1 mixed glioma 1 ependymoma 1 pilocytic astrocytoma
> 30	2 metastases	8 meningiomas	2 glioblastomas 1 lymphoma 1 metastasis 6 subependymomas

*   abbreviations: CPP = choroid plexus papillomas, PNET = primitive neuroectodermal tumor, SGCA = subependymal giant cell astrocytoma

tumor in this age group.

By location within third ventricle
- anterior third ventricle
  1. colloid cyst
  2. sellar mass
  3. sarcoidosis
  4. aneurysm
  5. hypothalamic glioma
  6. histiocytosis
  7. meningioma
  8. optic glioma

- posterior third ventricle
  1. pinealoma (dysgerminoma)
  2. meningioma
  3. arachnoid cyst
  4. vein of Galen aneurysm

By enhancement
    All lesions enhanced except: cysts (ependymal and arachnoid), dermoids and epidermoids. There are differences of opinion of the tendency for subependymomas to enhance, Jelinek et al.[104] found that they did not.

32.2.18.   Periventricular lesions

Periventricular solid enhancing lesions on CT (in decreasing frequency)
1. **lymphoma** (CNS involvement from systemic, or rarely primary brain): must be included in differential diagnosis of any solid enhancing periventricular brain tumor (*see page 461*). Very radiosensitive
2. ependymoma (usually invaginates)
3. metastatic Ca (especially malignant melanoma or choriocarcinoma)
4. ventriculitis
5. medulloblastoma (in peds), AKA cerebellar sarcoma in adults
6. pineal tumor (dysgerminoma type): usually midline, young patient
7. occasionally, glioblastoma can present like this

Periventricular low density on CT, or high signal on T2WI MRI
1. increased extracellular or intracellular water content (edema)
    A. in hydrocephalus: transependymal absorption of CSF
    B. necrosis from infarction
    C. edema from tumor
2. uncommon late variants of adrenoleukodystrophy
3. vascular disorders
    A. subacute arteriosclerotic encephalopathy (**Binswanger's disease**)[105, 106]
    B. cerebral embolism
    C. vasculitis
    D. amyloid angiopathy
    E. low flow states
4. demyelination: including multiple sclerosis
5. **leukoaraiosis**[107]: white matter disease that may be related to: Binswanger's encephalopathy, watershed infarction[108], normal aging[109], hypoxia, hypoglycemia[110]... CT or MRI demonstrates symmetric (or nearly so) periventricular white matter changes. May be asymptomatic or may present with findings including dementia
6. heterotopias: islands of grey matter in abnormal locations

32.2.19.   Meningeal thickening/enhancement

Two main categories of enhancement[111]:
1. dural enhancement: visible beneath the inner table of the skull. Does not follow the gyral convolutions. May be either:
    A. focal
        1. meningioma: recurrent or residual
    B. diffuse dural enhancement[112]: associated with extraaxial neoplastic processes in ≈ 65%. Clinically: H/A, multiple cranial nerve palsies, seizures; may be indistinguishable from leptomeningeal metastases
        1. intracranial hypotension: diffuse pachymeningeal enhancement on cerebral MRI in the <u>absence</u> of antecedent trauma or LP (or epidural

injection, etc.) *see page 178*
2. bacterial meningitis
3. primary CNS tumors: medulloblastoma, malignant meningioma
4. sarcoidosis
5. following craniotomy
6. metastases (mostly carcinomas):
    a. bony mets to skull: present in 10 of 13 patients
    b. dural metastases
    c. leptomeningeal
7. following subdural hemorrhage[113]
2. leptomeningeal: may be either:
   A. thin linear enhancement that closely follows the gyri
   B. small nodules attached to the brain

32.2.20. Ependymal and subependymal enhancement

Some overlap with periventricular enhancement. Ependymal enhancement often heralds a serious condition[114]. Main DDx is tumor vs. infectious process.
1. ventriculitis or ependymitis: ependymal enhancement occurred in 64% of cases of pyogenic ventriculitis in one series[115]. Infection may occur in the following settings
   A. following shunt surgery
   B. after intraventricular surgery
   C. with indwelling prosthetic devices
   D. with use of intrathecal chemotherapy
   E. with meningitis
   F. with viral ependymitis
   G. in some cases of CMV encephalitis in immunocompromised patients
   H. granulomatous involvements esp. in immunocompromised patients; e.g. tuberculosis, mycobacterium, syphilis
2. lymphoproliferative disorders
   A. CNS lymphoma: *see page 461*
   B. leukemia
3. metastasis
4. carcinomatous meningitis: typically also produces meningeal enhancement (*see page 491*)
5. multiple sclerosis: usually more *peri*ventricular (in the white matter)
6. transient enhancement reported in a child with ependymoma in the absence of tumor spread[116]
7. tuberous sclerosis: subependymal hamartomas appear as nodules which occasionally enhance (*see page 504*). These gradually calcify with age

Immunocompromised patients: DDX is mainly lymphoma vs. viral ependymitis[114]. The enhancement pattern is helpful[114]:
1. thin linear enhancement: suggests virus (CMV or varicella-zoster)
2. nodular enhancement: suggests CNS lymphoma
3. band enhancement: less specific (may occur with virus, lymphoma, or tuberculosis)

Immune competent patients[114]:
1. infection
   A. bacterial (pyogenic) ventriculitis
   B. tuberculous ventriculitis
   C. cystic lesions suggest cysticercosis
2. in the absence of constitutional symptoms
   A. lymphoma
   B. ependymoma
   C. germ cell tumor
   D. metastases
3. in the presence of appropriate constitutional symptoms: linear enhancement is rarely due to neurosarcoidosis or Whipple's disease, metastatic multiple myeloma (usually nodular)

32.2.21. Intraventricular hemorrhage

Etiologies:
1. most occur as a result of extension of intraparenchymal hemorrhages
    A. in the adult: especially thalamic or putaminal hemorrhages (*see page 849*)
    B. in newborns: extension of subependymal hemorrhage (*see page 861*)
2. pure intraventricular hemorrhage **(IVH)** is usually the result of a rupture of
    A. aneurysm: accounts for ≈ 25% of IVH in adults, and is second only to extension of intracerebral hemorrhage as the most common cause. IVH occurs in 13-28% of ruptured aneurysms in clinical series[117]. More common with the following aneurysms: a-comm, distal basilar artery or carotid terminus, VA or distal PICA (*see page 800* for patterns)
    B. vertebral artery dissection (or dissecting aneurysms): *see page 886*
    C. intraventricular AVM
    D. intraventricular tumor

32.2.22. Medial temporal lobe lesions

May be responsible for seizures, especially "uncal fits" (temporal lobe seizures).
1. hamartoma
2. mesial temporal sclerosis: should see atrophy of the parenchyma in this area with dilatation of the temporal horn of the lateral ventricle (*see page 257*)
3. glioma: may be low grade. Look for mass effect and possibly enhancement

32.2.23. Intranasal/intracranial lesions

Lesions within the nose that may communicate with the intracranial cavity:
1. infectious
    A. tuberculosis
    B. syphilis
    C. Hansen's disease (leprosy)
    D. fungal infections, especially:
        1. aspergillosis
        2. mucormycosis: seen primarily in diabetics or immunocompromised patients (*see page 586*)
        3. *Sporothrix schenckii*
        4. *Coccidioides*
    E. Wegener's granulomatosis: (*see page 61*) necrotizing granulomatous vasculitis of the upper and lower respiratory tracts with glomerulonephritis and nasal destruction[118]
    F. lethal midline granuloma: (*see page 62*) a locally destructive lymphomatoid infiltrative disease that may not have true granulomas, and may also cause local nasal destruction. However, renal and tracheal involvement do not occur as in Wegener's granulomatosis
    G. polymorphic reticulosis: may be a nasal lymphoma. Possibly the same disease as lethal midline granuloma (*see above*)
2. mucocele: a retention cyst of an air sinus that results from an occluded ostium and may cause expansive erosion of the involved sinus. Often enhances with IV contrast on CT, and may contain mucus or pus
3. neoplasms
    A. carcinoma of the nasal sinus
        1. squamous cell
        2. glandular
        3. undifferentiated nasal carcinoma: AKA lymphoepithelioma
    B. **esthesioneuroblastoma**[119] AKA olfactory neuroblastoma: named for the stem cell of the olfactory epithelium (esthesioneuroblast), a malignant tumor that arises from crest cells of the nasal vault, often with intracranial invasion. Very rare (≈ 200 reported cases). Presents with epistaxis (76%), nasal obstruction (71%), tearing (14%), pain (11%), diplopia, proptosis, anosmia and endocrinopathies[120]. Treatment: surgical resection followed by

XRT, and ± chemotherapy
C. metastatic tumors: very rare, possibly with renal cell carcinoma
D. benign tumors
    1. frontal meningioma: rarely erodes into nasal cavity
    2. rhabdomyoma
    3. benign hemangiopericytoma
    4. cholesteatoma
    5. chordoma
4. congenital lesions
    A. **encephalocele** (*see page 102*): a nasal polypoid mass in a <u>newborn</u> should be considered an encephalocele until proven otherwise. Classifications:
        1. cranial vault
        2. frontal ethmoidal
        3. basal
        4. posterior fossa
    B. **nasal glioma**: non-neoplastic glial tissue located within the nose, often conceptually and diagnosti-

Table 32-8 Encephalocele vs. nasal glioma

Finding	Encephalocele	Nasal glioma
pulsatile?	frequently (may not be if small)	no
changes with Valsalva maneuver	swells (Furstenberg sign)	no change
presence of hypertelorism	suggests encephalocele	does not correlate
attachment to CNS	stalk	none, or minimal
probe	can be passed lateral	cannot be passed lateral

cally confused with an encephalocele (*see Table 32-8*). The term "glioma" is a misnomer, and nasal glial heterotopia is preferred. Does not communicate with the subarachnoid space

32.2.24. Spinal epidural masses

See items marked with a dagger (†) under *Myelopathy* on page 902.

32.2.25. Destructive lesions of the spine

1. neoplastic (see *Differential diagnosis of spinal cord tumors*, page 506 for more):
    A. metastatic tumors with a predilection for bone: prostate, breast, renal cell, lymphoma, thyroid, lung... (see *Spinal epidural metastases*, page 516)
    B. primary bone tumors: chordomas (*see page 464*), osteoid osteoma (*see page 511*), hemangioma (*see page 512*)
2. infection:
    A. vertebral osteomyelitis: occurs mostly in IV drug abusers, patients with diabetes mellitus, and hemodialysis patients. May have associated spinal epidural abscess. Also see *Vertebral osteomyelitis*, page 243
    B. discitis (see *Discitis*, page 245)
3. chronic renal failure: some patients develop a destructive spondyloarthropathy that resembles infection[121, 122]
4. ankylosing spondylitis

DIFFERENTIATING FACTORS
   Of the many lytic or destructive lesions that involve the vertebra, destruction of the disc space is highly suggestive of <u>infection</u> which often involves at least two adjacent vertebral levels. Although tumors may involve adjacent vertebral levels and cause collapse of disc height, the disc space is usually not destroyed[123] (possible exceptions include: some vertebral plasmacytomas, a reported metastatic cervical carcinoma, and there may occasionally be destruction of the disc in ankylosing spondylitis[124]). Unlike pyogenic infections, the disc may be relatively resistant to tuberculous involvement in Pott's disease[125]. Also, since metastatic tumor involvement usually produces widespread bony involvement, it is less likely with involvement of a single bone.
   Paget's disease should be considered with a <u>dense</u> vertebra on x-ray in an older patient, commonly involving several contiguous involved vertebrae.

32.3. References

1. George W E, Wilmot M, Greenhouse A, *et al*.: Medical management of steroid-induced epidural lipomatosis. **N Engl J Med** 308: 316-9, 1983.
2. Kumar K, Nath R K, Nair C P V, *et al*.: Symptomatic epidural lipomatosis secondary to obesity: Case report. **J Neurosurg** 85: 348-50, 1996.
3. Haddad S F, Hitchon P W, Godersky: Idiopathic and glucocorticoid-induced spinal epidural lipomatosis. **J Neurosurg** 74: 38-42, 1991.
4. Nagashima C: Cervical myelopathy due to ossification of the posterior longitudinal ligament. **J Neurosurg** 37: 653-60, 1972.
5. Lucchesi A C, White W L, Heiserman J E, *et al*.: Review of arachnoiditis ossificans with a case report. **BNI Quarterly** 14: 4-9, 1998.
6. Marshman L A G, Hardwidge C, Ford-Dunn S Z, *et al*.: Idiopathic spinal cord herniation: Case report and review of the literature. **Neurosurgery** 44: 1129-33, 1999.
7. Fox M W, Onofrio B M: The natural history and management of symptomatic and asymptomatic vertebral hemangiomas. **J Neurosurg** 78: 36-45, 1993.
8. Harik S I, Raichle M E, Reis D J: Spontaneous remitting spinal epidural hematoma in a patient on anticoagulants. **N Engl J Med** 284: 1355-7, 1971.
9. Packer N P, Cummins B H: Spontaneous epidural hemorrhage: A surgical emergency. **Lancet** 1: 356-8, 1978.
10. Brem S S, Hafler D A, Van Uitert R L, *et al*.: Spinal subarachnoid hematoma: A hazard of lumbar puncture resulting in reversible paraplegia. **N Engl J Med** 303: 1020-1, 1981.
11. Rengachary S S, Murphy D: Subarachnoid hematoma following lumbar puncture causing compression of the cauda equina. **J Neurosurg** 41: 252-4, 1974.
12. Epstein N E, Danto J, Nardi D: Evaluation of intraoperative somatosensory-evoked potential monitoring during 100 cervical operations. **Spine** 18: 737-47, 1993.
13. Tobin W D, Layton D D: The diagnosis and natural history of spinal cord arteriovenous malformations. **Mayo Clin Proc** 51: 637-46, 1976.
14. Wirth F P, Post K D, Di Chiro G, *et al*.: Foix-Alajouanine disease. Spontaneous thrombosis of a spinal cord arteriovenous malformation: A case report. **Neurology** 20: 1114-8, 1970.
15. Rothman R H, Simeone F A, (eds.): The spine. 2nd ed., W.B. Saunders, Philadelphia, 1982.
16. Pruthi R K, Tefferi A: Pernicious anemia revisited. **Mayo Clin Proc** 69: 144-50, 1994.
17. Elia M: Oral or parental therapy for B12 deficiency. **Lancet** 352: 1721-2, 1998 (commentary).
18. Altrocchi P H: Acute spinal epidural abscess vs acute transverse myelopathy: A plea for neurosurgical caution. **Arch Neurol** 9: 17-25, 1963.
19. Sheremata W A, Berger J R, Harrington W J, *et al*.: Human T lymphotropic virus type I-associated myelopathy: A report of 10 patients born in the United States. **Arch Neurol** 49: 1113-8, 1992.
20. Deen H G: Diagnosis and management of lumbar disk disease. **Mayo Clin Proc** 71: 283-7, 1996.
21. Gritza T, Taylor T K F: A ganglion arising from a lumbar articular facet associated with low back pain and sciatica. **J Bone Joint Surg** 52: 528-31, 1970.
22. Kitigawa H, Kanamori M, Tatezaki S, *et al*.: Multiple spinal ossified arachnoiditis. A case report. **Spine** 15: 1236-8, 1990.
23. Thakkar D H, Porter R W: Heterotopic ossification enveloping the sciatic nerve following posterior fracture-dislocation of the hip: A case report. **Injury** 13: 207-9, 1981.
24. Johanson N A, Pellici P M, Tsairis P, *et al*.: Nerve injury in total hip arthroplasty. **Clin Orthop** 179: 214-22, 1983.
25. Burkman K A, Gaines R W, Kashani S R, *et al*.: Herpes zoster: A consideration in the differential diagnosis of radiculopathy. **Arch Phys Med Rehabil** 69: 132-4, 1988.
26. Bickels J, Kahanovitz N, Rupert C K, *et al*.: Extraspinal bone and soft-tissue tumors as a cause of sciatica. Clinical diagnosis and recommendations: Analysis of 32 cases. **Spine** 24: 1611-6, 1999.
27. Jones B V, Ward M W: Myositis ossificans in the biceps femoris muscles causing sciatic nerve palsy: A case report. **J Bone Joint Surg** 62B: 506-7, 1980.
28. Thompson R C, Berg T L: Primary bone tumors of pelvis presenting as spinal disease. **Orthopedics** 19: 1011-6, 1996.
29. Rumana C S, Baskin D S: Brown-Sequard syndrome produced by cervical disc herniation: Case report and literature review. **Surg Neurol** 45: 359-61, 1996.
30. Frymoyer J W: Back pain and sciatica. **N Engl J Med** 318: 291-300, 1988.
31. Deyo R A, Rainville J, Kent D L: What can the history and physical examination tell us about low back pain? **JAMA** 268: 760-5, 1992.
32. Janin Y, Epstein J A, Carras R, *et al*.: Osteoid osteomas and osteoblastomas of the spine. **Neurosurgery** 8: 31-8, 1981.
33. Calin A, Porta J, Fries J F, *et al*.: Clinical history as a screening test for ankylosing spondylitis. **JAMA** 237: 2613-4, 1977.
34. Crayton H E, Bell C L, De Smet A A: Sacral insufficiency fractures. **Sem Arth Rheum** 20: 378-84, 1991.
35. McCarron R F, Wimpee M W, Hudkins P G, *et al*.: The inflammatory effect of nucleus pulposus: A possible element in the pathogenesis of low-back pain. **Spine** 12: 760-4, 1987.
36. Hirsch C, Schajowicz F: Studies on structural changes in the lumbar annulus fibrosus. **Acta Orthop Scand** 22: 184-231, 1952.
37. Choice of lipid-regulating drugs. **Med Letter** 43 (1105): 43-8, 2001.
38. Jensen M C, Brant-Zawadzki M N, Obuchowski N, *et al*.: Magnetic resonance imaging of the lumbar spine in people without back pain. **N Engl J Med** 331: 69-73, 1994.
39. Bonney G: Iatrogenic injuries of nerves. **J Bone Joint Surg** 68B: 9-13, 1986.
40. Eskandary H, Hamzel A, Yasamy M T: Foot drop following brain lesion. **Surg Neurol** 43: 89-90, 1995.
41. Hawkins R J, Bilco T, Bonutti P: Cervical spine and shoulder pain. **Clin Orthop Rel Res** 258: 142-6, 1990.
42. Goldenberg D L: Fibromyalgia syndrome. **JAMA** 257: 2782-7, 1987.
43. Wolfe F, Smythe H A, Yunus M B, *et al*.: The American college of rheumatology 1990 criteria for the classification of fibromyalgia: Report of the multicenter criteria committee. **Arthritis Rheum** 33: 160-72, 1990.
44. Adler G K, Kinsley B T, Hurwitz S, *et al*.: Reduced hypothalamic-pituitary and sympathoadrenal responses to hypoglycemia in women with fibromyalgia syndrome. **Am J Med** 106: 534-43, 1999.
45. Stricker L J, Green C R: Resolution of refractory symptoms of secondary erythermalgia with intermittent epidural bupivacaine. **Reg Anesth Pain Med** 26: 488-90, 2001.

46. Davis M D, Sandroni P: Lidocaine patch for pain of erythromelalgia. **Arch Dermatol** 138: 17-9, 2002.
47. Cardoso E R, Peterson E W: Pituitary apoplexy: A review. **Neurosurgery** 14: 363-73, 1984.
48. Kapoor W N: Evaluation and management of the patient with syncope. **JAMA** 268: 2553-60, 1992.
49. Barron S A, Rogovski Z, Hemli Y: Vagal cardiovascular reflexes in young persons with syncope. **Ann Intern Med** 118: 943-6, 1993.
50. Smith D B, Hitchcock M, Philpot P J: Cerebral amyloid angiopathy presenting as transient ischemic attacks: Case report. **J Neurosurg** 63: 963-4, 1985.
51. Greenberg S M, Vonsattel J P, Stakes J W, et al.: The clinical spectrum of cerebral amyloid angiopathy: Presentations without lobar hemorrhage. **Neurology** 43: 2073-9, 1993.
52. Kaminski H J, Hlavin M L, Likavec M J, et al.: Transient neurologic deficit caused by chronic subdural hematoma. **Am J Med** 92: 698-700, 1992.
53. Moster M, Johnston D, Reinmuth O: Chronic subdural hematoma with transient neurologic deficits: A review of 15 cases. **Ann Neurol** 14: 539-42, 1983.
54. McLaurin R: Contributions of angiography to the pathophysiology of subdural hematomas. **Neurology** 15: 866-73, 1965.
55. Beal M F: Multiple cranial-nerve palsies - A diagnostic challenge. **N Engl J Med** 322: 461-3, 1990.
56. Krisht A F: Giant invasive pituitary adenomas. **Contemp Neurosurg** 21 (1): 1-6, 1999.
57. Manni J J, Scaf J J, Huygen P L M, et al.: Hyperostosis cranialis interna: A new hereditary syndrome with cranial-nerve entrapment. **N Engl J Med** 322: 450-4, 1990.
58. Chen J-R, Rhee R S C, Wallach S, et al.: Neurologic disturbances in paget disease of bone: Response to calcitonin. **Neurology** 29: 448-57, 1979.
59. Wilkins R H, Rengachary S S, (eds.). **Neurosurgery**. McGraw-Hill, New York, 1985.
60. Al-Mefty O, Fox J L, Al-Rodhan N, et al.: Optic nerve decompression in osteopetrosis. **J Neurosurg** 68: 80-4, 1988.
61. Salvarani C, Cantini F, Boiardi L, et al.: Polymyalgia rheumatica and giant-cell arteritis. **N Engl J Med** 347: 261-71, 2002.
62. Clark W C, Theofilos C S, Fleming J C: Primary optic sheath meningiomas: Report of nine cases. **J Neurosurg** 70: 37-40, 1989.
63. Strassburg H M: Macrocephaly is not always due to hydrocephalus. **J Child Neurol** 4 (Suppl): S32-40, 1989.
64. Section of Pediatric Neurosurgery of the American Association of Neurological Surgeons, (ed.) **Pediatric neurosurgery**. 1st ed., Grune and Stratton, New York, 1982.
65. Rushton A R, Shaywitz B A, Duncan C C, et al.: Computed tomography in the diagnosis of Canavan's disease. **Ann Neurol** 10: 57-60, 1981.
66. Carpenter M B: **Core text of neuroanatomy.** 2nd ed. Williams and Wilkins, Baltimore, 1978.
67. Rekate H, Grubb R, Aram D, et al.: Muteness of cerebellar origin. **Arch Neurol** 42: 637-8, 1985.
68. Ammirati M, Mirzai S, Samii M: Transient mutism following removal of a cerebellar tumor: A case report and review of the literature. **Childs Nerv Syst** 5: 12-4, 1989.
69. Apuzzo M L J: Surgery of masses affecting the third ventricular chamber: Techniques and strategies. **Clin Neurosurg** 34: 499-522, 1988.
70. Inoue Y, Tabuchi T, Hakuba A, et al.: Facial nerve neuromas: CT findings. **J Comput Assist Tomogr** 11: 942-7, 1987.
71. Tew J M, Yeh H S, Miller G W, et al.: Intratemporal schwannoma of the facial nerve. **Neurosurgery** 13: 186-8, 1983.
72. Enyon-Lewis N J, Kitchen N, Scaravilli F, et al.: Neurenteric cyst of the cerebellopontine angle. **Neurosurgery** 42: 655-8, 1998.
73. Ho V B, Smirniotopoulos J G, Murphy F M, et al.: Radiologic-pathologic correlation: Hemangioblastoma. **AJNR** 13: 1343-52, 1992.
74. Laurent J P, Cheek W R: Brain tumors in children. **J Pediatr Neurosci** 1: 15-32, 1985.
75. Onofrio B M, Mih A D: Synovial cysts of the spine. **Neurosurgery** 22: 642-7, 1988.
76. Piper J G, Menezes A H: Management strategies for tumors of the axis vertebra. **J Neurosurg** 84: 543-51, 1996.
77. Honma G, Murota K, Shiba R, et al.: Mandible and tongue-splitting approach for giant cell tumor of axis. **Spine** 14: 1204-10, 1989.
78. Osenbach R K, Youngblood L A, Menezes A H: Atlanto-axial instability secondary to solitary eosinophilic granuloma of C2 in a 12-year-old girl. Case report. **J Spinal Disord** 3: 408-12, 1990.
79. Verbiest H: *Benign cervical spine tumors: Clinical experience.* In **The cervical spine**, The Cervical Spine Research Society Editorial Committee, (ed.). J.B. Lippincott, Philadelphia, 2nd ed., 1989: pp 723-74.
80. Ciricillo S F, Rosenblum M L: Use of CT and MR imaging to distinguish intracranial lesions and to define the need for biopsy in AIDS patients. **J Neurosurg** 73: 720-24, 1990.
81. O'Neill B P, Illig J J: Primary central nervous system lymphoma. **Mayo Clin Proc** 64: 1005-20, 1989.
82. Davis D O: Sellar and parasellar lesions. **Clin Neurosurg** 17: 160-88, 1970.
83. Atchison J A, Lee P A, Albright L: Reversible suprasellar pituitary mass secondary to hypothyroidism. **JAMA** 262: 3175-7, 1989.
84. Taylor S L, Barakos J A, Harsh G R, et al.: Magnetic resonance imaging of tuberculum sellae meningiomas: Preventing preoperative misdiagnosis as pituitary macroadenoma. **Neurosurgery** 31: 621-7, 1992.
85. Symon L, Rosenstein J: Surgical management of suprasellar meningioma. **J Neurosurg** 61: 633-41, 1984.
86. Hoffman H J, Ostubo H, Hendrick E B, et al.: Intracranial germ-cell tumors in children. **J Neurosurg** 74: 545-51, 1991.
87. Abe T, Matsumoto K, Sanno N, et al.: Lymphocytic hypophysitis: Case report. **Neurosurgery** 36: 1016-9, 1995.
88. Mayfield R K, Levine J H, Gordon L, et al.: Lymphoid adenohypophysitis presenting as a pituitary tumor. **Am J Med** 69: 619-23, 1980.
89. Hungerford G D, Biggs P J, Levine J H, et al.: Lymphoid adenohypophysitis with radiologic and clinical findings resembling a pituitary tumor. **AJNR** 3: 444-6, 1982.
90. Daniels D L, Williams A L, Thornton R S, et al.: Differential diagnosis of intrasellar tumors by computed tomography. **Radiology** 141: 697-701, 1981.
91. Harsh G R, Edwards M S B, Wilson C B: Intracranial arachnoid cysts in children. **J Neurosurg** 64: 835-42, 1986.
92. Miller M E, Kido D, Horner F: Cavum vergae: Association with neurologic abnormality and diagnosis by magnetic resonance imaging. **Arch Neurol** 43: 821-3, 1986.
93. Sekhar L N, Moller A R: Operative management of tumors involving the cavernous sinus. **J Neurosurg** 64: 879-89, 1986.
94. Knosp E, Perneczky A, Koos W T, et al.: Meningiomas of the space of the cavernous sinus. **Neurosurgery** 38: 434-44, 1996.
95. Knosp E, Steiner E, Kitz K, et al.: Pituitary adenomas with invasion of the cavernous sinus space: A magnetic resonance imaging classification compared with surgical findings. **Neurosurgery** 33: 610-8, 1993.
96. Thomas J E, Baker H L: Assessment of roentgenographic lucencies of the skull: A systematic ap-

proach. **Neurology** 25: 99-106, 1975.

97. Horning G W, Beatty R M: Osteolytic skull lesions secondary to trauma. **J Neurosurg** 72: 506-8, 1990.
98. Le Roux P D, Griffin G E, Marsh H T, *et al.*: Tuberculosis of the skull - A rare condition: Case report and review of the literature. **Neurosurgery** 26: 851-6, 1990.
99. Lopez-Villegas D, Kulisevsky J, Deus J, *et al.*: Neuropsychological alterations in patients with computed tomography-detected basal ganglia calcification. **Arch Neurol** 53: 251-6, 1996.
100. Ang L C, Alport E C, Tchang S: Fahr's disease associated with astrocytic proliferation and astrocytoma. **Surg Neurol** 39: 365-9, 1993.
101. Bhimani S, Sarwar M, Virapongse C, *et al.*: Computed tomography of cerebrovascular calcifications in postsurgical hypoparathyroidism. **J Comput Assist Tomogr** 9: 121-4, 1985.
102. Morrison G, Sobel D F, Kelley W M, *et al.*: Intraventricular mass lesions. **Radiology** 153: 435-42, 1984.
103. D'Angelo V A, Galarza M, Catapano D, *et al.*: Lateral ventricle tumors: Surgical strategies according to tumor origin and development - a series of 72 cases. **Neurosurgery** 56: Supplement: Operative Neurosurgery (1): ONS36-45, 2005.
104. Jelinek J, Smirniotopoulos J G, Parisi J E, *et al.*: Lateral ventricular neoplasms of the brain: Differential diagnosis based on clinical, CT, and MR findings. **AJNR** 11: 567-74, 1990.
105. Kinkel W R, Jacobs L, Polachini I, *et al.*: Subcortical arteriosclerotic encephalopathy (Binswanger's disease). **Arch Neurol** 42: 951-9, 1985.
106. Roman G C: Senile dementia of the Binswanger type: A vascular form of dementia in the elderly. **JAMA** 258: 1782-8, 1987.
107. Hachinski V C, Potter P, Merskey H: Leuko-araiosis. **Arch Neurol** 44: 21-3, 1987.
108. Steingart A, Hachinski V C, Lau C, *et al.*: Cognitive and neurologic findings in subjects with diffuse white matter lucencies on computed tomographic scan (leuko-araiosis). **Arch Neurol** 44: 32-5, 1987.
109. Zatz L M, Jernigan T L, Ahumada A J: White matter changes in cerebral computed tomography related to aging. **J Comput Assist Tomogr** 6: 19-23, 1982.
110. Janota I, Mirsen T R, Hachinski V C, *et al.*: Neuropathologic correlates of leuko-araiosis. **Arch Neurol** 46: 1124-8, 1989.
111. Paakko E, Patronas N J, Schellinger D: Meningeal Gd-dtpa enhancement in patients with malignancies. **J Comput Assist Tomogr** 14 (4): 542-6, 1990.
112. River Y, Schwartz A, Gomori J M, *et al.*: Clinical significance of diffuse dural enhancement detected by magnetic resonance imaging. **J Neurosurg** 85 (5): 777-83, 1996.
113. Sze G, Soletsky S, Bronen R, *et al.*: MR imaging of the cranial meninges with emphasis on contrast enhancement and meningeal carcinomatosis. **AJNR** 10: 965-75, 1989.
114. Guerini H, Helie O, Leveque C, *et al.*: [diagnosis of periventricular ependymal enhancement in MRI in adults]. **J Neuroradiol** 30 (1): 46-56, 2003 (French).
115. Fukui M B, Williams R L, Mudigonda S: CT and MR imaging features of pyogenic ventriculitis. **AJNR Am J Neuroradiol** 22 (8): 1510-6, 2001.
116. Butler W E, Khan A, Khan S A: Posterior fossa ependymoma with intense but transient disseminated enhancement but not metastasis. **Pediatr Neurosurg** 37 (1): 27-31, 2002.
117. Mohr G, Ferguson G, Khan M, *et al.*: Intraventricular hemorrhage from ruptured aneurysm: Retrospective analysis of 91 cases. **J Neurosurg** 58: 482-7, 1983.
118. Brandwein S, Esdaile J, Danoff D, *et al.*: Wegener's granulomatosis: Clinical features and outcome in 13 patients. **Arch Intern Med** 143: 476-9, 1983.
119. Morita A, Ebersold M J, Olsen K D, *et al.*: Esthesioneuroblastoma: Prognosis and management. **Neurosurgery** 32: 706-15, 1993.
120. Hlavac P J, Henson S L, Popp A J: Esthesioneuroblastoma: Advances in diagnosis and treatment. **Contemp Neurosurg** 20 (8): 1-5, 1998.
121. Kuntz D, Naveau B, Bardin T, *et al.*: Destructive spondyloarthropathy in hemodialyzed patients: A new syndrome. **Arthritis Rheum** 27: 369-75, 1984.
122. Alcalay M, Goupy M-C, Azais I, *et al.*: Hemodialysis is not essential for the development of destructive spondyloarthropathy in patients with chronic renal failure. **Arthritis Rheum** 30: 1182-6, 1987.
123. Borges L F: Case records of the Massachusetts general hospital: Case 24-1989. **N Engl J Med** 320: 1610-8, 1989.
124. Cawley M D, Chalmers T M, Kellgren J H, *et al.*: Destructive lesions of vertebral bodies in ankylosing spondylitis. **Ann Rheum Dis** 31: 345-8, 1972.
125. Rothman R H, Simeone F A, (eds.): **The spine**. 3rd ed., W.B. Saunders, Philadelphia, 1992.

33. Index

A

A's and B's 862
abbreviations (located at beginning of book)
abdominal cutaneous reflex 704, **712**
  in multiple sclerosis 50
abducens palsy 586
  as false localizing sign 586
  due to brainstem compression 772
  due to clival fracture 665
  due to elevated ICP from tumor 404
  due to increased intracranial pressure 586
  following lumbar puncture 616
  in Gradenigo's syndrome 588
  in pseudotumor cerebri 495
  in trauma 637
ABELCET® (see amphotericin B)
abscess
  cerebral 217
    MR spectroscopy appearance 137
    Nocardia 223
    toxoplasmosis 232
    treatment 220
  spinal epidural 240
absence seizure
  absence status epilepticus 268
  definition 256, 257
acalculia 87
ACAS (see either asymptomatic carotid stenosis,
  or Asymptomatic Carotid Atherosclerosis Study)
ACDF (see anterior cervical discectomy)
acetaminophen 28
  and hepatic toxicity 28
acetazolamide
  for CSF fistula 177
  for hydrocephalus 186
  for Meniere's disease 592
  for pseudotumor cerebri 497
  for seizures 277
  IV 278
  side effects 278
achondroplastic dwarf 325
  and macrocephaly 920
  and myelopathy 902, 913
acid inhibitors 40
acoustic neuroma 429
  and hydrocephalus 430, 435
  and trigeminal neuralgia 379
  and vertigo 434
  bilateral in neurofibromatosis 2 430, 504

acoustic neuroma *(cont'd)*
  cranial nerve dysfunction post-op 436
  differential diagnosis
    of CPA lesion 922
    of tinnitus 921
  growth rate 431
  hearing loss with 430, 431
  recurrence following treatment 437
  stereotactic radiosurgery for 539, 541
    radiation dose 541
  treatment options 433
  vs. meningioma 923
acquired immunodeficiency syndrome (see
  AIDS)
acrocephaly 100
acromegaly 441
  and hyperostosis frontalis interna 483
  endocrine evaluation 447
  medical treatment 449
  reversibility of abnormalities 441
ACST (see Asymptomatic Carotid Surgery Trial)
ACTH (see corticotropin)
Activase® (see alteplase)
activity modifications for low back problems 297
Actonel® (see risedronate)
acupuncture 299
acute confusional state 44
acute corticosteroid myopathy 705
acute high-altitude sickness 687
acute idiopathic polyradiculoneuritis (see Guillain-Barré syndrome)
acute intermittent porphyria 13, 54
acute mountain sickness 687
acute subdural hematoma 672
acyclovir
  for herpes simplex encephalitis 227
  for herpes zoster 388
Adalat® (see nifedipine)
Adamkiewicz' artery 75
Addison's disease 8
Addisonian crisis (see adrenal crisis)
adenoma (see pituitary gland - adenoma)
ADH (see antidiuretic hormone)
adhesive arachnoiditis (see arachnoiditis)
Adie's pupil 583
admission criteria
  for alcohol withdrawal seizures 261
  head injury 638
admitting orders (see orders - admitting)
adrenal crisis (adrenal insufficiency) 11
  Addisonian crisis
  and macrocephaly 920

Amytal® (see amobarbital)
anal-cutaneous reflex 712
analgesics 27
    adjuvant medications 33
    for mild to moderate pain 30
    for moderate to severe pain 31
    for severe pain 31
    nonsteroidal anti-inflammatory drugs
        (NSAIDs) 28
    opioid 30, 33
anaphylaxis
    from chymopapain 306
    from IV contrast media 128
Anaprox® (see naproxen sodium)
anatomy
    cerebrovascular 76
    cortical surface *68*
    internal capsule 83
    parietal lobe 87
    spinal cord *73*
    surface anatomy 68
Ancef® (see cefazolin)
Anectine® (see succinlycholine)
anencephaly 111
    and organ donation 168
anesthesia dolorosa 384
anesthesiology 1
aneurysm clips
    and MRI 136
aneurysmal bone cyst
    sacral 906
    skull 931, 933
    spine
        differential diagnosis 512
        upper cervical 506
aneurysms 799
    AICA 815
    and fibromuscular dysplasia 63
    and polycystic kidney disease 801
    and pregnancy 825
    and subarachnoid hemorrhage 781
    angiogram for 784
    anterior cerebral artery 811
    anterior communicating artery (ACoA) 810
    associated systemic conditions 801
    basilar bifurcation/tip 815
    berry 800
    carotid terminus (bifurcation) 812
    cavernous carotid artery **818**, 820
    Charcot-Bouchard 853
    coiling 803
    DACA (see aneurysms - distal anterior cere-
        bral artery)
    dissecting (see dissection, arterial)
    distal anterior cerebral artery 811
    false aneurysms 820
        following carotid endarterectomy 876
    familial 801, **819**
    fusiform 800
    giant 821
    in infancy and childhood 799

aneurysms *(cont'd)*
    in moyamoya disease 892
    incidental 799, **816**
    infectious 821
    intraoperative rupture 808
        prevention 809
    location 800
    middle cerebral artery (MCA) 812
    miliary 853
    multiple 819
    mycotic 821
    operative techniques 805
    ophthalmic artery 812
    ophthalmic segment 812
    PICA 814
    posterior circulation 813
    posterior communicating artery (P-comm)
        811
    posttraumatic (see aneurysms - traumatic)
    presentation 800
    rebleeding 789
        intraoperative 808
        prevention 789
    recurrence after treatment 810
    rests 805
    saccular 800
    superior hypophyseal artery 813
    supraclinoid 812
    surgery for 805
        brain relaxation 806
        cerebral protection 806
            drugs for 808
        lumbar drainage 806
        timing of surgery 804
            basilar bifurcation aneurysms 815
    thrombosis
        spontaneous 802
        with detachable coils 803
    transmural pressure 790
    traumatic 666, **820**
    treatment options 802
        balloon embolization 803
        surgery 803, 805
        thrombosis with detachable coils 803,
            803
            dome-to-neck ratio 804
    trifurcation 812
    unruptured 816
    vein of Galen (see vein of Galen malforma-
        tion)
    vertebral artery 814
    vertebral-basilar junction 814
    with AVM 837
    wrapping 803
angioblastic meningioma 428
angioedema
    from contrast media reaction 129
    from propofol 808
angioendothelomatosis (see intravascular lym-
    phomatosis)

angiogram
  angiogram-negative SAH 822
  anterior cerebral artery *132*
  CT 785
  digital intravenous 871
  early draining vein 413
  emergency, in stroke 765
  following aneurysm surgery 808
  for aneurysms 784
  for brain death 166
  for carotid stenosis 870
  in gunshot wounds to the head 686
  in head trauma 641
  in hydranencephaly 181
  in intracerebral hemorrhage 857
  in meningiomas 428
  in non-missile penetrating head trauma 687
  in penetrating neck trauma 754
  in pregnancy 825
  in subarachnoid hemorrhage 784
  magnetic resonance angiography
    for carotid stenosis 870
    for cerebral aneurysms 785, 820
  middle cerebral artery *132*
  posterior fossa arterial *133*
  posterior fossa venous *134*
  radiation exposure 534
  risks **130**, 824, 870, 873
  spinal 823
  supratentorial venous system *133*
  tumor blush 413
angiographically occult vascular malformations
    840
angiography (cerebral) 130
  (see also angiogram)
angiolipoma 507
angioma (see venous angiomas)
angiomatous meningioma 427
angioplasty (see balloon angioplasty)
angiotensin-converting enzyme 57
angular artery 70
angular gyrus
  surface anatomy 70
anisocoria **582**
  from third nerve compression 583
  from uncal herniation 161, 583
  physiologic 582
ankle to brachial BP ratio 328
ankylosing spondylitis 291, **343**, 907, 909
  and lumbar spinal stenosis 327
  and upper cervical spine problems 336
annular tears 908
anosmia
  and postconcussive syndrome 682
  differential diagnosis 916
  in Foster-Kennedy syndrome 85, 427
  with basal skull fracture 665
  with CSF fistula 174
anosognosia 87
anoxic encephalopathy 145, 157, 162
Ansaid® (see flurbiprofen)

anterior approaches to the spine 600
  cervical 600
  lumbar 601
  thoracic 322, **600**
anterior cerebral artery 80
  angiogram *132*
anterior cervical discectomy 319
  Cloward technique 321
  complications 320
  fusion 320
  Smith-Robinson technique 321
anterior choroidal artery *78*, 79
  ligation for parkinsonism 365
  occlusion **778**
anterior cord syndrome 716
anterior interosseous nerve 552, 565
  neuropathy 569
anterior knee of Wildbrand 444, **813**
anterior lumbar interbody fusion 300
anterior spinal artery syndrome 716
anterior spine
  approaches 613
anterior tibial compartment syndrome 308
anthropoid posture 326
antibiotics
  for CSF fistula 177
  for specific organisms 210
  intrathecal 216
  prophylactic 211
    for external ventricular drains 650
    for gunshot wounds to the head 685
    with CSF shunt 194
      in pregnancy 204
  specific antibiotics
    cephalosporins 208
antibiotics antibiotics
  specific
    vancomycin 209
anticoagulation 21
  and acute subdural hematoma 672
  and intracerebral hemorrhage
    anticoagulation after the hemorrhage 858
    anticoagulation before the hemorrhage
      770, 854
  and risk of chronic subdural hematoma 674
  considerations in neurosurgery 21
  following craniotomy 21
  for cardioembolic stroke 774
  for stroke 770
  in spinal cord injury 705
  reversal of 24
anticonvulsants (see antiepileptic drugs)
antidepressants
  for low back pain 298
  for pain 33, 376
  for painful diabetic neuropathy 556
  for postherpetic neuralgia 389
antidiuretic hormone 12
antiepileptic drugs 268
  and birth defects 281
  and cerebral abscess 221

breakthrough bleeding *(cont'd)*
    following AVM surgery 839
    following carotid endarterectomy 876
bregma *69*, 69
Brevibloc® (see esmolol)
brevicollis 119
Brevital® (see methohexital)
broad-based disc herniation 290
Broca's (motor) aphasia 88
Broca's area *68*, 612
Brodmann's areas *68*, 68
bromfenac 28
bromocriptine
    for acromegaly 450
    for prolactinoma 448
bronchogenic cancer
    metastatic to brain 486
bronchospasm from contrast media reaction 129
Brooks fusion 624
Brown-Séquard syndrome **716**
    from cervical disc herniation 914
    in cervical spondylosis 333
    in radiation myelopathy 537
    with spinal cord tumor 510
Brudzinski's sign 212, **783**
bruit
    carotid 873
        loss of 879
        with carotid dissection 885
    cranial
        with AVM 836
        with carotid-cavernous malformation 845
        with dural AVM 843
Brun's syndrome 237
Bruns-Garland syndrome 556
BSAER 147
    during pentobarbital coma 663
    with acoustic neuroma 432
buffalo hump 440
bulbar-cervical dissociation 714, 717
bulbocavernosus reflex 712, 713
bulging lumbar disc 290
bundles of Probst 114
Buprenex® (see buprenorphine)
buprenorphine 33
burner (football injury) 743
burning hands syndrome 743
    differential diagnosis 912, 913
burr holes
    for chronic subdurals 675
    for trauma (emergency) 645
    Frazier 607, 619
burst fractures 745
    L5 748
    treatment 747
burst suppression
    and pentobarbital levels 663
    definition 145
    during aneurysm surgery 807
    for status epilepticus 267
    with etomidate 808

Butazolidin® (see phenylbutazone)
butorphanol 33
butterfly glioma 413, 415
butterfly vertebrae
    in lipomyelomeningocele 118

C

C1-2 arthrodesis 623
C1-2 puncture 618
C1-2 transarticular facet screws 624, **626**
C1-dens distance (see altantodental interval)
C4 cape 713
cabergoline
    for prolactinoma 449
cacosmia 257
CADASIL **64**
café au lait spots
    definition 502
    in neurofibromatosis 502
café-au-lait spots
    in McCune-Albright syndrome 484
caffeine
    as pain medication adjuvant 34
Calan® (see verapamil)
calcifediol 749
calcification
    basal ganglia 934
    choroid plexus 933
    in stroke 765
    intracranial (differential diagnosis) 933
    of subperiosteal hematoma 688
Calcimar® (see calcitonin)
calcitonin
    for fibrous dysplasia 484
    for odontoid fracture 729
    for osteoporosis 749
    for Paget's disease 342
calcitriol 749
calcium
    for osteoporosis 749
calcium antagonist (see calcium channel blockers)
calcium channel blockers
    for hypertension 5
    for vasospasm 787, 799
Calderol® (see calcifediol)
calorics (see oculovestibular reflex)
Campylobacter jejuni in Guillain-Barré 53
Canavan's disease 920
candelabra effect 167
candidiasis 239
candle guttering
    on myelography in arachnoiditis 316
    with tuberous sclerosis 505
capillary telangiectasia 840
Capoten® (see captopril)
capping (on myelography) 518
capsaicin
    for diabetic neuropathy 389

colloid cyst 457
   differential diagnosis 934
   treatment 458
      transcallosal approach 611
coloboma 103
coma 154
   approach to patient 156
   barbiturate 662
   definition 154
   differential diagnosis 155
   from infratentorial mass 160
   from subarachnoid hemorrhage 783
   from supratentorial mass 159
   hypoxic 162
   pseudocoma 156
   scales
      children's 154
      Glasgow 154
combined system disease **904**, 913
commissural myelotomy 392
common migraine 45
common peroneal nerve entrapment (see peroneal nerve - palsy)
communicating hydrocephalus 180
communicating syringomyelia 349
Compazine® (see prochlorperazine)
compensated hydrocephalus 181
complete spinal cord injuries 713
complex regional pain syndrome 396
complications
   with anterior cervical discectomy 320
   with carpal tunnel surgery 568
   with femoral arterial catheterization 559
   with lumbar laminectomy 307
compound skull fracture (see skull fractures - compound)
compression fracture
   cervical compression flexion fracture 734
   thoracolumbar 745
      in osteoporosis 748
      treatment 747
Concorde position 604
concussion 632
   definition 632
   grading 633
   multiple 634
   postconcussive syndrome 682
   second impact syndrome 633
   sports related 633
      return to play guidelines 633
conduction aphasia 88
conductive hearing loss 597
confusion
   following concussion 632
   in delerium 44
congenital brain tumors 480
congenital conditions (see developmental anomalies)
congenital hypermelanosis 920
congestive heart failure
   and mannitol 643

congophilic angiopathy 853
conjoined nerve root 905
conservative treatment for back pain 296
constitutional ventriculomegaly 920
contained (disc) herniation 289
contour lines (on lateral C-spine x-ray) 140
contralateral gaze 85
contrast agents
   and migraine H/A 45
   in neuroradiology 126
   inadvertent intrathecal injection of ionic agents 126
   ionic agents 126
   reactions (allergies) 128
   water-soluble 126
contrecoup injury of brain 632
contusio cervicalis posterior 716
contusion
   cerebral 632, 639, **669**
   spinal cord 732
conus medullaris
   lesions 517
   normal location in adult 615, 711
Cooley's anemia 27
copular point
   of PICA 81
cord sign 890
cordectomy
   for spasticity 369
   for syringomyelia 352
Cordis shunt 192
cordotomy 391, 396
   open (Schwartz technique) 392
   percutaneous 391
   sacral 390
core neuro exam (for coma) 157
corneal mandibular reflex 588
corneal reflex 164
coronal suture
   estimating position 620
   relative to lateral ventricles 71
   relative to motor strip 70
   synostosis of 100
coronal synostosis 100
coronary angiography/angioplasty as cause of peripheral neuropathy 559
corpectomy (see vertebral corpectomy)
corpus callosum
   agenesis 114
   callosotomy 284
      for Lennox-Gastaut syndrome 258
   in hydrocephalus 183, 184
   lesions (differential diagnosis) 927
corset brace 747
cortical blindness 202
   due to vascular encephalopathy 64
   following head injury 637
   in Creutzfeldt-Jakob disease 229
   peripartum 64
cortical stimulation 284
cortical surface anatomy 68

Cushing's triad **649**, 853
Cushing's ulcers 657
cutoff sign 765
CVA (see cerebrovascular accident)
cyanide toxicity from nitroprusside 4
cyanocobalamin (see vitamin B$_{12}$)
cyanotic heart disease
  and cerebral abscess 217
cyclobenzaprine 34
cyclooxygenase 28
cyclosporine
  for neurosarcoidosis 58
Cyklokapron® (see tranexamic acid)
cyproheptadine 451
cyst
  arachnoid 94
    intracranial 94, 96
  associated with gliomas 412
  colloid 457
  dermoid and epidermoid
    spine 118
  neurenteric **98**
    CP-angle 922
    spinal 902
  pineal 476
  posttraumatic leptomeningeal 668
  spinal
    ganglion 313
    juxtafacet 313
    meningeal 348
    pilonidal 118
    synovial 313
  with cerebellar (pilocytic) astrocytoma 419
cystic cerebellar astrocytoma 419
cystic medial necrosis 883
cysticercosis (see neurocysticercosis)
cystometrogram 92
  in cauda equina syndrome 305
cystourethrogram 92
Cytadren® (see aminoglutethimide)
cytokeratin stain 500
Cytotec® (see misoprostol)
cytotoxic cerebral edema **85**, 662

D

Dalmane® (see flurazepam)
dalteparin 23
danaparoid 23
Dandy's point 620
Dandy's syndrome 591
Dandy-Walker malformation **110**, 183
Dantrium® (see dantrolene)
dantrolene
  for spasticity 368
dapsone
  and peripheral neuropathy 54, 557
Daraprim® (see pyrimethamine)
Darvon®, Darvocet® (see propoxyphene)
Daumas-Duport astrocytoma grading 411

Daypro® (see oxaprozin)
DDAVP® (see desmopressin)
D-dimer 26
de Morsier syndrome (see septo-optic dysplasia)
de Quervain's syndrome 567
deafferentation pain
  following lumbar laminectomy 315
deafness 597
  in Chiari malformation 105
  in Klippel-Feil syndrome 120
  in Paget's disease 341
  (see also hearing loss)
Decadron® (see dexamethasone)
decerebrate posturing 155, 159
decompressive cervical laminectomy 335
decompressive craniectomy (see craniectomy -
      decompressive)
decorticate posturing 154, 159
dedifferentiation of astrocytomas 412
deep brain stimulation
  for pain 395
  for parkinsonism 366
deep tendon reflex (see muscle stretch reflex)
deep-vein thrombosis 25
  in spinal cord injuries 705
degenerated lumbar disc 290
degenerative disc disease 323
  and smoking 324
  definition 290
  MRI findings 294
Dejerine-Roussy syndrome 776
delayed acute subdural hematoma 673
delayed cervical instability 743
delayed deterioration
  after head injury 636
  following back surgery (discitis) 315
  with cryptococcal meningitis 239
delayed epidural hematoma 671
delayed ischemic neurologic deficit (DIND) 791
delerium 44
  with meperidine 152
delerium tremens 151
delta sign 890
Deltasone® (see prednisone)
demeclocycline for SIADH 14
dementia 44
  due to vitamin B$_{12}$ deficiency 904
  following radiation therapy 489, 535
  in ALS 52
  in NPH 200
  parkinson-dementia complex of Guam 48
  posttraumatic 682
dementia pugilistica 683
  risk factors 683
Demerol® (see meperidine)
demyelination
  in Charcot-Marie-Tooth 554
  in chronic immune demyelinating polyradic-
      uloneuropathy (CIDP) 54
  in diabetic amyotrophy 556
  tumefactive demyelinating lesions 51

differential diagnosis *(cont'd)*
    axis (C2) lesions 924
    Babinski sign 89
    back pain 907
    bladder dysfunction 90
    blindness
        binocular 918
        monocular 919
    brachial plexopathy 554
    burning hands syndrome 912, 913
    by location 922
    by signs and symptoms 902
    calcifications (intracranial) 933
    carpal tunnel syndrome 566
    cauda equina syndrome 305
    cavernous sinus lesions 929
    cerebellopontine angle (CPA) lesions 922
    cerebral metastases 488
    cervical radiculopathy 911
    chordomas
        cranial 465
        foramen magnum 924
    coma
        metabolic 155
        structural 155
    corpus callosum lesions 927
    cranial nerve palsies 917
    Creutzfeldt-Jakob disease 229
    diabetes insipidus (DI) 16
    diffuse demineralization of the skull 932
    diplopia 916
    dizziness 590
    drop attacks (see apoplexy)
    dural enhancement 936
    encephalocele 939
    encephalopathy 145, 915
    ependymal enhancement 937
    exophthalmos 919
    extra-axial fluid collections in children 678
    extraforaminal disc herniation 311
    facial nerve palsy 594
    facial sensory changes 921
    fasciculations 911
    femoral neuropathy 557, 907
    foot drop 909
    foramen magnum lesions 924
    foramen magnum tumors 492
    giant cell arteritis 59
    Guillain-Barré syndrome 54
    gyral enhancement 765
    hand atrophy/weakness 911
    headache 44
    headache of sudden onset 782
    hemiparesis/hemiplegia 914
    hydrocephalus 184
    infratentorial masses causing coma 160
    intracranial cysts 928
    intracranial/extracranial lesions 932
    intramedullary spinal cord tumor 510
    intraventricular lesions 934
    L4 radiculopathy 907

differential diagnosis *(cont'd)*
    L5 radiculopathy 910
    language disturbance 921
    lateral disc herniation 311
    leukoencephalopathy 926
    Lhermitte's sign 912
    lipomas (intracranial) 97
    localized increased density of calvaria 932
    low back pain 907
    low density lesion in AIDS 233
    lumbar stenosis 327
    lumbosacral plexus neuropathy 555
    lytic skull lesions 930
    macrocephaly 920
    macrocrania 920
    medial temporal lobe lesions 938
    Meniere's disease 592
    meningeal thickening/enhancement 936
    meralgia paresthetica 574
    metastases (cerebral) 488
    midline intracranial cavities 928
    multiple cranial neuropathies 917
    multiple intracranial lesions 925
    multiple sclerosis 49
    myelopathy 902
    nasal/intracranial lesions 938
    neck pain 912
    neurosarcoidosis 57
    new onset of focal deficit 763
    occipital neuralgia 563
    oculomotor palsy 585
    ophthalmoplegia 585
        painful 586
    orbital lesions 929
    osteoid osteoma 511
    osteolytic skull lesions 930
    painless ophthalmoplegia 587
    papilledema (unilateral) 581
    paraplegia 913
    Parinaud's syndrome 86
    Parkinson's disease 47
    paroxysmal headache 782
    pathologic lid retraction 919
    perioral numbness 921
    periventricular enhancement 937
    periventricular lesions 936
    peroneal nerve palsy 909
    pineal region tumors 476
    pituitary tumors 927
    pneumocephalus 667
    posterior fossa lesions 923
    proptosis 919
    pseudocoma 156
    pseudotumor cerebri 496
    pseudotumor of the orbit 929
    quadriplegia 913
    radiculopathy
        lower extremity 905
        upper extremity 911
    retinal hemorrhage 689
    ring enhancing lesions 926

doppler
   transcranial
      for brain death 166
      for vasospasm 793, 797
      ultrasound for carotid stenosis 870
Dorello's canal 588
dorsal column stimulation 395
dorsal rhizotomy 369
dorsal root entry zone (DREZ) lesions 395
   for postherpetic neuralgia 390
dorsal scapular nerve 553
Dostinex® (see cabergoline)
double lumen sign 884
double-crush syndrome 566
Down's syndrome
   and amyloid angiopathy 853
   and basilar impression 139
   and moyamoya disease 892
downbeat nystagmus 105, 580
doxacurium 38
doxepin
   as analgesic adjuvant 376
DPT (pediatric lytic cocktail) 37
dressing apraxia 88
DREZ (see dorsal root entry zone lesions)
drop attacks
   atonic seizures 256
   differential diagnosis (see apoplexy)
   in Lennox-Gastaut syndrome 258
   in Meniere's disease 592
   with colloid cysts 458
   with vertebrobasilar insufficiency 881
drop metastases 485
   with ependymomas 471, 472
   with medulloblastoma 473
   with pineal region tumors 476
   (see also metastases - spinal seeding)
droperidol 393
drug-induced neuropathy 557
drusen 497, 929
dry eye 594
DTs (see delerium tremens)
dual energy x-ray absorptiometry 749
Dublin measure of AOD 720
Duract® (see bromfenac)
Duragesic® (see fentanyl)
dural AVM 843
dural enhancement
   differential diagnosis 936
dural sinus thrombosis 888
   and idiopathic intracranial hypertension
      (pseudotumor cerebri) 496
   in transcallosal surgery 611
dural tail (with meningioma on MRI) 428
dural tear (see durotomy - unintended)
Duramorph® 393
Duret hemorrhages 160
durotomy
   to remove herniated disc 305
   unintended 307, **308**
      with surgery for lumbar stenosis 329

DVT (see deep-vein thrombosis)
Dyazide® (see hydrochlorothiazide)
dyes
   contrast agents in neuroradiology 126
   intraoperative 599
dynamic cerebral angiography
   for bow hunter's stroke 882
dysarthria
   following pallidotomy 367
   following thalamotomy 365
   in ALS 52
dysembryoplastic neuroepithelial tumors 409
dysphagia
   due to diffuse idiopathic skeletal hyperostosis
      347
   from ossification of the anterior longitudinal
      ligament 346
   from radiation therapy 537
   in ALS 52
   in Chiari type 2 malformation 108, 109
dysphasia
   following stereotactic biopsy 417
   with brain tumors 404
dystonia 370
   dystonia musculorum deformans 370

E

Eagle's syndrome 912
ε-aminocaproic acid (see epsilon-aminocaproic
   acid)
early draining vein 130, 413
early surgery for aneurysms 804
EC/IC bypass (see extracranial-intracranial bypass)
echinococcosis 238
echocardiography for cerebral embolism 773
eclampsia
   and encephalopathy 64
   and intracerebral hemorrhage **825**, 852
   and vasospasm 64
Ecstasy (street drug) 48
ectopic bone 755
EDAS (see encephaloduroarteriosynangiosis)
edema
   cerebral 85
      cytotoxic **85**, 662
      following head injury 636
      following radiation therapy 535
      from metastases 487
      high altitude 687
      ischemic 85
      vasogenic **85**, 661
         exacerbated by mannitol 661
      with acute subdural hematoma 672
   pulmonary
      from contrast media 129
      high altitude 687
      in spinal cord injury 703
      neurogenic 8

edema *(cont'd)*
  spinal cord
    following injury 714, 715, 742, 743
    following radiation therapy 521, 536
Edinger-Westphal nucleus 81, 581
EEG (see electroencephalogram)
Effendi grade (hangman's fracture) 725
Ehlers-Danlos syndrome 801
EKG changes after SAH 789
Elavil® (see amitriptyline)
electrocerebral silence on EEG 166
electrocorticography 283, 284
electrodiagnostics 145
electroencephalogram 145
  electrocerebral silence 166
  for brain death 166
  for hydranencephaly vs. hydrocephalus 180
  for withdrawal of anticonvulsants 280
  monitoring for vasospasm 793
  rebuildup in moyamoya disease 893
electromyography 147
  for low back problems 292
  H-reflex 293
  in ALS 52
  in diabetic amyotrophy 556
  in facial palsy 595
  in lumbosacral plexus neuropathy 555
  in peroneal nerve palsy 575
  to differentiate root from plexus lesion 910
  to localize S1 involvement 907
electroneuronography 666
electronystagmography 432
elevating head of bed
  following chronic subdural drainage 675
  to lower ICP 659
Elgiloy (aneurysm clip alloy) 136
Elliott's solution 174
embolism (cerebral)
  air 605
  amniotic fluid 774
  and atrial fibrillation 773
  and myocardial infarction 773
  and patent foramen ovale 773
  and prosthetic heart valves 773
  and stroke in young adults 774
  cardiogenic 773
  echocardiography, use of 773
  fat 774
  paradoxical 773, 774
  septic 217
  top o' the basilar 776
  with carotid angioplasty 878
embolization
  balloon
    for carotid-cavernous fistula 845
    of aneurysms 803
  of AVM 838
emergency burr holes 645
EMG (see electromyography)
emotional incontinence 778
  with pseudobulbar palsy 48

emotional lability (see emotional incontinence)
empty can test 911
empty delta sign 890
empty sella syndrome 499
  from chronic hydrocephalus 184
  primary 499
  secondary 454, **499**
empyema - subdural (intracranial) 223
enalapril 6
enaloprilat 4
encephalitis
  herpes simplex 225
  multifocal necrotizing (see encephalitis - herpes simplex)
  post-encephalitic parkinsonism 47
  varicella-zoster 227
  with CNS lymphoma 462
encephalocele 102, 939
encephaloduroarteriosynangiosis 894
encephalomyosynangiosis 894
encephalopathy
  AIDS 231
  and preeclampsia/eclampsia 64
  anoxic (see anoxic encephalopathy)
  bovine spongiform (BSE) 228
  chronic traumatic 683
  differential diagnosis 145, 915
  due to vascular autoregulatory dysfunction 64
  hypertensive 64
  uremic 64
  Wernicke's **151**, 266
encephalotrigeminal angiomatosis 505
enchondroma 506
end tidal pCO2 and air embolism 605
endocarditis (see bacterial endocarditis)
endocrine evaluation
  for pheochromocytoma/glomus jugulare 469
  for pituitary adenoma 444
    (table) 443
endocrinology 8
endodermal sinus cyst (see neurenteric cyst)
endolymphatic hydrops 591
endoneurium 560
endoscopic discectomy 307
endothelial cell proliferation
  and glioblastoma multiforme 411, 412
  and radiation myelopathy 537
  following stereotactic radiosurgery 538
endothelin receptor antagonists 794
enflurane 1
enoxaparin **23**, 26
enterogenous cyst (see neurenteric cyst)
entheses (in ankylosing spondylitis) 343
entrapment neuropathy 563
entrapped fourth ventricle 182
enuresis (in radiculopathy) 302
eosinophilic granuloma
  of the skull 482
    differential diagnosis 931
  of the spine 506

F

FABER test 303
facet injections
    for low-back pain 298
facet joint injections
    for low back pain 298
    for synovial cysts 314
facet syndrome 298
facial colliculus 594
facial diplegia 594
facial myokymia 371
facial nerve
    anastamosis for facial palsy 596
    palsy **593**
        Bell's palsy 595
        central vs. peripheral 594
        differential diagnosis 594
        in Guillain-Barré 53
        in Lyme disease 235
        posttraumatic 666
        treatment 596
        with cerebellar infarct 772
        with facial nerve neuroma 594
facial nerve neuroma 594, **922**
facial pain (see pain - craniofacial)
facial sensory changes 921
    following acoustic neuroma treatment 437
factor VII
    for intracerebral hemorrhage 857, 858
    to reverse antiplatelet drugs 22
Fahr's disease 934
failed back syndrome 310, **314**
faint 915
Fajersztajn's sign 303
falciform ligament 813
false aneurysms 820
    carotid 876
falx syndrome 673
famciclovir
    for herpes zoster 388
familial aneurysms 819
familial intracranial aneurysm syndrome 801
familial syndromes with CNS tumors 406
Famvir® (see famciclovir)
fanning of cervical spines 142
fascicles 560
fast spin echo (on MRI) 135
fastigium 71
fat
    on MRI 135
fat embolism syndrome 774
fat suppression MRI 135
febrile seizures 259, **264**
    and mesial temporal sclerosis 257
    definition 264
    preceding status epilepticus 264
fecal incontinence
    in cauda equina syndrome 305
felbamate 276

Felbatol® (see felbamate)
Feldene® (see piroxicam)
femoral neuropathy 557
    perioperative 559
    vs. L4 radiculopathy 907
    vs. plexus neuropathy 556
    vs. lumbosacral plexus neuropathy 555
femoral stretch test 303
fenoldopam 5
fenoprofen 28
fentanyl 2, **37**
    for pediatric sedation 37
    patch 32
    to control ICP 656, 658
festinating gait 47
fetal circulation 81, 130, 811
fetal hydantoin syndrome 281
fetal tissue transplantation
    for parkinsonism 365
FFP (see fresh frozen plasma)
FGFR genes (see fibroblast growth factor recep-
    tor genes)
fibrillary astrocytoma 410
fibrillation potentials on EMG 147
fibrin glue 178
fibrinoid necrosis 851
fibroblast growth factor receptor genes 102
fibromuscular dysplasia 63
    and arterial dissection 883
    and intracranial aneurysms 801
    and moyamoya disease 892
    and stroke in young adults 775
fibromyalgia 912
fibrous (fibroblastic) meningioma 427
fibrous dysplasia **483**
    differential diagnosis 930
fifth ventricle 928
filum terminale
    distinguishing features 121
    myxopapillary ependymoma 508
    tethering 120
finger drop 572
Finkelstein's test 567
Fischgold's lines 139, 140
Fisher SAH grade 792
Fishman's formula 173
fistula
    arteriovenous (direct) 835
    CSF (see cerebrospinal fluid - fistula)
fixed and dilated pupil (see pupillary dilatation)
Flagyl® (see metronidazole)
flail foot 909
FLAIR images (on MRI) 135
flame hemorrhages 890
flaring of cervical spines 142
Flexeril® (see cyclobenzaprine)
flexion compression fracture (see compression
    flexion fracture)
flexion-extension cervical spine x-rays 708
flexor synergy 89
floppy infant syndrome 281, 913

Frankfurt plane 70
Frazier burr hole 619
    emergency use of 607
free fat graft (epidural) 307
free fragment of disc material 290
free radical scavengers
    for intra-operative cerebral protection 806
    for vasospasm 794
Freedox® (see tirilazad)
Freidberg's test 906
fresh frozen plasma 20
fried egg cells 424
Froin's syndrome 510
Froment's prehensile thumb sign 569
frontal craniotomy 609
frontal eye field 69, **584**
frontal eye fields 85
frontal lobectomy 609
frontal sinus
    fractures 667
    infection and subdural empyema 224
frontal suture 100
Functional Independence Measure 901
fungal infections
    CNS 239
    superinfection 210
    vertebral osteomyelitis 244
furosemide
    for chronic SIADH 14
    for hydrocephalus 186
    for ICP management 658, 661
    for pseudotumor cerebri 498
    for pulmonary edema 129
    for SIADH 13
    prior to mannitol 643
Furstenberg sign 939
furuncle
    in spinal epidural abscess 241
fusiform aneurysms 800
fusion
    cervical spine 623
    lumbar spine 300
        bone graft extenders/substitutes 301
        brace therapy 329
        choice of technique 299
        correlation with outcome 301
        following discectomy 300
        for (chronic) low back pain 299
        pedicle screw fixation 300
        radiographic assessment 301
        with stenosis and spondylolisthesis 329
        with stenosis without spondylolisthesis
            329
F-wave response (on EMG) 148, 293

G

gabapentin 278
    for neuropathic pain 377
    for painful diabetic neuropathy 557

gabapentin *(cont'd)*
    for postherpetic neuralgia 388
    for trigeminal neuralgia 380
Gabitril® (see tiagabine)
gadopentetate dimeglumine
    in pregnancy 825
Gallie fusion 624
gangliogliomas 408, **466**
    brainstem 421
ganglion cyst (spinal) 313
ganglion impar (ganglion of Walther) 354
ganglioneuromas 466
Garamycin® (see gentamicin)
Gardner's syndrome 481
Gardner-Robertson hearing classification 432
Gardner-Wells tong placement 709
Gasserian ganglion (see trigeminal ganglion)
gastric emptying
    in head injury 680
Geipel hernia 313
gelastic seizures 97
gelatin sponge 600
Gelfoam® (see gelatin sponge)
gemistocytes 410
gemistocytic astrocytomas **410**, 412
generalized tonic-clonic seizure 256
geniculate neuralgia 386
gentamicin 210
    intrathecal 213
germ cell tumors 477
    differential diagnosis 927
germinal matrix hemorrhage 861
germinoma 477
Gerstmann's syndrome 87
GFAP (see glial fibrillary acidic protein)
"ghost-cell tumor" 463
giant aneurysms 821
giant cell arteritis 58
giant cell astrocytoma 505
giant cell tumor (of bone) **516**
    of the sacrum 906
    of the spine
        differential diagnosis 506
gigantism (from excess growth hormone) 441
Gill procedure 325
glabella 69, 69
Glasgow coma scale 154
Glasgow outcome scale 900
Gliadel® wafer (see carmustine (BCNU))
glial fibrillary acidic protein 412, **500**
    and oligodendrogliomas 424
glioblastoma multiforme 412
    in adult posterior fossa 923
    outcome 416
    treatment 415
glioma 409
    brainstem 420
    butterfly 413, 415
    definition 401
    hypothalamic 420
    low grade 408

growth hormone 441
  acromegaly **441**, 447
    biochemical "cure" 456
    treatment for 449
  and Creutzfeldt-Jakob disease 228
guanethedine block 397
Guglielmi detachable coils 803
guideline (practice guideline) - definition iii
Guidelines for the Management of Severe Head
    Injury 655
Guilford brace 741
Guillain-Barré syndrome **53**, 905
gunshot wounds
    to peripheral nerves 563
    to the brachial plexus 562
    to the head 684
      antibiotics for 685
      entrance/exit wound 685
      indications for angiography 686
    to the spine 753
Guyon's canal 571
gyral enhancement
    differential diagnosis 765
    on CT 765
    on MRI 765
gyri of Heschl 68

H

HACE (see high altitude cerebral edema)
hair-on-end skull 27, 932
Hakim shunt 192
Hakim-Adams syndrome (see normal pressure
    hydrocephalus)
halazepam 35
Haldol® (see haloperidol)
half-lives to steady state 270
Halifax clamps 624
hallucinosis 150
halo sign 176
haloperidol 37
    and parkinsonism 47
    for DTs 151
halothane 1
halo-vest brace 741
    and cerebral abscess 218
hamartomas
    hypothalamic 97
    with tuberous sclerosis 505
hamstrings 551
hanging drop technique 46
hangman's fracture 724
    Effendi grade 725
    Francis grade 727
    treatment 726
hard disc 331
harlequin eye sign 100
Harris-Benedict equation 680
head circumference (see occipital-frontal cir-
    cumference)

head fixation in surgery 600
head injury (see trauma - head)
headache 44
    following craniotomy 604
    from cranial defect 604
    in subarachnoid hemorrhage 782
    migraine 45
    paroxysmal 782
    post myelogram/LP 46
    spinal (see headache - post myelogram/LP)
    thunderclap 782
    warning (in subarachnoid hemorrhage) 782
    with brain tumors 405
    with giant cell arteritis 59
    with orgasm 782
    with unruptured aneurysms 782, 801
hearing classification 432
hearing loss 597
    American Acadamy of Otolaryngology hear-
        ing classification 432
    following loss of CSF 616
    following lumbar puncture 616
    following MVD for hemifacial spasm 373
    Gardener and Robertson classification 432
    with acoustic neuroma 430, 431
      following treatment 436
      sudden/spontaneous 430
    with glomus jugulare tumor 468
    with Meniere's disease 592
heart valves (prosthetic) (see prosthetic heart
    valves)
Heiss-Oldfield theory 350
helmets
    football, removal after injury 702
    motorcycle 673
hemangioblasomatosis 459
hemangioblastoma
    intracranial 459
      differential diagnosis 923
    spinal cord 509
hemangioma
    capillary
      orbital 929
      skull 481
      vertebral 512
    cavernous 923
      intracranial (see cavernous malforma-
          tion) 841
      orbital 929
      vertebral 512
    in Sturge-Weber 505, 929
    of the skull **481**, 931
      radiographic appearance 930
    vertebral 353, **512**, 903
      and spinal epidural hematoma 903
      treatment 513
hemangiopericytomas 428
hematocrit
    in hyperdynamic therapy 798
    in vasospasm 795
hematology 19

hematoma
  epidural
    cerebral 669
    spinal 903
  intracerebral 849
  post-op 602
  subdural 672
hemianopsia
  bitemporal 441, 444
  homonymous
    from occipital lobe lesions 85
    with parietal lobe tumors 405
    with pituitary tumors 444
  junctional scotoma 444, **813**
hemiballism 777
hemicraniectomy (for increased ICP) (see
    craniectomy - decompressive)
hemifacial spasm 371
hemiparesis
  differential diagnosis 914
  following pallidotomy 367
  infantile
    and seizure surgery 282
    from arterial dissection 885
  pure motor 776
hemiplegic migraine 45
hemispherectomy 283
hemodialysis following cerebral hemorrhage 858
hemogenic meningitis (see meningitis - he-
    mogenic)
hemorrhagic brain tumors 854
hemorrhagic contusion 639, **669**
hemorrhagic contusions 632
  excision to control ICP 659
hemorrhagic conversion of ischemic infarcts 773
hemostasis (surgical) 600
hemotympanum 637, 665
heparin 22
  and intracerebral hemorrhage 770
  and thrombocytopenia 22
  considerations in neurosurgery 21
  contraindications 21
  for cardioembolic stroke 774
  for carotid dissection 886
  for cerebrovascular venous thrombosis 891
  for DVT prophylaxis 26
  for DVT treatment 26
  for spinal cord injury 705
  for stroke 770
  low molecular weight **23**, 26
  mini-dose 26, 705
  reversal 24
hepatic toxicity
  from acetaminophen 28
  from labetalol 6
hereditary hemorrhagic telangiectasia (see Osler-
    Weber-Rendu syndrome)
hereditary motor and sensory neuropathy (see
    Charcot-Marie-Tooth syndrome)
hereditary neuropathy with liability to pressure
    palsies 554

herniation
  central 160
  following LP 616, 617
  herniation syndromes 159
  intervertebral disc (see intervertebral disc -
    herniation)
  spinal cord 903
  tonsillar 160
  uncal 161
  upward (cerebellar) **160**, 406
herniation (lumbar disc pathology) 290
herpes simplex encephalitis 145, **225**
herpes zoster 387
  and facial paralysis 596
  leukoencephalitis 227
  myelopathy 905
  ophthalmicus 387
    and stroke in young adults 774
  radiculopathy 906
herpetic ganglionitis 386
Hespan® (see hetastarch)
hetastarch 6
  and impaired coagulation **787**, 798
  for contrast media reaction 128
heterotopia 112
Heubner's artery 77, *131*, 131
  occlusion 778
Heyer-Schulte shunt 192
H-graft 624
hiccups
  from steroids 11
  treatment
    chlorpromazine (Thorazine®) 11
  with lateral medullary syndrome 777
high altitude cerebral edema 687
high altitude cerebral edema (HACE) 687
hippus 588
histamine
  release with morphine 2
  release with paralytics 38, 40
histamine$_2$ (H$_2$) antagonists
  for head trauma 657
histaminic migraine 45
histiocytosis X 482
  differential diagnosis 931
Hivid® (see zalcitabine)
HNPP (see hereditary neuropathy with liability
    to pressure palsies)
Hoffmann's sign 89
Hollenhorst plaques 870
hollow skull phenomenon (sign) on CRAG 167
Holmes-Adie's pupil 583
holoprosencephaly 112
Holter valve 193
Homans' sign 26
homocystinuria
  and arterial dissections 883
  and cerebrovascular venous thrombosis 888
  and strokes 775
homonymous hemianopsia (see hemianopsia -
    homonymous)

hyperhidrosis 352, 373
    facial 105
    with acromegaly 441
hyperkalemia
    following succinylcholine 38
hyperlordosis of the cervical spine 331
hypernatremia 15
hyperostosis cranialis interna 918
hyperostosis frontalis interna 483
hyperpathia
    with central cord syndrome 714
    with meralgia paresthetica 573
hypersensitivity vasculitis 63
hypertension
    and risk of stroke 764
    in Cushing's syndrome 440
    induced (to treat vasospasm) 797
    treatment 3
hypertensive encephalopathy 64
hypertensive hemorrhage 849
hyperthermia
    with hypothalamic lesion 457
hyperthyroidism 443
    and ophthalmopathy 929
    Graves' disease 929
    secondary 445
    treatment for TSH-secreting adenomas 451
hypertonic saline
    to lower ICP 661
hypertrichosis
    with diastematomyelia 122
    with tethered cord syndrome 120
hyperventilation
    and hypocalcemia 643
    for brain relaxation during surgery 806
    in coma 157
    in the E/R 643
    neurogenic 157
    producing symptoms in moyamoya disease
        893
    to lower ICP 659
hypocortisolism 11
hypofractionation 539
hypoglossal nerve
    anastamosis to facial nerve 596
    injury from carotid endarterectomy 877
hypogonadotropic hypogonadism
    following head injury 681
hypoid 130
hypokalemia
    hypokalemic alkalosis in Cushing's syn-
        drome 440
    in spinal cord injury 704
hyponatremia **12**, 14
    following SAH 788
    postoperative 12
hypophysitis 928
hypopituitarism
    and suprasellar germ cell tumors 927
    due to aneurysm 813
    due to pituitary tumor 438

hypopituitarism *(cont'd)*
    due to radiation therapy 535
    following head trauma 645
hypotension
    and ischemic optic neuropathy 203
    causing blindness 203
    causing spinal cord infarction 903
    during aneurysm surgery 807
    following head trauma
        etiologies 635
        prognostic significance 644
    following spinal cord injury (spinal shock)
        698, 703
    from contrast media reaction 128
    impact in severe traumatic brain injury 657
    orthostatic 48
    treatment 6
hypothalamic glioma 418, **420**
hypothalamic hamartomas 97
hypothermia
    and determining brain death 165
    and wound infection 216
    as cause of fixed pupils 158
    for cerebral protection
        during aneurysm surgery 807
        with closed head injury 658
hypothyroidism
    and pituitary tumors 445
    from aminoglutethimide 451
hypoxia
    following head trauma
        prognostic significance 644
    hypoxic coma 162
hypsarrhythmia 258

I

ibuprofen 29
    suspension 29
IDET (see intradiscal endothermal therapy)
idiopathic brachial plexus neuropathy 554
idiopathic cranial polyneuropathy 918
idiopathic intracranial hypertension 493
    and empty sella syndrome 494, 499
    without papilledema vi, 495
IDTA (see intradiscal endothermal therapy)
IGF-I (see somatomedin-C)
ileus
    following lumbar laminectomy (Ogilvie's
        syndrome) 308
    following spinal cord injury 703
iliac crest bone graft
    and meralgia paresthetica 574
iliopsoas 551
immunohistochemical staining patterns 501
impact damage in head injury 635
impedance
    during trigeminal rhizotomy 383
impedance plethysmography 26
Inapsine® (see droperidol)

intervertebral disc - herniation *(cont'd)*
    intravertebral disc herniation **313**
    lumbar 302
        and spondylolisthesis 324
        conservative treatment 296
        extreme lateral 311
        foraminal 311
        in asymptomatic patients 293
        in pediatrics 312
        indications for surgery 304
        intradural 312
        percutaneous procedures 306
        physical findings 302
        radiographic evaluation 293
        recurrent 317
        surgical treatment 304
        upper lumbar 310
    Schmorl's node **313**, 908
    sequestered 290
    surgical options 306
    syndromes
        cervical 318
        lumbar 304
    thoracic 322
  infection (discitis) **245**, 939
    sparing with tumors 939
  vacuum disc 289
intoxication
  cocaine 152
  ethanol 149
  opioid 151
intraarterial chemotherapy 407, 416
intracarotid amytal test 282
intracerebral hemorrhage 849
  and alpha-adrenergic agonists 852
  and cerebral amyloid angiopathy 853
  and leukemia 861
  and migraine 851
  and prosthetic heart valves 858
  and sympathomimetics 852
  and vasculitis 58
  angiogram, indications for 857
  anticoagulation
    following the hemorrhage 858
    preceding the hemorrhage 770, 854
  cerebellar
    following craniotomy 852
    treatment guidelines 860
  during percutaneous trigeminal procedures
    384
  etiologies 850
  following carotid endarterectomy 876
    emergency endarterectomy 879
  following craniotomy 852
  following evacuation of chronic subdural
    675, 676
  from brain tumors 854
  from depth electrodes 283
  grading system 856
  in the newborn 861
  in young adults 861
  lobar 850
    clinical syndromes 855

intracerebral hemorrhage - lobar *(cont'd)*
    mortality 860
    management 856
    MRI appearance 856
    postpartum 852
    rebleeding 855
    recurrent 853
    score 856
    stereotactic aspiration of 545
    surgical treatment 858
        STICH study 859
    tissue plasminogen activator
        injection into clot to treat 545
        intraventricular injection to treat 860
        preceding the hemorrhage 768, 851, 853
    traumatic 639, **669**
    treatment 856
    volume
        estimation 856
        prognostic value 859
    vs. ischemic infarct 764
    with aneurysmal rupture 800
    with ICP monitor 650
intracranial aerocele (see pneumocephalus)
intracranial cysts 928
intracranial hemorrhage (see intracerebral hem-
    orrhage)
intracranial hypertension (see intracranial pres-
    sure)
intracranial hypotension
  from overshunting 197
  spontaneous 178
intracranial pressure 647
  definitions 648
  elevation
    from histamine release 2
    with nipride 4
    with nitroglycerin 4
    with succinylcholine 38
  following SAH 790
  hypertension
    management 656
        hypothermia 658
        second tier therapy 658
        surgery for 656
    with cryptococcal meningitis 239
  hypotension 178, 197
  indications to treat 649
  management
    protocol 656
  monitoring 649
    and hemorrhage 650
    and infection 650
    and prophylactic antibiotics 650
    estimating ICP in infants 651
    fontanometry 651
    in gunshot wounds 686
    in multiple trauma 644
    indications 649
    monitor insertion technique 620
  normal values 648

intracranial pressure *(cont'd)*
   respiratory variations 653
   secondary rise 648
   waveforms 653
intradiscal electrothermal anuloplasty (see intradiscal endothermal therapy)
intradiscal endothermal therapy 306, **307**
intradiscal pressure 297, 306
intradiscal procedures 306
intradural disc herniation 312
intramedullary spinal cord tumors 508
intranasal/intracranial lesions 938
intraoperative aneurysm rupture 808
intraoperative dyes 599
intraoperative evoked potentials 146
   anesthesia requirements 3
intraoperative pneumoencephalogram 644
intraoperative ultrasound
   for spine fracture 748
intraosseous meningiomas 426
intraspinal narcotic administration 393
   implantable pump 394
intraspongious disc herniation (see Schmorl's
   node)
intrathecal drugs
   antibiotics
      for shunt infection 216
      gentamicin 210
      tobramycin 210
   baclofen 369
   contrast agents 126
      inadvertent use of ionic agent 126
      iohexol 127
   implantable pump 394
   methotrexate 464
      treatment for overdose 464
   morphine
      for pain 393
      for spasticity 368
   narcotics 393
      implantable pump 394
   steroids for postherpetic neuralgia 389
intravascular lymphomatosis 463
   and cauda equina syndrome 305
intravenous pyelography 92
intraventricular catheter 651, **651**, *652*
   insertion technique 651
   (see also ventricular catheterization)
intraventricular hemorrhage
   and vasospasm 791
   etiologies 938
   from closed head injury 640
   in the newborn 861
   with aneurysmal rupture **800**
      PICA aneurysms 814
   with intracerebral hemorrhage 858, 860
      in newborns 861
   yield of angiography 858
intraventricular lesions 934
   surgical approaches 610
intraventricular narcotic administration 394

intravertebral disc herniation 290, **313**
intubation
   in trauma 642
invasive pituitary adenoma 442
   treatment 453
inverse ptosis 584
inverted radial reflex 333
iodinated contrast
   adverse reactions 128
      with metformin (Glucophage®) 126
   agents used in neuroradiology 126
iodinated contrast allergy prep 128
iohexol 127
   for arteriography 127
   for myelography 127, 142
   intrathecal 127
ionic contrast agents 126
iophendylate meglumine 126
ioversol 127
   for arteriography 128
IPG (see impedance plethysmography)
iridoplegia, traumatic 582
ISAT (see International Subarachnoid Hemorrhage Aneurysm Trial)
ischemia (cerebral) (see cerebral ischemia)
ischemic cerebral edema 85
ischemic optic neuropathy 203
isoflurane 1
   and cerebral protection 807
   for status epilepticus 267
isolated angiitis of the CNS 62
isolated CNS vasculitis 62
isolated fourth ventricle 182
isolated posterior circulation 882
isoproterenol 7
Isoptin® (see verapamil)
isthmus
   of the axis (C2) *724*
Isuprel® (see isoproterenol)
IV solutions
   and elevated ICP 657
Ivalon® sponge (see polyvinyl formyl alcohol)
IVC (see ventricular catheterization)
ivory bone 340

J

J shaped sella turcica 139
jackknife spasms 258
Jackson classification 469
Jakob-Creutzfeldt disease (see Creutzfeldt-Jakob
   disease)
jaw claudication 59
jaw jerk 333
JC virus 231
Jefferson fracture 701, **723**
jejunal feedings 680
Jendrassik maneuver 304
jet ventilation 659
Jewett hyperextension brace 747

jugular foramen 72
  syndromes 86
jugular venous oxygen saturation 655
jumped facets (see locked facets)
junctional scotoma
  with ophthalmic artery aneurysms **813**
  with pituitary tumors 444
juvenile myoclonic epilepsy 257, 274
juvenile pilocytic astrocytoma 418
juxtafacet cyst (spinal) 313

K

kakosmia 257
Karnofsky scale 899
  and survival with astrocytoma 417
Keen's point 620
Kefzol® (see cefazolin)
Keppra® (see levetiracetam)
Kernig's sign 212, **783**
Kernohan grading system (for astrocytomas) 410
Kernohan's phenomenon 162, **670**
ketoconazole
  for Cushing's disease 450
ketoprofen 29
ketorolac tromethamine 29
ketotifen 502
keyhole foraminotomy
  for cervical radiculopathy 321
  in cervical myelopathy 335
Ki-67 (immunohistochemical stain) 500
kindling 258
Kleeblattschadel syndrome 102
Klippel-Feil syndrome 119
Klonopin® (see clonazepam)
Klumpke's palsy 561
Kocher's point 620
Korsakoff's syndrome/psychosis 151
kuru 228
kyphotic deformity
  following anterior cervical discectomy 321

L

l'etat lacunaire 776
labetalol **4**, 6
  for AVM surgery 839
  for glomus tumors 469
  in strokes 770
lacertus fibrosus compression of median nerve
    569
Lacricert® 607
lacunar strokes 776
  and arteriosclerotic parkinsonism 48
Ladd epidural monitor 651
lambda 69
lambdoid plagiocephaly 101
lambdoid synostosis 100
lamina cribrosa (of IAC) 72

laminectomy
  cervical 321, 335
    and subluxation 319
    and swan neck deformity 335
  lumbar
    and reflex sympathetic dystrophy 308
    and subluxation 328
    complications of epidural fat graft 307
    epidural fat graft 307
    for herniated disc 306
    post-op check 310
    post-op orders 309
    risks 307
    urgent (indications) 304
  thoracic 322
  wound infection 216
lamotrigine 278
language disturbance
  differential diagnosis 921
lansoprazole 787
Larodopa® (see levodopa)
Lasègue's sign 302
laser disc decompression 306
Lasix® (see furosemide)
lateral bending test 311
lateral canthal advancement 100
lateral cervical puncture 618
lateral cutaneous nerve of the forearm 553
lateral femoral cutaneous nerve 573
lateral fissure
  surface anatomy 70
lateral mass plates (see posterior cervical plates)
lateral massfracture of atlas 723
lateral medullary syndrome 777
  and vertebral artery dissection 887
  vs. brainstem compression 772
lateral oblique position 604
lateral recess syndrome 330
lateral rectus palsy 586
lateral ventricle
  surface anatomy 71
  surgical approaches 610
law of Laplace 197
lazaroids 662
Lazarus sign 165
lazy lambdoid 100
lead poisoning
  and macrocephaly 920
  and wrist drop 572
  from retained bullet 753
  vs. Guillain-Barré syndrome 54
LeFort fractures 667
left-right confusion 87
Lennox-Gastaut syndrome **258**, 264
lenticulostriate arteries 77, 78, *131*, 131
  lateral 131
lepirudin 23
leptomeningeal carcinomatosis (see carcinoma-
    tous meningitis)
leptomeningeal cysts 94
  posttraumatic 668

microaneurysms of Charcot-Bouchard 853
microcephaly **113**, 185
    and maternal cocaine abuse 113
    following CSF shunting 199
    with TORCH infections 920
microcystic meningioma 427
microfibrillar collagen 600
microglioma 461
micrographia 47
micro-metastases 489
microvascular decompression
    11th nerve for torticollis 371
    for hemifacial spasm 372
    for trigeminal neuralgia 381, **385**
midazolam 35, 37
    drip 36
    for EtOH withdrawal 150
    for status epilepticus 267
middle cerebral artery 80
    angiogram *132*
middle frontal gyrus
    approach to lateral or third ventricle 612
middle temporal gyrus *68*
    approach to amygdala 285
midline shift
    and coma 155
    with CVAs 765
migraine 45
    and intracerebral hemorrhage 851
    as a cause of stroke 775
    crash 782
    thunderclap headache 782
migrated disc (disc migration) 290
migration abnormalities 112
mild traumatic brain injury 632, 633
miliary aneurysms 853
Millard-Gubler syndrome 86
Miller-Fisher variant Guillain-Barré 54
mineralocorticoids 8, 11
mini-dose heparin 26, 705
Minnesota Multiphasic Personality Inventory
    and low back problems 296
    and nonepileptic seizures 262
miosis
    from narcotics 151, 157
    in Horner's syndrome 584
mirror motions 119
misoprostol 28
missile wounds
    to peripheral nerves 563
mithramicin (see plicamycin)
mitotane 451
mitral valve prolapse and stroke 774
Mivacron® (see mivacurium)
mivacurium 39
mixed gliomas 424
MMPI (see Minnesota Multiphasic Personality
    Inventory)
Möbius syndrome 917
Modic's classification of VB marrow changes
    290

modified ellipsoid volume 856
modified Rankin scale 900
Mollaret's meningitis 475
monoamine oxidase inhibitors
    interaction with meperidine 32
mononeuropathy
    definition 553
mononeuropathy multiplex
    definition 553
    ischemic 556
Monro-Kellie hypothesis 648
moon facies 440
Morgagni's syndrome 483
morphine 31
    disadvantages in neuro patients 2
    extended release oral forms 31
    for pulmonary edema 129
    intraspinal 393
    intrathecal 368, 393
Morquio syndrome 337, 902
motor cortex
    cortical anatomy *68*
    surface anatomy 70
motor neuron disease (see amyotrophic lateral
    sclerosis)
motor oil fluid 674
motor point block 368
motor strip *68*
motorcycle helmets 673
Motrin® (see ibuprofen)
moyamoya disease 892
    and arterial dissections 883
MPTP 47
MRA
    (see magnetic resonance angiography)
MRI (see magnetic resonance imaging)
MRS (see magnetic resonance spectroscopy)
MS (see multiple sclerosis)
MS Contin 31
Mt. Fuji sign 668
Much of CVS is poorly understood because of
    lack of a good endothelin 1 793
mucocele 938
mucormycosis **586**, 774, 917, 930
Müller's muscle 581, 584
multicentric (multifocal) gliomas 413
multifocal necrotizing encephalomyelitis (see
    encephalitis - herpes simplex)
multifocal varicella-zoster leukoencephalitis 227
multiple aneurysms 819
multiple concussions 634
multiple endocrine adenomatosis 438
multiple intracranial lesions 925
multiple myeloma 514
    and amyloidosis 560
    and carpal tunnel syndrome 560, 567
    of the skull 931
    of the spine 517
    workup for 515
multiple sclerosis 49
    and multiple primary gliomas 413

multiple sclerosis *(cont'd)*
   and trigeminal neuralgia 50, 378, 381
   and urinary bladder dysfunction 91
   MR spectroscopy appearance 137
   myelopathy 904
multiple system atrophy 48
Munchausen's syndrome
   and nonepileptic seizures 262
mural nodule
   in cerebellar astrocytoma 419
   in hemangioblastoma 460
Murphy's tit 819
muscle innervation 548
muscle relaxants 34
   for low back pain 297
muscle strength grading 548
muscle stretch reflex
   following lumbar spine surgery 310
   in alcohol withdrawal syndrome 150
   in amyotrophic lateral sclerosis 52
   in cauda equina syndrome 305
   in cervical spondylotic myelopathy 333
   in extreme lateral lumbar disc herniations
      311
   in Guillain-Barré syndrome 53
   in herniated cervical disc 318
   in herniated lumbar disc 304
   in herniated upper lumbar discs 311
   in lateral recess stenosis 330
   in lumbar spinal stenosis 326
   in multiple sclerosis 50
   in odontoid fracture 728
   in radiculopathy 289, 302
   in spinal cord injury 704, 712
   in trauma exam 638
   in whiplash associated disorder 699
musculocutaneous nerve 553
muzzle velocity 684
myalgia 908
myasthenia gravis
   and abducens palsy 586
   and painless ophthalmoplegia 587
Mycostatin® (see nystatin)
mycotic aneurysms 821
Mydfrin® (see phenylephrine - ophthalmic)
Mydriacyl® (see tropicamide)
mydriasis
   from cocaine abuse 152
   in botulism 913
   pharmacologic vs. third nerve compression
      583
   traumatic 582
   (see also pupillary dilatation)
myelitis 55
myelocele 111
myelography 142
   capping 518
   causing arachnoiditis 315
   emergency "blockogram" 518
   for drop metastases 472, 473
   for low back problems 295

myelography *(cont'd)*
   for spinal metastases 518
   for trauma 708
   in diagnosing arachnoiditis 315
   paintbrush effect 510, **518**
myeloma (see multiple myeloma)
myelomeningocele 115
   definition 114
   repair 116
myelopathy
   differential diagnosis 902
   due to cervical spondylosis 331
   from nonunion of odontoid fracture 730
   from Paget's disease 342
   radiation myelopathy (see radiation injury
      and necrosis)
   vs. myelitis 55
myelotomy
   Bischof's 369
   commissural 392
   for spasticity 369
   punctate midline 393
myocardial infarction in cerebral embolism 773
myoclonic status 268
myoclonus
   following intrathecal injection of ionic con-
      trast agent 126
   in Creutzfeldt-Jakob disease 229
   in hypoxic coma 162
   in metabolic coma 159
   in West's disease 258
   juvenile myoclonic epilepsy 257
   myoclonic status 268
myopathy
   steroid 11
Mysoline® (see primidone)
myxedema coma 454
myxopapillary ependymoma 471, **508**

N

NAA (see N-acetyl aspartate) on MRS
nabumetome 29
N-acetyl aspartate (NAA) on MRS 137
naevus flammeus 121
nafcillin
   for cerebral abscess 221
   for shunt infections 215
   for surgical prophylaxis 211
naked facet sign 737
nalbuphine 33
   following spinal narcotics 394
Nalfon® (see fenoprofen)
nalmefene 152
naloxone
   for opioid overdose 152
   for reversal of spinal narcotics 393
   for spinal cord injury 704
   in coma 156
Naprosyn® (see naproxen)

Numorphan® (see oxymorphone)
Nuromax® (see doxacurium)
nutrition in head injuries 679
nystagmus 580
    downbeat 580
        with Chiari I malformation 105
        monocular 585
        nystagmus retractorius 86, 580
        optokinetic 159
        seesaw 580
nystatin 210

O

OALL (see ossification - of the anterior longitu-
    dinal ligament)
oat cell lung cancer (see small cell lung cancer)
Obersteiner-Redlich zone 84, 371, 429
obesity
    and hyperostosis frontalis interna 483
    and idiopathic intracranial hypertension 493,
        496
    as a risk factor for neural tube defects 113
oblique cervical spine x-rays 707
obliteration of basal cisterns on CT
    following head injury 681
    in cerebellar infarct 772
obstructive hydrocephalus 180
obturator nerve entrapment 574
obturator neurectomy 368
obturator neuropathy
    following cardiac catheterization 559
occipital condyle fracture 721
occipital craniotomy 612
occipital nerve entrapment 563
occipital neuralgia 563
    with hangman's fracture 725
    with odontoid fractures 728
occipital neurectomy 564
occipital plagiocephaly 100
occipital vs. frontal skull fractures 639
occipital-frontal circumference 184
    graph
        children (inside front cover)
        for preemies 185
        related to weight and height 186
    measurement technique 185
occipitalization of the atlas
    and Chiari I malformation 104
occipital-parietal burr hole 619
occipito-atlantal dislocation (see atlanto-occipi-
    tal dislocation)
occipitoatlantal junction
    normal motion 624
    (see also atlanto-occipital dislocation)
occipitocervical fusion 624
occlusion syndromes 778
occlusive cerebrovascular disease 869
occlusive hyperemia 839
occult cerebrovascular malformations 840

octreotide
    for glomus jugulare tumors 470
    for growth hormone-secreting pituitary ade-
        nomas 450
    for TSH-secreting pituitary adenomas 451
ocular bobbing 158, 588
ocular dysmetria 580
ocular hemorrhage
    from subarachnoid hemorrhage 783
ocular pneumoplethysmography 871
Oculinum® (see botulinum toxin)
oculocephalic reflex 158, 164
oculomotor nerve compression
    as cause for anisocoria 583
oculomotor palsy 585
    from p-comm aneurysm 805
    (see also ophthalmoplegia)
oculosympathetic palsy 885
oculovestibular reflex 158, 164
odontoid process
    distance to C1 (see atlantodental interval)
    fractures 727
        compression screw fixation 624, **625**
        in rheumatoid arthritis 337
    retroversion 104
OFC (see occipital-frontal circumference)
Ogilvie's syndrome 308
olfactory groove meningiomas 427
olfactory hallucinations 257
olfactory neuroblastoma (see esthesioneuroblas-
    toma)
oligoastrocytomas 408, 424
oligoclonal bands
    in Lyme disease 236
    in multiple sclerosis **51**
oligodendroglioma 423
    treatment 424
olivopontocerebellar degeneration 47
Ommaya® reservoir insertion 621
Omnipaque® (see iohexol)
oncocytoma 443
ondansetron 787
Ondine's curse 391
operating microscope 599
operating room equipment 599
operations and procedures 599
OPG (see ocular pneumoplethysmography)
ophthalmic artery 79, 812
    aneurysms 812
    involvement in giant cell arteritis 59
ophthalmic nerve 378
ophthalmic segment aneurysms 812
ophthalmoplegia
    abducens palsy 586
    due to cavernous carotid artery aneurysms
        818, 918
    in Guillain-Barré 54
    multiple extraocular muscle involvement 586
    oculomotor palsy 585
    painful 586
    painless 587

opioid
   analgesics 30, 33
   effects on pupils 151, 157
   naloxone for overdose 152
   toxicity 151
   withdrawal syndrome 152
opisthion *69*, 69
OPLL (see ossification of the posterior longitudinal ligament)
opsoclonus 588
optic glioma 420
   in neurofibromatosis 503
optic nerve
   decompression
      for indirect optic nerve injury 645
      in osteopetrosis 918
   indirect injury 645
optic nerve sheath fenestration
   for cerebrovascular venous thrombosis 891
   for pseudotumor cerebri vi, 498
optic neuritis 50, 582
   vs. papilledema 581
option (practice option) - definition iii
Optiray® (see ioversol)
optokinetic nystagmus 87, 159
oral contraceptives
   and cerebrovascular venous thrombosis 888
   and idiopathic intracranial hypertension 496
   and seizure medication 281
   and stroke in young adults 775
orbital apex syndrome 586
orbital lesions 929
orbital pseudotumor (see pseudotumor - orbital)
orders
   admitting
      for minor head injury 642
      for moderate head injury 642
      subarachnoid hemorrhage 787
   post-op
      craniotomy 602
      lumbar laminectomy 309
      transsphenoidal pituitary surgery 454
      VP shunt 621
   pre-op
      craniotomy 602
      transsphenoidal pituitary surgery 454
organ donation 168
organ transplant patients
   and cerebral abscess 218
   and primary CNS lymphoma 462
Orgaran® (see danaparoid)
orthostatic hypotension 915
   with Shy-Drager syndrome 48
Orudis/Oruvail® (see ketoprofen)
os odontoideum 730
oscillopsia 588
   following vestibular neurectomy 591
Osler-Weber-Rendu syndrome 841
   and capillary telangiectasia 841
   and cerebral abscess 217
   and cerebral AVMs 835

Osler-Weber-Rendu syndrome *(cont'd)*
   and CVA in young adults 774
   and intracranial aneurysms 801
osmolality
   serum 11
      calculated 11
      in diabetes insipidus(DI) 16
      in SIADH 14
   urine
      in diabetes insipidus (DI) 17
      normal range 17
osmotic demyelination syndrome (see central
   pontine myelinolysis)
osmotic therapy 658
ossiculum terminale 730
ossification
   of the anterior longitudinal ligament 346
   of the posterior longitudinal ligament
      (OPLL) 331, **345**
      differential diagnosis 903
   of the yellow ligament 327
Ostac® (see clodronate)
osteitis deformans (see Paget's disease)
osteoblastic spinal lesions 518
osteoblastic spinal metastases 506
osteoblastoma 511
osteochondroma
   of the spine 506
osteoclastoma (see giant cell tumor)
osteoconduction 627
osteogenesis 627
osteogenic sarcoma
   of the spine 506
osteoid osteoma 511
osteoinduction 627
osteolytic skull lesions 930
osteoma (skull) 481
   differential diagnosis 932
osteomyelitis
   of the skull 217
   vertebral 243
osteopetrosis 918
osteoporosis
   and spine fractures 748
   from chronic heparin therapy 22
   in Cushing's syndrome 440
   in multiple myeloma 515
   steroid induced 11, 748
   treatment 749
   with prolactinomas 440
   with reflex sympathetic dystrophy 397
osteoporosis circumscripta (see Paget's disease
   of the skull)
osteosclerosis 918
otalgia 378
   in geniculate neuralgia 386
   in glossopharyngeal neuralgia 386
otitic hydrocephalus 496, 888
otorrhea, CSF 175
otoslcerosis 597
outcome assessment 899

overflow incontinence 90
overshunting 196
oxaprozin 29
oxazepam 35
for EtOH withdrawal 150
oxcarbazepine 274
oxidized cellulose 600
oxycarbazepine
for postherpetic neuralgia 388
Oxycel® (see oxidized cellulose)
oxycephaly 102
oxycodone 31, 32
for postherpetic neuralgia 387
OxyContin® 31
(also see oxycodone)
oxygen extraction fraction 659
OxyIR® 31
(also see oxycodone)
oxymorphone 32

P

pachygyria 112
Paget's disease **340**, 909, 939
and increased skull density 931
and lumbar spinal stenosis 327
as a cause of cranial neuropathies 918
as a cause of myelopathy 903
of the skull 931
of the spine 341
pain 376
back (see back pain)
causalgia 396
craniofacial 377
discogenic 296
from metastatic bone disease 27
in diabetic neuropathy 555
medication 27
meralgia paresthetica 573
neck (see neck pain)
neuropathic 376
nocturnal (see night pain)
procedures 390
commissural myelotomy 392
cordotomy 391
deep brain stimulation 395
dorsal root entry zone lesions 395
for trigeminal neuralgia 380
intraspinal narcotics 393
intraventricular narcotics 394
punctate midline myelotomy 393
spinal cord stimulation 395
reflex sympathetic dystrophy 396
visceral 27
pain pump (see intrathecal drugs - implantable
pump)
Paine retinaculatome 568
painful disc syndrome 296
painful ophthalmoplegia 586
paintbrush effect (on myelography) 510, **518**

palatal myoclonus 371
Palladone® (see hydromorphone)
pallidotomy
for Parkinson's disease 366
palmar cutaneous branch 565
palmaris longus tendon 565
Pamelor® (see nortriptyline)
pamidronate 342
Pancoast's tumor
and brachial plexopathy 554, 561
and Horner's syndrome 584
pancuronium **40**
effect on pupil 583
pre-treatment before succinylcholine 39
reversal 3
panhypopituitarism (see hypopituitarism)
Pantopaque 126
Pantopaque® (see iophendylate meglumine)
papaverine 808
intra-arterial for vasospasm 795
papillary meningioma (see malignant meningioma)
papilledema 580
from high altitude 687
unilateral
differential diagnosis 581
with idiopathic intracranial hypertension 495
para-articular heterotopic ossification 755
paradoxical air embolus 605
paradoxical embolism in cerebral embolism 773,
774
Parafon Forte® 34
paraganglioma 467
paralysis
from spinal cord injury
grading 704
upper vs. lower motor neuron 548
paralytics 38
early use in neurotrauma 642
paramedian pontine reticular formation 584
paraneoplastic syndrome 55
paraneoplastic syndromes 554
paraplegia
differential diagnosis 913
parasellar lesions 927
parasitic infections 236
parasympathetic
supply to bladder 90
supply to pupil 581
parietal boss 619
parietal craniotomy 611
parietal lobe syndromes 87
parietal thinning 931
Parinaud's syndrome **86**, 158, 161, 184, 776
park bench position 604
Parkinson, triangular space of 83
Parkinson's disease 47
secondary parkinsonism 47
treatment
surgical 49, **365**
deep brain stimulation 366

radiation therapy 534
    effect on IQ in children 535
    for cerebral metastases 489
    for chordoma 465
    for CNS lymphoma 464
    for low grade gliomas 414
    for malignant astrocytomas 415
    for malignant gliomas 415
    for meningiomas 429
    for multiple myeloma 515
    for pituitary adenomas 452
    for spinal metastases 520
    hyperfractionated 422
    stereotactic radiosurgery 537
    (see also radiation injury and necrosis)
radiculomedullary arteries 75
radiculopathy
    C5
        following cervical decompression 336
        from disc herniation 318
    C6
        mimicking MI 318
    C7
        from disc herniation 318
    cervical 318
        keyhole foraminotomy for 321
        mimicking MI 318
    definition 289
    differential diagnosis 905
    L4
        from disc herniation 304
        vs. femoral neuropathy 907
    L5
        and foot drop 909
        differential diagnosis 910
        from disc herniation 304
        from sacral fracture 753
    lumbar
        physical findings 302
        radiographic evaluation 293
    S1
        from disc herniation 304
        localizing 907
    upper lumbar 310
radiobiology 534
radiographic vasospasm 791
radionuclide cisternography
    for CSF leak 176
    for NPH **201**, 202
radionuclide shuntography 196
radiosensitive metastases 489
rads (equivalent in cGy) 534
Raeder's paratrigeminal neuralgia 588
raloxifene 750
Ramsay Hunt syndrome 386
Ramsay sedation scale (modified) 36
Ranawat grading scale 337
Ranchos Los Amigos cognitive scale 899
ranitidine - use with steroids 657
Rankin scale 900
rapacuronium 39

rapid sequence tranquilization 37
Raplon® (see rapacuronium)
Rathke's cleft cyst 439, **457**
rebleeding
    with aneurysms 789
    with angiogram negative SAH 822
    with AVMs 836
    with intracerebral hemorrhage 855
    with perimesencephalic nonaneurysmal SAH
        823
rebuildup in moyamoya disease 893
recombinant activated coagulation factor VII
    (see factor VII)
recombinant tissue plasminogen activator (see
    tissue plasminogen activator)
recommendations (practice recommendations) -
    definition iii
recurrent artery of Heubner 77
recurrent herniated lumbar disc 307, **317**
recurrent intracerebral hemorrhage 853
recurrent laryngeal nerve 320
recurrent meningitis 213
    with basal encephalocele 103
    with CSF fistula 174
    with dermal sinus 118, 119
red flags (in low back problems) 292
reflex sympathetic dystrophy 396
    following lumbar laminectomy and discecto-
        my 308
    upper extremity 912
        following anterior cervical discectomy
            321
        following brachial plexus gunshot wound
            562
        following carpal tunnel surgery 568
reflexes
    abdominal cutaneous
        in multiple sclerosis 50
        in spinal cord injury 704
    anal cutaneous 712
    cremasteric 704
    muscle stretch (see muscle stretch reflex)
    primitive 180
reflexology 699
Refludan® (see lepirudin)
refractory seizures 282
regeneration of peripheral nerves 560
regional brain syndromes 85
regional diagnoses 922
Regitine® (see phentolamine)
Reid's base line 70
Reiter syndrome 908
Relafen® (see nabumetome)
REM (see roentgen-equivalent man)
renal failure
    and destructive spondyloarthropathy 939
    from intrathecal contrast media 126
    with mannitol 661
renal-cell carcinoma
    metastatic to brain 487
    metastatic to spine 519

S

stereotactic radiosurgery *(cont'd)*
  for tectal gliomas 423
  for trigeminal neuralgia **382**, 538
  fractionated 539
  of the spinal cord or medulla 539
  premedication for 542
  target localization 540
  treatment morbidity and mortality 542
stereotactic surgery 545
  biopsy 546
    for pineal region tumors 478
    for suspected cerebral mets 488
    for suspected malignant glioma 417
    in AIDS 234
    indications 545
  for cerebral abscess 222
  for colloid cyst 459
  mesencephalotomy 390
  radiosurgery (see stereotactic radiosurgery)
steroid myopathy 705
steroids
  and osteoporosis 748
  effect on CT contrast enhancement 408
  effect on tissue plasminogen activator 11
  epidural
    following discectomy 307
    for low back problems 298
  equivalent doses 8
  following lumbar discectomy 307
  for Addisonian crisis 11
  for Bell's palsy 595
  for brain tumor 406
  for bronchospasm following IV contrast in-
    jection 129
  for carpal tunnel syndrome 567
  for cerebral abscess 221
  for cerebral metastases **488**, 490
  for cysticercosis 238
  for discitis 250
  for giant cell arteritis 60
  for gunshot wounds
    to the head 685
    to the spine 704
  for head injury 661
  for intracerebral hemorrhage 857
  for low back pain 298
  for myelitis 56
  for neurocysticercosis 238
  for orbital pseudotumor 587
  for pain 27, 33
  for pseudotumor cerebri 661
  for spinal cord injury 704
  for spinal metastases 518
  for stereotactic radiosurgery 542
  physiologic replacement 8
  replacement therapy 8
  side effects 10
  stress doses 10
  unmasking diabetes insipidus (DI) 17
  withdrawal 9
  (see also dexamethasone)

Stevens-Johnson syndrome
  with acetazolamide 278
  with carbamazepine 273
  with ethosuximide 276
  with lamotrigine 278
  with phenytoin 272
STICH study 859
Stimate® (see desmopressin)
stinger (football injury) 743
STIR image (on MRI) 135
STIR images (MRI)
  for vertebral factures 751
Stokes-Adams attacks 915
straight leg raising test 302
Strata (programmable) shunt valve 191
Streptase® (see streptokinase)
streptokinase
  for ischemic CVA 768
stress dose steroids 10
stress ulcers 657
stretch test
  cervical spine 734
  femoral 303
stridor from Chiari malformation 108
string of pearls sign
  on angiography
    with fibromuscular dysplasia 64
    with isolated CNS vasculitis 62
  on DWI MRI
    with occluded carotid artery 880
string sign 765, 884
stroke (see cerebrovascular accident)
Struther's ligament 569
stunned myocardium
  following SAH 789
Sturge-Weber syndrome 505
  and choroidal hemangioma 929
stylomastoid foramen 594
subacute combined columnal degeneration 904
subacute sclerosing panencephalitis 145
subarachnoid cyst (see arachnoid cyst)
subarachnoid hemorrhage 781
  admitting orders 787
  and cardiac problems 789
    cardiac arrhythmias 789
    stunned myocardium 789
  and coma 783
  and EKG changes 789
  and hydrocephalus 783, 786, **790**
  and neurogenic pulmonary edema 8, 788
  and ventricular catheterization 786
  angiogram negative 822
  clinical features 782
  differentiating from traumatic LP 173
  from AVM 781
  from cavernous carotid artery aneurysm 819
  from cocaine abuse 152
  grading scales 785
    Fisher grade (vasospasm) 792
    Hunt and Hess 785
    World Federation of Neurosurgeons 786

tic douloureux (see trigeminal neuralgia)
tick paralysis 54
Ticlid® (see ticlopidine)
ticlopidine 871
tiludronate 342
timing of aneurysm surgery 804
  basilar bifurcation aneurysms 815
Tinel's sign 561
  in carpal tunnel syndrome 566
  in peroneal nerve palsy 575
  in Tarsal tunnel 576
  with ulnar nerve entrapment in Guyon's canal 571
tinnitus
  differential diagnosis 921
  following concussion 682
  in idiopathic intracranial hypertension 495
  in Meniere's disease 592
tinzaparin **23**, 26
tirilazad mesylate
  for cerebral vasospasm 794
  for spinal cord injury 704
tissue plasminogen activator
  contraindications 768
  for cerebrovascular venous thrombosis 891
  for ischemic stroke (CVA) 768
  in stroke workup 776
  preceding intracerebral hemorrhage 768, 851, 853
  to lyse intracerebral hemorrhage 545
  to lyse intraventricular hemorrhage **860**
tissue transplantation
  donation following brain death 168
  for parkinsonism 365
titubition 405
tobramycin 210
Todd's paralysis **258**, 915
Tolectin® (see tolmetin)
tolmetin 29
Tolosa-Hunt syndrome 586, **587**
tonsillar herniation
  acute 160
  asymptomatic 106
  from LP shunt 189
  in Chiari malformation 104, **106**
  on MRI 105
top o'the basilar embolism 776
Topamax® (see topiramate)
topiramate 279
topotecan 407
Toradol® (see ketorolac tromethamine)
TORCH infections 920
torcular herophili 82
Torg ratio (see Pavlov's ratio)
Torkildsen shunt 182, **188**
torticollis 370
  congenital 100
  differential diagnosis 370
  due to atlantoaxial subluxation 722
Towne's view 139
toxic epidermal necrolysis with lamotrigine 278

toxicology (see neurotoxicology)
toxoplasmosis 231, **236**
  CT findings 232
  treatment in AIDS 233
t-PA (see tissue plasminogen activator)
tPA (see tissue plasminogen activator)
Tracrium® (see atracurium)
traction
  cervical **709**, 726
    (see also cervical traction)
  pelvic 298
train of four
  and reversal of neuromuscular blockade 3
tramadol 30
  for neuropathic pain 377
tram-tracking in Sturge-Weber 505
Trandate® (see labetalol)
tranexamic acid 789
transarticular facet screws (C1-2) 624, **626**
transcallosal approach 611
  for colloid cyst 459
  for pineal region tumors 479
transcortical approach to lateral ventricle 612
transcranial doppler
  for brain death evaluation 166
  for vasospasm 793, 797
transcranial motor evoked potentials 147
transcutaneous electrical nerve stimulation
  for back pain 298
  for occipital neuralgia 564
transependymal absorption of CSF 183, 196
  differential diagnosis 936
  in normal pressure hydrocephalus 201
transfer of trauma patients 637
transferrin (in CSF) 176
transient ischemic attack
  crescendo TIA 880
  definition 869
  differential diagnosis 915
  management 768
  with arterial dissection 883
  with vertebrobasilar insufficiency 881
transient monocular blindness (see amaurosis fugax)
transient neurologic deficit
  differential diagnosis 915
transient visual obscurations
  in idiopathic intracranial hypertension 495
transillumination of the skull 181, 678
transitional meningioma 427
transitional vertebrae 304
translabyrinthine approach to acoustic neuroma 434
transmissible spongiform encephalopathy agents 227
transmural pressure 790
transoral surgery 613
  odontoidectomy 613
  stereotactic biopsy 546
transsphenoidal surgery 454
  pre-op orders 454

---

tryptophan
  for pain 33
tuberculous meningitis 917
  and ophthalmoplegia 587
  and SIADH 13
  CSF findings 173
tuberculous spondylitis (see Pott's disease)
tuberculum sella meningiomas 427
tuberous sclerosis 504
tumefactive demyelinating lesions 51
tumor blush (on angiography) 413
tumor filter
  for CSF shunts 189
tumor markers 500
  in pineal region tumors 477
  Ki-67 500
  neuroendocrine tumors 500
tumor TIA 404, 487, 916
tumors
  brain
    and deep vein thrombosis 25
    and headaches 405
    astrocytoma 409
      cerebellar (pilocytic) 419
      classification 409
      fibrillary 410
      gemistocytic 410
      grading 410
      pilocytic 410, **417**
    congenital 480
    glioma 409
      low grade 408
    neonatal 480
    pediatric 480
    primary 408
    prophylactic anticonvulsants for 407
  brainstem glioma 420
  classification (CNS) 401
  foramen magnum 492
  glomus jugulare 468
  immunohistochemical staining patterns 501
  markers 477, 500
  metastases
    of CNS tumors through CSF 485
    of primary CNS tumors 485
    to brain 484
    to spine 516
    to upper cervical spine 517
  of the lateral ventricle 935
  of the third ventricle 610, 936
  posterior fossa 405
  primary brain 408
  primary spinal 506
  skull 480, 930
  spine 506
    and disc space involvement 939
    astrocytoma 508
    axis vertebra
      differential diagnosis 924
      metastases 517
    bone 511
    causing sciatica 906

21-aminosteroids
  following SAH 794
  for head injury 662
twilight state 264
Twining view of cervical spine 707
Twining's line 71
twist drill craniostomy for chronic subdurals 675
Tylenol® (see acetaminophen)
Tylox® (see oxycodone)

U

ulcerations (carotid) 870
ulcers
  antacids and H2 inhibitors for 40
  Cushing's 657
  prophylaxis 40
  steroid 10, 657
  stress **40**, 657
ulnar nerve 552
  entrapment 569
    treatment
      non-surgical 570
      submuscular transposition 570
      surgical options 570
  perioperative neuropathy 558
Ultane® (see sevoflurane)
Ultram® (see tramadol)
ultrasound
  for carotid stenosis 870
  for dural sinus thrombosis 891
  for low back pain 298
  for neonatal intracerebral hemorrhage 862,
    863
  intraoperative for spine fracture 748
uncal fits (see uncal seizures)
uncal herniation 161
  CT criteria 161
uncal seizures 257
  differential diagnosis 938
uncinate seizures (see uncal seizures)
undershunting 195
unintended durotomy (see durotomy - unintend-
    ed)
unruptured aneurysms 816
upgaze palsy
  differential diagnosis 86
  with Parinaud's syndrome 86
upper cervical spine abnormalities 336

upper lumbar disc herniation 310
upper motor neuron paralysis 548
upward cerebellar herniation 160
urea
     for cerebral salt wasting in SAH 788
     for hyponatremia 15
uremia
     and idiopathic intracranial hypertension 496
uremic encephalopathy 64
     and delerium 44
uremic neuropathy 560
urinary 17-hydroxycorticosteroids 446
urinary retention
     differential diagnosis 91
     in cauda equina syndrome 305
urine free cortisol 444
urine osmolality 17
     in diabetes insipidus (DI) 17
     normal range 17
urine specific gravity 17
urodynamic testing 92
urokinase
     for cerebrovascular venous thrombosis 891
     for intracerebral hematoma 545
urticaria 129
uveocyclitis
     with CNS lymphoma 462

V

"V" shaped pre-dens space 140
VA shunt (see ventriculo-atrial shunt)
vacuum disc 289
valacyclovir for herpes zoster 388
Valium® (see diazepam)
valproate 274
     and neural tube defects 113, 274
     for geniculate neuralgia 387
     for myoclonic status 268
     for status epilepticus 266
valproic acid (see valproate)
Valtrex® (see valacyclovir)
Vancocin® (see vancomycin)
vancomycin 209
     for cerebral abscess 221
     for meningitis 212
     for pseudomembranous colitis 209
     for shunt infections 215
     for subdural empyema 225
     for surgical prophylaxis 211
vanillylmandelic acid 469
varicella-zoster leukoencephalitis 227
vascular claudication 326
vascular dysautoregulatory encephalopathy 64
vascular malformations 835
     angiographically occult 840
     arteriovenous malformation (AVM) 835
vascular territories (cerebral) 76, 77
vasculitis (cerebral) 58
     drug induced 63

vasculopathy 58
     following stereotactic radiosurgery 542
vasodepressor syncope 915
vasogenic cerebral edema **85**, 661
vasopressin 19
     drip 798
     preparations 18
vasospasm 791
     and eclampsia 64
     diagnostic criteria 793
     following pretruncal nonaneurysmal SAH
          823
     optimal hematocrit 795
     protocol 796
     risk factors after SAH 792
     syndromes 791
     tests for diagnosing 793
     time course 792
     treatment 794
Vasotec® (see enalapril and enalaprilat)
vasovagal response
     differential diagnosis 915
     from contrast media reaction 128
VBI (see vertebrobasilar insufficiency)
vecuronium 39
vein of Galen malformation/aneurysms 836, **844**
veins
     basal vein of Rosenthal 82
     cerebral venous anatomy 82, *133*
     internal jugular 82
     supratentorial 82
     vein of Galen 82
     vein of Labbe 82
     vein of Trolard 82
Velcade® (see bortezomib)
venogram (see angiogram)
venous angiomas **839**, 840
venous anomaly (see venous angiomas)
venous infarction
     following transcallosal surgery 611
     with cerebrovascular venous thrombosis 889
     with subdural empyema 223
     with superior sagittal sinus occlusion 609
venous lakes (of the skull) 931
venous malformation (see venous angiomas)
venous system
     cerebral 82, *133*
ventricle
     fifth 928
     isolated fourth 182
     third 71
ventricles
     lesions/tumors within 934
     slit 197
     surface anatomy 71
ventricular access device 621
ventricular catheterization 620
     following SAH 786
     for brain relaxation during surgery 806
     infection of catheter 650
     insertion technique 619, 651

GARDNER/ROBERTSON HEARING (PAGE 432)

Class	Description	Audiogram (dB)	Speech discrimination
I	good-excellent	0-30	70-100%
II	serviceable	31-50	50-59%
III	nonserviceable	51-90	5-49%
IV	poor	91-max	1-4%
V	none	not testable	0

HOUSE-BRACKMANN GRADE (PAGE 431)

Grade	Function	Description
1	normal	normal function in all areas
2	mild dysfunction	slight weakness on close inspection
3	moderate dysfunction	obvious but not disfiguring
4	moderate-severe dysfunction	obvious weakness and/or disfiguring asymmetry
5	severe dysfunction	barely perceptible motion
6	total paralysis	no movement

MUSCLE STRENGTH (PAGE 548)

Grade	Strength
0	no contraction
1	flicker or trace contraction
2	movement with gravity eliminated
3	movement against gravity
4	movement against resistance
5	normal strength

4- slight resistance
4 moderate resistance
4+ strong resistance

LUMBAR DISC SYNDROMES (PAGE 304)

	L3-4	L4-5	L5-S1
Pain	anterior thigh	posterior LE	posterior LE, to heel
Weakness	quadriceps	EHL, anterior tibialis	gastrocnemius
Sensory loss	medial malleolus	dorsum of foot	lateral foot
Reflex	patellar	none	achilles

CERVICAL DISC SYNDROMES (PAGE 318)

	C4-5	C5-6	C6-7
Pain & sensory loss	shoulder	upper arm, thumb, radial forearm	index & middle fingers
Weakness	deltoid	biceps	triceps
Reflex change		biceps	triceps

KARNOFSKY SCALE (PAGE 899)

Score	Meaning
100	normal; no complaints, no evidence of disease
90	able to carry on normal activity; minor symptoms
80	normal activity with effort; some symptoms
70	cares for self; unable to carry on normal activity
60	requires occasional assistance; cares for most needs
50	requires considerable assistance and frequent care
40	disabled; requires special care and assistance
30	severely disabled; hospitalized, death not imminent
20	very sick; active supportive care needed
10	moribund; fatal processes are progressing rapidly

Handbook of Neurosurgery 6ed Quick Reference Tables 2

GLASGOW COMA SCALE (PAGE 154)

Points	Best eye	Best verbal	Best motor
6	-	-	obeys
5	-	oriented	localizes pain
4	spontaneous	confused	withdraws to pain
3	to speech	inappropriate	flexor (decorticate)
2	to pain	incomprehensible	extensor (decerebrate)
1	none	none	none

PREVERTEBRAL SOFT TISSUE (PAGE 141)

Space	Level	Maximum normal (mm) adults	Maximum normal (mm) peds
retropharyngeal	C1	10	unreliable
	C2-4	5 - 7	
retrotracheal	C5-7	22	14

STATUS EPILEPTICUS (PAGE 266)

Summary of medications for status epilepticus in average size adult (see text for details)

lorazepam (Ativan®) 4 mg IV slowly over 2 mins, may repeat after 5 mins

simultaneously load with phenytoin (@ < 50 mg/min) as follows:

1200 mg if not already on phenytoin

500 mg if on phenytoin (send level first)

phenobarbital IV (@ < 100 mg/min) until seizures stop, up to 1400 mg (watch BP)

if seizures continue > 30 mins, intubate and begin "general anesthesia"

HUNT-HESS SAH CLASSIFICATION (PAGE 785)

Grade	Description
0	unruptured aneurysm
1	asymptomatic, or mild H/A and slight nuchal rigidity
1a	no acute meningeal/brain reaction, but with fixed neuro deficit
2	Cr. N. palsy (e.g. III, IV), moderate to severe H/A, nuchal rigidity
3	mild focal deficit, lethargy or confusion
4	stupor, moderate to severe hemiparesis, early decerebrate rigidity
5	deep coma, decerebrate rigidity, moribund appearance

Add one grade for serious systemic disease (e.g. HTN, DM, severe atherosclerosis, COPD) or severe vasospasm on arteriography

FISHER GRADE (FOR VASOSPASM) (PAGE 792)

Group	Blood on CT
1	no blood detected
2	diffuse or vertical layers < 1 mm thick
3	localized clot and/or vertical layer ≥ 1 mm
4	intracerebral or intraventricular clot with diffuse or no SAH

SPETZLER-MARTIN AVM GRADING (PAGE 838)

Graded feature		Points
Size	small (< 3 cm)	1
	medium (3-6 cm)	2
	large (> 6 cm)	3
Eloquence of adjacent brain	non-eloquent	0
	eloquent	1
Venous drainage	superficial only	0
	deep	1

Spinal sensory and motor exam

← Spinal nerve root sensory distribution (see page 75)

→ Spinal nerve root motor distribution (see page 713)

Segment	Muscle	Action to test	Reflex
C1-4	neck muscles		
C3, 4, 5	diaphragm	inspiration, FEV1….	
C5, 6	deltoid	abduct arm > 90°	
	biceps	elbow flexion	biceps
C6, 7	extensor carpi radialis	wrist extension	supinator
C7, 8	triceps	elbow extension	triceps
	extensor digitorum	finger extension	
C8, T1	flexor digitorum profundus	grasp (flex DIP)	
	hand intrinsics	abduct little finger	
T2-9	intercostals		
T9, 10	upper abdominals	Beevor's sign	abdominal cutaneous
T11, 12	lower abdominals	Beevor's sign	abdominal cutaneous
L2, 3	iliopsoas	hip flexion	cremasteric reflex
L3, 4	quadriceps	knee extension	quadriceps (knee jerk)
L4, 5	medial hamstrings		± medial hamstrings
	tibialis anterior	ankle dorsiflexion	
L5, S1	lateral hamstrings	knee flexion	
	posterior tibialis	foot inversion	
	extensor hallucis longus	great toe extension	
S1, 2	gastrocnemius	ankle plantarflexion	achilles (ankle jerk)
S2, 3	flexor digitorum		
S2-4	bladder, lower bowel anal sphincter	clamp down during rectal exam	anal cutaneous reflex, bulbocavernosus

POSTERIOR

ANTERIOR

trigeminal nerve { V1, V2, V3 }

Redrawn from "Introduction to Basic Neurology", by Harry D. Patton, John W. Sundsten, Wayne E. Crill & Philip D. Swanson, ©1976, pp 173, W. B. Saunders Co., Philadelphia, PA, with permission

EYE CHART KEY
(hold at right angle to eye chart to keep from patient's view)

20/100	638
20/70	8745
20/50	63925
20/40	428365
20/30	374258
20/25	937826
20/20	428739